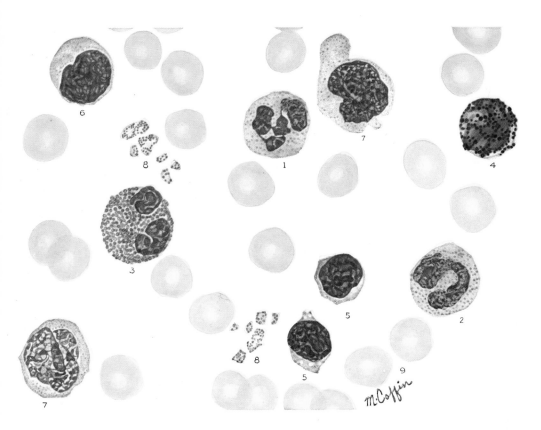

NORMAL CELLULAR CONSTITUENTS OF ADULT HUMAN BLOOD

1, Segmented (polymorphonuclear) neutrophil; 2, Band (stab) neutrophil; 3, Segmented eosinophil; 4, Basophil; 5, Small lymphocytes; 6, Large lymphocyte; 7, Monocytes; 8, Thrombocytes; and 9, Erythrocytes. (From Custer: An Atlas of the Blood and Bone Marrow, 2nd ed. W. B. Saunders Co., Philadelphia, 1974.)

With the assistance of

Charles E. Hess, M.D.

Associate Professor of Medicine,
University of Virginia School of Medicine

Daniel N. Mohler, Jr., M.D.

Professor of Medicine,
University of Virginia School of Medicine

Munsey S. Wheby, M.D.

Professor of Medicine,
Head, Division of Hematology
University of Virginia School of Medicine

BYRD STUART LEAVELL, M.D.

Professor of Medicine
School of Medicine, University of Virginia;
Hematologist and Attending Physician
University of Virginia Hospital
Charlottesville, Virginia

OSCAR ANDREAS THORUP, Jr., M.D.

Professor of Medicine and Associate Dean
School of Medicine, University of Virginia
Charlottesville, Virginia

Fundamentals of CLINICAL HEMATOLOGY

FOURTH EDITION

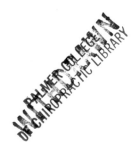

1976
W. B. SAUNDERS COMPANY
Philadelphia, London, Toronto

W. B. Saunders Company: West Washington Square
Philadelphia, PA   19105

1 St. Anne's Road
Eastbourne, East Sussex BN21 3UN, England

833 Oxford Street
Toronto, Ontario M8Z 5T9, Canada

Library of Congress Cataloging in Publication Data

Leavell, Byrd Stuart, 1910–

Fundamentals of clinical hematology.

Includes index.

1. Hematology.   I. Thorup, Oscar Andreas, joint author.
  II. Title.   III. Title: Clinical hematology. [DNLM:
  1. Hematologic diseases. WH100 L439f]

RB145.L45 1976   616.1′5   75–19845

ISBN 0–7216–5678–1

Listed here is the latest translated edition of this
book together with the language of the translation
and the publisher.

Spanish (*3rd Edition*) – NEISA, Mexico D. F., Mexico

Fundamentals of Clinical Hematology   ISBN   0-7216-5678-1

Last digit is the print number: 9   8   7   6   5   4   3   2   1

Dedicated to

Thomas Harrison Hunter, M.D.
Indomitable spirit, wise counsel, and constant friend

and

William Parson, M.D.
Master teacher, superb clinician, and dedicated
physician whose career of service to others has been
an inspiration to many.

NOTICE

Every effort has been made by the authors and the publisher of this book to insure that dosage recommendations are precise and in agreement with standards officially accepted at the time of publication. It does happen, however, that dosage schedules are changed from time to time in the light of accumulating clinical experience and continuing laboratory studies, particularly in the case of recently introduced products. The reader is urged, therefore, to check the product information sheet included in the package of each drug before it is administered, to be certain that there have been no changes in the recommended dosage or in the contraindications to its use.

PREFACE

The aim of the fourth edition of this text, like that of its predecessors, is to present a readable, concise yet comprehensive volume on clinical hematology to help students, residents and practicing physicians keep up with the increasing demands on them for self-study. Disease is viewed as an expression of derangement in normal metabolism. In order to provide a sound foundation for understanding the problems involved in hematological disorders, relevant physiological processes such as iron metabolism and blood coagulation are reviewed before the related clinical disorders are discussed. An attempt is made to relate each disease to a specific defect in metabolism or abnormality in some physiological process.

The general arrangement of the first three editions has been followed, but the continued increase in the knowledge of nearly every aspect of hematology has necessitated numerous changes. All of the chapters have been revised, and those on lymphoma, leukemia and plasma cell disorders have been rewritten. New chapters on the myeloproliferative disorders and the functions of lymphocytes have been added. Sections have been added which deal with disorders of the spleen and the hematological effects of alcohol. Advances in knowledge about blood platelets, lymphocytes, plasma proteins, treatment of leukemia and lymphomas and hemolytic anemias are exciting and these sections have been expanded.

Much effort has been made to present recent advances in the basic mechanisms in hematology, but the orientation of the volume remains clinical. Diagnosis and treatment are emphasized in order to make the book valuable to physicians in practice.

An extensive bibliography has again been included. It is hoped that the reading of the topics in the text will give an understanding of important fundamental aspects of the disorders and their management; the references and the bibliography should provide ready access to full and more detailed discussions of the different aspects of the disorders.

Our colleagues have been of great assistance to us. Dr. Daniel N. Mohler has revised the chapter on hemolytic anemia, and Dr. Munsey Wheby has revised the chapter on leukemia. Dr. Charles Hess has written the chapter on the lymphocytes and revised that devoted to the plasma cell disorders.

We are grateful to other friends who have been of assistance to us. These include Dr. Johnson T. Carpenter, Jr., Dr. Oliver B. Bobbitt, Dr. Thomas Bithell, Dr. David Teates, Dr. Diane Komp, Dr. William Constable, Dr. David Normansell, and all members of the faculty of the University of Virginia School of Medicine. We are indebted to Dr. John Kiraly, Dr. Howard Kirtland and Dr. Robert Laugen for their assistance in a variety of ways.

Preparation of the manuscript would have been very difficult without the help of Mrs. June Corbin, Mrs. Cindy Frazier and Mrs. Mary Lou Currier on this edition and that of Miss Barbara Marshall who has typed much of the text for all four editions.

Also, Mrs. Anne Russell of the Department of Medical Illustrations at the University of Virginia and her colleagues have again done much work for us.

The authors again express their appreciation for the invaluable assistance the staff of W. B. Saunders Company has given us in numerous ways on many occasions.

BYRD S. LEAVELL, M.D.

OSCAR A. THORUP, JR., M.D.

CONTENTS

CHAPTER 1

THE ORIGIN AND MORPHOLOGY OF BLOOD CELLS

The important contributions made by Ehrlich can be considered the beginning of modern hematology.[24] The staining methods which he introduced became the cornerstone of morphologic hematology and cytochemistry. With the use of the new technique Ehrlich described many cellular details and developed a classification of blood cells.

In recent years there have been enormous gains in the knowledge of the structure and function of cells as the result of information derived from electron microscopy, biochemical analysis of cell fractions, differential staining techniques, and immunologic methods. These have provided a better understanding of the derangements that occur in many hematologic diseases and have greatly expanded the methods used in the diagnosis of hematologic problems. Despite these advances, the study of the cells in the peripheral blood and in the bone marrow by means of light microscopy remains essential to the diagnosis of many hematologic disorders.

THE CELL

Most cells contain a nucleus and cytoplasm. Both are complex structures which have numerous vital functions. In general the nucleus controls the development, function, and division of the cell and the cytoplasm carries out most of its synthetic activity (Fig. 1–1).

The cell membrane. The cell membrane is one example of biologic membranes that control many vital functions. When studied with electron microscopy, membranes from bacteria, plants, and animals appear to consist of two dark lines separated by a lighter zone. Danielli and Davson[19] and Robertson[54] have proposed the general model of membrane structure that has been the one most widely accepted until recently. According to this hypothesis, all biologic

1

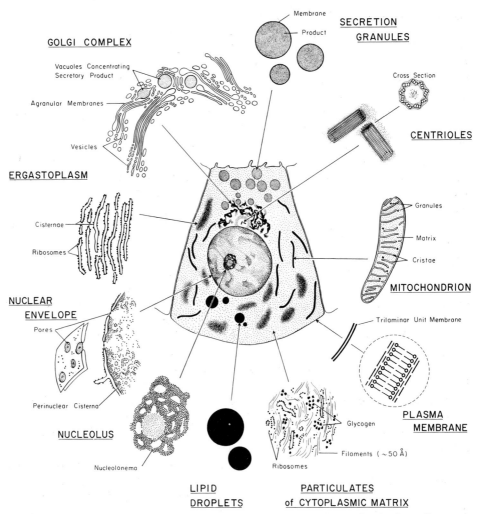

Figure 1–1   In the center of this figure is a diagram of the cell, illustrating the form of its organelles and inclusions as they appear by light microscopy. Around the periphery are representations of the finer structure of these same components as seen in electron micrographs. (From Bloom and Fawcett: A Textbook of Histology. 10th ed. Philadelphia, W. B. Saunders Co., 1975.)

membranes have the same basic structure, consisting of a bimolecular lipid leaflet sandwiched between layers that are nonlipid and largely protein; the lipid molecules have their polar groups facing outward and the long chain hydrocarbons inward. Position of the layers is maintained by ionic binding of hydrophilic head groups of the phospholipids to the protein layer. Although the membranes have a uniform appearance in section, chemical data indicate that membranes in different cells, and in different parts of the same cell, vary greatly in chemical composition and function.[38, 69] Among the diversified tasks assigned to membranes are the following: protein biosynthesis; energy transduction (especially nerves); transport of amino acids, sugar, and other small molecules; flow of water; maintenance of specific ion balance; pinocytosis; phagocytosis; and a variety of reactions in intermediary metabolism and controlled growth and division.[69] A more recent model that fits better with many of the observed data is the "fluid mosaic model."[8] Such a model allows for the considerable compositional differences between membranes that have been observed. It also can accommodate proteins that extend through the entire membrane, such as glycophorin in red cells. Furthermore, the concept is compatible with the free movement of membrane proteins that has been established by studies of antigen–antibody reactions involving fused membranes from two different species.[26] Nonhomogenous protein distribution is also recognized, and some evidence suggests that the distribution of the proteins may be important in growth and even in malignant transformation of some cells.

Nucleus. The nucleus, which is essential for growth and division of the cell, is found in nearly all cells; one exception is the mature erythrocyte. The most important constituent of the nucleus is deoxyribonucleic acid (DNA), which in combination with structural proteins forms the chromatin material of the nucleus. The appearance of the chromatin, which stains deeply with basic dyes because of its DNA content, varies with different stages of development of the cell. During interphase the chromatin consists of clumps of deeply staining material, heterochromatin, and a lighter staining portion, euchromatin. The DNA occurs in long thin threads in the form of a double helix that contains the genes and carries the biochemical, morphologic, and metabolic characteristics of the cell when it divides. The matrix of the chromatin in the nucleus has been referred to as nuclear sap, nuclear matrix, or nuclear ground substance.

Most cells contain from one to four blue staining nucleoli surrounded by aggregates of chromatin. The nucleoli stain blue because of the presence of ribonucleic acid (RNA). The nucleolus often is unusually large in rapidly growing cells. Although evidence indicates that the nucleolus is important in nucleic acid metabolism and protein synthesis, its precise function remains to be established.

Electron microscopy has shown that the nuclear envelope consists of two parallel membranes which enclose a narrow perinuclear space. Numerous "nuclear pores" are formed where the two membranes touch each other, but the extent that material passes from the nucleus to the cytoplasm through these pores is uncertain. The outermost layer of the nuclear membrane, where ribosomes are usually attached, is often continuous with the endoplasmic reticulum.

Cytoplasm. Electron microscopy has revealed that a large portion of the cytoplasm consists of fluid-filled channels of granular and agranular endoplasmic reticulum that are often continuous with the outer layer of the nuclear membrane. Much of the endoplasmic reticulum is given a granular appearance by adhering ribosomes. Each ribosome consists of two ribonucleoprotein particles of unequal size. Usually several ribosomes are attached to a single strand of messenger RNA (mRNA) to form a polyribosome. Protein synthesis begins with enzymatic activation of amino acids by the attachment of the AMP moiety of ATP to the amino acid,[63] and the subsequent transfer to a molecule of transfer RNA (tRNA or sRNA) specific for that particular amino acid. The molecules of tRNA are brought into line along the mRNA to form polypeptides in a sequence dictated by the code in the mRNA. The ribosome seems to read the message encoded into mRNA by moving along the mRNA from one end to the other. Ribosomes are situated near the endoplasmic reticulum in cells that produce protein destined to be secreted by the cell; the protein follows the reticular channels to the Golgi apparatus for further modification and temporary storage. The agranular reticulum, a tubular network without associated ribosomes, occupies varying amounts of cytoplasm in cells that differ greatly in function.

Mitochondria.   Mitochondria, which can be seen with light microscopy when stained supravitally with Janus green, occur in all aerobic cells of higher animals.[63] These organelles have two membranes. The inner membrane, which has many infoldings termed "cristae mitochondriales," surrounds a protein- and lipid-containing matrix. The membranes consist of 35 to 40 per cent lipid, mainly enzymatic. Although mitochondria are usually slender rods, the number, size, shape, and distribution of mitochondria vary widely in different kinds of cells.

The main function of the mitochondria concerns oxidative processes, particularly those involved in lipid metabolism, the Krebs cycle, and phosphorylation. Mitochondria have been referred to as "power plants" because they supply energy for many chemical reactions and transport systems. Through the breakdown of carbohydrates, fats, and proteins, high energy phosphates (ATP) are formed which are important in many cellular functions, including the transport of ions and molecules across subcellular and cellular membranes. Among the enzymes found in mitochondria are the cytochromes, coenzyme Q, flavoproteins, dehydrogenases, oxidative phosphorylation enzymes, Krebs cycle enzymes, glutamate dehydrogenase, and enzymes for protein and lipid synthesis.

Both DNA and RNA have been identified in mitochondria, and they constitute an extranuclear genetic system concerned with protein synthesis by a process that differs somewhat from cytoplasmic ribosomal synthesis: cyclophosphamide, for example, does not have the same inhibitory effect on protein synthesis in mitochondria that it has on cytoplasmic protein synthesis. Mitochondria are apparently formed by the growth and division of existing mitochondria.[63]

Lysosomes.   Lysosomes have been defined as a heterogeneous group of cytoplasmic organelles that mediate the digestive and lytic processes of the cell.[70] Lysosomes occur in most vertebrate cells; they contain a number of enzymes and other substances listed in Table 1–1. A number of histochemical and biochemical studies has resulted in the suggestion that any intracellular organelle contained in a single unit membrane and staining for acid phosphatase be considered a lysosome.

Several lysosomes that differ in function have been identified. One is the specific granule in leukocytes and macrophages that is so important in phagocytosis. The membrane of the lysosome fuses with the membrane of the "phagosome" formed by invagination of the cellular membrane when foreign bodies are engulfed; the subsequent discharge of enzymes from the lysosomes lyses the engulfed material. Because the enzymes remain confined within the fused membranes, the cell is not necessarily damaged by the reaction. Whereas granulocytes retain lysozyme within the cell, it is released from macrophages continuously, independent of phagocytosis or stimulation. The lysosomes may be important in the processing of antigens by macrophages, which is apparently

Table 1-1 *Enzymes and Other Substances Localized to Lysosomes*

ENZYMES	OTHER SUBSTANCES
Acid Phosphatase	Phagocytin
Acid ribonuclease	Cationic "inflammatory" protein
Acid deoxyribonuclease	Mucopolysaccharides and glycoproteins
Acid protease (or proteases); cathepsins	Plasminogen activator
Phosphoprotein phosphatase	Permeability-inducing protease
Beta-glucuronidase	Hemolysin (or hemolysins)
Beta-N-acetylglucosaminidase	Unidentified basic proteins
Alpha-mannosidase	
Beta-galactosidase	
Alpha$_1 \rightarrow {}_4$glucosidase	
Hyaluronidase	
Lysozyme	
Phospholipase, acid lipase	
Phosphatidic acid phosphatase	
Collagenase	
Arylsulfatases A and B	
Nonspecific esterases	

(From Weissman: N. Engl. J. Med., *273*:1085, 1965.)

a preliminary step for the stimulation of antibody production by antigens. Another form of lysosome is the "autophagic vacuole" that develops when a portion of the cytoplasm is destroyed in response to some injury. Cell death and destruction can be produced by the unrestricted release of the enzyme into the cytoplasm, or by phagocytosis by other cells. In surviving cells, both phagosomes and autophagic vacuoles can form "residual bodies" filled with debris that is often lipid.

The membranes of lysosomes, which resemble those surrounding mitochondria and erythrocytes, are affected in living cells by a number of substances including streptolysins O and S, x-rays, vitamin A, and bacterial endotoxins.[70] It appears likely that the labilizing effect of substances on lysosomes is a result of their effect on the membranes, because many exert similar effects on membranes of erythrocytes and mitochondria. The anti-inflammatory steroids, cortisone, prednisone, and others, have a stabilizing effect on lysosomes, which may explain in part the pharmacologic action of these compounds.[70]

Golgi apparatus. The Golgi apparatus is located near the nucleus. It can be seen by light microscopy when stained with osmium or silver compounds. Research with radioactive tracers, special staining methods, and electron microscopy has shown that the Golgi apparatus is the primary site for the synthesis of large carbohydrates and for "packaging" the secretions, external and internal, formed in the cell. Protein is synthesized from amino acids on the ribosomes and moves to the Golgi apparatus, where carbohydrates are added to the protein. The apparatus appears to contain a group of saccules; as these saccules move upward in the apparatus they accumulate more carbohydrate and more of the cell's secretion product. The topmost saccules bud off, eventually make their way through the cell membrane, and release their enclosed glycoprotein. Although the Golgi apparatus probably is not the exclusive site of the formation of carbohydrate side chains in glycoproteins and mucopolysaccharides, it appears to be the main organelle involved.[44]

THE BLOOD CELLS

Opinions about the origin of most of the blood cells have provoked disagreements and polemical outbursts over the years; even now, after many years of study and discussion, there is no unanimity of opinion on many points. Ehrlich recognized that the granulocytic series of cells arose from a nongranular precursor in the bone marrow, and thought that lymphocytes originated in the lymph glands.[24] This distinction formed the basis of his theory of the dual origin of white cells. Ehrlich considered this dualistic doctrine to be one of the most important results of his long-continued studies in hematology, but it was not accepted by many hematologists. The dualistic theory was supported by Banti, Turk, Naegeli, and others,[24, 49] and was opposed by the monophyleticists, Maximow, Jordan, Bloom, and others, who believed that myeloid tissue could arise postembryonically from lymphocytes.[11, 34, 41] Still another theory, the polyphyletic, has been advanced by Cunningham, Sabin, and Doan, who concluded that each type of adult cell has its own particular blast precursor.[18] Detailed discussions of the different theories of the origin of the various cells are presented in Downey's *Handbook of Hematology*[23] and in review articles.[18, 41, 47, 55]

Table 1–2   *Origin and Relationship of Blood Cells*

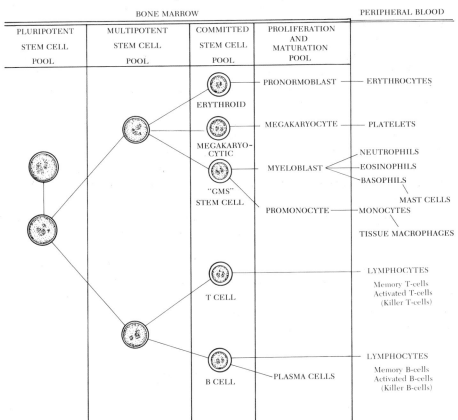

Much of the confusion regarding the identity of cells has been caused by lack of a uniform terminology. Different techniques and different types of material have been used by investigators who have given different names to the same cells and have employed the same term for different cells. Fortunately, unanimity of hematologic opinion as to the origin and relationship of the cells is not essential for the successful management of most clinical hematologic problems. There are enough points of agreement to allow the development of the workable concept of cellular relationships that is needed for an organized approach to clinical problems. A knowledge of morphology is necessary for the diagnosis of many hematologic diseases, and a terminology is essential for communication.

In selecting the terms to be used in this text the authors have chosen those that are used most commonly; in the classification of cells, the terms recommended by the Committee for Clarification of the Nomenclature of Cells and Diseases of the Blood-Forming Organs have been included in every instance.[16]

THE STEM CELL

The concept of the stem cell is generally accepted. Considerable recent evidence supports the view that the cell in question is morphologically indistinguishable from the small or medium-sized lymphocyte found in the bone marrow.[17] It has been demonstrated that it is these cells, separated from other marrow cells by glass wool column filters, which can incorporate tritiated thymidine into the nucleus, repopulate the marrow, and form spleen colonies in guinea pigs with the development of lines of erythroblasts, granulocytes, and megakaryocytes. Small lymphocytes found in the peripheral blood or lymph nodes, reticulum cells, granulocytic cells, and erythroblastic cells do not possess this capacity. In addition, a study reported that the injection of testosterone in rats led to a diminution in marrow and thymic lymphocytes associated with increased hematopoiesis and retained immunologic capacity; the observations were interpreted as a reflection of the accelerated differentiation of lymphoid cells in the marrow into erythroid and granulocytic cell lines, and those in the thymus into immunologically active cells.[25]

The concept of a single type of "stem" cell has been modified as a result of studies utilizing new techniques; different colony-stimulating units and committed cells have been recognized. In addition to the pluripotential stem cell able to reproduce itself or produce any of the marrow cell lines, "committed" stem cells able to produce only one type of cell, such as erythrocytes, have been found. Another, the "GMS" stem cell, can produce cells of either the granulocytic or the monocytic series, but no others. Still another "stem cell" seems able to form megakaryocytes, granulocytes, and erythrocyte precursors.

THE GRANULOCYTIC SERIES

The granulocytes (Fig. 1–2), which are motile and phagocytic, constitute the main defense of the body against bacterial infection. The kinetics and functions of these cells are discussed in Chapter 9.

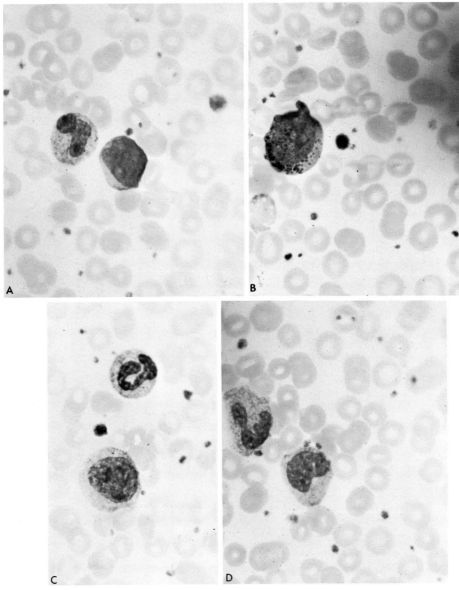

Figure 1–2   Early cells of the granulocytic series. *A*, Myeloblast. *B*, Progranulocyte. *C*, Myelocyte (early). *D*, Metamyelocyte.

Origin

Under normal conditions the older granulocytic cells, the bands and segmented cells, develop from the myelocytes in the bone marrow. Various cells have been considered to be the nongranular ancestors of the granular myelocytes.[18, 34, 41, 49] Although these theories differ in details, all agree that in the adult under normal circumstances the older cells of the granulocytic series arise in the bone marrow and are derived from the myelocytes and their precursors, which are either myeloblasts or cells that have an identical appearance in fixed smears.

Morphology

Myeloblast. The myeloblast occurs in normal bone marrow, but is not found in the circulating blood except in certain disease states. In fixed smears the diameter of myeloblasts ranges from 11 to 18 microns. With Wright's stain the nuclear material assumes a deep purplish blue color; the chromatin is finely divided, punctate, or strandlike, and appears condensed only around the rims of the nucleoli. The cytoplasm stains the same light blue color as the nucleolus, is variable in amount, and often forms little more than a rim about the nucleus. Myeloblasts generally give a negative reaction when a peroxidase stain is used, but some cells that are classed as myeloblasts with Wright's stain give a positive reaction with peroxidase stain. The staining properties of the cells are related to the nucleoproteins. Ribonucleic acid (RNA) occurs both in the nucleoli and in the cytoplasm; deoxyribonucleic acid (DNA) is found mainly in the nucleus. Protein synthesis in the cell is thought to be under the control of the nucleoproteins, and the presence of the nucleolus has been correlated with active cellular proliferation;[42, 71] cellular proliferation ceases when the nucleolus disappears and is replaced by the more deeply basophilic heterochromatin.[65]

Myeloblasts vary in size and other details. The nucleus is sometimes slightly indented, and in acute leukemia it is occasionally deeply indented or lobulated. Rieder cells are myeloblasts that have trifoliate or quadrifoliate nuclei. The cytoplasm of myeloblasts and monoblasts sometimes contains Auer bodies. These structures can be seen with Wright's stain and resemble a stained tubercle bacillus. Auer rods, which occur in the blasts of some patients with acute myeloblastic, acute myelomonocytic, and acute monocytic leukemia, are related to the azurophil granules and may result from the fusion of these granules. Auer rods and azurophil granules have in common the following: peroxidase positivity; Sudan black reaction; PAS positivity; the presence of RNA; negative reactions for alkaline phosphatase; similar ultrastructures as seen with the electron-microscopy.[1] When myeloblasts are stained supravitally with neutral red and Janus green, numerous small mitochondria can be seen in the cytoplasm. Myeloblasts do not stain with the nonspecific esterase or the periodic acid Schiff (PAS) stain.

Progranulocyte (promyelocyte). The progranulocyte is the next stage in development after the myeloblast, and some may resemble myeloblasts with the addition of azurophilic cytoplasmic granules. Other cells at this stage have a coarser nuclear structure than the myeloblast, are larger, and contain numerous azurophilic granules in the cytoplasm and in the region overlying the nucleus. Nucleoli may or may not be visible at this stage. The appearance and development of the granules appear to be closely related to the differentiation of the cytoplasmic proteins. Thorell has shown that the myeloblast has a high concentration of cytoplasmic polynucleotides and a prominent nucleolus.[65]

When the cell matures to the progranulocytic stage, the cytoplasmic polynucleo-tides decrease as the granules appear. Further development of the granules is associated with continued decrease in the polynucleotide content, and none is demonstrable by the time the myelocyte stage is reached. The nucleolus, which has been thought to have considerable influence over the differentiation of the cytoplasmic proteins, contains ribonucleic acid; this material decreases gradu-ally and is no longer detectable in the myelocytic stage. When the nucleolus disappears, further differentiation of the cytoplasmic protein cannot take place.

Myelocyte. Myelocytes are the first cells of the granulocytic series that contain specific granules, which are either neutrophilic, eosinophilic, or baso-philic. Both neutrophilic and eosinophilic granules give a positive peroxidase reaction. As the myelocyte develops from the progranulocyte it becomes smaller, and the nuclear chromatin becomes coarser. When supravital stains are used, numerous small mitochondria and a variable number of neutral red bodies can be demonstrated in the cytoplasm. The number, location, and arrangement of the neutral red bodies have been employed as a basis for classifying myelocytes according to different stages of development as myelo-cytes A, B, and C.[18]

Metamyelocyte (juvenile). As the myelocyte matures, the chromatin structure of the nucleus becomes coarser, specific granulation persists, and the nucleus becomes indented. At this stage the cell is termed a metamyelocyte.

Band cell (stab cell). According to the Committee on Nomenclature of Blood Cells (1949), any cell of the granulocytic series is classed as a band cell "which has a nucleus which could be described as a curved or coiled band, no matter how marked the indentation, if it does not completely segment the nucleus into lobes connected by a filament."[16]

Segmented cell (polymorphonuclear). These are the fully developed cells of the granulocytic series whose nuclei contain two or more lobes that are joined by a filamentous connection. The nuclear chromatin is coarse and has the appear-ance of blocks or knots connected by strands. The cytoplasm contains numerous granules that stain specifically with Wright's stain.

The neutrophil segmented cell (neutrophil) gives a positive peroxidase reaction. In supravital preparations numerous small refractile bodies fill the cytoplasm, and active ameboid movement is prominent. The granules do not stain with the nonspecific esterase stain but are positive with the periodic acid Schiff (PAS) stain.

Various abnormal forms of granulocytes have been described. Macro-polycytes, unusually large neutrophils with nuclei consisting of five to ten lobes, are seen in patients with a deficiency in vitamin B_{12} or folic acid. The Pelger-Huët anomaly, first described by Pelger in 1928,[51] is characterized by decreased segmentation of the nucleus and increased condensation of the nuclear chromatin. An abnormally large number of the cells (69 to 93 per cent) are two-lobed; they differ from band cells in that the individual lobes tend to be round and are joined by a narrow strand. The anomaly is inherited and involves the eosinophils and basophils as well as neutrophils. A similar "pseudo Pelger-Huët" anomaly is an acquired abnormality seen in some patients with severe infections and myeloproliferative disorders, particularly preleukemia. In these circumstances, segmentation is faulty and there is a predominance of two lobed band cells; cells with the "pince nez" nuclei are not so common.

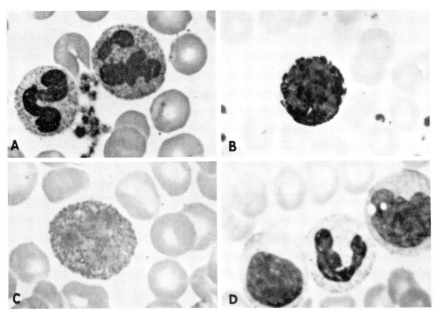

Figure 1-3 Later cells of the granulocytic series. *A,* Neutrophils. *B,* Basophil. *C,* Eosinophil. *D,* Comparison of lymphocyte, neutrophil, and monocyte.

A number of abnormalities have been described in the granules and cytoplasm of the granulocytes. Alder's constitutional granulation anomaly is characterized by the presence of large and numerous azurophil granulations in the neutrophils, eosinophils, and basophils; some of the monocytes and lymphocytes may be involved.[5] The heavy granulations may hide the nuclei of the cells. The blood of some but not all patients with gargoylism manifests this granulation anomaly.[29] "Toxic granulation" is the term given to changes in the granulocytes that occur in some patients with severe infections and other illnesses; the granules are dark and sometimes basophilic, and at times the cytoplasm is basophilic and vacuolated. Döhle inclusion bodies are round, blue-staining bodies sometimes seen in the cytoplasm of neutrophils; the bodies, which may measure 2 microns in diameter, are round or oval in shape; as many as three or four may be present in the periphery of the cell. They have been described in patients with various bacterial infections, and with burns.[68] The Chediak-Higashi syndrome, which is seen mainly in young children but also in young adults, is characterized by the presence of large eosinophilic, peroxidase positive inclusion bodies in myeloblasts and promyelocytes of the bone marrow; more mature cells of the granulocytic series contain abnormally large granules that stain normally.[13, 30] Patients with the syndrome have a predisposition to malignant lymphoma. The May-Heggelin anomaly is rare; it is characterized by Döhle bodies in the majority of the neutrophils, monocytes, and eosinophils associated with giant platelets, and, at times, thrombocytopenia.

The eosinophil segmented cell (eosinophil) is a fully developed cell. The nucleus does not stain as heavily as that of the neutrophil. The eosinophil is characterized by the presence of large granules that fill the cytoplasm and stain a bright yellowish red color with Wright's stain. When stained supravitally with neutral red and Janus green the granules appear large, very refractile, and yellow. These cells give a positive peroxidase reaction. Histochemical studies indicate that the eosinophil granules are composed of protein and surrounded by phospholipid.[10] Verdoperoxidase is also present.[2,3] Eosinophils contain about one-third of the histamine found in normal blood.[28]

The basophil segmented cell (basophil) is somewhat smaller than the neutrophil and eosinophil. The characteristic feature of this cell is the presence of large purplish black granules that almost completely fill the cell. The granules appear red when stained supravitally with neutral red. The cells are peroxidase negative. Basophils contain relatively large amounts of histamine,[14,15] about one-half of the histamine content of normal blood.[28] The presence of heparin has been suspected but not proved.

THE LYMPHOCYTIC SERIES

The lymphocytic series, which includes cells with diverse functions, is concerned with resistance to infection, antibody production, and tissue rejection. The cells have little motility. The functions of these cells are discussed in Chapter 14. A cell with the morphologic characteristics of the lymphocyte that arises in the bone marrow is thought to be a stem cell from which all the other blood cell lines develop.

Origin

Lymphocytes are produced in lymph nodes, in the periarterial pulp of the spleen, in nodules of the tonsils, in the mucous membranes of the gastrointestinal, genitourinary, and respiratory tracts, and in the lymph nodules in the bone marrow.[23,34,41,55] Various cellular origins of the lymphocytes have been suggested. Much evidence suggests that some lymphocytes are not irreversible "end cells" as the granulocytes are, but instead are cells that retain the potential for further differentiation, at least under special circumstances. The lymphocyte has been considered to be the source of plasma cells[41,62] and also of wandering tissue phagocytes.[41,53] The conclusion has also been reached that some lymphocytes act as stem cells.[21,34,35]

Morphology

Lymphoblast. The lymphoblast occurs in the peripheral blood rarely, if at all, except in cases of leukemia. It is distinguished from the myeloblast with difficulty, and the identity of a blast cell usually is assumed from the recognition of the older cells that accompany it. The nucleus of the lymphoblast is round and has a fine chromatin structure in which several nucleoli are often visible. The cytoplasm stains pale blue and contains no granules with Wright's stain but may have a granular appearance with PAS stain.

Prolymphocyte. Lymphocytic cells that are intermediate between lymphoblasts and lymphocytes are termed prolymphocytes. Although the nuclear chromatin appears coarser than that of the blast cells, it is finer than that of the lymphocytes. At times nucleoli or nucleolar remnants are visible. Usually the diameter of these cells is greater than 15 microns. The nucleus of some cells is indented or folded.

Lymphocyte. In dry smears the diameter of small lymphocytes varies from 7 to 10 microns, but the less common large lymphocytes may have a diameter of 20 microns. When Wright's stain is used, the nucleus of the small lymphocyte, which is usually round but sometimes indented, appears almost to fill the entire cell. The nucleus has a prominent membrane, stains deeply, and contains large masses of chromatin. No nucleoli can be identified. In the large lymphocytes the nuclear chromatin stains less deeply and appears some- what less compact. The cytoplasm, which is much more abundant in the larger lymphocytes, stains pale blue. A small number of reddish violet granules are scattered through the cytoplasm of many of the cells of this series. The lympho- cytes do not give a positive reaction with the peroxidase stain. When stained supravitally with Janus green and neutral red, the lymphocytes are seen to contain a variable number of short, rodlike mitochondria that usually appear clumped in one part of the cytoplasm, often opposite the nuclear indentation. A few small neutral red vacuoles are also seen. Lymphocytes do not take the non- specific esterase or the PAS stain.

Lymphocytes at times show definite staining abnormalities in disease states, particularly in virus infections. The cytoplasm of the larger cells is some- times deeply basophilic and opaque, and at other times it is almost colorless. Nuclear fenestrations and cytoplasmic vacuoles are often present.

THE MONOCYTIC SERIES

The monocytes are phagocytic cells related to the tissue macrophages. They function in the body defense against infection, particularly in the formation of granulomas and giant cells, and in the destruction of damaged tissue. They also play a role in immune reactions, probably by processing the antigen before it provokes a response from the lymphocytes.[48]

Origin

In 1924 Maximow stated that "of all the cells in the circulating blood, the monocytes offer the greatest difficulty to elucidation of their relationship and origin."[41] At various times monocytes have been considered to arise from lymphocytes,[11, 34] endothelial cells,[39] histiocytes,[6, 41] myeloblasts,[49] and mono- blasts.[56] A relationship between monocytes, histiocytes, and lymphocytes is shown by the study of the reaction in inflammation. Maximow considered it proved that the tissue macrophages (polyblasts, mononuclear–phagocytic ele- ments) arise partly through direct transformation of the free histiocytes of the tissue by mobilization, and also through changes that occur in monocytes and lymphocytes that migrate from blood vessels into the field of inflammation.

The present evidence discussed in Chapter 9 indicates that most if not all of the monocytes originate in the bone marrow, and then circulate in the peripheral blood for a short time until they migrate into the tissue and become phagocytic histiocytes; apparently the monocytes and myelocytes share a common ancestor stem cell.

Morphology

Monoblast.   According to the Committee on the Nomenclature of Blood Cells, the monoblast is any cell of the monocytic series that has a fine chromatin structure.[16] Nucleoli are usually visible, and such cells found in association with monocytes should be tentatively classed as monoblasts. These cells do not occur in the peripheral blood or bone marrow under normal conditions, but may be seen in patients with monocytic leukemia. The monoblast seen in acute monocytic leukemia is "negative" with peroxidase and Sudan black stains, "positive" with the nonspecific esterase.

Promonocyte.   Promonocytes are cells that have an indented nucleus and appear younger than the monocytes, in that the nuclear chromatin appears more finely divided and contains nucleoli or nucleolar remnants. These cells are thought to be intermediate between the blast cells and adult monocytes. They are not seen in the peripheral blood normally, but at times do occur in disseminated tuberculosis and other diseases involving the reticuloendothelial system, as well as in monocytic leukemia.

Monocyte.   The monocyte (Fig. 1–4) is usually larger than the other cells of the peripheral blood. In dried smears the diameter measures from 16 to 22 microns. When stained with Wright's preparation, the monocyte possesses an

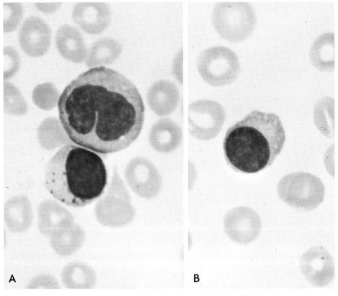

Figure 1–4   *A,* Monocyte and lymphocyte. *B,* Plasma cell.

abundant pale bluish gray cytoplasm which appears somewhat more opaque than the cytoplasm of the lymphocytes. The cytoplasm contains numerous fine reddish granules, and vacuoles are often present. The nucleus, which is often but not invariably indented, has a stringy chromatin structure that appears more condensed where the strands of chromatin meet. Monocytes and histiocytes are "positive" when stained with nonspecific esterase stain, "negative" with peroxidase. When these cells are stained supravitally with neutral red and Janus green, large numbers of short mitochondria can be seen in the cytoplasm. Neutral red regularly stains a group of cytoplasmic vacuoles near the indentation of the nucleus. This rosette of red vacuoles has been considered by some authors to be a characteristic peculiar to monocytes,[56] but others do not share this opinion. Although monocytes usually are easily distinguished from lymphocytes and myelocytes by their size and the appearance of the nucleus and cytoplasm, at times atypical cells are seen that cannot be identified with confidence by any of the staining methods; some such cells are considered to be "virocytes" and others are designated "lymphoreticular cells."

THE THROMBOCYTIC SERIES

The thrombocytes or blood platelets are an essential part of the hemostatic mechanism of the body; they are important in thrombosis and blood coagulation. The chemistry and function of these blood elements are discussed in Chapter 16.

Origin

Megakaryocytes are thought to arise from primitive mesenchymal cells by way of the hemocytoblast, the precursor of the megakaryoblast.[66]

Wright's hypothesis of the origin of the blood platelets as fragmented portions of the cytoplasm of the megakaryocytes of the bone marrow is generally accepted.[73] More recent studies that utilized antisera[7] and the electron microscope[4,31] support the same conclusion.

Morphology

Megakaryoblast. Megakaryoblasts, which are found only in the bone marrow in special circumstances, are larger than the other blast cells. The cytoplasm is pale blue. The nucleus, which is round or oval, has a finely divided chromatin structure, and a variable number of small nucleoli may be apparent.

Promegakaryocyte. Promegakaryocytes are considered to be intermediate between megakaryoblasts and megakaryocytes. The nucleus, which has a shape similar to that of the megakaryocyte, contains nucleoli surrounded by a rather coarse chromatin structure. The cytoplasm contains a number of fine purplish red granules.

Megakaryocyte. The megakaryocyte (Fig. 1–5) has now been demonstrated to circulate in small numbers in the venous blood of normal persons, and in

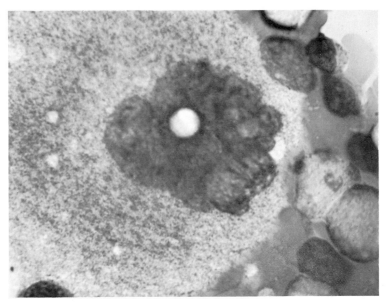

Figure 1–5 Megakaryocyte.

larger numbers in the venous blood of patients with cancer.[32,37] It has been demonstrated in dogs and in humans that the lungs trap the great majority of these large cells. It has been estimated that from 9 to 26 per cent of the platelets are released in the pulmonary capillaries by these mature megakaryocytes.[36] Megakaryocytes are found in the bone marrow. They are very large cells that often have a diameter that varies from 50 to 100 microns. The nucleus, which is usually polyploid, stains dark blue with Wright's stain and contains no visible nucleoli. The abundant cytoplasm stains light blue and contains numerous purplish red granules. These granules often appear in aggregates.

Thrombocyte (platelet). Thrombocytes, or blood platelets, are the smallest stained elements in the peripheral blood. Ordinarily they have a diameter of from 2 to 4 microns, but in some disease states, and on smears made from blood collected with an anticoagulant, the platelets appear much larger. In such circumstances they may approach the small lymphocyte in size, or may form a strand that stretches across an entire oil immersion field. These elements contain no nuclei, and when stained with Wright's stain appear to consist of a pale cytoplasm that contains numerous reddish purple granules.

THE PLASMACYTIC SERIES

The plasma cells are an important part of the body's defense mechanism and are the main sources of the plasma globulins. These cells are discussed in more detail in Chapter 14.

Origin

Michels reviewed the rather extensive literature on the plasma cell that appeared prior to 1931, and noted that at least four different cellular origins had been suggested.[45] These were: (1) histogenous origin from connective tissue cells, including tissue lymphocytes, fibroblasts, and resting wandering cells; (2) origin from emigrated lymphocytes; (3) origin from emigrated lymphocytes or pre-existing tissue lymphocytes; and (4) origin from immature blood cells such as myeloblasts or erythroblasts, through aberration. Sundberg reviewed the subject of the origin and function of the plasma cells[62] and pointed out that studies on the production of antibodies emphasize a close relationship between the plasma cells and the lymphocytes.

Morphology

Plasmablast (myeloma cell). Plasmablasts do not occur normally in the peripheral blood or in the bone marrow, and are seen only in plasmacytic leukemia or multiple myeloma. The nucleus, which is usually eccentric, has a fine chromatin structure and contains one or more large nucleoli. The cytoplasm stains blue and is more opaque than that of the myeloblast or lymphoblast.

Proplasmacyte. These cells are intermediate between the plasmablasts and the plasmacytes. The chromatin of the nucleus appears more coarse than that of the plasmablast but is definitely more immature than that of the plasmacyte. Usually a single nucleolus is present, but at times more than one are seen.

Plasmacyte (plasma cell, Marschalko's plasma cell). In fixed smears the plasma cells vary considerably in size, and diameters range from 10 to 20 microns. The characteristic feature of the cell is the eccentric location of the round or oval nucleus which has extremely coarse chromatin. The chromatin consists of blocks which stain deeply. The arrangement of the chromatin in the nucleus has been compared in appearance to the spokes of a wheel. The cytoplasm, which often has an irregular border, is abundant, stains dark blue, and is characterized by a perinuclear area of lighter staining. The cytoplasm is nonhomogeneous, and small vacuoles are often present. When supravital stains are used, numerous small mitochondria can be seen in the cytoplasm of the cell.

Plasmacytes usually are not seen in the peripheral blood but may appear in serum sickness, rubella, infectious mononucleosis, infectious hepatitis, multiple myeloma, plasma cell leukemia, and other conditions. Normally plasmacytes are present in the lymph nodes, the connective tissue, and the bone marrow.

THE ERYTHROCYTIC SERIES

The erythrocytes contain hemoglobin, which is essential for transport of the oxygen from the lungs to the tissues in the body. The production and function of these cells are discussed in Chapters 2 and 7.

Origin

Michels in 1931 published an extensive review of erythropoiesis.[46] He attributes the first observation of the red corpuscles to Jan Schwammerdam in 1658, and the first report of nucleated red corpuscles in the human species to Webber, who in 1838 observed them in a human fetus of 12 weeks. In 1857 Kölliker demonstrated erythropoiesis in the embryonic liver, and recognized that the non-nucleated red corpuscles arose from the nucleated forms. He recognized that the spleen was also an organ of erythropoiesis, but thought that nucleated red corpuscles did not occur in the blood or any of the organs of adults. Neumann in 1868 demonstrated that the mammalian red corpuscles arose throughout life from the nucleated elements in the bone marrow. He studied human cadaver material and observed erythropoiesis in many bones; he also noted that the red marrow increased at the expense of the yellow marrow to provide an additional source of erythrocyte production.

The identity of the precursors of the nucleated red cells has been a controversial subject. Maximow concluded that in the embryo the hemocytoblasts, which were derived from the mesenchyme, produce the nucleated precursors of the erythrocyte. He thought that hematopoiesis in the adult is homoplastic, that erythrocytes develop from nucleated precursors of fixed lineage, but he considered it possible that in abnormal conditions, when homoplastic production might be inadequate, heteroplastic formation might be called forth.[41] Jordan suggested that small lymphocytes that originate in the lymph nodes might leave the circulation in the bone marrow and serve as erythrocyte precursors.[34] Doan, Cunningham, and Sabin studied the bone marrows of pigeons recovering from starvation and the bone marrows of rabbits given repeated doses of dead typhoid bacilli[20] and concluded that the erythrocyte precursors arise from the endothelial cells of the capillaries and develop intravascularly, but that the granulocytes arise from reticular cells in the interspaces of the veins. Jordan and Johnson performed similar experiments on pigeons and concluded that, although erythropoiesis is mainly intravascular, the erythrocyte precursor is not an endothelial cell but instead is the hemocytoblast, which sometimes develops extravascularly and migrates into the vessels.[35] Bloom and Bartelmez[11] and Gilmour[27] also have concluded that in human embryos erythropoiesis is extravascular.

In the embryo the main site of erythropoiesis during the first two months is the yolk sac, where the first blood cells arise from mesenchymal cells.[11] In the next phase of development erythropoiesis is chiefly in the liver and, to a lesser extent, in the spleen until about the sixth month. Hematopoiesis appears in the bone marrow at about the fifth month, and increases in this tissue as it declines in the liver. After birth the bone marrow is essentially the only tissue concerned in the production of erythrocytes. In the first few years of postnatal life erythropoiesis is active in the marrow of practically all the bones, but in adults it is confined largely to the skull, thorax, vertebra, innominate bone, and the upper ends of the femur and humerus. In the normal bone marrow erythropoiesis is carried on mainly by division of the polychromatic and orthochromatic normoblast cells that comprise about 90 per cent of the erythrocyte precursors in the marrow. When erythropoiesis is accelerated, increased numbers of the earlier forms are evident. In disease states, when the hematopoietic tissue is displaced by metastatic cells or myelofibrosis, extramedullary erythropoiesis appears in the liver, spleen, and lymph nodes.

In postnatal life normally the blood cells are formed in the bone marrow and lymphoid tissues of the body. The bone marrow is the sole site of origin of the erythrocytic, granulocytic, and megakaryocytic cells. Transplant experiments indicate that formation of the microcirculation from reticular cells precedes hematopoietic repopulation.[64] Some of the lymphocytes also originate in the marrow; other morphologically similar cells that probably have different functions are produced in the thymus, lymph nodes, and other lymphoid tissue in the body. In certain hematologic disorders, extramedullary hematopoiesis appears in the spleen, liver, lymph nodes, and other tissues.

Morphology

The terminology used in discussion of the nucleated cells of the erythrocytic series has been the source of considerable confusion. Because different definitions have been given to the same term by different authors, the Committee for Clarification of the Nomenclature of Cells and Diseases of the Blood and Blood-Forming Organs has recommended an entirely new terminology for the nucleated cells of the erythrocytic series.[16] The terms recommended — rubriblast, prorubricyte, rubricyte, and metarubricyte — have not been used widely. The Committee felt that the recommended names indicated stages of differentiation in development of the adult erythrocyte. They recommended that the qualifying phrase "pernicious anemia type" be used to indicate the cells that showed the morphologic characteristics seen in patients with untreated pernicious anemia.

Usually the type of erythropoiesis is described as being either "normoblastic" or "megaloblastic." The term "megaloblast" has been used with different meanings in the literature. Ehrlich introduced the term to indicate the large nucleated precursor of the erythrocytes that is characterized by its much weaker affinity for nuclear stains.[24] He thought that the presence of this cell indicated an abnormal type of erythropoiesis that was seen in adults almost exclusively with pernicious anemia, and that it represented an embryonic type of cell. He considered it a line of cell maturation different from the "normoblastic" type which was seen in nearly all other types of anemia. The normoblastic type of maturation was characterized by erythrocyte precursors which contained a nucleus that gave an intense color with nuclear stains. Doan, Cunningham, and Sabin used the term "megaloblast" to indicate the first generation of cells in the red blood cell series that could be distinguished from endothelial cells in either the embryonic or adult types of erythropoiesis.[20] Thus, according to one usage of the term, "megaloblast" indicates an abnormal type of erythropoiesis that occurs only in special disease states when seen in postnatal human beings; according to the other usage, the term indicates a very young erythrocyte precursor that may occur whenever erythropoiesis is markedly increased but otherwise normal. The term "erythroblast" has been used by some authors to refer to all forms of nucleated red corpuscles, but Doan, Cunningham, and Sabin have used this term to indicate an intermediate stage in the development of the erythrocyte.[20] The term "megaloblast" is used in this text as it has been used by Ehrlich, Downey, Jones and Wintrobe.[23, 24, 33, 72]

Erythropoiesis is considered as being normal in type when the normoblastic series is present, and abnormal when the megaloblastic series is present. Similar stages in the development of the nucleated red cells can be recognized in both series. In normoblastic maturation the cells of the different stages are termed pronormoblast, basophilic normoblast, polychromatic normoblast, and orthochromatic normoblast. In the megaloblastic type of maturation the corresponding cells are termed promegaloblast, basophilic megaloblast, polychromatic megaloblast, and orthochromatic megaloblast.

Pronormoblast (rubriblast).   (Stage I). The pronormoblast is the youngest recognizable precursor of the erythrocyte. Its diameter varies from 12 to 19 microns. The nucleus, which is round and fills most of the cell, contains strands of chromatin and several nucleoli. The nongranular cytoplasm stains blue. Usually these cells can be distinguished from myeloblasts by the coarser staining of the nuclear chromatin and the more opaque cytoplasm. Thorell[65] has demonstrated that, during this and the next phase of development of the red blood cell, a considerable portion of the proteins is being formed. The production of protein is accompanied by a marked decrease in the cytoplasmic nucleotides; by the time the end of the basophilic normoblast stage is reached, the cytoplasmic nucleotides have practically disappeared and protein production is greatly reduced.

Basophilic normoblast (prorubricyte).   (Stage II).   The basophilic normoblast differs from the pronormoblast in that the nuclear chromatin is more coarse, distinct nucleoli are not seen, and the cytoplasm is more densely basophilic.

Polychromatic normoblast (rubricyte).   (Stage III).   This stage covers a relatively wide range in the maturation of the erythrocyte, from the beginning of recognizable hemoglobin in the cytoplasm to the complete disappearance of basophilia. During this time the nucleus becomes smaller and the nuclear chromatin becomes more condensed. This stage of development is characterized by a remarkable production of hemoglobin. Thorell has reported that the concentration of hemoglobin increases from 1×10^{-6} to 23×10^{-6} micrograms during this phase, and has suggested that it is at this time that the formation of the iron porphyrin component and its coupling to globin takes place.[65]

Orthochromatic normoblast (metarubricyte).   (Stage IV).   A normoblast is considered to reach the orthochromatic stage when the cytoplasm appears to contains its full complement of hemoglobin. The nuclear chromatin becomes more and more condensed, the nucleus diminishes in size and finally disappears. During this phase the quantity of hemoglobin of the cell reaches that contained at maturity, 28×10^{-6} micrograms. This is accompanied by a decrease in volume of the cell amounting to 25 to 33 per cent.

In normal persons, between 30 and 50 per cent of the normoblasts contain cytoplasmic aggregates of nonhemoglobin iron, ferritin, that stain with Prussian blue. These cells are called sideroblasts. Abnormal sideroblasts, "ringed sideroblasts," occur in some disorders of iron metabolism; these cells in which the iron has accumulated in the mitochondria may comprise more than 50 per cent of the nucleated red cells.[12]

Megaloblasts. The details, such as presence of nucleoli, basophilia, and degree of hemoglobinization, that distinguish a pronormoblast or a basophilic normoblast from a polychromatic normoblast provide the same criteria that are used for differentiating a promegaloblast from a polychromatic megaloblast and the other cells in this series. In distinguishing megaloblastic erythropoiesis from normoblastic erythropoiesis in the smear stained with Wright's stain, it is well to remember the admonition of Ehrlich and Lazarus, who wrote, "In order to gain a perfectly clear conception of the physiological and pathological import of the erythroblasts, it is absolutely necessary to consider, in the first place, only typical examples of both forms." There are, as would be expected, a large number of cells which cannot be classified either as normoblasts or as megaloblasts, since some of the characteristics which Ehrlich described for these cells are wanting.[24] Typical megaloblastic erythropoiesis is seen most often in patients with a deficiency of vitamin B_{12} or folate, or erythroleukemia (di Guglielmo's disorder), or during treatment with an antifolate compound or other chemotherapeutic agent.

The types of erythropoiesis are most easily distinguished at the third or "polychromatic" stage. Two details helpful in distinguishing megaloblasts from normoblasts at this stage are, first, an increase in the lighter staining parachromatin of the nucleus in the megaloblasts and, second, the appearance of hemoglobin in cells with nuclei that appear more immature than is ordinarily the case in the normoblastic type of erythropoiesis. The younger promegaloblasts and basophilic megaloblasts are also recognizably different from their normoblastic counterparts. The nucleus of the megaloblast stains lighter because the nuclear chromatin is usually more finely divided, and appears more separated because of the increase in parachromatin. In the orthochromatic stage the megaloblast is often larger than the corresponding normoblast; the increase in parachromatin usually remains evident until the nuclear chromatin becomes almost completely condensed and pyknotic in appearance.

Different degrees of megaloblastosis occur, and some hematologists employ a semi-quantitative gradation of from "one plus" to "four plus." "Megaloblastoid" is a term sometimes used to describe minor megaloblastic changes, usually an increase in the nuclear parachromatin, that occur in many patients with hematologic disorders, particularly myeloproliferative disorders, refractory anemia, and hemolytic anemia; the changes may be due to folate deficiency or some abnormality in folate–vitamin B_{12} metabolism, but often no satisfactory explanation is apparent.

Reticulocytes. Reticulocytes are young non-nucleated cells of the erythrocytic series that can be recognized only with supravital stains. These metabolically active cells contain mitochondria and polyribosomes. When brilliant cresyl blue is used, the reticulocyte appears to contain granules or a fibrillar network of RNA that stains light blue in color; the structures stained in this way are mainly ribosomes. When the preparation is counterstained with Wright's stain these structures appear darker and are recognized more easily. Normally reticulocytes constitute 1 per cent or less of the erythrocytes, from 25,000 to 50,000 per cu. mm. Determination of the number of reticulocytes in the peripheral blood affords one of the best measures of increased erythropoiesis, because the number of reticulocytes reflects the effective increase in bone marrow activity better than does the morphologic appearance of the bone marrow. The percentage of reticulocytes is nearly always increased after hemorrhage, during hemolysis, and after specific therapy is instituted for anemia. In patients with severe hemolytic anemia some of the reticulocytes in the peripheral blood contain granules of nonhemoglobin iron, ferritin, that stain with Prussian blue. The reticulocytes released into the circulation mature to become erythrocytes within several days unless they are destroyed.

Erythrocytes. The erythrocytes are adult members of the erythrocytic series. They are non-nucleated biconcave discs that stain a pink or pinkish gray color with Wright's stain. The diameters of the erythrocytes on dried films were found by Price-Jones to have a mean of 7.2 microns and to range from 6.7 to 7.7 microns.[52] When erythrocytes that have been stained with Wright's stain appear grayish blue the condition is termed "diffuse basophilia," and when bluish granules are evident in the cells "punctate basophilia" is said to be present. Both of these staining reactions are signs of immaturity and reflect the persistence of ribose nucleoprotein in the cells. Punctate basophilia, or "stippling," is increased after exposure to lead and other metals. Study of red cells in a film of peripheral blood stained with Wright's stain may disclose a number of variations in size and shape, but gives little inkling of the numerous variegated, bizarre, and beautiful shapes revealed by scanning electron microscopy.[9]

In disease states the erythrocytes are often abnormal. The cells may show marked abnormalities in shape (poikilocytosis) or size (anisocytosis). The deformity may vary from a slight irregularity to a marked elongation; cells of the latter variety are sometimes referred to as "pencil forms." Erythrocytes that have a diameter of less than 6 microns are termed "microcytes." Microcytes that occur in iron deficiency often exhibit a distinct increase in central pallor and are termed "hypochromic microcytes." In other disorders, such as familial spherocytosis, the diameter of the erythrocytes is less than normal, but the thickness of the cell is increased and the hemoglobin content is normal. Such cells, which are spoken of as "microspherocytes," appear small but stain deeply, and do not have the central pallor that is seen in the hypochromic microcytes and normal cells. Macrocytes, defined by some authors as cells with a diameter greater than 9 microns, occur in deficiencies of folic acid or vitamin B_{12}, myxedema, and other disorders. The presence of large oval macrocytes in the peripheral blood smear strongly suggests a deficiency of vitamin B_{12} or folate. "Target cells" ("Mexican hat cells"), which are thinner than normal and have a relatively large diameter, resemble the concentric circles of a rifle target in appearance. They occur in various types of anemia, such as sickle cell anemia, hemoglobin C disease, and the thalassemias, and also during jaundice and after splenectomy.

"Burr cells" (echinocytes) are erythrocytes which have numerous spinelike projections; they are seen in uremia and as artifacts. Acanthocytes (spur cells) occur as part of a rare syndrome comprising atypical retinitis pigmentosa,

---

Figure 1–6 *(opposite page—upper).* Normoblastic hyperplasia in hemolytic anemia.
Figure 1–7 *(opposite page—lower).* Megaloblastic hyperplasia in pernicious anemia. (From Heilmeyer and Bergemann: Atlas der klinischen Hämatologie und Cytologie. Berlin-Göttingen-Heidelberg, Springer, 1955.)

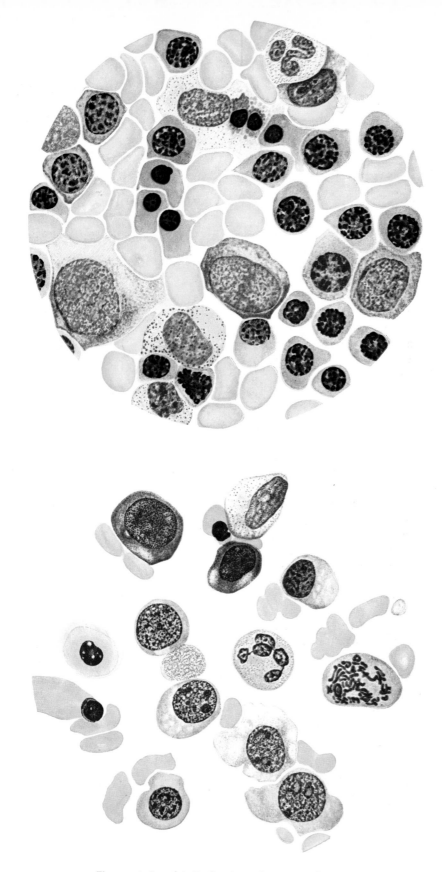

Figures 1–6 and 1–7   *See legends on opposite page.*

steatorrhea, ataxia, and absent serum beta-lipoprotein.[57, 59] "Spur cells," which have projections of varying size and shape, are seen in a variety of disorders including liver disease, microangiopathic hemolytic anemia, and thrombotic thrombocytopenic purpura; some of these abnormalities are the result of acquired damage to the red cell membrane, in some circumstances from a factor present in the plasma.[58, 61] Other forms of poikilocytes are "helmet cells" and shistocytes (cell fragments), most often seen in patients with impact hemolysis. "Howell-Jolly bodies" are sometimes seen in erythrocytes of patients with anemia. These particles usually occur singly. They are larger than the usual granules, and are thought to be nuclear particles because they take the nuclear stains. "Cabot rings," which may be single or double, occur in both nucleated and non-nucleated cells. Whether these structures, which sometimes appear bright red in smears prepared with Wright's stain, are derivatives of nuclear material, or products of cellular degeneration produced by toxic substances, is uncertain.

"Siderocytes" are erythrocytes that contain particles of nonhemoglobin iron. Siderotic granules resemble those seen in punctate basophilia when smears are prepared with Wright's stain, but the difference between the particles can be shown by the Prussian blue staining reaction. Siderocytes are seen most often in the peripheral blood in hemolytic anemia and after splenectomy. "Heinz bodies" are highly refractile particles of denatured hemoglobin, 1 to 3 microns in diameter, that can be visualized with supravital stains but not with Wright's stain. They occur in the peripheral blood of susceptible persons after exposure to certain drugs, particularly primaquine, acetanilid, and acetylphenylhydrazine. The observation that these bodies become more numerous after splenectomy suggests that the spleen may be able to remove these bodies from the intact cells.

Other abnormalities of the erythrocytes that can be seen on the stained smear are often of diagnostic significance. Erythrocytes that appear elongated with rounded ends are known as "ovalocytes" or "elliptocytes." Small numbers of such cells may occur on smears made from normal persons. This type of cell also develops as the result of a hereditary defect, in which case the vast majority of the cells have an oval or elliptical shape. The erythrocytes of patients with sickle cell anemia or sickle cell trait assume a crescent form when the hemoglobin is in the reduced state. In patients with sickle cell anemia some of these forms may be apparent in a fixed smear prepared with Wright's stain, but usually this deformity can be demonstrated only in moist preparations.

References

1. Ackerman, G. A.: Microscopic and histochemical studies of the Auer bodies in leukemic cells. Blood, 5:847, 1950.
2. Agner, K.: Verdoperoxidase. Acta Physiol. Scand., Suppl. 8, 2, 1941.
3. Agner, K.: Detoxicating effect of verdoperoxidase on toxins. Nature, 159:271, 1947.
4. Albrecht, M.: Studies on the evolution of thrombocytes, experiences with megakaryocytes in vitro. Int. Soc. Hem. Abstr. 437, p. 346, 1956.
5. Alder, A.: Über Konstitutonell Bedingte Granulation-veränderungen der Leukozyten. Deutsches Arch. klin. Med., 183:372, 1939.
6. Aschoff, L., and Kiyono, K.: Zur Frage der grossen Mononuklearen. Folia haemat. (1. Teil), 15:383, 1913.

7. Bedson, S. P., and Johnston, M. E.: Further observations on platelet genesis. J. Pathol. Bacteriol., *28*:101, 1925.
8. Berlin, R. D., Oliver, J. M., Ukena, T. E., and Yin, H. H.: The cell surface. N. Engl. J. Med., *292*:515, 1975.
9. Bessis, M.: Corpuscles. Springer-Verlag-Berlin, Heidelberg, New York, 1973.
10. Bloom, L. M., and Wislocki, G. B.: The localization of lipids in human blood and bone marrow cells. Blood, *5*:79, 1950.
11. Bloom, W., and Bartelmez, G. W.: Hematopoiesis in young human embryos. Am. J. Anat., *67*:21, 1940.
12. Cartwright, G. E., and Deiss, A.: Sideroblasts, siderocytes, and sideroblastic anemia. N. Engl. J. Med., *292*:185, 1975.
13. Chédiak, M.: Nouvelle anomalia leucocytaire de caractère constitutional et familial. Rev. Hematol., *7*:362, 1952.
14. Code, C. F.: The histamine-like activity of white blood cells. J. Physiol., *90*:485, 1937.
15. Code, C. F.: The source in blood of the histamine-like constituent. J. Physiol., *90*:349, 1937.
16. Condensation of the First Two Reports of the Committee for Clarification of the Nomenclature of Cells and Diseases of the Blood and Blood-Forming Organs. Blood, *4*:89, 1949.
17. Cudkowicz, G., Bennett, M., and Shearer, G. M.: Pluripotent stem cell function of the mouse marrow lymphocyte. Science, *144*:866, 1964.
18. Cunningham, R. S., Sabin, F. R., and Doan, C. A.: The development of leukocytes, lymphocytes, and monocytes from a specific stem-cell in adult tissues. Contrib. Embryol., Carnegie Inst., *16*:227, 1925.
19. Danielli, J. F., and Davson, H.: Contributions to theory of permeability of thin films. J. Cell Comp. Physiol., *5*:495, 1935.
20. Doan, C. A., Cunningham, R. S., and Sabin, F. R.: Experimental studies on the origin and maturation of avian and mammalian red blood-cells. Contrib. Embryol. Carnegie Inst., *16*:163, 1928.
21. Downey, H.: The occurrence and significance of the "myeloblast" under normal and pathologic conditions. Arch. Intern. Med., *33*:301, 1924.
22. Downey, H.: Origin of monocytes in monocytic leukemia and leukemic reticuloendotheliosis. Anat. Rec., *48*:16, 1931.
23. Downey, H.: Handbook of Hematology. Paul B. Hoeber, New York, 1938.
24. Ehrlich, P., and Lazarus, A.: Anemia, 2nd Ed. Rebman Ltd., London, 1910.
25. Frey-Wettstein, M., and Craddock, C. G.: Testosterone-induced depletion of thymus and marrow lymphocytes as related to lymphopoiesis and hematopoiesis. Blood, *35*:257, 1970.
26. Frye, L. D., and Edidin, M.: The rapid intermixing of cell surface antigens after formation of mouse-human heterokaryons. J. Cell Sci., *7*:319, 1970.
27. Gilmour, J. R.: Normal haemopoiesis in the intra-uterine and neonatal life. J. Pathol. Bacteriol., *52*:25, 1941.
28. Graham, H. T., Lowry, O. H., Wheelwright, F., Lenz, M. A., and Parish, H. H., Jr.: Distribution of histamine among leukocytes and platelets. Blood, *10*:467, 1955.
29. Griffiths, S. B., and Findlay, M.: Gargoylism: Clinical, radiological and haematological features in two siblings. Arch. Dis. Child., *33*:229, 1958.
30. Higashi, O.: Congenital gigantism of peroxidase granules. Tokoku J. Exp. Med., *59*:315, 1954.
31. Hiraki, K.: The function of the megakaryocyte: Observations both in idiopathic thrombocytopenic purpura and normal adults. Internat. Soc. Hem. Abstr. 436, p. 345, 1956.
32. Hume, R., West, J. T., Malmgren, R. A., and Chu, E. A.: Quantitative observations of circulating megakaryocytes in the blood of patients with cancer. N. Engl. J. Med., *270*:111, 1964.
33. Jones, O. P.: Cytology of Pathologic Marrow Cells with Especial Reference to Marrow Biopsies. *In* Downey, H. (ed.): Handbook of Hematology. Paul B. Hoeber, Inc., New York, 1938.
34. Jordan, H. E.: The significance of the lymphoid nodule. Am. J. Anat., *57*:1, 1935.
35. Jordan, H. E., and Johnson, E. P.: Erythrocyte production in the bone marrow of the pigeon. Am. J. Anat., *56*:71, 1935.
36. Kaufman, R. M., Airo, R., Pollack, S., and Crosby, W. H.: Pulmonary megakaryocytes: Their origin and significance. J. Clin. Invest., *44*:1063, 1965.
37. Kaufman, R. M., Airo, R., Pollack, S., Crosby, W. H., and Doberneck, R.: Origin of pulmonary megakaryocytes. Blood, *25*:767, 1965.
38. Korn, E. D.: Structure of biological membranes. Science, *153*:1491, 1966.
39. Mallory, F. B.: A histological study of typhoid fever. J. Exp. Med., *3*:611, 1898.
40. Marcus, A. J.: Platelet function. N. Engl. J. Med., *280*:1213, 1278, and 1330, 1969.
41. Maximow, A.: Relation of the blood cells to connective tissue and endothelium. Physiol. Rev. *4*:533, 1924.
42. Mazia, D., and Prescott, D. M.: Nuclear function and mitosis. Science, *120*:120, 1954.

43. McCulloch, E. A., Siminovitch, L., and Till, J. E.: Spleen-colony formation in anemic mice genotype WW$^{\text{V.}}$ Science, *144*:845, 1964.
44. Meuter, M., and Lebond, C. P.: The Golgi apparatus. Sci. Am., *22*:100, 1969.
45. Michels, N. A.: The plasma cell. Arch. Pathol., *11*:775, 1931.
46. Michels, N. A.: Erythropoiesis: A critical review of the literature. Folio haemat., *45*:75, 1931.
47. Miner, R. W. (ed.): Leukocyte functions. Ann. N.Y. Acad. Sci., *59*:667–1069, 1955.
48. Mosier, D. E.: A requirement for two cell types for antibody formation in vitro. Science, *158*: 1573, 1967.
49. Naegeli, O.: Blutkrankheiten und Blutdiagnostik. Verlag von Veit and Comp. Leipzig, *117*, 1908.
50. Osserman, E. F.: Lysozyme. N. Engl. J. Med., *292*:424, 1975.
51. Pelger, K.: Demonstratie van een paar zeldzaam voorkomende typen van bloedlichaampjes en bespreking der patienten. Nederl. tijdschr. geneesk., *72*:1178, 1928.
52. Price-Jones, C.: Red cell diameter in one hundred healthy persons and in pernicious anemia. The effect of liver treatment. J. Pathol. & Bacteriol., *32*:479, 1929.
53. Rebuck, J. W., and Crowley, J. H.: A method of study leukocyte functions in vivo. Ann. N.Y. Acad. Sci., *59*:757, 1955.
54. Robertson, J. D.: Ultrastructure of cell membranes and their derivatives. Biochem. Soc. Symp. (Cambridge, Engl.), *16*:3, 1959.
55. Sabin, F. R.: On the origin of the cells of the blood. Physiol. Rev., *2*:38, 1922.
56. Sabin, F. R., Doan, C. A., and Cunningham, R. S.: Discrimination of two types of phagocytic cells in connective tissue by the supravital technique. Contrib. Embryol., Carnegie Inst., *16*:125, 1925.
57. Salt, H. B., Wolff, O. H., Lloyd, J. K., Fosbrooke, A. S., Cameron, A. H., and Hubble, D. V.: On having no beta-lipoprotein. A syndrome comprising a-beta-lipoproteinaemia, acanthocytosis and steatorrhoea. Lancet, *2*:325, 1960.
58. Silber, R.: Acanthocytes, spurs, burrs and membranes. Blood, *34*:111, 1969.
59. Simon, E. R., and Ways, P.: Incubation hemolysis and red cell metabolism in acanthocytosis. J. Clin. Invest., *43*:1311, 1964.
60. Skendzel, L. P., and Hoffman, G. C.: Pelger anomaly of leukocytes: 41 cases in seven families. Am. J. Clin. Pathol., *37*:294, 1962.
61. Smith, J. A., Lonergan, E. T., and Sterling, K.: Spur-cell anemia. N. Engl. J. Med., *271*:396, 1964.
62. Sundberg, R. D.: Lymphocytes and plasma cells. Ann. N.Y. Acad. Sci., *59*:671, 1955.
63. Tapley, D. F., Kimberg, D. V., and Buchanan, J. L.: The mitochondrion. N. Engl. J. Med., *276*: 1124, 1182, 1967.
64. Tavassoli, M., and Crosby, W. H.: Transplantation of marrow to extramedullary sites. Science, *161*:55, 1968.
65. Thorell, B.: Studies on the formation of cellular substances during blood cell production. Acta med. Scand., Suppl. 200, 1947.
66. Tocantins, L. M.: The mammalian blood platelets in health and disease. Medicine, *17*:155, 1938.
67. Valentine, W. N., Pearce, M. L., and Lawrence, J. S.: Studies on the histamine content of blood. Blood, *5*:623, 1950.
68. Weiner, W., and Topley, E.: Döhle bodies in the leukocytes of patients with burns. J. Clin. Pathol., *8*:324, 1955.
69. Weinstein, R. S.: The structure of cell membranes. N. Engl. J. Med., *281*:86, 1969.
70. Weissman, G.: Lysosomes. N. Engl. J. Med., *273*:1084, 1143, 1965.
71. White, J. C.: The cytoplasmic basophilia of bone marrow cells. J. Pathol. Bacteriol., *59*:223, 1947.
72. Wintrobe, M. M.: Clinical Hematology, 4th Ed. Lea and Febiger, Philadelphia, 1956.
73. Wright, J. H.: The histogenesis of the blood platelets. J. Morphol., *21*:263, 1910.

CHAPTER 2

ERYTHROPOIESIS AND THE METABOLISM OF HEMOGLOBIN

ERYTHROPOIESIS

The primary task of the red blood cell is the transport of respiratory gases. (The important role played by 2,3-DPG, [2,3-diphosphoglycerate] in performing this function in different circumstances is discussed in Chapter 7.) To achieve this, there must be sufficient circulating erythrocytes to meet the metabolic needs of the body. There is a compensatory increase in the number of peripheral red blood cells when there is a decrease in the amount of oxygen reaching the tissue cells of the body. If there is a surfeit of oxygen available, a decrease in circulating erythrocytes occurs.

THE CONTROL OF ERYTHROPOIESIS

The physiologic control of the number of circulating erythrocytes is maintained by regulation of erythropoiesis and not by regulation of their peripheral destruction.

The sequence of events that occurs in erythropoiesis and the factors that regulate the process are an aspect of the fundamental biologic phenomena of cell reproduction and organ regeneration. The recognizable elements of the bone marrow are derived from pluripotential precursor cells which give rise to erythrocytic, granulocytic, and megakaryocytic cells. These stem cells have not been identified, but studies of regeneration after irradiation strongly suggest that these cells can circulate in the peripheral blood and repopulate the marrow.[17] The existence of another compartment of "committed cells" between the pluripotential cells and the recognizable elements of the marrow has been proposed.[112, 157]

27

Lajtha has proposed a model of stem cell kinetics which fits many experimental observations and the theoretical mathematical considerations concerned with this problem.[123, 124] According to this concept, in response to an appropriate stimulus, stem cells can either reproduce themselves or differentiate into precursors of the specific cell lines—erythrocytic, granulocytic, or megakaryocytic. If stem cells are removed from the compartment by death or differentiation, a feedback mechanism is triggered and stem cells divide to restore the stem cell population; the triggered cells cannot differentiate until they have completed the cell cycle. Such a mechanism would explain the maintenance of a stem cell pool in a relatively steady state in response to stimuli for differentiation or for replacement after damage to the cells. If the stimulus is for erythropoiesis, which may be an enzyme induction in the stem cell in response to erythropoietin,[124] the earliest recognizable specific red cell precursors, the pronormoblasts, are produced. These divide and mature, a process that is repeated by the intermediate basophilic and polychromatophilic normoblasts. The late orthochromatic normoblast does not divide but develops into a reticulocyte, the immediate precursor of the erythrocyte. The interval between mitosis of the cells is probably between 12 and 21 hours, and the average number of divisions during maturation in man is estimated at three or four.[4, 13, 121] Under normal conditions, about four days are required for the development of a pronormoblast into an erythrocyte. Iron is incorporated into all the erythrocyte precursors, but the intake is greatest in the pronormoblasts and least in the reticulocytes;[125] maximal hemoglobin production commences after the basophilic stage.

Erythropoietin

The theory that the well-known effect of hypoxia, the stimulation of erythropoiesis, was mediated by a humoral factor produced outside the erythropoietic tissue in response to the hypoxia was proposed by Carnot and DeFlandre in 1906.[25] In 1947 Grant and Root observed that the stimulation of erythropoiesis was not dependent on the oxygen saturation of the blood of the bone marrow.[68] Reissmann's demonstration in 1950 that hypoxia in only one of a parabiotic pair of rats caused increased erythropoiesis in both rats stimulated interest in a search for a plasma factor.[188] Erslev and others have amply demonstrated by numerous experiments and a variety of techniques that hemorrhage, hemolysis, hypoxia, and cobalt lead to the appearance of a plasma factor that stimulates erythropoiesis.[43] This factor, generally termed erythropoietin, has been the subject of comprehensive reviews.[53, 64, 228]

The erythropoietic factor is heat-stable and nondialyzable, contains sialic acid, and appears to be a glycoprotein that has an electrophoretic mobility characteristic of the alpha$_1$ or alpha$_2$ globulins. The mean half-life of erythropoietin in human plasma has been reported to be 24.9 hours.[196] Although this factor remains active in a pH range of 3 to 10, more erythropoietin is excreted into an alkaline urine. The mechanism responsible for this is unclear.[146] Erythropoietin is inactivated by proteolytic enzymes. The molecular weight has been reported to be 45,000.[53]

Jacobson and his collaborators have shown that the main, though not the sole, site of production of erythropoietin is the kidney; they suggest that 10 per cent of the erythropoietin may be formed elsewhere.[94, 95] An erythrocyte stimulating factor, which is released in response to hypoxia and is believed to be identical to erythropoietin, has been demonstrated in the plasma of nephrectomized rats.[54] Studies of anephric patients have shown that man can support red cell production at a reduced level in the absence of renal tissue.[158]

Failure to find large amounts of erythropoietin in the kidney prompted a search for a precursor. An enzyme has been found in the mitochondrial fraction of kidney homogenates of the cortex and medulla which yields erythropoietin on incubation with normal serum.[114] The enzyme, termed renal erythropoietic factor or REF, is believed to act on a substrate which is produced in the liver and is carried as an alpha 2-globulin in normal serum.[229, 261, 265, 266] Other recent investigations, however, support the concept that erythropoietin can be produced by the isolated perfused kidney in the absence of extrarenal substrate.[47] Little, if any, species specificity has been demonstrated.

The evidence indicates that the main action of erythropoietin is the stimulation of differentiation of committed stem cells into red cell precursors.[52] An increase in the synthesis of ribonucleic acid (RNA) in bone marrow cells in vitro is noted within 15 minutes of the addition of erythropoietin. This effect is abolished by actinomycin-D, which blocks DNA-dependent RNA synthesis.[109] The type of RNA produced is unknown,[85, 109]

The observation that stimulation of erythropoiesis causes the release of large reticulocytes with unusually dense reticulum probably indicates that such cells have been released earlier than normal. This has been interpreted as evidence that erythropoietin acts on differentiated red cell precursors to produce acceleration in the maturation of the erythrocytic series.[15] Stohlman has suggested that erythropoietin induces hemoglobin formation and can act either on the stem cell or on the early differentiated red cell precursors. When hemoglobin synthesis is accelerated, the critical hemoglobin concentration of the cell is reached more rapidly, a feedback mechanism shuts off further nucleic acid synthesis, and the terminal division is skipped. When this occurs, the intramedullary transit time of the erythroid cells is decreased; there is an early release of reticulocytes from the marrow,[53, 230] and macrocytes, which are short-lived, are produced.[230]

Evidence for the suppression of erythropoiesis through the action of inhibitors of erythropoietin[254] and/or stem cell function[49] has been presented. There is also a reduction in the response to hypoxia once the hematocrit rises above 60 per cent. The mechanism by which this is mediated is not clear, but it appears to be related to the elevated hematocrit per se.[105] Hypoxic stress stimulates the production of erythropoietin, a stimulus that is augmented or mediated by respiratory alkalosis, which is associated with an increased oxygen affinity of hemoglobin and decreased oxygen delivery to the tissues. The stimulus is reduced when 2,3-DPG in the red cell increases, or when the pH is reduced by a substance such as acetazolamide.[152]

Erythropoietin has been detected in the urine of normal persons,[50] and increased levels have been demonstrated in the plasma and urine in a variety of clinical states accompanied by anemia. Whether erythropoietin is the normal regulator of erythropoiesis or an emergency mechanism has not been established.

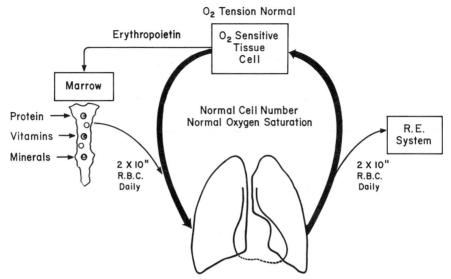

Figure 2–1   Schematic representation of the control of erythropoiesis under normal conditions.

Various observations support the concept that erythropoietin is increased in circumstances in which there is diminished oxygen-carrying capacity of the blood in relation to the need of the tissues. However, the demonstration that plasma erythropoietin levels are increased in subjects with compensated hyper-hemolysis, although there is no reduction in the oxygen-carrying capacity of the blood, indicates that there must be other regulators of erythropoietin pro-duction, possibly a feedback mechanism from the peripheral cells.[228, 230]

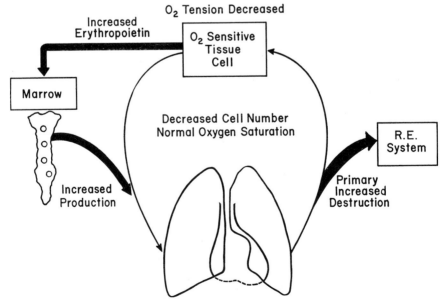

Figure 2–2   Schematic representation of the control of erythropoiesis with as yet uncompen-sated loss of red cells by increased destruction (or by bleeding).

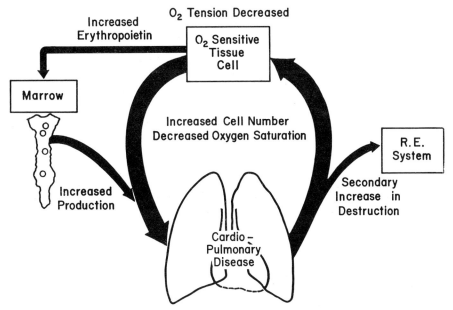

Figure 2–3 Schematic representation of the control of erythropoiesis in cardiopulmonary disease with decreased arterial oxygen saturation.

The mechanism by which androgenic steroids increase red cell mass and plasma volume is not clear.[213] The effect has been shown to be independent of the virilizing capacity of the hormone, and it occurs despite already-increased levels of erythropoietin.[3, 38, 56, 73, 153, 156]

Figures 2–1 to 2–4 indicate how a simple negative feedback system might operate to control erythropoiesis.

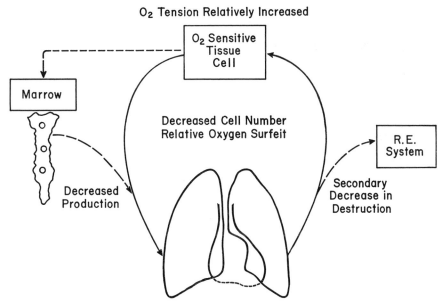

Figure 2–4 Schematic representation of the control of erythropoiesis under conditions of oxygen surfeit.

The physiologic control of erythropoiesis in the normal person, assuming an adequate supply of necessary protein, vitamins, and minerals, is depicted in Figure 2–1. The daily destruction of approximately 2×10^{11} erythrocytes must be compensated by the release of an equal number of erythrocytes from the marrow. Present evidence indicates that the kidney is the main but not the sole site of the production of an enzyme, REF, which, through its action on a circulating plasma globulin, liberates erythropoietin.[65, 94, 95, 159, 171]

Hemorrhage, or an increase in the rate of destruction of erythrocytes, results in anemia if it is uncompensated. The total quantity of oxygen reaching the tissue cells is reduced because of the decreased number of circulating erythrocytes. An increase in erythropoietin activity of the plasma has been demonstrated under such conditions, and is thought to be responsible for the increased erythropoiesis which compensates for the loss of red blood cells (Fig. 2–2).[43]

Decreased arterial oxygen saturation resulting from cardiopulmonary conditions has been found to increase erythropoietin activity and to be associated with increased erythropoiesis (Fig. 2–3). A secondary polycythemia results from the sustained stimulus.[30] A similar situation is thought to be obtained when cobaltous chloride is administered to a patient. Increased levels of erythropoietin have been demonstrated following administration of cobalt,[63] but the mechanism through which this effect is produced is unknown.[120]

A nonphysiologic increase in erythropoietin activity occurs in some patients. Certain tumors that arise in the kidneys and other organs are associated with erythrocytosis; tissue extracts prepared from some of these tumors contain erythropoietin or a substance with similar erythropoietic activity.[169] (See Chapter 11).

Anemia is associated with hypothyroidism in a high percentage of cases. Decreased oxygen demand by the tissue cells might be expected to be reflected by diminished erythropoietin production and anemia (Fig. 2–4). The red blood cell count stabilizes at a level sufficient to meet the diminished metabolic demands of the body. It has been shown, however, that further reduction of the circulating red blood cells by bleeding results in a prompt reticulocytosis, with a return of the red blood cell count to the prebleeding level in a normal period of time. These studies suggest that the anemia of myxedema occurs as the result of diminished metabolic demands rather than as an abnormality of the erythropoietic system.[130]

THE ROLE OF HEMOGLOBIN

Hemoglobin is formed by the developing erythrocyte in the bone marrow. The most rapid hemoglobin formation is in the class III (polychromatophilic) normoblast, when approximately 80 per cent of the hemoglobin carried by the mature cell is formed.[234] Though hemoglobin may be formed in the reticulocyte and, under exceptional circumstances, in the immature nonreticulated erythrocyte, its formation under normal conditions is confined to the developing normoblasts in the marrow.[140, 240]

The level of hemoglobin in the blood represents the balance between production and destruction of the hemoglobin molecule. In the normal person the hemoglobin level is constant, as production and destruction are nicely balanced.

The total quantity of hemoglobin in the blood may be determined by multiplying the concentration of hemoglobin by the blood volume, since hemoglobin production and destruction are in a state of equilibrium. If the concentration of hemoglobin is 15 gm. per cent (mean male equals 16.3 gm. per cent; mean female equals 14.5 gm. per cent),[37] and the total volume roughly 5000 ml., the total quantity of hemoglobin is calculated as follows:

$$\text{Total hemoglobin} = \text{concentration of hemoglobin (gm./ml.)} \times \text{blood volume (ml.)}$$
$$\text{Total hemoglobin} = 0.15 \times 5000 = 750 \text{ gm. hemoglobin}$$

The life span of the hemoglobin molecule is approximately 120 days; its destruction occurs coincident with that of the erythrocyte. If the total amount of hemoglobin in the body at any one time is 750 gm., and the life span of the red blood cell is 120 days, the amount of hemoglobin formed each day can be calculated, since 1/120 of the total amount must be formed daily.

$$\frac{\text{Total hemoglobin}}{\text{life span in days}} = \text{rate of production/day}$$

$$\frac{750}{120} = 6.25 \text{ gm. hemoglobin/day}$$

Under normal conditions the body produces approximately 6.25 gm. of hemoglobin per day. The maximal effort of the body in the event of hemolytic disease has been calculated to be approximately 40 gm. per day.[31] This means that the survival time of the erythrocyte may be reduced to 18 or 19 days without the occurrence of anemia if the bone marrow functions at maximal capacity.

$$\frac{\text{Total hemoglobin}}{\text{life span in days}} = \text{rate of production/day}$$

$$\frac{750 \text{ gm.}}{X} = 40 \text{ gm./day} \qquad X = 18.8 \text{ days}$$

When hyperhemolysis is compensated, excessive destruction of red blood cells exists without the development of anemia. It is generally felt that the increase in the production of red blood cells and hemoglobin is brought about by an increase in the mass of erythroid precursors, rather than by an increase in the rate of maturation in the individual red blood cell,[35] though the latter has not been ruled out as a contributing factor.

If the destruction of red blood cells exceeds the maximal effort of the bone marrow, anemia develops. The anemia becomes stabilized when erythrocyte production and erythrocyte destruction proceed at a constant rate. Although the values found for hemoglobin and red blood cells are not normal, they do not decrease progressively unless the life span of the cell is further shortened, or unless there is interference with marrow production. Laboratory findings in patients with sickle cell anemia illustrate these points. The life span of the erythrocyte is shorter than can be compensated for by maximal marrow production, and in usual circumstances the subnormal hemoglobin value stabilizes at a level that depends on the life span of the erythrocyte and the maximal marrow output. This anemia is made more severe by a sudden increase in hemolytic activity or by a decrease in erythrocyte production. Either mechanism results in a further reduction of circulating erythrocytes.

The Chemistry of Hemoglobin

In recent years much has been learned of the synthesis of cellular protein.[32, 162] The genetic information needed to produce a specific protein is coded in the order of the base pairs in the deoxyribonucleic acid (DNA) of the cell nucleus. The DNA molecule is a double-stranded helix. The strands are composed of alternating units of the sugar deoxyribose and a phosphate compound, and are bound together through each of the sugar units by the base pairs adenine and thymine or guanine and cytosine. The information is transferred by complementary base pairing of another macromolecule, ribonucleic acid (RNA), which is referred to as messenger RNA.[88] The process by which information is transferred from deoxyribonucleic acid (DNA) to ribonucleic acid (RNA) is referred to as transcription of the genetic message.

The RNA molecule is a single-stranded helix similar to DNA. Its structure differs from that of DNA in that the sugar in RNA is ribose, and where DNA contains the base thymine, RNA contains the base uracil. Messenger RNA leaves the nucleus, and by virtue of its chemical template makes possible the synthesis of a specific protein by the ribosomes in the cytoplasm of the cell. Ribosomes are composed of protein and a high molecular weight ribonucleic acid termed ribosomal RNA. In order for protein synthesis to proceed, amino acids of proper kind and amount must be delivered to the ribosomes. This is accomplished by another specialized form of low molecular weight RNA, which is termed soluble or transfer RNA. Each transfer RNA is specific for a certain amino acid, though each amino acid may bind to more than one type of transfer RNA. In order for the binding of amino acid and transfer RNA to occur, a specific amino acid activating enzyme and energy in the form of ATP must be present. The transfer RNA carries the amino acid to a specific site of the ribosome determined by the relationship of the order of base pairs on the messenger RNA to those of the transfer RNA. As the ribosome moves along the messenger RNA template, an ever-lengthening polypeptide of precisely ordered amino acids emerges. The completed polypeptide is then released to enter into the formation of a complete protein molecule. These events are depicted in a highly schematic fashion in Figure 2–5.

Hemoglobin has a molecular weight of 66,700[1, 93] and is thought to be ellipsoid in shape.[34, 89] The results of x-ray crystallographic studies have indicated that the hemoglobin molecule is composed of two identical half-molecules,[173] and this has been confirmed by the analysis of tryptic hydrolysates.[90] Each half-molecule has now been shown to contain two different peptide chains which have been designated α and β.[189] The sequence of the amino acids that comprise the α and β peptide chains is under genetic control, and their synthesis

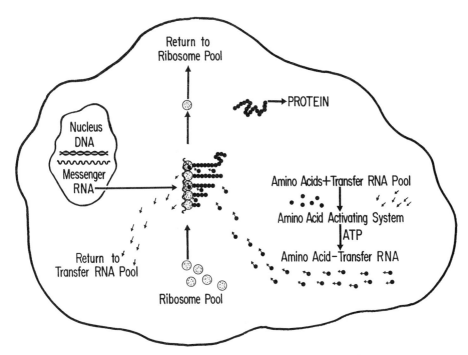

Figure 2–5 Diagram of protein production in a cell.

begins early in the development of the normoblast.[234] The importance of the proper organization of the amino acids during the synthesis of these proteins has been demonstrated by comparing the molecular structure of the hemoglobin from normal persons with that obtained from patients with one of the hemoglobinopathies.[90]

Of the approximately 30 peptide spots obtained from heat- and trypsin-digested hemoglobin by electrophoresis and chromatography, only one peptide from sickle cell hemoglobin differed from normal.[90] Analysis of the abnormal peptide revealed that a glutamic acid residue had been replaced by valine.[91] A similar study of the C hemoglobin molecule indicated that the same peptide was again abnormal, but in this instance the normal glutamic acid had been replaced by lysine.[87] In both instances the abnormal peptide was a component of the β peptide chain. Subsequent investigations of hemoglobins E, D, and I have revealed similar amino acid substitutions in other peptides of both the α and β chains.[92] These brilliant studies have revealed that a variation of only one amino acid out of more than 300 in the half-molecule can mean the difference between normal health, a moderate disability, and a fatal illness.

It has been suggested[92] that the chemical structure of the two genes that appear to be involved in the production of hemoglobin determines the amino acid sequence of the peptide chains. Any alteration of the chemical structure of the genes would alter in turn the sequence of the amino acids of the hemoglobin molecule. Since the genes are self-replicating macromolecules, any structural abnormality would be transmitted from one generation to the next.

Whether or not the effect of such an abnormality is clinically important depends on the portion of the peptide chain involved and the nature of the substitution.[92]

In addition to the protein moiety, the hemoglobin molecule contains four heme groups. The enzymes necessary for the initial and terminal synthetic steps of heme reside in the mitochondria, whereas those enzymes needed for the intermediate steps are present in the cytoplasm. The synthesis of the final tetrameric form of hemoglobin is accomplished in the cytoplasm. The polyribosomes synthesize α globin chains under the rate control of free α chains and release them spontaneously. The free α chains appear to bind the β chains while they are still on the polyribosomes, and free α β subunits are released into the cytoplasm. Heme is released from the mitochondria and combines with each chain of the dimer. Finally the two α β subunits unite to form the tetrad of hemoglobin.[143] Heme is fitted into a highly hydrophobic pocket on the surface of each globin chain, and is held in contact with histidine and other contiguous chemical groups in the pocket by van der Waal's forces.[249] Oxygen is carried in these pockets in a ligand with the ferrous ion of heme and the distal histidine residue.[89, 104, 170, 172, 174, 193, 234, 249]

Heme, a porphyrin ring structure containing a chelated iron atom, has been found to be part of the molecular structure of myoglobin, the cytochromes, peroxidase, and catalase as well as hemoglobin. Porphyrins are widely distributed in nature and are found in both plants and animals, where they serve many vital metabolic processes. Chlorophyll, which is essential for photosynthesis and thus for the existence of life on earth, is a magnesium porphyrin compound. A porphyrin structure with a complexed cobalt atom forms part of the vitamin B_{12} molecule.[84, 113, 217]

The chemistry of porphyrins.   Porphyrins differ from one another and are classified according to the nature and order of the side chains which may be substituted for the eight beta hydrogen atoms. One important group of porphyrins is that which has the same two side chains substituted for the replaceable hydrogen atoms in the 3 and 4 positions in each of the constituent pyrroles. Such an arrangement allows four possible isomers, the notations of which are I, II, III, IV. Uroporphyrin and coproprphyrin are examples of this group. Only types I and III are important to man.

The structural difference between uroporphyrin I and uroporphyrin III lies in the position of the acetic and propionic acid side chains in pyrrole ring IV (Fig. 2–6).

The structural difference between coproporphyrins I and II also lies in the position of the side chains located on pyrrole IV, and the difference between the uroporphyrins and coproporphyrins lies in the presence of a methyl group in the coproporphyrins in the position occupied by the acetic acid side chain in the uroporphyrins (Fig. 2–7).

Uroporphyrin and coproporphyrin each occur in both urine and feces, despite the impression to the contrary given by their names. The urine contains small amounts of uroporphyrin (5 to 10 micrograms per day) with both isomers present.[27] Larger quantities of coproporphyrin are found in the urine (100 to 300 micrograms per day), and the type III isomer predominates.[28, 185, 267] Inadequate data are available to determine a normal range of fecal uroporphyrin excretion. The quantity of fecal coproporphyrin excreted daily is from 150 to 400 micrograms.[130, 192]

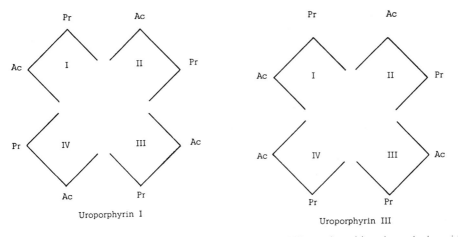

Figure 2–6 Schematic diagram of uroporphyrins I and III; acetic acid and propionic acid side chains.

When there are three different side chains substituted for the replaceable hydrogen atoms of the constituent pyrroles, a larger number of isomers are possible. Mesoporphyrin is a tetramethyl, diethyl, dipropionic acid porphyrin and 15 isomers have been enumerated. Protoporphyrin is similar but two vinyl are substituted for the two ethyl side chains. The isomer which is found in the hemoglobin molecule is classified as protoporphyrin IX, type III.

Porphyrin is composed of four monopyrroles. The elucidation of the synthesis of porphyrin has made it clear that glycine and succinyl-CoA are the basic building blocks.[183, 184, 218, 220, 223, 259] Succinyl-CoA, from the tricarboxylic acid cycle, with the addition of glycine forms α-amino, β-keto adipic acid, which is then decarboxylated to form δ-aminolevulinic acid. The formation of δ-aminolevulinic acid from succinyl-CoA and glycine requires pyridoxyl phosphate,[208] CoA,[193] ferrous iron,[20] and the enzyme δ-aminolevulinic acid synthetase (ALA synthetase) in mitochondria.[4, 58] The iron requirement may reflect an effect of the metal on the synthesis of the enzyme system, as intact cells are required to

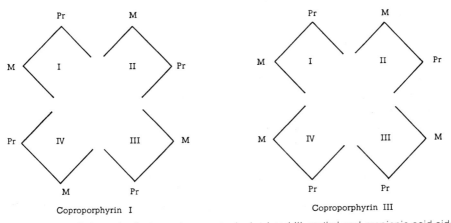

Figure 2–7 Schematic diagram of coproporphyrins I and III; methyl and propionic acid side chains.

show the effect and none is noted when iron is added to mitochondrial suspensions.[23, 238] Outside the mitochondria, two molecules of δ-aminolevulinic acid condense to form porphobilinogen, a monopyrrole, which contains acetic and propionic acid side chains.[215, 221, 222] This reaction has been shown to be catalyzed by the soluble enzyme δ-aminolevulinic acid dehydrase, which has been purified and found to contain —SH groups.[59, 207]

A cell-free extract of erythrocytes is capable of converting porphobilinogen to uroporphyrin.[12, 13, 31, 222] Two enzymes are required to catalyze this transformation. Uroporphyrinogen I synthetase (porphobilinogen deaminase) results in the formation of a linear tetrapyrrole which is then converted to type III isomer in the presence of the heat-labile uroporphyrinogen III cosynthetase (uroporphyrinogen isomerase). In the absence of the uroporphyrinogen III cosynthetase only the type I isomer is formed. The exact method by which the four pyrroles polymerize has not been settled, though a variety of possibilities have been suggested.[136, 147, 148, 258] It is felt that the macrocyclic structures which are formed from porphobilinogen are porphyrinogens, and that the porphyrins result from auto-oxidation of these compounds.[185, 193, 246] Although uroporphyrin is poorly utilized by hemolysates to form coproporphyrin, uroporphyrinogen III is easily transformed to coproporphyrinogen III by the soluble enzyme uroporphyrinogen decarboxylase.[164, 199] The decarboxylase is not specific, and decarboxylates the side chains of type I and III isomers at random. In contrast, the

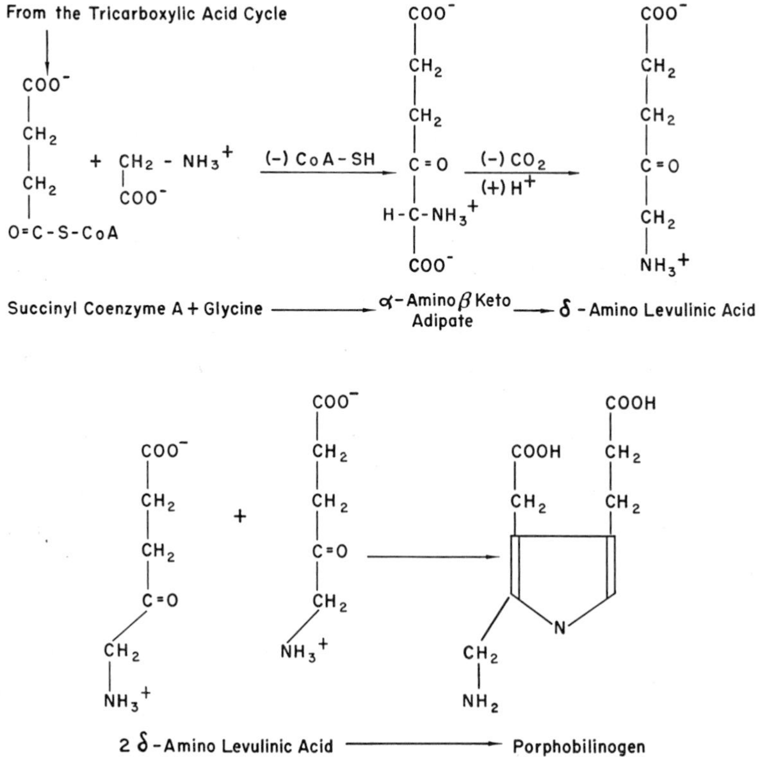

Figure 2–8 Formation of porphobilinogen from succinyl-coenzyme A and glycine.

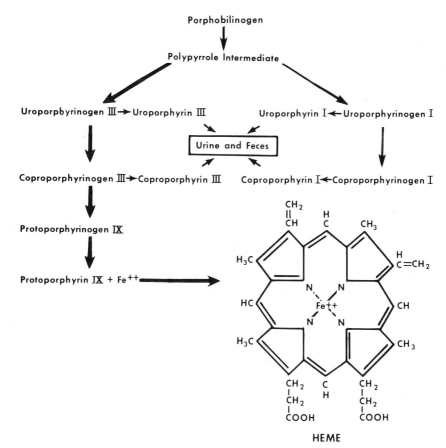

Figure 2-9 Formation of heme from porphobilinogen.

enzyme coproporphyrinogen oxidative decarboxylase is highly specific for the type III coproporphyrinogen isomer, and results only in the formation of protoporphyrinogen IX.[179] Protoporphyrinogen IX is converted to protoporphyrin IX by the enzyme protoporphyrinogen oxidase. The enzymes coproporphyrinogen oxidative decarboxylase and protoporphyrinogen oxidase are insoluble and located in the mitochondria.[48, 200] Ferrochetalase (heme synthetase) catalyzes the insertion of iron into protoporphyrin, although the reaction can occur in the presence of iron in the reduced state without ferrochetalase.[103, 104]

Following its formation in the mitochondria, heme diffuses into the extra-mitochondrial space where it combines with the completed α and β chains to form hemoglobin.[60, 180, 209, 263]

The intermediates in the biosynthesis of heme are then uro- and coproporphyrinogens and not uro- and coproporphyrins. It appears, however, that iron is incorporated into protoporphyrin and not protoporphyrinogen.[66]

Free protoporphyrin and coproporphyrin have been demonstrated in both the nucleated and non-nucleated erythrocytes. The concentration of both compounds increases just prior to reticulocytosis.[20, 211, 212] It has been suggested that they represent incomplete hemoglobin synthesis[267] or residuals left after hemoglobin synthesis.[161] The level of free erythrocyte protoporphyrin is from 13 to 139 micrograms per 100 ml. of erythrocytes.[241] Erythrocyte coproporphyrin concentration has been found to be from 0.5 to 1.5 micrograms per 100 ml. of erythrocytes.[20, 242]

Hemoglobin Catabolism

Senescent red cells are removed from the circulation by reticuloendothelial cells. The hemoglobin is liberated, but is not reutilized as such. Amino acids released from the degradation of globin return to the general amino acid pool.[77, 251, 252] The degradation of heme to bile pigment takes place in the microsomal fraction of the reticuloendothelial cells.[233] Heme is first transformed to biliverdin by a microsomal enzyme, heme oxygenase, with the release of iron. This is the rate limiting step in the breakdown of hemoglobin and requires molecular oxygen and NADPH. The iron is returned to the iron pool and reutilized in the formation of hemoglobin.

The biliveridin is next reduced to bilirubin by another microsomal NADPH-dependent enzyme, biliverdin reductase. The activity of both these enzymes is very high in the spleen and liver and can be induced in the other cells of the reticuloendothelial system. In macrophages harvested from experimental animals enzyme activity was capable of regulatory adaptation in response to the substrate load.[178, 233] In the rat, it has been possible to identify those liver cells which phagocytize red cells. This apparently distinct population correlated well with the level of microsomal hemeoxygenase. Data obtained in these studies suggest that the liver and spleen have comparable roles in red cell–hemoglobin degradation.[10] Bilirubin is then released from the reticuloendothelial cells into the plasma, where it is bound to albumin and transported to the parenchymal cells of the liver. There, in the liver microsomes, it is conjugated with glucuronic acid and excreted in the bile.[201, 202] Should the liver be unable to carry on this conjugation in the normal manner, a high "indirect acting" bilirubin level in the blood would result. Should there be obstruction of the excretion of the conjugated form via the biliary system, an increase in the "direct acting" bilirubin in the blood would result. Whether the bilirubin gives a "direct" or "indirect" van den Bergh reaction depends on the presence or absence of the glucuronic acid conjugation. The enzyme transferase found in the microsomes of the liver cells and uridine diphosphate glucuronic acid are both necessary for this reaction to occur. It has been suggested that the excess unconjugated bilirubin found in the newborn is due to inadequate development of the glucuronide conjugating system[19] (Fig. 2–10).

In the bowel the action of the intestinal bacteria on bilirubin leads to several degradation products which are known collectively as fecal urobilinogen. Approximately 50 per cent of the urobilinogen is reabsorbed from the gut and recirculated in the blood to be re-excreted by the liver. This is the source of urobilinogen in liver bile, and of the small amount lost through the kidney that is termed urinary urobilinogen. Normal daily excretion of urinary urobilinogen is from 0 to 3.5 mg.

The amount of fecal urobilinogen in the stool can be measured and has

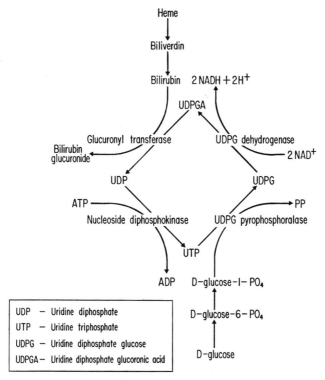

Figure 2–10 Diagram indicating relationship of glucose metabolism and heme degradation.

been found to vary from 40 to 280 mg. per day. Since the amount of fecal urobilinogen excreted depends on the amount of bilirubin secreted by the liver into the bile, it has been used as an index of hemoglobin breakdown. Hemoglobin from destroyed circulating red blood cells is not the only source of urobilinogen, however, and the excretion of fecal urobilinogen does not always measure red cell destruction accurately. Studying the excretion of stercobilin, one of the components of fecal urobilinogen, investigators have found that as much as 11 per cent must come from sources other than the breakdown of mature red blood cells.[138] Whether this represents a breakdown of developing cells while still in the marrow, or some nonhemoglobin porphyrin pathway, is not known. In certain disease states, the amount of nonhemoglobin stercobilin rises to as much as 50 per cent.[137, 139]

Should intravascular hemolysis occur, hemoglobin is released into the plasma, and is quickly bound by haptoglobin.[68, 163] Haptoglobin is an α-2-glycoprotein which combines stoichiometrically with hemoglobin, forming a stable complex.[96] As the plasma concentration of haptoglobin is 0.1 to 0.04 gm. per cent, approximately 100 mg. of hemoglobin is bound by 100 ml. of plasma.[128, 129] The haptoglobin-hemoglobin complex is too large to be filtered by the kidney, and does not appear in the urine. Heme and hemoglobin are removed from the plasma in the liver and degraded by the hepatic cells and not the Kupfer cells.[11]

When intravascular hemolysis continues for long periods, or the amount of free hemoglobin is sufficiently large, the binding capacity of plasma hapto-globin is exceeded and free hemoglobin appears in the urine. Free hemoglobin is cleared from the plasma faster than the haptoglobin-hemoglobin complex. Although the permeability of the glomerulus to free hemoglobin is relatively low, it is considerably greater than for albumin and other proteins of similar molecular weights. This may be explained in part by the fact that hemoglobin tends to dissociate into alpha-beta dimers at the physiologic pH and ionic strength of plasma.[21] Earlier work indicated that a negligible amount of hemo-globin was reabsorbed by the renal tubules,[126, 128] but recent studies show that the bulk of the hemoglobin filtered by the glomerulus in most clinical disorders with hemoglobinemia is reabsorbed by the proximal tubules. There iron is released and reabsorbed into the plasma for reutilization. The globin and porphyrin moieties also are rapidly catabolized and reutilized. Thus the proxi-mal tubular cell resembles the reticuloendothelial cell in its ability to conserve hemoglobin iron.[21]

Several types of haptoglobin have been identified by electrophoresis, and their transmission has been shown to be genetically determined.[163, 226] No selective advantage has been demonstrated and all have similar binding capa-cities. The half-life of haptoglobin appears to be in the order of 5.4 days.[97] The concentration of haptoglobin has been found to be decreased in all hemolytic states and in chronic hepatocellular disease. It is increased in the course of acute or chronic infection and in tissue destruction or proliferation.[163]

ABNORMAL PORPHYRIN METABOLISM

Characterization of the precursors and intermediates involved in the biosynthesis of heme has laid the foundation for the understanding of the several disorders associated with abnormal porphyrin metabolism.[40] Despite their rarity these disorders have evoked widespread interest, and have afforded unique opportunities for the study of porphyrin metabolism. Current interest centers on the relationship of porphyrin synthesis to other metabolic path-ways[118, 119, 161, 221] and mechanisms of detoxification of internal and external toxins. One of the difficult problems in the understanding of the pathophysi-ology of porphyria has been the failure to relate, in a constant fashion, the clinical symptoms of porphyria to the extent of pyrrole production. Granick[67] has suggested that heme synthesis is controlled by regulation of the production of ALA synthetase by a repressor-operator mechanism. The repressor is heme plus an aporepressor protein. The displacement of heme by a drug or steroid inactivates the repressor; the structural gene for ALA synthetase can then code more messenger RNA, and more enzyme is synthesized. Since the other enzymes in this system are not rate-limiting, this would lead to an overproduction of heme precursors. Labbe[117] has suggested that a biochemical lesion in the energy forming system in the mitochondria may lead secondarily to depression of the operator gene and overproduction of porphyrins. Thus, porphyrinogenesis would be secondary to some other metabolic defect.

Recently, human serum has been demonstrated to contain factors which stimulate and factors which inhibit porphyrin formation by cultured avian liver cells.[191]

There is no doubt that continued investigation of these disorders will widen our knowledge of mitochondrial and nuclear biochemistry and genetics.[194, 236]

The disease states which result from disordered porphyrin metabolism may be classified as follows:

    I. Disorders of porphyrin synthesis in the erythrocyte
        1. Porphyria (congenital) erythropoietica
        2. Protoporphyria (congenital) erythropoietica
    II. Disorders of porphyrin synthesis in the liver
        1. Porphyria hepatica
           a. Intermittent acute (Swedish porphyria)
           b. Hereditary coporporphyria
           c. Cutanea tarda
           d. Mixed (South African porphyria, porphyria variegata)
    III. Acquired (toxic) porphyria

Porphyria erythropoietica. Porphyria erythropoietica is a rare metabolic disorder of the erythrocyte which is probably transmitted as a recessive genetic abnormality.[239] Patients with this disorder appear to have both normal and abnormal erythroid cell lines in the marrow.[206] The nuclei, and to a lesser extent the cytoplasm, of cells of the affected line show a characteristic red fluorescence when studied with the fluorescence microscope. In addition they may have a dark nuclear inclusion body containing hemoglobin. As destruction of circulating erythrocytes cannot account for the quantity of porphyrin excreted by these patients, it has been postulated that uroporphyrin may be released into the plasma at a rapid rate during the maturation of the nucleated red cells in the marrow.[205] The red fluorescence which has been demonstrated in the spleen is thought to result from the local destruction of red blood cells containing the abnormal porphyrin. The isomers found in the urine and blood of these patients are copro- and uroporphyrin I. These porphyrins are not complexed with a metal, and the monopyrrole porphobilinogen is not found.

Recent studies have revealed that, when incubated with porphobilinogen, hemolysates prepared from the red cells of these patients had a greater porphyrin-forming ability than hemolysates prepared from normal red cells.[247] The finding of protoporphyrin IX indicated that isomerase was not lacking.[193, 247]

The suggestion has been made that excessive production of porphyrin precursors may overwhelm the normal isomerase activity, resulting in the production of the usual amount of type III porphyrins but excessive quantities of the type I isomers. A variety of genetic defects which might produce such a result have been suggested.[108, 247] The alternate formation of excessive quantities of uroporphyrin I which cannot be used in heme synthesis is believed responsible for the clinical manifestations of the disorder.[71, 139, 160, 259]

The clinical picture is characterized by photosensitivity which leads to erythema, blisters, ulcer formation, and ultimate mutilation of exposed areas. Hemolytic anemia is usually present, and thrombocytopenia may occur.[72] Splenomegaly is expected. Because of the deposition of uroporphyrin I in the bones and teeth, these structures are often red-brown and will fluoresce under a Wood's light.[2, 25, 78]

Treatment is nonspecific. Sunlight must be avoided. Splenectomy has relieved the hemolytic anemia in a number of patients.[206]

Erythropoietic porphyria has been found in cats, in cattle, and in the fox squirrel.[132, 133]

Congenital erythropoietic protoporphyria. Erythropoietic protoporphyria is an inborn error of metabolism characterized by a marked increase in the concentration of erythrocyte protoporphyrin IX and mild photosensitivity. Erythrocyte coproporphyrin III, fecal coproporphyrin, and fecal protoporphyrin concentration may be normal or increased, and plasma protoporphyrin may be elevated. The most severe skin lesions accompany the greatest increases of plasma and erythrocyte protoporphyrin.[175] Urinary porphyrin excretion is normal. There are two populations of red cells. Fewer than half the circulating cells exhibit fluorescence and photohemolysis.[100] Photohemolysis of the red cells of patients with erythropoietic protoporphyria occurs on exposure to long UV light in the 4000 Å range.[80] The radiation lesion has been estimated to be 10 Å in size and to result in the loss of intracellular potassium.[52] Lipid peroxidation, hydrogen peroxide formation, and loss of cell membrane-SH are all felt to play a role in photohemolysis.[62] The disorder appears in childhood and is believed to be transmitted as a Mendelian dominant.[75, 181, 262]

Patients with erythropoietic protoporphyria have abnormal sensitivity to light, and develop erythema, edema, and itching of the exposed skin.[144] Vesicle formation, hirsutism, and scarring have been reported[181] but are not characteristic.[75, 144] The one reported instance of hemolytic anemia was associated with hepatosplenomegaly, moderate leukopenia, and thrombocytopenia and it responded to splenectomy.[181]

The disorder appears to be the result of overproduction of normal protoporphyrin IX in the developing red cells in the marrow. A nonerythropoietic site for production of high plasma protoporphyrin levels has not been excluded.[187] The maximal skin sensitivity to monochromatic light has been shown to be 400 to 410 mμ, which corresponds to the Soret band of maximal light absorption by the porphyrin.[144] It has been suggested that the higher energy state attained by the porphyrins on exposure to light is in some way responsible for the skin damage.[19] A large amount of hyaline material has been shown to be invariably associated with the blood vessels of the upper corium in areas of exposed skin.[175] After exposure to 400 mμ light, a thickening of the walls of subepidermal small blood vessels was found. Some of these small vessels were occluded.[6] Electron microscopy has revealed that the amorphous material noted in the small blood vessels in the upper part of the dermis appeared to be derived from constituents of the blood or from the vessel wall.[198]

A recent report indicates that the anionic exchange resin cholestyramine may block enterohepatic circulation of protoporphyrin, prevent potential liver damage, and reduce skin photosensitivity. Further studies of these effects should prove interesting.[98, 106, 107]

Porphyria hepatica. The site of deranged porphyrin metabolism in this disorder is not the bone marrow but the liver.[206] Porphyria hepatica may be the result of a metabolic defect in the synthesis of heme proteins other than hemoglobin. Catalase synthesis has, for example, been shown to be abnormal in experimental porphyria.[204] Patients with hepatic porphyria have excessive production of porphyrin precursors ad the result of increased activity of δ-aminolevulinic acid synthetase.[149] These disorders are more common than the erythropoietic type.

Intermittent acute type.   The intermittent acute type of prophyria hepatica is a familial disorder inherited as an autosomal dominant. Evidence has been collected suggesting that it affected the royal houses of Stuart, Hanover, and Prussia, and may have been responsible for the illness of King George III.[141, 142, 260] It usually appears after puberty, though in rare cases it may be evident in childhood.[239] In this disorder the erythrocyte porphyrins are normal, but excessive quantities of zinc complexed uroporphyrin I and III and coproporphyrin III are found in the urine. The porphyrin precursor, porphobilinogen, is found in the urine during the acute attacks, and the finding of this monopyrrole is diagnostic. The liver contains large quantities of porphyrin precursors and increased amounts of porphyrin. Marrow porphyrins are normal. Hepatic δ-aminolevulinic acid synthetase levels have been found to be somewhat elevated.[264] Recent evidence indicates that reduced activity of hepatic uroporphyrinogen synthetase could be the fundamental defect. Reduction in this enzyme leads to the induction of δ-aminolevulinic acid synthetase as the result of a negative feedback from reduced heme synthesis.[149, 150, 151, 260] A method has been developed to measure uroporphrinogen synthetase activity in red cell hemolysates, and has revealed 50 per cent activity in patients with acute intermittent porphyria. This method offers promise for the detection of patients with latent disease.[144, 231]

Attacks of acute intermittent porphyria appear to be precipitated by any factors which increase the activity of hepatic ALA synthetase, which is the rate-limiting enzyme in the synthesis of heme.[150] Among the various factors reported to precipitate attacks of acute intermittent porphyria are pregnancy, endogenously derived 5 β steroids, contraceptive pills, various sedatives (especially barbiturates), tranquilizers, anticonvulsants, sulfa drugs, and methyl dopa.[102, 177] In normal women on contraception medication 64 per cent were reported in one study to have elevated ALA synthetase activity.[8, 39]

The clinical manifestations of the intermittent acute type of porphyria hepatica are varied, but abdominal colic (which can be of extreme severity), weakness and paresthesia of extremities, constipation, convulsions, coma, psychoses, and hypertension may occur. Fatalities are generally due to respiratory paralysis, but may occur during coma or from cachexia.[190] Hypochloremia or hyponatremia, noted during acute attacks, has been demonstrated to be the result of inappropriate secretion of antidiuretic hormone.[83, 135, 236]

Treatment includes avoidance of alcohol, barbiturates, or other liver toxins. Chlorpromazine has been reported to be effective in relief of symptoms,[246] and this has been confirmed.[239] Splenectomy is not indicated. The administration of hematin has been reported to relieve symptoms and chemical abnormalities, and warrants further investigation.[18, 244]

Hereditary coproporphyria.   There is persistent excretion of large amounts of coproporphyrin III in both urine and feces in this disorder, and porphyrin precursors occur in the urine during the acute episodes. The disorder is transmitted as a Mendelian autosomal dominant. Family studies have revealed that as many as 50 per cent of those with coproporphyria have no symptoms similar to those of acute intermittent porphyria. Photosensitivity is rare but has been noted. Acute attacks may be precipitated or exacerbated by the same drugs noted to affect the course of acute intermittent porphyria.[29, 61, 76]

Cutanea tarda type.   As its name suggests this disorder begins later in life, and its symptoms include photosensitivity. It is a familial disorder associated with parenchymal liver disease in a high percentage of cases. The photosensitivity is moderate in severity. The disease runs a mild course if the patients protect themselves from exposure to sunlight and hepatotoxins. A history of chronic alcoholism is not uncommon. The porphyrins excreted are the zinc complexed uroporphyrins I and III and coproporphyrin III. Porphyrins may be found in the blood and are elevated in the liver. Porphobilinogen is not found in the urine of these patients. The prognosis is generally good but depends on the degree of liver damage. Improvement has been reported following the administration of adenosine monophosphate, suggesting that some aberration in purine synthesis may play a role in this disorder.[55, 186]

Several investigators have noted a tendency to high serum iron and transferrin values in a number of patients with porphyria cutanea tarda.[41] Recently it has been demonstrated that iron absorption is increased in such patients, especially in those with cirrhosis, and after treatment with phlebotomy.[237] In vitro, iron has been demonstrated to block uroporphyrinogen III cosynthetase activity,[115] and focal areas of iron in hepatic siderosis may limit the decarboxylation of uroporphyrinogen.[99] Phlebotomy has resulted in markedly reduced porphyrin excretion and remission. Δ-aminolevulinic acid synthetase activity in liver biopsy specimens has been demonstrated to be reduced from a mean of 7 × normal to a mean of 3.5 × normal by phlebotomy.[155] Administration of iron results in a return of symptoms.[42] The precise role that iron may play in this disorder is unknown, but the effect of phlebotomy has been salutary.[7, 42]

Porphyria variegata (mixed type).   These patients have symptoms of both the cutanea tarda and the acute intermittent type of porphyria.[246] The high incidence of this disorder among the Boers of South Africa is responsible for the designation "South African porphyria." During the acute stage of the disorder, the urine contains δ-aminolevulinic acid, porphobilinogen, uroporphyrin, and coproporphyrin. The stool also contains large quantities of porphyrins. Between attacks the urine may be negative, but the stools continue to be positive.[235]

Acquired (toxic) porphyria.   Acquired porphyria with photosensitivity, marked porphyrinuria, and hepatomegaly has occurred as the result of the ingestion of the fungicide hexachlorobenzene.[24] The bullous lesions of the skin often progressed to ulceration and healed with scarring. Marked pigmentation in the upper keratin layer of the skin, and diffuse hypertrichosis with focal areas of alopecia, occurred in several cases. The urine contains increased amounts of uroporphyrin and coproporphyrin, but no porphobilinogen or δ-aminolevulinic acid. Feeding of hexachlorobenzene to rats will result in a similar disorder,[203] which can be ameliorated by the administration of adenosine monophosphate.[164]

A similar epidemic occurred in Japan as the result of the exposure of a large number of people to rice oil contaminated with polychlorobiphenyl.[232]

PORPHYRINURIAS

There are a number of conditions in which increased porphyrin excretion may occur.[2] The increased excretion of porphyrin in these varied disease states may reflect disordered hemoglobin or protein synthesis, or disordered synthesis of heme compounds other than hemoglobin.

1. Lead Poisoning

Lead poisoning results in a marked disturbance in heme synthesis. Urinary excretion of δ-aminolevulinic acid, uroporphyrin, and coproporphyrin is increased, and the concentration of free erythrocyte protoporphyrin is elevated.[16, 134, 253] A decrease in the activity of δ-aminolevulinic acid dehydrase is believed responsible for the accumulation of δ-aminolevulinic acid, and the increased excretion of porphyrins, despite a decrease in their synthesis, is postulated to be due to the interference by lead with the incorporation of iron into protoporphyrin.[75, 96]

2. Rheumatic fever coproporphyrin III[101]
3. Poliomyelitis—coproporphyrin III[248]
4. Liver disease[245]
    a. Alcoholic cirrhosis—coproporphyrin III
    b. Infectious hepatitis—coproporphyrin I
5. Anemia[206, 243, 245]
    a. Refractory—coproporphyrin III
    b. Hemolytic anemia—coproporphyrin I
    c. Pernicious anemia—coproporphyrin I
6. Idiopathic—coproporphyrin III[245]

ADDITIONAL FACTORS NEEDED FOR ERYTHROPOIESIS

In addition to protein, metals and certain vitamins must be present if normal erythropoiesis is to continue[26] (Fig. 2–11).

Iron.   The various details of iron metabolism are discussed in Chapter 5. Only a brief summary of this complex problem is presented at this time.

The daily diet of the average adult in the United States contains 12 to 15 mg. of iron, which is present mainly in the ferric form. Reduction to the ferrous form, the type of iron that is absorbed, is promoted by the acid reaction of the stomach and upper small intestine, by ascorbic acid, and by certain proteins. Iron is absorbed mainly in the upper portion of the small intestine, and the amount of iron that gains entrance to the body is largely controlled by regulation of the absorption of iron through the mucosa. Normally, less than 10 per cent of the ingested iron is absorbed. Various factors, such as the amount and form of iron in the intestine, the iron-phosphate ratio and possibly other details of the diet, the status of the iron stores, the degree of erythropoietic activity, and perhaps other factors, influence this absorptive mechanism. After absorption, the iron is transported in the plasma in the ferric state in combination with a beta-1 globulin fraction to the reticuloendothelial cells of the liver,

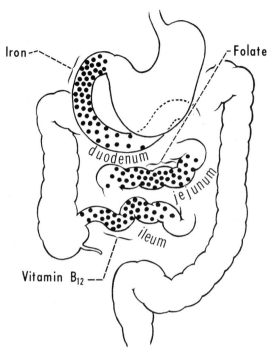

Figure 2–11 Main sites of absorption of some factors essential for normal erythropoiesis.

spleen, and bone marrow, where it is stored in the form of ferritin and hemosiderin or used in the production of hemoglobin. From these stores, the iron is mobilized for hemoglobin production in the bone marrow. The body has no means of excreting significant amounts of iron, and only minute amounts, about 1 mg. per day, are lost by cell desquamation and other means. Reduction of the amount of iron in the body occurs mainly as the result of bleeding and pregnancy.

Copper.   Although anemia due to copper deficiency is seen but rarely in adult humans, in experimental animals a deficiency of copper leads to the development of an anemia that is similar to iron deficiency anemia. The adult human body contains 100 to 150 mg. of copper.[257] The plasma level has been found to be 105 ± 16 micrograms per cent in males and 116 ± 16 micrograms per cent in females. Ninety per cent of the copper in the plasma is bound to the alpha-2 globulin ceruloplasmin.[86] Copper appears to function in the absorption, mobilization, and utilization of iron in hemoglobin synthesis and in the formation and maintenance of the cytochromes.[209, 257] The metal may exert an effect on hematopoiesis through an effect on the function of respiratory enzymes.

Cobalt.   Cobalt is known to play a role in animal nutrition, and the administration of cobalt is known to stimulate erythropoiesis in man and in animals.[166] However, the mechanism by which cobalt effects an increase in red blood cell production is not understood.[120] It has not been established that cobalt has any role in normal erythropoiesis aside from its importance as a part of the vitamin B_{12} molecule.

Pyridoxine.   For many years it was known that a deficiency of pyridoxine (vitamin B_6) in animals would produce a severe hypochromic microcytic anemia, but only recently has a similar disorder been described in man.[81] The deficiency, which is corrected by the administration of pyridoxine, is characterized by splenomegaly, hepatomegaly, hypochromic microcytic anemia, elevation of serum iron level, and saturation of the iron-binding capacity. The inability of these patients to metabolize iron normally is associated with disturbed tryptophan metabolism and the excretion of xanthurenic acid.

Vitamin B_{12} and folic acid.   Both vitamin B_{12} and folic acid are necessary for the normal maturation of the red cells. The average American daily diet probably contains approximately 20 micrograms of vitamin B_{12}, nearly all from animal protein. Different figures have been given for the daily folate intake, but it seems likely that the daily requirement for adults is 200 micrograms, for infants 50 micrograms, and for children 100 micrograms (Chap. 4). A deficiency of either results in a defect in nucleic acid metabolism that is reflected by the development of the megaloblastic type of erythrocyte maturation. Vitamin B_{12} has now been identified as the *extrinsic factor* of Castle. An *intrinsic factor* in the stomach, a mucoprotein, is necessary in order that the vitamin B_{12} ingested in the diet may be absorbed.[9, 27] The chemical characteristics of the intrinsic factor have been worked out in considerable detail.[70, 225, 256] An absence or deficiency of the intrinsic factor is responsible for pernicious anemia. Folic acid, also present in the diet, does not require the intrinsic factor for its absorption. The functions of these two vitamins are not completely understood. Both are concerned with the formation of purine or pyrimidine bases which are constituent parts of the nucleic acids. There seems to be a reciprocal relationship between vitamin B_{12} and folic acid in the synthesis of nucleic acid in many tissues of the body, particularly those with rapid turnover, such as the hematopoietic and gastrointestinal cells.[5, 154]

Ascorbic acid.   Ascorbic acid appears to participate in metabolic activities which affect both vitamin B_{12} and folic acid. It is important in the conversion of folic acid to folinic acid, and there is some evidence that it stimulates the formation of folic acid. This vitamin has intense reducing properties, and must play a significant role in oxidation-reduction reactions in the body.[61, 82]

Vitamin E (alpha-tocopherol).   Deficiency of this vitamin has been shown to produce anemia in several animal species, mainly through ineffective erythropoiesis.[224] Except for the possibility of a hemolytic anemia in premature infants,[167, 168] no deficiency has been clearly demonstrated in humans. The role of vitamin E deficiency in the anemia of protein-calorie malnutrition is still controversial.

Other vitamins may possibly play a role in erythropoiesis. Nicotinic acid is thought to be essential for the synthesis of coenzymes in the developing erythrocyte, but its role in hematopoiesis is not clearly established.[79] Riboflavin deficiency has been reported to be responsible for anemia in animals, but no anemia of this type has been recognized in man. It is thought to exert its influence by taking part in cellular oxidations.[227]

References

1. Adair, G. C.: A comparison of the molecular weights of the proteins. Proc. Cambridge Phil. Soc., 2:75, 1924.
2. Aldrich, R. F., Labbe, F. F., and Talman, E. K.: A review of prophyrin metabolism with special reference to childhood. Am. J. Med. Sci., 230:675, 1955.
3. Alexanian, R.: Erythropoietin and erythropoiesis in anemic man following androgens. Blood, 33:564, 1969.
4. Alpen, E. L., and Cranmore, D.: Observations on Regulation of Erythropoiesis and on Cellular Dynamics by Fe[59] Autoradiography. In Stohlman, F., Jr. (ed.): The Kinetics of Cellular Proliferation. Grune and Stratton, New York, 1959.
5. Angier, R. S., et al.: Synthesis of a compound identical with the L. casei factor isolated from liver. Science, 102:227, 1945.
6. Baart de la Faille-Kuyper, E. H., Rottier, P. B., and Baart de la Faille, H.: Epidermal changes in erythropoietic protoporphyria after irradiation with glass-filtered mercury light. Br. J. Dermatol., 80:747, 1968.
7. Baker, H., and Turnbull, A.: Porphyria cutanea tarda treated by repeated venesection: clinical and biochemical response. Proc. Roy. Soc. Med., 62:590, 1969.
8. Behm, A. R., and Unger, W. P.: Oral contraceptives and porphyria cutanea tarda. Can. Med. Assoc. J., 110:1052, 1974.
9. Berk, L., et al.: Observations on the etiologic relationship of achylia gastrica to pernicious anemia. N. Engl. J. Med., 239:911, 1948.
10. Bissell, D. M., Hammaker, L., and Schmid, R.: Liver sinusoidal cells. J. Cell Biol., 54:107, 1972.
11. Bissell, D. M., Hammaker, L., and Schmid, R.: Hemoglobin and erythrocyte catabolism in rat liver, separate roles of parenchymal and sinusoidal cells. Blood, 40:812, 1972.
12. Bogorad, L.: The enzymatic synthesis of uroporphyrinogens from porphobilinogen. Conference on Hemoglobin. Nat. Acad. Sci., Nat. Res. Council Publ. 557, 1958, p. 74.
13. Bogorad, L., and Granick, S.: The enzymatic synthesis of porphyrins from porphobilinogen. Nat. Acad. Sci. Proc., 39:1176, 1953.
14. Bond, V. P., Fliedner, T. M., Cronkite, E. P., Rubins, J. R., and Robertson, J. S.: Cell Turnover in Blood and Blood-forming Tissues Studied with Tritiated Thymidine. In Stohlman, F., Jr. (ed.): The Kinetics of Cellular Proliferation. Grune and Stratton, New York, 1959.
15. Borsook, H., Ratner, K., Tattrie, B., Teigler, D., and Lajtha, L. G.: Erythropoietin and the development of erythrocytes. Nature, 217:1024, 1968.
16. Boyett, J. D., and Butterworth, C. E.: Lead poisoning and hemoglobin synthesis. Am. J. Med., 32:884, 1962.
17. Brecher, G., and Cronkite, E. P.: Post-radiation parabiosis and survival in rats. Proc. Soc. Exp. Biol. Med., 77:292, 1951.
18. Bonkowsky, H. L., Tschudy, D. P., Collins, A., Doherty, J., Bossenmaier, I., Cardinal, R., and Watson, C. J.: Repression of the overproduction of porphyrin precursors in acute intermittent porphyria by intravenous infusions of hematin. Proc. Nat. Acad. Sci. U.S.A., 68:2725, 1971.
19. Brown, A. K., and Zuelzer, W. W.: Studies on the neonatal development of the glucuronide conjugating system. J. Clin. Invest., 37:332, 1958.
20. Brown, E. G.: Evidence for the involvement of ferrous iron in the biosynthesis of δ-aminolaevulinic acid by chicken erythrocyte preparations. Nature, 182:313, 1958.
21. Bunn, H. F., and Jandl, J. H.: The renal handling of hemoglobin. Tr. Assoc. Am. Physicians, 81:147, 1968.
22. Burnett, J. W., and Pathak, M. A.: Pathogenesis of cutaneous photosensitivity in porphyria. N. Engl. J. Med., 268:1203, 1963.
23. Burnham, B. F., and Lascelles, J.: Control of porphyrin biosynthesis through a negative-feedback mechanism. Biochem. J., 87:462, 1963.
24. Can, C., and Nigogosyan, G.: Acquired toxic porphyria cutanea tarda due to hexachlorobenzene (report of 348 cases caused by this fungicide). J.A.M.A., 183:88, 1963.
25. Carnot, P., and DeFlandre, C.: Sur l'activité du sérum hémopoiétique des differents organs au cours de la régénération du sang. Comp. Rend. Acad. Sci., 143:384, 1906.
26. Cartwright, G.: Dietary factors concerned in erythropoiesis. Blood, 2:111, 1947.
27. Castle, W. B.: The etiology of pernicious and related macrocytic anemias. Science, 82:159, 1935.
28. Comfort, A., Moore, H., and Weatherall, M.: Normal human urinary porphyrins. Biochem. J., 58:177, 1954.
29. Connon, J. J., and Turkington, V.: Hereditary coproporphyria. Lancet, 2:263, 1968.
30. Contopoulos, A. N., McCombs, R., Lawrence, J. H., and Simpson, M. E.: Erythropoietic activity in the plasma of patients with polycythemia vera and secondary polycythemia. Blood, 12:614, 1957.

31. Cookson, G. H., and Rimington, C.: Porphobilinogen. Biochem. J., *57*:476, 1954.

32. Crick, F. H. C., Barnett, L., Brenner, S., and Watts-Tobin, R. J.: General nature of the genetic code for proteins. Nature, *192*:1227, 1961.

33. Crosby, W. H., and Akeroyd, J. H.: The limit of hemoglobin synthesis in hereditary hemolytic anemia. Its relation to the excretion of bile pigment. Am. J. Med., *13*:273, 1952.

34. Cullis, A. C., Dintzis, H. M., and Perutz, M. F.: X-ray analysis of hemoglobin. Conference on Hemoglobin. Nat. Acad. Sci., Nat. Res. Council Publ. 557, 1958, p. 50.

35. Dacie, J. C.: The Hemolytic Anemias, 2nd Ed. Grune and Stratton, New York, 1960.

36. Dietrich, L. S., Nochol, C. A., Monson, W. J., and Elvehjem, C. A.: Observations on the inter-relation of vitamin B_{12}, folic acid, and vitamin C in the chick. J. Biol. Chem., *181*:915, 1949.

37. Drabkin, D. L.: Metabolism of hemin chromoproteins. Physiol. Rev., *31*:345, 1951.

38. Duarte, L., Medal, L. S., Labardini, L., and Arriaga, L.: The erythropoietic effects of anabolic steroids. Proc. Soc. Exp. Biol. Med., *125*:1030, 1967.

39. Editorial. The pill and porphyria. Br. Med. J., *3*:603, 1972.

40. Elder, G. H., Gray, C. H., and Nicholson, D. C.: The porphyrias: A review. J. Clin. Pathol., *25*:1013, 1972.

41. Epstein, J. H., and Pinski, J. B.: Porphyria cutanea tarda: Abnormal iron metabolism. Arch. Dermatol., *92*:357, 1965.

42. Epstein, J. H., and Redeker, A. G.: Porphyria cutanea tarda: A study of the effect of phlebotomy. N. Engl. J. Med., *279*:1301, 1968.

43. Erslev, A. J.: Humoral regulation of red cell production. Blood, *8*:349, 1953.

44. Erslev, A. J.: Physiologic control of red cell production. Blood, *10*:954, 1955.

45. Erslev, A. J.: The effect of anemic anoxia on the cellular development of nucleated red cells. Blood, *14*:386, 1959.

46. Erslev, A. J.: Erythropoietin in vitro. II. Effect on "stem cells." Blood, *24*:331, 1964.

47. Erslev, A. J.: Renal biogenesis of erythropoietin. Am. J. Med., *58*:25, 1975.

48. Falk, J. E., Dresel, E. I. B., and Rimington, C.: Porphobilinogen as a porphyrin precursor, and interconversion of porphyrins in a tissue system. Nature, *172*:292, 1953.

49. Field, E. O., Caughi, M. N., Blackett, N. M., and Smithers, D. W.: Marrow-suppressing factors in the blood in pure red cell aplasia, thymoma and Hodgkin's disease. Br. J. Haematol., *15*:101, 1968.

50. Finne, P. H.: Erythropoietin in concentrations of urine from healthy persons. Br. Med. J., *1*:697, 1965.

51. Fisher, J. W., Hatch, F. E., Roh, B. L., Allen, R. C., and Kelley, B. J.: Erythropoietin inhibitor in kidney extracts and plasma from anemic uremic human subjects. Blood, *31*:440, 1968.

52. Fleischer, A. S., Harber, L. C., Cook, J. S., and Baer, R. L.: Mechanism of in vitro photo-hemolysis in erythropoietic protoporphyria. (EPP). J. Invest. Dermatol., *46*:505, 1966.

53. Fried, W.: Erythropoietin. Arch. Intern. Med., *131*:929, 1973.

54. Fried, W., Kilbridge, T., Krantz, S., McDonald, T. P., and Lange, R. D.: Studies on extra-renal erythropoietin. J. Lab. Clin. Med., *73*:244, 1969.

55. Gajdos, A., and Gajdos-Török, M.: The therapeutic effect of adenosine-5-monophosphoric acid in porphyria. Lancet, *2*:175, 1961.

56. Gardner, F. H., Nathan, D. G., Piomelli, S., and Cummins, J. F.: The erythrocythaemic effects of androgen. Br. J. Haematol., *14*:611, 1968.

57. Giblett, E. R.: Haptoglobin: A review. Vox Sang., *6*:513, 1961.

58. Gibson, K. D., Laver, W. G., and Neuberger, A.: Initial stages in the biosynthesis of porphyrins. 2. The formation of δ-aminolevulinic acid from glycine and succinyl coenzyme A by particles from chicken erythrocytes. Biochem. J., *70*:71, 1958.

59. Gibson, K. D., Neuberger, A., and Scott, J. J.: The purification and properties of δ-amino-laevulinic acid dehydrase. Biochem. J., *61*:618, 1955.

60. Gibson, Q. H., and Antonini, E.: Rates of reaction of native human globin with some hemes. J. Biol. Chem., *238*:1384, 1963.

61. Goldberg, A., Rimington, C., and Lochhead, A. C.: Hereditary coproporphyria. Lancet, *1*:632, 1967.

62. Goldstein, B. D., and Harber, L. C.: Erythropoietic protoporphyria: lipid peroxidation and red cell membrane damage associated with photohemolysis. J. Clin. Invest., *51*:892, 1972.

63. Goldwasser, E., Jacobson, L. O., Fried, W., and Plzak, L. F.: Studies on erythropoiesis. V. The effect of cobalt on the production of erythropoietin. Blood, *13*:55, 1958.

64. Gordon, A. S.: Hemopoietine. Physiol. Rev., *39*:1, 1959.

65. Gordon, A. S., Piliero, S. J., Medici, P. T., Siegel, C. D., and Tannenbaum, M.: Attempts to identify the site of production of circulating erythropoietin. Proc. Soc. Exp. Biol. Med., *92*:598, 1956.

66. Granick, S.: Direct evidence for iron insertion into protoporphyrin to form heme. Fed. Proc., *13*:219, 1954.

67. Granick, S.: Hepatic porphyria and drug-induced or chemical porphyria. Ann. N.Y. Acad. Sci., *123*:188, 1965.

68. Grant, W. C., and Root, W. S.: The relation of O_2 in bone marrow blood to post-hemorrhagic erythropoiesis. Am. J. Physiol., *150*:618, 1947.

69. Grant, W. C., and Root, W. S.: Fundamental stimulus for erythropoiesis. Physiol. Rev., *32*:449, 1952.

70. Grasbeck, R.: Studies on the vitamin B_{12} binding principle and other biocolloids of human gastric juice. Acta med. Scand., Suppl. 314, 1956.

71. Gray, C. H., and Neuberger, A.: Studies in congenital porphyria. 1. Incorporation of ^{15}N into coproporphyrin, uroporphyrin and hippuric acid. Biochem. J., *47*:81, 1950.

72. Gross, S.: Hematologic studies on erythropoietic porphyria: A new case with severe hemolysis, chronic thrombocytopenia and folic acid deficiency. Blood, *23*:762, 1964.

73. Gurney, C. W., and Fried, W.: Further studies on the erythropoietic effect of androgens. J. Lab. Clin. Med., *65*:775, 1965.

74. Haeger-Aronsen, B.: Erythropoietic protoporphyria. A new type of inborn error of metabolism. Am. J. Med., *35*:450, 1963.

75. Haeger-Aronsen, B.: Studies on urinary excretion of δ-aminolevulinic acid and other haem precursors in lead workers and lead-intoxicated rabbits. Scand. J. Clin. Lab. Invest., *12* (Suppl. 47):1, 1960.

76. Haeger-Aronsen, B., Strathers, G., and Swahn, G.: Hereditary coproporphyria. Study of a Swedish family. Ann. Intern. Med., *69*:221, 1968.

77. Hahn, P. F., and Whipple, G. H,: Hemoglobin production in anemia limited by low protein intake. Influence of iron intake, protein supplements and fasting. J. Exp. Med., *69*:315, 1939.

78. Haining, R. G., Cowger, M. L., Shurtleff, D. B., and Labbe, R. F.: Congenital erythropoietic porphyria. Am. J. Med., *45*:624, 1968.

79. Handler, P., and Featherstone, W. P.: The biochemical defect in nicotinic acid deficiency. II. On the nature of the anemia. J. Biol. Chem., *151*:395, 1943.

80. Harber, L. C., Fleischer, A. S., and Baer, R. L.: Erythropoietic protoporphyria and photo-hemolysis. J.A.M.A., *189*:191, 1964.

81. Harris, J. W., Whittington, R. M., Weisman, R., Jr., and Horrigan, D. L.: Pyridoxine responsive anemia in the human adult. Proc. Soc. Biol. Med., *91*:427, 1956.

82. Harris, L.: Vitamin C. Br. M. Bull., *12*:57, 1956.

83. Hellman, E. S., Tschudy, D. P., and Bartter, F. C.: Abnormal electrolyte and water metabolism in acute intermittent porphyria. Am. J. Med., *32*:734, 1962.

84. Hodgkin, D. C., et al.: Structure of vitamin B_{12}. Nature, *176*:325, 1955.

85. Hodgson, G.: Synthesis of RNA and DNA at various intervals after erythropoietin injection in transfused mice. Proc. Soc. Exp. Biol. Med., *124*:1045, 1967.

86. Holmberg, C. G., and Laurell, C. B.: Investigations in serum copper. I. Nature of serum and copper and its relation to the iron-binding protein in human serum. Acta chem. Scand., *1*:944, 1947.

87. Hunt, J. A., and Ingram, V. M.: Allelomorphism and the chemical differences of the human hemoglobins A, S and C. Nature, *181*:1062, 1958.

88. Hurwitz, J., and Furth, J. J.: Messenger RNA. Sci. Am., *206*:41, 1962.

89. Ingram, D. J. E., Gibson, J. F., and Perutz, M. F.: Orientation of the four haem groups in haemoglobin. Nature, *178*:906, 1956.

90. Ingram, V. M.: A specific chemical difference between the globins of normal human and sickle-cell anaemia haemoglobin. Nature, *178*:792, 1956.

91. Ingram, V. M.: Gene mutation in human hemoglobin: The chemical difference between normal and sickle cell hemoglobin. Nature, *180*:326, 1957.

92. Ingram, V. M.: Constituents of human haemoglobin. Nature, *183*:1795, 1959.

93. Itano, H.: The Human Hemoglobins: Their Properties and Genetic Control. *In* Anfinsen, C. B., Jr., Anson, M. L., Bailey, K., and Edsall, J. T. (eds.): Advances in Protein Chemistry, vol. 12. Academic Press, New York, 1957.

94. Jacobson, L. O.: Sites of Formation of Erythropoietin. *In* Jacobson, L. O., and Doyle, M. A. (eds.): Erythropoiesis. Grune and Stratton, New York, 1962.

95. Jacobson, L. O., Goldwasser, E., Fried, W., and Plzak, L.: The role of the kidney in erythropoiesis. Nature, *179*:633, 1957.

96. Jandl, J. H., Inman, J. K., Simmons, R. L., and Allen, P. W.: Transfer of iron from serum iron-binding protein to human reticulocytes. J. Clin. Invest., *38*:161, 1959.

97. Jayle, M. F., and Moretti, J.: Haptoglobin: Biochemical, genetic and physiopathological aspects. Progr. Hematol., *3*:342, 1962.

98. Johns, W. H., and Bates, T. R.: Quantification of the binding tendencies of cholestyramine. J. Pharmacol. Sci., *58*:179, 1969.

99. Joubert, S. M., Taljaard, J. J. F., and Shanley, B. C.: Aetiological relationship between hepatic siderosis and symptomatic porphyria catanea tarda. Enzyme, *16*:305, 1973.

100. Kaplowitz, N., Javitt, N., and Harber, L. C.: Isolation of erythrocytes with normal proto-porphyrin levels in erythropoietic protoporphyria. N. Engl. J. Med., *278*:1077, 1968.
101. Kapp, E. M., and Coburn, A. F.: Studies on the excretion of urinary porphyrin in rheumatic fever. Br. J. Exp. Pathol., *17*:255, 1936.
102. Kappas, A., Bradlow, H. L., Gillette, P. N., and Gallagher, T. F.: Studies in porphyria. I. A defect in the reductive transformation of natural steroid hormones in the hereditary liver disease, acute intermittent porphyria. J. Exp. Med., *136*:1043, 1972.
103. Kassner, R. J., and Walchak, H.: Heme formation from Fe (II) and porphyrin in the absence of of ferrochelatase activity (BBA 27101). Biochim. Biophys. Acta, *304*:294, 1973.
104. Kendrew, J. C., and Perutz, M. F.: X-ray studies of compounds of biological interest. Ann. Rev. Biochem., *26*:327, 1957.
105. Kilbridge, T. M., Fried, W., and Heller, P.: The mechanism by which plethora suppresses erythropoiesis. Blood, *33*:104, 1969.
106. Kniffen, J. C.: Protoporphyrin removal in intrahepatic porphyrastasis. Clin. Res., *18*:77, 1970.
107. Kniffen, J. C., Noyes, W. D., and Porter, F. S.: Iron and cholestyramine in erythropoietic protoporphyria. Clin. Sci., *18*:38, 1970.
108. Kramer, S., Viljoen, E., Meyer, A. M., and Metz, J.: The anaemia of erythropoietic porphyria with the first description of the disease in an elderly patient. Br. J. Haematol., *11*:666, 1965.
109. Krantz, S. B., and Goldwasser, E.: On the mechanism of erythropoietin-induced differentiation. II. The effect on RNA synthesis. Biochem. Biophys. Acta, *103*:325, 1965.
110. Krueger, R. C., Melnick, I., and Klein, J. R.: Formation of heme by broken-cell preparations of duck erythrocytes. Arch. Biochem., *64*:302, 1956.
111. Krumdieck, N.: Erythropoietic substance in the serum of anemic animals. Proc. Soc. Exp. Biol. Med., *54*:14, 1943.
112. Kubanek, B., Tyler, W. S., Ferrari, L., Porcellini, A., Howard, D., and Stohlman, F., Jr.: Regulation of erythropoiesis. XXI. The effect of erythropoietin on the stem cell. Proc. Soc. Exp. Biol. Med., *127*:770, 1968.
113. Kuehl, F. A., Shunk, C. H,, and Folkers, K.: Vitamin B$_{12}$. J. Am. Chem. Soc., *77*:251, 1955.
114. Kuratowska, Z., Lewartowski, B., and Lipinski, B.: Chemical and biologic properties of an erythropoietin generating substance obtained from perfusate of isolated anoxic kidneys. J. Lab. Clin. Med., *64*:226, 1964.
115. Kushner, J. P., Lee, G. R., and Nacht, S.: The role of iron in the pathogenesis of porphyria cutanea tarda. An in vitro model. J. Clin. Invest., *51*:3044, 1972.
116. Labbe, R. F.: An enzyme which catalyzes the insertion of iron into protoporphyrin. Biochem. Biophys. Acta, *31*:589, 1959.
117. Labbe, R. F.: Metabolic anomalies in porphyria. The result of impaired biological oxidation. Lancet, *1*:1361, 1967.
118. Labbe, R. F., Talman, E. L., and Aldrich, R. A.: Porphyrin metabolism. II. Uric acid excretion in experimental porphyria. Biochem. Biophys. Acta, *15*:590, 1954.
119. Labbe, R. F., Talman, E. L., and Aldrich, R. A.: Purine metabolism in porphyria. Fed. Proc., *14*:241, 1955.
120. Laforet, M. T., and Thomas, E. D.: The effect of cobalt on heme synthesis by bone marrow in vitro. J. Biol. Chem., *218*:595, 1956.
121. Lajtha, L. G.: Bone marrow cell metabolism. Physiol. Rev., *37*:50, 1957.
122. Lajtha, L. G.: Stem Cell Kinetics and Erythropoietin. *In* Jacobson, L. O., and Doyle, M.A. (eds.): Erythropoiesis. Grune and Stratton, New York, 1962.
123. Lajtha, L. G.: Recent studies in erythroid differentiation and proliferation. Medicine, *43*:625, 1964.
124. Lajtha, L. G., Oliver, R., and Gurney, C. W.: Kinetic model of a bone-marrow stem-cell population. Br. J. Haematol., *8*:442, 1962.
125. Lajtha, L. G., and Suit, H. D.: Uptake of radioactive iron (^{59}Fe) by nucleated red cells. Br. J. Haematol., *1*:55, 1955.
126. Lathem, W., Davis, B. B., Zweig, P. H., and Dew, R.: Demonstration and localization of renal tubular reabsorption of hemoglobin by stop flow analysis. J. Clin. Invest., *39*:840, 1960.
127. Lathem, W., and Worley, W. E.: Distribution of extracorpuscular hemoglobin in circulating plasma. J. Clin. Invest., *38*:474, 1959.
128. Lathem, W., and Worley, W. E.: Renal excretion of hemoglobin: Regulatory mechanisms and differential excretion of free and protein-bound hemoglobin. J. Clin. Invest., *38*:652, 1959.
129. Laurell, C-B., and Nyman, M.: Studies of the serum haptoglobin level in hemoglobinemia and its influence on renal excretion of hemoglobin. Blood, *12*:493, 1957.
130. Leavell, B. S., Thorup, O. A., Jr., and McClellan, J. R.: Observations on the anemia in myxedema. Tr. Am. Clin. Climat. Assoc., *68*:137, 1957.

131. Lemberg, R., and Legge, J. W.: Hematin Compounds and Bile Pigments. Interscience Publishers, Inc., New York, 1949.
132. Levin, E. Y.: Comparative aspects of prophyria in man and animals. Am. N.Y. Acad. Sci., *241*:347, 1974.
133. Levin, E. Y., and Flyger, V.: Erythropoietic porphyria of the fox squirrel sciurus niger. J. Clin. Invest., *52*:96, 1973.
134. Lichtman, H. C., and Feldman, F.: In vitro pyrrole and porphyrin synthesis in lead poisoning and iron deficiency. J. Clin. Invest., *42*:830, 1963.
135. Lipschutz, D. E., and Reiter, J. M.: Acute intermittent porphyria with inappropriately elevated ADH secretion. J.A.M.A., *230*:716, 1974.
136. Lockwood, W. H., and Rimington, C.: Purification of an enzyme converting porphobilinogen to uroporphyrin. Biochem. J., *67*:8p, 1957.
137. London, I. M., and West, R.: The formation of bile pigment in pernicious anemia. J. Biol. Chem., *184*:359, 1950.
138. London, I. M., West, R., Shemin, D., and Rittenberg, D.: On the origin of bile pigment in normal man. J. Biol. Chem., *184*:351, 1950.
139. London, I. M., West, R., Shemin, D., and Rittenberg, D.: Porphyrin formation and hemoglobin metabolism in congenital porphyria. J. Biol. Chem., *184*:365, 1950.
140. London, I. M., Shemin, D., and Rittenberg, D.: Synthesis of heme in vitro by the immature non-nucleated mammalian erythrocyte. J. Biol. Chem., *183*:749, 1950.
141. Macalpine, I., and Hunter, R.: The "insanity" of King George III: A classic case of porphyria. Br. Med. J., *1*:65, 1966.
142. Macalpine, I., Hunter, R., and Rimington, C.: Porphyria in the royal house of Stuart, Hanover and Prussia: A follow-up study of George III's illness. Br. Med. J., *1*:7, 1968.
143. Maclean, N., and Jurd, R. D.: The control of haemoglobin synthesis. Biol. Rev., *47*:393, 1972.
144. Magnus, I. A., Jarrett, A., Prankerd, T. A. J., and Rimington, C.: Erythropoietic protoporphyria. A new porphyria syndrome with solar urticaria due to protoporphyrinemia. Lancet, *2*:448, 1961.
145. Magnussen, C. R., Levine, J. B., Doherty, J. M., Cheesman, J. Q., and Tschudy, D. P.: A red cell enzyme method for the diagnosis of acute intermittent porphyria. Blood, *44*:857, 1974.
146. Marver, D., and Gurney, C.: Renal erythropoietin excretion as a function of acid-base balance. Ann. N.Y. Acad. Sci., *149*:570, 1968.
147. Matheweson, J. H., and Corwin, A. H.: Biosynthesis of pyrrole pigments: A mechanism for porphobilinogen polymerization. J. Am. Chem. Soc., *83*:135, 1961.
148. Mauzerell, D.: The condensation of porphobilinogen to uroporphyrinogen. J. Am. Chem. Soc., *82*:2605, 1960.
149. Meyer, U. A.: Intermittent acute porphyria. Enzyme, *16*:334, 1973.
150. Meyer, U. A., and Schmid, R.: Hereditary hepatic porphyrias. Fed. Proc., *32*:1649, 1973.
151. Meyer, U. A., Strand, L. J., Doss, M., Rees, A. C., and Marver, H. S.: Intermittent acute porphyria—Demonstration of a genetic defect in porphobilinogen metabolism. N. Engl. J. Med., *286*:1277, 1972.
152. Miller, M. E., Rorth, M., Parving, H. H., Howard, D., Reddington, I., Valeri, C. R., and Stohlman, F., Jr.: pH effect on erythropoietin response to hypoxia. N. Engl. J. Med., *288*:706, 1973.
153. Mirand, E. A., Gordon, A. S., and Wenig, J.: Mechanism of testosterone action in erythropoiesis. Nature, *206*:270, 1965.
154. Moore, C. V., Bierbaum, O. S., Welch, A. D., and Wright, L. D.: The activity of synthetic Lactobacillus casei factor (folic acid) as an antipernicious anemia substance. J. Lab. Clin. Med., *30*:1056, 1945.
155. Moore, M. R., Turnbull, A. L., Barnardo, D., Beattie, A. D., Magnus, I. A., and Goldberg, A.: Hepatic δ-aminolaevulinic acid synthetase activity in porphyria cutanea tarda. Lancet, *2*:97, 1972.
156. Moores, R. R., Wright, C. S., Collins, L. R., Gardner, E., Jr., Lewis, J. P., and Smith, L. L.: Stimulation of erythropoietin by androgen in the human. Scand. J. Haematol., 5:6, 1968.
157. Morse, B. S., and Stohlman, F., Jr.: Regulation of erythropoiesis. XVIII. The effect of vincristine and erythropoietin on bone marrow. J. Clin. Invest., *45*:1241, 1966.
158. Naets, J. P., and Wittek, M.: Erythropoiesis in anephric man. Lancet, *1*:941, 1968.
159. Nathan, D. G., Schupak, E., Stohlman, F., Jr., and Merrill, J. P.: Erythropoiesis in anephric man. J. Clin. Invest., *43*:2158, 1964.
160. Neuberger, A., and Muir, H. M.: Biosynthesis of porphyrins and congenital porphyria. Nature, *165*:948, 1950.
161. Neve, R. A., and Aldrich, R. A.: Porphyrin metabolism III. Urinary and erythrocyte porphyrin in children with acute rheumatic fever. Pediatrics, *15*:553, 1955.

162. Nirenberg, M. W.: The genetic code: II. Sci. Am., *208*:80, 1963.
163. Nyman, M.: Serum haptoglobin: Methodological and clinical studies. Scand. J. Clin. Lab. Invest., Suppl. 39, 1959.
164. Ockner, R. K., and Schmid, R.: Acquired porphyria in man and rat due to hexachlorobenzene intoxication. Nature, *189*:499, 1961.
165. Olesen, H., and Fogh, J.: Apparent molecular weight of erythropoietin determined by gel filtration. Scand. J. Haematol., 5:211, 1968.
166. Orten, J. M., Underhill, F. A., Mugrage, E. R., and Lewis, R. C.: Blood volume studies in cobalt polycythemia. J. Biol. Chem., *99*:457, 1932-33.
167. Oski, F. A., and Barness, L. A.: Vitamin E deficiency: Previously unrecognized cause of hemolytic anemia in premature infants. J. Pediatr., *70*:211, 1967.
168. Oski, F. A., and Barness, L. A.: Hemolytic anemia in vitamin E deficiency. Am. J. Clin. Nutr., *21*:45, 1968.
169. Ossias, A. L., Zanjani, E. D., Zalusky, R., Estren, S., and Wasserman, L. R.: Case report: Studies on the mechanism of erythrocytosis associated with a uterine fibromyoma. Br. J. Haematol., *25*:179, 1973.
170. Pauling, L.: The oxygen equilibrium of hemoglobin and its structural interpretation. Proc. Nat. Acad. Sci., *21*:186, 1935.
171. Pavlovic-Kentera, V., Hall, D. P., Bragassa, C., and Lange, R. D.: Unilateral renal hypoxia and production of erythropoietin. J. Lab. Clin. Med., *65*:577, 1965.
172. Perutz, M. F.: Absorption spectra of single crystals of haemoglobin in polarized light. Nature, *143*:731, 1939.
173. Perutz, M. F., Liquori, A. M., and Eirich, F.: X-ray and solubility studies of the haemoglobin of sickle cell anaemia patients. Nature, *167*:929, 1951.
174. Perutz, M. F., Rossman, M. G., Cullis, A. F., Muirhead, H., Will, B., and North, A. C. T.: Structure of hemoglobin. Nature, *185*:416, 1960.
175. Peterka, E. S., Fusaro, R. M., and Goltz, R. W.: Erythropoietic protoporphyria. II. Histological and histochemical studies of cutaneous lesions. Arch. Dermatol., *92*:357, 1965.
176. Peterka, E. S., Fusaro, R. M., Runge, W. J., Jaffe, M. D., and Watson, C. J.: Erythropoietic protoporphyria. J.A.M.A., *193*:120, 1965.
177. Peters, H. A., Cripps, D. J., and Reese, H. H.: Porphyria: Theories of etiology and treatment. Int. Rev. Neurobiol., *16*:301, 1974.
178. Pimstone, N. R., Tenhumen, R., Sertz, P. T., Marver, H. S., and Schmid, R.: The enzymatic degradation of hemoglobin to bile pigment by macrophages. J. Exp. Med., *133*:1264, 1971.
179. Porra, R. J., and Falk, J. E.: The enzymatic conversion of coproporphyrinogen III into proto-porphyrin IX. Biochem. J., *90*:69, 1964.
180. Porra, R. J., and Jones, O. T. G.: An investigation of the role of ferrochelatase in the bio-synthesis of various haem prosthetic groups. Biochem. J., *87*:186, 1963.
181. Porter, F. S., and Lowe, B. A.: Congenital erythropoietic protoporphyria. I. Case reports, clinical studies and porphyrin analysis in two brothers. Blood, *22*:521, 1963.
182. Price, D. C., Epstein, J. H., Winchell, S., Sargent, T. W., Pollycove, M., and Cavalieri, R. R.: Iron kinetics in porphyria cutanea tarda. Clin. Res., *16*:124, 1968.
183. Radin, N. S., Rittenberg, D., and Shemin, D.: The role of glycine in the biosynthesis of heme. J. Biol. Chem., *184*:745, 1950.
184. Radin, N. S., Rittenberg, D., and Shemin, D.: The role of acetic acid in the biosynthesis of heme. J. Biol. Chem., *184*:755, 1950.
185. Raine, D. N.: An ether-soluble precursor of coproporphyrin in urine. Biochem. J., *47*:xiv, 1950.
186. Ratner, A. C., and Dibson, R. L.: Hepatic cutaneous porphyria: Response of a patient to treatment with adenosine-5-monophosphate. Arch. Dermatol., *89*:505, 1964.
187. Redeker, A. G., and Sterling, R. E.: The "glucose effect" in erythropoietic protoporphyria. Arch. Intern. Med., *121*:446, 1968.
188. Reissmann, K. R.: Studies on the mechanism of erythropoietic stimulation in parabiotic rats during hypoxia. Blood, 5:372, 1950.
189. Rhinesmith, H. S., Schroeder, W. A., and Pauling, L.: A quantitative study of the hydrolysis of human dinitrophenyl (DNP) globin: The number and kind of polypeptide chains in normal adult human hemoglobin. J. Am. Chem. Soc., *79*:4682, 1957.
190. Ridley, A.: The neuropathy of acute intermittent porphyria. Q. J. Med., *38*:307, 1969.
191. Rifkind, A. B., Sassa, S., Merkatz, I. R., Winchester, R., Harber, L., and Kappas, A.: Stimulators and inhibitors of hepatic porphyrin formation in human sera. J. Clin. Invest., *53*:1167, 1974.
192. Rimington, C.: Haems and porphyrins in health and disease. II. Acta med. Scand., *143*:177, 1952.
193. Rimington, C.: Biosynthesis of haemoglobin. Br. Med. Bull., *15*:19, 1959.

194. Rimington, C.: Porphyrin and haem biosynthesis and its control. Acta med. Scand., *179*:11, 1966.
195. Rodgers, G. M., Fisher, J. W., and George, W. J.: The role of renal adenosine 3',5'-monophosphate in the control of the erythropoietin production. Am. J. Med., *58*:31, 1975.
196. Rosse, W. F., and Waldmann, T. A.: The metabolism of erythropoietin in patients with anemia due to deficient erythropoiesis. J. Clin. Invest., *43*:1348, 1964.
197. Rudolph, W., Perretta, M.: Effects of erythropoietin on C14-formate uptake by spleen and bone marrow nucleic acids of erythrocyte-transfused mice. Proc. Soc. Exp. Biol. Med., *124*:1041, 1967.
198. Ryan, E. A., and Madill, G. F.: Electron microscopy of the skin in erythropoietic protoporphyria. Br. J. Dermatol., *80*:561, 1968.
199. Salomon, K., Richmond, J. E., and Altman, K. I.: Tetrapyrrole precursors of protoporphyrin IX. J. Biol. Chem., *196*:463, 1952.
200. Sano, S., and Granick, S.: Mitochondrial coproporphyrinogen oxidase and protoporphyrin formation. J. Biol. Chem., *236*:1173, 1961.
201. Schachter, D.: Nature of the glucuronide in direct-reacting bilirubin. Science, *126*:507, 1957.
202. Schmid, R.: Direct-reacting bilirubin, bilirubin glucuronide, in serum, bile, and urine. Science, *124*:76, 1956.
203. Schmid, R.: Cutaneous porphyria in Turkey. N. Engl. J. Med., *263*:397, 1960.
204. Schmid, R., and Schwartz, S.: Disturbance of catalase metabolism in experimental porphyria. J. Lab. Clin. Med., *40*:939, 1952.
205. Schmid, R., Schwartz, S., and Sundberg, R. D.: Erythropoietic (congenital) porphyria: A rare abnormality of the normoblasts. Blood, *10*:416, 1955.
206. Schmid, R., Schwartz, S., and Watson, C. J.: Porphyrin content of bone marrow and liver in the various forms of porphyria. Arch. Intern. Med., *93*:167, 1954.
207. Schmid, R., and Shemin, D.: The enzymatic formation of porphobilinogen from δ-aminolevulinic acid and its conversion to protoporphyrin. J. Am. Chem. Soc., *77*:506, 1955.
208. Schulman, M. P., and Richert, D. A.: Utilization of glycine, succinate and δ-aminolevulinic acid for heme synthesis. Fed. Proc., *15*:349, 1956.
209. Schultze, M. O.: The relation of copper to cytochrome oxidase and hematopoietic activity of the bone marrow of rats. J. Biol. Chem., *138*:219, 1941.
210. Schwartz, H. C., Goudsmit, R., Hill, R. I., Cartwright, S. F., and Wintrobe, M. M.: The biosynthesis of hemoglobin from iron protoporphyrin and globin. J. Clin. Invest., *40*:188, 1961.
211. Schwartz, S., Gliekman, M., Hunter, R., and Wallace, J.: Plutonium project report. CH3720 AECD-2109 (1945) GC770, V.632.
212. Schwartz, S., and Wikoff, H. M.: The relation of erythrocyte coproporphyrin and protoporphyrin to erythropoiesis. J. Biol. Chem., *194*:563, 1952.
213. Shahidi, N. T.: Androgens and erythropoiesis. N. Engl. J. Med., *289*:72, 1973.
214. Shanley, B. C., Zail, S. S., and Joubert, S. M.: Effect of ethanol on liver delta-aminolaevulinate synthetase in rats. Lancet, *1*:70, 1968.
215. Shemin, D.: The biosynthesis of porphyrins. Conference on Hemoglobin. Nat. Acad. Sci., Nat. Res. Council. Publ. 557, 1957, p. 66.
216. Shemin, D., Abramsky, T., and Russell, C. S.: The synthesis of protoporphyrin from δ-aminolevulinic acid in a cell-free extract. J. Am. Chem. Soc., *76*:1204, 1954.
217. Shemin, D., Corcoran, J. W., Rosenblum, C., and Miller, I. M.: On the biosynthesis of the porphyrinlike moiety of vitamin B_{12}. Science, *124*:272, 1956.
218. Shemin, D., and Kumin, S. J.: The mechanism of porphyrin formation. The formation of a succinyl intermediate from succinate. J. Biol. Chem., *198*:827, 1952.
219. Shemin, D., and Rittenberg, D.: The utilization of glycine for the synthesis of a porphyrin. J. Biol. Chem., *159*:567, 1945.
220. Shemin, D., and Rittenberg, D.: The biological utilization of glycine for the synthesis of the protoporphyrin of hemoglobin. J. Biol. Chem., *166*:621, 1946.
221. Shemin, D., and Russell, C. S.: δ-Aminolevulinic acid, its role in the biosynthesis of porphyrins and purines. J. Am. Chem. Soc., *75*:4873, 1953.
222. Shemin, D., Russell, C. S., and Aramsky, T.: The surrinate-glycine cycle. I. The mechanism of pyrrole synthesis. J. Biol. Chem., *215*:613, 1955.
223. Shemin, D., and Wittenberg, J.: The mechanism of porphyrin formation. The role of the tricarboxylic acid cycle. J. Biol. Chem., *192*:315, 1951.
224. Silber, R., and Goldstein, B. D.: Vitamin E and the hematopoietic system. Seminars Hematol., *7*:40, 1970.
225. Smith, E. L.: Vitamin B_{12}. Br. Med. Bull., *12*:52, 1956.
226. Smithies, O.: Zone electrophoresis in starch gels; group variations in the serum proteins of normal human adults. Biochem. J., *61*:629, 1955.

227. Spector, H., Maass, A. R., Michaud, L., Elvehjem, C. A., and Hart, E. B.: The role of ribo-flavin in blood regeneration. J. Biol. Chem., *150*:75, 1943.
228. Stohlman, F., Jr.: Erythropoiesis. N. Engl. J. Med., *267*:342, 1962.
229. Stohlman, F., Jr.: The kidney and erythropoiesis. N. Engl. J. Med., *279*:1437, 1968.
230. Stohlman, F., Jr., Lucarelli, G., Howard, D., Morse, B., and Leventhal, B.: Regulation of erythropoiesis. XVI. Cytokinetic patterns in disorders of erythropoiesis. Medicine, *43*:651, 1964.
231. Strand, L. J., Meyer, U. A., Felsher, B. F., Redeker, A. G., and Marver, H. S.: Decreased red cell uroporphyrinogen I synthetase activity in intermittent acute porphyria. J. Clin. Invest., *51*:2530, 1972.
232. Strik, J. J. T. W. A.: Species differences in experimental porphyria caused by polyhalogenated aromatic compounds. Enzyme, *16*:224, 1973.
233. Tenhunen, R., Marver, H. S., and Schmid, R.: The enzymatic conversion of hemoglobin to bilirubin. Proc. Nat. Acad. Sci., *61*:748, 1968.
234. Thorell, B.: Studies on the formation of cellular substances during blood cell production. Acta med. Scand., Suppl. 200, 1947.
235. Tiwari, G. N., Bahl, L., and Agrawal, S. P.: Porphyria variegaita. Ind. J. Pediatr., *40*:147, 1973.
236. Tschudy, D. P.: Biochemical lesions in porphyria. J.A.M.A., *191*:718, 1965.
237. Turnbull, A., Baker, H., Vernon-Roberts, B., and Magnus, I. A.: Iron metabolism in porphyria cutanea tarda and in erythropoietic protoporphyria. Q. J. Med., *42*:341, 1973.
238. Vogel, W., Richert, D. A., Pixley, B. Q., and Schulman, M. P.: Heme synthesis in iron deficient duck blood. J. Biol. Chem., *235*:1769, 1960.
239. Waldenstrom, J.: The porphyrias as inborn errors of metabolism. Am. J. Med., *22*:758, 1957.
240. Walsh, R. J., Thomas, E. D., Chow, S. K., Fluharty, R. G., and Finch, C. A.: Iron metabolism. Heme synthesis in vitro by immature erythrocytes. Science, *110*:396, 1949.
241. Ward, E., and Mason, H. L.: Free erythrocyte protoporphyrin. J. Clin. Invest., *29*:905, 1950.
242. Watson, C. J.: The erythrocyte coproporphyrin. Arch. Intern. Med., *86*:797, 1950.
243. Watson, C. J.: Porphyrin metabolism in anemias. Arch. Intern. Med., *99*:323, 1957.
244. Watson, C. J., Dhar, G. J., Bossenmaier, I., Cardinal, R., and Petryka, Z. J.: Effect of hematin in acute porphyic relapse. Ann. Intern. Med., *79*:80, 1973.
245. Watson, C. J., and Larson, E. A.: The urinary coproporphyrins in health and disease. Physiol. Rev., *27*:478, 1947.
246. Watson, C. J., deMello, R. P., Schwartz, S., Hawkinson, V. E., and Bossenmaier, I.: Porphyrin chromogens or precursors in urine, blood, bile and feces. J. Lab. Clin. Med., *37*:831, 1951.
247. Watson, C. J., Runge, W., Taddeini, L., Bossenmaier, I., and Cardinal, R.: A suggested control gene mechanism for the excessive production of type I and III porphyrins in congenital erythropoietic porphyria. Proc. Nat. Acad. Sci., *52*:477, 1964.
248. Watson, C. J., Schulze, W., Hawkinson, V., and Baker, A. B.: Coproporphyrinuria (Type III) in acute poliomyelitis. Proc. Soc. Exper. Biol. Med., *64*:73, 1947.
249. Weatherall, J. D., and Clegg, J. B.: The control of human hemoglobin synthesis and function in health and disease. Prog. Hematol., *6*:261, 1969.
250. Whang, J., Frei, E., III, Tjio, J. H., Carbone, P. P., and Brecher, G.: The distribution of the Philadelphia chromosome in patients with chronic myelogenous leukemia. Blood, *22*:664, 1963.
251. Whipple, G. H., and Robscheit-Robbins, F. S.: Amino acids and hemoglobin production in anemia. J. Exp. Med., *71*:569, 1940.
252. Whipple, G. H., and Madden, S. C.: Hemoglobin, plasma protein and cell protein—their interchange and construction in emergencies. Medicine, *23*:215, 1944.
253. Whitaker, J. A., and Viett, T. J.: Fluorescence of the erythrocytes in lead poisoning in children: an aid to rapid diagnosis. Pediatrics, *24*:734, 1958.
254. Whitcomb, W. H., Moore, M., Dille, R., Hummer, L., and Bird, R. M.: Erythropoietin and erythropoiesis inhibitor activity in man. J. Clin. Invest., *44*:1110, 1965.
255. White, W. F., Gurney, C. W., Goldwasser, E., and Jacobson, L. O.: Studies on erthropoietin. Progr. Hormone Res., *16*:219, 1960.
256. Williams, R. T.: Biochemistry of vitamin B_{12}. Biochem. Soc. Symposia, 13. Cambridge University Press, London, 1955.
257. Wintrobe, M. M., Cartwright, G. E., and Gubler, C. J.: Studies on the function and metabolism of copper. J. Nutr., *50*:395, 1953.
258. Wittenberg, J. B.: Formation of the porphyrin ring. Nature, *184*:876, 1959.
259. Wittenberg, J., and Shemin, D.: The location in protoporphyrin of the carbon atoms derived from the α-carbon atom of glycine. J. Biol. Chem., *185*:103, 1950.
260. Witts, L. J.: Porphyria and George III. Br. Med. J., *4*:479, 1972.
261. Wong, K. K., Zanjani, E. S., Cooper, G. W., and Gordon, A. S.: The renal erythropoietic factor. V. Studies on its purification. Proc. Soc. Exp. Biol. Med., *128*:67, 1968.

262. Wuepper, K. D., and Epstein, J. H.: Genetic study of erythropoietic protoporphyria (EPP). Clin. Res., *15*:256, 1969.

263. Yoneyama, Y., Okgama, H., Sugeta, Y., and Yoshikawa, H.: Formation in vitro of hemoglobin and myoglobin from iron protoporphyrin and globin in the presence of an iron chelating enzyme. Biochim. biophys. acta, *74*:635, 1963.

264. Zail, S. S., and Joubert, S. M.: Hepatic delta-aminolaevulinic acid synthetase activity in symptomatic porphyria. Br. J. Haematol., *15*:123, 1968.

265. Zanjani, E. D., Contrera, J. F., Cooper, G. W., and Gordon, A. S., and Wong, K. K.: Renal erythropoietic factor: Role of ions and vasoactive agents in erythropoietin formation. Science, *156*:1367, 1967.

266. Zanjani, E. D., Contrera, J. F., Gordon, A. S., Cooper, G. W., Wong, K. K., and Katz, R.: The renal erythropoietic factor (REF). III. Enzymatic role in the erythropoietin production. Proc. Soc. Exp. Biol. Med., *125*:505, 1967.

267. Zieve, L., Hill, E., Schwartz, S., and Watson, C. J.: Normal limits of urinary coproporphyrin excretion determined by an improved method. J. Lab. Clin. Med., *41*:663, 1953.

CHAPTER **3**

CLASSIFICATION, MECHANISMS, AND DIAGNOSIS OF ANEMIA

THE CLASSIFICATION OF ANEMIA

Problems related to anemia constitute a large segment of investigative hematology and an appreciable part of any clinical practice. The present chapter is devoted to the classification of anemia and to brief discussions of the underlying mechanisms that are involved in each type of anemia. The different mechanisms are discussed briefly at this time to emphasize the importance of these fundamentals and to provide a basis for the development of a unifying, systemic approach to the various clinical syndromes. Discussions of the pathophysiology of anemia in the individual syndromes are given in more detail in Chapters 4 through 8.

Anemia may be defined as a reduction in the circulation of either hemoglobin or erythrocytes. It occurs whenever the hematopoietic equilibrium is disturbed and the loss of erythrocytes or hemoglobin from the circulation exceeds production.

Anemia is usually classified according to etiology, pathophysiology, or morphologic characteristics. All classifications are important but none is entirely satisfactory. Classification according to etiology may be somewhat ambiguous because various details of a disease may be considered as "causes." Thus anemia may be "caused by" chronic blood loss; the blood loss may be due to several "causes," such as excessive vaginal bleeding and hemorrhoidal bleeding. Each of these types of bleeding may arise from one of several "causes," such as functional menorrhagia or uterine malignancy in one circumstance, and simple hemorrhoids associated with cirrhosis of the liver in the other. Difficulty in classification also arises if pathophysiology is viewed as a "cause" when anemia results from more than one factor, such as increased destruction and diminished production of erythrocytes.

Classification according to the morphologic characteristics of the erythrocytes is not entirely satisfactory either, because the same underlying disease may produce more than one type of anemia. "Aplastic" anemia may be normocytic or macrocytic; chronic bleeding may produce a simple microcytic type of anemia at one stage and a hypochromic microcytic type of anemia at another. Although each classification has shortcomings when used alone, all are very helpful in clinical hematology when they are used together. Determinations of the morphologic characteristics of the anemia and of the mechanism of its production are important steps toward the identification of the underlying cause, which is the objective of all diagnosis.

Morphologic classification. The morphologic classification of anemia is helpful in diagnosis, because the characterization of the anemia according to the size and hemoglobin content of the erythrocytes directs the future investigation toward a definite group of possible causative factors or clinical syndromes and eliminates others from consideration. In order to classify anemia morphologically, it is necessary to determine the size and hemoglobin content of the erythrocytes. With proper experience, abnormalities in these details can be detected when a well-prepared smear of the peripheral blood is examined carefully. In other circumstances the size and hemoglobin content of the erythrocytes can be determined most satisfactorily by the formulae devised by Wintrobe.[25]

$$\text{Mean Corpuscular Volume (MCV)} \atop \text{(in cubic microns, cu. } \mu) = \frac{\text{Vol. packed red cells (in cc. per 1000 cc. blood)}}{\text{R.B.C. (in mil. per cu.mm.)}}$$

$$\text{Mean Corpuscular Hemoglobin (MCH)} \atop \text{(in micromicrograms, } \mu\mu) = \frac{\text{Hb. (in gm. per 1000 cc. blood)}}{\text{R.B.C. (in mil. per cu.mm.)}}$$

$$\text{Mean Corpuscular Hemoglobin Conc. (MCHC)} \atop \text{(in per cent, \%)} = \frac{\text{Hb. (in gm. per 100 cc.)} \times 100}{\text{Vol. packed R.B.C. (in cc. per 100 cc. blood)}}$$

Anemia may be classified according to cell size and hemoglobin content, as shown in Table 3-1. The normal values found by the Wintrobe tube and with the automated Coulter counter differ slightly, as shown in Table 3-2. When this method of determining cell size and hemoglobin content is employed it must be remembered that obtaining a numerically expressed result does not insure accuracy; an error in any of the determinations necessary for the calculations

Table 3-1 *Classification of Anemia According to Size and Hemoglobin Content of the Erythrocytes*

Type	MCV (cu.μ)	MCHC (%)
1. Macrocytic	> 94	> 30
2. Normocytic	80-94	> 30
3. Simple Microcytic	< 80	> 30
4. Hypochromic Microcytic	< 80	< 30

(From Wintrobe, M. M.: The size and hemoglobin content of the erythrocyte. J. Lab. Clin. Med., *17*:899, 1932.)

Table 3-2 *Red Blood Cell Indices: Normal Values by Different Methods*

		MEAN	RANGE
MCV	(1)*	87	80-94
	(2)**	91	80-101
MCH	(1)	29	26-32
	(2)	31	27-34
MCHC	(1)	34	31-35
	(2)	34	32-36

*(1) Hemocytometer and Wintrobe tube.
**(2) Coulter Model S33.

will lead to an erroneous result. Furthermore, the result is an average figure that does not reveal the differences that may exist among the individual cells.

Classification according to mechanism. If "cause" of the anemia is thought of in the restricted sense of the immediate cause or "mechanism," a workable classification of anemia can be devised. Such a classification helps the physician focus on this aspect of the problem and provides a sound basis for further systematic investigation or treatment. A classification of anemia according to causative mechanisms is presented in Table 3-3.

MECHANISMS RESPONSIBLE FOR ANEMIA

DIMINISHED ERYTHROPOIESIS

When anemia results from diminished blood production, study of the peripheral blood usually reveals a normocytic or macrocytic anemia associated with a low or normal level of the reticulocytes. Leukopenia and thrombocytopenia are often present. If the diminished blood production is the result of vitamin B_{12} or folid acid deficiency, erythropoiesis is megaloblastic; if the anemia is due to other causes, erythropoiesis is normoblastic. Blood production may be inadequate because of a deficiency of the factors that are essential for erythropoiesis, or a failure of the bone marrow to utilize the essential substances although they are available.

Nutritional deficiency. The factors essential for normal erythropoiesis are metals (cobalt, iron, copper), protein (certain amino acids), and vitamins (vitamin B_{12}, folic acid, ascorbic acid, pyridoxine, niacin and possibly riboflavin, pantothenic acid, and thiamine).[26] A deficiency of any one of these factors might be expected to produce anemia. In adults, only deficiencies of folic acid, vitamin B_{12}, iron, and ascorbic acid are important in the production of anemia.[26] A lack of amino acids appears to be an unlikely cause of anemia in man since amounts of these substances sufficient for erythropoiesis become available from some body source even when the serum protein levels and the protein intake are exceedingly low.[8] Nevertheless, kwashiorkor, a disease in infants characterized by severe protein deficiency and anemia, has been cited as evidence that

Table 3–3 *Classification of Anemia According to Mechanism of Production*

MECHANISM	CAUSE	DISEASE OR CLINICAL SYNDROME
I. DIMINISHED ERYTHROPOIESIS		
A. Nutritional Deficiency		
1. Diet	Inadequate intake	Multiple deficiencies
2. Defective absorption Stomach	Failure to secrete intrinsic factor	Vitamin B_{12} deficiency (Pernicious anemia)
	Total gastrectomy	
	Partial gastrectomy	Iron deficiency
Intestine	Diarrhea	Folic acid, vitamin B_{12}, or iron
	Diverticula	deficiency (Sprue, malabsorption
	Fistulae	syndrome, or pernicious
	Stricture	anemia)
3. Increased demand	Pregnancy	(Folic acid, vitamin B_{12}, or iron deficiency)
	Growth	Iron deficiency
B. Bone Marrow Failure	Associated disease	Primary disease
	Drugs	Aplastic anemia
	Chemicals	Aplastic anemia
	Irradiation	Aplastic anemia
	Endocrine	Myxedema, pituitary disease
	Idiopathic	Aplastic anemia
II. BLOOD LOSS		
A. Acute	Trauma or disease	Shock or anemia
B. Chronic	Lesion of gastrointestinal tract or gynecologic disturbance	Iron deficiency anemia or primary disease

protein deficiency can cause anemia, because iron, folic acid, and infection do not appear to be factors, and protein feeding is followed by reticulocytosis and hematologic recovery. A deficiency of these essential factors may arise in various ways, such as faulty diet, defective absorption, or excessive demands for erythropoiesis.

Faulty diet is responsible for anemia in various parts of the world in usual or unusual circumstances; the intake of iron, folate, protein, or even vitamin B_{12} may be inadequate. In the United States dietary deficiency produces anemia in infants, but in adults, apart from food faddists or alcoholics, nutritional deficiency rarely causes anemia unless other factors operate to produce a conditioned or secondary deficiency. When anemia occurs in adults because of faulty diet, the anemia is usually the result of folic acid deficiency, possibly because of the large body reserves of vitamin B_{12} and iron. Finch has concluded that protein malnutrition is associated with a mild normochromic anemia. There is good evidence that marrow function remains intact but that there is a decrease in stimulation of the erythroid marrow. This decrease in erythropoietin stimulus is a natural consequence of the reduction in oxygen requirements in the protein-depleted individual.[15]

Defective absorption is a common cause of nutritional anemia in adults. In pernicious anemia vitamin B_{12} deficiency arises in this manner as a result of

Table 3-3 *Classification of Anemia According to Mechanism of Production*
(Continued)

MECHANISM	CAUSE	DISEASE OR CLINICAL SYNDROME
III. INCREASED HEMOLYSIS		
A. Hereditary Hemolytic Disorders	1. Erythrocyte membrane defects	1a. Hereditary spherocytosis b. Hereditary elliptocytosis c. Stomatocytosis d. Selective increase in membrane lecithin
	2. Pentose phosphate shunt-glutathione system enzyme deficiencies	2a. Glucose-6-phosphate dehydrogenase b. Others: 6-phosphogluconate dehydrogenase, glutathione reductase, glutathione synthetase, glutathione peroxidase
	3. Glycolytic enzyme deficiencies	3a. Pyruvate kinase deficiency b. Others: diphosphoglyceromutase, triosephosphate isomerase, phosphoglycerate kinase, glyceraldehyde-3-phosphate dehydrogenase, ATPase
	4. Hemoglobinopathy	4a. Sickle cell anemia b. Hemoglobin C disease c. Thalassemia d. Combinations: sickle cell–hemoglobin C disease, sickle cell-thalassemia disease, and others e. Unstable hemoglobins: Zurich, Köln, Genova, Sydney, Hammersmith, Gun Hill, and others

B. Acquired Hemolytic Disorders	1. Antibody mediated
	  a. Isoantibodies
	
	  b. Drug-induced antibodies
	
	  c. Autoantibodies
		
		1a. Transfusion reactions; erythroblastosis fetalis
		1b. Quinidine sensitivity, penicillin sensitivity, alpha methyl dopa sensitivity
		1c. Idiopathic; secondary-malignancies, connective tissue disease, mycoplasma pneumonia, paroxysmal cold hemoglobinuria

	2. Mechanical hemolysis	2a. March hemoglobinuria 2b. Cardiac hemolytic anemia 2c. Microangiopathic hemolytic anemia
	3. Infections	3a. Malaria 3b. Pneumococcal pneumonia 3c. Septicemia 3d. Viral and bacterial infections
	4. Chemical agents	
	5. Physical agents	
	6. Hypersplenism	
	7. Uncertain	7a. Paroxysmal nocturnal hemoglobinuria

defective gastric function and the failure to secrete the intrinsic factor that is essential for the normal absorption of vitamin B_{12}. A similar disorder is produced by total gastrectomy, a procedure that removes the tissue that secretes the intrinsic factor. In this circumstance the deficiency does not appear for several years after gastrectomy. Macrocytic anemia, associated with a megaloblastic type of erythropoiesis that is characteristic of vitamin B_{12} or folic acid deficiency, sometimes occurs in sprue or other diseases accompanied by severe diarrhea or other abnormalities which may lead to malabsorption. A similar anemia due to vitamin B_{12} deficiency that is refractory to oral treatment, yet responsive to parenteral therapy, has been reported in patients with diverticula, strictures, and fistulae of the small intestine. Iron deficiency anemia often occurs several years after partial gastrectomy. Investigation of such patients has shown that the iron deficiency in this circumstance is probably at least partly the result of an inability to absorb iron that is contained in food, although the ability to absorb medicinal iron may be normal.[31]

Excessive demands for erythropoiesis may produce a deficiency of essential factors if the reserve stores of the body have been depleted, even though the normal dietary intake has been maintained. During pregnancy anemia sometimes occurs because of iron deficiency that is the result of the added demands of fetal erythropoiesis; a similar type of anemia is seen in some children because of the increased need for iron to meet the increase in blood volume that accompanies body growth. A deficiency of folic acid, or more rarely of vitamin B_{12}, develops in some women during pregnancy, particularly in those who have a poor diet or suffer from severe gastrointestinal upsets. Depletion of the body reserves of folic acid may lead to megaloblastic erythropoiesis in severe hemolytic anemia. Infestation with *Diphyllobothrium latum* may be responsible for deficiency of vitamin B_{12}.

Bone marrow failure.   Even if adequate amounts of all the substances required for erythropoiesis are ingested and absorbed normally, erythropoiesis may be inadequate because of defective function of the bone marrow. Inadequate erythropoiesis is responsible for the occurrence of anemia in a number of circumstances, in the presence of chronic disease, after the ingestion of drugs, after exposure to chemicals, after irradiation, or in endocrine diseases; in many patients the disease is "idiopathic."

Diseases of long duration such as chronic infections, particularly if accompanied by fever, and various metabolic disorders, such as the uremic state, often depress erythropoiesis. The decreased marrow activity is reflected by diminished iron utilization and reduced production of young red cells. Although not all of the factors responsible for the depression of marrow activity are known, some important details have been established. The plasma of uremic rabbits has been shown to contain a lower than normal quantity of the erythropoietic factor, and uremic rabbits have been shown to be less responsive than normal to injection of plasma rich in erythropoietin.[14] Bone marrow cultures from uremic patients have been shown to have lower iron utilization than cultures from normal individuals.[24] In other diseases, such as carcinomatosis, disseminated tuberculosis, and leukemia, actual mechanical encroachment on the erythropoietic tissue may be a factor in the anemia, although it is rarely the sole mechanism.

Drugs act to depress the bone marrow in various ways. Anemia may occur alone, but more often it occurs in combination with leukopenia or thrombocytopenia. Some drugs depress the bone marrow, which is a tissue composed of rapidly dividing cells, by their pharmacologic action which interferes with nucleic acid metabolism and inhibits cell division or maturation. In this category are the various alkylating agents. Other drugs produce depression of hematopoiesis only in certain susceptible individuals. Marrow depression, which may be either temporary or permanent, may occur without warning. Reactions of this type have been reported to follow exposure to a variety of coal tar products, antibiotics, anticonvulsants, and heavy metals.

Chemicals that are employed in various industries and occupations may damage the bone marrow in the same manner as chemicals used as drugs. Usually an element of individual susceptibility is a factor. The chemicals that have been incriminated most often are organic solvents, particularly benzol and its derivatives. Exposure to chemicals often occurs through the use of cleaning agents, herbicides, or insecticide sprays.

Ionizing radiation from x-rays or radioactive materials causes anemia by depression of erythropoiesis if the bone marrow is exposed sufficiently. During roentgen ray therapy, or after the use of radioactive isotopes, the full hematologic effect may not be evident until several weeks after exposure. With the carefully calculated daily and total dosages that are used in radiation therapy, permanent damage rarely results because therapy is rarely continued for more than several weeks at a time. Although the exact mechanism of action of radiation is incompletely understood at present, it is known that cell multiplication is suppressed, possibly by inhibition of nucleic acid synthesis.[20]

Hormones. Both the pituitary gland and the thyroid gland are important in erythropoiesis. This is shown by the development of anemia after removal of either of the glands in animals, and by the occurrence of anemia in patients with hypopituitarism and myxedema. The anemia of myxedema, which is rarely severe, probably represents an adjustment to the decreased body metabolism comparable to the effect produced by exposure to increased oxygen tension, rather than a deficiency of the thyroid hormone per se.[5]

"Idiopathic" aplastic anemia. In some patients no explanation can be found for the bone marrow failure that is responsible for severe anemia. There is no history of unusual exposure to drugs, chemicals, or irradiation, and no evidence of an associated disease that might cause bone marrow depression. A congenital defect has been postulated for the disorder that occurs in infants and very young children, but aplastic anemia also develops in adults. The marrow hypoplasia is usually associated with pancytopenia, but in some patients anemia occurs alone; in others, the anemia is accompanied by either leukopenia or thrombocytopenia. A few patients later develop paroxysmal nocturnal hemoglobinuria.

BLOOD LOSS

Acute blood loss usually results in a normocytic, normochromic type of anemia. Although the total blood volume falls immediately after hemorrhage, the hematocrit determination may not reflect the degree of blood loss until 48 hours have elapsed. In persons with a responsive bone marrow, acute hemorrhage, which affords a well-known stimulus to erythropoiesis, is usually followed by an increase in platelets, leukocytes, and reticulocytes.

Chronic blood loss is a common cause of anemia. Bleeding of this type nearly always results in a deficiency of iron which, when severe, is characterized by a hypochromic microcytic anemia associated with normoblastic erythropoiesis in the bone marrow. In milder degrees of anemia due to deficiency of iron, hypochromia and microcytosis are absent.

INCREASED HEMOLYSIS

The normal survival time of the circulating erythrocyte as determined by the Ashby, chromium[51], N[15]-glycine, and diisopropylfluorophosphate methods is about 120 days.[2] Hemolytic anemia occurs whenever a decreased survival time of the erythrocytes is not balanced by increased erythropoiesis. A decrease in survival time of the erythrocytes to less than 20 days may be necessary to produce anemia if the bone marrow is functioning normally, since the bone marrow has the capacity to increase its production of erythrocytes sixfold.[10] Unless erythropoiesis is depressed for some reason, hemolytic anemia is characterized both by increased hemolysis and increased erythropoiesis.

Several different pathogenic mechanisms may cause a diminution in the survival time of erythrocytes. These mechanisms can be conveniently classified as "inherited" or "acquired." The defects may also be classified as "intracorpuscular" or "extracorpuscular." "Intracorpuscular" defects, which are intrinsic in the erythrocytes produced by the patient, result in a diminished survival time of the patient's erythrocytes in his own circulation and also after transfusion into a normal compatible recipient. "Extracorpuscular" factors are different in that they are part of the environment that the erythrocytes encounter in the patient's circulation; normal erythrocytes have a diminished survival when transfused into the patient, but the erythrocytes produced by the patient survive for the normal time when transfused into a normal recipient. Intracorpuscular defects are generally congenital, the result of some inherited disorder. Extracorpuscular defects are usually acquired as the result of some associated disease or disorder. In some patients the hemolytic anemia is the result of a combination of intracorpuscular and extracorpuscular abnormalities. Inherited or intrinsic abnormalities of the red cells that cause a shortened survival may be a defect in one of a number of enzymes necessary for the metabolic functions of the cell, a defect in the cell membrane, or the presence of an abnormal hemoglobin molecule, "hemoglobinopathy." The acquired disorders may have either extracorpuscular or intracorpuscular defects primarily, but in practically all cases abnormalities appear in the erythrocyte membrane before the cells are destroyed. Infectious agents, chemicals, and vegetable poisons produce hemolytic anemia in susceptible persons by damaging the erythrocyte or its precursor directly, or by stimulating the production of antibodies that damage the cells.

One of the most important contributions to hematology was made by Pauling, Itano, Singer, and Wells, who showed that the sickling phenomenon of sickle cell disease is a manifestation of a pathologic difference in the hemoglobin molecule that can be demonstrated by electrophoresis.[21] The difference between

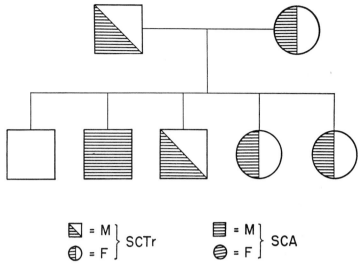

$$\boxed{\quad} = M \left.\right\} SCTr \qquad \boxed{\quad} = M \left.\right\} SCA$$

$$\ominus = F \qquad \qquad \ominus = F$$

Figure 3–1 Heredity in sickle cell disease. Study of the hemoglobin types in a family which illustrates the results that occurred from the mating of parents who were heterozygous for hemoglobin S.

these and normal hemoglobin molecules is in the globin portion and not in the heme fraction. The determination of the type of hemoglobin is genetically controlled. Normal adult hemoglobin contains two normal alpha chains and two normal beta chains and is written as alpha-2, beta-2 ($\alpha_2\beta_2$). Fetal hemoglobin is alpha-2, gamma-2 ($\alpha_2\gamma_2$), and A$_2$ hemoglobin is (alpha-2, delta-2) ($\alpha_2\delta_2$). Numerous abnormal hemoglobins have been reported, usually results of a genetic defect in the synthesis of the alpha or beta chains. These, which can be identified by hemoglobin electrophoresis or other special tests, are discussed in Chapter 7. When the abnormal hemoglobin occurs in the heterozygous state together with normal adult hemoglobin, a nonsymptomatic "trait" condition usually results. When the abnormal hemoglobin is present in the homozygous state, or when an individual is heterozygous for two abnormal hemoglobin types, a clinical disease characterized by a hemolytic disorder of the intracorpuscular type often occurs (Fig. 3–1).

Hemolytic anemia sometimes develops in patients who have splenomegaly when no autoantibodies or other abnormal hemolytic mechanisms can be demonstrated by the usual tests. The usual features of hemolytic anemia may be present, but on occasions during the management of a patient with anemia by means of transfusions, an increased demand for transfusions is the main clinical evidence of the hyperhemolysis. In some patients leukopenia and thrombocytopenia of considerable severity also occur. The reductions in the cellular elements of the circulating blood are associated with an apparently active bone marrow. Splenectomy is sometimes beneficial and the syndrome has been termed "hypersplenism." In some patients with tropical or non-tropical splenomegaly an increase in plasma volume, rather than a decrease in the circulating red cell mass, reduces hematocrit values in the peripheral blood.

The hemolytic anemias and the mechanism involved are discussed in detail in Chapter 7.

DIAGNOSIS OF THE
PATIENT WITH ANEMIA

The objectives in the management of the patient with anemia are, first, the discovery of its cause and, second, correction of the underlying defect. It is important to remember that the demonstration of "anemia" does not constitute a diagnosis but merely the recognition of a sign comparable to fever or edema. For this reason the seriousness of the anemia in any patient depends on the underlying cause of the anemia rather than its severity. A mild degree of anemia caused by a carcinoma of the gastrointestinal tract is a serious affair for the patient, but a severe degree of anemia from hemorrhoidal bleeding is not. Treatment of a patient with iron, or vitamins, or blood transfusions *without first making a diagnosis other than "anemia"* may jeopardize his chances of recovery. Anemia that is the result of iron deficiency secondary to blood loss from a carcinoma of the cecum may respond to iron salts orally or to blood transfusions, while the carcinoma changes from a curable to an incurable lesion. In situations in which the underlying cause cannot be corrected, accurate diagnosis is still essential for proper management. Unless this fact is recognized a patient with a macrocytic anemia may be "cured" of his anemia by treatment with the folic acid present in many multivitamin preparations, but the central nervous system lesions may progress and become irreversible if the patient is suffering from vitamin B_{12} deficiency.

A systematic investigation of the patient with suspected anemia nearly always provides the information necessary for the correct diagnosis and proper treatment. This investigation aims to provide answers to the following questions:

1. Does the patient have anemia?
2. What are the morphologic characteristics of the anemia?
3. What is the mechanism of the anemia?
4. What is the underlying cause or disease that is responsible for the abnormal mechanism?
5. What is the best form of treatment?

Although it is at times impossible to establish a complete diagnosis in a patient with anemia, in the vast majority of cases it is possible to classify the anemia according to the responsible mechanism, i.e., as being due either to deficient production, blood loss, or increased hemolysis. This is usually possible by the use of relatively simple laboratory procedures that can be performed in the physician's office or the hospital laboratory. If the physician understands the mechanism that is responsible for the anemia, he is in a position to manage the patient intelligently by administering the proper treatment or by planning any further investigation that may be necessary to identify the disorder that is responsible for the abnormal mechanism.

The answer to the question "Does the patient have anemia?" often cannot be gained from the history or the physical examination. Anemia of moderate severity may not be detected even by careful inspection of the skin and mucous membranes. In another circumstance a neurasthenic individual with pallor of the skin and mucous membranes may report all of the symptoms of anemia even though the blood is entirely normal. The presence of anemia can be

Table 3-4   *Lower Limits of Normal Hematocrit and Hemoglobin at Sea Level*

YEARS	SEX	HEMOGLOBIN (gm 100 ml.)	PACKED CELL VOLUME (%)
0.6–4	Both sexes	11	33
5–9	Both sexes	11.5	34.5
10–14	Both sexes	12	36
Adults	Men	14	42
	Women	12	36
	Pregnant women	11	33

(Reprinted from J.A.M.A., *203*:119, 1968.)

established only by laboratory procedures. The simplest and most reliable screening procedure is the hematocrit determination;[3] the normal range given for adult males is 40 to 54 per cent and for adult females 37 to 47 per cent. Other lower limits of normal hematocrit and hemoglobin are given in Table 3–4.[9] The hemoglobin determination, which has an accuracy comparable to that of the hematocrit if it is performed properly, is also advocated as a screening procedure by some authors.[4] In our experience the hematocrit determination has proved satisfactory, but even this procedure is far from infallible. Misleading values may be obtained if the blood is drawn from a vein subjected to too much stasis, if an improper amount of anticoagulant is used, or if centrifugation is faulty. The volume of packed cells is also influenced by the osmotic pressure in the plasma; low levels of serum electrolytes cause a rise in the hematocrit, and elevations cause a fall. Even if the techniques are not faulty, values in the normal range may be obtained occasionally in patients with either macrocytic anemia or iron deficiency anemia of mild degree. We have seen a patient with pernicious anemia and involvement of the central nervous system who had a hematocrit of 42 per cent, a hemoglobin of 14.3 gm. per 100 ml., and an erythrocyte count of 3.3 million per cu.mm. An analogous difficulty has been encountered in patients with iron deficiency when the hematocrit was 40 per cent, the hemoglobin 8.0 gm. per 100 ml, and the red blood count 5.0 million per cu.mm. Such unusual occurrences do not detract seriously from the usefulness of the hematocrit as a screening test, because the use of either the hemoglobin determination or erythrocyte count alone as a screening procedure is subject to the same limitations. An increased plasma volume which occurs in some patients with splenomegaly, and in some with increased plasma proteins, produces subnormal values of the hematocrit. In this circumstance determinations of the plasma volume and the total circulating red cell mass are necessary for an accurate evaluation.

In order to answer the question "What is the mechanism responsible for the anemia?" a careful history, a physical examination, and certain laboratory tests that reveal the morphologic and other characteristics of the blood are necessary. Laboratory procedures have assumed the most prominent place in the diagnosis of hematologic problems, but this does not mean that a carefully-taken history is unimportant. Without the benefit of a complete history the laboratory results may be puzzling or even misleading.

The history. When the history is obtained the patient should first be allowed to give his own account of his illness, and then he should be questioned about various details. A family history of anemia or splenectomy or a past history of recurrent episodes of anemia may be significant, particularly if the patient has hemolytic anemia. The dietary history is important in children, in cases of pregnancy, and in chronic illness, for it is in these circumstances that a dietary deficiency is most likely to become manifest. The history of the use of "tonics" and vitamins may help clarify an anemia that is difficult to classify because the hematologic features characteristic of the underlying disease or syndrome have been altered by such preparations. Repeated exposures to drugs or chemicals encountered in the patient's occupation or in the pursuit of a hobby may be a factor in the causation of anemia. A careful review of the body systems should be part of the history-taking because systematic questioning of this type may reveal important symptoms, such as paresthesias, mild ataxia, excessive menstrual bleeding, or even tarry stools, that have not been volunteered by the patient.

Physical examination. Although the physical examination alone rarely if ever suffices for the complete diagnosis of anemia, almost any part of the examination may contribute important information. The appearance of hemorrhages and exudates in the fundi may be the first indication that the patient has bacterial endocarditis, leukemia, uremia, or aplastic anemia. The presence of tumor masses, lymphadenopathy, hepatomegaly, or splenomegaly may bring the diseases of the reticuloendothelial system into consideration for the first time. Most hemolytic anemias, with the exception of sickle cell anemia, are associated with splenomegaly. Splenomegaly is unusual in untreated aplastic anemia, and the detection of an enlarged spleen makes some other diagnosis more likely. An appraisal of the nutritional state of the patient, the color of the tongue, the appearance of the papillae, the presence of fissuring of the lips, and the texture of the fingernails may give clues to the presence of a deficiency of folic acid, vitamin B_{12}, or iron. The detection of telangiectases on the skin or mucous membranes may give the first clue to an explanation of gastrointestinal hemorrhage. Even the general appearance of the patient, the tone of his voice, and his manner of speaking may lead to the recognition of myxedema as the cause of an undiagnosed case of anemia that has proved refractory to the usual forms of "antianemic" therapy. The demonstration of mild ataxia or decreased vibratory sense in the extremities may be the first indication that the patient has pernicious anemia, particularly if the hematologic picture has been altered by inadequate specific therapy or by coexisting iron deficiency.

Laboratory studies. Examination of the peripheral blood by laboratory methods is a most important step in the identification of the mechanism that is responsible for the anemia. If the hematocrit value is low, the following procedures are indicated: determination of the hemoglobin; erythrocyte count and determination of the red cell indices; leukocyte count; and a study of the stained blood smear. Study of a well-made and stained smear of the peripheral blood, which was once the main reliance of the hematologist, declined in popularity after determination of red cell indices, study of aspirated bone marrow, and other hematological examinations were introduced. Nevertheless, careful study of the leukocytes, erythrocytes, and platelets in the peripheral blood should be an important part of the examination of every patient suspected of having a hematologic disorder.

The leukocyte count can be estimated with considerable accuracy, and most cases of leukemia can be recognized by the number or immaturity of the leukocytes. In addition other abnormalities, although not diagnostic of a disease, give valuable information. Abnormalities of the lymphocytes suggest infectious mononucleosis or other viral infections. Multi-segmented polys or macropolycytes should make one suspect a deficiency of vitamin B_{12} or folate. Young cells of the granulocytic series accompanied by nucleated red cells and marked poikilocytosis, particularly the presence of teardrop forms, indicate myeloid metaplasia, leukemia or other disease of the bone marrow.

The appearance of the erythrocytes also deserves careful scrutiny. Sickle cells and ovalocytes are practically diagnostic; large oval macrocytes are almost pathognomonic for vitamin B_{12} or folate deficiency, as is the appearance of megaloblasts in the circulating blood. Microspherocytes, helmet cells, schistocytes, and polychromatophilic cells, indicate the presence of a hemolytic anemia of some sort; schistocytes, spur cells, and helmet cells in particular suggest a microangiopathic anemia that occurs in renal disease, carcinomatosis, prosthetic heart valves, and thrombotic thrombocytopenic purpura. A dimorphic population is seen in acquired sideroblastic anemia, and also in some patients who have been transfused. Marked poikilocytosis is strong evidence against aplastic anemia. Hypochromic microcytes and anisocytosis suggest iron deficiency but are not diagnostic, because they also occur in some patients with iron-loading anemia and defective hemoglobin metabolism. Target cells occur in hemoglobinopathies and in some patients with liver disease. Stomatocytes and spur cells are seen in patients with alcoholism and liver disease. Acanthocytosis is an inherited disorder characterized by cells similar to, if not identical with, spur cells. An MCHC of over 37 per cent suggests hereditary spherocytosis. Similar values which approach the limit of solubility of the abnormal hemoglobin occur in Hb C disease and SS disease, disorders in which further concentration or changes lead to hemoglobin crystalization. In patients who have had splenectomy the peripheral blood smear often is strikingly abnormal; target cells, nucleated red blood cells, Howell-Jolly bodies, siderocytes, and marked poikilocytosis occur. Similar findings have been seen in a patient with functional asplenia some years after Thorotrast administration. Rouleaux formation probably indicates hyperglobulinemia, and should be investigated.

Thrombocytopenia can be recognized in a peripheral smear, and a study of the other cellular elements may help to identify the cause as aplastic anemia, leukemia, or viral infection. Thrombocytosis and large, bizarre-shaped platelets suggest a myeloproliferative disorder. The platelets in Bernard-Soulier's disease are larger than normal and function abnormally. Study of the peripheral smear should be routine for any patient suspected of having thrombocytopenia because automatic counters, give erroneous normal results in some circumstances.

A stain for reticulocytes affords a generally reliable indication of the erythropoietic activity of the bone marrow. A count of over 100,000 per cu. mm. indicates hyperplasia, seen after hemorrhage and in hemolytic anemia; less than 20,000 per cu.mm. usually signifies hypoplasia. Special leukocyte stains, such as the peroxidase, Sudan black, nonspecific esterase, and the PAS, are helpful in distinguishing between the different types of acute leukemia.

With the results of the hemoglobin, hematocrit, and erythrocyte determinations, the mean corpuscular volume (MCV), mean corpuscular hemoglobin (MCH), and mean corpuscular hemoglobin concentration (MCHC) can be determined, and the anemia can be classified according to cell size and hemoglobin content as:

> macrocytic (MCV > 94 cu.μ) (MCHC > 30 per cent)
> normocytic (MCV 80-94 cu.μ) (MCHC > 30 per cent)
> microcytic (MCV < 80 cu.μ) (MCHC > 30 per cent)
> hypochromic (MCV > 80 cu.μ) (MCHC > 30 per cent)
> hypochromic microcytic (MCV < 80 cu.μ)[32] (MCHC < 30 per cent)

The method of calculating these values is given on page 60. The characterization of the anemia as macrocytic, normocytic, microcytic, or hypochromic microcytic provides a guide to other appropriate studies that may be necessary to determine the mechanism and cause of the anemia. The determination of the cell size and hemoglobin content by such calculations does not mean that a careful study of the blood smear is unimportant; study of the smear gives valuable information that may not be apparent in the calculations.

MACROCYTIC ANEMIA

If the patient is found to have macrocytic anemia of significant degree (MCV > 100 cu.μ), it is unlikely that acute hemorrhage has occurred, and for practical purposes chronic blood loss may be eliminated from consideration. The anemia is nearly always the result of diminished effective erythropoiesis and as a consequence the reticulocyte count is usually 1 per cent or less; often mild or moderate granulocytopenia and thrombocytopenia are present. Less often a hemolytic mechanism is responsible. Macrocytic anemia is most likely to be seen in the following circumstances: deficiency of vitamin B_{12} or folic acid. Mild degrees of macrocytosis also occur in some instances of "aplastic" anemia, myxedema, and hemolytic anemia. The procedures usually followed in the diagnosis of a patient with anemia of this type are shown in Illustrative Case 1 later in this chapter.

Deficiency of vitamin B_{12} and folic acid. If the macrocytosis is due to a deficiency of vitamin B_{12} there is usually leukopenia and thrombocytopenia, often of mild degree. If the anemia is moderate or severe in degree, the blood smear reveals considerable anisocytosis and poikilocytosis, and shows oval macrocytes and large multisegmented neutrophils. In the untreated patient the normal or subnormal reticulocyte count reflects the failure of a normal response to anemia. The slightly elevated level of indirect-reacting serum bilirubin and the increased fecal urobilinogen excretion reflect the increased destruction of erythrocytes in the peripheral circulation or in the bone marrow. The occurrence of the megaloblastic type of erythropoiesis in the bone marrow establishes almost unequivocally the presence of a deficiency of vitamin B_{12} or folic acid.

Since deficiencies of vitamin B_{12} and of folic acid can give identical hematologic pictures, further study is necessary to determine which is responsible. In this connection the gastric analysis is a very helpful procedure. With rare exceptions, patients with pernicious anemia do not secrete hydrochloric acid after the administration of histamine, and the presence of free HCl in the gastric analysis can be considered almost to exclude pernicious anemia from consideration. The other causes of vitamin B_{12} deficiency, such as total gastrectomy, intestinal shunts, fistulae, and malabsorption syndromes, are usually suggested by the history and confirmed by appropriate examinations. If the patient has evidence of posterolateral sclerosis associated with a normocytic or macrocytic anemia and histamine-fast achlorhydria, the diagnosis of pernicious anemia should be strongly suspected even though the marrow is not megaloblastic.

Folic acid administration can modify the appearance of the bone marrow and the peripheral blood in a patient with pernicious anemia, while allowing the central nervous system lesions to progress. For this reason, measurement of the level of vitamin B_{12} in the serum, or use of one of the tests of vitamin B_{12} absorption (such as the Schilling test) that utilize vitamin B_{12} labeled with radioactive cobalt, may be necessary to establish the diagnosis. If subnormal amounts of B_{12} are absorbed and excreted, the test is repeated and intrinsic factor is administered with the oral vitamin B_{12}. The addition of the intrinsic factor leads to substantial improvement in absorption of vitamin B_{12} in patients with pernicious anemia but has little or no effect in those with malabsorption syndrome, shunts, and fistulae. If the patient has anemia and a megaloblastic bone marrow due to a deficiency of vitamin B_{12}, the administration of vitamin B_{12} parenterally produces a conversion of the megaloblastic erythropoiesis to the normoblastic type, followed by a reticulocytosis and a rise of the hemoglobin and erythrocyte levels to normal.

When folic acid deficiency is responsible for the macrocytic anemia there is usually a history of inadequate diet or some disorder such as a malabsorption syndrome that produces a secondary deficiency. A dietary deficiency sufficient to produce this type of anemia is rare in the United States except in infancy, during pregnancy, in food faddists, and in alcoholics. Folic acid deficiency may produce the same hematologic picture as vitamin B_{12} deficiency, but the neurologic lesions that are so common in vitamin B_{12} deficiency are usually absent or mild in folic acid deficiency. The occurrence of a macrocytic anemia and a megaloblastic marrow in an adult who has retained the ability to secrete free HCl strongly suggests the possibility of folic acid deficiency. In folate deficiency serum folate levels are reduced whereas levels of vitamin B_{12} are normal. Concurrent antibiotic administration usually vitiates the results of these tests if the microbiologic assay method is used. Recent administration of other radioactive material may interfere with the Schilling test.

Aplastic anemia.   Mild or moderate macrocytosis is slightly more common than normocytic anemia in aplastic anemia. Although anemia of this type is usually accompanied by definite leukopenia and thrombocytopenia, anemia may occur alone. The term "chronic erythrocytic hypoplasia" is used to distinguish patients of the latter type. The reticulocyte count and serum bilirubin level are usually normal or subnormal; in chronic erythrocytic hypoplasia the reticulocyte count is often 0 or 0.1 per cent. A slight increase in the percentage of reticulocytes is occasionally seen, but when this occurs the absolute value (the number of reticulocytes per cu.mm.) is usually normal. The macrocytic anemia of aplastic anemia, even if severe, is rarely accompanied by a significant degree of poikilocytosis or anisocytosis. The bone marrow examination nearly always reveals the normoblastic type of erythropoiesis, but in rare cases a megaloblastic marrow occurs. Usually the marrow of patients with aplastic anemia is hypocellular, often markedly so, but a biopsy is necessary to determine cellularity and to establish the diagnosis. At times, the history of exposure to irradiation, chemicals, or drugs is helpful. On occasion, examination of the bone marrow in a patient with suspected aplastic anemia establishes a definite diagnosis of some other primary disease such as multiple myeloma, leukemia, carcinomatosis, or tuberculosis. In the majority of patients with aplastic anemia the cause remains obscure and the anemia is classified as "idiopathic." (See Illustrative Case 2.)

Myxedema. A mild or moderately severe macrocytic anemia occurs commonly in patients with myxedema. The red blood cell count usually is over 3.0 million per cu.mm. The peripheral blood shows no appreciable poikilocytosis or anisocytosis, and is generally normal in other respects. The erythropoiesis in the bone marrow is normoblastic and the cellularity is either normal or slightly reduced. The diagnosis of myxedema is usually suggested by the clinical features of the disease and is confirmed by the appropriate laboratory tests, such as determinations of the serum cholesterol level, basal metabolic rate, radioactive iodine uptake, and measurement of the plasma T_3, T_4 or TSH. When iron or vitamin B_{12} deficiency occur in the patient with myxedema, the anemia is more severe than in myxedema alone.

Hemolytic anemia. A macrocytic type of anemia is not uncommon in hemolytic disorders, particularly in the extracorpuscular or acquired type. The diagnosis of the patient with hemolytic anemia is considered in the discussion of hemolytic normocytic anemias, and in Illustrative Case 4.

NORMOCYTIC ANEMIA

If the patient is found to have a normocytic type of anemia (MCV 80 to 94 cu.μ), hyperhemolysis, acute blood loss, and deficient blood production must be considered.

Hyperhemolysis. A reticulocyte count greater than 4 per cent, or over 100,000 per cu.mm. in a patient who has neither had a recent hemorrhage nor received antianemic therapy should raise the suspicion of a hemolytic anemia. Often the reticulocyte count is over 10 per cent, and sometimes it is 30 per cent or more. Study of the stained smear often reveals suggestive evidence of a hemolytic process in the form of nucleated red cells, polychromatophilia, punctate basophilia, target cells, or spherocytes. Leukocytosis is often present. These abnormalities in the peripheral blood reflect the hyperplasia that is evident on examination of the bone marrow. At times the increase in erythropoiesis is so marked that a differential cell count of the marrow reveals that the myeloid-erythroid (M:E) ratio is 1:1 or less (normal 3:1 to 10:1). In some patients with hemolytic anemia striking hyperplasia occurs, and the early forms of normoblasts become so numerous that the normoblastic nature of the erythropoiesis may be misinterpreted as megaloblastic because of the morphologic similarities between the youngest cells of both series. Careful study of the cells at all different stages of development, particularly at the polychromatophilic stage, nearly always enables a correct interpretation of the marrow to be made; in some patients, however, the marrow actually becomes megaloblastic because of the development of folate deficiency.

Evidence of the hyperhemolysis is found in the moderate elevation of the indirect reacting bilirubin (1.0 to 4.0 mg. per 100 ml.) and in the increased fecal urobilinogen excretion.

Demonstration of a shortened erythrocyte survival time by means of tagged red cells is a useful way to establish the presence of hyperhemolysis in some circumstances. If a radioactive tag is employed, measurement of the accumulation of radioactivity in the spleen and liver gives some information from which inferences can be made about the site of destruction of the erythrocytes.

Although recognition of the hemolytic process is usually easy, it is sometimes difficult because all the signs of increased hemolysis and increased erythropoiesis may be absent or inconspicuous if the patient is seen during an "aplastic crisis," which occasionally develops during an intercurrent infection.

If the anemia is established as hemolytic in type, further tests are necessary to determine the nature of the hemolytic disorder. The diagnostic work-up on a patient of this type is described in Illustrative Case 4. At times study of parents or siblings is helpful in the diagnosis of a patient suspected of having hereditary spherocytosis, thalassemia, hemoglobinopathy, or an enzymatic defect.

Hemolytic anemia due to an extracorpuscular or acquired defect may be macrocytic or normocytic. In some patients the disease appears to be due to an autoimmune mechanism, and in others to some other mechanism. If the antiglobulin (Coombs) test is positive, autoimmune hemolytic disease is likely even though the osmotic fragility test reveals abnormal susceptibility to hypotonic saline. In such circumstances further study is necessary to determine whether the hemolytic process is "idiopathic" or "secondary" to some underlying disease, such as one of the lymphoma group, carcinoma, sarcoidosis, or one of the collagen disorders. A careful diagnostic study that may include roentgenographic examinations, serum protein studies, a search for L.E. cells, and biopsy of a lymph node or other tissue is often necessary. A diagnosis of the idiopathic type of disease is reached by exclusion. At times the diagnosis of autoimmune hemolytic disease as either idiopathic or symptomatic can be established only after a prolonged period of observation and repeated examinations. The macrocytic anemia of chronic liver disease is usually due to an extracorpuscular type of hyperhemolysis, but the Coombs test is usually negative. When the hemolytic anemia is due to chronic liver disease, abnormal liver function is found by tests and clinical evidence of liver disease usually is present. In other disease states a hemolytic element may be present, but is demonstrable only by careful study; in these patients the hemolytic process is usually mild, and inadequate blood production is the most important mechanism.

Examination of the urine for hemosiderin and of the plasma for hemoglobin, and measurement of the serum haptoglobin level, are important if intravascular hemolysis and hemoglobinuria are suspected. If positive, other more definitive tests are performed.

Acute blood loss. The anemia that follows acute blood loss is nearly always normocytic. If the acute hemorrhage is external and results from trauma or disease, its occurrence is generally recounted in the history. If the hemorrhage occurs from the gastrointestinal tract the event may not be noticed by the patient, and the finding of anemia may be the first clue to its occurrence. In some patients hemorrhages from a duodenal ulcer or a lesion of the small intestine recur over a period of years, and cause anemia that can be puzzling if the patient does not consult his physician until after the occult blood has disappeared from the feces. An elevated reticulocyte count in the absence of an increase in the serum bilirubin suggests recent hemorrhage if the patient has not recently been given specific therapeutic agents, such as iron or vitamin B_{12}. Leukocytosis and thrombocytosis in the peripheral blood, and marked normoblastic hyperplasia in the bone marrow, may also afford clues to a recent hemorrhage. The diagnosis of gastrointestinal bleeding is usually made from the history and by the detection of blood in the feces. The demonstration that a gastrointestinal lesion is the source of the bleeding is not always easy, and may not be possible without repeated roentgenographic study of the gastrointestinal tract or periodic observation of the patient. In the unusual circumstances in which the hemorrhage occurs into the muscles or other tissues as a result of trauma or ascorbic acid deficiency, reticulocytosis may occur in association with an elevation of the serum bilirubin and may erroneously suggest the presence of hemolytic anemia.

Deficient blood production.   Anemia that occurs in various chronic diseases is most often normocytic, but sometimes is mildly microcytic or hypochromic. If the anemia is due to diminished erythropoiesis alone or to mild hyperhemolysis associated with depressed erythropoiesis, as sometimes occurs in patients with malignancies and other diseases, only the erythrocytes are reduced. The leukocytes and platelets are usually normal unless altered by the primary disease. It is unusual for anemia of this type to be the primary problem in diagnosis because the underlying disease, such as chronic infection, arthritis, renal disease, malignancy, or endocrine disturbance, is usually apparent. More important is the fact that anemia of this type is sometimes the first clinical indication of the underlying disease. Some ambulatory patients with renal disease present as problems of anemia because the slowly progressing renal insufficiency has not been recognized or suspected; uremia probably is not the explanation of anemia unless the renal disease is chronic and severe.

The anemia in aplastic anemia is usually normocytic, but occasionally mildly macrocytic; it is associated with granulocytopenia, thrombocytopenia, reticulocytopenia, and a hypoplastic bone marrow. Pancytopenia also may occur in numerous disorders of the spleen and bone marrow in which ineffective erythropoiesis, an increased plasma volume, or increased cellular destruction may be present.

The diagnostic study of a patient of this type is shown in Illustrative Cases 2 and 3.

A normocytic anemia also occurs in some patients with mild anemia associated with iron deficiency. This may occur as an intermediate stage in the development of severe iron deficiency that is characterized by hypochromic microcytic anemia, or it may occur during the stage of incomplete recovery. In patients with this type of anemia the history often suggests iron deficiency, but the demonstration of a low level of serum iron or an increased iron-binding capacity or both, or the demonstration of reduced iron stores by examination of an appropriately stained specimen of marrow, or even a therapeutic trial with iron, may be necessary to establish the diagnosis.

SIMPLE MICROCYTIC ANEMIA

Simple microcytic anemia (MCV < 80 cu. μ, MCHC > 30 per cent) is most often seen in association with various chronic diseases, circumstances in which a normocytic anemia is more common. In chronic disease the granulocyte and platelet counts are usually normal and the reticulocyte count is low, less than 25,000 per cu.mm., unless there is some associated hemolysis. The serum iron and the total iron-binding capacity are both decreased while the storage iron in the marrow is increased.

HYPOCHROMIC MICROCYTIC ANEMIA

The finding of a hypochromic microcytic type of anemia (MCV < 80 cu. μ, MCHC < 30 per cent) almost invariably means iron deficiency (Illustrative Case 5). The erythrocytes on a stained blood smear have an increase in central pallor and show considerable poikilocytosis and anisocytosis. Elongated "cigar" forms, racquet cells, and microcytes are often numerous. The leukocytes and platelets are usually normal. The cellularity of the bone marrow may be subnormal, normal, or increased; erythropoiesis is normoblastic in type. The existence of iron deficiency can be established definitely by finding a subnormal level of the serum iron associated with an increase in the latent iron-binding capacity of the serum, or by the demonstration of depletion of the iron stores in the bone marrow.

The other diseases that may be confused with iron deficiency occur much less commonly and usually can be distinguished without difficulty. Pyridoxine deficiency and sideroachrestic anemia (iron-loading anemia) are usually hypochromic and microcytic, but the serum iron level is elevated and the storage iron is increased. In thalassemia the erythrocytes are hypochromic and microcytic, but the condition can generally be distinguished from iron deficiency by the family history, reticulocytosis, the presence of alkali resistant hemoglobin or hemoglobin A, the elevated level of the serum iron, and, if necessary, the failure to respond to therapy with iron preparations. When the serum iron level is low in thalassemia minor, as has been demonstrated in some cases, the differential diagnosis may be difficult and examination of the sternal marrow for stainable iron may be helpful.

When anemia is the result of iron deficiency it is important to determine the cause. Except in infants and young children, a dietary lack should not be accepted as an explanation of iron deficiency unless there are modifying factors. Among these are the increased need of iron during pregnancy and growth. However, iron deficiency may develop despite an adequate diet if absorption is impaired because of a malabsorption disorder or partial gastrectomy. In adult males, and in most postmenopausal women, unless there is some absorptive defect, iron deficiency anemia can be considered as practically synonymous with chronic blood loss. Blood loss usually occurs because of some ulcerated lesion in the gastrointestinal tract. Esophageal lesions, hiatus hernia, gastric carcinoma, benign gastric ulcer, duodenal ulcer, tumor of the small intestine, carcinoma of the colon, and hemorrhoids are all possible sources of chronic blood loss.

Should the examination reveal no significant source of bleeding the patient should be re-examined periodically and the roentgenographic studies repeated, because any of the lesions, particularly carcinoma of the cecum and stomach and tumors of the small intestine, may be a source of bleeding even though they are not recognized on the initial roentgenographic study. A diaphragmatic hernia can be responsible for chronic blood loss, but this lesion is found so frequently in patients in the middle-aged and older groups that it should not be accepted as the explanation of the anemia unless careful study of the remainder of the gastrointestinal tract has disclosed no other lesion. Although iron deficiency can occur as the result of repeated bleeding from the genitourinary or respiratory tract, bleeding from these sites of sufficient degree to cause anemia is unusual. When bleeding of this type occurs it is readily apparent to the patient. Hemosiderinuria associated with intravascular hemolysis may be severe enough to produce iron deficiency, and yet not be recognized by the patient.

In women menstruation and pregnancy afford added opportunities for the development of iron deficiency, since the increased need for iron in these circumstances may not be met by increased absorption of dietary iron. Even mildly excessive menstrual bleeding may lead to iron deficiency if the iron stores are low. If the individual has low iron stores early in life the iron reserves may not be restored to normal by the diet during growth and adolescence. In some premenopausal women it may be difficult to decide whether the number of pregnancies and the amount of menstrual bleeding can be accepted as a satisfactory explanation of iron deficiency. If there is any reasonable doubt, repeated tests for occult blood in the feces and study of the gastrointestinal tract for a possible source of bleeding are indicated.

EXAMINATION OF THE BONE MARROW

Aspiration of the bone marrow, introduced by Arinkin in 1929, has become a widely-used hematologic procedure. Details of different techniques for obtaining, preparing, and examining the marrow are described in monographs devoted to the subject[11, 18] (Fig. 3–2).

Technique. Various sites are used for the aspiration. The most satisfactory areas for routine use are the upper portion of the body of the sternum at the level of the third costal cartilage, the area just distal to the iliac crest, and the spinous processes of the third and fourth lumbar vertebrae. The sternal puncture is the easiest to perform, but because of the proximity of the sternum to the vital structures in the mediastinum it is more dangerous than the other sites if the needle is inserted too deeply. Puncture in this region is also more likely to cause apprehension in anxious patients. For these reasons the iliac crest is preferred. In children less than 2 years of age the proximal end of the tibia is usually the most satisfactory site; however, the iliac crest and the spinous processes can generally be employed successfully.

The skin over the aspiration site is shaved if necessary and then cleansed with soap and water, followed by iodine or some other skin antiseptic and alcohol. Sterile drapes are placed around the area. Sterile gloves and instruments are used. The skin and periosteum are infiltrated with 0.5 to 1.0 per cent

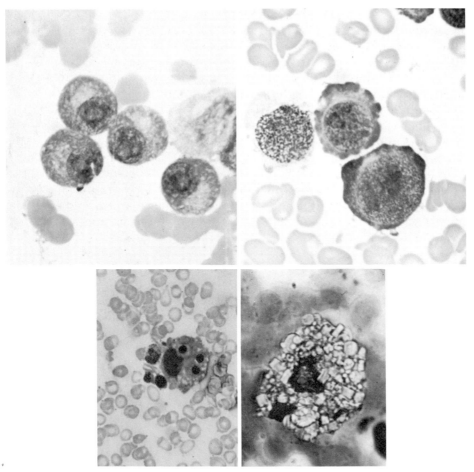

Figure 3–2 Bone marrow aspiration. *A,* Multiple myeloma. *B,* Megaloblastic erythropoiesis. *C,* Phagocytosis of cells by marrow histiocyte (histiocytic lymphoma). *D,* Cystinosis.

procaine solution by means of a hypodermic syringe and needle. Many different types of needles have been devised for the bone marrow puncture. A short needle that contains a stylet and has a guard set at 1.0 cm. from the tip of the needle (0.5 cm. for children) is usually satisfactory. The needle is pushed and rotated until a rather sudden decrease in resistance indicates that the marrow cavity has been entered. The stylet is then removed and a tightly-fitting 10 ml. syringe is attached to the needle. The plunger is withdrawn slowly until marrow appears in the syringe. With the needle in the proper position in the marrow cavity, some pain is usually experienced when the marrow is aspirated.

Thin preparations, made in the same way as a blood smear, from the first bit of marrow withdrawn usually are best, because the specimen is largely undiluted with blood. Some hematologists prefer to withdraw a larger specimen from the marrow and eject the material from the syringe into a watch glass. Particles of marrow are then picked up on an applicator stick or some other instrument, and touched to various areas of the clean slide. Such imprints give a better picture of the marrow architecture and of the fixed cells. However, preparations made in this manner usually contain a large number of damaged and unrecognizable cells. Bone marrow obtained by aspiration can be stained supravitally, with Wright's stain, with May-Grünwald-Giemsa stain, or by the peroxidase method. Marrow particles obtained by aspiration can also be fixed in paraffin and stained with hematoxylin and eosin.

A differential count is often performed on the nucleated cells in the marrow preparation. For a reproducible result it is usually necessary to count from 300 to 500 cells. The range of the different cells varies in normal marrows and the values given by different authors differ somewhat, as shown in Table 3–5. An accurate differential count is helpful in diagnosis on some occasions. It is also an excellent discipline for those in training because it forces a decision as to the identity of each cell. Nevertheless, it is time-consuming, and after a moderate amount of experience it is usually possible to gain the same information from a careful systematic study of the smear without actually doing a differential count.

Bone marrow biopsy.   The technique for bone marrow biopsy which we employ utilizes the standard adult Jamshidi biopsy needle. We prefer this needle to the modifications of the Vim-Silverman needle because, in our hands at least, it produces less crushing of the specimen. The preferred site for biopsy is the posterior inferior iliac spine, and physicians planning to perform marrow biopsies should familiarize themselves with the anatomy of the region.

Table 3–5   *Normal Adult Differential Marrow Cell Counts by Various Authors*

CELL TYPE	WINTROBE[27] (%) (RANGE)	CUSTER[11] (%) (RANGE)	ISRAELS[17] (%) (RANGE)	LEITNER[18] (%)	YOUNG AND OSGOOD[28] (%) (RANGE)
Myeloblasts	0.3–5.0	0.0–3.5	0.3–2.0	1.2	0.0–1.2
Progranulocytes	1.0–8.0	0.5–5.0	1.0–8.0	2.2	0.0–7.8
Myelocytes:					
Neutrophils	5.0–18.0	7.0–34.6	5.0–20.0	12.6	0.0–2.6
Eosinophils	0.5–3.0	0.3–3.0	....	1.4	0.0–0.4
Basophils	0.0–0.5	0.0–0.5	....	0.02	....
Metamyelocytes	13.0–32.0	15.1–37.0	13.0–32.0	11.0	1.8–11.8
Band cells			....	24.0	15.8–33.0
Segmented:					
Neutrophils	7.0–30.0	3.0–19.8	7.0–30.0	28.4	7.4–25.2
Eosinophils	0.5–4.0	0.1–3.0	0.5–4.0	1.8	0.0–1.0
Basophils	0.0–0.7	0.0–1.0	0.0–1.0	0.02	0.0–0.2
Lymphocytes	3.0–17.0	0.0–6.8	3.0–20.0	7.6	4.8–16.0
Plasmacytes	0.0–2.0	0.0–1.2	0.0–2.0	1.0	0.0–1.0
Monocytes	0.5–5.0	0.1–3.2	0.5–5.0	1.4	0.0–4.2
Reticulum cells	0.1–2.0	0.3–2.6	....	2.0	....
Megakaryocytes	0.03–3.0	0.05–1.5	Occas.	0.8	0.0–0.2
Pronormoblasts	1.0–8.0	0.0–0.0	0.5–4.0	0.8	....
Normoblasts (basophilic, polychromatic and orthochromatic)	7.0–32.0	17.5–42.0	19.0–35.0	27.6	5.4–24.2
Myeloid: erythroid ratio	about 3:1–4:1	2:1–6:1	4:1–20:1	3:1	2:1–8:1

The patient lies on one side or prone on a firm table or stretcher. The skin is prepared, and local anesthesia is given as described for the marrow aspiration. With the stylet in place, the biopsy needle is introduced and advanced to the cortical surface. The needle is then passed through the cortex with firm pressure and a rotary motion back-and-forth through an area of 90°. Once the tip of the needle is in the marrow space, the stylet is removed. Using the same back-and-forth rotary motion, the needle is advanced through the marrow until resistance is felt at the opposite cortical surface. The shaft of the needle is then moved slightly from side to side to break the marrow core, and the needle is removed with the same motion used in its insertion.

The sample is removed from the biopsy needle with the special stylet provided by pushing it through the distal (cutting) end and out the top. After removal of the specimen it is placed on a clean slide, and a smear is made by sliding the specimen along the surface with gentle pressure. The specimen is then placed in 10 per cent formalin for processing.

A small amount of bleeding is common at the biopsy site, but usually can be controlled with pressure. The biopsy causes greater discomfort than the aspiration; for this reason premedication with meperidine and a mild sedative is usually employed, although it may not always be necessary.

The biopsy should be preceded by the aspiration with a standard needle when both are to be done; the Jamshidi needle can be used for aspiration, but because of its size the specimen is often diluted.

In examining the bone marrow it is desirable to follow a definite plan. The slide is first examined with the low power objective. The cellularity of the specimen is noted, the number of megakaryocytes is estimated, and a search for sheets of malignant cells and other unusual cells is made, particularly near the edges of the preparation. The more suitably stained portions of the slide are examined under oil immersion. The erythrocyte precursors are studied, and the type of erythropoiesis is noted as megaloblastic or normoblastic. Attention is also paid to the number and maturity of these cells. Next, the granulocytic series is studied with particular reference to number and any increase in the younger forms, particularly myeloblasts and progranulocytes. The presence of any macropolycytes or giant metamyelocytes is also noted. Megakaryocytes are studied for number, maturity, and evidence of platelet formation. The plasma cells, reticulum cells, histiocytes, and other cells are studied similarly for number and immaturity, and for cytoplasmic inclusions. The number of lymphocytes is estimated, and the presence of any tumor cells or other abnormal or unidentified cells is noted.

After the marrow preparation has been studied in this fashion the various observations can be noted in the report. The cellularity is classed as normal, increased, or decreased. Erythropoiesis is classified according to the type of maturation as normoblastic or megaloblastic, and according to activity as normal, hypoplastic, or hyperplastic. The granulocytic maturation is classed as normal or abnormal, and any abnormality is specified. The megakaryocytes and platelet formation are classed as normal, reduced, or increased. Similarly the number and maturity of the lymphocytes, plasma cells, and reticulum cells are recorded. These observations form the basis for the conclusions that can be drawn from the marrow examination.

The value of bone marrow examination.   The bone marrow biopsy permits study of only a small, almost minute, piece of tissue from a large organ. It is not surprising that such a sample does not invariably reflect the status of the entire marrow, and that localized lesions such as metastatic malignancy and granulomas may not be seen. Nevertheless, it usually gives a reliable picture of many disorders of the hematopoietic system and frequently discloses the nature of localized lesions as well. Examination of the bone marrow may establish a diagnosis of certain diseases with assurance, it may render some particular diagnosis very unlikely, or it may give helpful information that is of indirect or limited value. The ease with which bone marrow can be obtained for examination has led to the use of this procedure in circumstances when other, simpler procedures, such as a careful study of a smear of peripheral blood, would suffice for a diagnosis. The decision as to the desirability of a bone marrow examination is based on the circumstances in the individual case.

Although the marrow examination may not be necessary in order to establish the diagnosis, the following diagnoses can usually be made by this method:

1. Multiple myeloma.
2. Leukemia, all types.
3. Untreated or partially-treated vitamin B_{12} or folic acid deficiency.
4. Storage disease, such as Gaucher's disease.
5. Metastatic malignancy (if "positive" cells are found).
6. Fungal disease (if "positive" cells are found).
7. Iron deficiency.
8. Iron overload.
9. Sideroblastic anemia.

In certain other diseases, when taken in conjunction with the peripheral blood, the bone marrow examination can often provide helpful information that is not diagnostic when taken alone. Among these are:

1. Aplastic anemia.
2. Idiopathic thrombocytopenic purpura.
3. Lymphosarcoma.
4. Hypersplenism.
5. Agranulocytosis.

It is sometimes difficult to exclude a diagnosis from further consideration because of the result of the bone marrow examination. "Myeloma cells" or a definite increase in plasma cells may not be found in multiple myeloma. Some patients with bone marrow failure have cellular specimens. Patients with pernicious anemia sometimes forget to relate that they have taken folic acid or received an injection of vitamin B_{12} from another physician. Aspiration occasionally yields a hypocellular or "aplastic" marrow in patients with leukemia. When the diagnosis remains in doubt, and when a hypocellular or acellular specimen is obtained by aspiration, a biopsy should be made. If abnormal bleeding is expected with operation, the iliac crest is the site of choice because bleeding can be more easily controlled than in the sternum or ribs. From the biopsy specimen both touch preparations for Wright's stain and paraffin sections for H and E and other stains can be made. A biopsy is necessary for staging the patient with lymphoma. Hodgkin's disease is rarely found by aspirate alone, and in other lymphomas a smear does not suffice to determine whether the mar-

Table 3–6 *Indications for Bone Marrow Examination*

A. Aspiration
    1. Unexplained anemia, leukopenia, or thrombocytopenia
    2. If necessary to evaluate storage or metabolism of iron
    3. Material for chromosome analysis
    4. Material for microbial culture

B. Biopsy
    1. Hypocellular specimens on aspirations
    2. Suspected leukemia
    3. As guide to treatment of acute leukemia
    4. Pancytopenia
    5. Idiopathic thrombocytopenia
    6. Suspected multiple myeloma or other plasma cell dyscrasia
    7. Suspected myelofibrosis
    8. Staging of lymphoma
    9. Suspected skeletal metastatic malignancy
   10. After diagnosis of carcinoma of breast, thyroid, and prostate, or oat cell carcinoma of lung
   11. Leukoerythroblastic anemia
   12. Unexplained splenomegaly
   13. Fever of undetermined origin
   14. Suspected widespread granulomatous or collagen vascular disease

row involvement by a lymphosarcoma is diffuse or nodular. Specimens obtained from the iliac crest with a Jamshidi needle and fixed in formalin have been satisfactory in our experience. Many pathologists and some hematologists prefer marrow sections to smears or imprints for routine study because sections give a better picture of the marrow architecture, cellularity, and iron content;[13] unfortunately, identification of individual cells in such preparations is less accurate than in touch preparations. Often both types of marrow examination are needed.

An unusual finding on a bone marrow examination is bone marrow necrosis.[7] The bone marrow appears cellular, but the cells are so weakly and poorly stained that they cannot be identified. In addition there is a large amount of background material which stains blue with Wright's stain. Sometimes the dye seems collected in small clumps. In some patients there is associated anemia, and and in others severe pancytopenia. Although the mechanism that produces the necrosis is unknown, interference with the marrow circulation and infarction have been postulated. The most common primary diseases are leukemia, sickle cell anemia, metastatic carcinoma, and septicemia. The marrow necrosis may occur shortly before death, but some patients recover within a few weeks.

The most common indications for bone marrow aspiration and/or biopsy are listed in Table 3–6.

ERRORS IN DIAGNOSIS

Some common errors in the diagnosis of anemia are:
In *adults:*
    1. Errors in reporting laboratory values on chart.
    2. Inadequate study of blood smear.
    3. Incorrect determination of erythrocyte indices.

4. Failure to do reticulocyte count.

5. Failure to check stools for occult blood.

6. Failure to investigate patients for neoplasm or other sources of bleeding.

7. Failure to check blood urea or blood urea nitrogen for renal insufficiency.

8. Failure to palpate enlarged spleen or nodes.

9. Failure to consider multiple myeloma as a cause for anemia in middle-aged and elderly patients.

10. Failure to consider myxedema as a cause of anemia.

In *children:*

Failure to consider possibility of hemolytic anemias of various sorts.

TREATMENT IN RELATION TO DIAGNOSIS

The purpose of the diagnostic study is to enable the physician to decide what is the best form of treatment for the patient. The most desirable form of treatment is the removal or correction of the cause. When this cannot be accomplished, therapy is directed toward the disordered mechanism. For either form of therapy it is important to establish an accurate diagnosis before treating the anemia unless the patient's condition demands immediate measures, such as transfusions. Premature treatment may be detrimental to the patient. The use of complex preparations that contain iron, vitamin B_{12}, folic acid, and other substances, under the impression that such therapy will afford adequate treatment for all types of anemia, may confuse the interpretation of the diagnostic studies without correcting the anemia. Even more important is the fact that treatment may produce a false sense of security when it corrects the anemia, which is but one aspect of the disorder, without affecting other more serious aspects of the disease. When no diagnosis has been established, often the best course is to withhold treatment until the nature of the anemia is better understood. It is rare that a delay in treatment until the necessary diagnostic studies are performed works to the disadvantage of the patient.

Illustrative Cases

CASE 1. MACROCYTIC ANEMIA

Initial Examination: Hematocrit, 25 per cent; RBC, 2.0 million/cu.mm.; Hemoglobin, 9.0 gm. per cent; Reticulocytes, 0.5 per cent. *Indices:* MCV, 125 cu.μ; MCH, 45 $\mu\mu$; MCHC, 35 per cent; WBC, 2500/cu.mm.; Platelets, 100,000/cu.mm.

Blood Smear: Oval macrocytes: polysegmented neutrophils, anisopoikilocytosis.

Mechanism: Deficiency of vitamin B_{12} or folate or faulty utilization.

Bone Marrow: Megaloblastic, cellular; giant band forms.

Other Examinations:

Other Examinations	Vitamin B$_{12}$ Deficiency		Folate Deficiency	Faulty Utilization
Serum folate	N		Low	N
Serum Vitamin B$_{12}$	Low		N	High
Gastric acidity	O	N	N	N
Schilling test				
No IF	O	O		
With IF	+	O		
Diagnosis:	Pernicious anemia	Small bowel disease	Inadequate diet Alcoholism Malabsorption Small bowel disease Excessive demands Pregnancy Hemolytic anemia Drugs Folate antagonists Diminished absorption	Dyserythropoiesis secondary to: Drugs Erythroleukemia (Positive PAS stain; myeloblasts increased)

Comments: Anemia may be normocytic if there is coexisting iron deficiency.

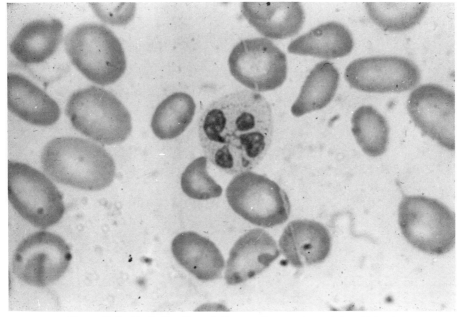

Figure 3–3 Illustrative Case 1. Macrocytic anemia, peripheral blood.

CASE 2. NORMOCYTIC ANEMIA; WITH PANCYTOPENIA

Initial Examination: Hematocrit, 25 per cent; RBC, 3.0 million/cu.mm.; Hemoglobin, 9.0 gm. per cent; Reticulocytes, 0.5 per cent. *Indices:* MCV, 83 cu.μ; MCH, 30 $\mu\mu$; MCHC, 36 per cent; WBC 2400/cu.mm.; Platelets, 40,000/cu.mm.

Blood Smear: No significant anisopoikilocytosis or young cells: favor marrow hypoplasia; anisopoikilocytosis, basophilia, young cells, large platelets: favor myeloproliferative disorder; nucleated red cells, young granulocytes, tear drop forms, basophilia favor myeloid metaplasia or leukemia.

Buffy Coat: Blasts, young cells: favor leukemia or myeloproliferative disorders.

Probable Diagnosis: Diminished red cell production.

Bone Marrow: Aspirate: Hypocellular (dilute or hypoplastic)
        Biopsy: Normoblastic (A) hypocellular; (B) cellular

	(A) *Hypocellular*	(B) *Cellular*
Diagnosis:	Bone marrow failure	Ineffective erythropoiesis
	Idiopathic	Leukemia
	Drugs	Multiple myeloma
	Irradiation	Myeloproliferative disorder
	Infection	Myelofibrosis (special stain)
		Preleukemia

Comment: Anemia in bone marrow failure is sometimes slightly macrocytic.

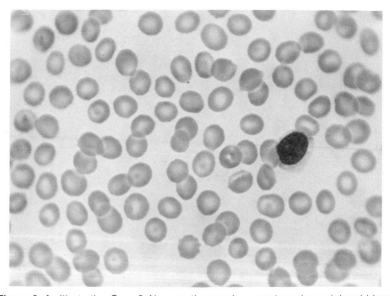

Figure 3–4 Illustrative Case 2. Normocytic anemia, pancytopenia, peripheral blood.

CASE 3. NORMOCYTIC ANEMIA; LEUKOCYTES, PLATELETS NORMAL

Initial Examination: Hematocrit, 25 per cent; RBC, 3.0 million/cu.mm.; Hemoglobin, 9.0 gm. per cent; Reticulocytes, 0.5 per cent. *Indices:* MCV, 83 cu. μ; MCH, 30 $\mu\mu$; MCHC, 36 per cent; WBC, 7000/cu.mm.; Platelets, 210,000/cu.mm.

Blood Smear: Normochromic erythrocytes, little or no anisopoikilocytosis, normal leukocytes: suggest chronic disease; hypochromia, anisopoikilocytosis: suggest iron deficiency, iron-loading, or dyserythropoiesis.

Probable Diagnosis: Diminished red cell production.

Bone Marrow: Cellular normoblastic:

    (A) Orderly: mild dyserythropoiesis.

Diagnosis:	Iron deficiency	Chronic disease	Sideroblastic anemia: congenital; acquired	Miscellaneous diseases, Multiple myeloma, Myxedema, etc.

Other Examinations:

Marrow hemosiderin	O	Incr.	Incr.	N
Serum iron	Low	Low	Incr.	N
TIBC	Incr.	Low	N	N
Transferrin saturation	Low	Low	Incr.	N
Ringed sideroblasts	O	O	Incr.	O

    (B) Disorderly: mild, dyserythropoiesis (congenital or acquired)

    (C) Erythrocytic hypoplasia (only rare RBC precursor)

                Pure red cell aplasia (PRCA) Thymoma; Autoimmune disorder

Comments: 1. Anemia in sideroblastic anemia may be macrocytic or dimorphic.

        2. Reticulocyte count in pure red cell aplasia (PRCA) is usually 0.1 per cent or less.

        3. Dyserythropoietic anemia is sometimes slightly macrocytic.

CASE 4. NORMOCYTIC ANEMIA; RETICULOCYTOSIS

Initial Examination: Hematocrit, 25 per cent; RBC, 2.7 million/cu.mm.; Hemoglobin, 8.0 gm. per cent; Reticulocytes, 10 per cent (270,000/cu.mm.). *Indices:* MCV, 90 cu. μ; MCHC, 32 per cent; MCH, 29 $\mu\mu$; WBC and platelets normal or increased.

Blood Smear: Polychromatophilia; Poikilocytosis, RBC autoagglutination, spherocytes: suggest RBC antibodies; Microspherocytes or elliptocytes: suggest hereditary disease; Target cells: suggest liver disease or hemoglobinopathy; Helmet cells, schistocytes, poikilocytosis: suggest mechanical hemolysis; Stomatocytes, spur cells: suggest alcoholism and liver disease; Erythrocytes normal except for polychromatophilia: consider hemorrhage.

Probable Diagnosis: Hemolytic anemia

Bone Marrow: Normoblastic hyperplasia (may show megaloblastosis if folate deficiency has developed)

Special Tests: *Diagnosis*

Coombs — Positive ⟶ (1) Gamma
  Negative
              Idiopathic
              Lymphoproliferative
              Connective tissue disease
              Drugs (penicillin, methyldopa)
              Erythroblastosis
        (2) Nongamma
              Mycoplasma pneumonia
              Cold agglutinin disease
              Infectious mononucleosis
              Drugs (quinidine type reaction)
              Paroxysmal nocturnal hemoglobinuria
                (PNH)
        (3) Gamma and nongamma
              Idiopathic
              Lymphoproliferative
              Connective tissue disease
              Paroxysmal cold hemoglobinuria
                (PCH)

Osmotic fragility — Positive ⟶ Hereditary spherocytosis
  Normal   Hereditary elliptocytosis
                                Immune hemolytic disease

Hemosiderinuria — Positive ⟶ Impact hemolysis
  (also decreased   March hemoglobinuria
   haptoglobin and   Valve prosthesis
   increased plasma   Microangiopathic anemia
   hemoglobin)   PNH
              Negative   PCH
                                Cold agglutinin disease
                                Mycoplasma pneumonia

Hemoglobin — Positive ⟶ SS disease
  electrophoresis   SC disease
                               Thalassemia (Incr. Hb A_2 and fetal Hb)
  Normal   Other hemoglobinopathies
                                 (Heat stable and unstable)

Ascorbate-cyanide — Positive ⟶ Enzyme deficiency
                                G6PD
                                6-PG
  Normal   Glutathione reductase
                                GSH peroxidase
                                GSH synthetase

Specific enzyme assays: pyruvic kinase and others

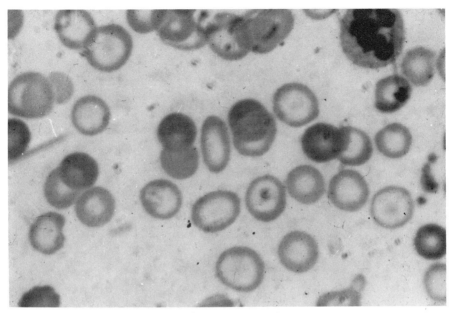

Figure 3–5 Illustrative Case 5. Hypochromic microcytic anemia.

CASE 5. HYPOCHROMIC MICROCYTIC ANEMIA

Initial Examination: Hematocrit, 25 per cent; RBC, 4.0 million/cu.mm.; Hemoglobin, 6.0 gm/100 ml.; Reticulocytes, 0.5 per cent. *Indices:* MCV, 62 cu. μ; MCH, 15 $\mu\mu$; MCHC, 24 per cent; WBC, 7200/cu.mm.; Platelets, 200,000/cu.mm.

Blood Smear: Hypochromic erythrocytes; anisopoikilocytosis; leukocytes not abnormal

Probable Mechanism: Iron deficiency or iron loading.

Bone Marrow: Cellular normoblastic

Other Examinations:	Iron deficiency anemia	Iron loading anemia
Storage iron	0	Incr.
Sideroblasts	0	Incr.—ringed
Serum iron	Low	High
Total iron binding	High	N
Transferrin saturation	Low	Incr.—75 per cent
Diagnosis:	Chronic blood loss	Congenital sideroblastic
	Excessive demands	Acquired sideroblastic
	Diminished absorption	Thalassemia
	Inadequate diet	
Additional Studies:	Stool exam	Family studies and Hb
	X-ray study GI tract	electrophoresis
Comment:	Reticulocytosis often present in thalassemia minor.	

References

1. Adams, E. B.: Anemia associated with protein deficiency. Seminars Hematol., 7:55, 1970.
2. Berlin, N. I., Waldmann, T. A., and Weissman, S. M.: Life span of red blood cell. Physiol. Rev., 39:577, 1959.
3. Biggs, R., and Macmillan, R. L.: The errors of some hematological methods as they are used in a routine laboratory. J. Clin. Pathol., 1:269, 283, 1948.
4. Block, M.: Importance and interpretation of routine blood counts. Rocky Mountain Med. J., 54:894, 1957.
5. Bomford, R.: Anaemia in myxoedema: and the role of the thyroid gland in erythropoiesis. Q. J. Med., 7:495, 1938.
6. Brain, M. C., Dacie, J. V., and Hourihane, D. O'B.: Microangiopathic haemolytic anemia: the possible role of vascular lesions in pathogenesis. Br. J. Haematol., 8:358, 1962.
7. Brown, C. H. III.: Bone marrow necrosis, a study of seventy cases. Johns Hopkins Med. J., 133:189, 1972.
8. Castle, W. B.: Erythropoiesis: Normal and abnormal. Bull. N.Y. Acad. Med., 30:827, 1954.
9. Committee on Iron Deficiency: Iron deficiency in the United States. J.A.M.A., 203:407, 1968.
10. Crosby, W. H., and Akeroyd, J. H.: Limit of hemoglobin synthesis in hereditary hemolytic anemia: Its relation to the excretion of bile pigment. Am. J. Med., 13:273, 1952.
11. Custer, R. P.: An Atlas of the Blood and Bone Marrow. W. B. Saunders Co., Philadelphia, 1949.
12. Dern, R. J., Weinstein, I. M., LeRoy, G. V., Talmage, D. W., and Alving, A. S.: The hemolytic effect of primaquine. I. The localization of the drug-induced hemolytic defect in primaquine-sensitive individuals. J. Lab. Clin. Med., 43:303, 1954.
13. Ellis, L. D., Jensen, W. N., and Westerman, M. P.: Needle biopsy of bone and marrow. Arch. Intern. Med., 114:213, 1964.
14. Erslev, A. J.: Erythropoietic function in uremic rabbits. Clin. Res. Proc., 5:141, 1957.
15. Finch, C. A.: Protein deficiency and anemia. Plenary session papers. Int. Soc. Hematol., 1968, p. 154.
16. Gurney, C. W., Goldwasser, E., Jacobson, L. O., and Pan, C.: Demonstration of erythropoietin in human plasma. J. Clin. Invest., 36:896, 1957.
17. Israels, M. C. G.: An Atlas of Bone-Marrow Pathology. Grune and Stratton, New York, 1948.
18. Leitner, S. J.: Bone Marrow Biopsy. J. A. Churchill, Ltd., London, 1949.
19. Miller, E. B., Singer, K., and Dameshek, W.: Use of the daily fecal output of urobilinogen and the hemolytic index in the measurement of hemolysis. Arch. Intern. Med., 70:722, 1942.
20. Mitchell, J. S.: Metabolic effects of therapeutic doses of X and gamma radiations. Br. J. Radiol., 16:339, 1943.
21. Pauling, L., Itano, H. A., Singer, S. J., and Wells, I. C.: Sickle cell anemia: A molecular disease. Science, 110:543, 1949.
22. Pirzio-Biroli, G., Bothwell, T. H., and Finch, C. A.: Iron absorption. II. The absorption of radio-iron administered with a standard meal in man. J. Lab. Clin. Med., 51:37, 1958.
23. Schilling, R. F.: Intrinsic factor studies. II. The effect of gastric juice on the urinary excretion of radioactivity after the oral administration of radioactive B_{12}. J. Lab. Clin. Med., 42:860, 1953.
24. Thorup, O. A., Strole, W. E., and Leavell, B. S.: The rate of removal of iron from culture medium by human bone marrow suspension. J. Lab. Clin. Med., 52:266, 1958.
25. Wintrobe, M. M.: The size and hemoglobin content of the erythrocyte. J. Lab. Clin. Med., 17:899, 1932.
26. Wintrobe, M. M.: Principles in the management of anemias. Bull. N.Y. Acad. Med., 30:6, 1954.
27. Wintrobe, M. M.: Clinical Hematology. 4th Ed. Lea and Febiger, Philadelphia, 1956.
28. Young, R. H., and Osgood, E. E.: Sternal marrow aspirated during life. Arch. Intern. Med., 55:186, 1935.

CHAPTER 4

DISORDERS OF VITAMIN B_{12} AND FOLIC ACID METABOLISM

Both vitamin B_{12} and folic acid (pteroylglutamic acid) are essential for normal metabolic processes. A deficiency of either substance causes a megaloblastic type of anemia associated with abnormalities in the maturation of granulocytes and gives rise to macrocytosis in the mucosa of the mouth, stomach, intestine, and vagina; an inadequate amount of vitamin B_{12} also leads to serious derangements of the nervous system. A deficiency of either vitamin B_{12} or folic acid usually is most apparent in the cells involved in erythropoiesis. The delay in cell division and maturation is reflected in the appearance of the nuclei of the erythrocyte precursors; the chromatin pattern of the nucleus remains dispersed while the cytoplasm enlarges and hemoglobinization progresses. These morphologic abnormalities, and the known importance of DNA and RNA metabolism in cell growth and division, suggest that a main function of these vitamins is concerned with DNA and RNA metabolism. The unraveling of the biochemical functions of these two vitamins and their relationship to each other is incomplete, but various details of their natural occurrence, absorption, transport, and storage have been established. In addition, a number of different clinical disorders which have in common a functional deficiency of one or the other of these vitamins have been recognized.

VITAMIN B_{12}

Vitamin B_{12}, which has a molecular weight of 1355 and the formula $C_{63}H_{88}O_{14}N_{14}Co$, is found in practically all animal tissue.[106] Beef liver has the highest concentration, 50 to 130 micrograms per 100 grams of fresh weight; beef kidney (20 to 50 micrograms) and herring (11 to 34 micrograms) are also rich sources. Beef muscle contains 2 to 8 micrograms; cheese (1.4 to 3.6 micrograms), egg yolk (1.2 micrograms), and milk (0.2 to 0.6 microgram) are relatively poor sources. In the United States the average daily diet probably contains over 5 micrograms. Vitamin B_{12} is synthesized exclusively by microorganisms, and these are the source of the vitamin found in various foodstuffs.

Intrinsic factor secreted by the stomach is essential for the absorption of vitamin B_{12} in foodstuffs. In man the factor is secreted only by the glands of the body of the stomach, probably by the parietal cells, and not in the pyloric end of the stomach or the small intestine, as is the case in swine. The factor, which is water-soluble but nondialyzable, is destroyed by heat or boiling and can be precipitated by ammonium sulfate, characteristics which indicate that it is a protein. In addition to amino acids it contains hexoses, hexose amines, and sialic acid. Although the intrinsic factor has not been purified, intrinsic factor activity has been demonstrated in a mucoprotein isolated from the acid glandular protein of the stomach, and in stomach mucosal fractions which have molecular

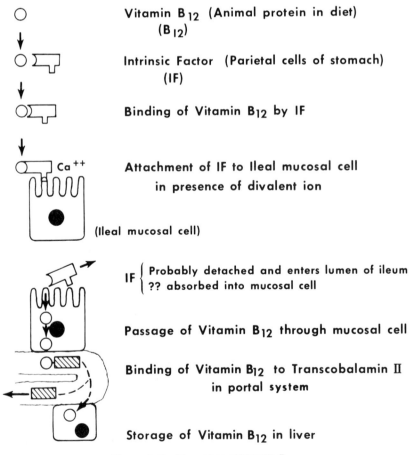

Vitamin B_{12} (Animal protein in diet)
(B_{12})

Intrinsic Factor (Parietal cells of stomach)
(IF)

Binding of Vitamin B_{12} by IF

Attachment of IF to Ileal mucosal cell
in presence of divalent ion

(Ileal mucosal cell)

IF { Probably detached and enters lumen of ileum
?? absorbed into mucosal cell

Passage of Vitamin B_{12} through mucosal cell

Binding of Vitamin B_{12} to Transcobalamin II
in portal system

Storage of Vitamin B_{12} in liver

Figure 4–1 Absorption of Vitamin B_{12}

weights that range from 5000 to 100,000.[36] Native intrinsic factor is thought to be a glycoprotein or mucopolysaccharide with a molecular weight of approximately 55,000.[41]

Vitamin B$_{12}$' is absorbed in the small intestine, mainly in the distal portion of the ileum, at a roughly neutral pH; both intrinsic factor (IF) and calcium ions are necessary for the absorption of physiologic amounts, but the mechanism by which intrinsic factor promotes absorption is uncertain (Fig. 4–1). The B$_{12}$-IF complex is resistant to digestion, a binding which may prevent utilization of the vitamin by the bacteria of the intestine before absorption occurs. The absorption of vitamin B$_{12}$ is accomplished by an interaction between the mucosal cell and the complex of vitamin B$_{12}$ and intrinsic fraction.[60] The role of calcium ions appears to be in the attachment of intrinsic factor to mucosal cells; vitamin B$_{12}$ first attaches to one of the active sites of the intrinsic factor and then the other active site of the IF attaches to the mucosal cell. As shown by studies in hamsters with vitamin B$_{12}$ ^{57}Co and electron microscopy, the receptor is located on the microvilli of the ileal cells; the attachment appears to be by adsorption rather than than by an energy-requiring enzymatic reaction.[26] Although it has been suggested that the IF molecule enters the mucosal cell by pinocytosis or by other means, the evidence indicates that the intrinsic factor is not absorbed as vitamin B$_{12}$ enters the cell. Intrinsic factor is necessary for the absorption of small quantities of vitamin B$_{12}$, but the vitamin can be absorbed in the absence of intrinsic factor when large amounts are ingested; when 30 micrograms is taken orally, 1 per cent appears in the urine,[41] and when 1000 micrograms is ingested, a prompt rise in the serum level occurs. It has been suggested that this occurs as a result of passive diffusion through the gut wall, but the size of pores of the absorptive cell, 4Å, compared to the size of the molecule of vitamin B$_{12}$, 8Å, has been cited as an objection to this explanation.[125]

After absorption, vitamin B$_{12}$ is transported in the plasma bound mainly to proteins which have different functions.[45, 46] Intrinsic factor does not pass through the mucosal cells into the portal blood; studies which employed catheterization of the portal vein and the ingestion of B$_{12}$ ^{57}Co disclose that the B$_{12}$-binding material has a molecular weight of approximately 100,000 and none of the immunologic characteristics of IF.[23] Vitamin B$_{12}$ in the plasma is taken up by transcobalamin II (TC II), a protein which has alpha$_2$-beta mobility.[41] The vitamin enters the blood from the intestine at a slow rate, first appearing three or four hours after a meal; absorption reaches a peak at from eight to 12 hours and continues for 24 hours. Nevertheless, the combination of TC II and vitamin B$_{12}$ is cleared rapidly from the plasma, and the level of vitamin B$_{12}$ bound in this way probably never exceeds 20 pg. per ml. of plasma; half an injected dose of TC II–vitamin B$_{12}$ leaves the plasma in less than 5 minutes, the vitamin being taken up mainly by the liver but also by other tissues. The source of TC II in man is unknown, but the observations on patients from whom large amounts of small intestine have been removed indicate that the intestinal tissue is not the source; in the mouse, TC II is produced in the liver. The plasma content of TC II is thought to be about 25 micrograms per liter, an amount able to bind approximately 986 pg. of vitamin B$_{12}$ per ml.; after oral absorption less than 2 per cent of the available TC II is bound to the vitamin B$_{12}$, but once attached the protein is not reused.

Transcobalamin I (TC I) also has a role in transport of vitamin B$_{12}$. The level of TC I is approximately 60 micrograms per liter, an amount that can combine with 700 to 800 pg. of vitamin B$_{12}$ per ml.: normally the binding capacity of TC I is about half saturated with vitamin B$_{12}$ from endogenous sources. It has been postulated that the leukocytes are the source of TC I, which appears to be the major mechanism for the binding of vitamin B$_{12}$, in the plasma and in its passage from cells. The level of TC I is greatly increased in myeloproliferative states, particularly chronic granulocytic leukemia. Other abnormalities that have been noted are decreased levels of TC II in chronic myeloproliferative states and in some patients with pernicious anemia; in pernicious anemia usually there is a normal amount of TC I which carries subnormal amounts of vitamin B$_{12}$.

Another plasma protein, TC III, acts as a binder for vitamin B$_{12}$ in vitro, but recent studies indicate that TC I and TC II are the only functional transport proteins of plasma B$_{12}$.[45] Although the binding capacity of the plasma for vitamin B$_{12}$ is usually unimpaired, in at least one study five of ten patients with untreated pernicious anemia were found to have deficient binding of radioactive B$_{12}$ to beta globulin; treatment with vitamin B$_{12}$ resulted in a more normal binding capacity. In one of the five patients, who had virtually no beta globulin binding of B$_{12}$ before treatment, the Schilling test gave a malabsorptive pattern; after treatment with vitamin B$_{12}$, both the beta globulin binding capacity and the ability to absorb oral vitamin B$_{12}$ when given with intrinsic factor returned.[74] Vitamin B$_{12}$ deficiency associated with a congenital deficiency of transcobalamin II has been reported, with correction by pharmacologic doses of vitamin B$_{12}$ given parenterally.[33]

The main storage site of vitamin B$_{12}$ in man is the liver, which in an adult may contain several milligrams, possibly 4;[106] at birth the liver contains about 25 micrograms.[4] The urinary excretion of vitamin B$_{12}$ by man on a normal diet is about 30 micromicrograms a day.[95] When vitamin B$_{12}$ is injected, appreciable amounts are excreted in the urine within eight hours; when 50 micrograms or more is given the quantity excreted in the urine increases with increasing doses. If 50 micrograms is injected, from 3 to 4 micrograms are excreted in eight hours; with the injection of 1000 micrograms, from 330 to 470 micrograms are excreted in the same period.

FOLIC ACID

Folic acid and PGA are the terms most commonly used to designate pteroylglutamic acid; before the chemical identity of the compound was established, other names such as vitamin M, vitamin B$_c$, and Lactobacillus casei factor were used. Folic acid occurs in nature chiefly in conjugated forms; leafy vegetables, liver, and yeast are rich sources. Significant amounts of the compound are produced in the intestinal lumen by the action of the bacteria normally found there.

The average daily diet in the United States contains 184 ± 67 micrograms of total folic acid activity as measured by the S. fecalis assay method.[12] This consists of three fractions in the following proportions: N^{10}-formyl-pteroyl-glutamic acid, 101 micrograms; citrovorum factor, 63 micrograms; PGA, 20 micrograms. The folate activity of four daily diets measured by L. casei assay was found to be 688 micrograms; fractionation gave percentages similar to those observed with S. fecalis. Repeated boiling of food in large quantities of water reduces or destroys its folate activity; probably pH changes in the gastro-intestinal tract also affect the availability of ingested dietary folate.[11] Patients may have tropical sprue and megaloblastic anemia despite a daily diet containing well over 1000 micrograms of folic acid activity. Since the anemia may respond to the oral administration of as little as 25 micrograms of PGA, apparently very little of the native folate in the food is absorbed by patients with the disease.[104] It has been suggested that some folic acid compounds found in the diet are active in bacteriologic assay but not in man.[12] The minimal daily requirement of folate activity (as PGA) for adults is probably 50 micrograms per day.[54]

Absorption, which occurs in the small intestine, does not require intrinsic factor. Human intestinal juice contains a conjugase capable of liberating folates from the bound form that is present in food; synthetic pteroylglutamic acid, and probably methyl- and formyl-folates, can cross the intestinal mucosa intact.[11] Folic acid is transported in the plasma where the normal level is reported to be between 5.9 and 21.0 nanograms per ml. (ng. per ml.). In pernicious anemia the level is normal; in folic acid deficiency it is reported to be less than 4.0 ng. per ml.[115] and less than 7 ng. per ml.[54] Each laboratory must establish its own normal range. The folic acid activity of serum is due largely to the monoglutamate form, N^5-methyl-tetrahydrofolic acid.[59] Microbiologic assay indicates that the total tissue store of the folate activity in man is 7.5 ± 2.5 mg.; the chief storage site of folic acid is the liver, which normally contains 3.5 to 7.5 mg.[54] Four and one-half months are required for a healthy adult to develop a megaloblastic anemia on a daily dietary intake of 5 micrograms of folate activity.

METABOLIC FUNCTIONS OF VITAMIN B$_{12}$ AND FOLIC ACID

The term "vitamin B$_{12}$" as used in the literature has two meanings.[40] It is used as a generic term for all the cobalamins active in man, but it is also used specifically for the commercially available cyanocobalamin, which is the form first isolated. The cobalamins are various derivatives of 5,6-dimethylimidazolyl-cobamide, and the coenzyme forms are therefore sometimes called "cobamide coenzymes." These coenzymes include a 5'-deoxyadenosylcobalamin and a methylcobalamin.

The cobalamins are among the most potent and important biologic compounds known because they appear to be involved in nearly every known metabolic system in man.[35] They are essential for normal growth, hematopoiesis, the production of epithelial cells, and for maintaining the function of the cells of

Table 4-1   *Metabolic Processes Dependent on Tetrahydrofolate*

PROCESS	INTERMEDIATE	GROUP TRANSFERRED
Methionine regeneration	5-Methyl-H_4folate	—CH_3
Thymine biosynthesis	5,10-Methylene-H_4folate	—CH_2—
Serine and glycine metabolism		
Purine biosynthesis	5,10-Methylidyne-H_4folate	—CH=
	10-Formyl-H_4folate	—CH=O
Histidine degradation	5-Formimino-H_4folate	—CH=NH

(Prepared by Dr. Robert W. McGilvery, Professor of Biochemistry, University of Virginia School of Medicine, Charlottesville, Virginia.)

the nervous system. The function of vitamin B_{12} is intimately related to that of the folate compounds, particularly in DNA synthesis.

The term "folic acid" is also employed generically for a group of closely related compounds as well as for a particular compound. The more systematic name, pteroylglutamic acid, has been proposed for the particular form involved in human metabolism, but folic acid, or folate, is still widely used in that sense.[68]

The active coenzyme form of pteroylglutamate, or folate, in the mammal is the reduced form, tetrahydrofolate, which is also known as "folinic acid" or "citrovorum factor." Tetrahydrofolate is commonly abbreviated as H_4folate. Tetrahydrofolate is involved in all the single-carbon transfer reactions except those utilizing CO_2 or methyl groups. Most of these reactions simply involve a transfer of one carbon unit from one compound to another via tetrahydrofolate, with one important exception. The transfer by which thymine is formed also involves the oxidation of the tetrahydrofolate to dihydrofolate. The various transfers are summarized in Table 4–1.

The conversion of dietary folate to H_4folate involves two reductases, with the intermediate formation of H_2folate. These enzymes are inhibited by folic acid antagonists, such as aminopterin and amethopterin (methotrexate), which therefore cause an effective deficiency of H_4folate. It is in this connection that the concomitant formation of H_2folate in thymine synthesis assumes especial importance, because the recovery of this product as H_4folate will be inhibited by these antagonists. The antagonists are therefore more likely to affect dividing cells in which DNA synthesis, and therefore thymine synthesis, is proceeding.

The interrelationship of the action of vitamin B_{12} and folate has been the subject of numerous studies. Many pieces of evidence, such as the appearance of blood cells in the stained smear, measurement of chemical compounds, the action of the compounds in bacteria, and the results of numerous other studies, have all pointed to some important role in DNA metabolism. It now appears that a vitamin B_{12} deficiency causes a secondary deficiency of folate because of the resultant accumulation of 5-methyl-H_4folate.[86] This "methyl trap" hypothesis was proposed by Herbert and others.[7, 116]

The connection between the two vitamins comes from a requirement for

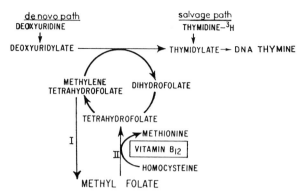

Figure 4–2 B_{12}, folic acid, methionine, and homocysteine interrelationships in thymidylate synthesis. I, 5,10-methylenetetrahydrofolic reductase; II, homocysteine transmethylase. (From Waxman, Metz, and Herbert: J. Clin. Invest., vol. 48, 1969, with permission of the authors and publisher.)

methylcobalamin as a coenzyme in the reaction by which a methyl group is transferred from 5-methyl-H_4folate to homocysteine; this reaction is an important means of regenerating methionine. If the cobalamins are deficient, 5-methyl-H_4folate accumulates. The accumulation occurs because the compound is formed irreversibly from 5,10-methylene-H_4folate, and there is no way to dispose of it except by the cobalamin-dependent transfer of the methyl group. The reactions involved are summarized in Figure 4–2.

The evidence supporting this concept is as follows. De novo DNA synthesis, as measured by the incorporation of deoxyuridine into the thymine of DNA, is defective in the marrow of patients with vitamin B_{12} deficiency. In some patients with pernicious anemia the apparent serum folate level is elevated, and this has been shown to be due to accumulation of 5-methyl-H_4folate. Added vitamin B_{12} corrects the abnormality in vitamin B_{12} deficient marrows, but not in the folate-deficient marrows, whereas folate (pteroylglutamate) corrects both types of deficiencies. Furthermore, a folate antagonist such as methotrexate blocks the corrective action of vitamin B_{12}. A series of experiments by Herbert and associates[117] led to the conclusion that inadequate synthesis of DNA in vitamin B_{12} deficiency is indeed due to a deficiency of tetrahydrofolate, because H_4folate must be continuously available to carry the one carbon unit necessary for de novo synthesis of thymine as its deoxynucleotide (Fig. 4–2). Thus, either folate deficiency from inadequate intake or from the action of antagonists, or vitamin B_{12} deficiency from whatever cause, may reduce H_4folate availability and impair or prevent de novo DNA synthesis.

Studies of phytohemagglutinin-stimulated cultured lymphocytes in normal persons, in patients with untreated pernicious anemia, and in those with treated pernicious anemia indicate that megaloblastosis and vitamin B_{12} deficiency are associated with low thymidylate synthetase activity.[51] It was postulated that, in the absence of this enzyme, folate was unable to function in the synthesis of DNA, and 5-methyl-tetrahydrofolate accumulated.

The important action of vitamin B_{12} in protecting the cells of the nervous system is not understood. The neurologic lesions do not respond to folate in the absence of vitamin B_{12}, and they may be the result of an impairment in other reactions requiring cobalamin coenzymes, such as the methylmalonyl coenzyme A isomerization that is involved in the metabolism of several amino acids and of fatty acids with odd-numbered chain lengths.

CLASSIFICATION OF MEGALOBLASTIC ANEMIAS

The most characteristic feature of deficiency of vitamin B_{12} or folic acid is the occurrence of a megaloblastic anemia. A deficiency can arise in various ways, as shown in Table 4–2. Probably the commonest cause of vitamin B_{12} deficiency is the deficiency of intrinsic factor that is found in pernicious anemia; folic acid deficiency is seen most often in persons with an inadequate intake associated with some other conditions, such as pregnancy or cirrhosis of the liver, and in patients with malabsorption syndrome. Very rarely a case of megaloblastic anemia is seen that cannot be fitted into one of the recognized causes; such cases are termed "idiopathic" for want of a better name. Vitamin B_{12} deficiency that results from inability to utilize the vitamin must be extraordinarily rare if it occurs; most of the reported instances have been shown to be instances of folic acid deficiency or of some block in nucleic acid metabolism.

Table 4–2   *Classification of Megaloblastic Anemias*

I. Vitamin B_{12} deficiency
  A. Inadequate intake
  B. Defective absorption
    1. Failure to secrete intrinsic factor
      a. Addisonian pernicious anemia
      b. Total gastrectomy
    2. Failure of absorption in the small intestine
      a. Malabsorption syndromes
      b. Blind loops and fistulas
      c. Fish tapeworm infestation
      d. Transcobalamin deficiencies

II. Folic acid deficiency
  A. Inadequate intake
  B. Defective absorption
    1. Malabsorption syndromes
    2. Blind loop syndrome
    3. Induced by drugs
  C. Inadequate utilization
    1. Ascorbic acid deficiency
    2. Therapy with folic acid antagonists
    3. Therapy with anticonvulsant drugs
    4. Therapy with pyrimethamine
  D. Excessive demands
    1. Pregnancy
    2. Infancy and growth
    3. Hyperhemolysis

VITAMIN B$_{12}$ DEFICIENCY

PERNICIOUS ANEMIA

Synonyms: Primary Anemia, Addison's Anemia, Biermer's Anemia.

Pernicious anemia is a disease that has intrigued numerous investigators for many years. The history of pernicious anemia is an "illustrative case" of the development and progress of medicine. First, centuries of almost complete ignorance, then the slow accumulation of clinical information from many scattered sources over a period of about a hundred years, a period which was followed by the rapid progress made in the past few decades. The disease affords an example of the successful combining of information gained from animal experiments with careful clinical observations to discover the clinical cure of a previously fatal disease. It is also an illustration of the way in which a significant contribution to clinical medicine stimulates further, more basic, investigation. This in turn leads to a better understanding of human physiology and chemistry that has a significance far beyond a particular disease.

History

The history of pernicious anemia has been reviewed by Haden[43] and by Castle.[13] Credit for reporting the first case of pernicious anemia is generally given to Combe for his report to the Medico-Chirurgical Society of Edinburgh on May 1, 1822. Thomas Addison of Guy's Hospital is given credit for recognizing the disease as a clinical entity. Addison described a progressive fatal type of anemia of unknown cause that occurred in both sexes, generally beyond the middle period of life. He observed the insidious onset, the increasing weakness, and pallor, and commented on the remarkable absence of wasting despite the fatal outcome of the extremely debilitating disease.[79] Biermer in 1871 independently described 15 cases of severe anemia, to which he gave the name "progressive pernicious anemia." Interest in the disease was stimulated and numerous papers followed. Ehrlich described the megaloblasts which he considered diagnostic of pernicious anemia[28] and provided a subject of interest and controversy for those interested in morphology that has continued to the present time. The importance of the gastric secretion of acid in various diseases was studied by Cahn and von Mering in 1886, and in 1921 Levine and Ladd demonstrated the almost constant occurrence of achlorhydria in pernicious anemia in a study of 107 patients with the disease. The relation of the gastric defect to the causation of pernicious anemia was demonstrated by Castle in 1929.[14, 17]

The studies of Whipple and Robscheit-Robbins demonstrated the importance of food factors, particularly liver, in correction of posthemorrhagic anemia in dogs, and suggested that such therapy deserved serious consideration in other more complex anemias, such as pernicious anemia.[120] Minot and Murphy's dramatic report on "The Treatment of Pernicious Anemia by a Special Diet" followed soon after.[83] The excellent results obtained with liver in this series of 45 patients with pernicious anemia were soon confirmed. The significance of this contribution has been emphasized by Haden: "There is nothing more dramatic in medicine than the effect of liver therapy on a patient with pernicious anemia. Only the use of sulfa drugs and other antibiotics such as penicillin afford such brilliant results."[43]

The use of whole liver by mouth led to the development of liver extracts of increasing potency that could be administered parenterally. The search for the active principle of liver extract culminated in the discovery of vitamin B_{12} by Smith[107] and by Rickes and colleagues in 1948.[96] The structural formula of vitamin B_{12} was determined by x-ray crystallographic analysis by Hodgkin in 1956.[63] Twenty-five years after it was identified, vitamin B_{12}, the most complicated vitamin thus far discovered and the only one containing cobalt, was synthesized in a monumental work that required 11 years of coordinated effort by 99 scientists from 16 countries.[81] Investigations by numerous workers have demonstrated important roles of vitamin B_{12} and folic acid in nucleic acid metabolism in the body.

Mechanism of Vitamin B_{12} Deficiency in Pernicious Anemia

The relationship between the abnormal gastric secretion and the effectiveness of the liver diet in pernicious anemia was shown by Castle and Townsend,[17] who utilized beef muscle, normal gastric juice, hydrochloric acid, and gastric juice from patients with pernicious anemia in their investigation. In a series of classic experiments they studied the hematologic effects of various combinations of these substances on patients with pernicious anemia in relapse. They demonstrated that patients with pernicious anemia lack a substance in the gastric juice that is necessary for the absorption of some factor present in meat that is essential for normal erythropoiesis. It was shown that this gastric factor, which could be destroyed by heat, is not hydrochloric acid. These studies thus established that the primary defect in pernicious anemia is the failure of the stomach to secrete a substance, probably an enzyme, that is necessary for the absorption of a dietary element essential to normal hematopoiesis. As a result of these observations it was postulated that an "extrinsic factor," present in the beef muscle, reacted with an "intrinsic factor," secreted in the normal gastric juice, to form an "erythrocyte maturation factor" which was the active principle that was stored in the liver. After vitamin B_{12} was isolated, Castle and co-workers repeated these experiments but substituted vitamin B_{12} for the beef muscle.[6] The results demonstrated that vitamin B_{12} is both an "extrinsic factor" and an "erythrocyte maturation factor." The function of the intrinsic factor is to make possible the absorption of vitamin B_{12} from the diet for utilization in the bone marrow and for storage in the liver.

Pernicious anemia and intestinal malabsorption of some sort are the two most frequent causes of vitamin B_{12} deficiency. The Schilling test usually distinguishes between the two. In a few patients with pernicious anemia, however, the absorption of the radioactive vitamin B_{12} does not improve after intrinsic factor (IF) has been added to the test dose.[10, 38, 101, 119] Malabsorption of vitamin

B$_{12}$ in the small intestine may be produced by three different mechanisms. One is small bowel disease, a situation that usually can be recognized by demonstrating either abnormalities of the small bowel on x-ray or other evidences of small bowel disease. Another is vitamin B$_{12}$ deficiency itself, which in some patients causes changes in the mucosal cells of the small bowel with impairment of their function; malabsorption of this type is usually corrected within one to ten months by treatment with vitamin B$_{12}$. The third mechanism of malabsorption occurs in the presence of antibodies to the intrinsic factor; these block the action of IF, which is essential for the absorption of vitamin B$_{12}$ in physiologic quantities. Pernicious anemia with coexisting malabsorption can be distinguished from vitamin B$_{12}$ deficiency, which results from malabsorption, by precise immunologic quantitation of the intrinsic factor; only in patients with pernicious anemia have antibodies against the intrinsic factor been demonstrated. Transient malabsorption of vitamin B$_{12}$ may result from reversible structural or functional changes in the gastric parietal cells or the ileal mucosa.[56]

The role of an autoimmune mechanism in pernicious anemia has attracted considerable attention.[30, 38, 39, 70, 71, 113] Autoantibodies to parietal cells have been found in the serum of approximately 90 per cent of patients with pernicious anemia; similar antibodies have been found in from 5 to 8 per cent of the normal population between the ages of 30 and 60, in 14 per cent of women over 60 years of age, and in as many as 60 per cent of patients with thyroid disease, idiopathic gastritis, and other disorders. Clinical pernicious anemia occurs in 12 per cent of patients with primary myxedema or Hashimoto's goiter.[15] Antibodies to intrinsic factor have been found in the serum of 60 per cent of patients with pernicious anemia, and in either the serum or gastric juice in 90 per cent; more important, these antibodies are very rarely found in other disorders or in the general population. Antibodies toward the parietal cells indicate only that gastritis of some sort is present, whereas the presence of antibodies to the intrinsic factor appears to be specific, or nearly so, for pernicious anemia. Up to the present time, however, neither antibody has been successfully incriminated in the production of the disease pernicious anemia. The occurrence of pernicious anemia in persons who have impaired antibody responsiveness and no demonstrable serum antibodies against parietal cells, intrinsic factor, or thyroid antigen indicates that these antibodies are not essential for the development of the disease.[22, 114] Because of these observations, the cellular immune mechanism would have to be involved in an immunologic explanation.[56] It is of considerable interest that prednisolone therapy has produced the reappearance of parietal cells associated with the secretion of hydrochloric acid and intrinsic factor, together with an increase in the absorption of vitamin B$_{12}$, in some patients with pernicious anemia; other changes found were a decrease in the antibody titer to intrinsic factor in the patient's serum; there was no change in the titer of the parietal cell antibodies. These results imply that the improvement noted in some patients with pernicious anemia after the administration of adrenocorticoid preparations is the result of stimulation of growth and function in the cells of the stomach, rather than an interference with the action of antibodies,[2, 69] but the alternative explanation cannot be excluded.

Clinical Manifestations

Pernicious anemia affects individuals of either sex; it occurs most often after the age of 40, and is rare before the age of 30. Although the disease is rare in Africans and in dark-skinned white races,[121] the incidence in blacks in the United States approaches that in whites.[61]

The clinical picture of pernicious anemia is variable. Patients with untreated pernicious anemia usually complain of an insidious onset of weakness, anorexia, pallor, "indigestion," and numbness and tingling in the extremities. In older persons dyspnea, palpitation, dizziness, and angina of effort often develop because of the effect of anemia on the circulatory system. Soreness of the tongue and diarrhea may be present. Although it is seldom severe, some loss of weight usually occurs; in a series of patients seen by the authors, the average weight loss before treatment was 25 pounds in blacks and 15 pounds in whites.[61]

In some patients with pernicious anemia, particularly since the advent of folic acid and the widespread use of multivitamin preparations, the hematologic abnormalities are mild or absent when neurologic manifestations are prominent. Subjective and objective neurologic findings have been reported in 80 per cent of patients, and were severe enough to cause some degree of incapacity in about 50 per cent.[100] The most common manifestations are paresthesias, incoordination, impairment of position and vibratory sense, and absence of reflexes. The symptoms range from subjective numbness and tingling of the extremities in the mildest form to an unsteady gait, difficulty in locomotion, and difficulty in buttoning the clothes in the more severely affected patients. In the most severe form of the disease the patient is unable to walk, and voluntary control of the bladder and rectum is impaired or lost. Some patients undergo marked personality changes associated with memory loss, impaired judgment, disorientation, hallucinations, and delusions.

A reversible type of malabsorption secondary to vitamin B$_{12}$ deficiency occurs frequently in patients with pernicious anemia; at times it is severe and is associated with nausea, vomiting, weight loss, hypoproteinemia, and leg edema.[76] The deficiency may be a consequence of the failure of the stomach to secrete intrinsic factor, or of the presence of antibodies to intrinsic factor, or of bacterial growth in the small bowel.

At times the diagnosis of pernicious anemia is suggested by aspects of the patient's appearance, such as gray hair, sallow skin, slight scleral icterus, and atrophy of the papillae of the tongue. The spleen is usually enlarged in hematologic relapse and is often palpable. In most patients neurologic examination reveals abnormalities of the peripheral nerves and posterolateral columns that are most marked in the lower extremities. The earliest signs are usually some loss of vibratory sense in the lower extremities, and impairment of sensation to pin prick and touch that may be either spotty or of the "stocking" type. With more severe changes the Romberg test is positive, position sense is impaired, and the deep tendon reflexes are lost at the ankles and knees. Further progression of the disease in the spinal cord is associated with the development of hyperreflexia and the presence of pathologic reflexes, such as an extensor plantar response. Paraplegia and loss of sphincter control are late manifestations. The neurologic dysfunctions in pernicious anemia have been classified as (1) cerebral, (2) olfactory, (3) peripheral nerve and posterior column of the spinal cord, and (4) peripheral nerve, posterior and lateral columns of the spinal cord.[100] The distinction between peripheral neuropathy, posterior column disease, and combined system degeneration is useful as an indication of the severity of the disease, but classification in this way is not always easy.

Laboratory Examination

In nearly every patient with uncomplicated and untreated pernicious anemia, macrocytic anemia occurs. Erythrocyte counts range from less than a million to near normal values. The MCV is nearly always over 100 cu. μ, and is often in the range of 120 to 130 cu. μ. The hemoglobin values are not reduced as much as the erythrocyte count, and the MCH is usually increased (over 33 $\mu\mu$). The blood smear shows considerable anisocytosis and poikilocytosis of erythrocytes that appear to be well filled with hemoglobin; oval macrocytes are usually present. If the anemia is severe, stippled red cells and nucleated red cells of the megaloblastic series may be seen. In the untreated patient the reticulocyte count is either normal or subnormal.

Leukopenia and thrombocytopenia occur commonly in pernicious anemia. Leukocyte counts of 3000 to 4000 per cu.mm. are common, and levels of 1600 to 2000 per cu.mm. sometimes occur. The leukopenia is due mainly to a reduction in the granulocytes. Some of the granulocytes show abnormalities such as hypersegmentation and an increase in size; these cells are called "macropolycytes." In patients with severe anemia the platelets often number less than 100,000 per cu.mm.

The gastric secretion in pernicious anemia is abnormal in several respects. The total quantity of the gastric juice is greatly reduced and achlorhydria is an almost constant finding. These abnormalities persist after treatment. Because exceptions occur so rarely, failure to secrete free hydrochloric acid after the injection of histamine subcutaneously can be considered an almost essential feature for the diagnosis of pernicious anemia.

The bone marrow in relapse is usually hypercellular. The characteristic feature is the occurrence of the megaloblastic type of erythropoiesis (Fig. 4–3). If anemia is severe, promegaloblasts and basophilic megaloblasts are increased in number and mitotic figures are numerous. The polychromatophilic megaloblasts, which are the easiest cells to identify in this series, persist even after the anemia in the peripheral blood has been abolished by transfusion. The erythrocyte precursors in the marrow are extremely sensitive to specific therapy, and the parenteral administration of even a few micrograms of vitamin B$_{12}$ or the ingestion of a few milligrams of folic acid is sufficient to change the megaloblastic picture in the marrow to a normoblastic one within a day or two. In such circumstances the appearance of the bone marrow may not be diagnostic. However, the morphologic abnormalities in the marrow in pernicious anemia are not confined to cells of the erythrocytic series. Deficiency of vitamin B$_{12}$ or folic acid also leads to the production of giant metamyelocytes and multisegmented macropolycytes. These abnormalities in the granulocytic series do not disappear as promptly as the megaloblasts do after specific therapy, and their presence may be helpful in

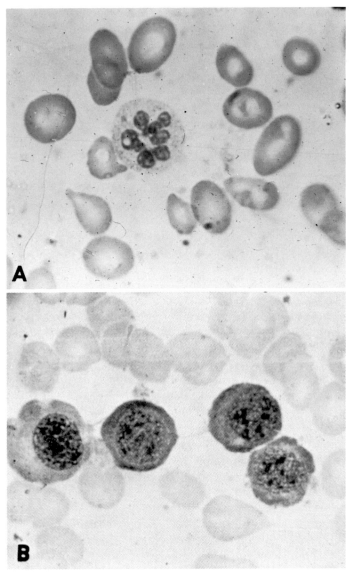

Figure 4–3   *A,* Peripheral blood and *B,* bone marrow from a patient with untreated pernicious anemia. The peripheral blood smear shows macrocytosis, anisocytosis, poikilocytosis, oval macrocytes, and a macropolycyte. The bone marrow shows the megaloblastic type of maturation.

diagnosis when the patient is seen for the first time soon after specific therapy has been started. The finding of multisegmented granulocytes in the smear of the peripheral blood is also one of the best screening procedures for a deficiency of vitamin B_{12} or folate.

Other laboratory tests in the untreated patient generally reveal an increased level of the indirect reacting bilirubin in the plasma (1.0 to 1.5 mg.), an elevation of the serum iron, an increase in fecal urobilinogen excretion, a decreased blood volume, and an increase in the plasma lactic acid dehydrogenase (400 to 4000 units). The levels of the serum iron and folate are often elevated in the untreated patient, but fall rapidly during the response to treatment with vitamin B$_{12}$. A diminution of the plasma protein is not unusual. The serum vitamin B$_{12}$ level is subnormal, less than 200 pg. per ml., and usually less than 100 pg. per ml.

Elevated serum muramidase activity occurs in patients with untreated megaloblastic anemia, presumably a reflection of the increased destruction of granulocytes in the marrow or circulation.[91]

Diagnosis

The diagnosis of pernicious anemia in the untreated patient is usually made without difficulty. The presence of macrocytic anemia associated with histamine-fast achlorhydria and a megaloblastic bone marrow practically establishes the diagnosis. The presence in the circulation of an antibody to intrinsic factor, found in two-thirds of patients with pernicious anemia, is essentially diagnostic, as is a serum vitamin B$_{12}$ level of less than 100 pg. per ml. or a saturation of the serum vitamin B$_{12}$-binding capacity of less than 10 per cent. The diagnosis is proved when the parenteral administration of vitamin B$_{12}$ produces the characteristic hematologic changes. These are the conversion of the megaloblastic type of erythropoiesis to the normoblastic type within a day or two, a rise in reticulocytes during the first week, and a return of the hemoglobin and red count to normal levels in succeeding weeks. The magnitude of the reticulocyte response depends on the degree of anemia, and varies inversely with the erythrocyte count. The maximal reticulocyte count (R) that is expected to follow the intramuscular injection of liver extract or vitamin B$_{12}$ in adequate amounts can be calculated from the formula:

$$R = \frac{82 - 22Eo}{1 + 0.5Eo}$$

where R represents the reticulocyte count in per cent and Eo represents the initial erythrocyte count in million per cu.mm.[65] For example, if the initial erythrocyte count is 1.5 million per cu.mm.:

$$R = \frac{82 - (22 \times 1.5)}{1 + (0.5 \times 1.5)} = \frac{82 - 33}{1 + 0.75} = \frac{49}{1.75} = 28 \text{ per cent}$$

In our experience it is not uncommon for the maximal reticulocyte count to fall slightly short of the expected maximum, even when the reticulocytes are counted twice a day (Fig. 4–4).

At times pernicious anemia must be differentiated from other conditions characterized by the megaloblastic type of erythropoiesis. The most common disorders in this category are folic acid deficiency of sprue and other dietary deficiencies, and vitamin B$_{12}$ deficiency secondary to intestinal fistulae, shunts, and diverticula. The fact that most conditions associated with folic acid deficiency do not produce histamine-fast achlorhydria often helps to distinguish pernicious anemia from folic acid deficiency. In addition, the disorders associated with folic acid deficiency are often manifested by rather severe gastrointestinal disturbance accompanied by only minor neurologic symptoms; the reverse is more likely to

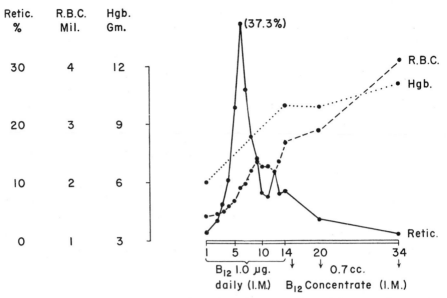

Figure 4–4   Reticulocyte response of a patient with untreated pernicious anemia to treatment with vitamin B$_{12}$. The maximal reticulocyte response, which was reached about the end of the first week in this patient, depends on the level of the erythrocytes before treatment.

be the case in pernicious anemia. In doubtful cases the determination of the serum B$_{12}$ level or the use of some test of vitamin B$_{12}$ absorption, such as the Schilling test, may be necessary in order to establish the diagnosis.[102, 105]

The Schilling test is performed by giving the patient a measured amount, usually 0.5 microcuries, of cyanocobalamin [57]Co orally; two hours later the patient is given an intramuscular injection of 1 mg. of nonradioactive cyanocobalamin; urine is collected for 24 hours and the amount of radioactive cyanocobalamin is determined. Normally more than 7 per cent of the ingested dose is excreted within 24 hours. Should the result be subnormal, the test is repeated with oral porcine intrinsic factor, 60 mg.; if excretion is then normal it is concluded that the patient has deficiency of intrinsic factor, in all probability pernicious anemia. If the absorption and excretion do not return to normal after the addition of intrinsic factor it is possible that the patient has a blind loop syndrome or some other disturbance in the bacterial flora of the intestine which leads to malabsorption of vitamin B$_{12}$. At times this can be established by repeating the test ten days after giving the patient tetracycline, 250 mg. four times a day. Other causes for low excretion of vitamin B$_{12}$ are incomplete urine collection, renal disease[105] and *Diphyllobothrium latum infestation.*

The term "achrestic anemia" was proposed for the group of patients with a megaloblastic bone marrow and a peripheral blood picture identical with that of pernicious anemia who responded poorly or not at all to parenteral therapy with liver extract of known potency.[66, 67] The report of Davidson suggests that at least some patients whose symptoms fit the description of achrestic anemia may well represent instances of folic acid deficiency.

When the patient with pernicious anemia has the neurologic features of the disease without the characteristic hematologic abnormalities, the diagnosis may be difficult. In such circumstances the patient usually has received vitamin B$_{12}$ or folic acid in an amount that is sufficient to convert the megaloblastic type of erythropoiesis to the normoblastic type and to raise the erythrocyte count to near normal levels. If examination of the peripheral blood and bone marrow does not suffice for the diagnosis, a gastric analysis should be made. If free hydrochloric acid is secreted after the histamine injection, the diagnosis of pernicious anemia can be discarded with considerable assurance. If histamine-fast achlorhydria is present, the Schilling test for vitamin B$_{12}$ absorption or some other similar test should be performed, since it will often clarify the diagnosis.

The tests of vitamin B$_{12}$ absorption are also helpful in the evaluation of patients without neurologic disease who have received treatment with vitamin B$_{12}$ or liver extract before the diagnosis was established. By such means the diagnosis can be verified or corrected without waiting months or years after specific therapy is withheld to see whether hematologic relapse occurs.

Both megaloblasts and sideroblasts appear in the marrow of some alcoholic patients; the abnormalities disappear rapidly when alcohol is withheld.[62]

Treatment

Prior to the report of Minot and Murphy in 1926 on the efficacy of liver, the treatment of pernicious anemia was unsatisfactory and the disease was invariably fatal.[83] Since that time more efficient preparations have been developed, but all are forms of substitution therapy that must be continued throughout the life of the patient. Vitamin B$_{12}$ is the essential factor, and the parenteral administration of as little as 1 microgram each day to a patient in relapse is sufficient to restore the blood to normal and prevent the development of neurologic lesions if these are not already present. In practice it is customary to administer larger amounts at longer intervals and to err toward an excessive dose, rather than risk an amount that may be suboptimal.

Although the selection of the details of the schedule may be somewhat arbitrary, some definite program of treatment should be followed. The following schedule has been found satisfactory for patients in relapse in our experience: vitamin B$_{12}$ 30 micrograms intramuscularly three times during the first week, then 30 micrograms once a week until the blood returns to normal. This schedule produces the expected reticulocyte response within the first week or ten days, and a return of the erythrocyte level to normal within six to ten weeks. Thereafter the patient receives injections of 60 micrograms every four weeks. A program of 30 micrograms every four weeks has maintained patients in hematologic remission and prevented the development of neurologic lesions, but in one reported series of 51 patients treated with 30 micrograms of vitamin B$_{12}$ parenterally each month, definite neurologic relapse occurred in the absence of hematologic relapse; three of these patients improved when the amount of vitamin B$_{12}$ was increased and one responded to liver extract.[103] Monthly injections of 250 or 500 micrograms have been recommended to sustain complete normality.[53] Such reports appear to confirm the clinical impression that not all patients with pernicious anemia require the same maintenance dosage. For this reason it is advisable to check the hematocrit levels every few months and the neurologic status at regular intervals so that the dosage of vitamin B_{12} can be adjusted if the therapy is not adequate. Because of the high excretion rate of injected vitamin B_{12}, from 50 to 98 per cent with doses 100 to 1000 micrograms, Herbert recommends that a monthly maintenance injection of at least 100 micrograms be employed; hydroxocobalamin has no advantage over cyanocobalamin in this type of therapy.[57] Although effective oral preparations are available, parenteral therapy is preferred because of greater reliability, less expense, and better supervision of the patient. Unless careful supervision is maintained some patients will develop hematologic or, more important, neurologic relapse as a consequence of inadequate therapy. In one report of 41 patients treated orally with vitamin B_{12} and folic acid, five failed to return, and in 14 others oral therapy was discontinued because of neurologic or hematologic relapse.[103]

When an elderly patient is severely anemic, the circulation is sometimes compromised by the low levels of the circulating hemoglobin. When this occurs, transfusions may be administered if it is considered inadvisable to wait for the erythropoietic effect of the vitamin B_{12}. The use of packed cells is preferred to whole blood because the former gives the desired increase in circulating hemoglobin without as great an increase in blood volume. Potassium depletion occurs in some patients, most often after therapy and just before reticulocytosis develops. The potassium needed in production of new cells may be the explanation. The potassium level should be monitored during therapy in all patients, particularly older persons with cardiovascular disease.[75]

When severe neurologic complications are present, vitamin B_{12} is often administered in amounts larger than those that are usually given to the patient with uncomplicated anemia. This practice is based on clinical observations which led to the belief that the optimal therapeutic dose of vitamin B_{12} may not be the same for both the hematopoietic and nervous systems. It has been recognized that there is little or no correlation between the severity of the anemia and the extent of the neurologic lesion, because some patients present with severe anemia and little or no neurologic involvement, and others have severe neurologic disease and only mild anemia. Although neurologic complications rarely if ever develop if a normal hematologic status is maintained with parenteral vitamin B_{12}, it has not been established that 1 microgram a day is the optimal initial treatment for the patient with existing neurologic involvement of significant degree. The neurologic response to therapy is much slower than the hematologic, and improvement may continue for several months after the blood has returned to normal. Some patients who show little neurologic improvement during the first month or two of therapy show gratifying improvement between the third and sixth months. Apparently little or no improvement can be anticipated after 10 to 12 months of therapy.

Because of these considerations we employ a larger dose of vitamin B_{12} in patients with neurologic involvement (100 micrograms three times a week for three months, then 100 micrograms weekly for three months), although it is recognized that the value of a dose larger than that necessary to produce hematologic remission has not been established. Although parenteral vitamin B_{12} is the most important treatment for patients with neurologic disease, physiotherapy is often very helpful in patients who are severely affected. It has been shown clearly that, although folic acid therapy may maintain the patient in a normal hematologic status, it does not prevent the development of neurologic lesions.[8, 99]

Vitamin B$_{12}$ appears to be a complete therapy in pernicious anemia. Dilute hydrochloric acid, folic acid, and liver extract are unnecessary. Likewise iron is not indicated unless there is an associated iron deficiency from some other cause.

Failure to respond to therapy, or the occurrence of a hematologic relapse while the patient is receiving adequate amounts of vitamin B$_{12}$, should raise the suspicion of the development of some infection, renal insufficiency, gastrointestinal bleeding, or the appearance of a carcinoma of the stomach. In former years the presence on the market of ineffective liver preparations was responsible for some therapeutic "failures."

Course and Prognosis

If the patient does not have significant neurologic involvement when he is first seen, the prognosis is excellent. He should be restored to his previous status, and with proper maintenance therapy his outlook should be that of his age group, with the possible exception of a greater likelihood of developing carcinoma of the stomach. The reported incidence of carcinoma of the stomach in patients with pernicious anemia varies considerably. One report placed the incidence in living patients at 1.7 per cent,[87] another roentgen study of 211 patients found gastric carcinoma in 8 per cent and benign polyps in 7.1 per cent.[97] Several reports place the frequency of carcinoma of the stomach at autopsy at from 8.4 per cent to 12.3 per cent,[72, 126] figures that are three to four times the incidence in individuals of the same age group who do not have pernicious anemia. The increased frequency of carcinoma suggests the desirability of periodic examinations in an effort to detect the carcinoma in an early stage. It has been recommended that the stool be examined for occult blood each month, that gastric cytology be studied every three to six months, and that suspicious cases have gastroscopy and roentgenographic study of the upper gastrointestinal tract.[126] In our experience these procedures have proved impractical as routine measures, and the problem of early recognition of the development of carcinoma remains a perplexing one.

If neurologic complications are present the prognosis is related to the extent and duration of the manifestations. If symptoms have been present for only a few months the outlook is excellent, particularly if the individual is less than 50 years old. Signs of an upper motor neuron lesion, such as the Babinski sign, usually persist despite treatment but sometimes disappear. Absent deep tendon reflexes usually return. Marked improvement may occur promptly, and maximal improvement occurs within 10 or 12 months. If paraplegia and loss of sphincter control have developed the outlook for recovery is poor. However, many patients who are severely ataxic and unable to walk improve after months of treatment and eventually recover sufficiently to resume most of their previous activities, even though subjective and objective neurologic abnormalities persist.

Before the advent of liver therapy, which was also before the use of antibiotics and frequent blood transfusions, 53 per cent of patients with megaloblastic anemia died within a month after admission to a hospital. A recent review of 108 patients with megaloblastic anemia in Scotland disclosed a mortality rate of 14 per cent compared to 1.6 per cent in those with iron deficiency; the main causes of death were cardiovascular disease and pulmonary edema, with and without transfusion.[75]

JUVENILE PERNICIOUS ANEMIA

Although pernicious anemia characteristically occurs in persons who are middle-aged or older, the clinical picture has been observed in children from a few months to 18 years of age. The most common symptoms are pallor, weakness, listlessness, and irritability; fever, anorexia, vomiting, diarrhea, glossitis, and weight loss also occur. Hepatosplenomegaly, jaundice, mental retardation, and neurologic abnormalities have been reported but are unusual. The hematologic features are the same as those seen in adult pernicious anemia; these are corrected by treatment with vitamin B_{12} or liver extract, but recur if treatment is discontinued. The disorder usually responds to the intramuscular injection of from 15 to 30 micrograms of vitamin B_{12} every two to four weeks.

The reported cases may be divided into several groups.[82] In one group of 20 patients, in 16 of whom the onset occurred before $2\frac{1}{2}$ years of age, histology of the gastric mucosa and secretion of acid were normal but secretion of the intrinsic factor was lacking; antibodies to intrinsic factor were not demonstrated in the serum. In one reported case of vitamin B_{12} malabsorption, the gastric biopsy and secretion of hydrochloric acid were normal; immunologically active intrinsic factor was secreted, but was functionally inadequate and did not facilitate the absorption of vitamin B_{12}; no serum antibodies against IF were demonstrated.[73]

In the second group of six patients, the disease became manifest later in childhood and was characterized by failure of secretion of the intrinsic factor associated with histamine-fast achlorhydria and atrophic gastritis; antibodies against intrinsic factor were demonstrated in four patients, all of whom had associated hypofunction of one or more endocrine glands. It has been suggested that the first group may represent a disease that results from a metabolic error with selective failure of intrinsic factor secretion; it may be distinct from and not genetically related to adult pernicious anemia. The second group more closely resembles the adult form of the disease. Autoimmunity, perhaps with genetic predisposition, has been postulated because of the familial incidence of pernicious anemia, myxedema, and immunoglobulin abnormalities found in some of the reported cases.[47, 108]

Another group of patients with deficiency of vitamin B_{12} has been considered by some authors to have a form of "juvenile pernicious anemia."[109] In 18 patients no abnormality was found in the secretion of acid or intrinsic factor, and biopsy of the gastric mucosa was normal; all had proteinuria. These patients apparently had a specific defect in the absorption of vitamin B_{12}. Since the absorption defect in these patients does not appear to be related to any lack of the intrinsic factor, use of the term "pernicious anemia" for this type of vitamin B_{12} deficiency appears incorrect. The eponym Imerslund's syndrome or Imerslund-Gräsbeck syndrome has been applied to this disorder, reported in at least 28 patients; it has been postulated that the malabsorption of vitamin B$_{12}$ is the result of an anomaly in the small intestine, a defect in the mechanism which releases vitamin B$_{12}$ from intrinsic factor.[32] A more recent study found no morphologically identifiable lesion in the ileal mucosal cells. If stimulated uptake of cyanocobalamin by homegenates of the biopsies and it was concluded that the defect lay somewhere after the attachment of IF to the ileal cell, and before the vitamin binds to transcobalamin II.[77]

Illustrative Cases

CASE 1

A 56-year-old white housewife was admitted to the hospital for the evaluation of progressive numbness and pain of two years' duration in the hands and feet. In the last few weeks before admission her gait had become unsteady. She had been taking "vitamin pills" as a tonic for many months. On an admission 13 years previously she was found to have histamine-fast achlorhydria and hypochromic anemia; the anemia responded to treatment with iron.

Physical examination. The patient was an obese white woman in no apparent distress. Pertinent abnormalities were found only on the neurologic examination. These were: absent gag reflex; moderate spastic paraparesis and increased tendon reflexes in the lower extremities; abnormal Babinski signs bilaterally; impairment of position sense in the hands and feet; and absence of vibratory sense in the feet and legs.

Laboratory examination. Admission blood studies disclosed the following: Hct. 42 per cent, Hb. 14.3 gm. per 100 ml., R.B.C. 4.3 million per cu.mm. There was moderate anisocytosis of the red cells; both microcytic and macrocytic forms were present. The urine, stool, and spinal fluid were normal. Gastric analysis on two occasions revealed the absence of free hydrochloric acid after the injection of histamine. Examination of the bone marrow showed a normoblastic type of erythropoiesis. A Schilling test for radioactive vitamin B$_{12}$ (B$_{12}$Co^{60}) absorption was performed. No significant absorption of vitamin B$_{12}$ occurred (0 per cent excretion). When the test was repeated with the addition of intrinsic factor, absorption of the orally-administered vitamin B$_{12}$ occurred (9 per cent excretion).

Diagnosis and treatment. A diagnosis of pernicious anemia with subacute combined degeneration of the spinal cord was made. The patient was treated with vitamin B$_{12}$ intramuscularly. During the next ten months her gait improved gradually and returned to normal. Impaired vibratory sense and paresthesias persisted.

Comment. The neurologic manifestations of pernicious anemia occurred in this patient in the absence of anemia. The diagnosis was suggested by the clinical features of neurologic disease associated with histamine-fast achlorhydria, and it was established by the demonstration of faulty vitamin B$_{12}$ absorption. It is probable that the essentially normal blood values and the normoblastic bone marrow were the results of folic acid contained in the multivitamin tablets which the patient had taken. This case also illustrates the well-recognized occurrence of histamine-fast achlorhydria some years before the onset of clinical pernicious anemia.

CASE 2

A 67-year-old white farmer was admitted to the hospital in August 1947 because of weakness, dizziness, exertional dyspnea, ataxia, and numbness of six months' duration in the hands.

Physical examination. The skin and mucous membranes were pale and the tongue was smooth. Vibratory sense was diminished in the legs, the knee jerks were diminished, and ankle jerks were absent. No pathologic reflexes were present.

Laboratory examination. Admission blood studies disclosed the following: Hb. 9.0 gm. per 100 ml.; R.B.C. 1.58 million per cu.mm.; Hct. 24 per cent (MCV 150 cu.μ, MCH 56 $\mu\mu$, MCHC 36 per cent); W.B.C. 2500 per cu.mm.; platelets 70,000 per cu-mm.; reticulocytes 0.6 per cent; differential count (per cent), granulocytes 36, lymphocytes 63. Examination of a smear of the peripheral blood revealed considerable anisocytosis and poikilocytosis; many macrocytes that were well-filled with hemoglobin were seen. Roentgenographic studies showed that the upper gastroinestinal tract and colon were normal. Gastric analysis revealed the absence of free HCl after the injection of histamine. Examination of the bone marrow disclosed that erythropoiesis was megaloblastic in character; giant band forms, large metamyelocytes, and macropolycytes were also present.

Diagnosis and treatment. A diagnosis of pernicious anemia was made and the patient was treated with daily intramuscular injections of 15 units of liver extract. After the first week, the dose was reduced to 15 units a week. Although the peak reticulocyte response of 7.8 per cent was well below the predicted maximum, the hemoglobin, red count, and hematocrit returned to normal within ten weeks. During the next seven years the patient progressed well on treatment with parenteral liver extract, 30 units per month, and later with vitamin B$_{12}$, 30 micrograms per month.

Course. In March 1954 a barium study of the stomach was made with normal results. In February 1955, when the patient was 75 years of age, he developed vague epigastric discomfort. A barium study about one month after the onset of symptoms revealed a filling defect in the antral portion of the stomach. Operation disclosed the presence of a carcinoma of the stomach that had already penetrated the serosal surface. A partial gastrectomy was performed and the patient was largely asymptomatic for about a year. After this time his health declined steadily until he died of his carcinoma in late 1956, one and one-half years after its discovery.

Comment. This case illustrates many interesting points that are considered typical of pernicious anemia. When first seen, the patient was an elderly man with a severe anemia without significant weight loss. The anemia was macrocytic, and was associated with leukopenia, thrombocytopenia, a megaloblastic bone marrow, and histamine-fast achlorhydria. The diagnosis of pernicious anemia was established by the response to specific therapy. Neurologic disease was never a problem. After being well for nearly eight years, the patient developed a carcinoma of the stomach which proved fatal in less than two years. The incidence of carcinoma of the stomach in patients with pernicious anemia has been reported to be several times that in the general population. The difficulty in dealing with the problem is shown by this patient. Radiographic study of the upper gastrointestinal tract was performed every 12 to 18 months, and yet the patient had an incurable carcinoma which was recognized only one month after the onset of vague gastrointestinal complaints.

LESS COMMON CAUSES OF VITAMIN B$_{12}$ DEFICIENCY

Dietary deficiency.   Vitamin B$_{12}$ deficiency that results solely from an inadequate intake is extremely rare in the Western world. The absorption of only a minute amount, about 1 microgram a day, is required by an adult. Very strict vegetarians are candidates for a deficiency of vitamin B$_{12}$, but rarely develop it.

Malabsorption.

Postgastrectomy.   Total gastrectomy, which removes the organ of secretion of the intrinsic factor, produces the clinical picture of pernicious anemia if the patient survives until the body stores of vitamin B$_{12}$ have been depleted. This usually requires three or four years. Patients who have had a total gastrectomy require the regular administration of vitamin B$_{12}$, just as do patients with pernicious anemia. Partial gastrectomy sometimes interferes with vitamin B$_{12}$ absorption, but rarely produces a clinical deficiency because the intrinsic factor is secreted in the cardiac portion of the stomach. Nevertheless, some patients, possibly because of partial atrophy of the gastric remnant, have suboptimal vitamin B$_{12}$ serum levels and should receive supplements of this factor. In one series of 187 patients studied from six to 20 years after partial gastrectomy, the incidence of vitamin B$_{12}$ deficiency was 3.5 per cent in those with duodenal ulcer and 22.8 per cent in those who had gastric ulcer.[93] In another series, low serum vitamin B$_{12}$ levels were found in 62 of 82 patients from one to 22 years after partial gastrectomy; in two-thirds of these the Schilling test was normal.[78]

Blind loops, and fistulae.   Impaired absorption of vitamin B$_{12}$ sometimes occurs in patients with ileitis and in those who have had extensive surgical resections of the small bowel, but this malabsorption is rarely severe enough to produce megaloblastic anemia. A more severe deficiency occurs in certain patients with fistulae, diverticula, blind loops, and strictures of the small intestine; in such patients the defective absorption appears to be related in some way to the bacterial flora of the intestine, since the ability to absorb vitamin B$_{12}$ is restored by treatment with tetracycline administered by the oral route but is not corrected by supplements of intrinsic factor.[49] Severe prolonged diarrhea, sprue, and other malabsorption syndromes are much more likely to produce severe folic acid deficiency accompanied by only mild and often insignificant vitamin B$_{12}$ deficiency.

Other uncommon causes of malabsorption of vitamin B$_{12}$ are folate deficiency and the ingestion of ethanol, neomycin, colchicine or para-amino salicylic acid.[24]

Fish tapeworm infestation.   A disease found mainly in Finland, Norway, and Sweden with the hematologic and neurologic manifestations identical to those seen in pernicious anemia occurs in some of the individuals who are infected with the fish tapeworm, Diphyllobothrium latum.[9] Approximately 2 per cent of those infested have anemia; in 50 per cent the serum B$_{12}$ level is low.[88] Apparently the tapeworms produce the deficiency by competing successfully for the available vitamin B$_{12}$ or by interfering with its absorption, because elimination of the parasites without other treatment is followed by recovery.

Transcobalamin Deficiency.   The clinical picture of vitamin B$_{12}$ deficiency occurred in two infants three and four weeks of age, despite normal serum levels of vitamin B_{12}. A deficiency of transcobalamin II was found in the infants and in several other members of the family; hematologic remission occurred in the infants following large doses of vitamin B_{12} parenterally, 2000 micrograms per week.[33, 44]

FOLATE DEFICIENCY

DIETARY DEFICIENCY

Folate deficiency associated with a megaloblastic anemia may be the result of an inadequate diet. Tropical macrocytic anemia is perhaps the best-known example, but a similar type of anemia occurs in other parts of the world where the diet is suboptimal, particularly when it is deficient in meat and leafy vegetables. Poverty and ignorance are probably the most important causes. At times a dietary deficiency may be produced by improper cooking of food that contains folate. In the Western world, even in vegetarians, dietary deficiency of folic acid is rarely a cause of anemia; anemia of this type occurs in pregnancy because the demands of folic acid are increased; megaloblastic anemia of folate deficiency is also seen in patients with portal cirrhosis who have a grossly deficient diet that consists mainly of carbohydrate in the form of alcohol. Treatment with a small amount of folic acid, 100 micrograms by mouth, has been recommended because a larger dose may obscure a coexisting deficiency of vitamin B_{12}.[53] Treatment with this dose of folic acid while the patient follows a diet low in folate (avoidance of liver, fresh fruits, fruit juices, and green vegetables) may be a diagnostic procedure; a reticulocyte response that peaks in ten days is a positive result.

MALABSORPTION SYNDROMES

Although some authors believe that idiopathic sprue (adult celiac disease, nontropical sprue), childhood celiac disease, and tropical sprue are but variants of the same disease, most writers distinguish tropical sprue from idiopathic sprue, and consider that the latter disorder may become manifest either in childhood as "celiac disease" or in adult life as "nontropical" sprue. In addition, the malabsorption syndrome may arise secondary to diseases of the small bowel. A classification is presented in Table 4–3.

If the absorption of vitamin B_{12} or folic acid is impaired sufficiently, a hematologic picture identical to that seen in untreated pernicious anemia occurs. When megaloblastic anemia occurs in patients with the malabsorption syndrome, a deficiency of folate usually is responsible; megaloblastic anemia rarely develops in the secondary malabsorption disorders. Iron deficiency anemia occurs in some patients with the malabsorption syndrome as a result of blood loss from the gastrointestinal tract, or from impaired absorption of iron.

In order to establish a diagnosis in a patient with suspected malabsorption

Table 4–3 *Malabsorption in the Small Bowel*

A. Primary malabsorption
  1. Nontropical sprue (idiopathic sprue, celiac disease, adult celiac disease, idiopathic steatorrhea)
  2. Tropical sprue

B. Secondary syndromes
  1. Lymphoma
  2. Whipple's disease
  3. Collagen disease
  4. Operative resection of the small bowel
  5. Others

syndrome, various examinations may be necessary. These include the following: measure of the amount of fat in the stools; determination of the levels of serum calcium, iron, cholesterol, and carotene; the d-xylose and vitamin A absorption tests; and roentgenographic study of the small intestine. Jejunal biopsy often provides very valuable information.

Nontropical Sprue

An increasing amount of evidence indicates that celiac disease in childhood and adult idiopathic steatorrhea (or nontropical sprue) are the same disease. The disorder is probably an inherited defect in absorption. In most patients improvement follows the exclusion of the gluten-containing foods, wheat, rye, and barley from the diet.

Nontropical sprue is usually a chronic disorder. Persistent or recurrent diarrhea occurs in the vast majority of patients, but malabsorption sometimes occurs in the absence of diarrhea. In one series of 94 patients with idiopathic sprue seen at the Mt. Sinai Hospital in New York[1] diarrhea, weakness, and weight loss each occurred in 80 per cent; about one-half had glossitis; flatulence, abdominal discomfort, anorexia, nausea, and vomiting were found in 20 to 30 per cent. In the same series about 25 per cent of the patients had tetany and abnormal bleeding (ecchymoses, epistaxis, melena, hematuria, menorrhagia, gingival bleeding) secondary to prothrombin deficiency; less than 20 per cent of the patients had paresthesias, bone pain, mental symptoms, and fever. The commonest abnormality seen on the physical examination was emaciation, which occurred in 65 per cent. Abdominal distention, edema, hepatomegaly, hypotension, tetany, and bleeding each had an incidence of from 20 to 35 per cent. Other abnormalities which had a frequency of about 10 per cent or less were pigmentation, lymphadenopathy, dry skin, splenomegaly, abdominal tenderness, absent reflexes, paresthesias, and sensory disturbances. Rarely, patients with long-standing disease develop signs of severe posterior column involvement that does not respond to treatment with vitamin B_{12}, folic acid, or liver extract.

Various types of anemia develop as the result of blood loss or defective absorption of factors essential for normal erythropoiesis. The reported incidence of macrocytic anemia in idiopathic sprue varies from 14 to 95 per cent, and the incidence of iron deficiency from 6 to 17 per cent.[1] In one series macrocytosis was present in 57.6 per cent, normal erythrocytes in 33 per cent, and hypochromic cells in 9.4 per cent. Hemoglobin levels of less than 10 grams per 100 ml. occurred in 51 per cent. In children the anemia is usually hypochromic and microcytic. Adults sometimes develop iron deficiency anemia in the absence of diarrhea, a circumstance in which malabsorption may not be suspected.

Although a deficiency of folate is usually responsible for the megaloblastic anemia, abnormalities in vitamin B_{12} absorption occur often and are sometimes of clinical importance. In a group of 25 patients with idiopathic sprue, 20 were found to have impaired absorption of vitamin B_{12} that did not improve when intrinsic factor was administered.[89] In another study, lowered serum vitamin B_{12} levels were found in about one-third of the patients with steatorrhea.[84] The absorption of vitamin B_{12} in the presence of added intrinsic factor has been found to improve after administration of corticosteroids.[37] Impaired absorption of folic acid has been shown to occur commonly in idiopathic steatorrhea.[34]

Treatment of the patient with nontropical sprue generally entails use of a gluten-free diet for at least six months, plus treatment for specific deficiencies. The administration of folic acid orally or intramuscularly in doses of 5 to 15 mg. a day usually produces a good hematologic response; smaller amounts, 0.5 to 1.0 mg. by mouth, are probably adequate.[53] Most patients are refractory to treatment with vitamin B_{12} parenterally,[55] but some respond at least partially. The response of the individual patient probably depends on the state of the vitamin B_{12} stores and the degree of folate deficiency; when both substances are deficient both folic acid and parenteral vitamin B_{12} are necessary. Gastrointestinal symptoms usually persist or recur, despite improvement in the blood, if treatment consists only of administration of both folic acid and vitamin B_{12}. The majority of patients become symptom-free on the gluten-free diet, but even in these patients the persistence of some malabsorptive defect has been demonstrated. The inability of the intestinal tract to absorb vitamin B_{12} and folic acid sometimes persists whether the patient is in remission or relapse;[1] continued treatment with these vitamins and also iron may be necessary. Acutely ill patients and those with the more severe or resistant forms of the disease are usually treated with prednisone, or a related compound, which produces striking improvement in all the manifestations of the disease. The initial dose of prednisone, 50 to 60 mg. a day, is usually necessary for a week or two; the amount is then reduced to a maintenance dosage, often no more than 5 mg. a day, which may be necessary for years.

Tropical Sprue

Tropical sprue is seen most frequently in people living in the Caribbean region and in parts of Asia. The nature of the disorder is puzzling because folate deficiency develops despite a diet that may be high in folate activity. The onset of tropical sprue may be sudden, but if the disorder has persisted for some time the clinical manifestations may closely resemble those usually seen in nontropical sprue; however, the disorders differ in some important details.

In tropical sprue, the usual hematologic picture is one that is indistinguishable from pernicious anemia and that responds to treatment with folic acid or vitamin B_{12} or both. In addition there are often striking improvement in appetite, weight, sense of well-being, and the gastrointestinal symptoms, a return of folate absorption to normal, and renewal of intestinal villi, changes that are rarely if ever seen in nontropical sprue. Although the appearance of the small intestinal mucosa improves in a prompt and striking manner after treatment with folic acid or vitamin B_{12}, it is incomplete; both the morphologic abnormalities in the villi and some degree of malabsorption persist.[112] These observations suggest that the deficiencies of folate and vitamin B_{12} found in patients with tropical sprue are the result of malabsorption rather than the cause; the nature of the basic lesion responsible for the malabsorption has not been determined. It has also been demonstrated that treatment with tetracycline and other antibiotics is often effective in tropical sprue, but ineffective in nontropical sprue.[42] The gluten-free diet which has been shown to be effective in the majority of patients with nontropical sprue has not been shown to be effective in tropical sprue.

Other Causes of Malabsorption

DRUGS

Oral contraceptives.   Malabsorption of folate has been reported after oral contraceptive therapy,[85, 118] but another study showed no effect on folate levels.[90] A study of patients taking orally-administered contraceptives for at least a year indicated that their serum folate level was lower than that in the controls, although the absorption of monoglutamic folate was equal in the two groups. The results suggest that orally-administered contraceptives interfere with the absorption of polyglutamic folate. Whether this effect is through enzyme inhibition or through some other mechanism is uncertain.[110] In one study, the serum folate level was accompanied by low levels of vitamin B_{12}; the latter were not altered by treatment with folate, and both the mechanism and the significance of the lowered levels remain unexplained.[118] "Megaloblastic" cervicovaginal cells were found in 19 per cent of women taking oral contraceptives, although levels of serum folate and vitamin B_{12} were normal. The abnormality in the cells disappeared after folate therapy.[122] The malabsorption is rarely severe enough to produce clinical disease.

Anticonvulsant drugs.   Over 50 cases of megaloblastic anemia associated with anticonvulsant drug therapy have been reported since Badenoch called attention to the entity in the English literature in 1954.[3, 31, 35, 52] Diphenylhydantoin sodium, primidone, phenobarbital derivatives, and more recently a preparation containing aspirin, salicylamide, and caffeine have been the associated drugs.[123] Nearly all the patients who developed the anemia had been taking the drugs for long periods, usually for years, but it has been reported after only six months of treatment. The peripheral blood is characterized by a macrocytic anemia, leukopenia with multisegmented granulocytes, and thrombocytopenia. Although the pathogenesis of the syndrome is not entirely understood, several explanations have been suggested. One postulates that the anemia is a manifestation of folate deficiency produced by the drug's acting as a competitive inhibitor of some enzyme system normally involving folic acid as a cofactor; another that the drug displaces folate from its plasma carrier; a third suggestion is that the drug, by inhibiting intestinal conjugases, in some way interferes with absorption of folate.[64, 98] In any event an inadequate dietary intake, particularly of folic acid and ascorbic acid, may be a contributing factor.

Recovery from the anemia has followed withdrawal of the drug; recovery also has followed treatment with even small amounts of folic acid, vitamin B$_{12}$, or a combination of the two vitamins. The anemia nearly always responds to the administration of folic acid, even if the anticonvulsant drug is continued. Mild or moderate deficiency of vitamin B$_{12}$ may occur in this group of patients, but significant vitamin B$_{12}$ deficiency is unusual. In one patient, however, the serum vitamin B$_{12}$ level was zero despite normal transcobalamin levels and a normal Schilling test.[27]

Folate antagonists. Megaloblastic anemia may be produced in patients with leukemia or other forms of lymphoma who are treated with antifolic compounds such as aminopterin, amethopterin, 6MP, 5-fluorouracil, and cytosine arabinoside; such patients may develop macrocytic anemia, megaloblastic bone marrow, and the other changes associated with folic acid deficiency, as well as gastrointestinal symptoms of glossitis and diarrhea.

Megaloblastosis has occurred during the administration of pyrimethamine; apparently the drug acts as an antifolate.[116]

Alcohol. Folate deficiency, megaloblastosis and anemia occur commonly in alcoholics, particularly those with liver disease and a poor diet.[29, 48] Megaloblastic hematopoiesis, which does not develop until the folate stores are depleted, apparently precedes abnormalities in the peripheral blood by one or two weeks (See Chapter 8).

INADEQUATE UTILIZATION OF FOLIC ACID

Associated Ascorbic Acid Deficiency

Megaloblastic anemia with the blood picture characteristic of vitamin B$_{12}$ or folate deficiency sometimes is seen in infants between the ages of two and 17 months.[127] The onset is insidious, with increasing pallor, failure to gain weight, recurrent fever, inconstant diarrhea, and, occasionally, episodes of abnormal bleeding. Premature infants are more liable to the disorder, which develops if the milk used for infant feeding has a low folate content; added factors of rapid growth and diarrhea may be contributory. A deficiency of ascorbic acid is also apparently a factor in the development of this syndrome; the powdered milk preparations used by patients with this disorder had a low content of ascorbic acid, and the disorder has almost disappeared since the foods have been fortified with ascorbic acid. The anemia responds to treatment with folic acid in doses of 10 to 30 mg. orally or parenterally, but at times simultaneous administration of ascorbic acid is necessary.

EXCESSIVE DEMANDS

Megaloblastic anemia develops when the demand for folate exceeds the supply. In pregnancy the daily requirement of folate is probably 400 micrograms, more than the usual American or European diet contains.[111, 124] The appearance of increased numbers of hypersegmented neutrophils in the peripheral blood is often the first evidence of folate deficiency.[20] When a physician prescribes a vitamin supplement to correct or prevent this deficiency during pregnancy he must be careful to select a preparation that contains adequate folate, because many multivitamin preparations contain no folate.

Severe hemolytic anemia may produce megaloblastic anemia because of the large amounts of folate required for the dividing marrow cells.

Folate deficiency and megaloblastic hematopoiesis have been observed in patients with chronic renal disease, particularly those who are receiving long-term hemodialysis. Serum vitamin B_{12} levels were normal and serum folate levels were low; it appeared that folate was removed by dialysis whereas vitamin B_{12} was not.[50]

References

1. Adlersberg, D.: The Malabsorption Syndrome. Grune and Stratton, New York, 1957.
2. Ardeman, S., and Chanarin, I.: Steroids and addisonian pernicious anemia. N. Engl. J. Med., *273*:1352, 1965.
3. Badenoch, J.: The use of labelled vitamin B_{12} and gastric biopsy in the investigation of anaemia. Proc. Roy. Soc. Med., *47*:426, 1954.
4. Baker, S. J., Jacob, E., Rajan, K. T., and Swaminathan, S. P.: Vitamin B_{12} deficiency in pregnancy and the puerperium. Br. Med. J., *1*:1658, 1962.
5. Baugh, C. M., and Krumdieck, C. L.: Effects of phenytoin on folic-acid conjugases in man. Lancet, *2*:519, 1969.
6. Berk, L., et al.: Observations on the etiologic relationship of achylia gastrica to pernicious anemia. X. Activity of vitamin B_{12} as food (extrinsic) factor. N. Engl. J. Med.,*239*:911, 1948.
7. Bertino, J. R., and Johns, D. G.: Folate metabolism in man. Plenary session papers. Int. Soc. Hematol., 1968, p. 133.
8. Bethell, F. H., and Sturgis, C. C.: The relation of therapy in pernicious anemia to changes in the nervous system. Early and late results in a series of cases observed for periods of not less than 10 years, and early results of treatment with folic acid. Blood, *3*:57, 1948.
9. Björkenheim, G.: Neurological changes in pernicious tapeworm anaemia. Acta Med. Scand., (Suppl. 260),*140*:1, 1951.
10. Brody, E. A., Estren, S., and Herbert, V.: Coexistent pernicious anemia and malabsorption in four patients, including one whose malabsorption disappeared with vitamin B_{12} therapy. Ann. Intern. Med., *64*:1246, 1966.
11. Butterworth, C. E., Jr.: The availability of food folate. Annotation. Br. J. Haematol., *14*:339, 1968.
12. Butterworth, C. E., Santini, R., and Frommeyer, W. B.: The pteroylglutamate components of American diets as determined by chromatographic fractionation. J. Clin. Invest., *42*:1929, 1963.
13. Castle, W. B.: A century of curiosity about pernicious anemia. Tr. Am. Clin. Climatol. Assoc., *73*:54, 1961.
14. Castle, W. B.: Observations on the etiologic relationship of achylia gastrica to pernicious anemia. I. The effect of the administration to patients with pernicious anemia of the contents of the normal human stomach recovered after the ingestion of beef muscle. Am. J. Med. Sci., *178*:748, 1929.
15. Castle, W. B.: Current concepts of pernicious anemia. Am. J. Med., *48*:541, 1970.
16. Castle, W. B., Rhoads, C. P., Lawson, H. A., and Payne, G. C.: Etiology and treatment of sprue —observations on patients in Puerto Rico and subsequent experiments on animals. Arch. Intern. Med., *56*:627, 1935.
17. Castle, W. B., and Townsend, W. C.: Observations on the etiologic relationship of achylia gastrica to pernicious anemia. II. Effect of the administration to patients with pernicious anemia of beef muscle after incubation with normal human gastric juice. Am. J. Med. Sci., *178*:764, 1929.
18. Chanarin, I., Anderson, B. B., and Mollin, D. L.: The absorption of folic acid. Br. J. Haemotol., *4*:156, 1958.

19. Chanarin, I., Dacie, J. V., and Mollin, D. L.: Folic acid deficiency in haemolytic anaemia. Br. J. Haematol., 5:245, 1959.
20. Chanarin, I., Rothman, D., Ardeman, S., and Berry, V.: Some observations on the changes preceding the development of megaloblastic anaemia in pregnancy with particular reference to the neutrophil leucocytes. Br. J. Haematol., 11:557, 1965.
21. Chesterman, D. C., Cuthbertson, W. F., Jr., and Pegler, H. F.: Vitamin B$_{12}$. Excretion studies. Biochem. J., 48:li, 1951.
22. Clark, R., Tornyos, K., Herbert, V., and Twomey, J. J.: Studies on two patients with concomitant pernicious anemia and immunoglobulin deficiency. Ann. Intern. Med., 67:403, 1967.
23. Cooper, B. A., and White, J. J.: Absence of intrinsic factor from human portal plasma during Co^{57}B$_{12}$ absorption in man. Br. J. Haematol., 14:73, 1968.
24. Corcino, J. J., Waxsman, S., and Herbert, V.: Absorption and malabsorption of vitamin B$_{12}$. Am. J. Med., 48:562, 1970.
25. Davidson, L. S. P.: Refractory megaloblastic anemia. Blood, 3:107, 1948.
26. Donaldson, R. M., Mackenzie, I. L., and Trier, J. S.: Intrinsic factor mediated attachment of vitamin B$_{12}$ to brush borders and microvillous membranes of hamster intestine. J. Clin. Invest., 46:1215, 1967.
27. Dvilansky, A., and Lehman, E.: Megaloblastic anemia after anticonvulsive therapy. N. Engl. J. Med., 287:990, 1972.
28. Ehrlich, P., and Lazarus, A.: Anemia. Rebman, Ltd., London, 1910.
29. Eichner, E. R., Pierce, H. I., and Hillman, R. S.: Folate balance in dietary-induced megaloblastic anemia. N. Engl. J. Med., 284:933, 1971.
30. Fisher, J. M., and Taylor, K. B.: A comparison of autoimmune phenomena in pernicious anemia and chronic atrophic gastritis. N. Engl. J. Med., 272:499, 1965.
31. Flexner, J. M., and Hartmann, R. C.: Megaloblastic anemia associated with anticonvulsant drugs. Am. J. Med., 28:386, 1960.
32. Francois, R., Revol, L., Germain, D., Bourlier, V., Karlin, Mme., Coeur, P., Pellet, H., and Manuel, Y.: Imerslund's syndrome. Ann. Pédiatr., 43:490, 1967.
33. Gimpert, E., Jakob, M., and Hitzig, W. H.: Vitamin B$_{12}$ transport in blood. I. Congenital deficiency of transcobalamin II. Blood, 45:71, 1975.
34. Girdwood, R. H.: A folic excretion test in the investigation of intestinal absorption. Lancet, 2:53, 1953.
35. Girdwood, R. H., and Lenman, J. A. R.: Megaloblastic anemia occurring during primidone therapy. Br. Med. J., 1:146, 1956.
36. Glass, G. B. J.: Gastric intrinsic factor and its function in the metabolism of vitamin B$_{12}$. Physiol. Rev., 43:529, 1963.
37. Glass, G. B. J.: Intestinal absorption and hepatic uptake of vitamin B$_{12}$ in diseases of the gastrointestinal tract. Gastroenterology, 30:37, 1956.
38. Goldberg, L. S., Bickel, Y. B., and Fudenberg, H. H.: Immunologic approaches to malabsorption of vitamin B$_{12}$. Arch. Intern. Med., 123:397, 1969.
39. Goldberg, L. S., and Fudenberg, H. H.: The autoimmune aspects of pernicious anemia. Am. J. Med., 46:489, 1969.
40. Goodman, L. S., and Gilman, A.: The Pharmacological Basis of Therapeutics. 3rd Ed. The Macmillan Co., New York, 1965.
41. Grasbeck, R.: Nature and action of intrinsic factor. Plenary session papers. Int. Soc. Hematol., 1968, p. 124.
42. Guerra, R., Wheby, M. S., and Bayless, T. M.: Long-term antibiotic therapy in tropical sprue. Ann. Intern. Med., 63:619, 1965.
43. Haden, R. L.: Pernicious anemia from Addison to folic acid. Blood, 3:22, 1948.
44. Hakami, N., Neiman, P. E., Canellos, G. P., and Lazerson, J.: Neonatal megaloblastic anemia due to inherited transcobalamin II deficiency in two siblings. N. Engl. J. Med., 285:1163, 1971.
45. Hall, C. A.: Transcobalamins I and II as natural transport proteins of vitamin B$_{12}$. J. Clin. Invest., 56:1125, 1975.
46. Hall, C. A.: Vitamin B$_{12}$ binding proteins of man. Ann. Intern. Med., 75:297, 1971.
47. Hall, C. A., and Beebe, R. T.: Early onset of pernicious anemia in two siblings: genetic and autoimmune aspects. Br. J. Haematol., 25:751, 1973.
48. Halsted, C. H., Robles, E. A., and Mezey, E.: Decreased jejunal uptake of labeled folic acid (3H-PGA) in alcoholic patients: roles of alcohol and nutrition. N. Engl. J. Med., 285:701, 1971.
49. Halsted, J. A., Lewis, P. M., and Gasster, M.: Absorption of radioactive vitamin B$_{12}$ in the syndrome of megaloblastic anemia associated with intestinal stricture or anastomosis. Am. J. Med., 20:42, 1956.
50. Hampers, C. L., Streiff, R., Nathan, D. G., Snyder, D., and Merrill, J. P.: Megaloblastic hemato-

poiesis in uremia and in patients on long-term hemodialysis. N. Engl. J. Med., *276*:551, 1967.

51. Haurani, F. I.: Vitamin B_{12} and the megaloblastic development. Science, *182*:78, 1973.
52. Hawkins, C. F., and Meynell, M. J.: Macrocytosis and macrocytic anemia caused by anticonvulsant drugs. Q. J. Med., *27*:45, 1958.
53. Herbert, V.: Current concepts in therapy. Megaloblastic anemia. N. Engl. J. Med., *268*:368, 1963.
54. Herbert, V.: Minimal daily adult folate requirement. Arch. Intern. Med., *110*:649, 1962.
55. Herbert, V.: The Megaloblastic Anemias. Grune and Stratton, New York, 1959.
56. Herbert, V.: Annotation. Transient (reversible) malabsorption of vitamin B_{12}. Br. J. Haematol., *17*:213, 1969.
57. Herbert, V.: Cyanocobalamin (vitamin B_{12}) injection intervals in pernicious anemia. J.A.M.A., *231*:765, 1975.
58. Herbert, V., and Castle, W. B.: Intrinsic factor. N. Engl. J. Med., *270*:1181, 1964.
59. Herbert, V., Larrabee, A. R., and Buchanan, J. M.: Studies on the identification of a folate compound of human serum. J. Clin. Invest., *41*:1134, 1962.
60. Herbert, V., Streiff, R. B., and Sullivan, L. W.: Notes on vitamin B_{12} absorption, auto-immunity and childhood pernicious anemia. Medicine, *43*:679, 1964.
61. Hicks, M., and Leavell, B. S.: Pernicious anemia in the American Negro. Ann. Intern. Med., *33*:1438, 1950.
62. Hines, J. D.: Reversible megaloblastic and sideroblastic marrow abnormalities in alcoholic patients. Br. J. Haematol., *16*:87, 1969.
63. Hodgkin, D., et al.: Structure of vitamin B_{12}. Nature, *178*:64, 1956.
64. Huffbrand, A. V., and Necheles, T. F.: Mechanism of folate deficiency in patients receiving phenytoin. Lancet, *2*:528, 1968.
65. Isaacs, R., and Friedman, A.: Standards for maximum reticulocyte percentage after intramuscular liver therapy in pernicious anemia. Am. J. Med. Sci., *196*:718, 1938.
66. Israels, M. C. G., and Wilkinson, J. F.: New observations on the aetiology and prognosis of achrestic anaemia. Q. J. Med., *9*:163, 1940.
67. Israels, M. C. G., and Wilkinson, J. F.: Achrestic anaemia. Q. J. Med., *5*:69, 1936.
68. IUPAC-IUB Commission on Biochemical Nomenclature: Tentative rules. J. Biol. Chem., *241*:2987, 1966.
69. Jeffries, G. H.: Recovery of gastric mucosal structures and function in pernicious anemia during prednisone therapy. Gastroenterology, *45*:371, 1965.
70. Jeffries, G. H.: Parietal cell antibodies. Editorial. Ann. Intern. Med., *63*:717, 1965.
71. Jeffries, G. H., Hoskins, D. W., and Sleisenger, M. H.: Antibody to intrinsic factor in serum from patients with pernicious anemia. J. Clin. Invest., *41*:1106, 1962.
72. Kaplan, H. S., and Rigler, L. G.: Pernicious anemia and carcinoma of the stomach — autopsy studies concerning their interrelationship. Am. J. Med. Sci., *209*:339, 1945.
73. Katz, M., Lee, S. K., and Cooper, B.: Vitamin B_{12} malabsorption due to a biologically inert intrinsic factor. N. Engl. J. Med., *287*:425, 1972.
74. Lawrence, C.: B_{12}-binding protein deficiency in pernicious anemia. Blood, *27*:389, 1966.
75. Lawson, D. H., Murray, R. M., and Parker, J. L. W.: Early mortality in the megaloblastic anemias. Q. J. Med., *41*:1, 1972.
76. Lindenbaum, J., Pezzimenti, J. F., and Shea, N.: Small-intestinal function in vitamin B_{12} deficiency. Ann. Intern. Med., *80*:326, 1974.
77. MacKenzie, I. L., Donaldson, R. M., Jr., Trier, J. S., and Mathan, V. I.: Mucosa in familial selective vitamin B_{12} malabsorption. N. Engl. J. Med., *286*:1021, 1972.
78. Mahmud, K., Ripley, D., and Doscherholmen, A.: Vitamin B_{12} absorption tests. J.A.M.A., *216*:1167, 1971.
79. Major, R. H.: Classic Descriptions of Disease. 3rd Ed. Charles C Thomas, Springfield, Ill., 1955.
80. Mason, J. D., and Leavell, B. S.: The effect of transfusions of erythrocytes on untreated pernicious anemia. Blood, *11*:632, 1956.
81. Maugh, T. H. II: Vitamin B_{12}: after 25 years, the first synthesis. Science, *179*:266, 1973.
82. McIntyre, O. R., Sullivan, L. W., Jeffries, G. H., and Silver, R. H.: Pernicious anemia in childhood. N. Engl. J. Med., *272*:981, 1965.
83. Minot, G. R., and Murphy, W. P.: Treatment of perncious anemia by special diet. J.A.M.A., *87*:470, 1926.
84. Mollin, D. L., and Ross, G. I. M.: Vitamin B_{12} deficiency in the megaloblastic anemias. Proc. Roy. Soc. Med., *47*:428, 1954.
85. Necheles, T. F., and Snyder, L. M.: Malabsorption of folate associated with oral contraceptive therapy. N. Engl. J. Med., *282*:858, 1970.
86. Nixon, R. F., and Bertino, J. R.: Interrelationships of vitamin B_{12} and folate in man. Am. J. Med., *48*:555, 1970.

87. Norcross, J. W., Monroe, S. E., and Griffin, B. G.: The development of gastric carcinoma in pernicious anemia. Ann. Intern. Med., 37:338, 1952.
88. Nyberg, W., Gräsbeck, R., Saarni, M., and Von Bonsdorff, B.: Serum vitamin B$_{12}$ levels and incidence of tapeworm anemia in a population heavily infected with *Diphyllobothrium latum.* Am. J. Clin. Nutr., 9:606, 1961.
89. Oxenhorn, S., Estren, S., Wasserman, L. R., and Adlersberg, D.: Malabsorption syndrome: Intestinal absorption of vitamin B$_{12}$. Ann. Intern. Med., 48:30, 1958.
90. Paine, C. J., Grafton, W. D., Dickson, V. L., and Eichner, E. R.: Oral contraceptives, serum folate, and hematologic status. J.A.M.A., 231:731, 1975.
91. Perillie, P. E., Kaplan, S. S., and Finch, S. C.: Significance of changes in serum muramidase activity in megaloblastic anemia. N. Engl. J. Med., 277:10, 1967.
92. Pritchard, J. A., Scott, D. E., and Whalley, P. J.: Folic acid requirements in pregnancy-induced megaloblastic anemia. J.A.M.A., 208:1163, 1969.
93. Pryor, J. P., O'Shea, M. J., Brooks, P. L., and Datar, G. K.: The long-term metabolic consequences of partial gastrectomy. Am. J. Med., 51:5, 1971.
94. Rabinowitz, J. C., and Himes, R. H.: Folic acid coenzymes. Fed. Proc., 19:963, 1960.
95. Register, U. D., and Sarett, H. P.: Urinary excretion of vitamin B$_{12}$ folic acid, and citrovorum factor in human subjects on various diets. Proc. Soc. Exp. Biol. Med., 77:837, 1951.
96. Rickes, E. L., Brink, N. G., Koniuszy, F. R., Wood, T. R., and Folkers, K.: Crystalline vitamin B$_{12}$. Science, 107:396, 1948.
97. Rigler, L. G., Kaplan, H. S., and Fink, D. L.: Pernicious anemia and the early diagnosis of tumors of the stomach. J.A.M.A., 128:426, 1945.
98. Rosenberg, I. H., Streiff, R. R., Godwin, H. A., and Castle, W. B.: Absorption of polyglutamic folate: participation of deconjugating enzymes of the intestinal mucosa. N. Engl. J. Med., 280:985, 1969.
99. Ross, J. F., Belding, H., and Paegel, B. L.: The development and progression of subacute combined degeneration of the spinal cord in patients with pernicious anemia treated with synthetic pteroylglutamic (folic) acid. Blood, 3:68, 1948.
100. Rundles, R. W.: Prognosis in neurologic manifestations of pernicious anemia. Blood, 1:209, 1946.
101. Schade, S. G., et al.: Occurrence in gastric juices of antibody to a complex of intrinsic factor and vitamin B$_{12}$. N. Engl. J. Med., 275:528, 1966.
102. Schilling, R. F.: Intrinsic factor studies. II. The effect of gastric juice on the urinary excretion of radioactivity after the oral administration of radioactive vitamin B$_{12}$. J. Lab. Clin. Med., 42:860, 1953.
103. Schwartz, S. O., Friedman, I. A., and Gant, H. L.: Long-term evaluation of vitamin B$_{12}$ in treatment of pernicious anemia. J.A.M.A., 157:229, 1955.
104. Sheehy, T. W., Rubini, M. E., Perez-Santiago, E., Santini, R. J., and Haddock, J.: The effect of "minute" and "titrated" amounts of folic acid on the megaloblastic anemia of tropical sprue. Blood, 18:623, 1961.
105. Silberstein, E. B.: The Schilling test. J.A.M.A., 208:2325, 1969.
106. Smith, E. L.: Vitamin B$_{12}$. Methuen & Co., London, 1960.
107. Smith, E. L.: Purification of antipernicious anemia factors from liver. Nature, 161:638, 1948.
108. Spector, J. I.: Juvenile achlorhydric pernicious anemia with IgA deficiency. J.A.M.A., 228:334, 1974.
109. Spurling, C. L., Sacks, M. S., and Jiji, R. M.: Juvenile pernicious anemia. N. Engl. J. Med., 271:995, 1964.
110. Streiff, R. F.: Folate deficiency and oral contraceptives. J.A.M.A., 214:105, 1970.
111. Strieff, R. R., and Little, A. B.: Folic acid deficiency in pregnancy. N. Engl. J. Med., 276:776, 1967.
112. Swanson, V. L., Wheby, M. S., and Bayless, T. M.: Morphologic effects of folic acid and vitamin B$_{12}$ on the jejunal lesion of tropical sprue. Am. J. Pathol., 49:167, 1966.
113. Taylor, K. B., Roitt, I. M., Doniach, D., Couchman, K. G., and Shapland, C.: Autoimmune phenomena in pernicious anaemia: gastric antibodies. Br. Med. J., 2:1347, 1962.
114. Twomey, J. J., Jordan, P. H., Jarrold, T., Trubowitz, S., Ritz, N. D., and Conn, H. O.: The syndrome of immunoglobulin deficiency and pernicious anemia: a study of ten cases. Am. J. Med., 47:340, 1969.
115. Waters, A. H., and Mollin, D. L.: Studies on folic acid activity of human serum. J. Clin. Pathol., 14:335, 1961.
116. Waxman, S., and Herbert, V.: Mechanism of pyrimethamine-induced megaloblastosis in human bone marrow. N. Engl. J. Med., 280:1316, 1969.
117. Waxman, S., Metz, J., and Herbert, V.: Defective DNA synthesis in human megaloblastic bone marrow: effects of homocysteine and methionine. J. Clin. Invest., 48:284, 1969.

118. Wertalik, L. F., Metz, E. N., LoBuglio, A. F., and Balcerzak, S. P.: Decreased serum B_{12} levels with oral contraceptive use. J.A.M.A., *221*:1371, 1972.

119. Wheby, M. S., and Bayles, T. M.: Intrinsic factor in tropical sprue. Blood, *31*:817, 1968.

120. Whipple, G. N., and Robscheit-Robbins, F. S.: Favorable influence of liver, heart, and skeletal muscle in diet on blood regeneration in anemia. Am. J. Physiol., *72*:408, 1925.

121. Whitby, L. E. H., and Britton, C. J. C.: Disorders of the Blood. 5th Ed. The Blakiston Co., Philadelphia, 1946.

122. Whitehead, N., Reyner, F., and Lindenbaum, J.: Megaloblastic changes in the cervical epithelium. J.A.M.A., *226*:1421, 1973.

123. Williams, J. O., Mengel, C. E., Sullivan, L. W., and Hag, A. S.: Megaloblastic anemia associated with chronic ingestion of an analgesic. N. Engl. J. Med., *280*:312, 1969.

124. Willoughby, M. L. N.: An investigation of folic acid requirements in pregnancy. Br. J. Haematol., *13*:503, 1967.

125. Wilson, T. H.: Membrane transport of vitamin B_{12}. Medicine, *43*:669, 1964.

126. Zamcheck, N., Grable, E., Ley, A. B., and Norman, L.: Occurrence of gastric cancer among patients with pernicious anemia at the Boston City Hospital. N. Engl. J. Med., *252*:1103, 1955.

127. Zuelzer, W. W., and Ogden, F. N.: Metaloblastic anemia of infancy. Am. J. Dis. Child., *71*:211, 1946.

CHAPTER 5

DISORDERS OF IRON METABOLISM

IRON METABOLISM

Iron is an essential element in many of the physiological processes in the body. It combines with protoporphyrin to form heme and with various proteins to form many important enzymes, such as catalase, cytochrome, and peroxidase. Since iron plays an essential role in hemoglobin metabolism, some knowledge of iron metabolism is necessary for the understanding and proper management of many of the problems of anemia seen in clinical practice. The history of iron in medicine has been reviewed by Fowler[58] and excellent summaries and monographs have been published.

The total quantity of iron in the body of an adult is determined largely by the size of the subject and the level of the circulating hemoglobin (Table 5–1). The normal range is from 3.0 to 5.0 gm. The iron is distributed as follows: hemoglobin, from 1.5 to 3.0 gm.; myoglobin, catalase, and cytochrome, about 300 mg.; plasma, 3 to 4 mg.; storage iron, 600 to 1600 mg.[47, 49, 69, 118, 166] A Committee on Iron Deficiency of the Council on Food and Nutrition in the United

Table 5–1 *Iron Values in the Human Adult, According to Various Authors*[47, 49, 64, 69, 118]

Daily dietary intake	12–15 mg.
Daily absorption	0.6–1.5 mg.
Total body iron	3.0–5.0 gm.
Hemoglobin iron	1.5–3.0 gm.
Storage iron	1.0–1.5 gm.
Parenchymatous iron	0.1–0.3 gm.
Daily loss, males	0.5–1.5 mg.
Daily loss, females	1.0–2.5 mg.
Daily loss, pregnant females	1.0 mg.

Table 5-2 *Estimated Dietary Iron Requirements*

	ABSORBED IRON REQUIREMENT (mg./day)	DAILY FOOD REQUIREMENT* (mg./day)
Normal men and nonmenstruating women	0.5–1	5–10
Menstruating women	0.7–2	7–20
Pregnant women	2–4.8	20–48†
Adolescents	1–2	10–20
Children	0.4–1	4–10
Infants	0.5–1.5	5–15‡

*Assuming 10 per cent absorption.
†This amount of iron cannot be derived from diet and should be met by iron supplementation in the latter half of pregnancy.
‡15 mg. is the maximum.
(Reprinted from J.A.M.A., *203*:407, 1968.)

States considered the following values to be normal: Total—70 kg. man, approximately 3.5 gm.; woman, 2.3 gm. Storage iron—men, 1000 mg.; women, 200 to 400 mg.[32] The daily iron requirement for members of both sexes of different ages has recently been estimated as shown in Table 5-2.[32]

The quantity of iron in the body is regulated by the amount of iron that is absorbed. There is no balanced mechanism of absorption and excretion like that which exists for many metals, such as calcium and sodium. This was first shown in 1937 by Widdowson and McCance.[165] They studied the urinary and fecal excretion of iron by two men and two women on a low iron intake, on a very high iron intake of 1000 mg. a day, and when they were again placed on a low iron intake. It was observed that on the low iron intake practically all of the ingested iron was recovered in the feces, and the subjects were considered to be "in balance." During the high iron intake period, when each subject ingested 1000 mg. per day for 36 to 40 days, it was calculated that each individual absorbed from 2000 to 5000 mg. of iron without any significant increase in the hemoglobin levels. When the subjects were again placed on a low iron intake of 7 to 10 mg. a day for a period of eight to ten days, they excreted all of the iron ingested during that time but none of the iron that was absorbed during the preceding period of high iron intake. From these studies it was concluded that the intestine cannot significantly alter the iron stores by varying the amount excreted in the feces; except in pregnancy and when bleeding occurs, the quantity of iron in the body is determined by the amount that is absorbed.

DIETARY SOURCES OF IRON

The amount of iron in the diet is only one factor that determines its usefulness; even more important is the facility with which it can be absorbed. The average daily diet of adults in the Western world contains from 10 to 30 mg. of iron. Muscle meats, eggs, legumes, wheat, and leafy vegetables contain more iron than fruit, potatoes, or rice; milk contains very little iron and refined sugar has none. Information about the availability of dietary iron has been provided by studies that utilized the incorporation of tracer iron into various foodstuffs.[29, 119, 140] These studies have shown that hemoglobin and liver are rich sources of iron; eggs and greens are relatively poor. Normal adults absorb from 5 to 10 per cent of the dietary iron, and adults with iron deficiency absorb from 10 to 20 per cent.[119, 125] About 1 mg. of iron is absorbed from an average daily diet by a normal adult; adults with severe iron deficiency anemia are unable to absorb more than 4 or 5 mg. of iron from a normal diet.[56] Comparable values have been found in children. In a group of normal children below 5 years of age, the mean absorption of tracer iron incorporated in eggs, cereal, rice, chicken liver, and whole milk was between 8 and 12 per cent. An average of 18 per cent was absorbed from eggs by children with iron deficiency. Children from 5 to 15 years of age and adults absorbed iron from eggs and whole milk less well than did the younger children. Absorption of 10 per cent of the iron contained in an optimal diet should meet the need for iron during the period of maximal growth.[140]

Iron absorption in humans has been difficult to measure accurately because of variations that exist between one normal person and another, and from day to day in the same person. Studies of absorption of food iron in 131 individuals made in a way designed to minimize these variations showed relatively low absorption of the iron (1.7 to 7.9 per cent) in wheat, corn, black beans, lettuce, and spinach, compared to the absorption from soy beans, fish, veal, and hemoglobin (15 to 20 per cent).[35]

ABSORPTION OF IRON

The quantity of iron that is absorbed after ingestion is determined by factors such as the amount and type of iron in the lumen of the intestine, the presence or absence of food, the nature of the food, the state of the iron stores in the body, the activity of the bone marrow, the secretions of the pancreas, and the function of the intestinal mucosa.

Both the quantity and the chemical state of the iron in the gastrointestinal tract influence absorption. Whippel[164] and others[15] have demonstrated that increasing the amount of iron ingested increases the amount that is absorbed, even though the percentage of absorption is smaller with larger amounts. Ferrous iron is absorbed better than ferric iron; in man and in most animals iron is absorbed mainly in the ferrous form.[118, 148]

The absorption of dietary iron has been studied by chemical analysis of the diet and feces,[92] by measuring the absorption of radioisotopic iron incorporated in foods such as eggs, muscle meat, vegetables, and bread during their production,[119] and by measuring the absorption of radioactive iron that has been mixed with food.[29, 125] Many factors influence the absorptive process. The presence of food affects the absorption of iron significantly; merely mixing ferrous salt with food before ingestion reduces the absorption of the iron by approximately 50 per cent,[29, 125, 146] possibly through the mechanical effect of the food. The iron–phosphorus ratio of the meal may be a factor; higher ratios favor absorption at certain levels of phosphorus in the diet. Large amounts of ascorbic acid and probably other reducing substances promote absorption.[119] Phytates inhibit movement of inorganic iron from the lumen because they bind the iron, but they are not an important factor in the absorption of food iron. Pancreatic secretions apparently inhibit iron absorption, and a deficiency may enhance absorption in certain disorders such as cirrhosis of the liver or chronic pancreatitis.[22]

Although iron probably can be absorbed from any part of the gastrointestinal tract, absorption is greatest in the duodenum, and diminishes progressively in the more distal portion of the bowel; the absorption of food iron occurs mainly if not exclusively in the duodenum.[19] The molecule of hemoglobin iron, an important dietary source of iron in meat, apparently enters the mucosal cell, where a substance that is presumably an enzyme, possibly xanthine oxidase, effects the release of iron and permits its passage from the mucosal cell into the plasma.[45]

The factors that control or influence the absorption of iron from the gut have been studied extensively. Iron deficiency, increased erythropoiesis, anoxia of high altitude, and ingestion of excessive amounts of iron all lead to increased iron absorption; increased iron stores, diminished erythropoiesis, and oxygen excess are associated with decreased absorption. An essential role in the absorptive process is played by the mucosal cell in the small intestine. The level of hemoglobin, the level of serum iron, the amount of unsaturated transferrin in the plasma, and the oxygen tension of the blood have been investigated as possible humoral factors that act as signals to the mucosal cell.

Several studies[146, 167] indicated that the relative saturation of transferrin exerts little or no control over iron absorption; another, which utilized the double isotope technique, supported the concept that the saturation of transferrin in the general circulation regulates the absorption of iron from the gastrointestinal tract.[66] The dilemma was resolved when still another study demonstrated that saturation or near-saturation of plasma transferrin in rats, dogs, and man did not significantly influence the amount of iron absorbed; the absorbed iron was deposited in the liver during the first circulation through the portal system and did not appear in the general circulation; this absorption was missed when only plasma iron in the peripheral circulation was studied.[162]

Other investigations have failed to demonstrate that the erythropoietin levels of the plasma,[98] the amount of iron stored in the liver, or the quantity excreted in the bile[161] exert any influence on iron absorption. Conflicting data have been presented concerning the influence of anemia and anoxia; observations on anemic patients with hypocellular marrows indicate that anemia per se does not lead to increased iron absorption,[125] but experiments on mice with marrow hypoplasia have shown that iron absorption increased after different types of anemia were produced, even when erythropoiesis was practically nil and adequate iron stores were maintained. Anoxia was also found to be a stimulus to iron absorption even though there was no demonstrable increase in erythropoiesis.[115] The balance of the evidence, however, seems to indicate that in man anemia and anoxia do not exert a direct effect, but may act indirectly.

The complexity of the absorptive process is also shown by studies on the influence of iron deficiency and achlorhydria. Iron deficiency is nearly always associated with an increased absorption of food iron and inorganic iron. Nevertheless the production of iron deficiency in rats has been followed by a significant change in the total acid secretion and acid concentration as compared to the normal animals.[121] Impaired iron absorption from labeled hemoglobin has been demonstrated in children with severe iron deficiency anemia, a defect that disappeared when the iron stores were replenished,[97] a similar defect was demonstrated in puppies, and the authors suggested that a decrease in the iron-containing or iron-dependent enzymes in the mucosa might produce secondary malabsorption. Although hydrochloric acid is not necessary for the absorption of inorganic ferrous iron, the acid apparently is important in the absorption of ferric iron (the type present in food). Studies on normal subjects and patients with pernicious anemia indicate that hydrochloric acid may facilitate the chelation of the ferric salts of ascorbate and other agents. Thus a deficiency in acid secretion may lead to faulty absorption of food iron by patients with achlorhydria as well as by those who have had a partial or total gastrectomy. Over a period of years such a defect may produce or contribute to iron deficiency.[138]

One concept that has been proposed to explain the regulation of iron absorption is the "mucosal block" theory, which assigns an important role to the ferritin mechanism. This theory was based mainly on two observations: first, the demonstration by Hahn et al.[65] that in dogs the oral administration of iron partially blocked the absorption of a second dose given several hours later; and second, Granick's observation that in guinea pigs oral iron stimulated the mucosal cells to produce a protein, apoferritin, which combines with iron to form ferritin.[62] It is possible that iron stimulates the production of apoferritin by binding to the apoferritin peptides on the polysomes, and thus relieves inhibition to apoferritin production.[36] According to the mucosal block theory, ferritin acted as a blocking agent. When the ferrous iron in the lumen of the intestine was in equilibrium with the ferric iron of the mucosal cells, no ferrous iron would be absorbed; after the ferric iron content of the cells was diminished by passage of iron from the mucosal ferritin into the blood stream, iron would pass from the lumen into the mucosa. At the time the theory was proposed it was known that any blocking mechanism which might exist was not completely effective, either in normal individuals or in patients with certain diseases, particularly hemochromatosis.[71, 164] Evidence against the existence of mucosal block as a physiologic mechanism was reported by Brown et al. in 1958.[19] Their studies confirmed the observation of Hahn et al. that in man a large dose of iron salt administered orally produces a partial and transient block to the absorption of a second dose of iron; however, they found that the amount of iron in the diet is too small to produce this effect. Other evidence against the mucosal block concept has been provided by animal experiments.[72] Heilmeyer gave guinea pigs 15 mg. of iron daily for 28 days and found that the amount of iron in the liver continued to increase over a period of 14 days, a time when the content of the ferritin in the stomach and small intestine was maximal. After the 14th day there was no further absorption, even though the ferritin in the mucosa of the stomach and small intestine diminished.

The function that is served by the build-up of ferritin in the mucosal cells is uncertain. Crosby and associates have reported that the ferritin iron in the epithelial cells is not absorbed but instead is sequestered and prevented from entering the circulation;[37] the iron is lost when the ferritin-containing cells are shed into the intestinal lumen. Conrad et al.[33] studied the effect of intravenously injected iron on the intestinal absorption of iron, and observed that radioactive

I
N
T
E
S
T
I
N
A
L

L
U
M
E
N

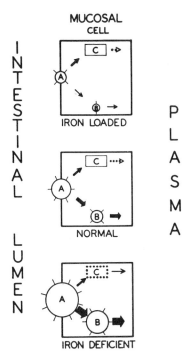

P
L
A
S
M
A

Figure 5–1 Proposed model of iron absorption. Each *square* represents a small intestinal epithelial mucosal cell. State of body iron is indicated. *A* represents the active transport mechanism for mucosal uptake of iron from intestinal lumen. *B* represents the active transport mechanism for mucosal transfer of iron to plasma. *C* represents the mechanism for temporary storage of iron. The sizes of *A* and *B* illustrate the relative transport rates. Both *A* and *B* are related to body iron requirements, but *A* is always greater than *B*. Iron is preferentially moved from *A* to *B* to plasma, but depending on the amount of iron available to *A* and the relationship of *A* to *B*, a variable portion of the iron transported by *A* moves to *C* for temporary storage. As indicated by the *dotted arrow* in normal and iron-loaded states, subsequent transfer of iron from *C* to plasma is very slow and may not occur before the cell is sloughed. *C* is *dotted* in the iron-deficient mucosal cell to indicate that the efficiency of *B* is such that storage may not occur unless large doses of iron are used. Within limits, these transport and storage mechanisms regulate the amount of iron absorbed. (From Wheby: Gastroenterology, vol. 50, 1966. Reprinted with permission of the author and the Williams and Wilkins Co.)

iron injected in this way was incorporated into the epithelial cells of the mucosa at the time the cells were formed in the crypts of Lieberkühn in normal and iron-loaded rats, but not in iron-deficient animals. They considered that the amount of this "messenger iron" in the cells might be the basis of control of iron absorption because the "messenger iron" seemed to reflect the status of the body stores; their studies indicated a correlation among the size of the dose of iron injected intravenously, the amount sequestered by the mucosal cells, and the amount of oral iron absorbed. The iron remained in the mucosal cells as they migrated toward the villous tip where they were shed. The authors concluded that the iron content of the intestinal epithelium plays an important role in the regulation of iron equilibrium in the body.

Many experiments indicate that the mucosal cell has a mechanism for transporting iron across the cell into the plasma and a mechanism for trapping iron in the mucosal cell. Although the importance of ferritin in these functions has not been defined, the model proposed by Wheby shown in Figure 5–1 provides a useful concept of the functioning of the mucosal cell. In iron deficiency the cell permits the rapid passage of dietary iron through the mucosal cell into the circulation. In iron storage disease the cell resists iron absorption but is not completely effective. In iron overload other cells, such as glandular epithelial cells and macrophages, also accumulate iron, and their subsequent desquamation increases the excretion of iron from the body.

The relationship between erythropoietic activity and absorption of iron from the gut has been studied in rats.[157] During eight days of low atmospheric pressure both erythropoiesis and iron absorption increased significantly; when the rats were restored to normal atmospheric pressure in a state of relative polycythemia, bone marrow activity and iron utilization immediately diminished, whereas deposition of iron in the mucosa of the intestine was elevated. Crosby has proposed the following sequence to explain the function of the intestinal mucosal cell in these circumstances.[38] When erythropoiesis increases because of hemorrhage or some other stimulus, more iron is utilized, plasma iron turnover accelerates, iron leaves the intestinal mucosal cells at a faster rate, and the iron content of the mucosa falls. The new epithelial cells that form in the crypts contain little iron and permit the passage of iron from the lumen; since such cells constitute practically the entire lining of the small intestine within two or three days, absorption increases until equilibrium is re-established. This hypothesis would explain the three- or four-day lag in increased iron absorption that follows bleeding, as well as the increase that occurs after bleeding and during hemolysis despite adequate or even excessive iron stores in the liver.

Although the exact mechanisms involved in the transfer of iron across the mucosal cell are unknown, iron transfer has been shown to be an active metabolic process. Dowdle et al.,[48] who utilized segments of small intestine from rats, have shown that the transport of iron across the mucosal cell can take place against a concentration gradient, is limited in capacity, and requires oxidative metabolism and the generation of phosphate bond energy. Other evidence indicates that the active transfer across the cell involves two steps, mucosal uptake and transfer to the serosal surface (or into the blood stream);[112, 113] both require oxidative metabolism. It also was observed that both divalent and trivalent iron are taken up at the mucosal surface, but that net transfer to the serosal surface (or blood stream), which is the slower step, is relatively specific for divalent iron (85 per cent). Wheby et al.[163] confirmed these findings; they injected radioiron salts into closed loops of the small intestine created in otherwise intact rats, and measured both the amount of radioactive iron in the intestinal wall after careful washing and that present in the whole carcass. They found two stages of mucosal absorption, a rapid uptake of iron from the lumen and a slower transfer of iron to the carcass; the second stage was restricted largely to the duodenal mucosa. Both steps varied inversely with the state of the body stores of iron. Absorption can be extremely rapid, as shown by the passage of radioiron through the mucosal cells within 15 seconds after injection in blind loops of iron-deficient rats; in other circumstances the mucosal cells act as temporary storage areas for the iron.

TRANSFERRIN AND THE TRANSPORT OF IRON

When it leaves the mucosal cells, iron in the ferric form is transported in the plasma attached to a beta-1-globulin, variously termed transferrin, siderophilin, iron-binding protein, or metal-binding globulin. The existence of a binding component in the serum was reported in 1945 by Holmberg and Laurell;[83] they concluded that the toxic effects of intravenously-administered iron occurred when the saturation limit of the plasma, about 300 micrograms per 100 ml., was exceeded and the surplus iron left the blood stream. In 1946, Schade and Caroline identified the protein fraction in human plasma that possesses the capacity to bind iron at physiologic pH as being a beta-1-globulin.[137] The protective effect of the protein binding of the iron in the blood has been demonstrated by means of intravenous injections of iron preparations. Poorly dissociated iron compounds, such as iron saccharide, can be given intravenously in large amounts, but easily dissociated iron compounds can be given only in small amounts, 5 to 10 mg. Larger amounts of easily dissociated iron compounds quickly saturate the total iron-binding capacity of the plasma, and the excess iron causes flushing, nausea, vomiting, shock, and even death.

Transferrin has a molecular weight of about 90,000. Each molecule combines with two molecules of ferric iron.[118] The biologic half-life of radioiodinated transferrin has been reported to be 12 days in a normal child and from 6.7 to 8.4 days in adults.[59, 94] The existence of variants in human transferrin that are under genetic control was first demonstrated by Smithies in 1957.[144] Since then at least 15 transferrins have been identified by starch gel electrophoresis.[4, 148] Only transferrin C is found in the majority of persons. The transferrin variants apparently do not differ in their ability to transport iron and deliver it to the tissues. Normally the transferrin in the plasma is about one-third saturated; the total iron-binding capacity is usually in the range of 300 to 359 micrograms per 100 ml., but the upper limit has been reported to be as high as 420.[118]

Transferrin functions not only for the transport of iron in the plasma, but also in the transfer of iron from the plasma to the developing erythrocytes. Jandl and Katz have shown that transferrin plays an important role in iron utilization by the developing normoblasts and reticulocytes, a process which involves the attachment of the transferrin molecule to the cell membrane.[89, 94, 96] The iron, which is tightly bound to the transferrin molecule, is transferred into the cell from the transferrin attached to the cell membrane in about one minute. The mechanism is energy-dependent. The rate of entry of transferrin-bound iron into erythroid cells is affected by several factors, one probably being the age

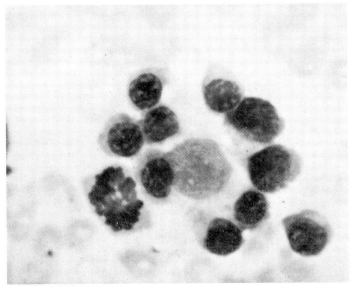

Figure 5–2   Macrophage surrounded by normoblasts in iron deficiency anemia; bone marrow aspiration. (Courtesy of Dr. S. G. Tan.)

of the cells; younger cells have a larger number of binding sites for transferrin molecules than do older cells. Another factor is the concentration of transferrin-bound iron in the surrounding medium; uptake increases as the absolute concentration of the transferrin-iron complex increases, and this is more important than its relative saturation. In addition, it has been proposed that the amount of heme in reticulocytes, and presumably in earlier cells, also regulates the entrance of iron into the cells by a feedback mechanism.[127] This interpretation is supported by the observations that the uptake of radioiron is decreased in reticulocytes incubated with heme, and that in the sideroblastic anemias, where heme synthesis is inhibited, excessive amounts of nonhemoglobin iron are found in the normoblasts and in the erythrocytes. Most of the iron is taken up by the pronormoblasts and basophilic normoblasts, and less by older nucleated cells, but some is taken up by reticulocytes.[102]

Electron microscopy has shown that early erythroid cells contain ferritin, and Bessis and Breton-Gorius have demonstrated that some ferritin is transferred directly from reticuloendothelial "nurse" cells to surrounding normoblasts; they termed the process ropheocytosis to indicate that the nutrient material is transferred by aspiration rather than by micropinocytosis.[5] The authors postulate that the iron in the marrow reticuloendothelial cells is largely that transported by transferrin, and to a lesser extent is derived from erythrophagocytosis in the marrow. Although the importance of these observations and their interpretation cannot be fully evaluated at present, the studies of Jandl and Katz,[90] and the demonstration that immature red cells assimilate iron from transferrin in vitro much more readily than do reticulum cells[101, 102] both favor the concept that the direct transfer of iron from the plasma to the young red cell is the normal mechanism. Also, it has been suggested that ferritin is being transferred from the normoblasts to the reticulum cells, rather than the reverse.[101] The nonessential role of the transferrin level in iron absorption and the apparent importance of transferrin for iron utilization in erythropoiesis were evident in studies of patients reported by Heilmeyer et al.; these patients, who had no demonstrable plasma transferrin, had a hypochromic anemia associated with greatly increased storage iron.[61, 74]

The normal plasma iron level in micrograms per 100 ml. has been reported to be 50 to 180, 80 to 160, and 43 to 210.[15, 24, 118] In the latter study the mean was 104.7 ± 3.4. In some series, the plasma iron values for males have been higher than those for females, but in others there has been no significant difference. In one series the mean for men was 119.6 ± 6.7 micrograms per 100 ml. (range 61 to 228) and for women 101.9 ± 5.5 micrograms per 100 ml. (range 35 to 246);[135] in another, the ranges were 81 to 162 micrograms per 100 ml. in men and 64 to 128 micrograms per 100 ml. in women.[75] Usually the level is highest in the morning and falls in the evening; in one study mean changes were 35.3 ± 6.0 in men and 16.1 ± 3.6 micrograms per 100 ml. in women. A mean serum level of 107.6 micrograms per 100 ml. has been reported in a group of boys and girls 4.5 to 8 years of age.[135] In children from 2 to 4.5 years old the mean in boys was 95.9 micrograms per 100 ml. and in girls 59.7 micrograms per 100 ml.

In one report of the serum iron values determined on several thousand presumably normal blood donors, serum iron levels of 200 micrograms per 100 ml. or more were found in 3.5 per cent; on retesting only rare elevations were

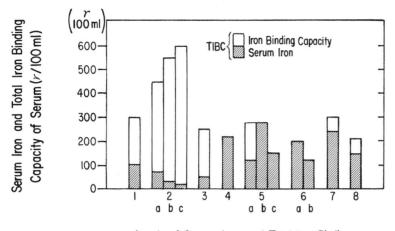

Levels of Serum Iron and Total Iron Binding
Capacity Observed in Patients with Various Disorders

Figure 5–3 1, Normal. 2, Iron deficiency (a, mild; b, moderate; c, severe). 3, Infection. 4, Viral hepatitis. 5, Bone marrow failure (a, untreated idiopathic; b, untreated drug-induced; c, idiopathic, over 300 blood transfusions). 6, Idiopathic hemochromatosis (a, untreated; b, treated). 7, Hereditary iron-loading anemia. 8, Untreated pernicious anemia.

found.[40] The results of the study confirmed the accuracy of the values obtained with automation and led to the conclusion that the report of an abnormally high level simply means that the determination should be repeated, preferably on a sample obtained late in the day, before the high value is taken as a reflection of disease.

Levels of iron and transferrin in the plasma vary in certain circumstances (Fig. 5–3). A rise in the plasma iron usually occurs in less than an hour after the ingestion of ferrous sulfate. The level is usually higher than normal in hemolytic anemia, untreated pernicious anemia, aplastic anemia, hemochromatosis, and hemosiderosis; in these disorders the total iron-binding capacity of the serum is not elevated but the percentage of saturation is increased. The serum iron level is also elevated in infectious hepatitis, and the rise appears to be correlated with the degree of parenchymal necrosis. In iron deficiency anemia the characteristic finding is a subnormal level of the plasma iron associated with an increase in the total iron-binding capacity. Similar changes usually occur during the latter part of pregnancy. The transferrin level is lower than normal in some patients with disturbed protein metabolism that occurs in certain disease states, such as nephrosis, uremia, liver disease, and starvation. In infections both the plasma iron and total iron-binding capacity are usually lower than normal; a decrease in the plasma iron has been observed within 24 hours after the production of fever.[24, 25] The low serum iron values seen in infection and malignancy are probably due to a reduced movement of iron from reticuloendothelial cells into plasma, rather than an acceleration of outflow of iron from the plasma to these storage cells; the utilization of iron that has gained access to the plasma appears to be unimpaired.[95] It has been suggested that the defect seen in iron metabolism that occurs in patients with inflammation and chronic disease may be the result both of destruction of erythrocytes and degradation of transferrin in the macrophage.[124] Such a process would account for the lowered serum transferrin level associated with normal synthesis that has been reported. Moderately lowered serum iron levels also occur in many patients with uremia or rheumatoid arthritis.

STORAGE OF IRON

The storage iron, usually from 600 to 1600 mg., constitutes from 16 to 23 per cent of the total in the body.[69, 118] This iron is stored as ferritin or hemosiderin chiefly in the phagocytic cells of the reticuloendothelial system in the liver, spleen, and bone marrow. The iron in both ferritin and hemosiderin can be utilized for hemoglobin formation. Several studies have shown that whereas erythrocytes are engulfed and degraded in the macrophages of the reticuloendothelial system, including the sinusoidal cells in the liver, in the rat, at least, the hepatic parenchymal cells remove and process circulating heme or hemoglobin.[9, 77]

Ferritin is a protein that has a molecular weight of about 560,000 and contains about 23 per cent iron in the form of ferric–hydroxy–phosphate;[5] the protein part of the complex is apoferritin. Studies of ferritin with the electron microscope have shown that the molecule is polygonal in shape, usually a regular hexagon, with a diameter of 100 to 110Å and sides measuring 70 to 80Å. The iron forms a central core of the protein shell. The apoferritin molecule is identical to the ferritin molecule except that iron is absent. Bessis and Breton-Gorius report that hemosiderin, which has been reported to contain from 1.5 to 37 per cent iron, is not a specific compound but a substance that contains a variable mixture of ferritin, apoferritin, and other material.[5]

Iron recently deposited in the tissues is utilized for erythropoiesis in preference to the older stores. When erythrocytes which have been tagged with radioiron and damaged by storage are injected into the circulation they are removed by the reticuloendothelial system at 20 to 40 times the normal rate; the tagged iron is promptly utilized for erythropoiesis, 85 per cent being used in 12 days.[123]

The incorporation of the plasma iron into the ferritin in the storage areas is an energy-dependent reaction involving ATP and ascorbic acid. Mazur et al. have used radioactive iron and slices of liver from rats to study the mechanism of the incorporation of plasma iron into hepatic ferritin.[114] They suggested that a complex is formed which involves 2 mols of ATP, 1 mol of ascorbic acid, and the iron-bound transferrin of the plasma. It was postulated that, on stimulation of the oxidation of ascorbic acid by ATP, the ferric iron bound to transferrin is reduced to ferrous iron and thus released from its bond to the protein for incorporation into ferritin.

The iron stores, which are estimated for clinical purposes by iron stains of marrow tissue and determinations of serum iron and transferrin levels, may be normal, subnormal, or increased. Subnormal stores occur most often in infants 12 to 24 months of age, and in situations in which there is uncompensated iron loss. Iron excess arises in two ways, either from excessive intestinal absorption or from hyperhemolysis. Excessive intestinal absorption of iron, which may occur as the result of either an intestinal defect (idiopathic hemochromatosis) or a diet high in iron (African Bantu), leads to the deposition of iron in the parenchymal cells. Excessive destruction of the red cells leads to the accumulation of excess iron in the reticuloendothelial cells, the clinical entity hemosiderosis. Iron overload also occurs in sickle cell anemia, thalassemia, "iron-loading" anemia, and refractory anemia associated with ineffective erythroid hyperplasia; in these patients the iron accumulation, which is augmented by increased intestinal absorption, may involve both epithelial cells and the reticuloendothelial cells.

The transfer of iron to the fetus takes place across the placenta, where the blood in the fetal circulation is separated from that of the mother only by the thin-walled villi that are in contact with a pool of maternal blood. The total amount of iron in the infant is approximately 300 mg.[128] The fetus acts as a parasite and is able to assimilate the required amount of iron even when the mother is deficient in iron. It accomplishes this in some manner other than simple diffusion, because iron from the maternal plasma is transferred to the fetal plasma even though the plasma level of the iron there is higher than in the maternal plasma; iron that enters the fetal circulation does not re-enter the maternal circulation. In the fetus the transferrin level is lower and the degree of saturation greater than in the mother.

EXCRETION OF IRON

The body normally conserves iron in a tenacious fashion. Only a very small amount is lost daily as a result of desquamation of cells of the skin and gastrointestinal tract, through the migration of leukocytes into the gastrointestinal tract, by the shedding of hair, and in the excretion of minute amounts of iron in the bile, urine, and sweat. Moore and Dubach found the fecal excretion of normal persons to be 0.3 to 0.5 mg. daily; in iron deficiency the amount may be only one-tenth as much.[118] The average man and the postmenopausal woman each lose about 0.5 to 1.5 mg. per day by various routes; menstruating women lose an average of about 1.0 to 2.5 mg. per day. During pregnancy an additional 1 mg. per day is lost, because the developing fetus is furnished a total of 0.3 to 0.5 gm., and other iron is lost as blood at the time of delivery. The normal loss of only 1.0 mg. per day means that years are required for a man or a postmenopausal woman with normal stores to develop iron deficiency solely because of a deficient diet. Iron deficiency in men and postmenopausal women is nearly always an indication of chronic blood loss. The conservation of iron is generally advantageous, but the inability of the physiologic mechanisms to rid the body of more than a small amount each day allows the accumulation of iron when excessive amounts gain access to the body as a result of blood transfusions, parenteral injection of iron, or abnormal absorption from the intestine. Crosby has placed the maximal limit of iron excretion through shedding iron-laden cells from the gastrointestinal tract at 5 mg. per day.[37]

FERROKINETICS

The availability of radioactive iron has made it possible to trace the pathways of iron in the body. Plasma iron can be labeled by the injection of a tracer amount of radioiron, and its clearance from the plasma can be followed by counting that which remains in the plasma at various intervals. From this determination, if the level of the serum iron is known, the plasma iron turnover can be calculated. The amount of iron that is utilized for effective hemoglobin synthesis can be measured by determining the amount that is incorporated in the circulating erythrocytes at various intervals of time. Normally, the halftime disappearance rate of iron injected intravenously is 90 to 100 minutes; 85 to 100 per cent of the injected iron can be accounted for in the circulating erythrocytes within a period of seven to ten days in normal subjects. The quantity of labeled iron in the sacral marrow, liver, and spleen can be ascertained by counting the gamma ray emission over these areas. Studies of this type by Huff,[86] Pollycove,[126] Finch,[14] and their associates form the main basis of our present concepts of internal iron metabolism.

The daily requirements of hemoglobin production of a normal adult human being can be calculated. If the hemoglobin level is 15 gm. per 100 ml., the total blood volume is 5000 ml., and the life span of the erythrocyte is 120 days, then the daily production of hemoglobin is 6.25 gm. $\left(\frac{15 \times 50}{120} = 6.25\right)$. Since each gram of hemoglobin contains 3.3 mg. of iron, the daily requirement of iron for hemoglobin production is about 21 mg. The average daily iron absorption, approximately 1 mg., just balances the daily loss from the body. The daily iron need for hemoglobin production is provided by the hemoglobin contained in the erythrocytes destroyed each day. This iron is mainly that transported from the reticuloendothelial cells to the erythropoietic tissue by the plasma, bound to transferrin. Since the total plasma iron amounts to 3 or 4 mg. it is evident that the total iron in the plasma must be renewed six or eight times in 24 hours.

The plasma iron turnover rate can be measured by the use of radioactive iron. A known amount of tagged iron is injected intravenously and the disappearance of the iron from the circulation is followed. If the level of the plasma iron and the blood volume are known, the turnover can be calculated. A simplified formula, which obviates determination of the blood volume, has been introduced by Bothwell and Finch:[14]

$$\text{Plasma iron turnover} \atop \text{(mg./day/100 ml. whole blood)} = \frac{\text{plasma iron (micrograms/100 ml.)}}{T\frac{1}{2} \text{ (minutes)}} \times \frac{100 - \text{Hct.}}{100}$$

($T\frac{1}{2}$ = time of clearance of 50 per cent of radioactivity from the plasma). The authors point out that important error may be introduced if the plasma volume or red cell mass is significantly abnormal. The presence of anemia does not lead to appreciable error, since the blood volume changes are in the range of 10 to 15 per cent. The formula is not suitable for use in patients with acute hemorrhage, burns, or salt depletion. Bothwell and Finch prefer to express the results in mg. per 100 ml. of whole blood per day, because it obviates the differences that result from body size as well as errors that may be introduced in measuring or assuming a figure for the blood volume. By this method the plasma iron turnover has been found to be about 0.6 mg. per 100 ml. of whole blood per day. With a blood volume of 5 liters the normal turnover is 30 mg. per day; if the total plasma iron is 3 or 4 mg., the complete turnover is at a rate of once every $2\frac{1}{2}$ to 3 hours.

The measured figure for plasma turnover of 0.6 mg. per 100 ml. of whole blood per day (30 mg. per day) is appreciably above the theoretical value calculated for hemoglobin production, 0.42 mg. per 100 ml. of whole blood per day (21 mg. per day). The figures indicate that about 30 per cent of the iron entering and leaving the plasma each day is not utilized for effective hemoglobin production. This means that there is appreciable movement of iron which apparently is not immediately involved in erythropoiesis. Efforts to interpret the results obtained by this type of study have led to the conclusion that the plasma iron is in equilibrium with one or more functional pools or compartments.[14, 87, 126, 142] Pollycove has suggested that the labile pool is in the marrow, but the anatomic site of the pool has not been established conclusively. Bothwell and Finch point out that the change in the slope of the iron disappearance curve to a less steep one after eight hours indicates that there are multiple components to the curve.[14] They also find good evidence of tissue exchange with a significant return of radioiron to the plasma. It is suggested that an appreciable portion of the plasma iron, 25 to 30 per cent, initially goes to tissue other than the marrow, mainly to the liver, while 10 per cent of the iron that goes to the marrow is involved in ineffective erythropoiesis, the erythrocytes being destroyed in the marrow without reaching the general circulation.

In addition to clarifying many aspects of normal iron metabolism, techniques that employ radioiron have led to a better understanding of the derangements that occur in certain diseases. By measuring the rate of clearance of iron from the plasma, the plasma iron turnover, and the incorporation of iron into circulating erythrocytes, the erythropoietic activity of the marrow can be estimated and its effectiveness determined. In patients with hypocellular inactive marrows, and in some with cellular marrows, both the clearance of iron from

METABOLIC PATHWAYS OF IRON

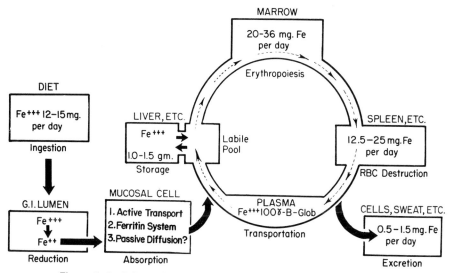

Figure 5–4 Schematic representation of the metabolic pathways of iron.

the plasma and its incorporation into circulating erythrocytes are diminished, and the iron going to storage is increased. In other patients with refractory anemia who have cellular marrows, and also in patients with pernicious anemia, the clearance of iron from the plasma is normal or increased, but the incorporation into circulating erythrocytes is greatly diminished; such results indicate ineffective erythropoiesis, either a diversion of iron to storage because of defective maturation or a premature destruction of the erythrocytes before they are released from the marrow.

ANEMIA OF IRON DEFICIENCY

Anemia that is the result of iron deficiency has been described under various names. Many of the terms that at present appear to be no more than different names for iron deficiency in special circumstances were used to indicate the various syndromes before the nature of the mechanism responsible for the anemia was appreciated. The following terms have been used: secondary anemia, idiopathic hypochromic anemia, chlorosis, chlorotic anemia, hypochromic anemia of pregnancy, hypochromic anemia of prematurity and adolescence, and iron deficiency anemia.

An interesting account of the history of iron in medicine has been published by Fowler.[58] According to this account the presence of iron in the blood was first discovered by Lemery and Geoffrey in 1713. This discovery did not come until sometime after iron deficiency had been described and iron had been used as a therapeutic agent. Iron deficiency anemia was first described by Johannes Lange of Basle in 1554 as "De Morbo Virgineo."[130] In this description of the syndrome that was later called "chlorosis," Lange noted that the disease was peculiar to virgins and described the change from rosiness of the cheeks to pallor, the pulsation of the temporal vessels, and the dyspnea on dancing and climbing stairs. Iron was first used to treat the anemia of chlorosis in the 1600s by Thomas Sydenham, one of the great English clinicians. In 1889 Hayem recognized that the anemia of iron deficiency is characterized by erythrocytes that are smaller than normal and that contain less than normal amounts of hemoglobin.[70]

MECHANISM OF DISEASE

Iron deficiency, which is probably the commonest type of anemia in the world, occurs in a number of clinical conditions, and various mechanisms may be involved. An improper diet is rarely the sole cause of iron deficiency except in infancy. Nevertheless, an inadequate intake may be an important factor in certain situations, particularly in infancy, during early childhood, in adolescence, and during pregnancy.

The anemia in infancy and childhood is mainly the result of a dietary iron deficiency; the amount of iron ingested is not adequate to provide for the increase in blood volume that is part of growth of the child. The state of the maternal iron stores has little or no effect on the development of anemia in the child because the fetus can obtain the needed iron, about 80 mg. per kg., even if the mother has iron deficiency. An unusual type of hypochromic microcytic anemia associated with virtual absence of marrow iron and excessive iron accumulation in the liver has been reported in two young children who had no defect in transferrin;[141] the mechanism is uncertain.

Mild or moderate anemia of iron deficiency is not uncommon in adolescence, but severe anemia ("chlorosis" of earlier times) is a rarity. The anemia, which is seen almost exclusively in girls, is usually explained by an iron intake that is insufficient to meet the requirements of rapid growth and the onset of menstruation.

Pregnancy is a common cause of iron deficiency anemia; the incidence varies in different parts of the world, but is probably about 25 per cent even in areas where nutritional problems are rare or minor. The development of the iron deficiency depends on several factors. One is the state of iron stores of the mother at the beginning of pregnancy; this is related to the economic status of the mother, the number of previous pregnancies, and the presence or absence of various diseases, particularly those associated with blood loss. Another factor is the iron intake of the mother, which is most important during the last half of pregnancy.

The commonest cause of iron deficiency anemia in both men and women is chronic blood loss. In adult males iron deficiency anemia is nearly always the result of chronic blood loss from the gastrointestinal tract. Any ulcerating lesion may be responsible—esophageal ulceration, hiatus hernia, gastric or duodenal ulcer, benign and malignant lesions of the stomach, small bowel, or colon, or hemorrhoids. The daily ingestion of aspirin may produce occult bleeding in the gastrointestinal tract. Blood loss from hookworm infestation is a major factor in iron deficiency in many parts of the world. A laudable and not uncommon cause of blood loss in certain conscientious individuals is excessive donation of blood. In women, in addition to gastrointestinal bleeding, excessive vaginal bleeding and pregnancy are common causes of iron deficiency. The state of the iron stores is important in the development of anemia from vaginal bleeding or pregnancy; the loss of small quantities of blood in normal menstruation may produce severe anemia in women whose iron stores are low, yet much more severe bleeding may produce only transient anemia if the reserves of iron are normal.

Intravascular hemolysis, with subsequent loss of iron as hemosiderin in the urine, produces iron deficiency and anemia if continued over a sufficiently long period. This occurs in some patients with prosthetic heart valves and is common in those with paroxysmal nocturnal hemoglobinuria.

Another cause of iron deficiency is impairment of the absorption of iron. This is seen most often in the United States in patients who have undergone partial gastrectomy. Such patients can absorb iron salts, but the absorption of dietary iron is markedly reduced and as a consequence the iron stores may become depleted over a period of years.[125] One report of 187 patients who had had partial gastrectomy for chronic peptic ulceration showed that 44 per cent developed iron deficiency anemia; there was a decline in hemoglobin levels for each five-year period of follow-up, but only approximately 10 per cent of the entire group had hemoglobin levels of less than 10 gm. per 100 ml. All responded to treatment with oral iron. Another interesting finding was that a coexisting deficiency of vitamin B_{12} was found in 3.8 per cent of patients operated on less than ten years previously, and in 15 per cent of those operated on more than 15 years previously.[129] As expected, the incidence was higher in those operated on for gastric ulcer (22.8 per cent) than in those with duodenal ulcer (3.5 per cent). Iron deficiency anemia usually develops in patients who have had total gastrectomy if they survive long enough. Poor absorption of iron also occurs in prolonged severe diarrhea and in the malabsorption syndromes.

Although probably not an important factor in the production of anemia, the life span of the red cell in patients with iron deficiency anemia was found to be shortened (46 to 85 days) when studied by the Ashby technique; erythrocytes from normal individuals survived normally when transfused into patients with iron deficiency anemia.[107]

Different morphologic varieties of anemia have been reported in kwashiorkor. A study of 22 African children indicates that, although hypochromia is common, there usually is stainable iron in the bone marrow; both plasma iron and iron-binding capacity are generally reduced.[1] The bone marrow in many patients shows some degree of megaloblastic change. On recovery from the disease, with improvement in the plasma proteins, the picture typical of iron deficiency develops in about one-half of the infants. It still remains uncertain how important infection, iron deficiency, and other dietary deficiencies are in the occurrence of anemia in this disease.

The relationship between the platelet count, iron deficiency, iron metabolism, and blood loss is a complex and intriguing problem. Thrombocythemia with platelet counts of over 1 million occur in patients with iron deficiency anemia and return to normal when anemia is corrected with iron therapy. We have also seen patients with severe iron deficiency, thrombocytopenia, and retinal hemorrhages. Recent studies have provided a better understanding of this problem.[30, 93] Studies on rats showed that the production of iron deficiency resulted in an increase in platelet production and platelet counts; survival time of the platelets was normal. Injection of iron was followed by a fall in platelet count and reduction to the normal range within 72 hours. Other studies have indicated that the increase in megathrombocytes is greater than the total increase. It has been postulated that a two-compartment iron system exists: in one the iron directly or indirectly inhibits the rise in platelet count above the steady state level; in the second iron is required for the synthesis of an integral portion of the platelet and for the maximum platelet production above steady state levels. Thrombocytopenia in severe iron deficiency may be the result of iron lack in the second "essential component" compartment.

CLINICAL MANIFESTATIONS

The symptoms that occur in the patient with iron deficiency anemia may be related to the primary disease or to anemia. Some patients consult a physician because they have noticed abnormal blood loss such as menorrhagia or rectal bleeding. Other patients, who have not noted any abnormal blood loss, visit a physician because of symptoms that are related to the anemia per se, such as weakness, easy fatigue, dyspnea on exertion, and palpitation. In addition to the usual symptoms of anemia, patients with iron deficiency sometimes complain of dysphagia, sore tongue, sore mouth, and brittle nails. Still other patients seek help because of symptoms that are caused by a lesion of the gastrointestinal tract, such as a duodenal ulcer or carcinoma of the bowel, and the presence of anemia is not suspected until a blood count is done. Some patients with iron deficiency anemia develop pagophagia, an extreme hunger for ice, and eat more than one or two trays of ice cubes a day; at times the symptom disappears on administration of iron before the anemia has been corrected. The eating of clay (pica) is sometimes considered to be a sign of iron deficiency, particularly in children, but the relationship is not as clear-cut as in pagophagia. In some groups clay-eating is part of the culture, and if the habit is carried far enough certain clays inhibit iron absorption.[3] In addition, the ingestion of laundry starch may be at least a contributing factor to the production of iron deficiency.[133]

Physical examination reveals no abnormality in some patients, and in others simply pallor of the skin and mucous membranes. At times fissuring at the angles of the mouth, atrophy of the papillae of the tongue, and glossitis are evident. In severe, long-standing iron deficiency the nails may be "spoon-shaped" and abnormally brittle. The spleen is often palpable in children and adults with iron deficiency, but does not extend more than a few centimeters below the left costal margin in the uncomplicated case. The splenomegaly may represent hyperplasia associated with the long standing hyperhemolysis linked with the shortened life span of the iron-deficient cells; the splenomegaly disappears after the iron deficiency is corrected. Throbbing headaches sometimes occur when the hemoglobin is greatly reduced, and disappear when the anemia is corrected. When the anemia is moderately severe an apical or precordial systolic murmur is usually present. Other cardiovascular abnormalities, such as cardiac dilatation and congestive failure, occur most often in younger children and in older persons with some coexisting heart disease.

Abnormalities other than anemia occur at times in patients with iron deficiency. Most common among these are fissuring about the mouth, trophic changes in the fingernails, koilonychia, and dysfunction of the esophagus. These abnormalities have been reported as manifestations of iron deficiency in the absence of anemia because these lesions have been found in nonanemic patients, and improvement in the lesions has followed promptly after the administration of iron salts. A similar response to treatment with iron has been reported in nonanemic patients who had normal levels of serum iron. Correction of achlorhydria, which is present in about 50 per cent of patients with iron deficiency anemia, has been reported after iron therapy,[67] but was not confirmed in a more recent study.[105] No improvement in the histologic appearance of the gastric mucosa or in the acid secretion occurred after a year of treatment with iron. Further evidence of a discrepancy between the iron content of the blood and that of the tissues, particularly iron-containing enzymes, is afforded by the work of Beutler, who found that, in rats that were made iron-deficient by bleeding and special diets, the decrease in the cytochrome C of the liver and kidney greatly exceeded the decrease in hemoglobin.[7, 8] Other studies have shown that not all iron-containing enzymes are so dependent on adequate supplies of iron. The concentration of catalase has been found to be normal in human red cells even under conditions of severe iron need.

The syndrome of postcricoid dysphagia, glossitis, koilonychia, and iron deficiency anemia, which has been called the Paterson-Kelly or Plummer-Vinson syndrome or sideropenic dysphagia, has been seen in patients with anemia or with iron deficiency without anemia.[27] In a study of 72 patients with a cricopharyngeal web these authors found that 63 suffered or had suffered from iron deficiency—some more than 15 years previously. Correction of the iron deficiency did not necessarily result in the disappearance of the web. It has long been thought that carcinoma of the esophagus was common in patients with this syndrome, and of these 72 patients four developed carcinoma of the esophagus, an incidence of 5 per cent, compared to five per million in the general population in England and Wales. The frequent association of thyroid disease, particularly myxedema, in patients with iron deficiency and webs led to the speculation that autoimmunity might be a factor.

LABORATORY EXAMINATION

The anemia of severe iron deficiency is characteristically hypochromic and microcytic (MCV is less than 80 cu. μ, MCH less than 30 $\mu\mu$, and MCHC less than 30 per cent). Very low values are often found. In the majority of patients with iron deficiency, study of a stained smear of the peripheral blood reveals that most of the erythrocytes are smaller than normal and show an increase in the central pallor that may be extreme (hypochromic microcytes); other erythrocytes appear normal in color, and some show polychromatophilia if erythropoiesis is active. Poikilocytosis often is evident and elongated "cigar

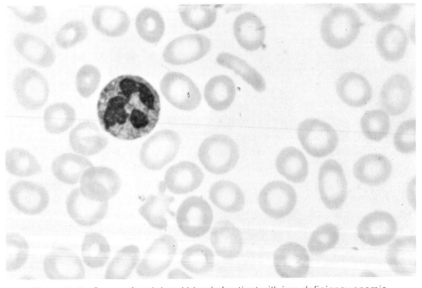

Figure 5–5   Smear of peripheral blood of patient with iron deficiency anemia.

forms" are seen frequently (Fig. 5–5). Occasionally nucleated red cells are present. The leukocyte count, platelet count, and reticulocyte counts are usually normal. Thrombocythemia with platelet counts of a million or more is present in some patients with iron deficiency; the count returns to normal with treatment that replenishes the iron stores. The converse of thrombocythemia, thrombocytopenia, which is sometimes accompanied by retinal hemorrhages, occurs in some patients with iron deficiency anemia, but the relationship to the iron deficiency is not clear.

Erythropoiesis is normoblastic in type; the cellularity of the marrow may appear normal, reduced, or increased. Numerous abnormalities occur in the normoblasts in iron deficiency.[78] These include not only reduced ragged cytoplasm, vacuolization, and delayed maturation of the cytoplasm, but also evidence of dyserythropoiesis, karyorrhexis, multinuclearity, nuclear budding, and abnormal mitosis.

In patients with less severe iron deficiency the anemia is not always hypochromic and microcytic; it may be hypochromic and normocytic, or normochromic and normocytic. In such patients other laboratory procedures may be helpful in establishing a diagnosis of iron deficiency. The presence of iron deficiency usually is accompanied by a reduction in the level of the serum iron, generally to less than 40 μg. per 100 ml. (normal 50 to 150), an increase in the latent iron-binding capacity of the serum to two or three times the normal value (normal 200 to 300 μg. per cent), and marked diminution or depletion of storage iron in the bone marrow. In iron deficiency the saturation of transferrin is often, but not invariably, less than 10 per cent; low saturations, 10 to 16 per cent, also occur in infections.

Study of bone marrow that is obtained by aspiration and stained for iron provides a reliable method of assessing the state of the iron stores, particularly if the stores are low;[52] preparations can be studied in the unstained state or after staining with Prussian blue.[122] The amount of iron in the storage cells is probably the most reliable index of the body stores of iron; nevertheless all the iron in the cells may not be used for hemoglobin production. The major portion of injected iron dextran is available for hemoglobin synthesis only after it has been processed by the reticuloendothelial system. Several weeks after injection, iron may be seen in the marrow reticuloendothelial cells, even though it has become progressively unavailable for hemoglobin synthesis.[76] The number and appearance of iron granules in the nucleated red cells give some indication of iron utilization. Normally one-third of the marrow normoblasts contain siderotic granules; these become small and virtually disappear in iron deficiency, and increase in some situations in which iron utilization is defective. These nonhemoglobin granules are thought to be aggregates of ferritin molecules.

When anemia is the result of iron deficiency the serum bilirubin is not elevated and the 24-hour fecal urobilinogen excretion is usually lower than normal because the mass of the circulating hemoglobin is reduced. The free erythrocyte protoporphyrin is increased in iron deficiency.[24] Achlorhydria occurs commonly in patients with this disorder.

The development of iron deficiency produces the following sequence of changes: (1) depletion of iron stores, which usually is evident in the bone marrow; (2) elevation of the iron-binding capacity of the serum; (3) fall in serum iron level; (4) development of normochromic or slightly hypochromic anemia; and (5) development of hypochromic microcytic anemia. The reverse sequence occurs when the deficiency is treated with oral iron.

DIFFERENTIAL DIAGNOSIS

The first step in making a diagnosis of this type of anemia is to establish the presence of iron deficiency, and the next is to determine the cause. If the anemia is hypochromic and microcytic, the commonly-seen iron deficiency must be distinguished from the uncommon thalassemia and the rare pyridoxine deficiency and other "iron-loading" disorders. Thalassemia is characterized by a family history of anemia, the occurrence of many target cells on the stained smear, and an elevated reticulocyte count; the spleen is usually enlarged and may extend below the level of the umbilicus. Determination of the serum iron level and examination of properly-stained marrow preparations fail to reveal any iron deficiency. Fetal hemoglobin and hemoglobin A_2 usually are increased. Pyridoxine deficiency and "iron-loading anemia," which are rare in man, are characterized by a hypochromic microcytic anemia; but even though the erythrocytes appear hypochromic, the level of the serum iron is elevated and administration of iron produces no improvement in the anemia. The demonstration of a lack or an excess of iron in the bone marrow preparations probably is the most reliable and simple means of distinguishing between iron deficiency anemia and other conditions associated with hypochromic cells. In the milder degrees of iron deficiency the anemia may be hypochromic, normochromic, normocytic, or slightly microcytic, rather than hypochromic microcytic. This is most likely to occur when severe deficiency has not developed or when the severe deficiency has been only partly corrected. In such circumstances the demonstration of a low serum iron level or an increase in the latent iron-binding capacity, or a histologic demonstration of low iron stores in the tissue, often establishes the presence of iron deficiency.

Once established, an effort must be made to find the cause of the deficiency. Faulty diet may be an acceptable explanation in infants and very young children, but in adults a search must be made for the cause of the blood loss. The absence of occult blood from a single specimen of feces does not exclude chronic or recurrent gastrointestinal bleeding from consideration. Unless the cause of the iron deficiency is clear-cut, most patients, particularly those who are middle-aged or older, will need a complete roentgenographic study of the entire gastrointestinal tract. Almost any ulcerative lesion in the esophagus, stomach, small intestine, or large bowel can be responsible for chronic bleeding and iron deficiency. Although hiatus hernia with ulceration often causes gastrointestinal bleeding and anemia, one should not conclude that the demonstration of a hiatus hernia in a patient with anemia has disclosed the source of the bleeding. Many middle-aged and older patients have an asymptomatic hiatus hernia. Examination of the small intestine and large bowel should be performed, and the hernia accepted as the cause of the bleeding only when no other likely site can be demonstrated. If a lesion of the gastrointestinal tract is suspected but not demonstrated at the time of the initial examination, the appropriate studies should be repeated because of the importance of demonstrating any lesion, particularly a neoplasm, that might require surgical correction. In women, particularly those of child-bearing age, the decision must be made whether or not the history of vaginal bleeding and pregnancies gives an adequate explanation of the anemia. Roentgenographic investigation of the gastrointestinal tract is often indicated, but the risk of irradiation of the ovaries or of an unsuspected early pregnancy should not be ignored. The ingestion of aspirin is a fairly common cause of bleeding, either from local irritation or through an effect on platelet aggregation.

TREATMENT, COURSE, AND PROGNOSIS

The most important aspect of the treatment of iron deficiency anemia is the correction of the cause. This is much more important than the correction of the anemia unless the patient is critically ill. The prognosis is related more to the underlying disease than to the severity of the anemia, which may have little or no influence on the outcome.

The feasibility and desirability of reducing the incidence of iron deficiency in different areas of the world by fortifying bread and other items in the diet with iron has been studied and discussed, but opponents and advocates have come to no agreement.[20, 39, 55] Chief objections have been that the proposed program has not been tested either for safety or efficacy;[39] iron given in this way might be deleterious to patients with hemochromatosis and other iron excess disorders. It could possibly even conceal chronic bleeding from a gastrointestinal lesion that requires more specific therapy.

In patients with anemia that is due to iron deficiency the administration of ferrous salts is followed by a reticulocytosis during the first week (Fig. 5–6). The magnitude of reticulocyte response, which usually is in the range of 4 to 10 per cent, depends on the initial hemoglobin level and not on the level of the erythrocyte count. Unless complicating factors are present, the reticulocytosis is followed by the return of the hemoglobin and red cells to normal levels within a period of six to 10 weeks. If the therapy with iron is successful the hemoglobin level should increase 2.0 gm. per 100 ml. in the first three weeks of treatment. The levels of iron and latent iron-binding capacity, and the storage iron in the marrow, which probably reflect the state of the stores of iron, return to normal much more slowly. Treatment probably should be continued until this occurs, but such complete therapy may require small amounts of iron salts orally for a long period, particularly if the patient is either a premenopausal woman or has had a partial gastrectomy. Prolonged treatment of this type is considered impractical by some.

The anemia of iron deficiency is usually corrected by the oral administration of 200 or 300 mg. of ferrous sulfate or ferrous gluconate three times a day. Various preparations contain between 35 and 70 mg. of iron per tablet; of the total dose of between 100 and 200 mg. of iron, probably no more than 20 or 30 mg. is absorbed. If a small amount of the drug is given initially and the dos-

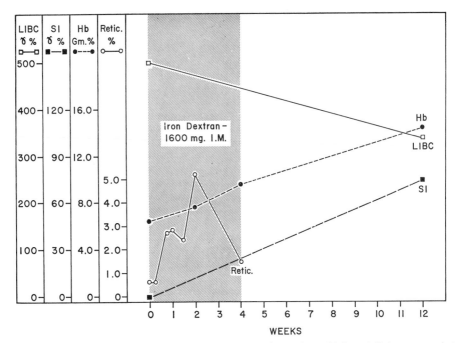

Figure 5–6 Chart showing hematologic response of a patient with iron deficiency anemia to treatment with iron. The reticulocyte peak, which is not as great as that seen after specific treatment in pernicious anemia, occurs before there is an increase in the levels of hemoglobin and serum iron and a decrease in the latent iron-binding capacity.

age increased gradually, gastrointestinal upsets rarely occur. Some patients tolerate one preparation better than another, and if one preparation is causing undesirable griping, diarrhea, or other symptoms, another compound should be substituted. Iron is less likely to cause gastrointestinal symptoms if it is given after meals. Although this is not an optimal time for iron absorption, adequate absorption usually occurs if the medication is given at this time. A single tablet of ferrous gluconate or ferrous sulfate at bedtime generally produces a satisfactory response and many patients find it simpler and more convenient to follow this schedule. The use of "sustained-release" preparations is not recommended; in one study no sustained release could be demonstrated, and indeed less iron was available than in usual preparations.[116]

Although iron salts administered orally correct the anemia in most patients, the method of treatment is not an efficient means of correcting the iron stores because iron absorption decreases when the blood returns to normal. In order to replenish the iron stores by the oral route it is often necessary to continue treatment for months or years. For this reason parenteral preparations are sometimes employed. Intravenous or intramuscular therapy with iron dextran is effective. Because it may be more dangerous, intravenous injection is used only in special circumstances. Intramuscular injections of 100 to 500 mg. may be given weekly or several times a week. The total amount given in a course of intramuscular treatment is usually between 1500 and 5000 mg., an amount sufficient to correct the anemia and replenish the iron stores. Reactions such as fever, pain at the injection site, discoloration of the skin and even vasomotor collapse may occur but are infrequent. The risk of late complications from the intra-muscular injections has not been determined precisely, but probably is slight.

Illustrative Cases

CASE 1

A 74-year-old white housewife was admitted to the hospital for evaluation of anemia and weight loss of 20 pounds during the preceding year. About $1\frac{1}{2}$ years prior to admission she had an episode of constipation, cramping midabdominal pain, and vomiting. Roentgenographic examinations of the gallbladder and upper gastrointestinal tract were negative. Her attacks recurred with increasing frequency, and about six weeks before admission they were occurring once or twice a week. At this time the patient was found to be anemic and was treated with iron.

Physical examination. The skin and mucous membranes were pale. The right side of the abdomen was moderately tender and a firm, movable 6 by 10 cm. mass was felt in the right lower quadrant. The liver edge was palpable 2 cm. below the right costal margin.

Laboratory studies. Admission blood studies disclosed the following: Hct. 26 per cent, Hb. 6.7 gm. per 100 ml., R.B.C. 3.4 million per cu.mm., W.B.C. 4900 per cu.mm.; serum iron 11.5 μg. per 100 ml.; unsaturated iron-binding protein 455 μg. per 100 ml. The feces gave a strongly positive benzidine reaction.

Barium enema examination revealed a 5-or 6-cm. constricted area in the ascending colon and another filling defect in the sigmoid colon. After blood transfusions operation was performed. A carcinoma of the ascending colon and a carcinomatous polyp in the descending colon were found. Both lesions were resected and convalescence was uneventful.

Three months later the Hct. was 43 per cent, Hb. 12.6 gm. per 100 ml., R.B.C. 4.4 million per cu.mm., plasma iron 99 μg. per 100 ml., and unsaturated iron-binding protein 270 μg. per 100 ml.

Comment. At the time of admission this patient had evidence of severe iron deficiency in the form of hypochromic microcytic anemia associated with a decrease in the level of serum iron and an increase in the unsaturated iron-binding capacity. The most important aspect of the diagnosis in a patient with anemia of this type is the demonstration of the cause of the anemia. Usually, as was the case in this patient, the iron deficiency is the result of chronic blood loss. In adult males and elderly women chronic unrecognized blood loss is nearly always the result of a lesion in the gastrointestinal tract. This patient had two primary malignant lesions in the colon. It appears likely that the lesion in the ascending colon was responsible for the blood loss, and the tumor in the sigmoid colon was responsible for the symptoms of partial intestinal obstruction. In all probability a more thorough examination at the time her symptoms began, a year and a half before admission, would have revealed a lesion in the colon. Fortunately this patient appeared to have no metastases when her bowel resections were performed, despite a delay in in diagnosis that might well have been fatal.

CASE 2

This 69-year-old white housewife was admitted with the chief complaint of "anemia" of two years' duration. She related that for two years she had felt weak, nervous, and slightly dizzy. She had been treated irregularly during this time with liver extract and iron. Despite this therapy some degree of anemia persisted and she was referred for further study. Careful questioning elicited no history of weight loss, gastrointestinal symptoms, or abnormal bleeding.

Physical examination. The patient was well developed, well nourished, and somewhat obese. General examination revealed no specific abnormalities, but the pelvic examination revealed an erosion of the cervix.

Laboratory examination. Admission blood studies: Hb. 9.1 gm. per 100 ml.; R.B.C. 3.8 million per cu.mm.; Hct. 31 per cent; reticulocytes 1.9 per cent. The leukocyte count, platelet count, and differential count were normal. Bone marrow examination disclosed a hypercellular marrow with a normoblastic type of erythropoiesis. Repeated stool examinations were consistently positive for occult blood.

Gastrointestinal x-ray study revealed a hiatus hernia that was about 10 cm. in the greatest diameter. Barium enema examination revealed a lesion at the hepatic flexure which was associated with some narrowing over an area of 2 or 3 cm. Proctoscopic examination disclosed no lesion. Biopsy of the cervix was reported as showing an epidermoid carcinoma.

Treatment and course. The patient was transfused with 3 units of blood, and was operated upon nine days after admission. A right colectomy was performed and the patient stood the procedure well. At the time of operation there was no evidence of metastases from the lesions in bowel or cervix. Histologic study of the bowel tumor revealed mucinous adenocarcinoma grade III extending through the thickness of the wall. The regional lymph nodes were free of tumor. The patient's convalescence from the laparotomy was uneventful, and 16 days after her right colectomy radium was applied to the cervix. She received 6000 mg. hours using six sources, and the following month she received 6000 R of external radiation.

Comment. This patient illustrates many instructive points. She was treated for two years for anemia with iron and liver extract without any effort being made to discover the cause of the anemia. This treatment altered the morphologic characteristics of the red blood cells without correcting the anemia. This case illustrates the importance of determining the cause of the anemia before treatment. When the gastrointestinal tract was investigated two possible bleeding sites were found. The hiatus hernia was found first, but this lesion occurs so frequently in this age group that it was thought important to study the lower gastrointestinal tract. This was done and the carcinoma of the colon was discovered. Fortunately the lesion was operable despite the duration of the illness. The finding of a carcinoma of the cervix on the routine examination emphasizes the importance of a complete examination in all patients.

ANEMIAS ASSOCIATED WITH ABNORMAL UTILIZATION OF IRON

"Iron-loading anemia," "sideroblastic anemia," and "sideroachrestic anemia" are diagnostic terms that have been applied to patients who have anemia associated with an abnormality in iron metabolism. These patients seem to be different from patients with thalassemia and the other known hemoglobinopathies. Knowledge of the pathologic physiology in these patients is incomplete; in some even the natural history of disease is unknown. Because of these inadequacies, many questions remain and the anemias cannot be classified in a satisfactory manner. Some patients appear to fit into a well-defined syndrome, but others manifest features found in several different syndromes. An example is the patient who appears to have a hereditary form of the disorder, yet responds partially to treatment with pyridoxine. The bone marrow of patients with these disorders contains many sideroblasts, but whether the presence of "ringed sideroblasts" is a sine qua non for the inclusion in this group of diseases is uncertain; some patients have iron overload and anemia, but a careful search of the marrow does not reveal any typical ringed sideroblasts.

The characteristics of sideroblastic anemia are listed in Table 5–3.

The increase in size and amount of nonhemoglobin iron in the perinuclear area has been explained by studies with electron microscopy which have disclosed the accumulation of excessive amounts of iron in the mitochondria.[6] This accumulation is related to the defect in heme synthesis which exists in these disorders. Mitochondria are concerned in the first step in porphyrin synthesis, and also in the last step (Fig. 5–7). In the first step, which requires pyridoxal-5-phosphate and the Krebs cycle, glycine combines with succinyl CoA to form delta-aminolevulinic acid. The last step, coupling of protoporphyrin and iron to form heme, requires heme synthetase and also pryidoxal phosphate, which probably is necessary for the release of iron from the mitochondria. Iron may accumulate in excess because of some defect in the control of the entrance of iron into the cell, or as a result of defective utilization because of some metabolic block. Excessive amounts of iron from whatever cause might damage the mitochondria or other organelles in the cell. (See Chapter 2.)

The mitochondrial accumulation of particles of iron, usually small and few in number, has also been reported in patients with thalassemia, mechanical hemolytic anemia, and porphyria cutanea tarda, and in those receiving chlor-

Table 5–3 *Characteristics of Sideroblastic Anemia*

1. Hypochromic and microcytic or normocytic anemia.
2. Marked anisocytosis and poikilocytosis.
3. Normal or elevated serum iron levels.
4. Refractory to therapy with iron.
5. Erythroid hyperplasia of the bone marrow.
6. Increased sideroblasts in the marrow.
7. Ringed sideroblasts.
8. Reduced incorporation of iron into red cells.
9. Normal or slightly reduced red cell survival time.
10. Hemosiderosis and/or hemochromatosis.

SYNTHESIS OF HEME

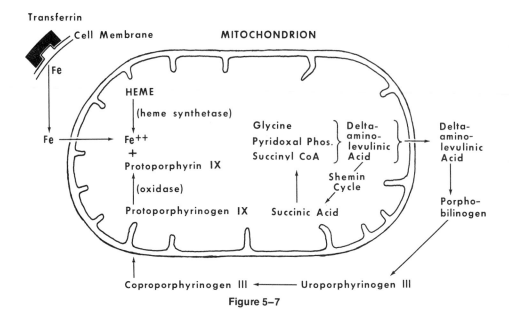

Figure 5–7

amphenicol.[60] It is possible that both a metabolic block and deranged ingress of iron into the cell are factors.

Sideroblasts with iron-loaded mitochondria, "ringed" sideroblasts, are abnormal and are associated with sideroblastic anemia. From 40 to 70 per cent of the normoblasts in idiopathic sideroblastic anemia are "ringed" sideroblasts. The percentage is less in drug-induced sideroblastic anemia (alcohol, isoniazid, cycloserine pyrazinamide, chloramphenicol, and lead);[23] these agents all partially inhibit the activity of ALA synthetase.

The studies of patients with iron-loading[73] have shown enzymatic defects located at different steps in the synthesis of heme; the different defects can produce identical or similar clinical pictures. In pyridoxine-responsive anemia there is iron-loading and, in addition, a diminution in the free erythrocyte protoporphyrin and coproporphyrin; this can be explained if there is a block in the first stage of porphyrin metabolism, the union of glycine and succinyl-CoA to form delta-aminolevulinic acid, a reaction that requires pyridoxal phosphate. The existence of such a block or blocks appears to be confirmed by Vogler and Mingioli, who studied hemoglobin synthesis in reticulocytes of patients with pyridoxine responsive anemia with the use of labeled glycine and delta-aminolevulinic acid; when labeled glycine was added no increase in heme was found, but when labeled delta-aminolevulinic was added increased heme production followed.[155, 156] Their later studies disclosed a defect in the incorporation of glycine into heme, the rate being only from 11 to 25 per cent of normal. The incorporation of delta-aminolevulinic acid into heme was only 46 to 81 per cent of normal. These observations suggested two defects in the synthesis of heme, the major one occurring prior to the formation of ALA, and the minor one somewhere between the synthesis of ALA and heme. Studies after repeated phlebotomies disclosed that, when the iron stores were reduced to normal, incorporation of delta-aminolevulinic acid by the patient's reticulocytes equaled the normal rate, although glycine incorporation was still reduced. These results indicated that excess of iron was a significant factor in reduced heme synthesis activity in patients whose primary defect was probably defective ALA synthetase activity.[156]

According to Heilmeyer,[73] in the congenital form of sideroachrestic anemia there are iron-loading and an increase in erythrocyte coproporphyrin associated with a normal or reduced level of erythrocyte protoporphyrin; this combination suggests a block in heme synthesis at the step between the formation of coproporphyrinogen and protoporphyrin IX, probably a failure of the oxidase enzyme. In the acquired type of sideroachrestic anemia, characterized by the increase in the iron associated with increase in coproporphyrin and protoporphyrin, there appears to be a defect in the union of iron and protoporphyrin IX, probably a deficiency in the enzyme heme synthetase. In lead intoxication, and in anemia associated with INH therapy, there are increases in coproporphyrin and protoporphyrin which suggest a block in the combining of iron with protoporphyrin to form heme; in addition, there probably are defects or partial blocks earlier in the metabolic pathway.

There may well be blocks at other steps in the metabolic pathway in other patients who fit into this syndrome. Heilmeyer, London, and others have produced evidence to indicate that heme, protoporphyrin, and coproporphyrin all may act by feedback mechanisms to slow down the first stage of porphyrin metabolism when the other substances are present in increased amounts. The production of globin and heme ordinarily proceed at approximately the same rate. An imbalance in these reactions is a possible explanation for the defect in iron metabolism found in beta thalassemia: with the slow production of the beta chain, globin production lags, and consequently iron, plus the other compounds, protoporphyrin and coproporphyrin, accumulate.

A clinical classification of the sideroblastic anemias is presented in Table 5–4. Pyridoxine-responsive anemia and the anemia responsive to crude liver extract are placed in separate categories, because of the unpredictable response to treatment with pyridoxine seen in patients with either hereditary or acquired disease.

Table 5–4 *Classification of Sideroblastic Anemia*

A. Primary
  1. Hereditary
  2. Acquired

B. Secondary
  1. Associated with chemicals (isoniazid, cycloserine, lead, possibly others)
  2. Associated with other diseases (rheumatoid arthritis, polyarteritis nodosa, leukemia and other myeloproliferative disorders, myeloma, carcinoma, alcoholism, hemolytic anemia)

C. Unclassified
  1. Pyridoxine responsive anemia
  2. Anemia responsive to crude liver extract

(Modified from Mollin, D. L.: Br. J. Haematol., *11*:41, 1965.)

HEREDITARY SIDEROBLASTIC ANEMIA
(CONGENITAL SIDEROACHRESTIC ANEMIA,
HEREDITARY IRON-LOADING ANEMIA)

The first description of the hereditary hypochromic type of anemia has been credited to Cooley[34] and Rundles and Falls.[134] This disorder has been reported in siblings and in patients who have a family history of anemia. Nearly all of the reported cases have been males, but females are not exempt. The anemia is usually noticed in childhood or in the early adult years, and hemochromatosis often develops during the third and fourth decade. Early in the disorder patients often present with a history of weakness or easy fatigue; if hemochromatosis has developed, abdominal pain, heart failure, or thrombophlebitis are commonly seen. Physical examination usually discloses poor physical development associated with mild enlargement of the liver and spleen; sometimes increased pigmentation of the skin is apparent.

Laboratory examinations show that classically the anemia is moderately severe, hypochromic and microcytic (MCV, 53 to 68 cu. μ; MCH, 18 to 20 $\mu\mu$; MCHC, 33 per cent), although in some cases included in this category it has been normocytic or macrocytic. The leukocyte count is normal; the differential count usually is normal but sometimes the lymphocytes are slightly increased. The platelet count is normal or diminished, but, in patients who have had splenectomy, counts of a million or more are common. Reticulocyte counts are usually normal, but counts as high as 15 per cent have been noted. The stained smear of the peripheral blood presents a striking appearance because of the presence of marked anisochromia, anisocytosis, poikilocytosis, and leptocytosis. If the spleen has been removed many of the hypochromic erythrocytes contain iron-staining granules (siderocytes). Examination of the bone marrow reveals a very hyperplastic marrow with erythropoiesis of the normoblastic type; many young forms are present. If stains for iron are used, many of the nucleated cells are seen to be sideroblasts, normoblasts with granules of nonhemoglobin iron in the cytoplasm: they constitute from 80 to 95 per cent of the total (normal, 30 per cent). Ringed sideroblasts are considered by some to be almost pathognomonic of the disorder,[151] but they also occur in patients considered to have other disorders of iron metabolism.

The morphologic evidence of the disturbance in iron metabolism is confirmed by special studies. The serum iron is normal or increased, with values of 125 to 300 micrograms per 100 ml. reported. The degree of saturation of the transferrin may be normal, but usually is greatly increased. Studies with radioactive iron have disclosed rapid clearance of the iron from the plasma, associated with decreased utilization of the iron as measured by its appearance in the circulating erythrocytes; the picture is that of ineffective erythropoiesis. Iron absorption from the gastrointestinal tract must be increased early in the disorder, but radioiron studies have given variable results; later in the disease absorption may diminish because of a build-up in tissue iron. Other evidence of abnormal hemoglobin metabolism in these patients is an increase in the coproporphyrin concentration and a decreased or normal protoporphyrin level in the erythrocytes.

Investigations have failed to disclose any evidence of significant hyperhemolysis. Fecal urobilinogen excretion is normal, serum bilirubin is normal or slightly increased, and red cell survival as measured by chromium-tagged cells has been reported as normal or only slightly decreased. Electrophoresis has shown no increase in the A_2 hemoglobin, and determinations of the fetal hemoglobin have been normal.

Treatment with iron, cobalt, vitamin B_{12}, and adrenocortical steroid is of no value; occasionally splenectomy is beneficial. The main therapeutic measures are pyridoxine, phlebotomies, and chelating agents. The administration of pyridoxine to some patients is followed by a partial hematologic response associated with symptomatic improvement. Such improvement warrants inclusion of the patient in the "pyridoxine-responsive anemia" group according to Horrigan and Harris.[84] Probably all patients thought to have the disorder should be given a trial on pyridoxine hydrochloride, 100 to 200 mg. a day. If phlebotomies can be tolerated they are advisable. Removal of iron in this way is the most effective means of preventing the development of severe hemochromatosis later in life, and removal of some of the tissue iron sometimes leads to improvement in erythropoiesis. Some patients with this disorder to not tolerate phlebotomy; an effective chelating agent would be valuable in treatment for these.

ACQUIRED SIDEROBLASTIC ANEMIA

Patients who have been reported as examples of "acquired sideroblastic anemia," "refractory anemia with sideroblastic bone marrow," "refractory normoblastic anemia," "refractory sideroblastic anemia," and as early examples of the DiGuglielmo syndrome appear to have the same, or a very closely related, syndrome that may be of diverse etiology.

The common features of the disorder, which usually appears in middle-aged or elderly males, are a moderately severe anemia associated with normoblastic hyperplasia of the bone marrow; the granulocyte and platelet counts may be normal or reduced, and show no constant pattern. In one series approximately one-third of the patients were female. The anemia is the result of ineffective erythropoiesis; studies with radioactive iron have shown rapid clearance of the plasma iron, but diminished utilization of the iron for the circulating erythrocytes. The serum iron level usually is increased, often over 200 micrograms per 100 ml., and saturation of the iron-binding capacity is increased, sometimes reaching 100 per cent. Appropriate stains disclose greatly-increased stores of iron in the marrow and a high percentage of sideroblasts; "ringed" sideroblasts often are present. The circulating erythrocytes usually are normocytic or slightly macrocytic, MCV 80 to 114 cu. μ, and normochromic; some patients had a hypochromic microcytic anemia, and some appeared to have a mixture of large and small cells. The reticulocyte count is normal or slightly increased, and hemolysis of circulating red cells, as gauged by chromium survival studies, is only slightly increased. Little PAS material is seen in the normoblasts, which may be helpful in distinguishing this disease from erythroleukemia.[100]

The clinical course is often relatively benign, but some patients develop hepatosplenomegaly and other features of hemochromatosis. Leukemia has developed in a number of our patients; an increase in myeloblasts and promyelocytes or other cells of the granulocytic series sometimes is evident months or years before the appearance of frank leukemia. Terminal acute leukemia has also followed acquired sideroblastic anemia which appeared first after several years' treatment of multiple myeloma with chemotherapeutic agents. One review, however, places the evidence of acute leukemia at only 5 or 7 per cent in nearly 100 patients;[100] the median survival time was 10 years.

Treatment of the anemia by means other than transfusion is rarely effective. Nevertheless we give patients a trial on pyridoxine 200 mg./day orally for a month, or oxymetholone 100 mg./day for three months; if megaloblastosis is present, folate is given. The literature contains the report of at least one response to immunosuppressive therapy in six months.[168] Because of the possible damaging effects of long-standing iron overload, an attempt to reduce the tissue iron by phlebotomy, which is rarely tolerated well, is still advisable.

Secondary Sideroblastic Anemia Associated with Chemicals

A number of substances are known to inhibit heme synthesis.[73] Among the most important in clinical medicine are the antituberculous drugs and lead.

A relatively small number of patients with tuberculosis treated with isoniazid, cycloserine, or pyrazinamide, known to act as antagonists to pyridoxal-5-phosphate, have developed sideroblastic anemia.[73, 117] The disappearance of the anemia when the drugs were discontinued indicates that the drugs played an essential role. The stimulation of erythropoiesis and the improvement in the peripheral neuritis that follows the administration of pyridoxine while patients are being treated with INH point toward a deficiency or defective utilization of pyridoxine. Apparently incorporation of iron into protoporphyrin is defective.[73] Why only a small percentage of patients treated with these drugs develop the abnormality remains unclear.

The anemia of lead poisoning is usually mild, hemolytic and slightly hypochromic; basophilic stippling is present in the erythrocytes and reticulocytosis of varying degree is present. Sideroblasts are increased in the marrow. Other abnormalities are increased amounts of protoporphyrin and coproporphyrin in the erythrocytes accompanied by increased urinary excretion of delta-aminolevulinic acid, protoporphyrin III, and uroporphyrin.[106] The swelling and disintegration of the mitochondria that have been revealed by electron microscopy are associated with some abnormality in the synthesis of hemoglobin involving several enzymatic reactions.[106] There is evidence that lead inhibits the synthesis of delta-aminolevulinic acid, the conversion of this substance to porphobilinogen, and the conversion of coproporphyrinogen III to protoporphyrin IX; in addition, movement of iron from the stroma of the cells into the mitochondria and its union with protoporphyrin to form heme are inhibited. Thus it appears that the presence of lead inhibits, but does not block completely, nearly every step in the synthesis of heme.

Sideroblastic Anemia Associated with Other Diseases

Sideroblastic anemia has been observed in a number of diseases (see Table 5-4); often the clinical picture and the hematologic abnormalities are not striking. The ringed sideroblasts usually disappear on successful treatment of the underlying disease, or with the administration of pyridoxine and folic acid.[117] Ringed sideroblasts occur in hemolytic anemia when there is some associated defect in hemoglobin synthesis; they are seen in thalassemia and some acquired disorders, but not in hereditary spherocytosis.

Varying numbers of ringed sideroblasts, with or without anemia, have been observed in a number of diseases: few (1 to 4 per cent) in Di Guglielmo's syndrome, collagen disorders, megaloblastic anemia, malignant neoplasm, acute and chronic infections, uremia, liver disease, hemochromatosis, acquired hemolytic anemia, leukemia, and lymphoma; moderate numbers (5 to 21 per cent) in thalassemia major, myeloproliferative disorders, and lymphoma and leukemia after treatment; large numbers (37 to 77 per cent) in refractory normoblastic anemia and severe infection accompanied by leukopenia.[16] In two patients with lymphoma, the ringed sideroblasts appeared for the first time after treatment with alkylating agents, and in one with chronic leukemia after treatment with 6-mercaptopurine. A reversible type of sideroblastic anemia has been reported in severe alcoholics with liver disease and folate deficiency.[79]

The puzzling relationship of sideroblastic anemia to the Di Guglielmo syndrome and leukemia has been reviewed by Dameshek.[43] The frequent development of leukemia in patients who have acquired sideroblastic anemia, "refractory normoblastic anemia," or "aplastic anemia with a hypercellular marrow" has been noted many times (Chapter 10).

PYRIDOXINE-RESPONSIVE ANEMIA

The first report of a patient with pyridoxine-responsive anemia was by Harris et al. in 1956, and since that time an increasing number of reports of similar patients have appeared although the disorder must still be considered a rare one.[44, 53, 68, 130, 152] One review included 72 patients.[84]

This disorder has been reported in patients from 8 to 87 years of age. About 80 per cent were males. Hepatomegaly, splenomegaly, and diffuse skin pigmentation have been noted in about 50 per cent. Most patients have been well nourished; none has had other evidence of pyridoxine deficiency such as dermatitis, neuropathy, glossitis, or convulsions.

The reported hemoglobin levels have ranged from 3.8 to 11 gms. per 100 ml. Typically the erythrocytes are hypochromic and microcytic, but in some patients they are hypochromic and normocytic or macrocytic; normochromic cells have been seen in a few patients. In the peripheral blood smear anisocytosis, poikilocytosis, and target cells are prominent; siderocytes are often increased. The reticulocytes are normal or low. The number of leukocytes and platelets show no consistent variations but may be abnormal.

In about 80 per cent of the reported patients the bone marrow examination has disclosed normoblastic hyperplasia. Iron stains demonstrate a striking increase of iron in the reticuloendothelial cells and normoblasts. The number of sideroblasts is greatly increased and "ringed" sideroblasts have been observed. In a minority of the patients megaloblastic hyperplasia has been observed; in these macrocytosis is the rule and microcytosis the exception.

Characteristically the level of serum iron is increased, usually over 200 micrograms per 100 ml., and the iron-binding capacity is 80 to 100 per cent saturated. Studies with radioactive iron have shown accelerated plasma clearance of injected iron and increased plasma iron turnover associated with subnormal or minimal incorporation of the radioiron into erythrocytes.

Other studies have shown a slight or moderate decrease in erythrocyte survival time as determined by the ^{51}Cr method. Negative Coombs tests and a slight increase in the osmotic resistance to hypotonic saline have been reported. The free erythrocyte protoporphyrin is not inceased as it is in iron deficiency.

The cause of the pyridoxine responsiveness in this group of patients has not been determined. The familial incidence of the disorder indicates that heredity may be an etiologic factor. There is no evidence of dietary deficiency in any of the patients reported, except in one that was experimentally induced. Likewise, there is no evidence of malabsorption in most of the reported patients. Further evidence against the presence of a true deficiency of pyridoxine is the large amount of pyridoxine that is necessary to produce the remission, 10 to 100 mg. intramuscularly, or 200 mg. orally. Discontinuance of the pyridoxine has resulted in hematologic relapse in the reported patients who had previously responded, but the remission may be prolonged. The incompleteness of the remission in the majority of the reported patients suggests that a deficiency of pyridoxine is not the only defect. Response to treatment is often manifested by a reticulocytosis of from 2 to 50 per cent in from four to ten days, followed by a fall in the serum iron level.

ANEMIA RESPONSIVE TO CRUDE LIVER EXTRACT

Two patients have been reported with hypochromic microcytic anemia, hyperferremia, anisocytosis, poikilocytosis anisochromasia, and leptocytosis accompanied by bone marrow hyperplasia of the normoblastic type, who responded to crude liver extract administered orally but not to iron, vitamin B_{12}, or folic acid.[85] At the time of the report the effect of pyridoxine had not been determined in these patients, although it was thought that pyridoxine was not a component of the liver extract which proved effective in their case. Crude liver extract was found to be ineffective in many of the pyridoxine-responsive anemia patients who responded only partially and has also been found to be ineffective in at least some of the patients classified in the refractory group of sideroblastic anemias.

IRON OVERLOAD

Excessive iron is stored in the body in special circumstances. Ingestion of large amounts of iron, abnormally high intestinal absorption, and excess parenteral iron, usually administered in the form of transfusions, lead to excessive

Table 5–5   *Classification of Disorders Associated with Excess Body Iron*

I. Increased Total Body Iron

   A. Hemochromatosis
      1. Idiopathic (Genetic)
      2. Secondary
         a. Hepatic cirrhosis
         b. Excessive ingestion of iron
            (1) South African Bantu
            (2) Kaschin-Beck Disease
            (3) Chronic ingestion of medicinal iron
         c. Refractory and sideroblastic anemias

   B. Hemosiderosis secondary to transfusions

II. Local Increase in Iron

   A. Reticuloendothelial
      1. Redistribution of iron associated with anemias
      2. Gaucher's Disease

   B. Hepatic cirrhosis

   C. Congenital atransferrinemia

   D. Renal hemosiderosis

   E. Idiopathic pulmonary hemosiderosis

accumulation of iron. The most common clinical conditions associated with iron excess are idiopathic hemochromatosis, iron overload in the Bantu, hemosiderosis, and the group of anemias associated with abnormal utilization of iron.

A classification of conditions associated with iron excess is shown in Table 5–5.

Idiopathic hemochromatosis. Idiopathic hemochromatosis is characterized by the slow increase of an excessive amount of iron in the body; the total of non-hemoglobin iron is greatly increased, being in the range of 20 to 40 grams compared to the normal of about 1.0 gram. Excessive iron deposits are found in the parenchymal cells of the liver, pancreas, heart, and adrenal glands; less striking increases are found in the skin, synovial membranes, kidneys, spleen, and other organs. Portal cirrhosis and pancreatic fibrosis usually occur. Pituitary or adrenal failure as a result of iron deposition may be serious.[147] The clinical symptoms usually appear between the ages of 40 and 60; over 90 per cent of the patients are men. The commonest symptoms are those associated with diabetes mellitus (weakness, weight loss, or hyperpigmentation of the skin) or those associated with heart failure or cirrhosis of the liver. Iron deposits in the myocardium usually are present in the patients with heart failure; the hyperpigmentation of the skin, which occurs in about 90 per cent of patients, is due mainly to increased melanin, since excessive iron deposits are demonstrated only in about one-half of those with hyperpigmentation. Hepatomegaly is an almost constant finding on physical examination; splenomegaly and spider telangiectases occur in about one-half; ascites, signs of heart failure, and testicular atrophy occur in one-third or less. Arthropathy — polyarthritis, hypertropic arthritis, monarticular synovitis, or arthralgias — occurs in from 40 to 50 per cent of patients. It usually appears together with other evidence of the disease, but on occasion is the first manifestation. Unfortunately, like the sterility suffered by some patients, the arthropathy is not reversed by a phlebotomy regimen.[41] Death is usually the result of heart failure (30 per cent), hepatic coma (15 per cent), hematemesis (15 per cent), hepatoma (14 per cent), or pneumonia (13 per cent).[54]

The disease is associated with an increased absorption of iron from the intestinal tract, but this apparently does not exceed 2 to 4 mg. a day. Neither the cause of the increased absorption nor the relationship of the iron deposits to the scarring of the organs is established with certainty. Although the portal cirrhosis is considered by some to be primary,[108] most authors have concluded that the disorder is the result of an inherited defect in the absorption of iron.[50, 54] It is probable that a defect in the function of the intestinal mucosa is responsible for the increased absorption because the intake of iron, the plasma transferrin, iron transport, and iron utilization apparently are normal. Evidence that supports the hereditary nature of the disease is the occurrence of the disorder in families and the demonstration of increased levels of serum iron in relatives who did not have the clinical disease.[46] In some patients, folate deficiency has seemed to produce an elevation of the serum iron and the deposition of iron in hepatic cells.[63] The relationship of the tissue iron to the tissue damage has been the subject of some controversy. The failure to produce the disease by administering excessive amounts of iron orally has led to the concept that both the tissue damage and the increased iron absorption and deposition are the result of an unknown defect.[18] Nevertheless, a clinical picture of hemochromatosis has been reported in a 70-year-old woman who took 1000 gm. of elemental iron over a 10-year period; autopsy confirmed the diagnosis.[91] At present the observations on patients with idiopathic hemochromatosis in the preclinical stage, which have disclosed that iron stores are excessive before cirrhosis develops,[13] similar observations on patients with hereditary iron-loading anemia, and the clinical improvement that follows removal of iron all support the concept that iron deposition is responsible for the tissue damage.

Congenital iron overload in infants, associated with hypotonia and minor anomalies without associated anemia or hyperhemolysis, has been reported.[154] The hypothesis was advanced that the children were born with excessive iron which was the result of a genetically-determined defect in the infants. The disorder ended fatally in both infants; no abnormalities of iron metabolism were demonstrated in either the father or the mother.

The best screening procedures for diagnosis are determinations of the serum iron and iron-binding capacity. In over 80 per cent of the patients in one report, the serum iron level was over 180 micrograms and the saturation of the transferrin was over 80 per cent.[50] Others state that usually the serum iron level is over 200 micrograms per 100 ml. and that the transferrin is completely saturated or almost so, the main exceptions being when infection or neoplasm had occurred.[14] If the screening tests suggest hemochromatosis, a needle biopsy of the liver is usually done; study of the tissue allows a definitive diagnosis. Because of the familial incidence of the disease, any brothers and sons the patient may have should be studied for early detection of the disorder at a time when treatment will be easier and more beneficial.[139]

The patient with hemochromatosis may have from 20 to 25 gm. of excess iron in the body, an amount requiring approximately 100 phlebotomies of 500 ml. of whole blood (200 to 250 mg. of iron). If the patient can tolerate two phlebotomies a week (and many do), the objective, which is to produce iron deficiency with a hemoglobin of from 11 to 12 gm./100 ml., can be reached in a year's time. When the anemia persists without phlebotomy it can be inferred that the excess iron has been removed; at that point a liver biopsy is advisable to determine the state of the stores. If the iron stores are depleted, removal of one 500-ml. unit of blood every two to four months usually suffices for maintenance. This regimen has produced remarkable results, even disappearance of hepatic cirrhosis and severe heart disease, and improvement in the diabetes mellitus and skin pigmentation[41, 51] leaving hepatoma as the commonest cause of death.

Iron overload in the Bantu. Iron overload of a particular kind occurs almost exclusively among the Bantu in Africa.[11, 14] The disease becomes manifest in late adolescence and is most severe between the ages of 40 and 60. The Bantu ingest excessive amounts of iron, sometimes as much as 100 mg. a day, not only because of the type of diet they consume but also because iron utensils are used in cooking and in the preparation of alcoholic drinks; although the positive daily balance is not often more than 2 or 3 mg., this increment is large enough to explain the heavy deposits found in middle age.[12] The disease is caused by excessive iron intake and not by an abnormality in intestinal function. In most patients iron deposits are confined to the liver and to the reticuloendothelial system, and the distribution differs from that found in hemochromatosis; the total amount of tissue iron is probably about 15 grams or less, and 10 grams or more of this may be in the liver. In the liver there is an association between severe hepatic siderosis and significant portal fibrosis or cirrhosis, particularly when the iron content of the liver is over 2 per cent by dry weight. In patients who develop cirrhosis, other aggravating factors, such as alcoholism and malnutrition, may be important.

Hemosiderosis. Post-transfusional hemosiderosis is an important development in some patients with chronic bone marrow failure or hemolytic anemia who require frequent blood transfusions. Usually the iron is stored in the reticuloendothelial cells and is not found in the parenchymal cells; with this distribution hepatomegaly, splenomegaly, and hyperpigmentation of the skin often develop, but are not accompanied by any serious disturbances in function. A second more serious form of this disorder has been recognized in which there is an accumulation of iron in parenchymal cells which is often associated with tissue damage and fibrosis; iron may be deposited in the parenchymal cells by transfer from the reticuloendothelial cells or by an increase in the intestinal absorption of iron.[21] Increased absorption is favored by hyperactive erythropoiesis, and accumulation of iron in the liver is favored by a saturated state of the iron-binding capacity; in the latter circumstance most of the iron absorbed in the gut is promptly deposited in the liver and does not gain access to the general circulation. Treatment with chelating agents may be helpful in some patients with this disorder who cannot be treated effectively with phlebotomies because of the anemia.

Idiopathic pulmonary hemosiderosis is a rare disorder characterized by widespread pulmonary capillary hemorrhages, hemoptysis, sudden falls in the hemoglobin level, hypochromic anemia, and reticulocytosis.[145] At times episodes of massive hemorrhage, dyspnea, cyanosis, and fever occur. It is seen most often in males, in childhood or early adult life. Later in the course of the disease, pulmonary hemosiderosis, fibrosis, dyspnea, and hepatosplenomegaly occur; cor pulmonale develops only occasionally. The cause of the disease is unknown; defects in the pulmonary epithelial cells and macrophages have been suggested;[99] iron is trapped in the macrophages which accumulate in the alveoli of the lungs. The disorder may be accompanied by gamma-A-immunoglobulin deficiency, and possibly is a part of a generalized disorder of the lymphoreticular system.

Congenital atransferrinemia is a rare genetic disorder in which the plasma transferrin level is markedly reduced or absent.[61, 74] The clinical picture is that of severe hypochromic anemia, low serum iron and iron-binding capacity, normoblastic hyperplasia of the marrow, hepatomegaly, and generalized hemosiderosis. In this condition iron is absorbed from the gut, but cannot be used for hemoglobin production in the normal way. One of the reported cases apparently responded to the injection of human iron-free transferrin.[61]

Acute Iron Intoxication

Acute iron intoxication, rarely seen except in children who have ingested a large number of iron tablets, is potentially serious; mortality rates as high as 50 per cent have been reported in untreated patients.[88] Treatment with BAL, EDTA, and exchange transfusion have been occasionally successful. The most promising treatment utilizes deferoxamine, a chelating agent. Some children have survived who were treated with gastric lavage followed by the instillation of 7000 mg. of deferoxamine methane sulfonate in 50 ml. of distilled water in the stomach; the same preparation was given intravenously, 15 mg. per kg. per hour over a 12-hour period.

One report recommends the following treatment for acute iron intoxication:[31]

1. General measures
    a. Induction of emesis
    b. Gastric lavage
    c. Suction and maintenance of clear airway
    d. Control of shock with I.V. fluids, blood, oxygen, vasopressor agents
    e. Correction of acidosis.
2. Intramuscular deferoxamine mesylate (Desferal) 1.0 gm. I.M., followed by 0.5 gm. I.M. q 4 hr. for two doses, or more if necessary (not to exceed 6.0 gm. in 24 hours).
3. Intravenous deferoxamine is recommended only if the patient is in cardiovascular shock. The rate of infusion should not be more than 15 mg. per kg. per hour I.V. slowly, followed by 0.5 gm. q 4 hr. for two doses or more (not to exceed 6.0 gm. in 24 hours).
4. Deferoxamine is contraindicated in patients with severe renal disease or anuria.

In another report of acute iron poisoning in 27 children seen over a 10-year period, there were no deaths.[57] Primary therapy was gastric lavage with a phosphate salt to bind all unabsorbed iron. Deferoxamine mesylate was used only when free iron was demonstrated in the serum by a rapid method.

References

1. Adams, E. B., and Scragg, J. N.: Iron in the anemia of kwashiorkor. Br. J. Haematol., *11*:676, 1965.
2. Aisen, P.: The role of transferrin in iron transport. Br. J. Haematol., 26:159, 1974.
3. Ansell, J. E., and Wheby, M. S.: Pica: its relation to iron deficiency. Va. Med. Mon., 99:951, 1972.
4. Bearn, A. G., and Parker, W. C.: Some Observations on Transferrin. *In* Gross, F. (ed.): Iron Metabolism. Springer-Verlag, Berlin, 1964.
5. Bessis, M. D., and Breton-Gorius, J.: Iron metabolism in the bone marrow as seen by electron microscopy: a critical review. Blood, *19*:635, 1962.
6. Bessis, M. C., and Jensen, W. N.: Sideroblastic anaemia, mitochondria and erythroblastic iron. Br. J. Haematol., *11*:49, 1965.
7. Beutler, E.: Iron enzymes in iron deficiency. I. Cytochrome C. Am. J. Med. Sci., *234*:517, 1957.
8. Beutler, E., and Blaisdell, R.: Iron enzymes in iron deficiency. II. Catalase in human erythrocyte. J. Clin. Invest., *37*:833, 1958.
9. Bissell, D. M., Hammaker, L., and Schmid, R.: Hemoglobin and erythrocyte catabolism in rat liver: separate roles of parenchymal and sinusoidal cells. Blood, *40*:812, 1972.
10. Bjorkman, S. E.: Chronic refractory anemia with sideroblastic bone marrow. Blood, *11*:250, 1956.
11. Bothwell, T. H.: Iron Overload in the Bantu. *In* Gross, F. (ed.): Iron Metabolism. Springer-Verlag, Berlin, 1964.
12. Bothwell, T. H.: Pathophysiological and clinical aspects of iron overload. Series Haematol., *6*:56, 1966.
13. Bothwell, T. H., Cohen, I., Abrahams, O. L., and Perold, S. M.: A familial study in idiopathic hemochromatosis. Am. J. Med., 27:730, 1959.
14. Bothwell, T. H., and Finch, C. A.: Iron Metabolism. Little, Brown & Co., Boston, 1962.
15. Bothwell, T. H., Pirzio-Biroli G., and Finch, C. A.: Iron absorption: I. Factors influencing absorption. J. Lab. Clin. Med., *51*:24, 1958.
16. Bowman, W. D., Jr.: Abnormal ("ringed") sideroblasts in various hematologic and non-hematologic disorders. Blood, *18*:662, 1961.
17. Brown, E. B., Jr., Dubach, R., and Moore, C. V.: Studies in iron transportation and metabolism. XI. Critical analysis of mucosal block by large doses of inorganic iron in human subjects. J. Lab. Clin. Med., *52*:335, 1958.
18. Brown, E. B., Jr., Dubach, R., Smith, D. E., Reynafarje, C., and Moore, C. V.: Studies in iron transportation and metabolism. X. Long-term iron overload in dogs. J. Lab. Clin. Med., *50*:862, 1957.
19. Brown, E. B., Jr., and Justus, B. W.: In vitro absorption of radioiron by everted pouches of rat intestine. Am. J. Physiol., *194*:319, 1958.
20. Butterworth, C. E., Jr.: Iron "undercontamination?" J.A.M.A., *220*:581, 1972.
21. Byrd, R. B., and Cooper, T.: Hereditary iron-loading anemia with secondary hemochromatosis. Ann. Intern. Med., 55:103, 1961.
22. Callender, S. T.: Digestive Absorption in Iron. *In* Gross, F. (ed.): Iron Metabolism. Springer-Verlag, Berlin, 1964.
23. Cartwright, G. E., and Deiss, A.: Sideroblasts, siderocytes, and sideroblastic anemia. N. Engl. J. Med., *292*:185, 1975.
24. Cartwright, G. E., Huguley, C. M., Jr., Ashenbrucker, H., Fay, J., and Wintrobe, M. M.: Studies on free erythrocyte protoporphyrin plasma iron and plasma copper in normal and anemic subjects. Blood, *3*:501, 1948.
25. Cartwright, G. E., et al.: Anemia of infection. II. The experimental production of hypoferremia and anemia in dogs. J. Clin. Invest., *25*:81, 1946.
26. Catovsky, D., Shaw, M. T., Hoffbrand, A. V., and Dacie, J. V.: Sideroblastic anaemia and its assocation with leukaemia and myelomatosis: a report of five cases. Br. Jr. Haematol., *20*:385, 1971.
27. Chisholm, M., Ardran, G. M., Callender, S. T., and Wright, R.: A follow-up study of patients with post-cricoid webs. Q. J. Med., *40*:409, 1971.
28. Chisholm, M., Ardran, G. M., Callender, S. T., and Wright, R.: Iron deficiency and autoimmunity in post-cricoid webs. Q. J. Med., *40*:421, 1971.
29. Chodos, R. B., Ross, J. F., Apt, L., Pollycove, M., and Halkett, J. A. E.: Absorption of radio-iron labelled foods and iron salts in normal and iron-deficient subjects and in idiopathic hemachromatosis. J. Clin. Invest., *36*:314, 1957.
30. Choi, S. I., and Simone, J. V.: Platelet production in experimental iron deficiency anemia. Blood, *42*:219, 1973.

31. Ciba Pharmaceutical Co.: Deferoxamine mesylate (Desferal Mesylate). Clin. Pharmacol. Ther., *10*:595, 1969.
32. Committee on Iron Deficiency: Iron deficiency in the United States. J.A.M.A., *203*:407, 1968.
33. Conrad, M. E., Weintraub, L. R., and Crosby, W. H.: The role of the intestine in iron kinetics. J. Clin. Invest., *43*:963, 1964.
34. Cooley, T. B.: A severe type of hereditary anemia with elliptocytosis: interesting sequence of splenectomy. Am. J. Med. Sci., *209*:561, 1945.
35. Cook, J. D., Layrisse, M., and Finch, C. A.: The measurement of iron absorption. Blood, *33*: 421, 1969.
36. Crichton, R. R.: Ferritin: structure, synthesis and function. N. Engl. J. Med., *284*:1413, 1971.
37. Crosby, W. H.: The control of iron balance by the intestinal mucosa. Blood, *22*:441, 1963.
38. Crosby, W. H.: Intestinal response to the body's requirement for iron. J.A.M.A., *208*:347, 1969.
39. Crosby, W. H.: The iron-enrichment-now brouhaha. J.A.M.A., *231*:1054, 1975.
40. Crosby, W. H., Likhite, V. V., O'Brien, J. E., and Forman, D.: Serum iron levels in ostensibly normal people. J.A.M.A., *227*:310, 1974.
41. Crosby, W. H., and Southgate, M. T.: Hemochromatosis (iron-storage disease). J.A.M.A., *228*:743, 1974.
42. Dameshek, W.: The Di Guglielmo syndrome. (Edit.) Blood, *13*:192, 1958.
43. Dameshek, W.: Sideroblastic anaemia: is this a malignancy? Br. J. Haematol., *11*:52, 1965.
44. Dawson, D. W., Leeming, J. T., Oelbaum, M. H., Pengelly, C. D. R., and Wilkinson, J. F.: Pyridoxine-responsive hypochromic anemia. Lancet, *2*:10, 1961.
45. Dawson, R. B., Rafal, S., and Weintraub, L. R.: Absorption of hemoglobin iron: the role of xanthine oxidase in the intestinal heme-splitting reaction. Blood, *35*:94, 1970.
46. Debre, R., Dreyfus, J. C., Frezal, J., Labie, D., Lamy, M., Maroteaux, P., Schapira, F., and Schapira, G.: Genetics in hemochromatosis. Ann. Hum. Genet., *23*:16, 1958.
47. Demulder, R.: Iron. Arch. Intern. Med., *102*:254, 1958.
48. Dowdle, E. B., Schacter, D., and Schenker, H.: Active transport of Fe[59] by everted segments of rat duodenum. Am. J. Physiol., *198*:609, 1960.
49. Drabkin, D. L.: Metabolism of the hemin chromoproteins. Physiol. Rev., *31*:345, 1951.
50. Dreyfus, J. C., and Schapira, G.: The Metabolism of Iron in Haemochromatosis. *In* Gross, F. (ed.): Iron Metabolism. Springer-Verlag, Berlin, 1964.
51. Dymock, I. W., Cassar, J., Pyke, D. A., Oakley, W. G., and Williams, R.: Observations on the pathogenesis, complications and treatment of diabetes in 115 cases of hemochromatosis. Am. J. Med., *52*:203, 1972.
52. Ellis, L. D., Jensen, W. N., and Westerman, M. P.: An evaluation of depleted stores in a series of 1,332 needle biopsies. Ann. Intern. Med., *61*:44, 1964.
53. Erslev, A. J., Lear, A. A., and Castle, W. B.: Pyridoxine-responsive anemia. N. Engl. J. Med., *262*:1209, 1960.
54. Finch, S. C., and Finch, C. A.: Idiopathic hemochromatosis, an iron storage disease. Medicine, *34*:381, 1955.
55. Finch, C. A., and Monsen, E. R.: Iron nutrition and the fortification of food with iron. J.A.M.A., *219*:1462, 1972.
56. Finch, C. A., et al.: Iron metabolism: The pathophysiology of iron storage. Blood, *5*:983, 1950.
57. Fischer, D. S., Parkman, R., and Finch, S. C.: Acute iron poisoning in children. J.A.M.A., *218*: 1179, 1971.
58. Fowler, W. M.: Chlorosis—an obituary. Ann. Med. Hist., *8*:168, 1936.
59. Gitlin, D., Janeway, C. A., and Farr, L. E.: Studies on the metabolism of plasma proteins in the nephrotic syndrome. I. Albumin, gamma-globulin and iron-binding globulin. J. Clin. Invest., *35*:44, 1956.
60. Goodman, J. R., and Hall, S. G.: Accumulation of iron in mitochondria of erythroblasts. Br. J. Haematol., *13*:335, 1967.
61. Goya, N., Miyazaki, S., Kodate, S. and Ushio, B.: A family of congenital atransferrinemia. Blood, *40*:239, 1972.
62. Granick, S.: Protein apoferritin and ferritin in iron feeding and absorption. Science, *103*:107, 1946.
63. Greenberg, M. S., and Grace, N. D.: Folic acid deficiency and iron overload. Arch. Intern. Med., *125*:140, 1970.
64. Gubler, C. J.: Absorption and metabolism of iron. Science, *123*:87, 1956.
65. Hahn, P. F., Balem, W. F., Ross, J. F., Balfour, W. M., and Whipple, G. H.: Radioactive iron absorption by the gastro-intestinal tract. J. Exp. Med., *78*:169, 1943.
66. Hallberg, L., and Solvell, L.: Absorption of a single dose of iron in man. Acta Med. Scand., *168*(Suppl. 358):19, 1960.
67. Hallen, L.: Part II. Gastric Secretion. Acta Med. Scand., (Suppl. 90):398, 1938.
68. Harris, J. W., Whittington, R. M., Weisman, R. J., and Horrigan, D. L.: Pyridoxine responsive anemia in human adult. Proc. Soc. Exp. Biol. Med., *91*:427, 1956.

69. Haskins, D., Stevens, A. R., Jr., Finch, S., and Finch, C. A.: Iron metabolism: iron stores in man as measured by phlebotomy. J. Clin. Invest., *31*:543, 1952.
70. Hayem, G.: Maladies du Sang. Masson et Cie., Paris, 1900.
71. Hegsted, D. M., Finch, C. A., and Kinney, T. D.: The influence of diet on iron absorption: II. The interrelation of iron and phosphorus. III. Comparative studies with rats, mice, guinea pigs and chickens. J. Exp. Med., *90*:147, 1949; *90*:137, 1949; *96*:115, 1952.
72. Heilmeyer, L.: *In* Wallerstein, R. O., and Mettier, S. R. (eds.): Iron in Clinical Medicine. University of California Press, Berkeley, Calif., 1958.
73. Heilmeyer, L.: Disturbances in Heme Synthesis. Charles C Thomas, Springfield, Ill., 1966.
74. Heilmeyer, L., Keller, W., Vivell, O., Keiderling, W., Betke, K., Wohler, F., and Schultze, H.: Kongenitale Atransferrinamie bei eine sieben jahre alten Kind. Dtsch. Med. Wochenschr., *86*:1745, 1961.
75. Heilmeyer, L., and Ploetner, K.: Das Serumeisen und die Eisenmangelkrankheit, Pathogenese, Symptomatologic und Therapie. Jena, 1937.
76. Henderson, P. A., and Hillman, R. S.: Characteristics of iron dextran utilization in man. Blood, *34*:357, 1969.
77. Hershko, C., Cook, J. D., and Finch, C. A.: Storage iron kinetic II uptake of hemoglobin iron by hepatic parenchymal cells. J. Lab. Clin. Med., *80*:624, 1972.
78. Hill, R. S., Pettit, J. E., Tattersall, M. H. N., Kiley, N., and Lewis, S. M.: Iron deficiency and dysenthropoiesis. Br. J. Haematol., *23*:507, 1972.
79. Hines, J. D., and Cowan, D. H.: Studies on the pathogenesis of alcohol-induced sideroblastic bone marrow abnormalities. N. Engl. J. Med., *283*:441, 1970.
80. Höglund, S.: Studies in iron absorption. VI. Transitory effect of oral administration of iron on iron absorption. Blood, *34*:505, 1969.
81. Höglund, S., and Reizenstein, P.: Studies in iron absorption. IV. Effect of humoral factors on iron absorption. Blood, *34*:488, 1969.
82. Höglund, S., and Reizenstein, P.: Studies in iron absorption. V. Effect of gastrointestinal factors on iron absorption. Blood, *34*:496, 1969.
83. Holmberg, C. G., and Laurell, C. B.: Studies on the capacity of serum to bind iron. A contribution to our knowledge of the regulation mechanism of serum iron. Acta Physiol. Scand., *10*:307, 1945.
84. Horrigan, D. L., and Harris, J. W.: Pyridoxin responsive anemias: An analysis of 62 cases. Adv. Intern. Med., *12*:103, 1964.
85. Horrigan, D. L., Whittington, R. M., Weisman, R., and Harris, J. W.: Hypochromic anemia with hyperferricemia responding to oral crude liver extract. Am. J. Med., *22*:99, 1957.
86. Huff, R. L., et al.: Plasma and red cell iron turnover in normal subjects and in patients having various hematopoietic disorders. J. Clin. Invest., *29*:1041, 1950.
87. Huff, R. L., and Judd, O. J.: Kinetics of Iron Metabolism. Advances in Biological and Medical Physics. Vol. IV. Academic Press, New York, 1956.
88. Jacobs, J., Greene, H., and Gendel, B. R.: Acute iron intoxication. N. Engl. J. Med., *273*:1124, 1965.
89. Jandl, J. H., Inman, J. K., Simmons, R. L., and Allen, D. W.: Transfer of iron from the serum iron-binding protein to human reticulocytes. J. Clin. Invest., *38*:161, 1959.
90. Jandl, J. H., and Katz, J. H.: Plasma-to-cell cycle of transferrin. J. Clin. Invest., *42*:314, 1963.
91. Johnson, B. F.: Hemochromatosis resulting from prolonged oral iron therapy. N. Engl. J. Med., *278*:1100, 1968.
92. Johnston, F. A., Frenchman, R., and Boroughs, E. D.: The iron metabolism of young women on two levels of intake. J. Nutr., *38*:479, 1949.
93. Karpatkin, S., Garg, S. K., and Freedman, M. L.: Role of iron as a regulator of thrombopoiesis. Am. J. Med., *57*:521, 1974.
94. Katz, J. H.: Iron and protein kinetics studied by means of doubly labelled human crystalline transferrin. J. Clin. Invest., *40*:2143, 1961.
95. Katz, J. H.: The delivery of iron to the immature red cell—a critical review. Series Haematol., *6*:15, 1966.
96. Katz, J. H., and Jandl, J. H.: The Role of Transferrin in the Transport of Iron into the Developing Red Cell. *In* Gross, F. (ed.): Iron Metabolism. Springer-Verlag, Berlin, 1964.
97. Kimber, R. C., and Weintraub, L. R.: Malabsorption of iron secondary to iron deficiency. N. Engl. J. Med., *279*:453, 1968.
98. Krantz, S., Goldwasser, J., and Jacobson, L. O.: Studies on erythropoiesis. XIV. The relationship of humoral stimulation to iron absorption. Blood, *14*:654, 1959.
99. Krieger, I., and Brough, J. A.: Gamma-A deficiency and hypochromic anemia due to defective iron mobilization. N. Engl. J. Med., *276*:886, 1967.
100. Kushner, J. P., Lee, G. R., Wintrobe, M. M., and Cartwright, G. E.: Idiopathic refractory sideroblastic anemia. Clinical and laboratory investigation of 17 patients and review of the literature. Medicine, *50*:139, 1971.

101. Lajtha, L. G.: *In* Stohlman, F. R., Jr. (ed.): Kinetics of Cellular Proliferation. Grune and Stratton, New York, 1959.
102. Lajtha, L. G., and Suit, H. I.: Uptake of radioactive iron (Fe) by nucleated red cells in vitro. Br. J. Haematol., *1*:55, 1955.
103. Lange, J.: De Morbo Virgineo. Medicinalium epistolarum miscellaneo. Wechelus, Basle, 1554, p. 74. (Quoted from Major, R. H.: Classic Descriptions of Disease. 3rd Ed. Charles C Thomas, Springfield, Ill., 1959, p. 487.)
104. Layrisse, M., Cook, J. D., Martinez, C., Roche, M., Kuhn, I., Walker, R. B., and Finch, C. A.: Food iron absorption: a comparison of vegetable and animal foods. Blood, *33*:430, 1969.
105. Lees, F., and Rosenthal, F. D.: Gastric mucosal lesions before and after treatment in iron deficiency anemia. Q. J. Med., *27*:19, 1958.
106. London, I. M.: Biosynthesis of hemoglobin and its control in relation to some hypochromic anemias in man. Series Haematol., *2*:1, 1965.
107. Loria, A., Sanchez-Medal, L., Lisker, R., de Rodriguez, E., and Labardini, J.: Red cell life span in iron deficiency anemia. Br. J. Haematol., *13*:294, 1967.
108. MacDonald, R. A.: Idiopathic hemochromatosis. Arch. Intern. Med., *107*:606, 1961.
109. MacDonald, R. A., and Mallory, G. K.: Hemochromatosis and hemosiderosis. A study of 211 autopsied cases. Arch. Intern. Med., *105*:686, 1960.
110. MacGibbon, B. H., and Mollin, D. L.: Sideroblastic anemia in man: observations on seventy cases. Br. J. Haematol., *11*:59, 1965.
111. Magnus, E. M.: Folic acid activity in serum and red cells in patients with vitamin B_{12} deficiency: relation to treatment. Br. J. Haematol., *11*:188, 1965.
112. Manis, J. G., and Schachter, D.: Active transport of iron by intestine: effects of oral iron and pregnancy. Am. J. Physiol., *203*:81, 1962.
113. Manis, J. G., and Schachter, D.: Active transport of iron by intestine: features of a two-step mechanism. Am. J. Physiol., *203*:73, 1962.
114. Mazur, A., Green, S., and Carleton, A.: Mechanism of plasma iron incorporation into hepatic ferritin. J. Biol. Chem., *235*:595, 1960.
115. Mendel, J. A., Weiler, R. J., and Mangalik, A.: Studies on iron absorption. II. The absorption of iron in experimental anemias of diverse etiology. Blood, *22*:450, 1963.
116. Middleton, E. J., Nagy, B., and Morrison, A. B.: Studies on the absorption of orally administered iron from sustained-release preparations. N. Engl. J. Med., *274*:136, 1966.
117. Mollin, D. L.: Introduction: sideroblasts and sideroblastic anemia. Br. J. Haematol., *11*:41, 1965.
118. Moore, C. V., and Dubach, R.: Metabolism and requirements of iron in the human. J.A.M.A., *162*:197, 1958.
119. Moore, C. V., and Dubach, R.: Observations on the absorption of iron from foods tagged with radioiron. Tr. Assoc. Am. Physicians, *64*:245, 1951.
120. Murray, M. J., and Stein, N.: The effects on iron absorption of gastro-intestinal secretions from patients with iron-deficiency anemia and haemochromatosis. Br. J. Haematol., *15*:87, 1968.
121. Murray, M. J., and Stein, N.: Effect of iron stores on gastric acid secretion by rats. Br. J. Haematol., *15*:401, 1968.
122. Nixon, R. K., and Olson, J. P.: Diagnostic value of marrow hemosiderin patterns. Ann. Intern. Med., *69*:1249, 1968.
123. Noyes, W. D., Bothwell, T. H., and Finch, C. A.: The role of the reticuloendothelial cell in iron metabolism. Br. J. Haematol., *6*:43, 1960.
124. O'Shea, M. J., Kershenobich, D., and Tavil, A. S.: Effects of inflammation on iron and transferrin metabolism. Br. J. Haematol., *25*:707, 1973.
125. Pirzio-Biroli, G., Bothwell, T. H., and Finch, C. A.: Iron absorption. II. The absorption of radioiron administered with a standard meal in man. J. Lab. Clin. Med., *51*:37, 1958.
126. Pollycove, M.: Iron Kinetics. *In* Wallerstein, R. O., and Mettier, S. R. (eds.): Iron in Clinical Medicine. University of California Press, Berkeley, Calif., 1958.
127. Ponka, P., and Neuwirt, J.: Regulation of iron entry into reticulocytes. I. Feedback inhibitory effect of heme on iron entry into reticulocytes and on heme synthesis. Blood, *33*:690, 1969.
128. Pribilla, W., Bothwell, T. H., and Finch, C. A.: Iron Transport to the Fetus in Man. *In* Wallerstein, R. O., and Mettier, S. R. (eds.): Iron in Clinical Medicine. University of California Press, Berkeley, Calif., 1958.
129. Pryor, J. P., O'Shea, M. J., Brooks, P. L., and Datar, G. K.: The long-term metabolic consequence of partial gastrectomy. Am. J. Med., *51*:5, 1971.
130. Raab, S. O., Haut, A., Cartwright, G. E., and Wintrobe, M. M.: Pyridoxine-responsive anemia. Blood, *18*:285, 1961.
131. Rath, C. E., and Finch, C. A.: Chemical, clinical, and immunological studies on the products of human plasma fractionation. XXXVIII. Serum iron transport measurement of serum iron-binding capacity in man. J. Clin. Invest., *28*:79, 1949.

132. Rather, L. J.: Hemochromatosis and hemosiderosis. Am. J. Med., *21*:857, 1956.
133. Roselle, H. A.: Association of laundry starch and clay ingestion with anemia in New York City. Arch. Intern. Med., *125*:57, 1970.
134. Rundles, R. W., and Falls, H. F.: Hereditary (sex-linked) anemia. Am. J. Med. Sci., *211*:641, 1946.
135. Rustung, E.: Studies of serum iron. Acta Derm. Venereol. *29*(Suppl. 21):1, 1949.
136. Sano, S., and Granick, S.: Mitochondrial coproporphyrinogen oxidase and protoporphyrin formation. J. Biol. Chem., *236*:1173, 1961.
137. Schade, A. L., and Caroline, L.: An iron-binding component in human blood plasma. Science, *104*:340, 1946.
138. Schade, S. G., Cohen, R. J., and Conrad, M. E.: Effect of hydrochloric acid on iron absorption. N. Engl. J. Med., *297*:672, 1968.
139. Scheinberg, I. H.: The genetics of hemochromatosis. Arch. Intern. Med., *132*:126, 1973.
140. Schulz, J., and Smith, N. J.: A quantitative study of the absorption of iron salts in infants and children. Am. J. Dis. Child., *95*:109, 1958.
141. Shahidi, N. T., Nathan, D. G., and Diamond, L. K.: Iron deficiency anemia associated with an error of iron metabolism in two siblings. J. Clin. Invest., *43*:510, 1964.
142. Sharney, L., Schwartz, L., Easserman, L. R., Port, S., and Leavitt, D.: Pool systems in iron metabolism: with special reference to polycythemia vera. Proc. Soc. Exp. Biol. Med., *87*:489, 1954.
143. Sheldon, J. H.: Haemochromatosis. Oxford University Press, London, 1935.
144. Smithies, O.: Variations in human serum beta globulins. Nature, *180*:1482, 1957.
145. Soergel, K. H., and Sommers, S. C.: Idiopathic pulmonary hemosiderosis and related syndromes. Am. J. Med., *32*:499, 1962.
146. Steinkamp, R., Dubach, R., and Moore, C. V.: Studies in iron transportation and metabolism. VIII. Absorption of radioiron from iron-enriched bread. Arch. Intern. Med., *95*:181, 1955.
147. Stocks, A. E., and Martin, F. I. R.: Pituitary function in haemochromatosis. Am. J. Med., *45*:839, 1968.
148. Tompsett, S. L.: Factors influencing the absorption of iron and copper from the alimentary tract. Biochem. J., *34*:961, 1940.
149. Tranchida, L., Palutke, M., Poulik, M. D., and Prasad, A. S.: Primary acquired sideroblastic anemia preceding monoclonal gammopathy and malignant lymphoma. Am. J. Med., *55*:559, 1973.
150. Turnbull, A., and Giblett, E. R.: The binding and transport of iron by transferrin variants. J. Lab. Clin. Med., *57*:450, 1961.
151. Verloop, M. C., Plodem, W., and Leunis, J.: Hereditary Hypochromic Hypersideraemic Anaemia. *In* Gross, F. (ed.): Iron Metabolism. Springer-Verlag, Berlin, 1964.
152. Verloop, M. C., and Rademaker, W.: Anaemia due to pyridoxine deficiency in man. Br. J. Haematol., *6*:66, 1960.
153. Verwilghen, R., Reybrouck, G., Callens, L., and Cosemans, J.: Antituberculous drugs and sideroblastic anaemia. Br. J. Haematol., *11*:65, 1965.
154. Vitale, L., Opitz, J. M., and Shahidi, N. T.: Congenital and familial iron overload. N. Engl. J. Med., *280*:642, 1969.
155. Vogler, W. R., and Mingioli, E. S.: Heme synthesis in pyridoxine-responsive anemia. N. Engl. J. Med., *273*:347, 1965.
156. Vogler, W. R., and Mingioli, E. S.: Porphyrin synthesis and heme synthetase activity in pyridoxine-responsive anemia. Blood, *32*:979, 1968.
157. Weintraub, L. R., Conrad, M. E., and Crosby, W. H.: Regulation of the intestinal absorption of iron by the rate of erythropoiesis. Br. J. Haematol., *11*:432, 1965.
158. Weintraub, L. R., Dawson, R. B., and Rafal, S.: Absorption of hemoglobin iron: release of iron from heme by intestinal xanthine oxidase. J. Clin. Invest., *47*:101a, 1968 (Abs. #299).
159. Weintraub, L. R., Weinstein, M. B., Huser, H., and Rafal, S.: Absorption of hemoglobin iron: role of heme-splitting substance in intestinal mucosa. J. Clin. Invest., *47*:531, 1968.
160. Wheby, M. S.: Regulation of iron absorption. Gastroenterology, *50*:888, 1966.
161. Wheby, M. S., Conrad, M. E., Hedberg, S. E., and Crosby, W. H.: The role of bile in the control of iron absorption. Gastroenterology, *42*:319, 1962.
162. Wheby, M. S., and Jones, L. G.: Role of transferrin in iron absorption. J. Clin. Invest., *42*:1007, 1963.
163. Wheby, M. S., Jones, L. G., and Crosby, W. H.: Studies on iron absorption. Intestinal regulatory mechanism. J. Clin. Invest., *43*:1433, 1964.
164. Whipple, G. H., and Robscheit-Robbins, F. S.: Iron and its utilization in experimental anemia. Am. J. Med. Sci., *191*:11, 1936.
165. Widdowson, E. M., and McCance, R. A.: The absorption and excretion of iron before, during and after a period of very high intake. Biochem. J., *31*:2029, 1937.

166. Widdowson, E. M., McCance, R. A., and Spray, C. M.: The chemical composition of the human body. Clin. Sci., *10*:113, 1951.
167. Yuile, C. L., Hayden, G. W., Bush, J. A., Tesluk, H., and Stewart, W. B.: Plasma iron and saturation of plasma iron. Binding protein in dogs as related to the gastrointestinal absorption of radioiron. J. Exp. Med., *92*:367, 1950.
168. Zervas, J., Geary, C. G., and Oleesky, S.: Sideroblastic anemia treated with immunosuppressive therapy. Blood, *44*:117, 1974.

CHAPTER 6

BONE MARROW FAILURE

CLASSIFICATION

The disorder characterized by pancytopenia, which is usually diagnosed "aplastic anemia," "refractory anemia," or "chronic bone marrow failure," is probably a syndrome rather than a disease entity. The syndrome is sometimes present at birth, but it may appear at any age. In some patients it develops after exposure to a drug or another chemical compound, but in others it appears under no suspicious circumstances. The severity of the anemia, leukopenia, and thrombocytopenia varies in different patients and may vary at different times in the same patient. The cellularity of the bone marrow and the results obtained with the ferrokinetic studies may be different in patients who have similar abnormalities in the peripheral blood.[67] It is likely that different mechanisms are at fault in different patients; more precise information may establish that the syn-

---

Table 6–1 *Classification of Bone Marrow Failure (Aplastic Anemia)*

    I. Hereditary (Congenital)
       A. Hypoplastic Anemia (Blackfan and Diamond[18])
       B. Pancytopenia
          1. With congenital deformities (Fanconi[21])
          2. Without congenital deformities (Estren and Dameshek[20])
       C. Congenital dyserythropoietic anemia

    II. Acquired (Chemicals, Infections, or Idiopathic)
       A. Erythrocytic Hypoplasia
       B. Pancytopenia
          1. With hypocellular marrow
          2. With cellular marrow
             a. Inactive erythropoiesis
             b. Ineffective erythropoiesis

---

drome includes several different diseases with different enzymatic or molecular defects.

Although an entirely satisfactory classification is not possible at present, a workable one is presented in Table 6–1. The relationship of this group to refractory sideroblastic anemia (Chapter 5) and Di Guglielmo's disease (Chapter 10), which are not included in the classification, is uncertain. Whether the syndromes characterized by pancytopenia are related to erythrocytic hypoplasia is unknown. The difference in the hematologic features, the more frequent association with thymoma, the better prognosis with supportive measures, and the better response to therapeutic agents, all warrant placing the patients with erythrocytic hypoplasia in a separate group. In addition, some separation of the pancytopenia groups according to the microscopic appearance of the bone marrow and the ferrokinetic characteristics appears desirable in order to recognize the differences, even though their cause is poorly understood.

APLASTIC ANEMIA

Ehrlich described the first case of aplastic anemia in 1888.[23] This patient was a 21-year-old white woman who died about one month after the onset of an illness characterized by menorrhagia, retinal hemorrhages, and marked pallor. The peripheral blood, which showed marked anemia and leukopenia, was considered unusual in that no nucleated red cells were seen despite the severe anemia. This apparent lack of increase in blood production in response to the anemia was explained by the fatty, inactive appearance of the bone marrow at autopsy. Following Ehrlich's description similar cases of this acute fatal illness were reported. It was recognized also that a clinical picture identical with these "idiopathic" cases occurred as a result of exposure to toxic agents such as benzene, arsenicals, and roentgen rays. The concept of the disorder was broadened further by the inclusion of patients with the clinical picture and peripheral blood characteristic of "aplastic" anemia, even though the bone marrow showed normal or increased cellularity.[87] Many such patients are now thought to be examples of ineffective erythropoiesis of some type rather than aplasia. In addition, cases have been considered to belong in this category if the anemia resulted from a failure of erythropoiesis when the anemia occurred alone or was associated with either neutropenia or thrombocytopenia.

MECHANISM OF THE ANEMIA

The primary defect in patients with this type of anemia is the failure of the bone marrow to produce erythrocytes, and usually granulocytes and platelets, in normal numbers in spite of adequate amounts of all the known hematopoietic factors. The defect may be either an unresponsiveness of the erythropoietic tissues to adequate stimuli or the lack of some necessary stimulus. The presence of a defective response of the erythropoietic tissue is indicated by the reports of apparently adequate amounts of erythropoietin in the plasma of patients with hypoplastic anemia. The evidence available at present indicates that the defect in most patients is an inability of the erythropoietic tissue to respond to adequate stimuli. In most cases the pancytopenia is the result of the failure of the hematopoietic stem cell rather than any fault in the stroma or environment; successful bone marrow transplantation in man and animals strongly supports this interpretation. In certain circumstances, however, radiation, particularly doses in excess of 4000 R, can so damage the stroma cells and the microenvironment that repopulation could not be accomplished even by normal stem cells.[16]

CAUSATIVE AGENTS

The defective erythropoiesis may be the result of various forms of injury to the blood-forming tissue. In some patients the failure of erythropoiesis is clearly due to the effect on the bone marrow tissue of agents that are known to produce cellular damage if given in sufficient quantity. Included in this category are x-rays, chemicals, such as benzene, and drugs, such as nitrogen mustard, urethane, and the antimetabolites (antifolic compounds, 6-mercaptopurine). Prolonged nitrous oxide anesthesia (five or six days) may also belong in this category.[36, 48] In other circumstances the damage to the bone marrow occurs as a result of some individual idiosyncrasy to drugs or chemicals that are ordinarily innocuous. Occasionally an infection appears to be the precipitating factor. Many times no adequate explanation for the aplasia is apparent and the case is classified as "idiopathic."

Total body radiation, administered therapeutically or received accidentally, may result in severe or even fatal aplastic anemia; less than 0.1 per cent of persons will survive an exposure of 700 rads, and 300 rads constitute the LD_{50}. In addition, heavy partial body radiation, such as that currently used in the treatment of lymphomas and other malignancies, may induce marrow hypoplasia. Nevertheless, 3500 or 4000 rads may be given to much of the body, including the neck, mediastinum, para-aortic, and inguinal areas, with only temporary marrow depression.

Since the first reports of an association between infectious hepatitis and aplastic anemia in 1955,[50, 73] nearly 200 patients have been reported.[11, 32] Most were between 2 and 20 years of age, but some were middle-aged. At least three-quarters were male. Although aplastic anemia appeared during an attack of hepatitis, it usually developed after the hepatitis had subsided, sometimes after an interval as long as 26 weeks. The development of aplastic anemia is not related to the severity of the hepatitis; the aplastic anemia has been unusually severe and only 10 per cent of the reported patients have survived. For this reason early bone marrow transplantation within weeks of onset has been advocated if appropriate arrangements can be made.[11] How infectious hepatitis causes aplastic anemia is not apparent. Autoimmunity has not been a frequently recognized mechanism in aplastic anemia; failure of the liver to detoxify substances appears to be an unlikely explanation because many of the patients have normal liver function tests at the time the aplastic anemia first appears, sometimes months after the hepatitis. Another suggested explanation is that the

Table 6-2 *Drugs or Chemicals Most Often Associated with Pancytopenia*

1. Chloramphenicol
2. Phenylbutazone
3. Solvents (including benzene)
4. Sulfonamides
5. Insecticides (gamma benzene hexachloride, chlordane)
6. Methylphenylethylhydantoin
7. Gold
8. Mepazine
9. Chlorpromazine
10. Oral hypoglycemic agents

hepatitis induces a genetic alteration in the hematopoietic cells, a theory consistent with the delayed appearance and severity of the aplasia.

Almost any drug or chemical may produce anemia or pancytopenia in a susceptible patient, but some are much more likely to do so than others. From a series of nearly 600 patients with aplastic anemia and pancytopenia compiled by the Registry on Blood Dyscrasias of the American Medical Association, the ten most common offenders are listed in Table 6-2.[77] Chloramphenicol was by far the commonest suspect, being the only drug administered in 113 cases. In another 150 patients the drug had been administered in association with other drugs with known or uncertain toxicity. The next most common drug, phenylbutazone, was reported in only 13 patients alone and in only 13 others in association with other drugs. In a recent report of 80 patients in Scandinavia, 29 of whom gave a history of exposure to a drug that might have been responsible, oxyphenbutazone and related compounds were the commonest suspects.[8] These were: oxyphenbutazone (Tandearil), ten cases; phenylbutazone (Butazolidin), four; chloramphenicol, four; sulfonamide, two; no other drug more than once.

A report from California gives the following estimate of the incidence of aplastic anemia: (1) incidence in the U.S.A., two per one million population per year; (2) incidence in California, between one in 400,000 and one in 700,000; (3) incidence after chloramphenicol, between one in 24,000 and one in 132,000; (4) deaths after chloramphenicol, 4.5 grams, one in 36,000; 7.5 grams, one in 21,000; (5) incidence after phenylbutazone, one in 124,000; (6) incidence after Atabrine in World War II, one in 50,000.[93] The best estimates placed the incidence of aplastic anemia as one per 100,000 in patients receiving chloramphenicol.[5]

A report of the published and unpublished cases of chloramphenicol toxicity covered 576 patients; in 70 per cent the associated disorder was pancytopenia, an estimated incidence of one in 20,000 taking the drug. The disease occurred in both members of three sets of twins treated with the drug. The review contained the distressing information that chloramphenicol had been used for typhoid or paratyphoid infections in only 5 per cent of the reported cases with toxic drug reactions; in nearly every instance it had been used in a situation which reflected doubtful judgment, such as in 29 per cent for respiratory infections, 14 per cent for urinary tract infection without culture, 4 per cent for acne, 4 per cent for whooping cough, 4 per cent as "prophylaxis," 2 per cent for "FUO," and 10 per cent for infections of unknown cause.[66]

Observations on patients who developed anemia or pancytopenia after administration of chloramphenicol, and also studies on patients who were receiving this drug but had not developed abnormalities in the peripheral blood, indicate that the hematologic effects observed are the result of several factors. These are: (1) the qualitative action of the drug on cells of the hematopoietic system; (2) the quantity of the drug administered; and (3) an individual factor in the patient receiving the drug.[5, 62, 71, 74, 99] The ability of chloramphenicol to inhibit erythropoiesis was shown when it was demonstrated that a dose of 50 to 60 mg. per kg. for several days could inhibit the therapeutic response to specific treatment with vitamin B_{12} and iron.[74] Another investigation of the toxic effect of the drug indicates that bone marrow depression is a pharmacologic property of the drug. Bone marrow depression occurred regularly with blood levels of 25 micrograms per ml. which accompanied a daily dose of 50 mg. per kg. of body weight; a daily dose of 25 to 30 mg. per kg. produced adequate blood levels and was recommended. These studies indicate that chloramphenicol causes first depression of erythropoiesis and then depression of the other elements in the marrow. Depression of erythropoiesis is manifested by a rise in the serum iron level, a decrease in the iron utilization, and a fall in the circulating reticulocytes; vacuolization appears in the cytoplasm and nucleus of normoblasts in the bone marrow. Serial studies of the bone marrow of patients receiving chloramphenicol suggest that the marrow passes through a reversible phase of depression from which it recovers promptly, within one week if the drug is discontinued, and sometimes even if it is continued. This stage may be followed by a more severe depression which persists while the drug is being administered; recovery from the phase may be slow, or even absent, in some patients after the drug is discontinued. In the reported patients prolonged administration of the drug or high dosage levels are found much more often than "hypersensitivity" reactions to administration of the drug in very small doses or for very short periods, such as a day or two.[5, 13]

The mechanism by which chloramphenicol affects the bone marrow is uncertain. A direct effect is manifested by vacuolization of the red cell precursors, diminished iron uptake, and inhibition of the incorporation of heme in normoblasts and amino acids in the leukocytes.[6] In addition, Weisberger and colleagues report that small amounts of chloramphenicol may block or reduce protein synthesis.[96] A series of experiments demonstrated that therapeutic concentrations of chloramphenicol inhibited the accelerated incorporation of ^{14}C formate into reticulocyte ribosomes that was induced by added RNA or polyuridylic acid, and suggested that chloramphenicol blocked the binding of messenger RNA to the ribosome and spared the ribosome-bound RNA; the structural similarity between chloramphenicol and pyrimidine nucleotides raised the possibility that they might be competitive.

Another hypothesis concerning the action of the marrow cells has been advanced by Yunis and associates, who have reported that small amounts of chloramphenicol, 20 micrograms per ml., inhibit the incorporation of ^{14}C leucine into the protein of mitochondria from human bone marrows;[58, 100] altered configuration of the mitochondria exposed to the drug was shown by electron microscopy. The mammalian mitochondria are much more sensitive to the drug than are the mammalian cytoplasmic ribosomes; the latter are much less sensitive than bacterial ribosomes. The observations support the hypothesis that the reversible bone marrow depression that is produced by chloramphenicol results from inhibition of the mitochrondrial function.

The observation that reticulocytopenia, inhibition of iron utilization, morphologic changes in the marrow, mild anemia, thrombocytopenia, and alteration in serum iron all reverted to normal when the drug was withdrawn has led to different opinions about the relation of these effects of the drug to the development of clinical aplastic anemia.

Yunis and co-workers have emphasized that two different types of marrow depression occur: the pharmacologic, which occurs in many patients and produces the commonly observed changes, and the pathologic, which occurs in a small percentage of patients and leads to persisting marrow aplasia, even after small doses. They have shown that, when ^{14}C formate uptake by marrow tissue was measured, there was a significantly lower uptake in formation of DNA and RNA in the marrow obtained from patients who had recovered from chloramphenicol-induced aplastic anemia as compared to the marrow of normal subjects.[98] The difference disappeared when the chloramphenicol concentration reached 250 micrograms per ml. The results suggested some abnormality in nucleic acid metabolism in the marrow of patients who had recovered from the dyscrasia. An apparently discordant result has been obtained in a study of colony formation in vitro, where marrow from a patient with aplastic anemia after treatment with chloramphenicol, and from a recovered patient, both manifested increased resistance to the inhibiting effect of chloramphenicol.[41]

The infrequent development of aplastic anemia in patients receiving chloramphenicol, the poor correlation between the dose of the drug and the development of aplastic anemia, the low incidence and good prognosis of the disease in blacks, and the occurrence of dyscrasias in some patients who received only small amounts of the drug for short periods, all point toward some idiosyncrasy, possibly a hereditary defect, in those who develop aplastic anemia. The development of pancytopenia in the absence of demonstrable antibodies is best explained by some effect on the stem cell. Observations made on identical twins who developed aplastic anemia following the administration of chloramphenicol support this concept.[63] The similarities in the course of the disease in both patients suggested a genetic factor. During development of the disease in one patient, the authors observed that the youngest cells in the marrow disappeared first and were the first to reappear during recovery, a sequence which suggested that the failure of differentiated forms to develop from a damaged precursor cell was the primary event. The possibility that a drug causes aplastic anemia by an effect on an enzyme system in the stem cell is analogous to the effect produced by certain drugs in patients with varying degrees of G6PD deficiency; both the inherited defect and the drug are required to produce the clinical syndrome.

Weisberger has suggested that the toxicity of chloramphenicol is the result of impaired metabolism of the drug.[96] Evidence advanced to support this concept is the observation that patients who have erythropoietic depression after taking the drug have a high serum level of free chloramphenicol; normally the free form is "detoxified," at least in part, by glucuronyl transferase in the liver. The increased incidence of toxicity in premature infants and other patients with liver disease supports the idea of a deficiency in this mechanism. The impaired clearance of chloramphenicol after an intravenous test dose was considered a reliable indicator of subsequent erythropoietic toxicity, and the only test currently available able to predict toxic effects;[84] an abnormal test or an abnormally high level of free chloramphenicol in the serum may be a contraindication to further use of the drug, or at least an indication for careful monitoring of the blood counts.

Whether or not the disastrous effects that chloramphenicol produces in a small percentage of patients are primarily the result of defective liver function, a subnormal enzyme system in the stem cell, or some other mechanism has not been established. Nevertheless, the delay of several months in the development of aplastic anemia in some patients after cessation of the drug, the sequential changes that have been observed in the blood and marrow, and the sequela of paroxysmal nocturnal hemoglobinuria that occurs occasionally, all point to a major effect on the stem cell.

Idiopathic cases. In a large percentage of patients with this syndrome no acceptable cause for the marrow failure can be found. These cases are classified as "idiopathic." Although the mechanism of the anemia in this group is obscure, various possible explanations have been advanced. Bomford and Rhoads suggested that erythropoiesis might be damaged as a result of the failure of the liver to inactivate completely hormones and other chemicals in the body, with the result that a chemical compound toxic to the bone marrow might be produced by the abnormal metabolism of normal or innocuous compounds.[7] Another possibility, damage to the bone marrow by an autoimmune process, has been suggested as a result of the recognition of the role of antibodies in the production of hemolytic anemia, erythrocytic hypoplasia, and thrombocytopenia purpura.[17, 29, 30, 46] Autoantibodies against erythrocytes, leukocytes, and platelets have been reported in a patient with aplastic anemia who had never been transfused. An increase in the circulating blood of cells with the morphologic characteristics of the young lymphocytes which are undergoing DNA synthesis, has been found in patients with idiopathic aplastic anemia, but not in those who gave a history of exposure to toxic agents.[14] The similarity of the findings in this group to those in hemolytic anemia was interpreted as evidence to support the autoimmune hypothesis. A possible etiologic relationship between leukemia and aplastic anemia must also be considered, because leukemia sometimes develops in patients with aplastic anemia, and both diseases have been reported to occur after exposure to benzol[9] or radiation. Still another possibility, which is suggested by the racial incidence and reports of a familial tendency, is the occurrence of a hereditary defect in the bone marrow that renders it more susceptible to either exogenous or endogenous toxins in later life.[62]

Some cases of "idiopathic" aplastic anemia may be the result of the gradual failure of an enzyme system in the stem cell. It is also possible, but not proved, that an enzyme system which is inherently weak or becomes so for some reason may, because of this deficiency, be badly or irreparably damaged not only by drugs but also by the ingestion of minute amounts of chemicals found in food from preservatives, herbicides, or pesticides. Unapparent viral infections, such as anicteric hepatitis, also may be responsible in some instances.

Hemolytic aspects. Although the main feature of this syndrome is deficient erythropoiesis, hyperhemolysis, as manifested by an increased fecal urobilinogen excretion, is found in some patients. This occurs most often in patients who have cellular marrows. Studies that employ radioactive iron indicate that most such patients have ineffective erythropoiesis rather than an absence of erythropoiesis;

iron is utilized in erythropoiesis, but excessive hemolysis occurs in the marrow before the cells are released into the circulation. This increased intramedullary hemolysis is responsible for the evidences of hemolytic anemia in some patients with "aplastic" or "refractory" anemia. In other patients a decreased survival time of the circulating erythrocytes may be the only evidence of hemolysis.[94] When hyperhemolysis is present in patients who have not been transfused, it is usually of such minor degree that anemia would not develop if the bone marrow were able to function normally. Increased hemolysis is seen most often in aplastic anemia in patients who have received numerous transfusions, when splenomegaly and hepatomegaly are often present.

CLINICAL MANIFESTATIONS

Aplastic anemia may occur at any age. In one series about one-half of the patients developed the disorder after the age of 50 years;[62] men were affected more often than women, possibly as a result of a higher incidence of occupational exposure to chemicals. In another series of 408 patients who had aplastic anemia following chloramphenicol therapy, 62 per cent were females; the peak incidence of the disease occurred between the ages of 3 and 7.[5] In this series, the amount of chloramphenicol ingested and the period during which it was taken varied considerably. Ten per cent developed the dyscrasia within four days of beginning therapy and 22 per cent developed it while taking the drug, even though only 9 per cent had a previous exposure to the drug. The median time for development of symptoms was 38 days after the drug was stopped, but in 10 per cent aplasia did not develop until 130 days after the last dose of the drug. Aplastic anemia is rare in the black as compared to the white, and this is especially true of the "idiopathic" type.

The onset of the disorder is generally gradual and is characterized by increasing weakness and other evidences of anemia, such as exertional dyspnea, palpitation, and pallor. Weight loss is infrequent and night sweats are rare. In about one-third of the patients abnormal bleeding is the initial complaint. Although the onset is usually insidious, sometimes the disorder begins abruptly with marked weakness, fever, other evidence of infection, and hemorrhagic manifestations.

The most striking abnormality found on the physical examination is the pallor of the skin and mucous membranes. There is no yellowish tinge of the skin or sclerae. Grayish brown pigmentation of the skin and testicular atrophy occur in an appreciable percentage of patients with this disease; these abnormalities are found particularly in those who have been transfused, and it seems likely that they are due at least in part to transfusion hemosiderosis. In about one-half of the patients there is evidence of abnormal bleeding in the skin, mucous membranes, or retinae at the time of the initial examination. Although enlargement of the spleen, liver, and lymph nodes is unusual in the untreated patients, and indeed is strong evidence against the diagnosis in such circumstances, these organs have been found to be enlarged in about one-third of one group of patients who had been under observation and treatment for some time, probably because of the transfusions they had received.

LABORATORY EXAMINATION

In a series of 50 patients studied at the University of Virginia Hospital the following peripheral blood conditions were noted: pancytopenia 37; anemia alone 7; anemia with leukopenia 4; anemia and thrombocytopenia 2.[62] The anemia was macrocytic (MCV > 94 cu. μ) in 60 per cent and normocytic in the remainder. A mild reticulocytosis of 2 to 5 per cent occurred at some time during the course of the disease in 21 patients, but an absolute increase in reticulocytes was rarely seen. Only nine patients had reticulocyte counts that were persistently 0.1 per cent or less. In the same series of 50 patients, 41 had leukopenia. There was a relative lymphocytosis in 37, and an absolute lymphocytosis (over 3000 per cu.mm.) in six. Only five had an absolute decrease in lymphocytes (less than 1500 per cu.mm.). The platelet counts varied from practically zero to normal levels, but were markedly reduced in most patients.

The smear of the peripheral blood of patients with aplastic anemia manifests little poikilocytosis although the cells may be slightly macrocytic; significant poikilocytosis suggests some other diagnosis, such as hemolytic anemia, vitamin deficiency, iron deficiency, or myeloid metaplasia.

The marrow specimen obtained by aspiration or surgical biopsy usually shows decreased cellularity. In the authors' series the marrow was hypocellular in 74 per cent, normal in 16 per cent, and hypercellular in 10 per cent. Similar discrepancies between the cellularity and function of the bone marrow have been reported by others.[7, 70, 87] In Best's series of chloramphenicol-treated patients, the bone marrow was examined in 129 patients; 3 per cent were hypercellular and 7 per cent had normal cellullarity; in 12 per cent one cell line was depressed, in 5 per cent two cell lines, and in 74 per cent all three cell lines were depressed (hypoplastic or aplastic).[5] In the bone marrow of many patients with this disease there is an increase in mononuclear cells that generally are classed as lymphocytes, although their identity and origin are uncertain. The differential count of the cells in the bone marrow often reveals increased percentages of plasma cells and reticulum cells.

The results of other laboratory procedures are often interesting and sometimes are helpful in diagnosis. The level of the serum iron may be increased and the latent iron-binding capacity may be saturated even before the patient has received any blood transfusions. The serum bilirubin level usually is normal but increased fecal urobilinogen excretion has been observed in some patients. Liver function tests usually are normal unless the patient has received a large number of transfusions which lead to increased iron deposition in the liver.

DIFFERENTIAL DIAGNOSIS

The disease which causes the most difficulty in differential diagnosis is leukemia. Even though careful studies of the blood and bone marrow do not reveal leukemia when the patient is first seen, the possibility that the patient may still develop evidence of leukemia at a later date continues to be a source of concern. The detection of significant enlargement of the spleen before the patient has been transfused should always raise the suspicion that the patient has leukemia, myelofibrosis, or some disease of the lymphoma group rather than aplastic anemia. The distinction between leukemia and aplastic anemia can usually be made as a result of the bone marrow examination and a careful study of the peripheral blood. When a normocellular or hypercellular marrow specimen is obtained by aspiration or biopsy, it probably means that the patient has ineffective erythropoiesis rather than aplastic anemia, but it may signify that the aplasia is spotty rather than general, or that the marrow is beginning to recover.

Any significant increase in very young cells in the marrow or peripheral blood should raise the suspicion of leukemia even though a definite diagnosis cannot be made. Hypercellularity of the marrow and the presence of abnormal normoblasts with increased nuclear parachromatin suggests "preleukemia" and the need for careful follow-up studies. If what is considered a satisfactory marrow sample is not obtained after needle aspiration, biopsy should be done to obtain a sample; some patients with leukemia have packed marrows or marrows that contain considerable reticulum tissue and yield only a very hypocellular or acellular specimen on aspiration. Although leukemia sometimes becomes manifest only months or years after the appearance of anemia, the distinction can be made in most patients after a relatively short period of observation. In the 14 autopsies in one series, the diagnosis of aplastic anemia was confirmed in all but one patient.[62] In this patient, who had aplastic anemia while under observation for five years, the presence of acute myeloblastic leukemia became manifest six weeks before death. When leukemia appears some years after the onset of the anemia in a patient diagnosed as having aplastic anemia, a question of the relationship of the two diagnoses arises. The question is whether the patient has both aplastic anemia and leukemia, possibly from the same or related causative factors, or only leukemia that has masqueraded as aplastic anemia.

Aplastic anemia must be distinguished from pernicious anemia, which may present with marked pancytopenia before treatment, but this usually is not difficult because of the differences in appearance of the skin and the tongue, and the absence of central nervous system involvement in aplastic anemia. Most patients with aplastic anemia retain the ability to secrete hydrochloric acid, and this finding is sufficient practically to exclude pernicious anemia from consideration. Examination of the bone marrow, even though hypocellular, generally permits the identification of erythropoiesis as the normoblastic type rather than the megaloblastic type seen in untreated pernicious anemia. Examination of the smear of peripheral blood also helps to distinguish between the two diseases; even when the anemia is severe and macrocytic in aplastic anemia, a smear of the peripheral blood usually shows but little poikilocytosis and anisocytosis.

At times the problem of the differential diagnosis between the idiopathic aplastic anemia and anemia associated with generalized carcinomatosis may arise. The finding of young leukocytes and nucleated red cells in the peripheral blood suggests the possibility of carcinomatosis of the bone marrow. The presence of metastases can be established sometimes by a bone marrow aspiration which reveals the malignant cells, and at other times by a radiographic study of the skeleton which discloses evidence of osseous involvement.

TREATMENT

The most desirable form of treatment of aplastic anemia caused by drugs and chemicals is prevention. Regular blood counts should be made on patients taking drugs that are known to produce blood dyscrasias. McCurdy has recommended that patients receiving chloramphenicol should receive serial reticulocyte counts. If the reticulocyte count drops abruptly or falls below 0.5 per cent, bone marrow examination should be made;[59] if erythropoietic activity is diminished or vacuoles are present in the young normoblasts, the drug should be discontinued. Unfortunately, careful and repeated assessment of the blood and marrow while the drug is being administered may not indicate the patients who will develop aplastic anemia later. A drug, such as chloramphenicol, which is known to be potentially dangerous should not be used if a safer one will be effective. Some unfortunate instances of aplastic anemia have occurred in patients who were treated with potentially dangerous drugs for minor illnesses which probably would have ended in recovery if treated with safer preparations or simple supportive measures.

The present-day treatment of aplastic anemia leaves much to be desired, although various measures such as removal of the patient from exposure to drugs or chemicals that might be toxic, attempts to supply the various cellular elements by transfusions, efforts to stimulate the proliferation of stem cells or hyperplasia of the remaining hematopoietic cells, and attempts to reconstitute bone marrow by grafting are sometimes successful.

Transfusion of red cells usually presents no major problem and may be given on an out-patient basis as often as symptoms warrant. Some older patients with vascular disease and angina may require a hemoglobin level of 10 gm. per 100 ml. whereas others are comfortable with a lower level. Nevertheless, even the transfusion of red cells is not without dangers such as febrile reactions to the leukocytes in the preparation, infectious hepatitis, and exogenous hemochromatosis. Transfusion of granulocytes is feasible with the newer methods of separation, and in all probability will be used more and more because it can be lifesaving in certain situations when the patient's granulocytes are practically nonexistent. Transfusion of unmatched platelets soon results in the production of antibodies toward the platelets which sharply diminishes their usefulness. If platelets matched for the HL-A antigens are available they may survive for nearly a week when transfused, and platelets from the same donor may be used successfully for months or even years. Unfortunately this arrangement for platelet transfusion is available to only certain patients because of the logistic problems involved. When suitably matched platelets are not available, fresh platelet packs from unmatched donors are used in emergencies in the hope that even the short platelet survival time in a patient may be sufficient to avert some serious complication.

The optimism for treatment with androgens, particularly large doses of oxymetholone, generated by the early reports of successes[2, 75, 80] has dimmed considerably. In these early accounts remissions were reported in nearly one-half of the patients treated, and in 70 per cent of those treated for more than two months. Undesirable effects such as hirsutism, hoarseness, weight gain, and hepatotoxicity, which at times was serious or even fatal, did not seem to constitute a real contraindication to oxymetholone in the usual recommended dose of 1 to 2 mg. per kg. per day. Unfortunately, later reports have shown remissions in only 10 to 25 per cent of the patients treated.[4] A review of the published results suggests that the patients who are less seriously affected are more likely to have a remission after androgens; these are patients who have only hypoplasia of the marrow, not aplasia, and who do not have severe reductions in granulocytes or platelets. In patients with severe marrow aplasia, granulocyte counts less than 500 per cu.mm., and platelet counts of less than 20,000 per cu.mm., treatment has rarely been successful.

How androgens exert their effect in some patients with aplastic anemia remains unclear. It seems unlikely that the known effect of androgens in increasing the production of erythropoietin is the important one, because patients with aplastic anemia have high levels of circulating erythropoietin even in relapse. The long lag phase required for the response in some patients is also unexplained. Experimental studies have shown that in animals androgens produce an increase in the incorporation of radioactive iron into red cells, followed by an increase of the red cell mass. In addition, in vitro studies of the marrow cultures from children showed that in about one-half testosterone produced an increase in the uptake of labeled thymidine within a few hours, evidence of DNA synthesis.[42]

The place of prednisone and related compounds in the treatment is uncertain. It is most often used when bleeding is a problem, and treatment with 10 to 60 mg. a day may be beneficial. Whether this result is a reflection of some increased production or survival of platelets that is not apparent in the circulation, or some improvement in resistance of the capillaries, is uncertain. Occasionally, in aplastic anemia and chronic erythrocytic hypoplasia, therapy with prednisone is followed by a remission. The result may be related to its effect on the immune mechanism and antibodies or, less likely, to a myelostimulatory action which has been seen in animals.

Splenectomy has been effective in some patients,[33] but only a few respond well and the operation cannot be considered a standard form of treatment.

The results of grafting of allogeneic marrow are much better than they were a few years ago. One report by Thomas and associates[83] disclosed that, of 24 patients with severe aplastic anemia who had received a graft, 11 were alive with functioning grafts without evidence of graft–versus–host disease for intervals that had lasted from five months to nearly three years after grafting. Ten had returned to normal activity. All patients received grafts from HL-A identical siblings, and the recipients were prepared by cyclophosphamide or total body radiation before grafting, and then treated with intermittent methotrexate therapy for 100 days after grafting. Deaths in the series were due to sepsis, the pregraft preparation or graft rejection. These authors emphasize that previous transfusions, particularly of leukocytes and platelets from donors who were not HL-A matched, increased the likelihood of the failure of engraftment or rejection after the graft. Grafts from persons other than identical twins or HL-A matched siblings have been failures thus far. In another review of the subject, Thomas and associates report successful grafting in 33 of 34 patients with aplastic anemia who survived the grafting procedure long enough to be evaluated. Sixteen were alive with functioning grafts more than four months later. Deaths were caused by graft–versus–host disease and infections.[86]

Because these recent results are so much better than the early experience with grafts, and the prognosis is so poor in patients with aplastic anemia following hepatitis, it has been advocated that marrow transplantation be given an early trial in such patients before they have become too ill and the conventional methods of treatment have reduced the likelihood of success of the graft.[11] Likewise the high-risk, poor-prognosis group of patients, those with neutrophil counts of < 200 cu.mm., platelet count < 20,000 cu.mm., and 70 per cent of nonmyeloid nucleated cells in the marrow, should be considered as urgent cases for early marrow grafting before other conventional treatment has reduced the chance of successful graft.[22]

Antibiotic drugs are used when infection is present, but their use over a long period as prophylactic agents is inadvisable because of the possible development of resistant strains of bacteria and fungus infections. When patients have severe granulocytopenia, any unnecessary trauma to the skin or mucous membranes, even rectal examination and rectal temperature-taking, is to be avoided whenever possible. Because of the likelihood of gram-negative septicemia if the granulocyte count is less than 500 per cu.mm., it is probably advisable to begin treatment for these organisms without awaiting the results of the blood cultures if the patient is febrile or acutely ill. Whether treatment with antibiotics to "sterilize" the colon is a worthwhile procedure to prevent septicemia, perirectal abscess, and other lesions is unsettled.

CLINICAL COURSE AND PROGNOSIS

Aplastic anemia is a serious disorder, but the outlook for survival with the treatment available has improved considerably. In one series of 62 patients reported in 1919, only three survived for more than a year.[81] In 1941, Bomford and Rhodes reported that, in their series of 66 patients, 15 recovered completely; many of these cases developed as the result of toxic exposure to chemicals.[7] In a series of 62 patients seen at the University of Virginia Hospital, 40 have died and 22 are living. Of the 40 patients who died, 50 per cent survived for one year, 35 per cent for three years, 20 per cent for five years, and 10 per cent for ten years. Of those who are still alive, over 50 per cent have survived for five years or more (Fig. 6–1). Similar results have been reported by others.[51, 76] A report from Scandinavia disclosed that only 16 of a series of 80 patients were alive three years after diagnosis; in this series, a history of exposure to drugs that might have been causative was obtained more frequently in patients under 50 years of age.[8] In recovery from aplastic anemia the increase in platelets lags behind that of the other blood elements; thrombocytopenia of varying degree may remain after the other values have returned to normal, as shown in Figure 6–2, which illustrated the course of a patient (Case 1) who recovered from aplastic anemia which developed after administration of chloramphenicol and sulfonamide.

The prognosis is best when the offending agent can be recognized and eliminated, giving the marrow a chance to recover before it has been damaged too severely. The outlook is better in patients who have erythrocytic hypoplasia than in those who have pancytopenia. Patients who have a severe pancytopenia

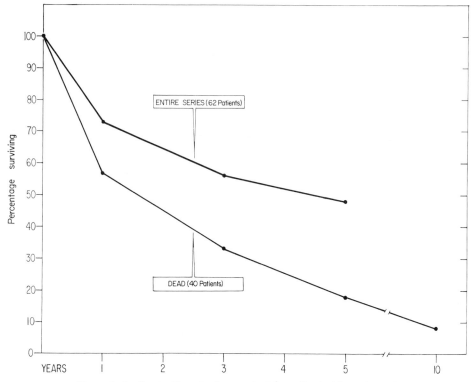

Figure 6-1 Survival in aplastic anemia, from estimated time of onset.

associated with what appears to be a totally aplastic marrow have a very poor prognosis. Most such patients do not respond to any form of treatment, and supportive measures such as transfusions, platelet packs, and antibiotics rarely prolong survival more than a few months. Contrary to the experience of some,[51, 92] in our patients a hypocellular or acellular marrow, severe reticulo-cytopenia (0.1 per cent or less), thrombocytopenia (less than 10,000 per cu.mm.), and severe leukopenia (leukocytes less than 1000 per cu.mm.) have indicated a worse-than-average prognosis.

The clinical course of the disease is extremely variable. Some patients have an acute illness with septicemia, fever, prostration, and bleeding; the outlook for such patients is poor and death usually occurs within a matter of a few days, weeks, or months. Fortunately, many patients have a longer and more benign course extending over a period of years. Death in these patients is most often the result of hemorrhage, either gastrointestinal or intracranial; infections such as septicemia or pneumonia also are often terminal complications. Serious infections are more likely to occur in patients who have an absolute neutrophil count of less than 500 cu.mm.; in addition, infection almost invariably causes a further fall in the neutrophil count, often accompanied by a reduction in the platelet and reticulocyte counts.[92] Some patients die from coexisting disorders, such as vascular disease, or from complications of therapy, and a few develop leukemia as a terminal event. More recently, the development of paroxysmal nocturnal hemoglobinuria has been recognized as a sequela to aplastic anemia in some patients.[28, 52]

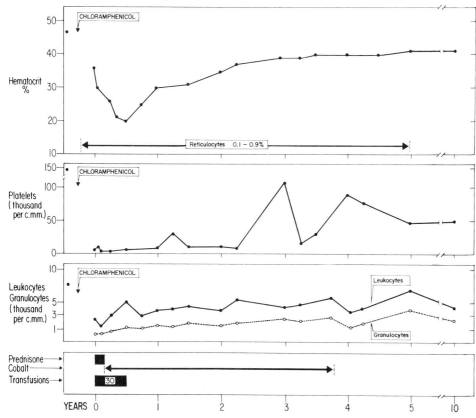

Figure 6–2 Course of aplastic anemia following treatment with chloramphenicol in a woman aged 62 at onset.

Paroxysmal nocturnal hemoglobinuria, a rare disorder, developed in 15 per cent of 46 patients with aplastic anemia seen by Lewis and Dacie;[52] the same authors found that, of 60 patients with PNH, 15 had earlier been diagnosed as having aplastic anemia. PNH may develop as long as six years after the diagnosis of aplastic anemia is made.[28] The disorder is characterized by intravascular hemolysis associated with ahaptoglobinemia, reduced red cell acetylcholinesterase, hemosiderinuria, leukopenia, variable degrees of thrombocytopenia, episodes of abdominal pain, and venous thrombosis. Presumably there is an acquired defect in the red cell membrane which permits hemolysis to be produced by complement in vivo without the action of antibody. Maximum lysis occurs at pH 6.8 when complement-sensitive sites in the cell are most exposed. The most acceptable explanation for the development of this disorder in patients with aplastic anemia is that the stem cell has undergone a somatic mutation which has resulted in the development of two red cell populations, one with a membrane defect that makes it extremely sensitive to complement and susceptible to hyperhemolysis, and the other with a normal life span. A further interesting but unfortunate association has been the development of acute myeloblastic leukemia in several patients with paroxysmal nocturnal hemoglobinuria.[40, 43, 44]

APLASTIC ANEMIA IN CHILDREN

The syndrome of aplastic anemia, both congenital and acquired, occurs in children as well as adults. In 1927 Fanconi described three siblings with bone marrow hypoplasia, pancytopenia, and congenital anomalies.[26] In 1967 he reviewed the abnormalities seen in 129 patients with this syndrome.[27] Listed as the chief criteria for Fanconi's anemia were the following: (1) pancytopenia; (2) hyperpigmentation; (3) malformation, especially of the skeleton; (4) small stature since birth; (5) hypogonadism; and (6) familial occurrence (which need not be evident). Of the skeletal manifestations, abnormalities in development of the thumb and the radius are most common; manifestations of anemia and thrombocytopenia usually do not appear until seven or eight years after birth. Early in the disease, hyperactive megaloblastic or "megaloblastoid" marrow may be present. Other common symptoms and signs found in 129 cases include microsomy in 60 per cent, microcephaly in 40 per cent, malformation of the kidneys in 28 per cent, strabismus in 22 per cent, and mental retardation in 17 per cent. Both hypoplastic and normally cellular marrows have been found in patients thought to have this syndrome.[20] Other syndromes that have been described in infants are the familial hypoplastic anemia characterized by pancytopenia without associated congenital anomalies,[25] and a type of hypoplastic anemia which affects the red cell series solely or predominantly.[21]

Aplastic anemia in children, defined as physiologic and anatomic failure of the bone marrow with marked decrease of blood-forming elements in the marrow, peripheral pancytopenia, and no splenomegaly, hepatomegaly, or lymphadenopathy, differs in some respects from the disorders in adults.[79] The prospect for remission when treated only by supportive measures is very poor, even worse than for adults. The history of exposure to a possible toxic chemical is obtained in a high percentage of cases; in one group of 17 children from five months to 13 years of age with aplastic anemia, a history of exposure to naphthalene, chloramphenicol, or DDT was obtained in 12. Withdrawal of the suspected agent and administration of testosterone and corticosteroids produced a remission in a high percentage of patients; nine of 17 patients treated with these preparations (testosterone or methyl testosterone, 1 to 2 mg. per kg. of body weight per day, and triamcinolone, 8 to 20 mg. per day) obtained complete remissions after being treated for 2½ to 15 months. When the drugs were discontinued, a partial hematologic relapse occurred for about two months; this was followed by spontaneous recovery by the third month. Similarly gratifying responses to this regime occurred in six of seven patients from 2 to 10 years of age who had congenital aplastic anemia. The response in this group differed from that of the acquired group in that the platelet response was incomplete; furthermore, persistent pancytopenia recurred in several patients when the drugs were discontinued, and maintenance dosage of the drug was found to be necessary. Despite these encouraging early results, it has been reported that in children treated in this way the overall mortality rate remained more than 50 per cent.[2] Further experience with androgen therapy in children with acquired aplastic anemia[54] has been very disappointing compared to earlier, more optimistic reports.[2] In a group of 58 children under 16 years of age seen at the Childrens' Hospital in Boston and treated with androgen, corticosteroids and supportive measures, the mortality rate was a dismal 71 per cent, and the median survival less than six months. Repeated platelet transfusions may be valuable in children; such treatment may prevent fatal hemorrhage and enable the patient to survive until remission occurs.[49]

The clinical course of acquired aplastic anemia in children treated with supportive care has been reported.[38] The study included 33 children, from 10 months to 14 years old, seen between the years 1951 and 1968. They were treated with supportive measures but without androgens; 16 patients (48.4 per cent) died, 15 have recovered, and two are still being transfused. The report emphasizes that the approximately 50 per cent survival is the same as that seen after treatment with corticosteroids and testosterone. This group of patients also provided some interesting figures concerning the time of recovery and those who survived; the mean time of recovery from anemia was ten months; from leukopenia, 12 months; and from thrombocytopenia, 18.9 months.

PURE RED CELL APLASIA
(PURE RED CELL ANEMIA)

Erythrocytic hypoplasia, which may be congenital or may develop at any time from childhood to old age, is characterized by normocytic (or slightly

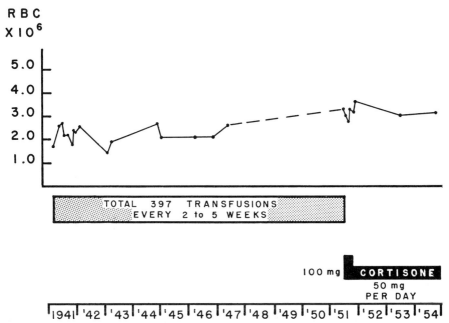

Figure 6–3 Chart showing responses of a patient with pure red cell anemia to treatment with cortisone. Although this patient required an average of 400 ml. of blood per week for 10½ years, no further transfusions were necessary after the institution of treatment with cortisone. (From Mohler and Leavell: Ann. Int. Med., vol. 49, 1958.)

macrocytic) anemia, usually severe, associated with normal leukocyte and platelet counts. The reticulocytes, although sometimes slightly increased, usually are greatly reduced and often number less than 0.1 per cent. Normoblasts may not be found in an examination of the bone marrow and at best are scarce. In these patients the danger is severe anemia; hemorrhage and infections usually are not problems. Nevertheless, some patients who appear to have simple erythrocytic hypoplasia at onset later develop thrombocytopenia or pancytopenia and become vulnerable to the complications seen in aplastic anemia. Most patients with erythrocytic hypoplasia require periodic transfusions to maintain a satisfactory red cell volume (Fig. 6–3). In some, however, treatment with corticosteroids produces a gratifying response manifested by reticulocytosis, increased normoblasts in the bone marrow, and a return of the peripheral blood count to normal; at times relapse occurs when the drug is discontinued, and readministration of the steroid may or may not produce another remission. In acquired erythrocytic hypoplasia, some instances are classified as "idiopathic," and others are associated with thymoma or follow exposure to drugs.

The association of erythrocytic hypoplasia and thymoma was first reported by Matras and Priesel in 1928.[18] Since that time, more than 50 patients, all but one over 40 years of age, have been reported.[39] Thymomas have been found in 50 per cent of adults with pure red cell anemia, and erythrocytic hypoplasia occurs in less than 10 per cent of patients with thymoma; the meaning of the association is uncertain. There is no convincing evidence that the thymus is concerned in erythropoiesis; in accord with the concept that nearly any abnormality of the thymus can lead to an abnormality in the immune mechanism, it has been suggested that the thymoma may be responsible for an autoimmune mechansim directed against either the red cell precursors or erythropoietin.

The studies of Krantz and colleagues have led to a much better understanding of this disorder.[45] Studies with the marrow culture technique demonstrated that normoblasts from patients with PRCA synthesized heme from 1.5 to 5.5 times better when incubated with normal plasma or saline than when incubated with the patients' plasma, and heme synthesis in normal marrow cells was reduced to 6 to 17 per cent of the control level when incubated with plasma from patients with PRCA for two to three days. These results led to a search for an inhibitor, and it was demonstrated that the gamma-G-globulins from patients with PRCA acted as inhibitors when active disease was present but failed to have this effect after recovery. It was further shown that plasma of some patients with PRCA was cytotoxic for erythroblasts; the active factor was present in the gamma-G-globulin fraction and was dependent on complement, which indicated that it was either an antibody or an immune complex.

These observations strongly suggest that, in acquired PRCA, the aplasia of the erythrocytic series is caused by an antibody or immune complex that is cytotoxic for erythroblasts. They also probably explain the effectiveness of treatment with immunosuppressive drugs and prednisone. The congenital form of PRCA may be a reflection of a similar immunologic defect. Marrow cells from patients with the congenital type have responded to erythropoietin and normal serum;[64] also, treatment with 6-mercaptopurine was followed by remission in two patients.[45]

Although the prognosis for patients with pure red cell anemia or chronic erythrocytic hypoplasia is not good, improvement has followed thymectomy, splenectomy, and treatment with prednisone and immunosuppressive agents. Remission in the anemia occurs only in the 25 or 30 per cent of patients with PRCA and thymoma after thymectomy. Some patients have responded to treatment with corticosteroids, some to splenectomy, and some to corticosteroids only after splenectomy.[45]

If thymoma can be demonstrated, thymectomy probably is indicated. This decision and the subsequent care of the patient require good cooperation between the thoracic surgeon, the neurologist, and the hematologist. Because of the frequency of associated myasthenia gravis in patients with thymoma and the operative risks involved in the former disease, recognized or unrecognized, careful neurologic assessment is necessary in every patient. Improvement after thymectomy may be prompt or may not occur until after several months; in the interim, transfusions of packed red cells should be given as often as necessary. If no improvement has occurred after several months, a trial of prednisone, 60 mg. per day, is indicated. If no improvement occurs within a few months of prednisone treatment, an immunosuppressive agent such as Cytoxan or 6-mercaptopurine should be added; response to one of the agents may occur only after several months.[45, 57]

Pure red cell anemia occurs in association with carcinoma. In some patients the presence of anemia and a good response to prednisone has preceded the recognition of the carcinoma by over a year.[61]

Pure red cell aplasia associated with drug therapy has been reported in 40 patients.[68] Twenty-one cases followed treatment with chloramphenicol. Other drugs that have been connected with aplasia of the red cells are sulfathiazole, arsphenamine, penicillin, phenobarbital, Chenopodium, isoniazid, tolbutamide, diphenylhydantoin sodium, phenylbutazone, and chlorpropamide. Ten of 12 patients reported in detail recovered when the drug was stopped, and one recovered when riboflavin was given with the drug.[97]

INEFFECTIVE ERYTHROPOIESIS

Ineffective erythropoiesis is characterized by the combination of anemia, hyperplasia of the erythrocytic series in the bone marrow, low or slightly elevated total reticulocyte count, increased plasma iron turnover associated with decreased erythrocyte incorporation of iron, and often mild increases in the unconjugated bilirubin in the plasma. The hyperplasia of the erythrocyte precursors is accompanied by hyperhemolysis of the erythrocytes and their precursors in the marrow, with the result that a reduced number of red cells reach the extramedullary circulation; in addition, some of those that reach the peripheral circulation are defective and doomed to premature destruction in the spleen and elsewhere.

In a number of disorders the ineffective erythropoiesis is accompanied by varying degrees of granulocytopenia and thrombocytopenia. This association occurs in vitamin B_{12} or folate deficiency, and in some myeloproliferative disorders, particularly myeloid metaplasia, preleukemia, leukemia, and erythroleukemia; considerable anisopoikilocytosis of the erythrocytes is often evident. In addition, at least some reported instances of "refractory normoblastic anemia" and "aplastic anemia with cellular marrow," as well as acquired sideroblastic anemia, are problems of ineffective erythropoiesis (Fig. 6–4).

Ineffective erythropoiesis also occurs with abnormalities confined to the erythrocytic series. The genetic disorders include the thalassemia syndromes, the congenital sideroblastic anemias, and the congenital dyserythropoietic anemias.

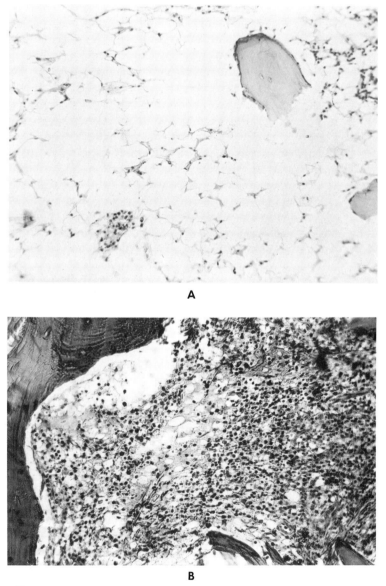

A

B

Figure 6–4 Bone Marrow: A. Aplastic anemia B. Ineffective erythropoiesis.

Table 6–3 *Congenital Dyserythropoietic Anemia*

Type   I. Macrocytic "megaloblastoid" anemia with erythroblastic internuclear chromatin bridges, and serum test negative.

Type II. Normoblastic anemia with multinucleated erythroblasts. "HEMPAS" (positive acidified serum test).

Type III. Macrocytic anemia with erythroblastic multinuclearity and "gigantoblasts."

CONGENITAL DYSERYTHROPOIETIC ANEMIA

The dyserythropoietic anemias first described by Heimpel and Wendt[35] have been classified as Types I, II, or III, as shown in Table 6–3. The red cell precursors in the marrow are strikingly abnormal when examined by light or electron microscopy. Dyserythropoiesis is manifested by an asynchrony of nuclear and cytoplasmic maturation. Among the abnormalities seen are: nuclear lobulation; binuclearity and multinuclearity with internuclear bridging; nuclear fragmentation with karyorrhexis and pyknosis; mitotic abnormalities; and megaloblastic changes. The cytoplasm of the cells often is vacuolated; basophilic stippling and excess iron may be evident in the lysosomes and mitochondria.[53] The circulating red cells manifest marked anisocytosis and poikilocytosis.

The Type I disease may be inherited as an autosomal recessive and may not be recognized until late in life.[55] The Type II congenital disorder, in addition to the nuclear abnormalities, is further characterized by demonstrating an abnormality in the red cell membranes, a positive acid serum test; the disorder has been called "HEMPAS" (Hereditary Erythroblastic Multinuclearity Associated with a Positive Acidified-Serum Test).[15] In some patients Gaucher-like histiocytes are found in the marrow.[24] The Type III anemia is characterized by a macrocytic anemia with erythroblastic multinuclearity and "gigantoblasts." Still another variant of congenital dyserythropoietic anemia, one associated with lipid abnormalities in the erythrocytes, has been reported in a mother and two daughters.[95]

Those who have reported all these different types consider that they are not instances of erythroleukemia or sideroblastic anemia.

Illustrative Cases

Case 1

APLASTIC ANEMIA

A 61-year-old white housewife had numerous urinary tract infections which were treated with sulfonamides over a period of years. On two occasions in the spring of 1959 she took 1.0 gm. of chloramphenicol, and in

September, 4.0 gm.; she had a small but undetermined quantity of sulfonamide in the spring and in October. In June her hematocrit was 43 per cent,
white blood count 4200 per cu.mm., platelets and differential count normal.
On December 7, 1959 she noticed ecchymoses of the skin; at that time the
hematocrit was 36 per cent, white blood count 2600 cu.mm., and platelets
5000 per cu.mm. A bone marrow aspiration was hypocellular.

Prednisone was prescribed with some symptomatic improvement in her
purpura, but on January 19, 1960 she was admitted to the hospital acutely ill
with chills, temperature (103° F.), and hypotension; septicemia was suspected but not proved. Her hematocrit was 26 per cent, white blood count
1500 (20 per cent granulocytes), platelets 2500 per cu.mm. The bone marrow
was very hypocellular. She responded to antibiotics and transfusions, but
similar febrile episodes, gastrointestinal bleeding, and periarticular ecchymoses occurred during the next two months. During this time she received
15 transfusions. She then began to improve, less frequent transfusions became necessary, and none was needed after July, 1960. The course of her
blood counts is shown in Figure 6–2.

In June, 1972, 13 years after the onset of aplastic anemia, the patient
developed gross hematuria; at the time her platelet count was 60,000 per
cu.mm. Diagnostic studies indicated a malignant tumor at the upper pole of
the left kidney; metastatic malignant cells were found in the bone marrow.
Despite radiation the patient died in November, 1972. Autopsy confirmed
widespread metastatic carcinoma in the skeleton and lungs. Bone marrow
from the ribs and vertebrae was markedly hypocellular with scattered metastatic carcinoma cells and large numbers of plasma cells. How much the
radiotherapy six weeks prior to death contributed to the hypoplasia of the
bone marrow is uncertain.

Comment. This patient developed aplastic anemia following repeated
treatments with sulfonamide and chloramphenicol. Frequent transfusions
were necessary for the first six months of the illness but none was necessary
after that time. She was treated with prednisone, androgen, and cobalt; her
improvement began while on the last drug, but it is doubtful if any of the
agents were responsible. The blood counts improved gradually; the hematocrit and leukocyte count returned to normal, but thrombocytopenia persisted
for 13 years.

CASE 2

PURE RED CELL APLASIA

A white government official, who had been admitted to the hospital
several times between 1920 and 1950 because of hemorrhages from a
duodenal ulcer, was admitted in January 1956 at the age of 82 because of
mild congestive heart failure, and was found to have a normochromic,
normocytic type of anemia. Admission blood studies showed the following:
Hb. 6.5 gm. per 100 ml., R.B.C. 2.5 million per cu.mm., Hct. 20 per cent,
W.B.C. 5500 per cu.mm., reticulocytes 0.6 per cent, differential count (per
cent), segmented leukocytes 50, lymphs. 37, monocytes 10, basophils 2.
The platelets were normal in number. The serum iron was 127 μg. per 100 ml.
and the unsaturated iron-binding protein was 185 μg. per 100 ml. Blood urea
was normal. The bone marrow obtained by aspiration appeared active and

normoblastic. No cause for the anemia was found and he was treated with blood transfusions.

Treatment and course. The anemia recurred and failed to respond to oral iron, folic acid, vitamin B_{12}, or cobaltous chloride. In July 1956 examination of the bone marrow disclosed almost complete absence of erythropoiesis and slightly depressed myelopoiesis. During the period from January to July he received transfusions amounting to an average of 1500 ml. of whole blood every month. In August 1956, when the R.B.C. was 1.4 million per cu.mm., Hb. 3.9 gm. per 100 ml., Hct. 11 per cent, and reticulocytes 0 per cent, prednisone was started in a dose of 20 mg. daily. Striking improvement followed and the bone marrow reverted toward normal. On a maintenance dose of 10 to 15 mg. of prednisone a day the hematocrit remained in the range of 38 to 41 per cent for 6½ months without transfusions.

Unfortunately an exacerbation of a previously mild diabetes occurred, and the symptoms of peripheral neuritis became so severe that prednisone was discontinued in February 1957. The neurologic symptoms subsided, but on April 9, 1957 the hematocrit had fallen to 16 per cent. Subsequently the anemia failed to respond to prednisone, testosterone, or cobalt, and transfusions were required regularly until his death at home in March 1961. The leukocyte and platelet counts remained normal and the reticulocyte count was usually zero. Extensive studies failed to reveal any apparent cause for this anemia. An autopsy was not performed.

Comment. This elderly government official had aplastic anemia of the chronic erythrocytic hypoplasia type. This syndrome is characterized by anemia with almost complete absence of reticulocytes and erythrocytic hypoplasia in the bone marrow; the levels of the leukocytes and platelets in the circulating blood are normal. Anemia of this type generally pursues a chronic course refractory to all therapy except transfusions, but in some patients it responds to treatment with prednisone, thymectomy, or other measures. The symptoms generally are due to anemia; bleeding and infections are rarely serious problems.

References

1. Ajlouni, K., and Doebin, T. D.: Syndrome of hepatitis and aplastic anemia. Br. J. Haematol., *27*:345, 1974.
2. Allen, D. M., Fine, M. H., Necheles, T. F., and Dameshek, W.: Oxymetholone therapy in aplastic anemia. Blood, *32*:83, 1968.
3. Al-Mondhiry, H., Zanjani, E. D., Spivack, M., Zalusky, R., and Gordon, A. S.: Pure red cell aplasia and thymoma, loss of serum inhibitor of erythropoiesis following thymectomy. Blood, *38*:576, 1971.
4. Alexanian, R., Nadell, J., and Alfrey, C.: Oxymetholone treatment for the anemia of bone marrow failure. Blood, *40*:353, 1972.
5. Best, W. R.: Chloramphenicol-associated blood dyscrasias (a review of cases submitted to the A.M.A. Registry). J.A.M.A., *201*:181, 1967.
6. Bithell, T. C., and Wintrobe, M. M.: Drug-induced aplastic anemia. Semin. Hematol., *4*:194, 1967.
7. Bomford, R. R., and Rhoads, C. P.: Refractory anemia. I. Clinical and pathological aspects. Q. J. Med., *10*:175, 1941.
8. Bottiger, L. E., and Westerhelm, B.: Aplastic anemia. Acta Med. Scand., *192*:315, 1972.
9. Bowditch, M., and Elkins, H. B.: Chronic exposure to benzene (benzol). J. Indust. Hyg. Toxicol., *21*:321, 1939.

10. Brown, C. H., III: Bone marrow necrosis: a study of seventy cases. Johns Hopkins Med. J., *133*:189, 1972.
11. Camitta, B. M., Nathan, D. G., Forman, E. N., Parkman, R., Rappaport, J. M., and Orellana, T. D.: Posthepatic severe aplastic anemia–an indication for early bone marrow transplantation. Blood, *43*:473, 1974.
12. Chervenick, P. A., and Boggs, D. R.: Patterns of proliferation and differentiation of hematopoietic stem cells after compartment depletion. Blood, *37*:568, 1971.
13. Cone, T. E., Jr., and Abelson, S. M.: Aplastic anemia following two days of chloramphenicol therapy. Case report of a fatality in a 6-year-old girl. J. Pediatr., *41*:340, 1952.
14. Cooper, I. A., and Firkin, B. G.: The presence of deoxyribonucleic and (DNA) synthesizing cells in patients with refractory anemia. Blood, *24*:415, 1964.
15. Crookston, J. H., Crookston, M. C., Burnie, K. L., Francombe, W. H., Dacie, J. V., Davis, J. A., and Lewis, S. M.: Hereditary erythroblastic multinuclearity with a positive acid serum test: a type of congenital dyserythropoietic anemia. Br. J. Haematol., *17*:11, 1969.
16. Crosby, W. H.: Experience with Injured and Implanted Bone Marrow; Relation of Function to Structure. *In* Stohlman, F., Jr. (ed.): Hemopoietic Cellular Proliferation. Grune & Stratton, New York, 1970, p. 87.
17. Dale, D. C., Reynolds, H. Y., Pennington, J. E., Elin, R. J., Pitts, T. W., and Graw, R. G., Jr.: Granulocyte transfusion therapy of experimental pseudomonas pneumonia. J. Clin. Invest., *54*:664, 1974.
18. Dameshek, W., Brown, S. M., and Rubin, A. D.: "Pure" red cell anemia (erythroblastic hypoplasia) and thymoma. Semin. Hematol., *4*:222, 1967.
19. Davis, S., and Rubin, A. D.: Treatment and prognosis in aplastic anemia. Lancet, *1*:871, 1972.
20. Dawson, J. P.: Congenital pancytopenia associated with multiple congenital anomalies (Fanconi type). Pediatrics, *15*:325, 1955.
21. Diamond, L. K., and Blackfan, K. D.: Hypoplastic anemia. Am. J. Dis. Child., *56*:464, 1938.
22. Editorial: Bone marrow grafting for aplastic anemia. Lancet, *1*:22, 1975.
23. Ehrlich, P.: Ueber einen Fall von Anäme mit Bermerkungen über regenerative Veränderungen des Knochenmarks. Charité-Ann., *13*:300, 1888.
24. Enquist, R. W., Gockerman, J. P., Jenis, E. H., Warkel, R. L., and Dillon, D. E.: Type II congenital dyserythropoietic anemia. Ann. Intern. Med., *77*:371, 1972.
25. Estren, S., and Dameshek, W.: Familial hypoplastic anemia of childhood. Am. J. Dis. Child., *73*:671, 1947.
26. Fanconi, G.: Familiäre infantile perniziösaartige Anämie perniözioses Blutbild und Konstitution. Jahrb. f. Kinderh., *117*:257 1927.
27. Fanconi, G.: Familial constitutional panmyelocytopathy, Fanconi's anemia (F.A.). Semin. Hematol., *4*:233, 1967.
28. Gardner, F. H., and Blum, S. F.: Aplastic anemia in paroxysmal nocturnal hemoglobinuria, mechanisms and therapy. Semin. Hematol., *4*:250, 1967.
29. Gardner, F. H., and Pringle, J. C., Jr.: Androgens and erythropoiesis. Arch. Intern. Med., *107*:846, 1961.
30. Gasser, C.: Pure red cell anemia due to auto-antibodies; immune type of aplastic anemia (erythroblastopenia). Le sang, *26*:6, 1955.
31. Grumet, F. C., and Yankee, R. A.: Long-term platelet support of patients with aplastic anemia. Effect of splenectomy and steroid therapy. Ann. Intern. Med., *73*:1, 1970.
32. Hagler, L., Pastore, R. A., Bergin, J. J., and Wrensch, M. R.: Aplastic anemia following a viral hepatitis: report of two fatal cases and literature review. Medicine, *54*:139, 1975.
33. Heaton, L. D., Crosby, W., and Cohen, A.: Splenectomy in the treatment of hypoplasia of the bone marrow with a report of twelve cases. Ann. Surg., *146*:637, 1957.
34. Heimpel, H., Forteza-Vila, J., Queisser, W., and Spiertz, E.: Electron and light microscopic study of the erythroblasts of patients with congenital dyserythropoietic anemia. Blood, *37*:299, 1971.
35. Heimpel, H., and Wendt, F.: Congenital dyserythropoietic anemia with karyorrhexis and multinuclearity of erythroblasts. Helv. Med. Acta, *37*:103, 1968.
36. Henriksen, E.: Tetanus og N_2O−narkose Svaer knoglemarvsintoxication some følge af protraheret kvaelstrofforiltenarkose. Nord. Med., *56*:1418, 1956.
37. Herzig, R. H., Poplack, D. G., and Yankee, R. A.: Prolonged granulocytopenia from incompatible platelet transfusions. N. Engl. J. Med., *290*:1220, 1974.
38. Heyn, R. M., Ertel, I. J., and Tubergen, D. G.: Course of acquired aplastic anemia in children treated with supportive care. J.A.M.A., *208*:1372, 1969.
39. Hirst, E., and Robertson, T. I.: The syndrome of thymoma and erythroblastopenic anemia. Medicine, *46*:225, 1967.
40. Holden, D., and Lichtman, H.: Paroxysmal nocturnal hemoglobinuria with acute leukemia. Blood, *33*:283, 1969.

41. Howell, A., Andrews, T. M., and Watts, R. W. E.: Bone marrow cell resistant to chloramphenicol in chloramphenicol-induced aplastic anemia. Lancet, *1*:65, 1975.
42. Jacobson, W., Sidman, R. L., and Diamond, L. K.: The effect of testosterone on the uptake of triatiated thymidine by the bone marrow of children. Ann. N.Y. Acad. Sci., *149*:389, 1968.
43. Jenkins, D. E., and Hartmann, R. C.: Paroxysmal nocturnal hemoglobinuria terminating in acute myeloblastic leukemia. Blood, *33*:274, 1969.
44. Kaufmann, R. W., Schechter, G. P., and McFarland, W.: Paroxysmal nocturnal hemoglobinuria terminating in acute granulocytic leukemia. Blood, *33*:287, 1969.
45. Krantz, S. B.: Pure red cell aplasia. Br. J. Haematol., *25*:1, 1973.
46. Krantz, S. B., and Kao, W.: Studies on red cell aplasia. I. Demonstration of a plasma inhibitor to heme synthesis and an antibody to erythroblast nuclei. Acad. Sci. U.S.A., *58*:493, 1967.
47. Krantz, S. B., and Kao, V.: Studies on red cell aplasia. II. Report of a second patient with an antibody to erythroblast nuclei and a remission after immuno-suppressive therapy. Blood, *34*:1, 1969.
48. Lassen, H. C. A., Henriksen, E., Neukirch, F., and Kristensen, H. S.: Treatment of tetanus. Severe bone-marrow depression after prolonged nitrous-oxide anaesthesia. Lancet, *270*: 527, 1956.
49. Levin, R. H., Barrett, P. V. D., Cline, M. J., Berlin, N. I., and Freireich, E. J.: Platelet therapy and red cell defect in aplastic anemia. Arch. Intern. Med., *11*:278, 1964.
50. Levy, R. N., Sawitsky, A., Florman, A. L., and Rubin, E.: Fatal aplastic anemia after hepatitis. N. Engl. J. Med., *273*:1118, 1965.
51. Lewis, S. M.: Course and prognosis in aplastic anemia. Br. Med. J., *1*:1027, 1965.
52. Lewis, S. M., and Dacie, J. V.: The aplastic anaemia-paroxysmal nocturnal haemoglobinuria syndrome. Br. J. Haematol., *13*:236, 1967.
53. Lewis, S. M., and Verwilghen, R. L.: Annotation: dyserythropoiesis and dyserythropoietic anemia. Br. J. Haematol., *23*:1, 1972.
54. Li, F. P., Alter, B. P., and Nathan, D. G.: The mortality of acquired aplastic anemia in children. Blood, *40*:153, 1972.
55. Maldonado, J. E., and Taswell, H. F.: Type I dyserthropoietic anemia in an elderly patient. Blood, *44*:495, 1974.
56. Maloney, M. A., and Patt, H. M.: Origin of repopulating cells after localized bone marrow depletion. Science, *165*:71, 1971.
57. Marmont, A., Peschle, C., Sanguineti, H., and Condorelli, M.: Pure cell aplasia (PRCA): response of three patients to cyclophosphamide and/or antilymphocytic globulin (ALG) and demonstration of two types of serum IgG inhibitors to erythropoiesis. Blood, *45*: 247, 1975.
58. Martelo, O. J., Manyan, D. R., Smith, U. S., and Yunis, A. A.: Chloramphenicol and bone marrow mitochondria. J. Lab. Clin. Med., *74*:927, 1969.
59. McCurdy, P. R.: Chloramphenicol bone marrow toxicity. J.A.M.A., *176*:106, 1961.
60. McGuire, L. B.: Aplastic anemia in an adult with two remissions on androgen. Va. Med. Mon., *91*:207, 1964.
61. Mitchell, A. B. S., Pinn, G., and Pegrun, G. D.: Pure red cell aplasia and carcinoma. Blood, *37*:594, 1971.
62. Mohler, D., and Leavell, B. S.: Aplastic anemia. An analysis of 50 cases. Ann. Intern. Med., *49*:326, 1958.
63. Nagoa, T., and Maure, A. M.: Concordance for drug-induced aplastic anemia in identical twins. N. Engl. J. Med., *281*:7, 1969.
64. Ortega, J. A., Shore, N. A., Dukes, P. P., and Hammond, D.: Congenital hypoplastic anemia inhibition of erythropoiesis by sera from patients with congenital hypoplastic anemia. Blood, *45*:83, 1975.
65. Oski, F. A., and Stockman, J. A., III: Anemia in early infancy. Br. J. Haematol., *27*:195, 1974.
66. Polak, B. C. P., Wesseling, H., Schut, D., Herxheimer, A., and Meyler, L.: Blood dyscrasias attributed to chloramphenicol. Acta Med. Scand., *192*:407, 1972.
67. Pollycove, M., and Lawrence, J. H.: Ferrokinetics of refractory anemia. Proceedings of the Eighth International Congress of Hematology, 1960, p. 42.
68. Recker, R. R., and Hynes, H. E.: Pure red blood cell aplasia associated with chlorpropamide therapy. Arch. Intern. Med., *123*:445, 1969.
69. Reynafarje, C., and Faura, J.: Erythrokinetics in the treatment of aplastic anemia with methandrostenolone. Arch. Intern. Med., *120*:654, 1967.
70. Rhoads, C. P., and Miller, D. K.: Histology of the bone marrow in aplastic anemia. Arch. Pathol., *26*:648, 1938.
71. Rich, M. L., Ritterhoff, R. J., and Hoffman, R. J.: A fatal case of aplastic anemia following chloramphenicol (Chloromycetin) therapy. Ann. Intern. Med., *33*:1459, 1950.
72. Rubin, D., Weisberger, A. S., Botti, R. E., and Storaasli, J. P.: Changes in iron metabolism in early chloramphenicol toxicity. J. Clin. Invest., *37*:1286, 1958.

73. Rubin, E., Gottlieb, C., and Vogel, P.: Syndrome of hepatitis and aplastic anemia. Am. J. Med., *45*:88, 1968.
74. Saidi, P., Wallerstein, R. O., and Aggeler, P. M.: Effect of chloramphenicol on erythropoiesis. J. Lab. Clin. Med., *57*:247, 1961.
75. Sanchez-Medal, L., Gomez-Leal, A., Duarte, L., and Rio, M. G.: Anabolic androgenic steroids in the treatment of acquired aplastic anemia. Blood, *34*:283, 1969.
76. Scott, J. L., Cartwright, G. E., and Wintrobe, M. M.: Acquired aplastic anemia: an analysis of thirty-nine cases and review of the pertinent literature. Medicine, *38*:119, 1959.
77. Semi-annual Tabulation of Reports Compiled by the Registry on Blood Dyscrasias (March 20, 1963). Am. Med. Assoc., Chicago, 1963.
78. Shahidi, N. T.: Androgens and erythropoiesis. N. Engl. J. Med., *289*:72, 1973.
79. Shahidi, N. T., and Diamond, L. K.: Testosterone-induced remission in aplastic anemia on both acquired and congenital types. N. Engl. J. Med., *264*:953, 1961.
80. Silinik, S. J., and Firkin, B. G.: An analysis of hypoplastic anemia with special reference to the use of oxymetholone (Adroyd) in its therapy. Australian Ann. Med., *17*:224, 1968.
81. Smith, L. W.: Report on an unusual case of aplastic anemia. Am. J. Dis. Child., *17*:174, 1919.
82. Stohlman, F., Jr.: Aplastic anemia. Blood, *40*:282, 1972.
83. Strob, R., Thomas, E. D., Buckner, C. D., Clift, R. A., Johnson, F. L., Fefer, A., Glucksberg, H., Giblett, E. R., and Neiman, P.: Allogenic marrow grafting for treatment of aplastic anemia. Blood, *43*:157, 1974.
84. Suhrland, L. G., and Weisberger, A. S.: Delayed clearance of chloramphenicol from serum in patients with hematologic toxicity. Blood, *34*:466, 1969.
85. Thomas, E. D., et al: Aplastic anemia treated by bone marrow transplantation. Lancet, *1*:284, 1972.
86. Thomas, E. D., Storb, R., Clift, R. A., Fefer, A., Johnson, F. L., Neiman, P. E., Lerner, K. G., Glucksberg, H., and Buckner, C. D.: Bone marrow transplantation. N. Engl. J. Med., *292*:832, 895, 1975.
87. Thompson, W. P., Richter, M. N., and Edsall, K. S.: An analysis of so-called aplastic anemia. Am. J. Med. Sci., *187*:77, 1934.
88. Tsai, S. Y., and Levin, W. C.: Chronic erythrocytic hypoplasia in adults. Am. J. Med., *22*:322, 1957.
89. Twomey, J. J., Douglass, C. C., and Sharkey, O., Jr.: The monocytopenia of aplastic anemia. Blood, *41*:187, 1973.
90. van der Weyden, M., and Firkin, B. G.: The management of aplastic anemia in adults. Br. J. Haematol., *22*:1, 1972.
91. Vilter, R. W., Jarrold, T., Will, J. J., Mueller, J. F., Friedman, B. I., and Hawkins, V. R.: Refractory anemia with hyperplastic bone marrow. Blood, *15*:1, 1960.
92. Vincent, P. C., and Gruchy, G. C.: Complications and treatment of acquired aplastic anemia. Br. J. Haematol., *13*:977, 1967.
93. Wallerstein, R. O., Condit, P. K., Kasper, C. K., Brown, J. W., and Morrison, F. R.: Statewide study of chloramphenicol therapy and fatal aplastic anemia. J.A.M.A., *208*:2045, 1969.
94. Wasserman, L. R., Stats, D., Schwartz, L., and Fudenberg, H.: Symptomatic and hemopathic hemolytic anemia. Am. J. Med., *18*:1961, 1955.
95. Weatherly, T. L., Flannery, E. P., Doyle, W. F., Shohet, S. B., and Garratty, G.: Congenital dyserythropoietic anemia (CDA) with increased red cell lipids. Am. J. Med., *57*:912, 1974.
96. Weisberger, A. S.: Mechanisms of action of chloramphenicol. J.A.M.A., *209*:97, 1969.
97. Yunis, A. A., Arimura, G. K., Lutcher, C. L., Blasquez, J., and Halloran, M.: Biochemical lesion in Dilantin-induced erythroid aplasia. Blood, *30*:587, 1967.
98. Yunis, A. A., and Bloomberg, G. R.: Chloramphenicol toxicity: clinical features and pathogenesis. Prog. Hematol., *4*:138, 1964.
99. Yunis, A. A., and Harrington, W. J.: Patterns of inhibition by chloramphenicol of nucleic acid synthesis in human bone marrow and leukemic cells. J. Lab. Clin. Med., *56*:831, 1960.
100. Yunis, A. A., Smith, U. S., and Restrepo, A.: Reversible bone marrow suppression from chloramphenicol. Arch. Intern. Med., *126*:272, 1970.

CHAPTER 7

HEMOLYTIC ANEMIA

The erythrocytes normally have a life span of about 120 days. When the erythrocyte is destroyed or disintegrates, the iron of the hemoglobin is stored in the cells of the reticuloendothelial system. In these same cells heme is converted into the unconjugated form of bilirubin, which is then transported in the plasma to the liver where the bilirubin is conjugated and excreted through the biliary system; in the bowel, bilirubin is converted into fecal urobilinogen.

Whether the senescent red cells are phagocytized by the reticuloendothelial cells or are fragmented in the circulation before the particles are engulfed by these cells has not been established. Whatever the actual mechanism, reticuloendothelial cells in any part of the body, particularly the bone marrow, the liver, the spleen, and the lymph nodes, participate in the process. Splenectomy in an otherwise normal individual produces no significant increase in the life span of the erythrocytes; this indicates that the spleen is not essential for the physiologic destruction of the cells. The concept has evolved that the erythrocyte is destroyed because its metabolic activity fails, its reserves are exhausted, and it is no longer able to maintain itself. The abnormalities which have been detected in older cells, such as increases in density, osmotic fragility, mechanical fragility, loss of pliability, and negative charge, are probably manifestations of underlying changes in the metabolic status of the cells. The aging process in the red cells appears to be primary; when this has reached a certain point, the cells, or their disintegrating fragments, are taken up by reticuloendothelial cells in any part of the body.

Hemolytic anemias are characterized by a shortened life span of the red cells. An increase in the number of cells destroyed is usually accompanied by enlargement of the spleen, a rise in the level of unconjugated bilirubin in the plasma, and elevation of the fecal urobilinogen excretion. Considerable hemolysis may occur without an increase in serum bilirubin because of the ability of the liver to increase the clearance of plasma bilirubin six- to eightfold in the absence of coexisting liver dysfunction. Thus, a bilirubin above 4.0 mg. per 100 ml. suggests coexisting liver dysfunction or biliary obstruction.[4] Compensatory erythroid hyperplasia occurs in the marrow, and increased numbers of reticulocytes appear in the peripheral blood. In stained smears of the peripheral blood there is usually visible evidence of hereditary or acquired abnormality in the structure of the erythrocytes in the form of spherocytosis, poikilocytosis, anisocytosis, or basophilic stippling.

In most patients with hemolytic anemia, red cell destruction is primarily extravascular in the reticuloendothelial system. In a limited number of hemolytic disorders, red cells are destroyed intravascularly, with resulting hemoglobinuria. Hemoglobin released in the plasma is bound by an α_2 globulin, haptoglobin, which is capable of binding two molecules of hemoglobin. When the threshold of haptoglobin binding is exceeded, in the range of 90 to 130 mg. of hemoglobin per 100 ml. of plasma, hemoglobin appears in the urine. Other indications of intravascular hemolysis are increases in plasma hemoglobin, methemalbumin, and lactic dehydrogenase, decreased or absent haptoglobin, and hemosiderinuria. Staining for hemosiderin in the urine sediment is a sensitive indicator of intravascular hemolysis, and may remain positive long after gross hemoglobinuria has cleared.

ERYTHROCYTE METABOLISM AND METHEMOGLOBINEMIA

The red blood cell is the site of numerous metabolic activities designed to maintain cellular integrity and to transport oxygen and carbon dioxide. Four main areas of red cell metabolism which are crucial to normal red cell survival and function may be identified. These are the red cell membrane, the pentose phosphate shunt–glutathione system, glycolysis by the Embden-Meyerhof pathway, and hemoglobin. Abnormalities in any of these areas of metabolism will result in impaired red cell survival and function.

THE RED CELL MEMBRANE

The details of the structure and organization of the erythrocyte membrane are still a subject of controversy, although many advances in our understanding of plasma membranes have been made in recent years. The membrane appears to be composed of a fluid lipid matrix consisting of equal amounts of cholesterol and phospholipid with a mosaic of heterogeneous proteins interspersed throughout. The proteins have their polar groups exposed to the plasma and their nonpolar groups immersed in the lipid membrane. Some proteins traverse the entire membrane, whereas others penetrate only to the outer or inner surface of the membrane.[15, 19, 40, 45, 46, 56, 57]

Two of the most important protein constituents of the membrane are glycophorin and spectrin. Glycophorin, which is the principal membrane glycoprotein, accounts for approximately 10 per cent of membrane protein, and appears on the external surface of the membrane. The molecule is about 60 per cent carbohydrate and contains most of the membrane sialic acid, which gives the red cell its negative charge. Many of the blood group antigens and a variety of receptors are located on the membrane in the glycophorin fraction.[31]

Spectrin is a large molecular weight protein (approximately 140,000) found on the inner surface of the membrane, and it accounts for about 20 per cent of the stromal protein.[30] It forms microfilaments in the membrane which are responsible for the normal red cell's biconcave shape and deformability. The integrity of the red cell membrane requires the phosphorylation of spectrin by a protein kinase, present in the membrane that is catalyzed by cyclic nucleotides.[18] In addition to protein kinases the membrane contains the following enzymes: glyceraldehyde–3–phosphate dehydrogenase, aldolase, 3-phosphoglycerate kinase, adenylate kinase, ATPase, and cholinesterase.[13, 15, 41]

Two essential attributes of the red cell membrane are its deformability and permeability characteristics. The red cell, which averages about 7 microns in diameter, must traverse passages less than 3 microns in diameter in the microcirculation of the bone marrow and spleen.[54, 58] In order to accomplish this feat the membrane must remain pliable, because any decrease in deformability will lead to sequestration and destruction by the reticuloendothelial system.[54]

The permeability properties of the erythrocyte membrane are important in controlling the volume of the red cell and in preventing colloid osmotic hemolysis. Because the red cell contains a relatively high concentration of molecules, such as hemoglobin, phosphorylated intermediates, and glutathione, which do not cross the red cell membrane, there is a slightly positive osmotic gradient towards the inside of the erythrocyte.[25] If this osmotic force were unopposed, water would enter the cell in excess of its capacity, and hemolysis would ensue. The erythrocyte protects itself from osmotic lysis by active cation transport and a relative impermeability to cations. The red cell membrane is freely permeable to water and the anions, chloride and bicarbonate, which traverse the membrane in less than a second.[59]

In contrast, the exchange of sodium ions and potassium ions proceeds much more slowly, with a halftime of over 30 hours.[59] This allows the red cell "time" to adjust its volume by the active transport of the sodium ion together with water out of the cell. The intracellular:extracellular ratio for K^+ is 25:1, and for Na^+ is 1:12.[53] The passive movements of these cations is in the direction of their electrochemical gradients, with Na^+ leaking into the cell and K^+ leaking out. These electrochemical gradients are maintained by active transport, with Na^+ being pumped out while K^+ is pumped in. The energy for active transport is provided by ATP, which is derived from glycolysis. The energy is released by action of ATPase residing in the red cell membrane.[12, 19] The volume control of the red cell depends on a combination of the permeability of the membrane and the rate of the cation pump. Any disturbance which increases permeability or curtails the production of ATP for active transport may lead to colloid osmotic hemolysis.

PENTOSE PHOSPHATE SHUNT–GLUTATHIONE SYSTEM

Approximately 90 per cent of the glucose utilized by the mature red cell is converted to lactate by the anaerobic enzymatic steps of the Embden-Meyerhof pathway, and the remaining 10 per cent is metabolized by the oxidative pentose phosphate pathway.[33] The pentose phosphate shunt is important to the red cell as the pathway for the generation of NADPH (Fig. 7–1). NADPH, together with reduced glutathione (GSH), is the main line of defense of the red cell against oxidative injury.[24] When the red cell is exposed to a variety of oxidant drugs, which function as electron transport agents in oxidation-reduction reactions, or after a number of infections, hydrogen peroxide is formed. This is reduced by the following series of interrelated reactions:[8, 32]

1. Red cell + oxidant $\longrightarrow$ H_2O_2

2. $H_2O_2 + 2\ GSH \xrightarrow[\text{peroxidase}]{\text{glutathione}}$ $2H_2O + GSSG$

3. $GSSG + NADPH + H^+ \xrightarrow[\text{reductase}]{\text{glutathione}}$ $2\ GSH + NADP^+$

4. $G\text{–}6\text{–}P + NADP^+ \xrightarrow[\text{dehydrogenase}]{\text{glucose–6–phosphate}}$ $6\text{–}PG + NADPH + H^+$

(G–6–P = glucose–6–phosphate; 6–PG = 6–phosphogluconate)

In order for glutathione peroxidase to remain effective in reducing H_2O_2 to H_2O, a continuous supply of GSH must be available. This is accomplished by the reduction of GSSG to GSH by glutathione reductase, which in turn requires NADPH as a cofactor. A deficiency of glutathione peroxidase, glutathione reductase, or glucose–6–phosphate dehydrogenase, or an inability to synthesize glutathione, leads to defective reduction of H_2O_2. When H_2O_2 accumulates, hemoglobin is irreversibly oxidized and precipitated as Heinz bodies.[24] Rifkin has shown that the precipitated Heinz bodies are attached to the red cell membrane; being rigid bodies they interfere with the deformability of the membrane, which leads to the cell's sequestration and lysis by the spleen and reticuloendo-thelial system.[38, 39] The formation of Heinz bodies appears to be the common pathway of hemolysis in anemias secondary to defects in the pentose phosphate shunt–glutathione systems, unstable hemoblogins, and thalassemia.

Although the red cell is rich in catalase, which also decomposes H_2O_2, it does not appear to be as physiologically important to the red cell in reducing low levels of H_2O_2 as glutathione peroxidase,[32] since a hereditary deficiency of cata-lase[1] is not associated with hemolytic anemia, whereas a deficiency of glutathione peroxidase is.[36, 48–49]

GSH may also be important in maintaining red cell integrity by reducing sulfhydryl groups of hemoglobin, membrane proteins, and enzymes when they become oxidized.

GLYCOLYSIS

Figure 7–1 shows the anaerobic metabolism of glucose by the Embden-Meyerhof pathway and the aerobic metabolism of glucose by the pentose phosphate shunt. In contrast to nucleated cells which contain mitochondria and metabolize glucose via the Krebs cycle, yielding 38 moles of ATP per mole of glucose utilized, the mature red cell contains no mitochondria and the yield of ATP is only 2 moles per mole of glucose metabolized.[33]

The energy of ATP is used by the red cell primarily for the active transport of Na^+ and K^+ and is important in controlling the volume of the cell.[34] ATP also has a role in maintaining the permeability, shape characteristics, and deformability of the red cell membrane.[26, 54–55] Any deficiency in the supply of ATP resulting from a lack of the substrate glucose, or from a deficiency of some enzyme in the Embden-Meyerhof pathway, will lead to failure of the cation pump and, ultimately, to colloid osmotic hemolysis. ATP is also necessary for the phosphorylation of the filamentous membrane protein spectrin which is crucial to red

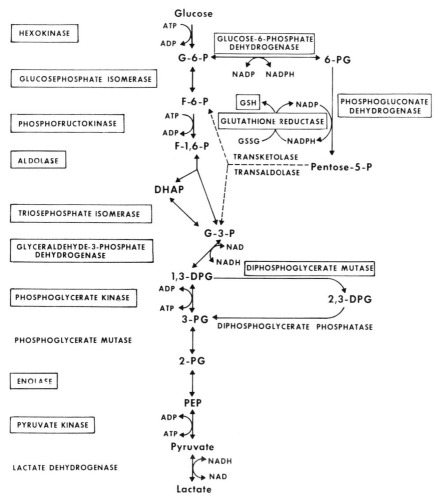

Figure 7–1   Glycolytic and pentose phosphate shunt pathways. Deficiencies of the enclosed enzymes have been associated with hereditary hemolytic anemia.

cell shape and deformability.[18] When ATP is depleted the red cell undergoes a disk-to-sphere transformation and becomes trapped in the microcirculation.[29, 35] In addition, decreased erythrocyte ATP levels lead to less bound Ca^{++} with a concomitant increase in membrane Ca^{++}, resulting in increased membrane rigidity and permeability.[26]

The erythrocyte is unique among cells utilizing anaerobic glycolysis in that it contains an unusually large amount of 2,3-diphosphoglycerate (2,3 DPG) and no glycogen.[2] It has been shown by Chanutin and Curnish[67] and by Benesch and Benesch[3] that 2,3-DPG plays a key role in controlling oxygen-hemoglobin dissociation. This compound has a strong affinity for hemoglobin, and in the presence of high levels of 2,3-DPG oxygen is released more readily to the tissues. It has been demonstrated that patients with anemia, or living at high altitudes, respond with an increase in 2,3-DPG which renders their hemoglobin more efficient in delivering oxygen to the tissues.[37] On the other hand, patients with hexokinase deficiency have lower than normal levels of 2,3-DPG with an increased affinity of their hemoglobin for oxygen.[11]

Another important function of the glycolytic pathway is the generation of NADH, which is the physiologic cofactor for the reduction of methemoglobin to oxyhemoglobin.[21–22]

HEMOGLOBIN

Although many abnormal hemoglobins have been described in man, only a few of these have been of pathologic importance in the genesis of hemolytic anemia. These have usually involved amino acid substitutions which render the hemoglobin susceptible to structural change under certain conditions, such as the molecular stacking with tactoid formation, which occurs with sickle hemoglobin when oxygen tension is reduced, and the precipitation of unstable hemoglobins with Heinz body formation upon exposure to oxidant drugs. These changes impair membrane deformability and lead to red cell destruction.

The function of the erythrocyte is to carry oxygen from the lungs to the cells of the body and to transport carbon dioxide to the lungs. Under normal circumstances the hemoglobin molecule in the mature erythrocyte is in a stable state, and there is no degradation or resynthesis during the life span of the cell. However, hemoglobin does change constantly, from the reduced to the oxidized state. When the iron is in the reduced form, hemoglobin can bind and transport oxygen. Ferric or oxidized hemoglobin, which is known as methemoglobin, is not able to function as an oxygen transport system.

Two methemoglobin reductase systems are of importance in maintaining hemoglobin in the reduced state. Both pathways are dependent on carbohydrate metabolism for the regeneration of reduced pyridine nucleotides, and are referred to as NADH methemoglobin reductase[43] and NADPH methemoglobin reductase.[20] The NADH dependent system appears to be the major pathway under physiologic conditions.[21–22] These reactions function so efficiently that not more than 1 per cent of the hemoglobin in the erythrocyte is in the oxidized state.[20]

Methemoglobinemia. Methemoglobinemia of greater than 1.5 to 2.0 gm. per 100 gm. hemoglobin will produce cyanosis, and concentrations in the order of 70 gm. per 100 gm. hemoglobin are probably lethal.[5, 22] Significant amounts of methemoglobin may occur in a variety of disorders.

1. A genetically determined abnormality in the NADH methemoglobin reductase system is not uncommon.[6, 17, 42] The condition appears benign, though patients may complain of mild dyspnea on exertion and have slight compensatory erythrocytosis. The blood may contain 20 to 45 per cent methemoglobin. Family studies indicate a recessive autosomal mode of inheritance. The condition requires no therapy, but the cyanosis will respond to methylene blue, which activates the NADPH methemoglobin reductase system.

A severe degree of NADH reductase deficiency has been found in association with mental retardation.[23]

A form of methemoglobinemia transmitted by an autosomal dominant gene has been described in which erythrocyte NADH and NADPH methemoglobin reductase concentrations and hemoglobin structure appear normal but erythrocyte glutathione synthesis appears to be depressed.[51] The reduction in glutathione concentration is believed to affect the function of the sulfhydryl-dependent enzyme glyceraldehyde-3-phosphate dehydrogenase, reducing the availability of NADH to the NADH-dependent methemoglobin reductase system.[52]

2. A genetically determined altered structure of the hemoglobin molecule may result in methemoglobinemia, and the abnormal hemoglobin has been designated hemoglobin M.[44] A number of variants of hemoglobin M have been described.[22] The mechanism by which methemoglobin accumulates in these patients has not been completely elucidated. It has been suggested that the ferric iron in methemoglobin M forms a complex with a ligand provided by the abnormal amino acid substitution in the hemoglobin molecule, and that this complex resists enzymatic reduction.[16, 28] The abnormality appears to be transmitted as an autosomal characteristic, and the homozygous state is probably incompatible with life. In the heterozygous state only 25 to 35 per cent of the hemoglobin is methemoglobin, suggesting a lowered rate of synthesis.

3. Toxic methemoglobinemia.

An elevated level of methemoglobin is also found following the introduction into the body of compounds that preferentially oxidize hemoglobin and exceed the capacity of the normal blood cell reducing systems. Among the most important offenders are nitrites, sulfonamides, and aniline derivatives.[14, 50] Methemoglobinemia with cyanosis has also been observed in individuals taking the antimalarial drugs, primaquine and chloroquine. Such individuals have been found to be heterozygous for NADH methemoglobin reductase deficiency.[9]

Sulfhemoglobin is another compound that is not capable of carrying oxygen. Its formation represents an irreversible change in hemoglobin, and it persists until the destruction of the red blood cell. It is unaffected by methylene blue or ascorbic acid. Some source of sulfur, such as a sulfur-containing drug or chronic constipation, plus the ingestion of a drug which will oxidize hemoglobin, is thought necessary for its production. The syndrome of enterogenous cyanosis is probably related to the formation of either methemoglobin or sulfhemoglobin secondary to disturbed bowel function.[14]

CLASSIFICATION

Any process that shortens the life span of the erythrocyte results in hyper-hemolysis; if erythropoiesis is unable to compensate for the increased hemolysis, anemia appears. A diminished life span of the erythrocytes has been demonstrated in almost every type of anemia found in association with disease. In many instances the shortening of the life span is slight, not more than the normal marrow can compensate for if it functions normally. If the degree of hemolysis is minor, the anemia is more properly considered a reflection of inadequate marrow response. The term "hemolytic anemia" is usually reserved for those patients in whom hemolysis is the major mechanism of the anemia. The term "hemolytic disease" is a broader one that includes patients without anemia who have appreciable hemolysis. Since the normal bone marrow is capable of increasing its production rate about six- to eightfold,[10] it is possible for red cell survival to decrease from the normal 120 days to as little as 15 to 20 days without anemia developing.

A number of different abnormalities affect the red cell and cause hemolytic anemia. As knowledge about the nature of these disorders increases, more precise names will come into use and a more satisfactory classification will become possible.

For the present it is convenient to classify hemolytic disorders according to whether they are hereditary or acquired, as shown in Table 7–1.

HEREDITARY HEMOLYTIC DISORDERS
Erythrocyte Membrane Defects

HEREDITARY SPHEROCYTOSIS

History

Vanlair and Masius first described spherocytosis of red cells in 1871.[80, 122] Minkowski reported the first detailed clinical description of "congenital hemolytic icterus" in 1900.[14] Seven years later Chauffard pointed out two of the characteristic features of the disease: reticulocytosis and increased fragility of the red cells in hypotonic saline.[68–69] The importance of the spleen in the pathogenesis of the anemia and the curative role of splenectomy were recognized in the early studies of Heilmeyer[90] and Dacie,[73] and emphasized by the detailed observances of Emerson[82–83] and Young.[122]

Mechanism of Disease

Hereditary spherocytosis is believed to be inherited as an autosomal dominant.[121, 122] According to this concept at least one parent and one-half the offspring

Table 7–1 *Classification of Hemolytic Disease*

I. Hereditary hemolytic disorders
   A. Erythrocyte membrane defects
      1. Hereditary spherocytosis
      2. Hereditary elliptocytosis
      3. Hereditary stomatocytosis
      4. Selective increase in membrane lecithin
      5. Lecithin–cholesterol acyl transferase deficiency
   B. Pentose phosphate shunt–glutathione system enzyme deficiencies
      1. Glucose-6-phosphate dehydrogenase
      2. Others: 6-phosphogluconate dehydrogenase, glutathione reductase, glutathione peroxidase, glutathione synthetase, glutamyl-cysteine synthetase
   C. Glycolytic enzyme deficiencies
      1. Pyruvate kinase
      2. Others: diphosphoglyceromutase, triosephosphate isomerase, glucosephosphate isomerase, phosphoglycerate kinase, phosphofructokinase, hexokinase, glyceraldehyde-3-phosphate dehydrogenase, aldolase, enolase
   D. Miscellaneous enzyme deficiencies
      1. ATPase
      2. Adenylate kinase
      3. Ribose phosphate pyrophosphokinase
   E. Hemoglobinopathies
      1. Sickle cell anemia
      2. Hemoglobin C disease
      3. Thalassemia
      4. Combinations: sickle cell–hemoglobin C disease, sickle cell-thalassemia disease, sickle cell–hemoglobin D disease, and others
      5. Unstable hemoglobins: Zurich, Köln, Genova, Sydney, Hammersmith, Gun Hill, and others
II. Acquired hemolytic disorders
   A. Antibody-mediated
      1. Isoantibodies
         a. Transfusion reactions
         b. Erythroblastosis fetalis
      2. Drug-induced antibodies
         a. Quinidine
         b. Penicillin
         c. Methyldopa
      3. Autoantibodies
         a. Idiopathic
         b. Secondary–lymphoproliferative disease, connective tissue disease, mycoplasma pneumonia, paroxysmal cold hemoglobinuria
   B. Paroxysmal nocturnal hemoglobinuria
   C. Mechanical hemolysis
      1. March hemoglobinuria
      2. Cardiac hemolytic anemia
      3. Microangiopathic hemolytic anemia
   D. Infections
      1. Malaria
      2. Bacterial infections
      3. Viral infections
   E. Chemical agents
   F. Physical agents
   G. Hypersplenism
   H. Hypophosphatemia
   I. Liver disease
   J. Renal disease

of the patient should be affected. However, apparent exceptions have been observed in families that were studied carefully.[122] It is likely that hereditary spherocytosis is a heterogeneous disorder, and more than one closely related genetic membrane defect may lead to a similar clinical picture.

Patients with hereditary spherocytosis manifest the evidences of a hemolytic process, such as increased fecal urobilinogen excretion, elevation of the indirect-reacting serum bilirubin in the plasma, splenomegaly, reticulocytosis, and normoblastic hyperplasia in the bone marrow. Although the anemia is cured by splenectomy, an intracorpuscular defect has been shown by Dacie and Mollison[75] to be the primary factor in the increased hemolysis. They demonstrated that erythrocytes from normal donors survived from 100 to 130 days when transfused into patients with hereditary spherocytosis; in contrast, erythrocytes that were obtained from a patient with hereditary spherocytosis four days prior to splenectomy and one year after splenectomy disappeared from the circulation in 14 days and 19 days respectively when transfused into normal recipients. The importance of both the intracorpuscular defect and the spleen in the hyperhemolysis in this disease was further demonstrated by Emerson.[82] He observed that erythrocytes from a patient with hereditary spherocytosis, both before and after splenectomy, had shortened survival times when transfused into a normal recipient; erythrocytes from the same patient had a normal survival time when transfused into an otherwise normal recipient whose spleen had been removed because of trauma.

Ever since the increased osmotic fragility of the erythrocytes in hereditary spherocytosis was first described, efforts have been made to find some link between this peculiarity and the increased destruction of the erythrocytes in vivo. Haden demonstrated that the increased susceptibility of the erythrocytes in the disease to hypotonic saline is related to their increased thickness and "microspherocytic" shape.[87] The observation that microspherocytosis and increased osmotic fragility persisted after splenectomy suggested that the defects in the red cell were the result of an inherited abnormality of the erythrocyte.[87] Ham and Castle found that sterile incubation caused an increase in the spheroidicity and osmotic fragility of human erythrocytes, and postulated that abnormally susceptible erythrocytes would be hemolyzed more easily than normal cells by erythrostasis in the spleen, which might be compared to incubation in vitro.[88] This concept implies selective sequestration of the abnormal "spherocytes" in the spleen, because normal erythrocytes survive normally in patients with hereditary spherocytosis.[75, 83, 108] Such selective sequestration has been demonstrated in experiments that utilized mixtures of different types of cells that could be identified by differential agglutination. Identifiable normal erythrocytes were transfused into patients with hereditary spherocytosis prior to splenectomy; when the spleen was studied after its removal it was found that the patient's cells had been selectively retained by the spleen.

Although selective sequestration by the spleen of the abnormal red cells in hereditary spherocytosis has been clearly demonstrated, the mechanism by which this is accomplished is not entirely clear. In experiments that utilized millipore filters with 5-micron pores, Jandl and his associates observed that only the most spheroidal cells were retained by the filter.[99] A spherical erythrocyte is considerably less deformable than a biconcave one, and it is not surprising that many of these cells are trapped by the microcirculation of the spleen where they may be required to pass through apertures less than 3 microns in diameter.[58] However, the spherical shape of the cell does not appear to be the entire answer. Crosby and Conrad showed that flattening of the spherocyte by producing iron deficiency did not prevent sequestration of the cells by the spleen and did not improve red cell survival.[71] A possible explanation for this observation may come from the work of LaCelle and Weed,[100] who have used a micropipette technique to measure the deformability of the red cell membrane. They have found an increased rigidity of the membrane of red cells from patients with hereditary spherocytosis even before the cell becomes spherical.

Although the basic red cell lesion has not yet been determined in hereditary spherocytosis, a number of metabolic abnormalities have been demonstrated which help to explain the cells' particular vulnerability to erythrostasis both in vitro and in vivo. Jacob and Jandl,[92, 94] amplifying the observations of earlier workers,[64, 89] have shown an increased permeability to the passive influx of sodium. The red cell compensates for this leak by increasing the rate of active transport of sodium out of the cell with a concomitant increase in glucose and ATP utilization.[92, 94, 104] This mechanism is effective as long as sufficient glucose is available to the cell. In the spleen where erythrostasis occurs, glucose may fall to inadequate levels.[97-98] ATP generation declines, sodium leaks into the cell faster than it can be pumped out, and eventually osmotic swelling and lysis occurs.

When red cells from patients with hereditary spherocytosis are incubated in the absence of glucose for prolonged periods they first begin to swell, a change which can be explained by the permeability lesion described above; later the cells lose volume, become smaller, and assume the microspheroidal shape characteristic of the disease. This change requires another explanation. A spherocyte is formed when there is an alteration in the ratio of surface area to volume. Since the spherocyte in hereditary spherocytosis is a small one, it must follow that the cell has lost surface area. This has been shown to be the case by Reed and Swisher,[112] who have demonstrated excessive membrane lipid loss upon incubation. The composition of lipid in the membrane of red cells in hereditary spherocytosis is normal,[76] and when lipid is lost from the membrane the proportions of the various lipids in the membrane remain the same, indicating that whole fragments of the membrane are lost.[112, 118] This has been shown directly by electron microscopy of incubated red cells,[117] and accounts for the loss of surface area with subsequent microspherocytosis.[118] Cooper and Jandl have proposed that fragmentation is a late irreversible event signaling the imminent demise of the cell, whereas an earlier selective loss of membrane cholesterol may lead to reversible sphering.[97] They infused ^{51}Cr-labeled red cells from a patient with hereditary spherocytosis into patients with obstructive jaundice, and observed improvement in osmotic fragility and red cell survival. Since bile acids in the plasma of patients with obstructive jaundice block the transfer of cholesterol from red cells to plasma, they postulated that an increase in membrane cholesterol was responsible for the observed improvement in red cell survival.[70]

Weed and his associates have emphasized the role of calcium in membrane rigidity.[26, 55, 100] As intracellular calcium increases, an actomyosin-like protein on the inner surface of the membrane undergoes a sol-to-gel transformation which

is reversed by ATP. They have postulated that the red cell membrane in hereditary spherocytosis may have an increased affinity for calcium, since the spherocytic red cell is more sensitive to falling levels of ATP and increase in calcium
than the normal red cell.

Jacob and his associates have focused attention on a possible defect in the
microfilamentous membrane protein, spectrin, in the pathogenesis of the abnormal spherocyte. They have shown that treatment of normal red cells with vinblastine or heating produces erythrocytes that mimic those seen in hereditary
spherocytosis in all respects, presumably through the denaturation of spectrin
which is essential for normal red cell shape and deformability.[93] For the proper
function of spectrin, phosphorylation by ATP is required in a reaction catalyzed
by cyclic nucleotides.[18] The phosphorylation of spectrin by protein kinase is
diminished in the red cell membranes from patients with hereditary spherocytosis
and this suggests that a genetically-altered spectrin may be responsible for the
shortened red cell survival in this disease.[86, 95]

From these observations it can be seen how the spleen is ideally suited to
bring out the red cell defects in hereditary spherocytosis. When erythrostasis
occurs, ATP depletion follows, leading to intracellular accumulation of sodium,
loss of membrane lipid, sphering, enhancement of calcium effect on membrane
protein, alteration in spectrin, rigidity of the membrane, and ultimately sequestration by the microcirculation of the spleen.

Clinical Manifestations

Hereditary spherocytosis is the most common hereditary hemolytic anemia
among patients of northern European descent. In the United States the incidence is about 22 per 100,000.[105] It occurs in both sexes, but is rare in blacks.[66]
Clinical evidence of the disease may appear soon after birth or not until after
middle age.

The severity of the disease varies greatly in different patients. In some the
clinical manifestations are so mild that the disease is asymptomatic, and the patients lead an active normal life. In such individuals the diagnosis can be established only after a careful study of the blood because the anemia may be mild,
or even absent, if the bone marrow is able to compensate for the increased
hemolysis. The only clue to a hemolytic disorder may be an increase in reticulocytes and erythroid hyperplasia of the bone marrow. More often the patient has
the symptoms of a mild chronic illness; in others an attack of cholelithiasis calls
attention to the disease. Some patients do not realize that they have been feeling
subnormal until after splenectomy produces an increased sense of well-being.

In many patients the course of the disease is associated with episodes of
severe illness, the so-called "crisis." These attacks are characterized by the
sudden onset of fever, abdominal discomfort, nausea, vomiting, and rapidly-
increasing weakness and pallor. Tachycardia and low blood pressure are usually
present and shock may develop. Some patients appear severely ill and lethargic
and lapse into unconsciousness. It was formerly thought that the episode of
crisis was caused by a marked increase in the severity of hemolysis, but studies of

such episodes indicate that the majority are the result of a combination of decreased erythropoiesis and a continuation of the usual degree of hemolysis. Owren has described the occurrence of an "aplastic crisis" characterized by rapidly-increasing anemia, leukopenia, and thrombocytopenia that accompanied a fall in the reticulocyte count, a decrease in the plasma bilirubin, and the development of an aplastic picture in the bone marrow.[108] The occurrence of episodes of this type in several members of a family at the same time suggests that some intercurrent infection is the causative factor. Other attacks labeled as crisis that are associated with increasing jaundice may be, in reality, attacks of biliary colic and infection. In these circumstances the features of obstructive jaundice and infection are superimposed on those of hyperhemolysis. Cholelithiasis occurs in over one-half the patients over the age of 10, and in only about 5 per cent of those under 10 years of age.[63] In one group of 14 patients over 11 years of age, cholelithiasis occurred in 12.[122]

The most constant abnormality found on physical examination is splenomegaly of mild or moderate degree. In most patients the spleen is firm and does not extend below the level of the umbilicus, but in some patients it fills the entire left half of the abdominal cavity. The liver is often palpable but is rarely significantly enlarged. The patient with hereditary spherocytosis has been described as "more jaundiced than sick," but the degree of clinical jaundice is usually mild unless there is associated liver disease or dysfunction of the biliary tract. Both the pallor and the jaundice may be so mild as to be overlooked on the physical examination. In patients with hereditary spherocytosis, growth and development are usually normal. Abnormalities such as tower skull, polydactyly, skeletal defects, leg ulcers,[114] and infantilism have been reported in this disease, but appear to be uncommon.[121]

Laboratory Examination

The anemia is usually moderate and hematocrits of 30 to 35 per cent are common. The hematocrit may be normal if the hemolytic process is fully compensated, or markedly reduced if there is an episode of crisis.

The MCV is usually normal or slightly reduced, the result of the presence of both small spherocytes and large young red cells. The MCHC is characteristically increased because the hemoglobin is densely packed in the microspherocytes that have lost more surface area than cellular contents by fragmentation. Figure 7–2 shows a stained blood smear revealing many characteristic microspherocytes. A reticulocytosis of from 5 to 20 per cent or more is found regularly, unless erythropoiesis is depressed because of an aplastic crisis or for some other reason. During an aplastic crisis reticulocytes may disappear from the peripheral blood.[108] In the usual patient the bone marrow undergoes hyperplasia of the normoblastic type. During an aplastic crisis the marrow may be either aplastic or unusually cellular; the appearance depends on whether the specimen is obtained near the onset of crisis or during the recovery phase.

Study of the patient discloses other features common to hemolytic anemias of all types, such as an elevation of the level of serum bilirubin, an increase in the excretion of fecal urobilinogen and urinary urobilinogen, and normal or ele-

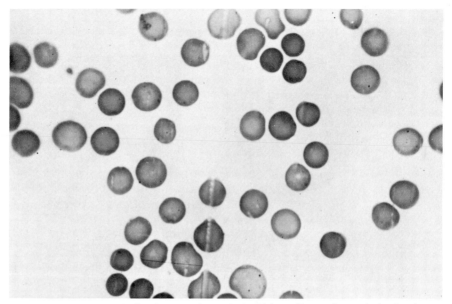

Figure 7–2 Peripheral blood smear of a patient with hereditary spherocytosis showing many microspherocytes.

vated levels of the serum iron. In one series, the serum bilirubin level ranged from 0.4 to 5.7 mg. per 100 ml., but in 80 per cent it was below 3.0 mg.[122] Levels higher than 4.0 mg. per 100 ml. are unusual, and concomitant biliary tract or liver disease should be suspected under such circumstances.

Increased fragility of erythrocytes in hypotonic saline solutions has been recognized as a characteristic feature of hereditary spherocytosis. When normal erythrocytes are tested in saline solutions, hemolysis begins in concentrations of about 0.45 per cent and is complete at 0.30 per cent. In most patients with hereditary spherocytosis hemolysis begins at concentrations of from 0.50 per cent to 0.75 per cent, and is complete at 0.40 per cent. The results may be expressed quantitatively.[74, 122] When incubated for 24 hours at 37° C., erythrocytes from patients with hereditary spherocytosis show a greater increase in osmotic fragility than do normal cells[122] (Fig. 7–3). In mildly-affected cases the abnormal osmotic fragility may not be evident until after incubation, and for this reason an incubated osmotic fragility is preferred. The autohemolysis test performed by incubating whole blood under sterile conditions for 48 hours is abnormal, and is corrected to nearly normal by the addition of glucose.[74] Normally less than 2 per cent hemolysis occurs in the autohemolysis test, whereas in hereditary spherocytosis usually 20 to 30 per cent of the red cells hemolyze (Fig. 7–4).

Differential Diagnosis

The diagnosis may be difficult if the patient is seen for the first time during an episode of aplastic crisis or during an attack of biliary colic, when the hemo-

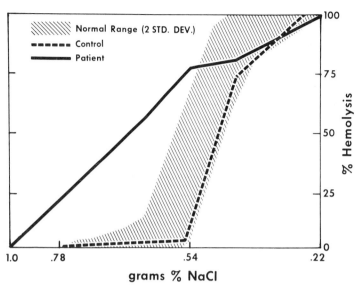

Figure 7–3   Typical incubated osmotic fragility curve of a patient with hereditary spherocytosis compared to a normal control.

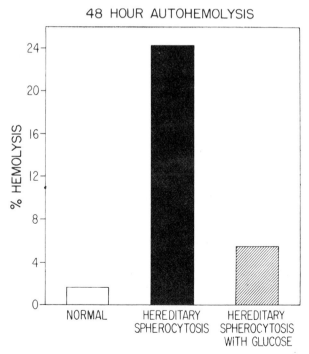

Figure 7–4   Typical autohemolysis pattern in a patient with hereditary spherocytosis compared with a normal control.

lytic nature of the underlying disorder may not be suspected. As a rule the presence of mild anemia, splenomegaly, and slight icterus suggests the diagnosis. The presence of hyperhemolysis is confirmed if reticulocytosis, increased urobilinogen excretion, and elevation of the indirect-reacting bilirubin in the blood are found.

Hereditary spherocytosis is generally distinguished from other types of hemolytic anemia by the family history and the hypotonic fragility test. However, the presence of microspherocytes and increased osmotic fragility does not establish the disorder as hereditary spherocytosis, for these sometimes occur in other types of hemolytic anemia. Increased osmotic fragility has been found in immune hemolytic anemia, myelofibrosis, leukemia, erythroblastosis fetalis, ovarian tumors, lymphomas, uremia, pneumonia, and after the administration of hemolytic poisons such as acetylphenylhydrazine, sulfanilamide, and arsenic. Nonspecific spherocytosis can usually be distinguished from hereditary spherocytosis by the autohemolysis test. Spherocytosis which occurs secondary to antibody injury, uremia, and other disorders will be accompanied by an increase in autohemolysis but, unlike hereditary spherocytosis, this will not be improved by the addition of glucose. At times study of the blood of siblings and parents is necessary to establish the diagnosis of hereditary spherocytosis in an individual patient. The Coombs antiglobulin test, hemoglobin electrophoresis, and the alkali denaturation test are often helpful in distinguishing hereditary spherocytosis from other hemolytic anemias, such as the hemoglobinopathies and immune hemolytic disease.

Treatment

Splenectomy was first performed by Wells in 1887 on a patient with this disease, some years before its nature was recognized.[74] It has been established since then that the procedure almost invariably relieves the anemia and jaundice.[74, 122] The serum bilirubin level returns to normal promptly and the erythrocyte count generally becomes normal in from two to four weeks (Fig. 7–5). Although spherocytosis is less marked after splenectomy, both the spherocytosis and increased osmotic fragility persist after operation,[74, 122] and although the length of red cell survival improves, it does not become entirely normal.[67] Operation appears to be indicated in virtually all patients with this disease except those with the mildest form of the disorder, unless there are other contraindications to surgery. Splenectomy may be done in infancy if the anemia is severe, but postponement to late childhood if possible is recommended because of the increased severity of infection in some children under two years of age.[65] following this operation. If the patient has cholelithiasis, cholecystectomy may be performed at the time of splenectomy, but at times it may be more prudent to perform the operations separately.

Folic acid, iron, and vitamin B_{12} are without value in the uncomplicated case of hereditary spherocytosis. Transfusions may be necessary during episodes of "crisis," particularly if splenectomy must be done at such a time, but these do not constitute a regular form of treatment.

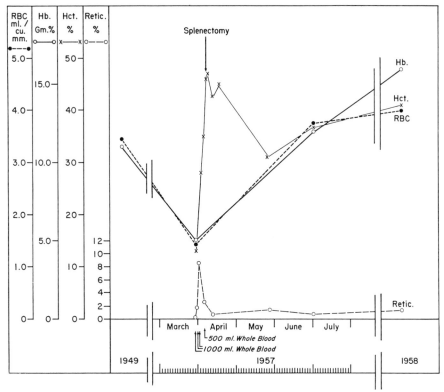

Figure 7-5 Hereditary spherocytosis, showing results of splenectomy. The patient was admitted during an "aplastic crisis" when the reticulocytes were nearly zero; despite transfusions the reticulocytes rose within a few days.

Illustrative Case

This white woman was first admitted to the University of Virginia Hospital in March, 1957, at the age of 38, for fever, weakness, and anemia. She had been told at another hospital in 1940 that she was anemic and should have a splenectomy, but she declined to have the operation. She had noted intermittent episodes of jaundice all her life. Her brother and daughter had a similar anemia for which splenectomy had been performed. On admission she was acutely ill and febrile. Physical examination was normal except for an enlarged spleen palpable 4 cm. below the left costal margin.

Laboratory examination. Admission blood studies: Hct. 13 per cent, Hb. 5.2 gm. per 100 ml., MCV 89, MCH 35, MCHC 40, W.B.C. 5400 per cu.mm., serum bilirubin 1.0 mg. per 100 ml.; no reticulocytes were seen. Spherocytes were seen on peripheral blood smear. Erythroid hyperplasia was evident in the bone marrow. Osmotic fragility was increased, as was the autohemolysis test which was improved by glucose.

Course. Splenectomy was performed and results are shown in Figure 7–5. Her gall bladder was also removed and showed chronic cholecystitis, but no stones were found. She is no longer anemic.

Comment. The diagnosis of hereditary spherocytosis was readily established in this patient by the presence of spherocytes on the blood smear, increased osmotic fragility, abnormal autohemolysis test improved by glucose, splenomegaly, and family history of hemolytic anemia which responded to splenectomy.

She also represents the problem these patients may have with aplastic crises accompanied by a marked fall in hematocrit, which may be life-threatening. This is one of the main reasons for recommending splenectomy when this diagnosis is made.

HEREDITARY ELLIPTOCYTOSIS

Elliptocytosis in man was reported first by Dresbach in 1904; the cells were seen in a healthy 22-year-old mulatto male.[79] The disorder is inherited as an autosomal dominant,[72] and affects 0.02 to 0.05 per cent of the general population. It is usually manifested as an asymptomatic trait, but about 12 per cent of persons with elliptocytosis have evidence of increased hemolysis, and some have frank hemolytic anemia.[61, 109, 119] The disorder is usually recognized by the elliptical appearance of the erythrocytes. Although small numbers of elliptocytes, rod cells, or oval cells may be observed in a variety of hematologic disorders, they are not seen in the large numbers characteristic of hereditary elliptocytosis where regularly more than 25 per cent of the cells are rod-shaped or oval, and usually between 50 to 90 per cent abnormal cells are present.[62] Poikilocytes, microcytes, and other abnormal forms occur only when there is increased hemolysis. The MCV, MCH, and MCHC usually are normal. No abnormality of the hemoglobin has been demonstrated by electrophoresis. Patients with hemolytic anemia have a moderately severe anemia, hemoglobin in the range of 7.5 to 9.2 grams per 100 ml., accompanied by normal leukocyte and platelet counts. Hemolysis and hyperbilirubinemia severe enough to require exchange transfusion has been noted in newborns, at which time the red cells more closely resemble pyknocytes than elliptocytes.[60] The osmotic fragility test and the autohemolysis test have been abnormal in some patients and normal in others. These tests are more likely to be abnormal when there is frank hemolysis.[119] An increased membrane permeability to the passive influx of sodium, similar to that seen in hereditary spherocytosis, has been described,[124] and a more rapid than normal decline in red cell ATP and 2,3 DPG has been reported.[77] It has also been observed by electron microscopy and shadow casting that the hemoglobin of elliptocytes is aggregated in a bipolar arrangement.[111] Splenomegaly occurs in patients with anemia, and studies with tagged erythrocytes have indicated a shortened survival time associated with an increased uptake of radioactivity over the spleen.[72] Splenectomy usually relieves the anemia although the abnormal appearance of the erythrocytes persists.[115]

OTHER ERYTHROCYTE MEMBRANE DEFECTS

Hereditary stomatocytosis in association with hemolytic anemia and abnormal red cell osmotic fragility has been reported in a number of different families.[101, 102, 107, 120, 123] The characteristic feature that all patients with this disorder have in common is a morphologic alteration of their red blood cells, consisting of a slit or mouthlike opening in the central part of the red cell on dried smears and bowl-shaped erythrocytes on wet preparations. Such red cells have been called stomatocytes. Wiley and his associates have pointed out the importance of red cell hydration in determining erythrocyte morphology on dried smears. When the cells are overhydrated, stomatocytes are plentiful,[107, 123] but when they are dehydrated only target cells are seen on the dried smear, although bowl shapes appear in wet preparations.[120] It is important, therefore to examine red cell morphology in both wet and dry states and to consider the possibility of hereditary stomatocytosis in patients with unexplained hereditary hemolytic anemia who have target cells on the blood film. Patients with stomatocystosis and hemolytic anemia probably represent a heterogeneous group of red cell disorders rather than a specific biochemical entity, as there has been decreased glucose-6-phosphate dehydrogenase in one family,[101] low erythrocyte glutathione in another patient,[103] and marked increase in permeability to univalent cations in three other families.[103, 106, 121] The increase in cation permeability and osmotic fragility is similar to that seen in hereditary spherocytosis, but differs in that the red cells of patients with stomatocytosis do not display membrane lipid loss and do not become spherocytes. In one of the families reported by Oski and his associates,[107] the hemolytic process was quite mild in the face of a much more severe cation leak than is seen in hereditary spherocytosis, emphasizing the importance of additional membrane lesions in hereditary spherocytosis. Acquired reversible stomatocytosis with hemolytic anemia has been observed in some patients as a complication of alcohol ingestion.[78]

Jaffé and Gottfried have reported an hereditary hemolytic anemia in a large family from the Dominican Republic.[96] The disorder is inherited as an autosomal dominant and is characterized by an increased content of the phospholipid, lecithin, in the red cell membrane. Both unincubated and incubated osmotic fragility of the erythrocytes were less than normal. The accumulation of lecithin (phosphatidyl choline) in these cells has been shown to be due to defective transfer of esterified membrane fatty acid from phosphatidyl choline to phosphatidylethanolamine, associated with increased cation permeability and glycolysis resulting in increased vulnerability of these red cells to the stress of erythrostasis.[140] Wiley and his colleagues have noted the similarity of their patients with hereditary stomatocytosis to those reported by Jaffé[96] and Shohet,[113] in that all patients had an increase in membrane phosphatidyl choline. Other patients with hereditary stomatocytosis have been reported to have increased red cell lipid,[107, 122] but individual phospholipids were not measured.

A mild anemia with slight hemolysis and a reduced compensatory bone marrow response has been reported secondary to a complete absence of lecithin: cholesterol acyl transferase.[84, 116] There was a marked increase in erythrocyte cholesterol and a decrease in phosphatidylethanolamine and sphingomyelin.[143]

Another type of hereditary stomatocytosis has been reported in patients of Mediterranean origin who have a mild hemolytic anemia with normal osmotic fragility and no cellular electrolyte changes.[81, 91, 106] In still another group, dehydrated red cells were present with a decrease in total cation content, but no stomatocytes were observed on dry or wet preparations.[85]

It is clear that hereditary stomatocytosis is a syndrome which may include a variety of different red cell membrane defects.

PENTOSE PHOSPHATE SHUNT-GLUTATHIONE SYSTEM ENZYME DEFICIENCIES

GLUCOSE-6-PHOSPHATE DEHYDROGENASE DEFICIENCY

History

In 1926, Cordes noted that the antimalarial drug pamaquine caused hemolytic anemia in some patients.[149] Earle, in 1948, made the observation that only the erythrocytes of blacks hemolyzed after taking pamaquine.[154] The Korean War in the early 1950s focused major attention on this problem, when large numbers of American blacks stationed in Korea developed acute hemolytic anemia after taking primaquine for treatment or prophylaxis of malaria. A study group was formed under the direction of Alving that was responsible for contributing much of the early information to the understanding of this type of hemolytic anemia.[152, 153] They quickly learned that patients who had had hemolysis while taking pamaquine also had hemolysis after taking primaquine.[159] They demonstrated that Heinz body formation was a prominent part of the hemolytic process,[132] and in 1956 a deficiency of red cell glucose-6-phosphate dehydrogenase (G-6-PD) was shown to be the basic red cell defect.[145] A number of detailed reviews is available.[127, 130, 146, 166, 170, 195]

Clinical Manifestations

Glucose-6-phosphate dehydrogenase deficiency is transmitted on the X chromosome with full expression in the hemizygous male and partial expression in the heterozygous female.[147] In the United States the disorder is found most frequently in blacks. Approximately 10 to 13 per cent of male American blacks have G-6-PD deficiency, 20 per cent of female blacks are carriers, and 3 per cent of black women react to oxidant drugs.[194] Less than 1 per cent of whites of Northern European origin have the deficiency, but the disorder is prevalent among whites in the Mediterranean area, being as high as 48 per cent in Sardinian males.[194] The disorder is world-wide and it has been estimated that over 100 million people have this deficiency.[146] Since the areas of highest incidence correspond to areas where there is a high incidence of malaria, it has been postulated that G-6-PD deficiency confers some resistance against the malarial parasite.[127, 171]

When a patient with G-6-PD deficiency is exposed to an oxidant drug or some other type of oxidant stress, the following sequence of events occurs: acute hemolysis is evident between the second and fourth day and is accompained by hemoglobinuria. The hematocrit continues to fall for seven to 12 days, and approximately 30 to 50 per cent of the red cell mass is destroyed. During this time Heinz bodies are seen and the bilirubin may be elevated. As the reticulocyte response reaches its peak (around 10 to 12 days) the hematocrit begins to rise again and gradually returns to normal levels in four to five weeks, even though the offending drug is continued.[152] It has been shown with radioiron labeling that, in black patients, the older population of red cells are hemolyzed and the younger red cells are relatively resistant to this type of drug-induced hemolysis.[131] This correlates well with G-6-PD activity, which decreases as red cells age in black patients. In contrast, hemolysis is not self-limited in the more severe type of deficiency seen in patients of Mediterranean origin.[184]

Table 7–2 lists some of the drugs which have been reported to produce hemolysis in G-6-PD-deficient patients. All of these drugs are oxidants in that they have the ability to transport electrons and serve as catalysts in oxidation-reduction reactions. Most of the offending drugs are aromatic amines.[127] Although ingestion of the fava bean produces acute hemolytic anemia in people of Mediterranean origin with G-6-PD deficiency, favism has not been reported in blacks with the deficiency.[162]

Hemolytic anemia may be precipitated in G-6-PD-deficient patients, not only by oxidant drugs but also by infection. In a series of hemolytic episodes in G-6-PD-deficient patients reviewed by Burka and his colleagues,[142, 143] infection alone was a more frequent cause of hemolysis than drugs alone. The episodes were associated with both bacterial and viral infections, and were particularly common with infectious hepatitis.[179, 183] In addition, diabetic acidosis may induce a hemolytic episode.[155]

Whites from the Mediterranean area and blacks who have G-6-PD deficiency

Table 7–2 Some Drugs Which Produce Hemolysis of G-6-PD-Deficient Red Cells

1. Antimalarials—primaquine, pamaquine, pentaquine, quinocide, quinacrine, quinine
2. Sulfonamides—sulfanilamide, sulfapyridine, sulfisoxazole, sulfamethoxy-pyridazine, sulfacetamide, sulfoxone, salicylazosulfapyridine
3. Nitrofurans—nitrofurantoin, furaltadone, nitrofurazone, furazolidine
4. Analgesics—acetanilid, acetophenetidin, aspirin, antipyrine, aminopyrine
5. Diuretics—thiazides, acetazolamide
6. Hypoglycemic agents—tolbutamide, chlorpropamide
7. Sulfones—thiazosulfone, diaminodiphenylsulfone (DDS), sulfoxone
8. Miscellaneous—chloramphenicol, para-aminosalicylic acid (PAS), vitamin K, naphthalene (moth balls), fava beans, probenecid, isoniazid, quinidine, dimercaprol (BAL), neoarsphenamine

are not anemic, and have no difficulty unless they are exposed to oxidative stress. On the other hand, whites of Northern European origin usually have a mild hemolytic anemia at all times which is made worse by oxidants.[170, 173] These cases would have been classified as congenital nonspherocytic hemolytic anemia before the specific red cell enzyme deficit was established.

Laboratory Examination

In the black and the Mediterranean white, routine hematologic tests are normal except during a hemolytic episode brought on by exposure to some oxidant or acute infection. During that time, signs of hemolysis are present, including hemoglobinuria and bilirubinemia. The red cells usually show Heinz bodies early in the course of the hemolytic episode. In patients with congenital nonspherocytic hemolytic anemia secondary to G-6-PD deficiency, the usual findings of chronic hemolysis are present.

Much of the laboratory evaluation in G-6-PD deficiency has been directed towards detecting individuals with the deficiency, in order to avoid exposure to offending agents and to diagnose the cause of acute hemolysis in a likely candidate, such as a black male.

Although a number of screening tests have been proposed, the most useful in the authors' hands have been the methemoglobin reduction test[141] and the cyanide–ascorbate test.[161] The methemoglobin reduction test has the advantage of employing simple reagents, sodium nitrite and methylene blue, and may be read visually. It is not sensitive enough, however, to pick up heterozygous females, and is often equivocal after an acute hemolytic episode when most of the older red cells with the lowest G-6-PD levels have been lysed. In this situation the test must be repeated several months later. The cyanide–ascorbate test has the advantage of screening not only for G-6-PD deficiency but also for other enzymes in the pentose phosphate shunt–glutathione system; glutathione reductase, glutathione synthetase, and glutathione peroxidase. All of these enzymes are necessary for the effective reduction of the hydrogen peroxide generated by ascorbic acid. The test can also be read visually and has the advantage of detecting most of the heterozygous females. It is also usually positive during an acute hemolytic episode. For these reasons we feel that this is the screening test of choice. If this test is positive then a specific enzyme assay should be carried out to determine which enzyme is deficient.

Variants of Glucose-6-Phosphate Dehydrogenase

More than 80 mutants of G-6-PD have been described.[167, 170, 208] Different types of G-6-PD have been distinguished electrophoretically and by enzyme kinetics. About one-half of the reported variants have normal or only slightly-reduced enzyme activity and have no clinical manifestations of disease.[207] The two major electrophoretic types are A+ and B+. Whites have only type B+; 82 per cent of blacks have type B+ and 18 per cent have A+. Black females may have both types. Yoshida and his colleagues have shown that the faster moving A+

differs from B$^+$ only by the substitution of aspartic acid for asparagine.[206] Whites of Mediterranean origin with G-6-PD deficiency have deficiency of the B$^-$ type. In blacks, although type B$^+$ is the most common, the common deficiency is of A$^-$-type and rarely of the B$^-$ type. No biochemical difference has been found between A$^+$- and A$^-$- types, except that the A$^-$-type enzyme in deficient blacks is degraded more rapidly than normal. This may account for the older red cells showing the more marked deficiency. In blacks with the A$^-$-type of G-6-PD deficiency only the erythrocyte is affected, whereas many of the mutants in whites involve other tissues including leukocytes[148, 181] and platelets.[182]

OTHER DEFICIENCIES OF THE PENTOSE PHOSPHATE SHUNT–GLUTATHIONE SYSTEM

Although a number of patients have been described with erythrocyte 6-phosphogluconate dehydrogenase deficiency, sufficient clinical information has not been reported to determine whether they had mild hemolysis or were susceptible to oxidative stress.[140] On the other hand, patients with deficiencies of glutathione reductase,[144, 204] glutathione synthetase,[135, 174, 180] γ-glutamyl-cysteine synthetase,[166] and glutathione peroxidase[36, 48, 136] who have chronic hemolytic anemia and susceptibility to oxidants have been reported. These are very rare and probably transmitted as an autosomal recessive, except for gluta-thione reductase deficiency, which has been reported to be relatively common in Germany, but not in the United States, and is thought to be transmitted as an autosomal dominant.[204] However, Beutler has pointed out that flavin compounds stimulate glutathione reductase activity, and that some patients who were thought to have hereditary glutathione reductase deficiency were in reality suffering from riboflavin deficiency.[128]

GLYCOLYTIC ENZYME DEFICIENCIES

In 1953 Dacie and his colleagues popularized the concept of the congenital nonspherocytic hemolytic anemias characterized by the absence of sphero-cytes or abnormal hemoglobin, accompanied by normal osmotic fragility of fresh red cells.[150] The next year Selwyn and Dacie divided this group of patients into types I and II based on the autohemolysis test; type I patients had normal or slightly-increased autohemolysis which was improved by glucose, and type II had increased autohemolysis which was not improved by the addition of glu-cose.[187] It is apparent now that G-6-PD deficiency corresponds to type I and pyruvate kinase deficiency to type II. As more specific defects in red cell metab-olism become delineated in patients with hereditary hemolytic anemia, the de-scriptive term "congenital nonspherocytic hemolytic anemia" should drop from usage.[151]

Pyruvate Kinase Deficiency

In 1961, Valentine and his associates[203] demonstrated a deficiency in red cell pyruvate kinase to be the cause of hereditary hemolytic anemia corresponding generally to the type II congenital nonspherocytic hemolytic anemia described by Dacie. This was the first time a specific enzyme defect had been discovered in the main pathway of glycolysis, the Embden-Meyerhof pathway. It is the most common of the glycolytic enzyme deficiencies associated with hemolytic anemia. Over 135 documented cases have been reported.[139, 164, 191–193, 202]

The patients have ranged in age from birth to 65 and have been predominantly of Northern European ancestry, although many other ethnic groups have been affected. The deficiency is transmitted as an autosomal recessive, with heterozygous family members having about one-half the normal amount of enzyme activity but showing no signs of disease. The great variation in the severity of the anemia in homozygous patients suggests genetic polymorphism, but this has not been clearly established.[209] Splenectomy often ameliorates the anemia, particularly in severe cases, although the hemolytic anemia persists at a lesser degree of severity.[139]

Osmotic fragility of fresh erythrocytes is normal, but increases greatly after incubation. Autohemolysis is markedly abnormal and is not improved by the addition of glucose, but it is lessened by adding ATP. The reticulocyte count is often between 20 and 50 per cent, and may be even higher after splenectomy, since there is selective destruction of reticulocytes by the spleen.[164, 172] In the more severe cases the erythrocyte membrane appears to be damaged, with crenated red cells that resemble acanthocytes appearing on the peripheral blood smear.[176] A simple screening test is available to detect erythrocyte pyruvate kinase deficiency.[129]

Although most patients with pyruvate kinase deficiency hemolytic anemia have low red cell ATP levels as a result of their metabolic block, the severity of the anemia does not correlate well with ATP levels or enzyme activity, and the specific sequence of biochemical events leading to red cell destruction remains to be clarified.[196, 209]

OTHER GLYCOLYTIC ENZYME DEFICIENCIES

Since pyruvate kinase deficiency hemolytic anemia was described in 1961, patients with hereditary hemolytic anemia secondary to nine additional enzyme deficiencies involving the anaerobic glycolytic pathway have been described:[197] 2,3-diphosphoglyceromutase,[138] triosephosphate isomerase,[185–186, 188] hexokinase,[165, 175, 201] glucosephosphate isomerase,[125, 126, 134, 178] phosphoglycerate kinase,[169, 199] phosphofructokinase,[195, 205] aldolase,[133] enolase,[189] and glyceraldehyde-3-phosphate dehydrogenase.[177] The position of these enzymes in the Embden-Meyerhof pathway is shown in Figure 7–1. In addition to deficiencies of these glycolytic enzymes, deficiencies of ATPase,[156, 158] adenylate kinase,[137, 190] and ribosephosphate pyrophosphokinase[198, 200] have been reported in association with hemolytic anemia.

Most of these enzyme deficiencies have been shown to be transmitted as an autosomal recessive and are consequently rare, there being only a few families reported with each type of deficiency. The hereditary erythrocyte enzyme deficiencies have been reviewed.[162]

HEMOGLOBINOPATHIES

More than 100 abnormal hemoglobins have been described in man, but relatively few have been associated with clinical disease. Heller has proposed a classification of the hemoglobinopathies based on their functional characteristics:[334]

Group 1. Abnormal hemoglobins without physiologic aberrations. This constitutes the largest group, and although these hemoglobin mutants are of genetic and biochemical interest they are without clinical significance.

Group 2. "Aggregating" hemoglobins. Hemoglobins S and C fall into this group, as structural changes occur in the red cell because of tactoid formation of hemoglobin S and crystal formation of hemoglobin C.

Group 3. "Unbalanced" synthesis of hemoglobins. This group consists of the thalassemia syndromes in which one type of hemoglobin chain is synthesized in excess of other hemoglobin chains, with the excess chains precipitating as Heinz bodies.

Group 4. Unstable hemoglobins. These hemoglobins, which usually involve an amino acid substitution in the region of heme attachment, are susceptible to oxidative denaturation with precipitation as Heinz bodies. Hemoglobins Zurich, Köln, Seattle, and many others belong to this group.

Group 5. Hemoglobins with abnormal heme function. This group includes the M hemoglobins that are associated with methemoglobinemia; hemoglobins Chesapeake, Rainier, and, others which have an increased affinity for oxygen with compensatory polycythemia; and hemoglobin Kansas and others which have a decreased affinity for oxygen.

SICKLE CELL ANEMIA

History

The first case of sickle cell anemia was described by Herrick in 1910.[241] This patient, a 20-year-old black male from the West Indies, had most of the classic clinical and hematologic features of the disease. In addition to the usual morphology of many of his erythrocytes, which had the shape of a sickle, this patient had cardiac enlargement, icterus, anemia, normoblasts in the peripheral blood, and leukocytosis. Huck established the fact that the sickling property resides in the cell and not in the plasma.[246] Ponder showed that red cells washed free of hemoglobin do not sickle,[273] and Harris showed that stroma-free solutions of deoxygenated sickle hemoglobin form sickle tactoids.[237] Hahn and Gillespie demonstrated that sickling is a reversible reaction related to the degree of oxygenation of the hemoglobin in the erythrocyte.[236] A most important contribution was made by Pauling, Itano, Singer, and Wells in 1949 when they established that sickle cell anemia is a molecular disease.[266–267] They demonstrated that hemoglobin obtained from patients with sickle cell anemia differed electrophoretically from that present in erythrocytes of normal individuals, and concluded that the abnormality resided in the protein portion of the molecule. The nature of the defect was further characterized by Ingram, who showed that the molecule of sickle cell hemoglobin differs from a molecule of normal hemoglobin only by having glutamic acid replaced by valine in the beta chain.[248] The studies of Neel and others have shown that the molecular abnormality of hemoglobin is genetically controlled.[263] The complete amino acid sequence of the alpha and beta chains of sickle and normal hemoglobin have been described.[243]

Mechanism of the Anemia

The sickling property is a gene-transmitted abnormality that is heterozygous in persons with sickle cell trait and homozygous in individuals with sickle cell anemia.[263] The consequence of this defect is found in the globin portion of the hemoglobin molecule and not in the heme portion.[266-267] Sickle cell hemoglobin and normal hemoglobin differ in that the beta peptide chain in each half of the sickle cell hemoglobin molecule contains valine in the sixth position, where glutamic acid is found in normal hemoglobin.[248] Thus it appears that, of almost 300 amino acids present in each half of the hemoglobin molecule, hemoglobin S and hemoglobin A differ in only one amino acid. The substitution of valine for glutamic acid, with the resultant loss of the carboxyl group, explains the electrophoretic differences in these two hemoglobins. In addition, efforts have been made to explain the unusual chemical and clinical manifestations of the disease by this molecular peculiarity.

The sickle cell hemoglobin tends to polymerize and form tactoids under conditions of lowered oxygen tension[272] and lowered pH.[237] Sickling of erythrocytes is reversible and is thought to be the result of realignment of the hemoglobin molecules in the cell envelope, rather than the actual crystallization of the hemoglobin molecules.[237] Murayama, using scale models of the hemoglobin molecule, has proposed the following explanation for the molecular stacking of deoxygenated S hemoglobin. The substitution of valine for glutamic acid in the sixth position of the beta chain allows an intramolecular hydrophobic bond to form between the valines in the first and sixth positions at the amino terminal end of the beta chain. This cyclization of the two ends of the beta chain forms a "key" arrangement which fits into a complementary site in the alpha chains of an adjacent molecule so that molecular stacking occurs. When S hemoglobin is oxygenated, the two beta chains move closer together by approximately 7Å, leading to disruption of the "lock" and "key" arrangement and unsickling of the S hemoglobin. Based on electron microscopy, Murayama has also proposed that when hemoglobin S sickles, microtubules are formed, consisting of six monofilaments of hemoglobin twisted around a hollow center.[261, 262]

Erythrocytes from patients with sickle cell anemia will sickle in the physiologic ranges of oxygen concentration, but a marked lowering of the oxygen tension is necessary to produce sickling in individuals with the sickle cell trait. It has been assumed that this difference between erythrocytes that contain only sickle hemoglobin and those that contain both normal and sickle hemoglobin forms the basis for the different clinical manifestations of sickle cell anemia and sickle cell trait. Individuals who have the sickle cell trait are essentially asymptomatic, and remain so unless the oxygen saturation of the blood is reduced to an abnormal degree or acidosis develops. Patients who are homozygous for hemo-globin S have sickle cell anemia, a chronic illness characterized by anemia and the occurrence of infarctions in various organs of the body.

The anemia, which is hemolytic in type, is the result of the intracorpuscular defect. Erythrocytes from normal individuals survive for about 120 days when transfused into patients with sickle cell anemia, but erythrocytes from patients with sickle cell anemia have a much shorter survival time when transfused into normal recipients. Studies that utilized the analysis of ^{15}N-hemin disappearance and fecal stercobilin ^{15}N appearance indicate complete random destruction of the red cells, a shortened survival time of the erythrocytes (16 days in one pa-tient), and no evidence of more than one population of cells.[249] It has been sug-gested that the excessive destruction of the erythrocytes is the result of the increase in mechanical fragility that has been demonstrated when the erythro-cytes assume the sickle cell form.[237] According to this explanation, the erythro-cytes become sickled under the oxygen tensions that occur in the body normally, and in this form both the mechanical fragility of the cells and the amount of trauma that they encounter in the circulation are increased.

A serious complication of sickle cell anemia is the "hypoplastic or aregenera-tive crisis."[279] Systemic infections may depress erythropoiesis, and although they are of little note in persons with a normal red cell life span, they may be life-threatening in patients with a shortened red cell life span. The transient marrow aplasia may be responsible for a sudden increase in the severity of the anemia.

The development of the lesions that occur in the various organs of the body is usually attributed to thrombosis and infarction or to ischemic necrosis and hemorrhage;[227, 254] either ischemia or thrombosis would be favored by the pack-ing and stasis of the sickle-shaped erythrocytes in the capillaries under conditions of lowered oxygen tension. It has been suggested that the assumption of the sickle form is associated with an increase in viscosity which leads to a "vicious cycle" of increased deoxygenation, increased sickling, and increased stasis.[235]

Clinical Manifestations

Sickle cell trait and sickle cell anemia have been found almost entirely in the black race. The incidence of the sickling trait varies in different parts of the world and is about 9 per cent in American blacks. Sickle cell anemia has a frequency of about one-fortieth that of the trait.[260]

Sickle cell anemia is characterized by the occurrence of symptoms in virtually any part of the body. These symptoms are sometimes bizarre and vary greatly from patient to patient, and from time to time in the same patient. Most patients with sickle cell anemia, both children and adults, continue in a mild state of chronic illness with stable levels of erythrocytes and serum bilirubin, but nearly all patients at one time or another experience episodes of more severe symptoms, the attacks of so-called "crisis." Different types of attacks have been described as "crisis."

The aregenerative type of hypoplastic crisis, manifested by erythrocytic hypoplasia or aplasia in the marrow, marked decrease in the number of reticulo-cytes in the circulating blood, and a rapidly-increasing anemia, usually follows bacterial or viral infection and need not be associated with any pain. The factors which are responsible for the bone marrow failure, which often is associated with a precipitous fall in the hemoglobin level, are not understood. The authors have observed the same patient with sickle cell anemia during several attacks of pneumococcal pneumonia; on some occasions a hypoplastic crisis developed, and at other times pneumococcal pneumonia was not associated with significant change in the values of the circulating blood.

Another type of attack called "crisis" is that associated with localizing signs of disease. These are thought to be the result of erythrostasis and anoxia or infarction. Infarction of the spleen, kidney, bone, and lungs, and localized neurologic lesions, are examples of this type. Patients with sickle cell anemia also have other illnesses, such as acute appendicitis, renal colic, and gall bladder disease, that must be distinguished from the episodes of "crisis."

A third type of painful "crisis" is the most puzzling of all. The onset is quite sudden and may occur when a patient awakes in the morning or after an afternoon nap. The attack usually begins with aching pain in one or both knees or legs. It increases steadily in severity and in extent and often progresses to the back, the abdomen, both arms, the neck, and the head. The pain may involve almost the entire body within ten minutes or after several hours; at times it does not progress beyond one or several extremities, or one side of the body. Sometimes the attacks are mild and last but a day or two. More often the pain is severe and may not be completely relieved by aspirin or narcotics. The frequency of these attacks varies greatly; attacks occur in some patients every few weeks, in some several times a year, and in others only at intervals of years. Nearly all patients emphasize the suddenness of the onset of the attack. Respiratory infections, insect bites, fever, a feeling of nervousness, and various indications precede some attacks, but in others the patient feels perfectly well and is engaged in nothing more strenuous than talking with members of the family when the attack begins abruptly. Fever is not invariably present, peripheral blood counts remain unchanged, and the patient manifests no cyanosis, shock, or localized vascular insufficiency.

The most common cutaneous manifestations of the disease are indolent ulcers or scars on the lower legs, which can be found on about 75 per cent of the older children or adults with the disease. Ulceration is rare in very young children.[85, 227] The ulcers, which have sharply defined edges, are usually single but may be multiple and bilateral (Fig. 7–6).

Various types of cardiac abnormalities have been reported in from 50 to 91 per cent of the patients.[283] The commonest of these is an apical systolic murmur which occurs in the majority. Although they are rare, mitral, aortic, and pulmonic diastolic murmurs have been reported. Cardiac enlargement, which often involves both ventricles, is a common finding and has been attributed to the chronic anemia.[284] Cor pulmonale occurs in some patients, possibly as a result of repeated pulmonary infarctions and pulmonary hypertension.[284] Electrocardiographic abnormalities, such as a prolonged PR interval and minor changes in the ST segment and T wave, occur but are nonspecific.

Symptoms referable to the genitourinary tract are not common but may be dramatic and serious. Episodes of hematuria may occur as a complication of both sickle cell trait and sickle cell disease.[210, 255] The bleeding is usually unilateral and

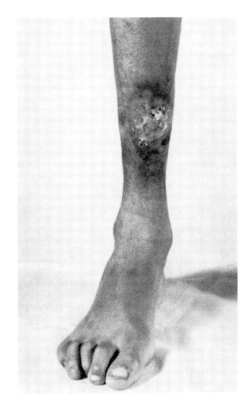

Figure 7–6 Typical leg ulcer in sickle cell anemia.

recurrent, and may be marked. Some patients have been operated upon for suspected tumor because of unilateral hematuria associated with an abnormal intravenous pyelogram. A defect in the capacity of the kidney to concentrate the urine has been noted in most patients with sickle cell anemia and in many with sickle cell trait.[271, 280] The defect may be temporarily corrected by transfusion with normal red blood cells in young patients, but this is not often true in adults who have had time to develop irreversible structural damage to the renal medulla. The pathogenesis of hematuria and hyposthenuria is incompletely understood. Sickling of the erythrocytes of patients with sickle cell disease and sickle cell trait is thought to occur in the medullary capillaries as the result of a combination of reduced oxygen tension and hyperosmolality (and perhaps reduced pH). The resulting engorgement and vascular obstruction is particularly evident in the peritubular areas, and local ischemia is believed to lead to degeneration of the tubular epithelium, extravasation of blood around the collecting tubules, and in some instances to papillary necrosis.[210, 237, 271] Chronic renal insufficiency may occasionally be seen in older patients. Glomerular congestion and enlargement early in the course of the disease, followed by progressive ischemia, fibrosis, and obliteration of the glomeruli, is believed responsible for the progressive decline in glomerular filtration rate late in the course of the disorder.[215]

Priapism has been reported in a number of patients; it sometimes persists for from 10 to 36 days and is often followed by complete impotence.

Nearly all patients with sickle cell anemia at one time or another complain of gastrointestinal symptoms such as anorexia, nausea, vomiting, or jaundice. Severe pain may occur in any part of the abdomen, and at times it is difficult to decide whether surgical intervention is indicated. Such pains may be due to infarction of the spleen or some other organ, or may be related to cholelithiasis, which has been reported to have an incidence of 25 per cent. In a group of 47 patients ranging in age from 12 to 58 years with sickle cell anemia, study suggested that one-third of the patients over 10 years of age had gall stones and chronic cholecystitis, although less than 10 per cent had signs or symptoms attributable to this complication.[213] Elective cholecystectomy has been recommended in patients who have gall stones, because the risk of operation does not seem great and it is difficult to distinguish jaundice with cholangitis and gall stones from that caused by sickling and hepatic stasis.[213] Some patients with sickle cell anemia develop right upper quadrant pain, tenderness, rapid and marked enlargement of the liver, and greatly elevated direct-acting serum bilirubin. In such patients it may be difficult to decide whether it is an attack of severe fulminating hepatitis, possibly from transfusions, hepatic vein thrombosis, or generalized hepatic congestion with sickle cells that has developed.

A wide variety of central nervous system manifestations has been reported in patients of all ages.[247] These include hemiplegia, aphasia, dysphagia, nystagmus, drowsiness, coma, headache, convulsions, and stiff neck. Electroencephalographic abnormalities are common in children.[242] Evidence of the neurologic involvement may subside completely, but some patients die during these episodes and others develop a spastic paralysis that persists. The lesions in the central nervous system are presumed to be the result of vascular accidents or circulatory disturbances of a transient nature.

Characteristic conjunctival vascular abnormalities consisting of comma-shaped capillary segments seemingly isolated from the rest of the vascular network are often seen with a hand lens or slit lamp in patients with sickle cell anemia.[231, 265] Funduscopic examination of the retina of patients with sickle cell anemia or sickle cell trait may reveal marked tortuosity and dilatation of the retinal vessels (Fig. 7–7). In addition, one may find neovascularization and microaneurysms, stasis, or thrombosis of retinal vessels and retinal hemorrhages.[257]

Sickle cell anemia is often accompanied by symptoms or signs referable to the joints and skeleton. Pain in the joints is common, but actual swelling of the joints is rare. Skeletal abnormalities are usually demonstrable only by roentgenograms; the commonest manifestations are "fish tailing" of the vertebral bodies and radiolucent areas of necrosis in these or other bones.[228, 258] The "hair on end" appearance of the skull sometimes occurs but is not common. Other abnormalities that can be demonstrated radiologically in some patients are gallstones, pulmonary infarcts, and cardiac enlargement. In young children attacks of dactylitis, particularly in the hands, are common.

Bone marrow infarction, recognized by the necrotic appearance of the marrow aspirate, has long been considered a possible source of pulmonary and cerebral emboli; more recently it has been suspected to be a cause of painful crisis.[220]

Sickle cell anemia in infants is an especially serious disease. In one report, 10 of 64 patients died during the first year of life; the causes of death were

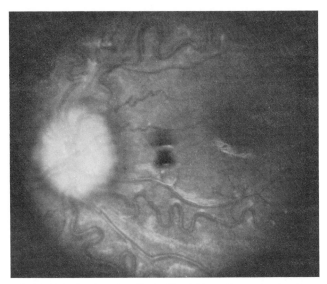

Figure 7–7 Ophthalmic fundus of patient with sickle cell anemia showing marked tortuosity and dilatation of retinal vessels.

pneumonia, crisis, sepsis with meningococcus, pseudomonas, and salmonella organisms, and diarrhea.[274] The disease was first manifested by dactylitis, particularly in the hands but also in the feet, with or without any x-ray abnormalities, infection, or crisis, and with nonspecific symptoms termed a "failure to thrive." Fulminant pneumococcemia may terminate fatally within a few hours after onset.[252] Predisposing factors may be a deficiency of pneumococcal serum opsonizing activity[282] and functional asplenia,[270] which have been reported in sickle cell anemia. Intravascular coagulation has been present in some of the children with septicemia. Sudden death in children also occurs during crisis.[250] Extreme pallor, weakness, lethargy, tachycardia, and cold clammy skin are the most common manifestations of shock. The principal finding at autopsy has been severe congestion of internal organs, especially the liver and spleen, with sickled erythrocytes. Treatment of the so-called "splenic sequestration crisis" consists primarily of correction of the hypovolemia by blood transfusion.[322]

Although the presence of sickle cell trait usually is associated with no manifestation of disease, important exceptions occur. Hematuria, which may be persistent and very troublesome, occurs in patients with sickle cell trait. Patients with sickle cell trait flying at high altitudes have developed splenic infarction; others have died suddenly while involved in very strenuous physical exercise.[251] In the last two conditions, anoxia, dehydration, and acidosis are probably responsible for the attacks.

Salmonella osteomyelitis has been reported in a number of patients with sickle cell anemia, and it has been established that there is an increased incidence of this infection in the disease.[245] Bacteremia and multiple foci of involvement, particularly in the long bones, occur. Pus may collect beneath the skin or in the joints after spontaneous rupture of a subperiosteal abscess through the periosteum. The reason for the increased susceptibility of patients with sickle cell anemia is not clear; a possible factor may be that the macrophages have a diminished capacity to phagocytize and kill salmonella organisms as a result of erythrophagocytosis by the reticuloendothelial cells.[232, 253] Local ischemia or infarction and splenic atrophy with functional asplenia may also be important.

Functional asplenia, possibly the result of a diversion of splenic blood flow through intravascular shunts, has been reported in children with splenomegaly; splenic function was restored when transfusions raised the level of normal cells to 50 per cent, probably by reducing the blood viscosity.[268]

Laboratory Examination

In the usual patient with sickle cell anemia, the hemoglobin and erythrocyte count are reduced to about one-half the normal values. The anemia is normocytic and normochromic unless complicating factors are present. On the stained smear of peripheral blood a few sickled forms may be seen, but the most prominent features are marked anisocytosis, poikilocytosis, and the presence of target cells; nucleated red cells are often present (Fig. 7–8). Fragmented cells and other abnormalities usually seen in impact hemolysis have been observed in patients with sickle cell anemia and pulmonary emboli.[212] The leukocyte count is usually between 12,000 to 16,000 per cu.mm.; the reported counts have ranged from 4000 to 69,000 per cu.mm.[240, 276] The platelet count is usually normal, but counts over 1 million per cu.mm. sometimes occur.

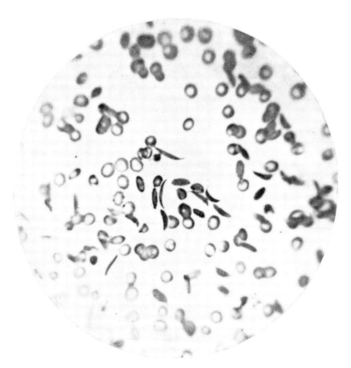

Figure 7–8   Erythrocytes in sickle cell anemia; Wright's stain. (Courtesy of Dr. B. E. Washburn and the Virginia Medical Monthly, vol. 15, 1911.)

The laboratory evidences of a hemolytic process are found unless a hypo-plastic phase is present. The reticulocyte count is often over 20 per cent, and although the level of the indirect-reacting bilirubin in the serum is increased, it usually does not exceed 3.0 mg. per 100 ml. unless there is some associated hepatic or biliary complication. The daily fecal urobilinogen excretion varies spontaneously, and decreases after transfusions of whole blood. The plasma iron level is normal or elevated and the latent iron-binding capacity is normal.

Examination of the bone marrow usually reveals erythrocytic hyperplasia of the normoblastic type associated with hyperplasia of the myeloid cells. Occasion-ally, a long-continued marrow hyperplasia leads to folate deficiency which may be manifested by the megaloblastic type of erythropoiesis. During a hypoplastic crisis, acute transient marrow aplasia has been reported. Sickling of the adult erythrocytes and of the nucleated red cells may be observed in material obtained from the marrow. Long filamentous erythrocytes are observed more often in the marrow preparations than in preparations made from the peripheral blood.

The sedimentation rate in patients whose red cells sickle is not increased as much as is usually the case in patients with a comparable degree of anemia. Prolonged stasis of venous blood causes an increased retardation of the sedi-mentation rate because sickling occurs.

The erythrocytes of sickle cell anemia are abnormally resistant to hypotonic saline; in one series the average figure for beginning hemolysis was 0.35 per cent, and for completion was 0.22 per cent.[226] Some of the cells are not hemolyzed in distilled water. The mechanical fragility of the cells is normal when they are in the discoid form, but becomes increased if sickling is produced by exposure to carbon dioxide.[225]

The characteristic sickling phenomenon can be demonstrated in moist sealed cover slip preparations that were first introduced by Emmel.[230] The un-desirable features of the cover slip method are the time required for the sickling to take place, even in patients with sickle cell anemia, and the occurrence of false negative results. At least 14 other tests that produce sickling have been described.[256] The sodium metabisulfite method has proved to be satisfactory in our experience (Fig. 7–9).[490] The use of hemoglobin electrophoresis has proved to be essential in distinguishing patients with sickle cell anemia from those who have the sickle cell trait combined with some unrelated anemia, and from those patients who are heterozygous for two abnormal hemoglobins.[350] It is essential to use electrophoresis in the further investigation of patients who have abnormal results of screening tests, such as Sickledex(R), which are based on the ab-normal solubility of hemoglobin S.

Differential Diagnosis

There is usually no difficulty in establishing the diagnosis of sickle cell anemia if the possibility is considered. A positive test for sickling indicates that the individual has either sickle cell trait or sickle cell anemia. The demonstra-tion of the sickling phenomenon in a patient who has anemia does not establish the diagnosis of sickle cell anemia, because the sickle cell trait is common in blacks who may have anemia from some other cause. An incorrect diagnosis

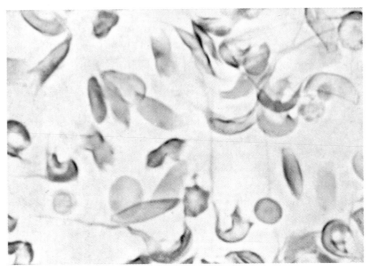

Figure 7–9 Sickle cell preparation with sodium metabisulfite.

of sickle cell anemia may be made in patients with sickle cell trait who have chronic blood loss or pernicious anemia, unless proper studies are carried out. Unless the patient has been transfused recently, the diagnosis of sickle cell anemia can nearly always be established or excluded by hemoglobin electrophoresis. The discovery of a relatively mild degree of anemia associated with a positive sickling test in a patient who has significant splenomegaly should arouse the suspicion that the patient has a combination of sickle cell trait plus some other hemoglobin abnormality, such as hemoglobin C, rather than sickle cell anemia. Hemoglobin electrophoresis is the most valuable method of distinguishing sickle cell anemia from sickle cell–hemoglobin C disease and other disorders that are due to the occurrence of sickle cell hemoglobin with some other abnormal hemoglobin. The differentiation of sickle cell anemia from sickle cell–thalassemia and from sickle cell–hemoglobin D disease is discussed in later sections of this chapter. When the second amino acid substitution of hemoglobin Memphis occurs in conjunction with homozygous hemoglobin S, there is an ameliorating effect on the blood viscosity of sickle cell disease, so that painful crises are rare.[341] Amino acid analysis is necessary to establish the diagnosis, since the electrophoretic pattern is that of homozygous hemoglobin S.[340–341]

If the diagnosis of sickle cell anemia is not considered, the disease may be mistaken for acute rheumatic fever when the patient presents with anemia, joint complaints, fever, cardiac enlargement, and cardiac murmurs. The absence of the severe pains, swelling, and tenderness of the joints that usually are seen in rheumatic fever may help to distinguish between these two diseases. In other patients with signs of acute intra-abdominal disease, it may be difficult to make the correct diagnosis because patients with sickle cell anemia sometimes develop acute surgical emergencies just as any other patients do, but they also develop signs of acute intra-abdominal disease as the result of sickle cell anemia alone. Both possibilities must be considered when the patient is seen, and the decision must be made on the basis of the evidence available at that time. Sickle cell anemia must be differentiated from other diseases that cause ulcers of the extremities and from those that produce symptoms or signs of involvement of the central nervous system. Sickle cell anemia has been confused at times with rheumatoid arthritis, osteomyelitis, poliomyelitis, meningitis, cerebrovascular accident, infectious hepatitis, and other diseases.[256]

Course and Prognosis

Sickle cell anemia is a serious disorder and few patients survive the third decade. Many die during childhood, and rarely will a patient live to a ripe old age.[221] Death comes most often from infections such as pneumonia and chronic pyelonephritis with renal failure. Other causes of death are heart failure, bone marrow and fat emboli,[276] shock with abdominal crisis, complications in the central nervous system, tuberculosis, and sarcoidosis.[234, 244]

The occurrence of pregnancy has been considered a serious matter in patients with sickle cell anemia who reach childbearing age. The incidence of spontaneous abortion, stillbirth, and death soon after birth is probably increased. Hazards to the mother are heart failure, pulmonary embolism, shock, cerebrovascular accidents, and uremia.[256] Pyelonephritis occurs frequently. Pregnancy appears to be a greater problem in sickle cell–hemoglobin C disease than in sickle cell anemia.[281]

In some patients with sickle cell anemia physical development is greatly retarded, and hypogonadism occurs. In other patients the growth and development seem to follow a normal pattern. The reason for these differences in patients with sickle cell anemia is not apparent, but the differences in development are not due solely to differences in the severity of the anemia.

Treatment

The treatment of sickle cell anemia is generally unsatisfactory. Transfusions are the only means available at present of returning the blood to normal levels. Transfusions are not used to maintain the blood in the normal range because patients with this disease adjust very well to their lowered hemoglobin levels. Transfusions are valuable during periods of aplastic crisis, abdominal crisis, and at any other time when the patient is severely ill. They are also advantageous in carrying patients through pregnancy or operations, because multiple transfusions depress erythropoiesis and reduce the number and percentage of sickle cells in the peripheral circulation (Fig. 7–10).[229] Partial exchange transfusions, which combine the removal of the patient's blood with replacement of normal packed cells, raise the hemoglobin level and lower the concentration of sickle cells more quickly than transfusion alone. Exchange is particularly desirable in patients who have frank or incipient heart failure, and can be accomplished without an increase in blood volume. Whether or not such a treatment, when carried out at regular intervals, will reduce the frequency of attacks of crisis remains uncertain. The value of these measures in crisis and in pregnancy has been confirmed by several reports.[216, 275]

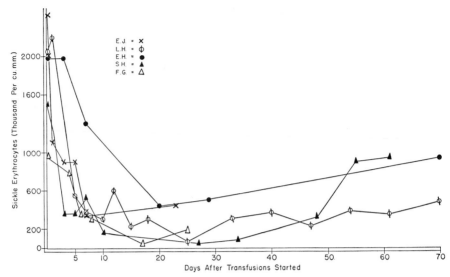

Figure 7-10 The effect of transfusion on the number of circulating sickle cells in sickle cell anemia. (From Donegan, MacIlwaine, and Leavell: Am. J. Med., vol. 17, 1954.)

Splenectomy is sometimes beneficial in children. The beneficial effect seems to be related to the size of the spleen.[278] In most adults with the disease the spleen is markedly reduced in size, probably because of repeated infarctions, and splenectomy has little place in the treatment.

Various measures have been used in an effort to reduce the sickling, and thereby relieve or reduce the severity of the clinical symptoms in these patients. In this category are cortisone, ACTH, tolazoline, sodium bicarbonate, aceta-zolamide, and urea. None of these agents can be considered to be of proved value at the present time. Double blind studies have failed to show any value in phenothiazine,[259] low molecular weight dextran,[211] or urea.[223, 224]

Patients are often critically ill during episodes of "crisis." At such times blood transfusions, antibiotics, and measures to relieve pain are necessary. The short-term use of antibiotics appears justified even though the presence of an infection cannot be established, because these episodes are so often preceded by an infection. Oxygen is of no value in the treatment of sickle cell crisis unless pulmonary disease is present, because the hemoglobin is fully oxygenated in the lungs.

It has been pointed out that the hyposthenuria associated with sickle cell disease and sickle cell trait requires careful attention to fluid balance. Clinical hydration is maintained as long as free access to fluids is allowed and no stressful situation occurs. Negative water balance may occur early in the course of sickle cell crisis and will respond to fluid therapy. The possible role of negative fluid balance in sickle cell crisis remains to be determined.[239]

Hematuria should be treated conservatively, with blood replacements as needed. Surgery should be avoided.

Priapism, a painfully serious complication that often leads to impotence, has been treated successfully in at least two patients with a derivative of venom of the pit viper (Arvin), which leads to defibrination.[214]

Cyanate, a substance which inhibits sickling in vitro[219] and lengthens the survival in vivo of sickle cell erythrocytes,[233] is being used in clinical trials in sickle cell anemia, but not enough evidence is available to assess its effectiveness on toxicity.

In view of the fact that treatment has not been very effective in sickle cell anemia, more emphasis should be placed on its possible prevention. Although this disease occurs once in 500 births in blacks and has a median survival of only 20 years, only recently has attention been given to public education of the populations affected,[277] Because of the availability of simple tests to detect those with sickle cell trait, it should be possible greatly to reduce the incidence of the disease by education and genetic counseling.

Illustrative Case

This patient, a black male, was first admitted to the hospital at the age of 12 because of fever, cough, and pleuritic pain of one week's duration. For some years he had been troubled with recurring chronic ulcers in the lower tibial region. A brother 10 years of age had a similar illness characterized by recurring attacks of fever and chronic ulceration of the legs. One sister had died ten days previously of unknown cause. The patient's father, mother, and four siblings were alive and well.

Physical examination. Temperature 105, pulse 120, respirations 26, and blood pressure 105/55. The patient was alert, thin, and appeared acutely ill. The veins in both fundi were extremely tortuous. A systolic murmur was present. Above the left internal malleolus there was an ulcer 4 cm. in diameter.

Laboratory examination. Admission blood studies: Hb. 4.0 gm. per 100 ml. R.B.C. 1.4 mil. per cu.mm., W.B.C. 22,000 per cu.mm., reticulocytes 0.1 per cent. The leukocyte differential count was normal, but a few sickled erythrocytes and many target cells were present on the fixed stained smear. A moist coverslip preparation was positive for sickling. A chest roentgenogram showed increased bronchial markings and an infiltrate in the left lower lobe.

Treatment and course. A diagnosis of sickle cell anemia with pneumonia was made. The patient was given blood transfusions and penicillin and made an uneventful recovery. Before discharge from the hospital on the 16th day, the leukocyte count had fallen to 11,000 per cu.mm. and the reticulocyte count had risen to 5.4 per cent despite numerous transfusions.

This patient was observed for eight years, during which time his course was characterized by chronic ill-health and exacerbations of acute illness. The erythrocyte count was usually in the range of 1.5 to 2.0 mil. per cu.mm. and the reticulocyte count was usually 25 or 30 per cent. The growth and development were subnormal. The extremities were long and thin, the trunk was short, and no secondary sex characteristics developed. At the age of 20 he weighed but 80 pounds and appeared to be about 10 years of age. He was hospitalized on four occasions because of pneumonia. In some of these attacks the reticulocyte count was 0.1 per cent and the serum bilirubin was less than 1.0 mg per 100 ml.; in others the reticulocyte count was 18 per cent and the serum bilirubin was 3.0 mg. per 100 ml. Repeated roentgenograms revealed progressive enlargement of the heart. In December 1954, when he was 21 years old, this patient was hospitalized with congestive heart failure and severe anemia. He failed to respond to the usual measures and died in acute heart failure.

Postmortem. The testes appeared to be prepubertal, and a section through the prostate gland disclosed only a few glands and those appeared immature. The heart was moderately hypertrophied. The right atrium and ventricle were markedly dilated. The pulmonary artery was greatly dilated from its point of origin, but no thrombi were demonstrated in the larger branches. Microscopic examination of the lungs disclosed emphysema, thickening of the walls of the smaller pulmonary artery that produced complete obliteration of the lumen in some areas, and multiple small granulomatous lesions. The lymph nodes from various parts of the body were enlarged and contained innumerable discrete epithelioid cell granulomas. These granulomatous lesions were diagnosed as Boeck's sarcoid. The spleen was scarred and contracted and weighed only 28 grams. The bone marrow was hyperplastic.

Comment. Many of the commonest features of sickle cell anemia were evident in this young black who had a severe hemolytic anemia, chronic ill health, and retarded physical development. He had ulcerations of the lower legs, a systolic murmur over the precordium, and a tortuous "corkscrew" appearance of the retinal veins. During his first admission he apparently had an episode of "aplastic crisis." Other attacks of pneumonia of equal severity did not produce such depression of the bone marrow. He died at the age of 21 of heart failure associated with cor pulmonale. As is often the case, the spleen was scarred and smaller than normal. The presence of Boeck's sarcoid that was demonstrated at the postmortem examination was not suspected ante mortem.

HOMOZYGOUS HEMOGLOBIN C DISEASE

Hemoglobin C was first described by Itano and Neel.[337] Instances of homozygous hemoglobin C disease have been reported by a number of observers.[331, 348, 351, 353, 355] The disease occurs almost exclusively in blacks, in whom the incidence of hemoglobin C trait has been found to be about 2 or 3 per cent.[350] The patients reported have presented a fairly uniform clinical picture characterized by splenomegaly, mild or moderately severe hemolytic anemia, and recurrent jaundice. A report of the disease in one patient who was 74 years of age indicates that the disorder is consistent with a normal life span.[355]

The hemoglobin values in the reported cases have varied from 8.7 to 12.5 gm. per 100 ml.[354] The most prominent feature of the stained smear is the presence of numerous target cells that often constitute from 50 to 100 per cent of the erythrocytes. The osmotic fragility of the red cells is decreased. Hemoglobin electrophoresis discloses the presence of only hemoglobin C. Mild reticulocytosis is often present. The erythrocytes have a decreased life span and the fecal urobilinogen excretion is increased.[354] Intraerythrocytic hemoglobin crystals have been observed in patients, particularly after splenectomy (Fig. 7–11).[331, 355] The mechanism of the anemia is the crystalization of hemoglobin, which de-

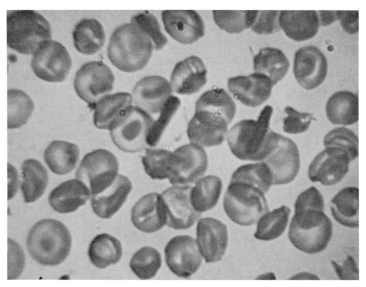

Figure 7–11 Target cells and hemoglobin crystals in an isotonic saline suspension of erythrocytes from the peripheral blood of a patient with homozygous hemoglobin C disease after splenectomy. Note persistence of the cellular membrane about the hemoglobin crystal in the center of the picture.

creases red cell deformability and increases blood viscosity.[325, 342] The amino acid substitution is lysine for glutamic acid at the sixth position of the amino terminal end of the beta chain.[329]

THALASSEMIA

Synonyms: Mediterranean Anemia, Cooley's Anemia

History

Archeologic data, based on characteristic skeletal changes, indicate that thalassemia may have originated over 50,000 years ago in a valley south of Italy and Greece now covered by the Mediterranean.[321] Thalassa is the Greek word meaning sea.

Thalassemia, or "Cooley's anemia", was first recognized as a clinical entity by Cooley and Lee, who described five cases of this disorder in 1925.[291] A similar but much less severe disease found in adolescents and adults was reported in 1940 by Wintrobe, Matthews, Pollack, and Dobyns.[317] As a result of studies on the genetics of the disease, Valentine and Neel concluded that these disorders were related and suggested that the term "thalassemia major" be used to denote the severe form of the disease, which appeared to be the homozygous condition, and the name "thalassemia minor" be given to the milder form, which appeared to be the heterozygous state.[315]

Mechanism of Disease

The thalassemia syndromes may be currently viewed as a result of a bio-chemical defect in the synthesis of hemoglobin. No amino acid substitution has been demonstrated, and the hemoglobin once formed is normal in structure.[299] The explanation for decreased hemoglobin synthesis in thalassemia is unclear, but most likely involves a reduction in the messenger RNA that directs the synthesis of a specific hemoglobin chain.[290, 302, 304, 316] Severe forms of alpha thalassemia may result from deletion of the gene that directs alpha chain synthesis.[307, 314]

Four pairs of genes are responsible for the synthesis of the various subunits of hemoglobin: alpha (α) chains, beta (β) chains, gamma (γ) chains, and delta (δ) chains. Dimers of these different type chains combine with another type of dimer to form the particular four-chain hemoglobin molecule. In the adult, hemoglobin A ($\alpha_2\beta_2$) accounts for about 95 per cent of the hemoglobin, hemoglobin A_2 ($\alpha_2\delta_2$) for 1 to 3 per cent, and hemoglobin F ($\alpha_2\gamma_2$) for less than 2 per cent.[302] A deficiency in the synthesis of any one of these chains may lead to one of the thalassemia syndromes. It is convenient to classify thalassemia by the deficient subunit.

Beta thalassemia. A defect in the synthesis of beta chains is by far the most common type of thalassemia.[316] When the patient inherits the abnormal gene from both parents and is homozygous for the defect, severe anemia, thalassemia major, results. When the patient is heterozygous for the defect, the anemia is mild and is termed thalassemia minor. For reasons which are not entirely clear, some homozygous patients have a milder-than-usual course, and some heterozygous patients have a more severe course than usual. Such patients are said to have thalassemia intermedia.

In thalassemia major there is a marked diminution in beta chain synthesis, and there appears to be a compensatory increase in hemoglobin F, which ranges from 20 to 90 per cent.[302, 316] Most patients with thalassemia minor have normal or only slightly increased hemoglobin F, but have a significant increase in hemoglobin A_2 in the range of 3 to 7 per cent.[302, 316] A few patients with thalassemia minor have increased hemoglobin F rather than A_2, and probably represent a variant.[302, 316]

It is heterozygous beta thalassemia that interacts with other types of beta chain hemoglobinopathies. Such double heterozygotes may synthesize very little hemoglobin A, which results in the clinical picture of the homozygote for the other abnormal hemoglobin. This is the case in sickle cell–thalassemia disease, in which nearly all of the hemoglobin may be hemoglobins S and F.

Another variant of beta thalassemia is hemoglobin Lepore, which is manifested by a mild hypochromic anemia and red cell morphology characteristic of thalassemia.[308] In this circumstance there is not only decreased synthesis of beta chains, but also a structural alteration in the beta chain which is an amalgam of the N–terminal end of a delta chain and the C–terminal end of a beta chain.[286] Hemoglobin Lepore is associated with a decrease in hemoglobin A, slight increase in hemoglobin F, and a normal or decreased amount of hemoglobin A_2. Hemoglobin Lepore appears to be very similar to hemoglobin Pylos.[295]

Hereditary persistence of fetal hemoglobin (HPFH). This condition, though neither a form of thalassemia nor a cause of hemolytic anemia, may be confused with beta thalassemia when it coexists with anemia of some other cause. A distinguishing feature is that the fetal hemoglobin is found in all the patient's red cells in HPFH, whereas in thalassemia syndromes and some other conditions of hematologic stress, it is found in only a small proportion of the total population of red cells.[316]

Alpha thalassemia. Patients heterozygous for alpha thalassemia have a clinical picture similar to that in heterozygous beta thalassemia, displaying a mild microcytic hypochromic anemia with erythrocytosis and poikilocytosis.[302, 304, 316] They differ from those with beta thalassemia in that there is no enhanced production of hemoglobin A_2 or F because there is diminished production of alpha chains, which those hemoglobins contain.[300] Alpha thalassemia does not interact with beta chain hemoglobinopathies such as hemoglobin S or C, but does with hemoglobinopathies involving the alpha chain, hemoglobins I[285] and Q.[292]

Homozygous alpha thalassemia usually is not compatible with life; the infant is stillborn or dies shortly after birth. Studies of the blood of such infants have shown a hemoglobin composed of four gamma chains (γ_4), which is referred to as Bart's hemoglobin. This hemoglobin has virtually no Bohr effect and binds oxygen nearly irreversibly at the oxygen tension of tissues.[297] Infants with alpha thalassemia trait may also have small amounts of Bart's hemoglobin at birth, but it disappears as gamma chain synthesis ceases.[293, 297]

Hemoglobin H disease is another form of alpha thalassemia occurring in families with heterozygous alpha thalassemia. The clinical picture most nearly resembles that of thalassemia intermedia.[296] Hemoglobin H is composed of a tetramer of four beta chains (β_4), and is probably a result of the increased synthesis of beta chains over alpha chains with polymerization of the excess beta chains to form hemoglobin H.[296] This hemoglobin migrates more rapidly than hemoglobin A on starch block electrophoresis, and may account for from 10 to 34 per cent of the total hemoglobin.[310] Like Bart's hemoglobin, it has a high affinity for oxygen that inhibits its capacity to deliver oxygen to the tissues.[289, 296] Hemoglobin H is also unstable and susceptible to oxidation with precipitation of hemoglobin into large Heinz bodies which may be seen with supravital stains on blood smears, particularly after splenectomy. There is evidence[298] of duplication of the alpha chain locus in man, so that variations in the severity of alpha thalassemia may result from inheritance of varying numbers of the same gene for thalassemia, as well as from different genes producing disease of different severity.

Delta and gamma thalassemia. Although the clinical syndromes of thalassemia consist of the alpha and beta types, a decrease in the synthesis of gamma and delta chains has been described, but has no clinical sequelae.[294, 304]

Mechanism of the Anemia

Nathan and his associates[304, 305] have stressed the role of unbalanced hemoglobin synthesis in the pathogenesis of the hemolytic anemia seen in thalassemia. They view the relative overproduction of normal chains as a more important cause of pathology in thalassemia than the underproduction of other hemoglobin chains. In beta thalassemia the alpha chains, which are produced in excess, polymerize to form an unstable hemoglobin that readily precipitates to form Heinz bodies—the inclusion bodies that have been observed in thalassemic cells.[287, 304] The precipitation of rigid Heinz bodies renders the red cell vulnerable to fragmentation and sequestration in any area of restricted passage in the microcirculation, particularly the spleen.[312] It has also been shown that the precipitation of Heinz bodies in thalassemic red cells causes increased membrane permeability to cations, which aggravates their susceptibility to lysis.[305] In alpha thalassemia, a similar situation exists when excess beta chains polymerize to form hemoglobin H, with subsequent Heinz body formation.

In addition to the increased destruction of thalassemic red cells in the circulation, there is also evidence for ineffective erythropoiesis with destruction of red cell precursors within the bone marrow and defective iron utilization.[316]

Clinical Manifestations

Thalassemia occurs mainly in families of Mediterranean origin, particularly those from Italy, Greece, Sicily, and Syria, but it also is seen in blacks and in Southeast Asia.[303] In a large Italian population in Rochester, N. Y., the incidence of thalassemia minor has been estimated at one in 25 persons, and of thalassemia major as one of 2368 births.[306]

Thalassemia minor, the heterozygous form of the disease, is largely asymptomatic. It is the type seen most often in adults. In its mildest form, which may be found by chance or in the study of the family of a patient with the major form of the disease, the only apparent abnormality in the routine laboratory tests may be the presence of target cells. Other patients with this mild form of the disease have more pronounced hypochromic microcytosis and mild reductions in hemoglobin and hematocrit associated with an elevated red cell count. In patients with thalassemia minor, appropriate studies often demonstrate an increased osmotic resistance of the red cells associated with an increase in hemoglobin A_2. Splenomegaly, slight reticulocytosis, and mild icterus are sometimes present. The occurrence of "intermediate" forms of thalassemia with moderately severe anemia is not well understood. It appears likely that many instances of the intermediate form are in reality cases in which the heterozygous thalassemia gene is associated with some other unrecognized hemoglobin abnormality.

Thalassemia major, the homozygous form of the disease is a severe disorder that generally becomes manifest early in childhood, nearly always in the first decade. Pallor and easy fatigue often appear in the first few years of life. As the disease progresses, the diagnosis may be suggested by the patient's appearance. The head often appears unduly large. The prominence of the malar eminences associated with depression of the bridge of the nose and the muddy yellowish color of the skin was termed "Mongolian" by Cooley and Lee.[291] Marked splenomegaly and hepatomegaly are usually present. The abdomen often protrudes because the spleen may fill the left half of the abdominal cavity. Chronic leg ulcers sometimes occur, but are not common.[311] Evidence of abnormalities of the cardiovascular system in the form of cardiac enlargement, edema, pleural effusions, and ascites is not unusual. Skeletal defects may be prominent but they are not pathognomonic of thalassemia. The changes in the skull consist of a thinning of the inner and outer table associated with a widening of the diploë, which may contain prominent vertical striations that produce the "hair on end" appearance of the skull. Alterations in the long bones, which are less striking, consist of widening of the medullary canals, thinning of the cortices, osteoporosis, and heavy trabeculations near the ends of the shaft. Because of defective iron utilization coupled with increased iron absorption and blood transfusion therapy, iron overload with the clinical picture of hemochromatosis is a common complication.

Thalassemia major must be considered a fatal disease at present because the majority of patients do not survive to adult life. The prognosis appears worse if the disease becomes manifest early in life. Death is usually caused by an intercurrent infection or complications of iron overload.

Laboratory Examination

Thalassemia major is characterized by a microcytic hypochromic type of anemia.[316] The anemia is usually severe, but the erythrocyte count may range from 1.0 mil. per cu.mm. to 4.0 mil. per cu.mm. The MCV is often less than 60 to 70 cu. μ. The reduction in the MCHC is not as pronounced as the decrease in the MCH.[311] Osmotic fragility of red cells may be decreased. Stained films of the peripheral blood show a severe degree of poikilocytosis, anisocytosis, and polychromatophilia. The erythrocytes appear small and hypochromic. Many stippled cells and "target" cells are present. Nucleated red cells, which are almost invariably present, are often numerous and sometimes outnumber the leukocytes. Reticulocytosis is usually present and is accompanied by normoblastic hyperplasia in the bone marrow. Leukocyte counts in the range of 10,000 to 25,000 per cu.mm. are common, and immature forms sometimes appear in the peripheral blood. The platelet count is generally normal.

In thalassemia minor the erythrocyte count is often normal or increased, even though the hemoglobin and hematocrit are reduced. In some such cases there may be a mild reticulocytosis and slight hyperbilirubinemia. Target cells, anisocytosis, poikilocytosis, polychromatophilia, and stippling are evident in the blood smear, and are much more prominent than one would expect from the degree of anemia that is present.

Other features common to most hemolytic anemias are usually present in thalassemia major. These are: elevation of the indirect-reacting bilirubin in the serum; increased excretion of urobilinogen in the feces and urine; elevation of the serum iron; and decrease in the latent iron-binding capacity. In addition, the erythrocytes are abnormally resistant to hemolysis in hypotonic saline; hemolysis may not be complete at 0.2 per cent saline or even in distilled water.

One of the characteristic hematologic features of thalassemia major is the presence of large amounts of hemoglobin F.[311] Hemoglobin of this type constitutes from 50 to more than 90 per cent of the hemoglobin in some patients with thalassemia major.[301] The presence of hemoglobin A_2, usually in increased amounts, is found in nearly all patients with thalassemia minor when hemoglobin electrophoresis is performed on starch slabs.[301] A few patients have normal amounts of hemoglobin A_2 and increased hemoglobin F, and even fewer have increased amounts of both.

Diagnosis

The appearance of the typical patient with thalassemia major may suggest the diagnosis. In thalassemia major the diagnosis usually is not difficult because of the evident hepatosplenomegaly, the presence of anisopoikilocytosis, target cells, and normoblasts on the blood smear, evidence of hemolysis, and the presence of increased amounts of hemoglobin F.

Although the diagnosis of thalassemia major is rarely difficult, the distinction between the milder forms of thalassemia and other types of hemolytic anemia and hemoglobinopathies is not always easy. The occurrence of hypochromic microcytosis – with or without anemia – target cells, nucleated red cells, and stippled cells in the peripheral blood of a young person with hepatosplenomegaly suggests the diagnosis. At other times, the presenting problem may be a hypochromic microcytic anemia that must be distinguished from iron deficiency. In doubtful cases either the determination of the plasma iron level, which is low in iron deficiency and normal or high in thalassemia, or an evaluation of iron stores in the bone marrow, is helpful. The finding of microcytic erythrocytosis in a patient is sometimes the first indication that the patient has thalassemia minor. The demonstration of increased resistance of the erythrocytes in the hypotonic saline test supports the diagnosis. The demonstration of an increase of hemoglobin A_2 by electrophoresis is helpful in establishing the diagnosis. The recognition of the presence of a thalassemia gene in patients who have some other inherited hemoglobinopathy may be very difficult. For example, a person who is heterozygous for hemoglobin S and the β-thalassemia gene may appear to have sickle cell anemia clinically, and show only hemoglobins S and F on electrophoresis because of the suppression of hemoglobin A. Studies of other members of the family may be necessary to establish the true nature of the disorder.

Therapy

Patients with thalassemia minor rarely need treatment. In thalassemia major, blood transfusions are the only effective means of correcting the anemia. The question of how vigorous transfusion therapy should be has not been determined. Some hematologists feel that the hemoglobin should be maintained in the range of 7 gm. per cent to avoid symptoms of anemia, and give as few transfusions as possible to avoid adding to the problem of iron overload. Others feel that thalassemic children do better if their hemoglobin level is maintained in the range of 10 gm. per cent. Wolman and others have presented evidence that children whose blood levels are maintained at a level nearer normal have an improved rate of growth, less bone malformation, and decrease in hepatosplenomegaly and cardiomegaly, and in general they are more active and feel better.[288, 309, 318, 320] Although this is accomplished at the expense of increasing the iron burden, this is balanced to some degree by diminished iron absorption and better tissue oxygenation, which may be a factor in the toxicity of iron to tissues.

The removal of excess storage iron by iron-chelating agents such as desferrioxamine has been tried by a number of investigators in thalassemic patients. Although initially a significant excretion of chelated iron in the urine occurs, this soon diminishes to the point that the relatively small loss of iron over an extended period does not merit the time, expense, and toxicity of administering chelating agents.[316]

Splenectomy may be helpful in patients in whom significant red cell sequestration by the spleen is demonstrated, and in patients in whom marked splenomegaly causes discomfort. Although splenectomy may often decrease the blood transfusion requirement, other clinical problems are not benefited and the patient's life is not prolonged. Also, Smith and his co-workers have emphasized the increased incidence of severe infections after splenectomy, particularly in children under two years of age.[313]

Other important features in the management of thalassemia include prompt treatment of infection, which is a frequent complication in this disorder, and folic acid therapy when folic acid deficiency occurs as a result of increased utilization of folate by a hyperactive bone marrow.[316]

Illustrative Case

A 5½-year-old white male was admitted to the hospital for transfusion therapy. Anemia, first noted at 4 months of age, was treated with iron. It was not until he was 21 months old that the diagnosis of thalassemia major was established. At that time the hemoglobin was 5.6 gm. per 100 ml., hct. 20 per cent, and reticulocytes 11.5 per cent. There was an increase in both fetal and A_2 hemoglobins. The liver was felt 7 cm. below the right costal margin and the spleen at the level of the iliac crest. A program of blood transfusions every four weeks was instituted in an effort to keep the patient's hemoglobin near normal levels. On this regimen the patient did well, with nearly normal growth and development.

Laboratory Examination. At the time of admission to the University of Virginia Hospital, the hemoglobin was 9.0 gm. per cent and hematocrit 25 per cent. Leukocyte and platelet counts were normal. Microcytosis, hypochromia, target cells, anisocytosis, and poikilocytosis were seen on the peripheral blood smear. The serum iron was 147 micrograms per cent and total iron-binding capacity 196 micrograms per cent, with 75 per cent saturation. Serum folate was 1.6 nanograms per ml. The bone marrow examination disclosed erythroid hyperplasia with increased iron stores and slight megaloblastic changes.

Family Studies. Both parents, a brother, and a sister of the patient have mild anemia with target cells and hypochromia on the blood smear. All have increased levels of hemoglobin A_2 but normal hemoglobin F, consistent with the diagnosis of thalassemia minor.

Comment. Although the patient was undoubtedly anemic at birth, the correct diagnosis of thalassemia was not made until he was nearly 2 years of age. Iron therapy for a year-and-a-half aggravated the iron overload problem.

Once thought of, the diagnosis of thalassemia major was readily made on the basis of a microcytic hypochromic hemolytic anemia, target cells, high serum iron, elevated fetal hemoglobin, hepatosplenomegaly, and findings of thalassemia minor in the parents and siblings. The patient developed folic acid deficiency with a megaloblastic marrow, a not uncommon complication of a chronically hyperactive bone marrow. The patient has done well with a vigorous transfusion program, but the long-term effects of the increased iron burden remain to be seen.

COMBINATIONS AND OTHER HEMOGLOBINOPATHIES

SICKLE CELL–HEMOGLOBIN C DISEASE

Hemoglobin C was first recognized as a new hemoglobin in a study of patients who were diagnosed as atypical sickle cell anemia, but instead proved to have sickle cell-hemoglobin C disease.[337] The presence of both hemoglobin C and hemoglobin S was demonstrated by electrophoresis. In the reported patients, the major portion of the hemoglobin has been of the C type.[357]

The clinical features of this disease have been described by several authors.[339, 351] The disease is generally much milder than sickle cell anemia, but severe episodes of crisis may occur in some patients; pregnancy may be associated with serious complications. In adults the spleen is usually considerably enlarged, in contrast to sickle cell anemia, in which a small spleen is an almost constant feature. The anemia is usually mild or moderate in degree and the hematocrit and hemoglobin values range from 70 to 100 per cent of normal, except during episodes of crisis. The reticulocyte count is normal or slightly increased.[351] On fixed stained smears of the peripheral blood, from 50 to 100 per cent of the erythrocytes appear as target cells, and intraerythrocytic hemoglobin crystals have been described in patients who have had splenectomy.[330] Sickling can be demonstrated in moist preparations. The osmotic fragility of the erythrocytes is decreased. The diagnosis is established by electrophoresis, which reveals the presence of both hemoglobin S and hemoglobin C. Exchange transfusion during the last trimester of pregnancy has been reported to be effective in lessening its complications.[275]

SICKLE CELL–THALASSEMIA DISEASE

Sickle cell–thalassemia disease probably was first described by Silvestroni and Bianco in 1946, before electrophoretic studies of hemoglobin were made.[346] The majority of patients with this disease are whites of Greek or Italian stock and blacks.[357] It has been possible to demonstrate that the patient with this disease is a double heterozygote for the two abnormal genes present in the parents.[344]

The disease resembles sickle cell anemia, but the severity of the anemia, the frequency of painful crisis and leg ulcers, and the degree of splenomegaly vary greatly from one patient to another. The hematologic characteristics are microcytic hypochromic anemia, erythrocytic sickling in moist preparations, and the presence of numerous target cells on the fixed smear. Reticulocytosis is usually present. It is the beta type of thalassemia that interacts with S hemoglobin, since both genes affect the beta chain. In some patients virtually all the hemoglobin is S and F, so that family studies are necessary to establish the diagnosis of sickle cell–thalassemia disease.

SICKLE CELL–HEMOGLOBIN D DISEASE

Hemoglobin D was described first by Itano.[336] It has been found to be more common among nonblacks in some parts of the world, but is more common in blacks than in whites in the United States, where the incidence in blacks has been reported to be 1:1000[352] and 4:1000.[327]

Sickle cell–hemoglobin D disease has been the subject of several reports.[324, 352] The patients who have this disorder are normally developed, often remain asymptomatic for long periods, and may have little or no anemia. The concentration of hemoglobin S may vary from 25 to 75 per cent in these patients.[324] Attacks that resemble mild episodes of sickle cell crisis occur. Differentiation of this disorder from sickle cell anemia may be difficult because in both diseases sickling occurs in preparations of fresh blood, and filter paper electrophoresis at pH 8.6 shows only a single concentration peak that has the mobility of S hemoglobin. In some instances the differentiation can be made by comparing the solubilities of the reduced forms of the hemoglobin, because the solubility of reduced hemoglobin D is normal whereas that of reduced hemoglobin S is decreased.[336] Differential solubility studies may not be conclusive, and in such circumstances electrophoresis on agar at pH 6.2 may be utilized to differentiate the two hemoglobins.[352] Homozygous hemoglobin D disease has also been reported.[328]

Less Common Syndromes

Thalassemia–hemoglobin C disease and thalassemia–hemoglobin E disease are similar clinically and hematologically. Splenomegaly, mild hypochromic anemia, target cells, and increased resistance to hypotonic saline occur in both diseases.[326, 349, 356, 357]

Hemoglobin Memphis has a glutamine for glutamic acid substitution at the 23rd position in the alpha chain.[340–341] Patients doubly heterozygous for this hemoglobin and hemoglobin S are clinically indistinguishable from the usual patient with sickle cell trait. However, when hemoglobin Memphis occurs in combination with homozygous hemoglobin S, the clinical picture is considerably milder than that usually seen in sickle cell disease.[340] The anemia is not much different, but painful crises are rare. This has been attributed to a decrease in viscosity conferred by the alpha chain substitution. The electrophoretic pattern is that of hemoglobin SS, and amino acid analysis is necessary to establish the diagnosis.

Two abnormal hemoglobins which sickle and migrate electrophoretically as hemoglobin C have been described. They have the usual valine for glutamic acid substitution of hemoglobin S, but in addition they have a second amino acid substitution in the beta chain. In hemoglobin Harlem, the second substitution is asparagine for aspartic acid at the 73rd position;[322] in hemoglobin

Georgetown the second substitution has not been established.[333, 343] Only heterozygous patients with these hemoglobinopathies have been observed. They have no clinically-apparent disease, except those individuals who are heterozygous for hemoglobin Harlem and have a renal concentrating defect.[322]

UNSTABLE HEMOGLOBINS

Carrell and Lehman[323] have used the term "unstable hemoglobin hemolytic anemia" to refer to a group of similar disease syndromes. The clinical picture is characterized by a congenital hemolytic anemia, red cell inclusions which are typical Heinz bodies, excretion of a dipyrrole of the bilifuscin-mesobilifuscin type in the urine, and splenomegaly. The hemoglobin is heat-labile and precipitates when a hemolysate is incubated at 50° C. for several hours. In the past, most of these disorders have probably been called congenital Heinz body hemolytic anemia.

Many abnormal hemoglobins of this type have been described (hemoglobins Zurich, Köln, Genova, Sydney, Hammersmith, Gun Hill, Seattle, Olmsted, Santa Ana, and others).[323, 332, 335, 338] These abnormal hemoglobins have in common an amino acid substitution in the region where heme is attached to globin, which has been referred to as the "heme pocket." The comparatively high stability of normal hemoglobin is dependent on the interaction of the globin molecule with the heme groups, and amino acid substitutions in that area render the molecule unstable.[323, 329, 334, 345, 346]

The anemia in these patients is usually mild except upon exposure to oxidant drugs. Such exposure causes an acute hemolytic episode similar to that seen in glucose-6-phosphate dehydrogenase deficiency. The main treatment is avoidance of oxidant drugs, but splenectomy has also been of benefit in some of these patients.[323] The amino acid substitution is usually "silent," in that electrophoretic mobility is normal and amino acid analysis must be carried out to establish the diagnosis. However, a presumptive diagnosis may be made by demonstrating heat-labile hemoglobin plus Heinz bodies in the red cells. Several reviews of the unstable hemoglobins and other hemoglobinopathies are available.[323, 329, 334, 335, 345]

ACQUIRED HEMOLYTIC DISORDERS

Antibody Mediated

Transfusion reactions are discussed in Chapter 18.

ERYTHROBLASTOSIS FETALIS

History

In 1932 Diamond, Blackfan, and Baty recognized that hydrops fetalis, hemolytic anemia of the newborn, and icterus gravis neonatorum were closely related and dependent on the same underlying process.[367] These disorders are now grouped together under the term erythroblastosis fetalis. Levine and Stetson established an immunologic basis for the anemia in 1939 by demonstrating materno-fetal blood group incompatibility,[375] and in 1940 Landsteiner and Wiener reported their studies of the Rh antigen in human erythrocytes.[371] The following year Levine and his co-workers presented evidence that Rh incompatibility between mother and infant accounted for most of the cases of erythroblastosis.[374, 376] Additional data supporting this concept were reported in 1943 by Mollison, who showed that Rh-positive red cells were eliminated rapidly after transfusion into infants with erythroblastosis during the first 14 days of life, whereas Rh-negative red cells had a normal survival.[380] The value of the exchange transfusion with Rh-negative blood was demonstrated by Wallerstein in 1946.[388] The importance of this form of treatment in preventing the most serious complication of the disease, kernicterus, was shown in 1950 by Allen, Diamond, and Vaughan.[359] A major advance in erythroblastosis occurred in 1961 when Finn and his associates showed that the disorder could be prevented by the administration of anti-D gammaglobulin to the mother shortly after delivery.[368] This successfully inhibited the production of anti-Rh antibodies by the mother exposed to her infant's Rh positive red cells, and protected subsequent pregnancies.

Mechanism of Disease

The anemia in erythroblastosis fetalis is hemolytic in type.[358, 376, 380] The destruction of the fetal red cells is caused by the presence in the fetal circulation of isoantibodies that are formed in the mother in response to a blood group antigen that the mother lacks. Agglutinogens A, B, and D are strongly antigenic and the others are less so. Allen and Diamond state that A and B incompatibilities are responsible for about two-thirds of the cases of erythroblastosis fetalis, D (Rh) for about one-third, and other blood factors for 2 to 3 per cent.[358] Nevertheless, Rh incompatibility is more important clinically because it causes disease of greater severity.[384] The occurrence of ABO hemolytic disease is virtually limited to group A or B offspring of group O mothers.[392] A possible explanation for difference in response of the group O mothers has been afforded by studies of the size of the antibodies.[384] Group O mothers form not only IgM isohemagglutinins but also IgG isohemagglutinins which traverse the placental barrier, whereas group A and B mothers tend to form only IgM isohemagglutinins, a size that is unlikely to enter the fetal circulation. Immunization with Rh antigen results first in the appearance of IgM antibodies, but on continued immunization the IgG antibodies appear. There is considerable individual difference in the ability to form antibodies, and less than 10 per cent of the Rh-negative mothers who have Rh-positive husbands become sensitized; even if the husband is homozygous Rh-positive (DD), the wife may have many children without becoming sensitized.[384]

The method of sensitization of the mother to the fetal red cells in the cases of Rh (D) incompatibilities is an intriguing problem. Although the administration of incompatible blood by transfusion or by intramuscular injection may be responsible for sensitization in women prior to pregnancy, the isoantibody formation in mothers is usually the result of pregnancy. Allen and Diamond report that quantities of blood as small as 0.1 to 1.0 ml. may be sufficient to produce sensitization. Using an acid elution technique to demonstrate fetal hemoglobin in erythrocytes, it has been demonstrated that small quantities of fetal red cells gain access to the maternal circulation throughout pregnancy. This occurs most frequently during the last trimester.[365] Post partum, approximately 50 per cent of the mothers can be shown to have fetal red cells in their circulation. In a small percentage transplacental bleeding is sufficient to lead to anemia in the newborn infant, or to stillbirth.[365]

Kernicterus, circumscribed areas of yellow coloring in the brain that involve the nuclear areas particularly, is one of the most serious manifestations of erythroblastosis fetalis. It causes death within seven days in 70 per cent of the babies who have this complication.[369] The brain damage, which is not present at birth, has been shown to be related to the level of the serum bilirubin, since kernicterus occurs in 50 per cent of babies whose level of the serum bilirubin is over 30 mg. per 100 ml. In newborn babies, the ability of the liver to convert indirect-reacting bilirubin (unconjugated bilirubin) to the direct-reacting form (bilirubin-glucuronide) for excretion is poorly developed, and the deficiency is even more marked in premature infants.[362] When this mechanism is defective, even though the level of serum bilirubin may not be greatly elevated at birth, the level of the serum bilirubin rises rapidly after birth if hemolytic anemia is present. Unconjugated bilirubin has been identified as the pigment present in the brain in infants dying with kernicterus.

It has been suggested that in patients with early kernicterus and relatively low serum bilirubin levels, methemalbumin may interfere with the ability of the bilirubin to bind to the serum proteins.[383] Brown, Zuelzer, and Robinson have demonstrated that the serum bilirubin concentration is not always a gauge of the diffusible or total body bilirubin.[363] If the bilirubin cannot bind with the protein in the vascular spaces, the plasma level may be low even though bilirubin has diffused into the cells in appreciable quantities. This shift may be of special importance in premature infants who have lower serum albumin levels than full-term infants.[363]

Clinical Manifestations

Erythroblastosis is reported to occur in about 1 per cent of pregnancies.[358] About one-fifth of the affected infants die in utero, or are born critically ill with anemia at the time of birth.

Many erythroblastotic infants appear normal at birth. Jaundice is said to be usually absent at birth, because of the ability of the mother to excrete fetal bilirubin.[358] However, jaundice may appear within two or three hours and may increase rapidly thereafter unless treatment is instituted. Petechial hemorrhages sometimes develop soon after birth. Hepatomegaly and splenomegaly occur almost invariably in Rh disease. When erythroblastosis is due to A or B incompatibility the spleen is often enlarged, but to a lesser degree than in Rh disease. Pulmonary edema, pleural effusions, ascites, and edema may be manifestations of heart failure. Kernicterus, which usually becomes manifest late in the second day of life, is rare in the absence of considerable jaundice.[369] Any infant with erythroblastosis should have frequent and careful neurologic examinations. In the early stages kernicterus may be accompanied by no more than minimal neurologic signs that are easily missed. When the kernicterus is more pronounced, the affected infant has a high-pitched cry, irritability, tremor, and an overactive but incomplete Moro reflex; opisthotonos, twitching, convulsions, and respiratory distress may also occur. If the child has kernicterus and survives, sequelae, such as deafness, mental retardation, athetoid movements, and spastic ataxia, develop. In the more severely-affected infant with a cord blood hemoglobin of less than 7.5 gm. per 100 ml., pulmonary hemorrhage is a common cause of death.[372]

Laboratory Examination

Anemia is considered to be present if the hemoglobin level of the cord blood is less than 14.0 gm. per 100 ml.,[381, 384] if the hemoglobin level of the venous blood is less than 15 gm. per 100 ml.,[358] or if the hemoglobin level of capillary blood is less than 16.0 gm. per 100 ml. on the first day.[381] A hemoglobin level of less than 9.0 gm. per 100 ml. at birth indicates anemia of severe degree. Reticulocytosis is usually present. A high percentage of reticulocytes indicates a severe hemolytic process even if associated with a normal level of hemoglobin. Nucleated red cells are commonly present in the peripheral blood, but may be absent in one-third of the cases on the first day.[381] Spherocytosis usually is not found when Rh antibodies are present, but is a characteristic feature with ABO incompatibility. Polychromatophilia is marked. Elevated leukocyte counts are the rule and have little prognostic value. Thrombocytopenia often occurs in severe cases.

The normal level of serum bilirubin in cord blood is considered to be from 0.8 to 2.6 mg. per 100 ml.,[381] and a level above 4 mg. per 100 ml. is unusual in erythroblastosis.[384] The level of indirect-reacting serum bilirubin in normal newborn babies at 48 hours rarely exceeds 13 mg. per 100 ml. In erythroblastosis the level of the serum bilirubin may be normal at birth and rise rapidly thereafter. For this reason frequent determinations are most important in the management of these patients.

Diagnosis

Erythroblastosis fetalis must be distinguished from other causes of anemia, such as hereditary spherocytosis, G-6-PD deficiency, and hemorrhage, and from other causes of jaundice, such as infectious hepatitis, bacterial infections, syphilis, cytomegalic inclusion disease, and fungus infection, that occur during the first days of life.[358, 387] Nucleated red cells occur in the peripheral blood in a number of disorders, but the occurrence of large numbers of normoblasts or reticulocytes usually indicates the presence of hemolytic disease of some type.

The possibility of erythroblastosis, particularly Rh disease, should be suspected in pregnant women who give a history of a normal pregnancy followed by pregnancies that ended with jaundiced infants, abortion, or stillbirth. In about 40 to 50 per cent of the cases of ABO hemolytic disease, the firstborn child is affected.[392] The presence of marked edema or pallor at birth, or the appearance of jaundice during the first 24 hours, may be the first indication of the disease in the infant. However, all the abnormal clinical findings characteristic of the disease are sometimes absent at birth, and for this reason the laboratory examinations are often of greater importance than the clinical features.

Every effort is made to make an antenatal diagnosis of erythroblastosis by the use of appropriate laboratory procedures whenever possible. All pregnant women should be typed to determine the ABO, and Rh grouping routinely; if the prospective mother is Rh-negative, the father should be tested for Rh type, and the mother should be tested for possible Rh sensitization at seven months and within two or three weeks of delivery.[358, 381, 384] If anti-Rh antibodies are not detected at that time erythroblastosis is unlikely; if antibodies are present, regardless of the titer, the physician is alerted for the possibility of the disease. A positive Coombs (antiglobulin) test on the fetal red cells (cord blood or infant's blood) establishes the diagnosis. If the husband is Rh-positive the wife should be checked carefully for sensitization in each pregnancy, because a normal course in preceding pregnancies is no guarantee that isoimmune disease will not develop in subsequent pregnancies.

Although ABO incompatibility between mother and fetus exists in 20 per cent of pregnancies erythroblastosis fetalis occurs in only 5 per cent of these (1 per cent of the total). A possible explanation for the lower incidence and milder nature of ABO disease as compared to anti-Rh disease is that the antigens A and B occur on other tissue cells of the fetus as well as on the erythrocytes. In such a circumstance the other tissue cells may take up the antibodies and spare the erythrocytes. Rh antigens apparently are largely or exclusively confined to the erythrocytes, and consequently in this situation the red cells alone suffer from the reaction with antibodies.[358] Erythroblastosis due to ABO incompatibility is rarely associated with severe anemia. Marked hepatomegaly or splenomegaly is unusual. The most significant clinical feature is the occurrence of jaundice during the first 24 hours. When erythroblastosis is suspected, an antiglobulin (Coombs) test should be done on the baby's blood, and tests for ABO and Rh factors should be done on the blood of the mother and the baby. The occurrence of A, B, or Rh incompatibility between mother and child, accompanied by reticulocytosis and elevated serum bilirubin in the child, is strong presumptive evidence of erythroblastosis.[358] Although the direct Coombs test is regularly strongly positive in infants with Rh hemolytic disease, it is frequently only weakly positive or even negative when erythroblastosis is due to ABO incompatibility.[386] This has been attributed to a paucity of A and B antigenic sites on fetal red cells, since antibody eluted from fetal cells can be made to react strongly with adult red cells.[386]

Prevention

A major advance in the management of Rh hemolytic disease has been the observation that the administration of an appropriate dose of anti-Rh D gamma globulin to an Rh-negative mother within 72 hours of delivery of an Rh-positive infant will prevent sensitization to the Rh antigen in nearly all patients so treated. The failure rate is in the order of 1 per cent or less.[364, 385, 387, 390, 391]

The background for this form of treatment rests on observations by Nevanlinna and Vaino[382] that the risk of Rh hemolytic disease is much less in those instances in which the mother and fetus are ABO incompatible. This naturally-occurring protection is thought to be due to antibody destruction of fetal red cells before the mother has sufficient exposure to the Rh antigen to become immunized. In a similar fashion the passive administration of anti-Rh gamma globulin prevents sensitization of the Rh-negative mother by Rh-positive fetal red cells.

This type of prophylaxis is of no benefit to the mother who has already been sensitized by previous pregnancies or by blood transfusions.[387, 390] Mothers who have a significant anti-Rh titer and give birth to a Coombs-positive infant, therefore, should not be treated with anti-Rh D gamma globulin, as this will not prevent an anamnestic response to antigenic challenge. All other Rh-negative mothers who are in danger of becoming sensitized should receive adequate amounts of anti-Rh gamma globulin soon after delivery.[364, 385, 391] As more and more Rh-negative mothers receive proper prophylaxis, the incidence of erythroblastosis fetalis should be greatly reduced. There is some evidence that intravenous prophylaxis is more effective than the intramuscular route.[390]

Treatment

Infants with erythroblastosis should be treated in a hospital that is properly equipped and staffed to follow the course of the disease and carry out exchange transfusion at any time of day or night. Once the diagnosis of hemolytic disease of the newborn has been established, the treatment will depend on the severity of the disease. Mild forms of the disease may need no treatment other than careful observation. Therapy is directed toward preventing kernicterus that is due to the toxic action of the unconjugated bilirubin on cells in the brain. The indications for exchange transfusions in erythroblastosis fetalis listed by Allen and Diamond are:[358, 384]

1. Anemia: hemoglobin of less than 13 gm. per 100 ml. on venous blood or less than 15 gm. per 100 ml. in capillary blood;

2. Increased serum bilirubin (indirect-reacting type): over 7 mg. per 100 ml. on cord blood; a rapidly-rising serum level; exchange transfusion is performed as often as necessary to keep the serum level less than 20 mg. per 100 ml.;

3. Prematurity, except in the mildest cases;

4. History of a previous baby with kernicterus;

5. Reticulocyte count above 15 per cent;

6. Maternal anti-Rh titer of 1:64 or higher.

Zuelzer and Cohen state that, as a general rule, exchange transfusion is performed if the serum bilirubin level in full-term infants exceeds the following: 10 mg. per 100 ml. in the first 24 hours; 14 mg. per 100 ml. in the second 24 hours; 17 mg. in the third or fourth day.[392]

The exchange transfusion performs several important functions. In addition to lowering the level of serum bilirubin in the infant's blood, it removes cells that are susceptible to hemolysis, lowers the antibody content of the blood, and supplies albumin that enables the infant's blood to bind a larger amount of bilirubin. Repeated exchange transfusions may be required to keep the serum bilirubin level below 20 mg. per 100 ml. Following an exchange transfusion the infant is observed carefully, and the serum bilirubin level is measured as often as is considered necessary. The mortality rate of exchange transfusion is said to be between 1 and 2 per cent for term infants and about 4 per cent for premature infants.[392] This factor must be considered when deciding whether to do exchange transfusion; it is particularly pertinent when the procedure is considered for nonerythroblastotic infants who are jaundiced.

Fresh blood is used for transfusion whenever possible. It is preferable to obtain the blood for transfusion prior to the birth of the infant. In cross-matching for transfusion the prospective donor cells should be tested against the mother's serum.[358,381,384] Prospective donors should be of the same Rh and ABO groups as the mother; Rh-negative blood of the mother's group is used if it is fairly certain that the disease is due to anti-Rh agglutinins. Group O blood is used when the destruction is thought to be due to anti-A or anti-B agglutinins.[381] ABO agglutinins in the donor blood incompatible with the baby's cells should be of low titer and should be neutralized with A and/or B specific substances. If no compatible donor can be found, the mother's red cells, separated from her plasma that contains the antibodies, may be used.[384] When the mother's blood is not available for cross-matching, it is best to select a group O, Rh-negative donor to cross-match with the baby's blood.

If edema of congestive heart failure secondary to anemia is present, phlebotomy is often necessary in order to lower the venous pressure. The oxygen-carrying capacity of the blood can be increased by means of transfusion with packed red cells, which only partially replaces the blood volume.

Induction of labor at about the 34th week has been recommended for those infants who, on the basis of amniocentesis studies, antibody titers, and previous history, are predicted to have severe disease, in an effort to prevent stillbirth.[358,384] Before advising this course the dangers of prematurity must be considered.

Amniocentesis and intrauterine transfusion have a useful place in the management of severe erythroblastosis.[361,379,387] Amniocentesis is carried out to detect those severely-affected infants who are unlikely to survive until the 34th week; in these cases intrauterine transfusion at an earlier date is their main chance for survival. Amniotic fluid should be examined only when anti-Rh antibody is already known to be present, since there is a risk of sensitizing an unsensitized mother with this procedure. If antibody is present, or if there is a history of an erythroblastotic infant, amniocentesis should be performed beginning at the twenty-third to the twenty-fifth week of gestation.[379]

Since early delivery and exchange transfusion carry less risk, intrauterine transfusion should be reserved for the more severely-affected infant.[361] The over-all survival rate with intrauterine transfusion, taking into account those infants dying in the neonatal period, is only 40 per cent.[361,387] The timing of the procedure is important because, once the infant becomes hydropic, transfusion usually is of no benefit.

Several examinations of the amniotic fluid are necessary to gauge whether the bilirubin-like pigment in the fluid is increasing. Based on criteria established by Lilley[377, 378] and modified by others,[361, 387] a decision as to which fetuses should have intrauterine transfusion can be made by measuring the pigment in the amniotic fluid.

Other approaches to the treatment of hyperbilirubinemia of the newborn are the use of phototherapy[360, 373] and phenobarbital.[324a, 366, 389] Phototherapy is based on the observation that the plasma level of indirect bilirubin decreases when an infant is exposed to light of the wavelengths between 300 and 600 mμ, which causes the oxidative breakdown of bilirubin. Since there is no good evidence at present that phototherapy significantly reduces the incidence of subsequent neurologic damage, retarded motor development, or kernicterus in the human, and since the long-term possible toxic effects are as yet unknown, this type of therapy should be used with the same kind of caution reserved for any new drug that becomes available for the treatment of newborn infants. Although it may have a role in the treatment of the jaundice of prematurity and of infants with mild hemolytic disease secondary to ABO incompatibility, it should not be used in the infant with Rh erythroblastosis, since this might delay indicated exchange transfusion.[360]

Phenobarbital lowers the serum bilirubin by accelerating the conjugation and transport of bilirubin by the liver. It has been used in an effort to ameliorate neonatal jaundice by administering the drug both to the mother during the last few weeks of pregnancy and to the newborn infant.[366, 389] There are conflicting reports concerning the efficacy of this form of therapy, and more information is needed before its proper role as a therapeutic agent in jaundice of the newborn can be determined.

Illustrative Case

The patient was the product of the seventh pregnancy of a 38-year-old white female. The mother was type A, Rh-negative and father was type A, Rh-positive. There had been two previous neonatal deaths due to erythroblastosis. Saline antibodies were positive in 1:4 dilution and indirect Coombs test was positive in dilution of 1:64. Pregnancy was uneventful; labor lasted 6 hours and 21 minutes and terminated in a normal spontaneous delivery.

The baby appeared to be in fair condition in the delivery room. He was well-developed and weighed 2700 gm. The skin was grayish in color, and was covered with multiple small ecchymoses. The umbilical cord was icteric. The baby was active when stimulated and cried vigorously. The spleen edge extended 5 cm. below the left costal margin and the liver 7 cm. below the right costal margin.

Laboratory examination and treatment. Initial blood examination: total bilirubin 4 mg per 100 ml., Hct. 25 per cent; Hb. 7.0 gm. per 100 ml.; W.B.C. 13,000 per cu.mm.; nucleated red cells 150 per 100 leukocytes. Direct Coombs test was positive.

A diagnosis of erythroblastosis was made and an exchange transfusion was performed. After exchange transfusion the serum bilirubin level was 2.4

mg. per 100 ml. and the hematocrit 29 per cent. The leukocyte count was 4800 per cu.mm. Five hours later another exchange transfusion was performed at a time when the serum bilirubin had risen to 6 mg. per 100 ml. and the nucleated red cell count had reached 337 per 100 leukocytes. After the second exchange transfusion serum bilirubin level was 2.7 mg. per 100 ml. and the hematocrit was 36 per cent. No further exchange transfusions were necessary and the patient was discharged on the thirteenth day, at which time he was eating well and appeared healthy. At this time the hematocrit was 46 per cent, the white count was 12,000 per cu.mm., and the blood smear contained 5 nucleated red cells per 100 white cells.

Comment. This patient illustrates many of the common features of erythroblastosis. The father was Rh-positive, the mother was Rh-negative. Two siblings had died previously in the neonatal period because of erythroblastosis. The disease was anticipated in this patient. At birth, pallor, ecchymoses, splenomegaly, and hepatomegaly were present; the antiglobulin test was positive. Because of the previous history in the family and the severe anemia, exchange transfusion was performed even though the serum bilirubin level was only slightly elevated at the time of birth. The necessity of the second exchange is debatable. Although the level of the serum bilirubin level was not greatly elevated, exchange transfusion was considered to be the safest course, mainly because of the rate of increase in the bilirubin level. The patient made an uneventful recovery.

IMMUNE DRUG-INDUCED HEMOLYTIC ANEMIA

Drug-induced Coombs positive hemolytic anemia is being recognized with increased frequency. In a recent survey by Garratty and Petz of 200 patients with acquired immune hemolytic anemia, 16 per cent of cases were caused by drugs.[454] In a series of 84 patients with all types of immune hemolytic anemia, Bell and his associates found that 24 per cent of the cases were associated with the anti-hypertensive drug methyldopa.[397] Hemolytic anemias induced by drugs are important as they afford insight into the various mechanisms by which exogenous agents may induce red cell antibodies. Three types of antibody induction are exemplified by reactions to the drugs: quinidine, penicillin, and methyldopa[407, 454, 481, 482] (Table 7–3).

QUINIDINE TYPE (IMMUNE-COMPLEX MECHANISM)

This type of drug-induced anemia was first described following the use of stibophen (Fuadin) for the treatment of schistosomiasis.[413, 428] The immune mechanism involved has been clarified by Shulman in his studies on patients with quinidine-related hemolysis.[471] He has presented evidence in favor of the concept that the positive Coombs test is caused by the attachment of antigen–antibody complexes to the red cell. The drug is a hapten that serves as an antigen when it is bound to some plasma protein. The antibody is directed against the protein-bound circulating drug, and then as a secondary effect the antigen-antibody complex combines with the red cell surface, usually with the

Table 7–3 *Immune Drug-Induced Hemolytic Anemia*

PROTOTYPE DRUG	MECHANISM	TYPE OF ANTIBODY
Quinidine	Antigen-antibody complex	IgM
Penicillin	Hapten binding to red cell	IgG
Methyldopa	Induction of anti-Rh IgG autoantibodies	IgG

fixation of complement. The antigen-antibody complex dissociates from the red cell, leaving only complement behind, so that a nongamma (anticomplement) Coombs serum may be necessary to detect this type of drug reaction.

Quinidine is much more likely to produce immune thrombocytopenia than immune hemolytic anemia.[399] Shulman has proposed that the type of antibody that a patient has against quinidine determines whether he will develop thrombocytopenia or anemia.[471] People more commonly respond with IgG antibody, and the target for this drug-antibody complex is the platelet. The rare patient who develops IgM quinidine antibodies has a hemolytic anemia because the IgM-drug complex is attracted to the red cell. As further substantiation of this concept, patients have been reported who have had both IgG and IgM antibodies against quinidine and have had both thrombocytopenia and hemolytic anemia.[421, 471]

Other drugs which are thought to produce immune hemolytic anemia by the immune–complex mechanism are shown in Table 7–4. Although the antibody involved with most of these drugs is IgM, in some IgG antibodies have been incriminated (aminopyrine, dipyrone, melphalan, the sulfonylureas, and insulin). This type of immune mechanism is an uncommon cause of immune hemolytic anemia; only a few cases have been reported with each drug. The clinical picture is usually one of an acute hemolytic anemia with intravascular

Table 7–4 *Drugs That Have Been Reported to Cause a
Positive Coombs Test with Hemolytic Anemia*

IMMUNE-COMPLEX MECHANISM	HAPTEN-CELL MECHANISM	AUTOIMMUNE MECHANISM
Quinidine[421, 471]	Penicillin[453, 475]	Methyldopa[402, 481, 482]
Quinine[450]	Cephalothin[426, 448]	L-dopa[422, 476]
Stibophen[413, 428]		Mefenamic acid[459, 469]
Sulfonamides[409]		*Chlorpromazine[438]
P-aminosalicylic acid (PAS)[443, 470]		*Diphenylhydantoin[467]
Phenacetin[443, 450, 470]		*Mephenytoin[473]
Aminopyrine[481]		*Methysergide[472]
Isoniazid[460]		
Chlorpropamide[442]		
Tolbutamide[398]		
Indomethacin[410]		
Phenylbutazone[412]		
Chlordiazepoxide[410]		
Dipyrone[436]		
Melphalan[416]		
Insulin[419]		
Rifampicin[454, 456]		

*Immune mechanism not established but autoimmunity suggested.[481]

hemolysis and hemoglobinuria.[481] The anemia subsides promptly when the offending drug is discontinued, although the anticomplement Coombs test may remain positive for several weeks.

PENICILLIN TYPE (HAPTEN–CELL MECHANISM)

Although circulating antibodies to penicillin occur frequently in patients receiving this antibiotic, Coombs-positive hemolytic anemia secondary to penicillin is rare and occurs only under special circumstances.[407, 481]

The breakdown derivatives of penicillin, benzylpenicilloyl acid, and benzylpenaldic acid are firmly bound to the red cell by covalent bonds.[437] In this situation the red cell is normal, and antibodies reacting with penicillin injure the carrier red cell leading to hemolysis. In order for this to become clinically significant, large amounts of penicillin must be given before sufficient penicillin is bound to red cells to cause a positive Coombs test. In most of the recorded cases, penicillin was administered intravenously at dosages greater than 10 million units a day.[453, 475] Also, the type of antibody response against penicillin is important. In most patients, circulating antibodies to penicillin are of the IgM class, and it is only the rare patient who responds to penicillin with a high titer of IgG antibody who develops a Coombs-positive hemolytic anemia.[407, 481] However, it should be kept in mind, particularly in the cases of patients who are taking large doses of penicillin for subacute bacterial endocarditis or lung abscess, and whose anemia begins to get worse rather than better.

Although cross-reactions with penicillin antibodies have been reported with ampicillin, methicillin, and cephalothin,[451] hemolytic anemia has been observed in only a few patients receiving large doses of cephalothin.[426, 448] On the other hand, cephalothin may cause a positive direct Coombs test by altering the red cell membrane so that nonimmune adherence of serum proteins and immunoglobulins occurs.[454, 474, 476] This nonimmune reaction does not cause hemolysis but may lead to difficulties in cross-matching blood for transfusions. This type of nonspecific Coombs reaction may be positive in 4 to 40 per cent of patients taking cephalothin, depending on what type of Coombs antisera is used.[454, 474] Other cephalosporin drugs have also been reported to cause a nonspecific positive direct antiglobulin test which has not been associated with hemolysis.[454]

Unlike the quinidine immune-complex type of hemolytic anemia, that associated with penicillin does not usually involve intravascular hemolysis as only IgG is present on the red cell membrane.[481] Rarely, the IgG antipenicillin antibodies do form immune complexes which fix complement[434] and may lead to severe intravascular hemolysis.[458] Evidence of hemolysis disappears quickly when penicillin is discontinued, but the Coombs test remains positive for 60 to 80 days.[481]

METHYLDOPA TYPE (AUTOIMMUNE MECHANISM)

The association of Coombs-positive hemolytic anemia with methyldopa (Aldomet) therapy was first recognized by Carstairs, Worlledge, Dacie, and associates in 1966.[402, 483] They noted that several patients who had what appeared to be typical idiopathic autoimmune hemolytic anemia were taking methyldopa.

They then surveyed a group of hypertensive patients taking methyldopa, and found that 20 per cent of them had a positive Coombs test but most of them did not have hemolytic anemia, the incidence of clinical hemolysis being about 1 per cent.[481] These observations have been amply confirmed by others,[440] and a review of the published data on 1395 hypertensive patients taking methyldopa revealed an over-all incidence of 15 per cent with a positive direct Coombs test, and slightly less than 1 per cent with overt hemolytic anemia.[481] The incidence of a positive Coombs test is dose-related in those patients with a positive test without hemolysis, being 11 per cent in those taking less than 1.0 gm. per day and 36 per cent in those taking over 2.0 gm. per day.[402, 481] There is no dose relationship in those patients having hemolytic anemia after taking the drug, and many of them were taking less than 1.0 gm. per day.[481, 483] This type of immune drug-induced hemolytic anemia is more common than the quinidine and penicillin types combined.[481]

It usually takes from three to six months of methyldopa therapy for the Coombs test to become positive, and this delay is not shortened when a previously Coombs-positive patient is restarted on the drug. The Coombs test gradually becomes negative when the methyldopa is stopped, but this may take anywhere from one month to two years, depending on the initial strength of the Coombs test. However, there does not appear to be any correlation between the rate of recovery and the total dose of methyldopa or the length of therapy. The clinical and hematologic findings are identical to those of a patient with idiopathic autoimmune hemolytic anemia.[481]

In contrast to the quinidine and penicillin types of immune hemolytic anemia, which require the presence of the drug for a positive Coombs test, methyldopa induces a positive Coombs test that remains positive long after the drug is discontinued. Furthermore, antibodies eluted from the patient's red cells will react with normal red cells without the presence of methyldopa, and the reaction is not blocked by methyldopa or its derivatives.[440]

The antibody on the red cell after methyldopa therapy is identical to the type usually seen in idiopathic autoimmune hemolytic anemia. It is of the IgG class, being most active at 37° C, and having Rh specificity.[423, 440] The antibodies are also heterogenous as with the idiopathic type.[396] One difference between the Coombs test in the idiopathic variety and that induced by methyldopa is that, with rare exceptions,[423, 452] only IgG is present on the red cell in the drug-induced type, whereas IgG plus complement is found in nearly one-third of the patients with idiopathic autoimmune hemolytic anemia.[410]

Methyldopa is not unique in producing this type of immune hemolysis. L-dopa, used for the treatment of parkinsonism, causes a positive direct Coombs test in approximately 10 per cent of the patients taking this drug,[481] but it has rarely been associated with hemolytic anemia.[422, 476] Also, mefenamic acid, used in the treatment of rheumatoid arthritis, has produced a similar type of immune hemolysis in a few patients.[459, 469] The other drugs listed in Table 7–4 under the autoimmune mechanism have been suspected to be of this type, but not enough serologic data are available to establish the type of immune mechanism.[481]

The mechanism whereby methyldopa induces autoantibodies against the red cell is unclear. There is no evidence to suggest that there are cross-reacting antibodies between methyldopa or its metabolites with the Rh locus on the red cell, or that the drugs alter this locus in such a way as to make it antigenic. Large amounts of the drug in vitro will produce nonspecific adherence of immuno-globulin to the red cell membrane after prolonged incubation, but this does not explain the Rh-specific antibodies which occur or the long period before these antibodies disappear after the drug is discontinued.[425]

Since a number of other presumed autoantibodies have been associated with the administration of methyldopa, such as antinuclear factor,[420, 481] rheumatoid factor,[481] leukoagglutins,[449] platelet agglutinins,[449] and possibly liver antibodies,[401, 444] it is probable that the drug alters immune balance in such a way as to break tolerance to a number of autoantigens. There is also a suggestion that there may be a genetic predilection for this type of immune reaction, in that the occurrence of a positive Coombs test after methyldopa is infrequent in blacks, orientals, and Indians.[441] The recent demonstration that methyldopa causes an increase in lymphocyte cyclic AMP,[446] a mediator known to be important in immunoregulation,[400] could lead to an explanation of how this drug might disrupt normal immune balance.

The fact that methyldopa and mefenamic acid can induce a Coombs-positive hemolytic anemia identical to that seen in idiopathic autoimmune hemolytic anemia has important implications for our understanding of the idiopathic type. It is likely that other drugs and exogenous agents such as bacteria and viruses may also induce red cell autoantibody formation.

AUTOIMMUNE HEMOLYTIC ANEMIA

History

The first recognizable description of this type of "acquired" hemolytic anemia has been credited to Hayem,[408] and its history has been reviewed by Dameshek and Schwartz.[411] The discovery of the antiglobulin or Coombs test in 1945 by Coombs, Mourant, and Race[404] was followed by a marked increase in interest in this syndrome, which has led to numerous studies on the demonstration, production, action, and nature of "autoantibodies." A number of excellent reviews have been published.[403, 408, 410, 455]

Patients with autoimmune hemolytic anemia have the usual manifestations of a hemolytic process, such as shortened erythrocyte survival time, increased fecal urobilinogen excretion, elevated serum bilirubin, anemia, reticulocytosis, and splenomegaly. The distinguishing feature is the positive Coombs antiglobulin test, which identifies antibodies on the red cell surface. The disorder occurs during the course of some diseases, particularly those of the lymphoproliferative group, but also appears in patients in whom no primary disease can be demonstrated. In the former circumstance the disorder is classified as secondary or symptomatic; in the latter, patients are classified as "primary" or "idiopathic."

Pathogenesis

The type of antibody attached to the red cell determines the mechanism of hemolysis. IgM antibodies have been referred to as saline antibodies, complete antibodies, agglutinins, and hemolysins. Because they are large, they can combine with antigen sites on adjacent red cells, causing agglutination in saline or in the circulation. IgM antibodies fix complement which, if present in sufficient amounts, causes lysis of red cells in saline and intravascular hemolysis in vivo; such antibodies are called hemolysins. Those causing only agglutination are referred to as agglutinins. Red cells agglutinated by IgM antibodies in the circulation are removed primarily by the liver and to a lesser extent by the spleen.[431] Examples of IgM antibodies are the major blood group antibodies, anti-A and anti-B and cold agglutinins.

IgG antibodies have been referred to as incomplete or sensitizing antibodies. Although they have two combining sites like IgM antibodies, because of their smaller size and the normal distance between negatively charged red cells, they coat the red cell surface but do not cause agglutination in saline or in the general circulation. The major importance of the development of the Coombs antiglobulin test is in the detection of this type of red cell antibody.[404] IgG antibodies usually neither fix complement nor lead to intravascular hemolysis or agglutination. Red cells coated with IgG antibodies are removed from the circulation primarily by the spleen.[433] Although only one molecule of IgM is necessary to fix complement, two molecules of IgG situated close together on the red cell surface are required. Complement usually is not fixed by IgG antibodies directed against widely-spaced antigens such as in the Rh system. These antibodies will fix complement if present in high titer or directed against an antigen densely spaced on the cell surface.[464] Red cells coated with IgG antibodies do not agglutinate in saline, but do when suspended in a high protein media such as albumin. In the spleen, where the plasma protein concentration is higher than in the general circulation, IgG-coated red cells begin to agglutinate and are sequestered.[433]

Another important factor in the destruction of IgG-coated erythrocytes by the spleen is that mononuclear cells in the spleen, as well as circulating monocytes, have a receptor for IgG.[439] These cells also have a receptor for the third component of complement, but not for other immunoglobulins or plasma proteins.[431] When IgG-coated red cells become attached to splenic phagocytes, the erythrocytes may be lysed or, more commonly, a portion of the red cell membrane may be removed, leading to erythrocyte fragmentation, spherocytosis, and ultimately sequestration and lysis by the spleen. In most cases of idiopathic autoimmune hemolytic anemia, the antibody involved is IgG.[408, 410, 417, 455] IgA antibodies are rarely involved in Coombs-positive hemolytic anemia.[403]

The antibodies involved in Coombs-positive hemolytic anemia may also be classified according to whether they react optimally at 37° C (warm antibodies) or at lower temperatures (cold antibodies).[408, 410] The IgG antibodies seen in idiopathic autoimmune hemolytic anemia, Rh isoantibodies, and those induced by methyldopa are of the warm variety, whereas the IgM red cell antibodies found after mycoplasma pneumonia and chronic cold hemagglutinin disease are examples of cold antibodies.[410] These cold antibodies fix complement, and at 37° C, or room temperature, the IgM antibody which fixed complement at a lower temperature dissociates from the red cell, leaving only complement on the red cell surface. It is therefore important to use a nongamma (anticomplement)

Coombs serum when checking for red cell antibodies at room temperature, in order not to miss cold antibodies.

For a number of years there was controversy as to whether the globulins on the red cell surface were really antibodies to red cells, because these globulins reacted with nearly all red cells they were tested against with no apparent specificity. Then it was learned that the antigens involved were very common ones ("public antigens") which occur on the red cells of all but a few individuals.[477] In idiopathic autoimmune hemolytic anemia and in methyldopa-induced hemolytic anemia, the IgG antibodies have been found, with only rare exceptions, to be directed against antigens of the Rh system.[408, 410, 440] When Weiner and Vos used Rh null red cells (cells containing no Rh locus) to test for antibody specificity in idiopathic autoimmune hemolytic anemia, they found specificity to the Rh locus in about 70 per cent of the sera.[478] In high titer cold agglutinin hemolytic anemia following mycoplasma pneumonia, the antibodies have anti-I specificity, in infectious mononucleosis they have anti-i specificity, and in paroxysmal cold hemoglobinuria the Donath-Landsteiner antibody is directed against the P antigen.[408, 410]

Although a number of hypotheses have been proposed, there is no completely satisfactory one to explain why a patient develops autoantibodies against his own red cells. The main theories expounded are: (1) alteration of red cell antigen; (2) cross reaction with a red cell antigen; and (3) induction of lymphoid cells to produce antibodies against normal red cells.

It is possible that viruses, bacteria, or drugs such as methyldopa might alter red cell antigens, particularly the Rh locus, so that the red cells become antigenic for normal lymphoid cells. There is no experimental evidence to support this theory, and the fact that eluted antibodies react as strongly with normal cells from other donors as with the patient's red cells makes this explanation unlikely.

The observation that mycoplasma infection produces a Coombs-positive hemolytic anemia, and that syphilis is associated with most cases of the Donath-Landsteiner antibody in paroxysmal cold hemoglobinuria, has raised the possibility that antibodies against mycoplasma and the spirochete may cross-react with I and P antigens of the red cell, and in a similar fashion other exogenous agents may produce cross-reactions.[406] Again, there is little experimental evidence to substantiate this hypothesis, and the fact that autoantibodies persist long after the exogenous agent presumably is gone casts doubt on this theory.

Small amounts of autoantibodies are present normally, and it is possible that some exogenous agent interferes with the normal immune regulatory system in such a way that autoantibody titers increase sufficiently to cause clinically-apparent disease. The observation that most secondary immune hemolytic anemias are associated with lymphoproliferative disorders has led to the theory of a mutation of a clone of lymphocytes which make antibodies against normal red cell antigens. The fact that this type of antibody, as well as that studied in chronic cold hemagglutinin disease, is usually homogeneous, in terms of immunoglobin light chains and subclasses of heavy chains, supports the concept that the antibodies are monoclonal in origin and may have arisen from a mutant strain of lymphocytes.[410] In contrast, the antibodies observed in idiopathic autoimmune hemolytic anemia[395, 418] and methyldopa-induced anemia[396] are heterogeneous with respect to light chains and subclasses of heavy chains. This

Table 7-5   *Incidence of Types of Coombs Positive Hemolytic Anemia*

	PER CENT OF TOTAL PATIENTS			
	Dacie[410]		*Bell*[397]	
TYPE OF DISORDER	*1947–1968*		*1967–1973*	
Warm (IgG)	70		68	
Idiopathic	37		21	
Secondary	33		47	
Drugs (methyldopa, etc.)		4		24
Lymphoproliferative		12		14
SLE and related disorders		12		7
Infections		4		–
Cold (IgM)	30		32	
Idiopathic (cold hemagglutinin disease)	13		10	
Secondary	16		22	
Lymphoproliferative		2		7
SLE and related disorders		1		4
Infections (mycoplasma, etc.)		8		8
Paroxysmal cold hemoglobinuria		5		2

suggests that normal lymphoid tissue is responding to chronic exogenous antigenic stimulation or that the normal suppression of humoral antibodies has been abrogated.

Clinical Manifestations

Autoimmune hemolytic anemia may arise in association with some other disease, in which case it is termed "secondary" or "symptomatic." It may also occur when no other disease is demonstrable, and is then classified as "primary" or "idiopathic." Table 7–5 compares the different types of Coombs positive hemolytic anemia in a large series of 295 patients studied by Dacie and his colleagues over a 20-year-period[410] with a smaller but more recent group of 84 patients studied by Bell.[397] In both groups a warm antibody of the IgG type was present in about 70 per cent of the patients. Idiopathic cases accounted for 50 per cent of Dacie's patients, but only 31 per cent of Bell's. The main difference between the two series was the larger percentage of cases secondary to drugs in the more recent series, since the relationship to methyldopa-induced warm autoantibodies had only been known for a few years when Dacie's series was published. On the other hand, another large series of 234 patients reviewed in 1969 by Pirofsky revealed only 18 per cent to be idiopathic, and just 3 per cent of the cases to be attributable to drugs.[455] As was the case with the two series shown in Table 7–5, most of the secondary cases were related to lymphoproliferative disorders, connective tissue disorders, or infections.[455]

The idiopathic disorder occurs at any age in either sex, but females are affected more often than males. The severity and duration of the disease may vary greatly. At times the onset of the disease is sudden and the course is rapid and fulminating. In such patients the course is characterized by high temperature, rapidly-progressing weakness, and dyspnea. Anemia becomes more severe, icterus is usually apparent, and hemoglobinuria sometimes occurs. More often the course of the disorder is a chronic one that persists with varying degrees of severity over a period of months or years. Spontaneous remissions sometimes occur. When the disorder is associated with the cold type of autoantibodies, Raynaud's phenomenona and hemoglobinuria may appear on exposure to cold.

In secondary autoimmune hemolytic disease, the clinical features are those of the underlying disorder plus those associated with the hemolytic anemia. At times the hemolytic element may be so severe that it dominates the clinical picture, and at other times it may be merely an incidental finding. When hemolytic anemia follows mycoplasma pneumonia, the anemia, which may be severe, usually appears suddenly at the end of the second or third week of illness and disappears spontaneously in one or two weeks.[408] In diseases such as lymphocytic lymphoma the hemolytic anemia may precede other evidence of the primary disease by months, or it may not appear until after the underlying disease has been under observation and treatment for several years.

The main abnormalities on physical examination in the idiopathic cases are pallor and splenomegaly. In addition, patients with the secondary type may manifest evidence of the underlying disease, such as lymphadenopathy, hepatomegaly, or evidence of disease in the skin, lungs, and gastrointestinal tract.

Laboratory Examination

Any degree of anemia may occur in either the idiopathic or secondary forms of disease, depending on the severity of the hemolytic process. The anemia is usually macrocytic (MCV > 94 cu.μ) because of reticulocytosis, but a stained smear of the peripheral blood often reveals many microcytes, polychromatophilia, poikilocytosis, and the presence of normoblasts. Spherocytosis is often present, and correlates with an increased osmotic fragility. Autoagglutination may be observed with cold-reacting antibodies, and can be distinguished from rouleau formation by its disappearance upon warming the blood. Reticulocytosis is usually present, but reticulocytopenia occurs in some patients. Leukocytosis is common during periods of active hemolysis and the count may exceed 30,000 per cu.mm.; the increase is mainly in the granulocytic series, and myelocytes may be found in the peripheral blood. Neutropenia sometimes occurs in chronic cases but is unusual during episodes of crisis. Erythrophagocytosis by monocytes is sometimes evident on plain smears or on smears made from the buffy coat, and may suggest the diagnosis. The platelet count is usually normal or moderately reduced, but severe thrombocytopenia is found in some patients, which may also be on an immune basis as described by Evans.[390]

The autohemolysis test shows increased hemolysis after incubation which is not decreased by glucose and may be increased further by the addition of glucose.[408] Hemoglobin electrophoresis reveals the normal A type of hemoglobin. Serum bilirubin is frequently increased and haptoglobin decreased or absent.

Of fundamental importance in the diagnosis of autoimmune hemolytic anemia is the demonstration of a positive direct Coombs test. The direct Coombs test is the demonstration of gamma globulin or complement attached to washed red cells, and the indirect Coombs test is the demonstration of antibodies in the patient's serum which react with other individuals' red cells and may be either autoantibodies or isoantibodies. In autoimmune hemolytic anemia the direct Coombs test is regularly positive, and in some patients, usually those with more severe anemia, the indirect Coombs test is also positive. The severity of the hemolytic process correlates fairly well with the amount of antibody present on the red cell.[463]

There is a small group of patients who have the clinical characteristics of autoimmune hemolytic anemia and respond well to corticosteroid therapy, but in whom a positive Coombs test cannot be demonstrated. In some instances this may be because there are too few IgG molecules on the red cells to be detected by the routine Coombs test[423] but enough to decrease significantly red cell survival.[447] In other instances the cause of the hemolysis may be the rare IgA type which may not be detected with standard Coombs sera.[403]

One type of Coombs serum may be prepared by immunizing rabbits against whole human serum, in which case it is referred to as broad spectrum and detects all the immunoglobulins and complement to some extent. More specific and sensitive Coombs sera may be prepared by immunizing a rabbit against one of the purified immunoglobulins or complement. Since IgA is rarely involved in immune hemolytic anemia, and IgM is usually detected only when the test is performed at low temperatures, common practice is to use anti-IgG Coombs serum (often referred to as gamma) and anticomplement Coombs serum (often referred to as nongamma).[403, 464]

When these two types of Coombs sera are used, most cases of autoimmune hemolytic anemia fall into one of three patterns: IgG, IgG plus complement, or complement alone.[410, 417] In idiopathic autoimmune hemolytic anemia due to warm antibodies, Dacie and Worlledge found a pattern of IgG in 55 per cent, IgG plus complement in 38 per cent, and 7 per cent with complement alone.[410, 417] When the hemolytic anemia is caused by a cold antibody either spontaneously (chronic cold hemagglutinin disease) or secondary to a lymphoma, usually only complement can be detected on the red cell.[410, 417] In the hemolytic anemia associated with lupus erythematosus, complement is regularly found on the red cell in addition to IgG, whereas in the hemolytic anemia induced by methyldopa only IgG is found.[403] It should be pointed out that when the Coombs test is performed on large numbers of hospitalized patients or normal blood donors, a significant number will show complement-only reactions and have no evidence of excessive hemolysis.[410]

Treatment and Prognosis

Treatment of the patient with autoimmune hemolytic disease is directed toward both the hemolytic anemia and the underlying disease. Blood transfusion, adrenocorticosteroid preparations, immunosuppression, and splenectomy are the most important measures for the treatment of the anemia. Blood transfusions may be lifesaving during episodes of crisis, and may be necessary periodically in patients with the chronic type of disorder who have failed to respond satisfactorily to splenectomy or steroids. The use of packed red cells for transfusions after the plasma and leukocytes have been removed from the blood often reduces the incidence of febrile transfusion reactions. Cross-matching is often difficult because of the presence of the abnormal antibody in the patient's serum, and transfusions should be avoided if possible. In patients for whom no compatible donor blood can be found and whose need for transfusion is urgent, the least incompatible blood available should be used. The transfusion should be given slowly with careful monitoring.

Splenectomy induces a complete remission in about 40 to 65 per cent of patients. It is more likely to be helpful in cases of the idiopathic variety than in the secondary group. Although the response to splenectomy is unpredictable, and relapse may occur at any time after an apparently good postoperative response,[485] the use of ^{51}Cr to measure splenic sequestration is valuable in selecting patients who are most likely to respond to splenectomy.[432] In a series of 45 patients reported by Allgood and Chaplin, 68 per cent obtained a complete remission after splenectomy, and 44 per cent remained cured without supplementary corticosteroid therapy.[393] They noted that a negative indirect Coombs test and IgG type antibody predisposed to a favorable response to splenectomy, and others have noted[417] that a good response to previous corticosteroid therapy makes a satisfactory response to splenectomy more likely. They also pointed out that, although significant splenic sequestration of ^{51}Cr-labeled red cells presaged a good result from splenectomy, the lack of significant red cell sequestration did not preclude a good response.[393]

Treatment with the adrenocortical steroid drugs produces improvement in many patients with this type of anemia. There is evidence that corticosteroids decrease hemolysis by reducing the phagocytosis of antibody-coated cells in the spleen[394] and by decreasing the concentration of antibody on the red cell and in the serum.[463] In the group of patients reported by Allgood and Chaplin, 84 per cent obtained an initial partial or complete remission following a single course of steroid therapy, but only 16 per cent were able to maintain the remission when steroids were discontinued.[393] Because of the high frequency of relapse when steroids are discontinued and the many deleterious side-effects of prolonged steroid therapy, splenectomy should not be delayed in those patients in whom large doses of corticosteroids are necessary to control the hemolytic process.

Immunosuppressive therapy with such drugs as azathioprine, 6-mercaptopurine, chlorambucil, and cyclophosphamide has met with variable success in the treatment of autoimmune hemolytic anemia.[405, 410, 465, 468] This type of therapy is usually reserved for the more refractory patient who has not responded to splenectomy or to corticosteroid therapy. Although such therapy has been effective in some patients, it carries the risk of bone marrow depression associated with these drugs. Other therapeutic approaches include thymectomy, antithymocyte antiserum, heparin, and ε-aminocaproic acid, which have been used in a few patients with some success.[455]

In patients with chronic cold hemagglutinin disease with high titers of cold agglutinins, corticosteroid therapy and splenectomy have rarely been of any benefit.[410, 417, 466] Immunosuppressive therapy has been successful in lowering the antibody titer and improving the anemia in some of these patients.[430] Dacie reported a good response to chlorambucil therapy in three of nine patients with chronic cold hemagglutinin disease.[410]

In the very acute type of illness, a more aggressive plan of treatment is often necessary. In this circumstance numerous blood transfusions, intravenous steroids, and splenectomy all may be utilized in the space of a few days.

If the hemolytic anemia is of the secondary variety, appropriate therapy should be directed at the primary disease as soon as feasible. If this is one of the connective tissue diseases, corticosteroid therapy of the hemolytic process may be all that is necessary. If the underlying disorder is a carcinoma or an ovarian tumor, definitive surgical treatment is usually indicated. If lymphocytic lymphoma is present the anemia may improve following treatment with chemotherapy, but simultaneous therapy with prednisone or some related compound is usually necessary, at least in the beginning of the course of therapy.[461] Therapy of the lymphoma with x-ray or chemotherapeutic agents may also cause an exacerbation of the hemolytic process.[461]

The prognosis of patients with the secondary type of anemia is mainly that of the underlying disease. The prognosis is generally favorable when the disorder follows a virus infection, and is poor when it is associated with malignancy or one of the connective tissue diseases. Patients with a negative indirect Coombs test and IgG antibodies on their red cells generally respond better to therapy and have a more favorable prognosis than those patients whose red cells are also coated with complement.[393] The presence of complement is more likely to be associated with underlying disease than is the presence of IgG alone.[417] The commonest causes of death are cardiac failure caused by anemia, acute renal failure, septicemia, and pulmonary emboli.[393] Pirofsky observed an over-all mortality rate of 64 per cent in 226 patients with adequate follow-up, but only 38 per cent in those with the idiopathic variety. In those with the secondary form the prognosis was governed largely by the type of underlying disease.[455] The occurrence of severe anemia, reticulocytopenia, thrombocytopenia, and leukopenia appear to be associated with a poor prognosis.

Illustrative Case

This 53-year-old white housewife had been under observation for five years as a tuberculosis suspect, but the diagnosis was never established. On a periodic chest roentgenogram it was noted that hilar adenopathy had developed, and the patient was admitted to the hospital for investigation. She admitted occasional vague chest pains and an irregular cough but denied weight loss, pruritus, or other symptoms.

Physical Examination. The posterior cervical and axillary lymph nodes were enlarged and measured 0.5 to 1 cm. in diameter. The spleen was felt two fingerbreadths below the left costal margin. Physical examination was otherwise within normal limits.

Laboratory Examination. Admission blood studies: Hb. 7.1 gm. per cent; hematocrit 27 per cent; R. B. C. 1.9 million per cu.mm.; retics. 22.3 per cent; W. B. C. 18,000 per cu.mm. Differential count (per cent): bands 4 segmented 50, lymphocytes 40, monocytes 1, eosinophils 4, basophils 1. The serum protein was 8.9 gm. per 100 ml., albumin 3.5 gm. per 100 ml., globulin 5.4 gm. per 100 ml. The direct antiglobulin (Coombs) test was positive and the Wassermann test was anticomplementary. Blood cultures, tuberculin skin test, platelet counts, and examination for L. E. cells were normal. Plasma electrophoresis indicated increased total protein, increased gamma globulin, decreased albumin, and beta globulin with two peaks; the pattern was considered suggestive of Boeck's sarcoid. Bone marrow aspiration revealed marked normoblastic hyperplasia; plasma cells and eosinophils appeared to be slightly increased.

Regular roentgenograms and laminograms of the chest suggested a slight enlargement in the right hilus area. On bronchoscopy no mass was visualized. Biopsies of the right prescalene node and right axillary node were interpreted as "hyperplastic lymphadenitis."

Treatment and Course. The patient was thought to have a hemolytic anemia of the autoimmune type. Although sarcoid, lymphosarcoma, and disseminated lupus were suspected as underlying primary diseases, no diagnosis could be established. Accordingly the patient was given prednisone, 20 mg. every eight hours beginning on June 24. On June 26 this was reduced to 10 mg. four times a day, and at discharge on July 3 the dose was reduced to 5 mg. three times a day. There was a striking improvement in her blood count, and on September 16 her hematocrit was 42 per cent and the reticulocyte count had fallen to 1.5 per cent. On November 4, one month after her prednisone dosage had been reduced to 2.5 mg. three times a week, the patient was asymptomatic and the hematocrit was 39 per cent.

Comment. This patient had evidence of a hemolytic anemia, and the positive direct Coombs test indicated that the anemia was of the extracorpuscular or autoimmune type. No primary diagnosis was established and the case might be considered to be "idiopathic." However, various features strongly suggest the presence of some underlying disease, and in this circumstance the patient must be examined periodically for additional evidence of some primary disorder. The anemia has responded well to treatment with prednisone for two years, although the Coombs test remains positive.

PAROXYSMAL COLD HEMOGLOBINURIA

Paroxysmal cold hemoglobinuria is a rare disorder. The sudden attacks of intravascular hemolysis and hemoglobinuria that occur on exposure to cold are due to the presence of an autohemolysin in the serum. The attacks are precipitated by chilling of the body, and hemolysis occurs during the subsequent warming. Donath and Landsteiner demonstrated that hemolysis occurs in paroxysmal cold hemoglobinuria because of the presence of an autohemolysin in the patient's blood.[414] The hemolysin in the patient's plasma unites with the patient's erythrocytes in the presence of complement at low temperatures. In the presence of the complement, hemolysis occurs on warming. The antibody usually is not active at body temperature or at room temperature.[427] The Wassermann reaction is reported to be positive in over 90 per cent of patients with the disorder, and unquestionable clinical evidence of syphilis is found in about 30 per cent.[336, 408] The disorder has also been observed to follow such infections as measles, mumps, chicken pox, and infectious mononucleosis.[484] The Donath-Landsteiner hemolysin is an IgG antibody which has anti-P specificity.[410, 429] It bears no relationship to the Wassermann antibody.[410]

The attacks are precipitated by exposure to cold, but there is a wide range of variability in the amount of chilling that is necessary, and hemolysis is more severe and frequent when the antibody is of high thermal amplitude.[457] The interval between the chilling and the onset of symptoms may vary from a few minutes to seven or eight hours. The prodromal period is apt to be associated with malaise, headache, abdominal cramps, and pains in the back and legs. The actual paroxysm is usually manifested by a shaking chill followed by a temperature rise to 102° or 104° F that lasts for several hours. After the chill the voided urine usually appears dark red or brown; urine of this character may be passed in only the first or first few specimens after the chill, or over a period of two or three days. Severe, reversible acute renal failure may develop during an attack.[445] During the episode mild jaundice, splenomegaly, and hepatomegaly are often demonstrable. Severe leukopenia that is the result of the virtual disappearance of the granulocytes from the peripheral blood also occurs.[462]

Treatment during the attack consists of keeping the patient in a warm environment and administering transfusions when necessary. Between episodes exposure to cold is avoided and any underlying disease is treated. Many patients remain asymptomatic during these intervals.

The diagnosis is made by the history and by abnormalities that can be demonstrated in the laboratory tests. The degree of the anemia and the evidence of blood regeneration depend on the severity of the hemolysis. Hemoglobinemia, hemoglobinuria, and a positive antiglobulin test can be demonstrated during an attack. More specific tests establish the diagnosis. In various modifications of the Donath-Landsteiner test, hemolysis is demonstrated after the blood has been chilled and rewarmed in vitro.[408, 490] Paroxysmal cold hemoglobinuria must be distinguished from the hemoglobinuria that follows exposure to cold in patients with cold agglutinins; the latter disorder occurs in association with mycoplasma pneumonia, and hemolysis occurs only when the agglutinin is present in high titer.

PAROXYSMAL NOCTURNAL HEMOGLOBINURIA

Paroxysmal nocturnal hemoglobinuria (PNH), or the Marchiafava-Micheli syndrome, is a rare disorder of unknown cause that occurs in both sexes.[409, 427, 462, 487, 494, 496, 500, 516] Although the disease has been reported in patients ranging in age from 5½ to 52 years of age, it usually appears during the third or fourth decade.[462, 516] The disease is characterized by intravascular hemolysis and hemoglobinuria that is usually more marked during or immediately after sleep, chronicity, spontaneous remissions and exacerbations, thrombotic complications and refractoriness to therapy. It has been demonstrated that the increased hemolysis is due to an acquired intracorpuscular defect, since erythrocytes from patients with paroxysmal nocturnal hemoglobinuria have a diminished survival time when transfused into normal subjects, but erythrocytes from normal individuals survive normally when transfused into patients with paroxysmal nocturnal hemoglobinuria.[409]

The exact nature of the red cell defect in PNH is yet to be defined. The most characteristic abnormality, one leading directly to hemolysis, is an increased sensitivity to complement. Rosse has demonstrated three populations of red cells in patients with PNH in terms of the red cell sensitivity to complement in vitro. One population has normal sensitivity to complement, another population is 1.5 to 5 times as sensitive to lysis by complement as normal cells, and the third population is markedly sensitive to complement, being 20 times more sensitive than normal red cells.[464, 513] These three populations have also been demonstrated in vivo by red cell survival curves, and the degree of hemolysis seen clinically correlates with the complement-sensitive populations.[464, 513] Yachnin has shown that complement may become attached to PNH red cells and the complement sequence be completed without the presence of antibody,[518] probably by the activation of the alternate pathway of complement which may be initiated by a number of conditions (endotoxin, low ionic strength, low pH) leading to the fixation of C3.[497]

Acetylcholinesterase activity of PNH red cells is very low or absent.[499, 500] This is probably a secondary rather than a primary defect, since in vivo experiments with acetylcholinesterase inhibitors have shown no detrimental effect,[511] and familial deficiency of erythrocyte acetylcholinesterase is not associated with hemolysis or positive serologic tests for PNH.[506] Neutrophil alkaline phosphatase is low or absent,[494] and PNH leukocytes and platelets have also been demonstrated to have increased sensitivity to complement.[486]

Normal red cells can be made to take on many of the characteristics of PNH red cells by in vitro treatment with large amounts of sulfhydryl-containing compounds, such as glutathione, cysteine, and aminoethylisothiouronium (AET), including complement sensitivity, low acetylcholinesterase, and electron microscopic changes of the red cell membrane.[516] This suggests that some alteration in erythrocyte membrane sulfhydryl groups may be responsible for enhanced sensitivity to complement, but as yet this remains speculative.

The diagnosis of PNH is usually based on a positive acidified serum or Ham test.[409, 490] This test is very specific, and when done properly rarely gives either false positive or false negative results.[409, 500] An interesting exception is a hereditary anemia referred to as HEMPAS (hereditary erythroblastic multinuclearity with a positive acidified serum test).[492] These patients' red cells are particularly sensitive to an isoagglutinin present in most normal sera, and consequently give a positive Ham test with most, but not all, sera. The acidified serum test will be negative when autologous serum is used, because the antibody is not present in the patient's serum. The sugar water test is negative.

The sugar water or sucrose test of Hartmann and Jenkins[501] is a sensitive test in the diagnosis of PNH, and is based on the enhancement of complement by low ionic strength solutions. This test also has high specificity for PNH when properly performed.[502] Inulin, an activator of the alternate pathway of complement, has also been used in a simple and rapidly-performed test which so far appears to be specific for PNH.[488]

In addition to the tests mentioned above, it is important to test the urine for hemosiderin. Although hemoglobinuria may not be present in a substantial number of patients, because the amount of hemoglobin filtered may be small and readily reabsorbed, hemosiderinuria from the tubule deposits of iron is regularly present. Whereas hemosiderinuria may be present in a variety of hemolytic disorders associated with intravascular hemolysis, its absence speaks strongly against the diagnosis of PNH.[516]

Many cases of PNH are preceded by a period of pancytopenia before the anemia becomes frankly hemolytic.[409, 487, 494, 496, 510, 516] In at least 25 per cent of PNH patients aplastic anemia has been diagnosed previously, and the diagnosis of PNH should always be considered and tested for in such patients.[510, 516] It is tempting to speculate that the abnormal population of PNH red cells arises as a mutation following bone marrow injury. Since PNH has been recorded to follow familial aplastic anemia,[493] drug-induced aplastic anemia,[510] and idiopathic aplastic anemia,[510] it is likely that the mutation is related to disordered hematopoiesis which follows bone marrow hypoplasia, rather than being due to any specific etiologic agent.

The treatment of PNH has been unsatisfactory.[503] The administration of alkali and splenectomy have been of no benefit. A combination of iron and androgen therapy has been reported to improve the anemia,[500, 503] but not infrequently iron therapy may lead to an acute worsening of the anemia because of an increase in reticulocytes, which are more sensitive to the hemolytic action of complement.[507, 515] Corticosteroids have been shown to be helpful in some patients, but large doses may be necessary and severe relapses may occur when the dosage is lowered or discontinued.[495] Blood transfusions should be used as infrequently as possible because of the risk of hepatitis, and because they frequently cause a hemolytic reaction when whole blood is used. Since the activation of the complement system by isoantibodies to leukocytes and platelets may play a role in increasing hemolysis, washed red cells with removal of most of the leukocytes and platelets should be used when transfusion is necessary.[516] Another approach to the treatment of PNH has been bone marrow transplantation when an HL-A identical sibling has been available.[517]

The course of the disease is a chronic one which may continue for many years in some patients,[491] although the median survival is slightly less than five years.[516] Infections, antisera, a number of drugs, and menstruation may precipitate hemolytic crises. In fatal cases, death is caused not only by anemia and infections during acute episodes, but also by thromboses of cerebral, coronary, portal, hepatic, and pulmonary vessels.[409, 516] The disorder may terminate in acute myeloblastic leukemia,[504-505, 508] and has also been reported in association with myelofibrosis[498, 509] and erythroleukemia.[489]

MECHANICAL HEMOLYSIS

Mechanical damage to the red cell as a cause of hemolytic anemia can be divided into three categories: (1) erythrocyte injury secondary to impact of red cells in the microcirculation against a flat surface, as in march hemoglobinuria; (2) erythrocyte damage secondary to valvular heart disease; and (3) red cell damage secondary to obstructive disease of small blood vessels.

MARCH HEMOGLOBINURIA

Although hemoglobinuria occurring in a soldier after a long and strenuous march was reported as long ago as 1881 by Fleicher,[525] it was not until 1964 that Davidson[526] focused attention on trauma to red cells in the superficial capillaries of the feet against a hard flat surface as the cause of hemolysis. He noted that the common denominator in such cases was walking or running on a hard surface, and that equally strenuous exercise such as swimming, cycling, or running on a soft surface did not cause hemoglobinuria. He and others also demonstrated that this type of hemoglobinuria could be prevented by putting rubber insoles into the runners' shoes.[526, 527]

In addition to marathon runners,[531] this type of impact hemolysis has been reported in a young man indulging in vigorous karate exercises involving considerable trauma to the ulnar surfaces of his hands,[539] and in conga-drum players.[533]

Since most individuals do not have hemoglobinuria after walking or running on a hard surface, an intrinsic red cell defect that is brought out by this kind of stress has been looked for, but none has been found.[538] Chaplin and his associates reported the case of a young man who had hemoglobinuria and a congenital heart lesion with chronically-depressed haptoglobin levels. They postulated that the relatively low haptoglobin levels made the patient more prone to exceed the capacity of haptoglobin after traumatic intravascular hemolysis, with hemoglobinuria occurring as a consequence.[524]

Unlike the other types of mechanical hemolysis to be described, the blood smear in march hemoglobinuria does not show red cell fragmentation. The hemoglobinuria must be distinguished from myoglobinuria, which also may occur after strenuous exercise.

CARDIAC HEMOLYTIC ANEMIA

Many patients with valvular heart disease, both those with prosthetic valve replacements and those who have had no operation, have a decreased red cell survival because of trauma to erythrocytes as they pass through the heart.[534] In many patients the degree of hemolysis is slight and easily compensated for by increased red cell production, so that anemia is mild or absent. Hemolysis in such patients usually goes unrecognized unless special studies are made. On the other hand, hemolysis is marked in some patients, resulting in severe anemia with hemoglobinuria and the expected adverse effects on cardiac function.

Table 7–6 lists the types of cardiac abnormalities that have been associated with mechanical hemolysis. Although many types of operative procedures and prosthetic devices have been associated with hemolysis, replacement of the aortic valve by a prosthesis has been the most common offender. In one series of 317 operative cases involving the aortic valve, approximately 10 per cent developed clinically significant hemolytic anemia.[536] Traumatic hemolysis has also been reported with rupture of an aneurysm of the sinus of Valsalva.[529]

Although the mechanism whereby turbulence of blood across a diseased or

Table 7–6   *Types of Cardiac Abnormalities Associated with Mechanical Hemolysis*

OPERATED PATIENTS	UNOPERATED PATIENTS
Aortic valve replacement	Aortic disease
Mitral valve replacement	Stenosis
Repair of atrial septal defect	Insufficiency
Repair of tetralogy of Fallot	Coarctation
Repair of atrioventricular canal defect	Mitral disease
	Insufficiency

artificial heart valve leads to red cell fragmentation and intravascular hemolysis is not entirely clear, in most instances there is a significant regurgitation jet stream resulting from separation, tearing, or malposition of the artificial valve. This usually occurs in the high flow aortic area, but has also been observed with faulty mitral prosthetic valves[542] and with severe mitral insufficiency without surgery.[543] The damage to the red cells is apparently caused by turbulent flow and shearing forces as erythrocytes become adherent to fibrin deposits on the prosthetic or diseased valve. Nevaril and his associates have shown in vitro that a shearing force of 3000 dynes per cm^2 causes erythrocyte fragmentation and hemolysis, a shear stress similar to that which has been estimated to occur across an insufficient aortic valve.[535]

The diagnosis of traumatic hemolysis in cardiac patients is not difficult to make if one is aware of the possibility of its occurrence and looks for laboratory abnormalities that accompany intravascular hemolysis. There is increased plasma hemoglobin, decreased plasma haptoglobin, increased serum lactic dehydrogenase, and hemosiderinuria. The appearance of schistocytes (distorted and fragmented red cells) on the peripheral blood smear indicates traumatic damage to erythrocytes in the circulation (Fig. 7–12). The number of fragmented red cells present correlates well with the severity of the hemolytic process, and in some patients with mild hemolysis no distorted cells may be seen.[528]

Prolonged hemosiderinuria and hemoglobinuria may lead to iron deficiency which aggravates the anemia.[530] As the anemia becomes more severe, cardiac output is increased, which heightens the degree of turbulence across the valve and makes the traumatic hemolysis worse. For this reason any iron deficiency

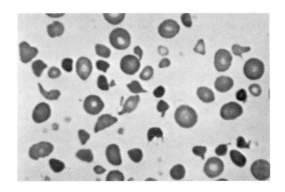

Figure 7–12 Peripheral blood smear showing schistocytes and red cell fragmentation. (From Davidsohn and Henry: Todd-Sanford Clinical Diagnosis by Laboratory Methods. Philadelphia, W. B. Saunders, 1969.)

should be treated promptly. At times, correcting the iron deficiency is enough to lead to a compensated hemolytic state, but usually it is necessary to repair the defective valve in order to correct both the anemia and cardiac dysfunction.

MICROANGIOPATHIC HEMOLYTIC ANEMIA

The term "microangiopathic hemolytic anemia" was used in 1962 by Brain, Dacie, and Hourihane to describe hemolytic anemia occurring in a variety of disorders which have in common disease of the small blood vessels.[519-522] They were struck by the similarity between the blood smears in these patients and those previously described in patients with traumatic hemolysis secondary to valvular heart disease. In both instances burr cells, helmet cells, fragmented cells, and spherocytes were noted. (Fig. 7-13.)

They postulated that the mechanism of hemolysis was trauma to red cells by turbulent flow across abnormal valves in one, and squeezing through partially-obstructed and abnormal small vessles in the other.

Table 7-7 lists the types of disorders which have been associated with microangiopathic hemolytic anemia.[521] They all have in common disease of the microcirculation with partial obstruction to the flow of erythrocytes. In nearly all instances the renal vasculature is involved,[520] but obstruction of other vessels may also cause fragmentation and traumatic lysis of erythrocytes. This has been observed in patients with disseminated carcinoma with small vessel involvement,[521] purpura fulminans,[532] hemangiomas,[521] and pulmonary hypertension.[540] Also fragmented red cells on the blood smear may be a clue to the diagnosis of disseminated intravascular coagulation.

Microangiopathic hemolytic anemia has been produced experimentally in animals by inducing the generalized Shwartzman reaction,[521] by the injection of thrombin,[521] by rapid defibrination from injecting a purified coagulant fraction of Malayan pit-viper venom (Arvin),[537] and by producing malignant hypertension with a combination of salt overload and the administration of desoxycorti-

Table 7-7   *Causes of Microangiopathic Hemolytic Anemia*

Thrombotic thrombocytopenic purpura
Purpura fulminans
Hemolytic-uremic syndrome of childhood
Acute glomerulonephritis
Renal cortical necrosis
Polyarteritis
Wegener's granulomatosis
Malignant hypertension
Pulmonary hypertension
Eclampsia
Lupus erythematosus
Scleroderma
Amyloidosis
Carcinomatosis involving small blood vessels
Rejection of renal homografts
Hemangiomas
Disseminated intravascular coagulation

costerone.[541] In these models, red cells have been observed to become enmeshed in fibrin clots, to be adherent to fibrin deposited on vessel walls, and at times to become adherent to damaged endothelium. This red cell adherence, plus the force of blood flow through partially occluded small vessels, leads to shear stresses which cause erythrocyte fragmentation and traumatic hemolysis (Fig. 7–13).[523]

The importance of a careful examination of the peripheral blood smear in any patient with anemia needs repeated emphasis. This simple procedure is particularly valuable in patients with impact hemolysis, in whom the characteristic finding of fragmented and distorted red cells may provide the first clue to the nature of the pathologic mechanism of the anemia and the type of underlying disease. It is important to make the diagnosis of microangiopathic hemolytic anemia not only as a clue to the underlying disease, which may be treated, but also as an indication for heparin therapy, which in some instances may prevent progressive and irreversible impairment of renal function,[519-521] or ameliorate diffuse intravascular coagulation.

INFECTIONS

Hemolytic anemia may be caused by a variety of infections. The acute intravascular hemolysis which occurs in some patients with mycoplasma pneumonia with a high titer of cold agglutinins has been discussed previously in this chapter. As was previously pointed out in the section on glucose–6–phosphate dehydrogenase deficiency, patients with this enzyme deficiency frequently have associated hemolysis with infection, particularly hepatitis, even when no oxidant drugs are administered.[142]

It is not uncommon for malaria to be associated with hemolytic anemia,[547] and in some patients, particularly those taking quinine, the Coombs test has been positive.[544] It is important to distinguish between those patients who have intravascular hemolysis, "blackwater fever," as a result of red cell injury from the malaria parasite (usually *P. falciparium*), and those patients with G–6–PD deficiency who have hemolysis after receiving an oxidant drug like primaquine for the treatment of the disorder.[547] Less commonly, hemolytic anemia has been reported to occur in toxoplasmosis,[555] *Clostridium welchii* infections,[546] cholera,[548] typhoid fever,[560] bartonellosis,[561] and relapsing fever.[545]

Although a relatively large number of bacteria and viruses have been incriminated as possible causative agents in hemolytic anemia, most of the reports are in the older literature and the association is not well documented.

CHEMICAL AGENTS

Therapeutic drugs are not included in this section and have been discussed under drug-induced immune hemolysis and as oxidant agents under glucose–6–phosphate dehydrogenase deficiency.

Arsine gas (AsH_3) exposure, which may occur during the smelting and refining of metals and in forestry workers when arsenic-containing chemicals are used, can cause a severe hemolytic anemia.[552, 554] The stained blood smears show basophilic stippling, anisocytosis, poikilocytosis, and red cell fragments. The unstained smear may show a blue–green cast to the nuclei of the leukocytes.[552] The hemolysis is usually intravascular. The mechanism of the hemolysis is poorly understood, but may involve the production of hydrogen peroxide during the oxidation of arsine and/or the binding of membrane sulfhydryl groups.[552]

Another metal known to produce a hemolytic anemia is copper.[551] Release of inorganic copper into the blood stream in Wilson's disease has been associated with hemolysis,[549] and contamination of the dialysis fluid with copper during hemodialysis has produced acute intravascular hemolysis.[557, 559] Contamination of dialysis fluid by chlorinated water, which leads to the formation of chloramine, an oxidant, has also caused hemolytic anemia.[550]

PHYSICAL AGENTS

Physical impediments to the flow of erythrocytes with resulting trauma and hemolysis by such agents as prosthetic heart valves have been discussed under the section dealing with mechanical hemolysis.

Red cells may also be injured by extensive thermal burns and subsequently

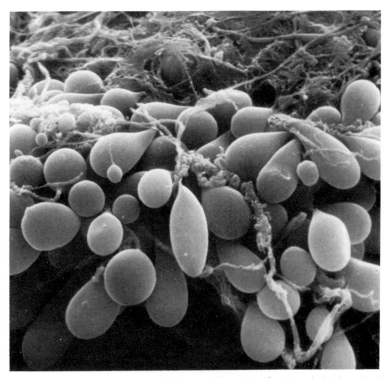

Figure 7–13 Possible mechanism of shistocyte formation. Section of clot from in vitro model showing effect of fibrin strands on red cell. Dense fibrin bonds formed from accumulation of finer strands. Red cells in contact with fibrin are deformed and fragmented. × 5100. Scanning electron microscope. (Prepared By Bull, B. S. personal communication.)

hemolyzed.[562] The blood smear shows many spherocytes, some fragmented cells, there is increased osmotic fragility of the red cells, and intravascular hemolysis with hemoglobinuria may occur.[562] It can be demonstrated both in vitro and in vivo that heating red cells to temperatures above 47° C. causes membrane damage, leading to red cell sphering and decreased survival.[556] The degree of anemia is related to the surface area of the body involved and the severity of the burn.

HYPOPHOSPHATEMIA

Hypophosphatemia may occur as a complication of metabolic acidosis in diabetics and alcoholics. In the presence of profound hypophosphatemia (serum phosphorus less than 1.0 mg. per 100 ml.), hemolytic anemia has been reported.[553, 558] The blood smear of these patients showed microspherocytes, polychromasia, fragmented cells, and target cells. When the low phosphorus was corrected, the hemolysis subsided and the red cell morphology returned to normal. Metabolic studies showed a decrease in red cell ATP and 2,3 diphosphoglycerate, an increase in membrane lipid, and an increase in red cell rigidity.[553, 558] The hemolytic mechanism of the anemia was documented by demonstrating a decreased red cell survival.[553, 558]

References

ERYTHROCYTE METABOLISM AND METHEMOGLOBINEMIA

1. Aebi, H., Heiniger, J. P., and Suter, H.: Some properties of red cells and other tissues from normal and acatalatic humans. Biochem. J., 89:63, 1963.
2. Bartlett, G. R.: Human red cell glycolytic intermediates. J. Biol. Chem., 234:445, 1959.
3. Benesch, R., and Benesch, R. E.: The effect of organic phosphates from the human erythrocyte on the allosteric properties of hemoglobin. Biochem. Biophys. Res. Commun., 26:162, 1967.
4. Berk, P. D., Martin, J. F., Blaschke, T. F., Scharschmidt, B. F., and Plotz, P. H.: Unconjugated hyperbilirubinemia. Ann. Intern. Med., 82:552, 1975.
5. Bucklin, R., and Myint, M. K.: Fatal methemoglobinemia due to well water nitrates. Ann. Intern. Med., 52:703, 1960.
6. Cawein, M., Behlen, C. H. II, Lappat, E. J., and Cohen, J. E.: Hereditary diaphorase deficiency and methemoglobinemia. Arch. Intern. Med., 113:578, 1964.
7. Chanutin, A., and Curnish, R. R.: Effect of organic and inorganic phosphates on the oxygen equilibrium of human erythrocytes. Arch. Biochem. Biophys., 121:96, 1967.
8. Cohen, G., and Hochstein, P.: Glucose-6-phosphate dehydrogenase and detoxification of hydrogen peroxide in human erythrocytes. Science, 134:1756, 1961.
9. Cohen, R. J., Sachs, J. R., Wicker, O. J., and Conrad, M. E.: Methemoglobinemia provoked by malarial chemoprophylaxis in Vietnam. N. Engl. J. Med., 270:1127, 1968.
10. Crosby, W. H., and Akeroyd, J. H.: The limit of hemoglobin synthesis in hereditary hemolytic anemia. Am. J. Med., 13:273, 1952.
11. Delivoria-Papadopoulos, M., Oski, F. A., and Gottlieb, A. J.: Oxygen-hemoglobin dissociation curves: effect of inherited enzyme defects of the red cell. Science, 165:601, 1969.
12. Dunham, P. B., and Gunn, R. B.: Adenosine triphosphatase and active cation transport in red blood cell membranes. Arch. Intern. Med., 129:241, 1972.
13. Fajnhole, N., Condrea, E., and DeVries, A.: Activation of enzymes in red blood cell membranes by a basic protein isolated from cobra venom. Biochim. Biophys. Acta., 255:850, 1972.
14. Finch, C. A.: Methemoglobinemia and sulfhemoglobinemia. N. Engl. J. Med., 239:470, 1948.
15. Firkin, B. G., and Wiley, J. S.: The red cell membrane and its disorders. Progr. Hematol., 5:26, 1966.

16. Gerald, P. S., and George, P.: Second spectroscopically abnormal mehtemoglobin associated with hereditary cyanosis. Science, *129*:393, 1959.
17. Gibson, Q. H., and Harrison, D. C.: Familial idiopathic methaemoglobinemia. Five cases in one family. Lancet, *253*:941, 1947.
18. Guthrow, C. D., Jr., Allen, J. E., and Rasmussen, H.: Phosphorylation of an endogenous membrane protein by an endogenous, membrane-associated cyclic adenosine 3', 5'-monophosphate-dependent protein kinase in human erythrocyte ghosts. J. Biol. Chem., *247*: 8145, 1972.
19. Hoffman, J. F.: The red cell membrane and the transport of sodium and potassium. Am. J. Med., *41*:666, 1966.
20. Huennekens, F. M., Liu, L., Myers, H. A. P., and Gabrio, B. W.: Erythrocyte metabolism. III. Oxidation of glucose. J. Biol. Chem., 227:253, 1957.
21. Jaffé, E. R.: Hereditary methemoglobinemias associated with abnormalities in the metabolism of erythrocytes. Am. J. Med., *41*:786, 1966.
22. Jaffé, E. R., and Heller, P.: Methemoglobinemia in man. Progr. Hematol., *4*:48, 1964.
23. Jaffé, E. R., Neumann, G., Rothberg, H., Wilson, F. T., Webster, R. M., and Wolff, J. A.: Hereditary methemoglobinemia with and without mental retardation. A study of three families. Am. J. Med., *41*:42, 1966.
24. Jandl, J. H.: The Heinz body hemolytic anemias. Ann. Intern. Med., *58*:702, 1963.
25. Jandl, J. H.: Analytical review: leaky red cells. Blood, *26*:367, 1965.
26. LaCelle, P. L.: Alteration of membrane deformability in hemolytic anemia. Semin. Hematol., *7*:355, 1970.
27. Lewis, S. M., Osborn, J. S., and Stuart, P. R.: Demonstration of an internal structure within the red blood cell by ion etching and scanning electron microscopy. Nature, *20*:614, 1968.
28. Liddell, J., and Lehmann, H.: Defects of hemoglobin and of methemoglobin reductase. Ann. N.Y. Acad. Sci., *123*:207, 1965.
29. Lux, S. E., and John, K. M.: Alteration of the physical state of spectrin in ATP-depleted red cells. Blood, *44*:909, 1974.
30. Marchesi, V. T., and Steers, E., Jr.: Selective solubilization of a protein component of the red cell membrane. Science, *159*:203, 1968.
31. Marchesi, V. T., Tillack, T. W., Jackson, R. L., Segrest, J. P., and Scott, R. E.: Chemical characterization and surface orientation of the major glycoprotein of the human erythrocyte membrane. Proc. Natl. Acad. Sci., *69*:1445, 1972.
32. Mills, G. L., and Randall, H. T.: Hemoglobin catabolism. II. The protection of hemoglobin from oxidative breakdown in the intact erythrocyte. J. Biol. Chem., *232*:589, 1958.
33. Murphy, J. R.: Erythrocyte metabolism. II. Glucose metabolism and pathways. J. Lab. Clin. Med., *55*:286, 1960.
34. Murphy, J. R.: Erythrocyte metabolism. V. Active cation transport and glycosis. J. Lab. Clin. Med., *61*:567, 1963.
35. Nakao, M., Nakao, T., Yamazoe, S., and Yoshikawa, H.: Adenosine triphosphate and shape of erythrocytes. J. Biochem., *49*:487, 1961.
36. Necheles, T. F., Maldonado, N., Barquet-Chediak, A., and Allen, D. M.: Homozygous erythrocyte glutathione-peroxidase deficiency: clinical and biochemical studies. Blood, *33*:164, 1969.
37. Oski, F. A., Gottlieb, A. J., Delivioria-Papadopoulous, M., and Miller, W. W.: Red-cell 2,3-diphosphoglycerate levels in subjects with chronic hypoxemia. N. Engl. J. Med., *280*: 1165, 1969.
38. Rifkind, R. A.: Destruction of injured red cells in vivo. Am. J. Med., *41*:711, 1966.
39. Rifkind, R. A., and Davon, D.: Heinz body anemia—an ultrastructural study. I. Heinz body formation. Blood, *25*:885, 1965.
40. Robertson, J. D.: The structure of biological membranes. Arch. Intern. Med., *129*:202, 1972.
41. Schrier, S. L.: Organization of enzymes in human erythrocyte membranes. Am. J. Physiol., *210*:139, 1966.
42. Scott, E. M.: The relation of diaphorase of human erythrocytes to inheritance of methemoglobinemia. J. Clin. Invest., *39*:1176, 1960.
43. Scott, E. M., and McGraw, J. C.: Purification and properties of diphosphopyridine nucleotide diaphorase of human erythrocytes. J. Biol. Chem., *237*:249, 1962.
44. Singer, K.: Hereditary hemolytic disorders associated with abnormal hemoglobins. Am. J. Med., *18*:633, 1955.
45. Singer, S. J.: The molecular organization of membranes. Ann. Rev. Biochem., *43*:805, 1974.
46. Singer, S. J., and Nicholson, G. L.: The fluid mosaic model of the structure of cell membranes. Science, *175*:720, 1972.
47. Solomon, A. K.: Red cell membrane structure and ion transport. J. Gen. Physiol., *43*:1, 1960.
48. Steinberg, M., Brauer, M. J., and Necheles, T. F.: Acute hemolytic anemia associated with erythrocyte glulathione-peroxidase deficiency. Arch. Intern. Med., *25*:302, 1970.

49. Steinberg, M. H., and Necheles, T. F.: Red blood cell glutathione peroxidase deficiency. Biochemical studies on the mechanism of drug-induced hemolysis. Am. J. Med., *50*:542, 1971.
50. Ternberg, J. L., and Luce, E.: Methemoglobinemia: a complication of silver nitrate treatment of burns. Surgery, *63*:328, 1968.
51. Townes, P. L., and Lovell, G. R.: Hereditary methemoglobinemia: a new variant exhibiting dominant inheritance of methemoglobin A. Blood, *18*:18, 1961.
52. Townes, P. L., and Morrison, M.: Investigation of the defect in a variant of hereditary methemoglobinemia. Blood, *19*:60, 1962.
53. Valberg, L. S., Holt, J. M., Paulson, E., and Szivek, J.: Spectrochemical analysis of sodium, potassium, calcium, magnesium, copper, and zinc in normal human erythrocytes. J. Clin. Invest., *44*:379, 1965.
54. Weed, R. I.: The importance of erythrocyte deformability. Am. J. Med., *49*:147, 1970.
55. Weed, R. I., LaCelle, P. L., and Merrill, E. W.: Metabolic dependence of red cell deformability. J. Clin. Invest., *48*:795, 1969.
56. Weinstein, R. S.: The structure of cell membranes. N. Engl. J. Med., *281*:86, 1969.
57. Weinstein, R. S., and McNutt, N. S.: Ultrastructure of red cell membranes. Semin. Hematol., *7*:259, 1970.
58. Weiss, L., and Tavassoli, M.: Anatomical hazards to the passage of erythrocytes through the spleen. Semin. Hematol., *7*:372, 1970.
59. Whittam, R.: Transport and Diffusion in Red Blood Cells. Edward Arnold Ltd., London, 1964.

HEREDITARY SPHEROCYTOSIS AND OTHER ERYTHROCYTE MEMBRANE DEFECTS

60. Austin, R. F., and Desforges, J. F.: Hereditary elliptocytosis: an unusual presentation of hemolysis in the newborn associated with transient morphologic abnormalities. Pediatrics, *44*:196, 1969.
61. Baker, S. J., Jacob, E., Rajan, K. T., and Gault, E. W.: Hereditary haemolytic anaemia associated with elliptocytosis: a study of three families. Br. J. Haematol., *7*:210, 1961.
62. Bannerman, R. M., and Renwick, J. A.: The hereditary elliptocytoses; clinical and linkage data. Ann. Hum. Genet., *26*:23, 1962.
63. Bates, G. C., and Brown, C. H.: Incidence of gallbladder disease in chronic hemolytic anemia (spherocytosis). Gastroenterology, *21*:104, 1952.
64. Bertles, J. F.: Sodium transport across the surface membrane of red blood cells in hereditary spherocytosis. J. Clin. Invest., *36*:816, 1957.
65. Burman, D.: Congenital spherocytosis in infancy. Arch. Dis. Child., *33*:335, 1958.
66. Butterworth, C. E., Kracke, R. R., and Riser, W. H., Jr.: Hereditary spherocytic anemia in the Negro. Blood, *5*:793, 1950.
67. Chapman, R. G.: Red cell life span after splenectomy in hereditary spherocytosis. J. Clin. Invest., *47*:2263, 1968.
68. Chauffard, A.: Pathogenie de l'ictère congénital des adults. Sem. Med., *27*:25, 1907.
69. Chauffard, A., and Fiessinger, N.: Ictère congénital hémolytique avec lesions globulaires. Bull. Mem. Soc. Med. Hop. Paris, *24*:1169, 1907.
70. Cooper, R. A., and Jandl, J. H.: The role of membrane lipids in the survival of red cells in hereditary spherocytosis. J. Clin. Invest., *48*:736, 1969.
71. Crosby, W. H., and Conrad, M. E.: Hereditary spherocytosis: observations on hemolytic mechanisms and iron metabolism. Blood, *15*:662, 1960.
72. Cutting, H. O., McHugh, W. J., Conrad, F. G., and Marlow, A. A.: Autosomal dominant hemolytic anemia characterized by ovalocytosis. Am. J. Med., *39*:21, 1965.
73. Dacie, J. V.: Familial haemolytic anaemia (acholuric jaundice), with particular reference to changes in fragility produced by splenectomy. Q. J. Med., *36*:101, 1943.
74. Dacie, J. V.: The congenital anaemias. Part I in The Haemolytic Anaemias: Congenital and Acquired. 2nd Ed. Grune & Stratton, New York, 1960.
75. Dacie, J. V., and Mollison, P. L.: Survival of normal erythrocytes after transfusion to patients with familial hemolytic anaemia. Lancet, *1*:550, 1943.
76. DeGier, J., Ban Deenen, L. L. M., Verloop, M. L., and Van Gastel, Z.: Phospholidid and fatty acid characteristics of erythrocytes in some cases of anemia. Br. J. Haematol., *10*:246, 1964.
77. deGruchy, G. C., Loder, P. B., and Hennesy, I. V.: Haemolysis and glycolytic metabolism in hereditary elliptocytosis. Br. J. Haematol., *8*:168, 1962.

78. Douglass, L. L., and Twomey, J. J.: Transient stomatocytosis with hemolysis: a previously unrecognized complication of alcoholism. Ann. Intern. Med., 72:159, 1970.

79. Dresbach, M.: Elliptical human red corpuscles. Science, 19:469, 1904.

80. Dreyfus, C.: Chronic hemolytic jaundice. Bull. N. Engl. Med. Center, 4:122, 1942.

81. Ducrou, W., and Kimber, R. J.: Stomatocytes, haemolytic anaemia and abdominal pain in Mediterranean migrants. Med. J. Aust., 2:1087, 1969.

82. Emerson, C. P.: Influence of the spleen on the osmotic behavior and the longevity of red cells in heriditary spherocytosis: a case study. Boston Med. Q., 5:65, 1954.

83. Emerson, C. P., Jr., Shenn, S. C., Ham, T. H., and Castle, W. B.: The mechanism of blood destruction in congenital hemolytic jaundice. J. Clin. Invest., 26:1180, 1947.

84. Gjone, E., Torsvik, H., and Norum, K. R.: Familial plasma cholesterol ester deficiency: a study of the erythrocytes. Scand. J. Clin. Lab. Invest., 21:327, 1968.

85. Glader, B. E., Fortier, N., Albala, M. M., and Nathan, D. G.: Congenital hemolytic anemia associated with dehydrated erythrocytes and increased potassium loss. N. Engl. J. Med., 291:491, 1974.

86. Greenquist, A., and Shohet, S. B.: ATP dependent phosphorylation of membrane protein in normal and hereditary spherocytosis red cells. Blood, 42:997, 1973.

87. Haden, R. L.: The mechanism of the increased fragility of the erythrocytes in congenital hemolytic jaundice. Am. J. Med. Sci., 188:441, 1934.

88. Ham, T. H., and Castle, W. B.: Relation of increased hypotonic fragility and erythrostasis to the mechanism of hemolysis in certain anemias. Tr. Assoc. Am. Physicians, 55:127, 1940.

89. Harris, E. J., and Prankerd, T. A.: The rate of sodium extrusion from human erythrocytes. J. Physiol., 121:470, 1953.

90. Heilmeyer, L.: Spherocytosis as a manifestation of pathological spleen function. Dtsch. Arch. Klin. Med., 179:292, 1940.

91. Jackson, J. M., and Knight, D.: Stomatocytosis in migrants of Mediterranean origin. Med. J. Aust., 1:939, 1969.

92. Jacob, H. S.: Abnormalities in the physiology of the erythrocyte membrane in hereditary spherocytosis. Am. J. Med., 41:734, 1966.

93. Jacob, H. S.: The abnormal red-cell membrane in hereditary spherocytosis: evidence for the causal role of mutant microfilaments. Br. J. Haematol., 23(Suppl):35, 1972.

94. Jacob, J. S., and Jandl, J. H.: Increased cell membrane permeability in the pathogenesis of hereditary spherocytosis. J. Clin. Invest., 43:1704, 1964.

95. Jacob, H. S., Yawata, Y., Matsumoto, N., Abman, S., and White, J.: Cyclic nucleotide-membrane protein interaction in the regulation of erythrocyte shape and survival: Defect in hereditary spherocytosis. Erythrocyte Structure and Function. Brewer G. J. Ed., Alan R. Liss, Inc., New York, 1975, p. 235.

96. Jaffé, E. R., and Gottfried, E. L.: Hereditary nonspherocytic hemolytic disease associated with altered phospholipid composition of erythrocytes. J. Clin. Invest., 47:1375, 1968.

97. Jandl, J. H.: Hereditary Spherocytosis. In Beutler, E. (ed.): Hereditary Disorders of Erythrocyte Metabolism. Grune & Stratton, New York, 1968.

98. Jandl, J. H., and Aster, R. H.: Increased splenic pooling and the pathogenesis of hypersplenism. Am. J. Med. Sci., 253:383, 1967.

99. Jandl, J. H., Simmons, R. L., and Castle, W. B.: Red cell filtration and the pathogenesis of certain hemolytic anemias. Blood, 18:133, 1961.

100. LaCelle, P. L., and Weed, R. I.: Abnormal membrane deformability. A model for the hereditary spherocyte. J. Clin. Invest., 48:48a, 1969.

101. Lock, S. P., Smith, R. S., and Hardisty, R. M.: Stomatocytosis: a hereditary red cell anomaly associated with haemolytic anaemia. Br. J. Haematol., 7:303, 1961.

102. Meadow, S. R.: Stomatocytosis. Proc. Roy. Soc. Med., 60:13, 1967.

103. Miller, D. R., Rickles, F. R., Lichtman, M. A., LaCelle, P. L., Bates, J., and Weed, R. I.: A new variant of hereditary hemolytic anemia with stomatocytosis and erythrocyte cation abnormality. Blood, 38:184, 1971.

104. Mohler, D. N.: Adenosine triphosphate metabolism in hereditary spherocytosis. J. Clin. Invest., 44:1417, 1965.

105. Morton, N. E., MacKinney, A. A., Kosower, N., Schilling, R. F., and Gray, M. P.: Genetics of spherocytosis. Am. J. Hum. Genet., 14:170, 1962.

106. Norman, J. G.: Stomatocytosis in migrants of Mediterranean origin. Med. J. Aust., 1315, 1969.

107. Oski, F. A., Naiman, J. L., Blum, S. F., Zarkowsky, H. S., Whaun, J., Shohet, S. B., Green, A., and Nathan, D. G.: Congenital hemolytic anemia with high-sodium, low-potassium red cells. N. Engl. J. Med., 280:909, 1969.

108. Owren, P. A.: Congenital hemolytic jaundice. The pathogenesis of the "hemolytic crisis." Blood, 3:231, 1948.

109. Ozer, F. L., and Mills, G. L.: Elliptocytosis with haemolytic anemia. Br. J. Haematol., *10*: 468, 1964.
110. Pearson, H. A.: The genetic basis of hereditary elliptocytosis with hemolysis. Blood, *32*:972, 1968.
111. Rebuck, J. W., and Van Slyck, E. J.: An unsuspected ultrastructural fault in human ellipto-cytes. Am. J. Clin. Pathol., *49*:19, 1968.
112. Reed, C. F., and Swisher, S. N.: Erythrocyte lipid loss in hereditary spherocytosis. J. Clin. Invest., *45*:777, 1966.
113. Shohet, S. B., Nathan, D. G., Livermore, B. M., Feig, S. A., and Jaffé, E. R.: Hereditary hemo-lytic anemia associated with abnormal membrane lipid. II. Ion permeability and transport abnormalities. Blood, *42*:1, 1973.
114. Taylor, E. S.: Chronic ulcer of the leg associated with congenital hemolytic jaundice. J.A.M.A., *112*:1575, 1939.
115. Torlontano, G., Fontana, L., De Laurenzi, A., Papa, G., and Proietti, M.: Hereditary ellipto-cytosis. Acta Haematol., *48*:1, 1972.
116. Torsvik, H., Gjone, E., and Norum, K. R.: Familial plasma cholesterol ester deficiency. Clinical studies in a family. Acta Med. Scand., *183*:387, 1968.
117. Weed, R. I., and Bowdler, A. J.: Metabolic dependence of the critical hemolytic volume of human erythrocytes: relationship to osmotic fragility and autohemolysis in hereditary spherocytosis and normal red cells. J. Clin. Invest., *45*:1137, 1966.
118. Weed, R. I., and Reed, C. F.: Membrane alterations leading to red cell destruction. Am. J. Med., *41*:681, 1966.
119. Weiss, H. J.: Hereditary elliptocytosis with hemolytic anemia. Am. J. Med., *35*:455, 1963.
120. Wiley, J. S., Ellroy, J. C., Shuman, M. A., Shaller, C. C., and Cooper, R. A.: Characteristics of the membrane defect in the hereditary stomatocytosis syndrome. Blood, *46*:337, 1975.
121. Young, L. E.: Hereditary spherocytosis. Am. J. Med., *18*:486, 1955.
122. Young, L. E., Izzo, M. J., and Platzer, R. F.: Hereditary spherocytosis. I. Clinical hematologic and genetic features in 28 cases with particular reference to the osmotic and mechanical fragility of incubated erythrocytes. Blood, *6*:1073, 1951.
123. Zarkowski, H. S., Oski, F. A., Shaafi, R., Shohet, S. B., and Nathan, D. G.: Congenital hemolytic anemia with high sodium, low potassium red cells. I. Studies of membrane permeability. N. Engl. J. Med., *278*:573, 1968.
124. Zipursky, A., Peters, J. C., Rowland, M. R., and Israels. L. G.: An abnormality in erythrocyte sodium transport in hereditary elliptocytosis. J. Pediatr., *67*:939, 1965.

Enzyme deficiency hemolytic anemia

125. Arnold, H., Blume, K-G., Engelhardt, R., and Lohr, G. W.: Glucosephosphate isomerase de-ficiency. Evidence for in vivo instability of an enzyme variant with hemolysis. Blood, *41*:691, 1973.
126. Baughan, M. A., Valentine, W. N., Paglia, D. W., Ways, P. O., Simons, E. R., and DeMarsh, Q. B.: Hereditary hemolytic anemia associated with glucose phosphate isomerase (GPI) deficiency—a new enzyme defect of human erythrocytes. Blood, *32*:236, 1968.
127. Beutler, E.: Glucose-6-phosphate Dehydrogenase Deficiency. *In* Stanbury, J. B., Wyngaarden, J. B., and Frederikson, D. S. (eds.): The Metabolic Basis of Inherited Disease. 3rd Ed. McGraw-Hill, New York, 1972.
128. Beutler, E.: Effect of flavin compounds on glutathione reductase activity: in vivo and in vitro studies. J. Clin. Invest., *48*:1957, 1969.
129. Beutler, E.: A series of new screening procedures for pyruvate kinase deficiency, glucose-6-phosphate dehydrogenase deficiency, and glutathione reductase deficiency. Blood, *28*:553, 1966.
130. Beutler, E.: Abnormalities of the hexose monophosphate shunt. Semin. Hematol., *8*:311, 1971.
131. Beutler, E., Dern, R. J., and Alving, A. S.: The hemolytic effect of primaquine. IV. The relationship of cell age to hemolysis. J. Lab. Clin. Med., *44*:439, 1954.
132. Beutler, E., Dern, R. J., and Alving, A. S.: The hemolytic effect of primaquine. VI. An in vitro test for sensitivity of erythrocytes to primaquine. J. Lab. Clin. Med., *45*:40, 1955.
133. Beutler, E., Scott, S., Bishop, A., and Margolis, N.: Red cells aldolase deficiency and hemolytic anemia; a new syndrome. Clin. Res., *21*:727, 1972. Abstr.
134. Beutler, E., Sigalore, W. H., Muir, W. A., Matsumoto, F., and West, C.: Glucose-P-isomerase (GPI) deficiency: GPI Elyria. Ann. Intern. Med., *80*:730, 1974.
135. Boivin, P., Galand, C., André, R., and Debray, J.: Anémies hémolytiques congénitales avec déficit isolé en glutathion réduit par déficit en glutathione synthétase. Nouv. Rev. Fr. Hematol.. *6*:859, 1966.

136. Boivin, P., Galand, C., Hakim, J., and Gueroult, N.: Anémie hémolytique avec déficit en-glutathione-peroxydase chez un adulte. Enzymol. Biol. Clin., *10*:68, 1969.

137. Boivin, P., Galand, C., Hakim, J., Simony, D., and Seligman, M.: Une nouvelle erythro-enzymopathie. Anemie hemolytique congenitale non spherocytaire et deficit hereditaire en adenylate-kinase erythrocytaire. Presse Med., *79*:215, 1971.

138. Bowdler, A. J., and Prankerd, T. A. J.: Studies in congenital nonspherocytic haemolytic anaemias with specific enzyme defects. Acta Haematol., *31*:65, 1964.

139. Bowman, H. S., and Procopio, F.: Hereditary non-spherocytic hemolytic anemia of the pyruvate-kinase deficient type. Ann. Intern. Med., *58*:567, 1963.

140. Brewer, G. J., and Dern, P. J.: A new inherited enzymatic deficiency of human erythrocytes: 6-phosphogluconate dehydrogenase deficiency. Am. J. Hum. Genet., *16*:472, 1964.

141. Brewer, G. J., Tarlov, A. R., and Alving, A. S.: Methemoglobin reduction test: a new simple in vitro test for identifying primaquine sensitivity. Bull. W. H. O., *22*:633, 1960.

142. Burka, E. R.: Infectious disease: a cause of hemolytic anemia in glucose-6-phosphate dehydro-genase deficiency. Ann. Intern. Med., *70*:222, 1969.

143. Burka, E. R., Weaver, Z. III., and Marks, P. A.: Clinical spectrum of hemolytic anemia associ-ated with glucose-6-phosphate dehydrogenase deficiency. Ann. Intern. Med., *64*:817, 1966.

144. Carson, P. E., Brewer, G. J., and Ickes, C. E.: Decreased glutathione reductase with suscepti-bility to hemolysis. J. Lab. Clin. Med., *58*:804, 1961.

145. Carson, P. E., Flanagan, C. L., Ickes, C. E., and Alving, A. S.: Enzymatic deficiency in primaquine-sensitive erythrocytes. Science, *24*:484, 1956.

146. Carson, P. E., and Frischer, H.: Glucose-6-phosphate dehydrogenase deficiency and related disorders of the pentose phosphate pathway. Am. J. Med., *41*:744, 1966.

147. Childs, B., Zinkham, W., Browne, E. A., Kimbro, E. L., and Torbert, J. V.: A genetic study of a defect in glutathione metabolism of the erythrocyte. Johns Hopkins Med. J., *102*:21, 1958.

148. Cooper, M. R., De Chatelet, L. R., McCall, C. E., La Vior, M. F., Spurr, C. L., and Balhner, R. L.: Complete deficiency of leukocyte glucose-6-phosphate dehydrogenase with defec-tive bactericidal activity. J. Clin. Invest., *51*:759, 1972.

149. Cordes, W.: Experiences with plasmochin in malaria: preliminary reports. 15th Annual Report, United Fruit Co., 1926.

150. Dacie, J. V., Mollison, P. L., Richardson, N., Selwyn, J. G., and Shapiro, L.: Atypical congenital hemolytic anemia. Q. J. Med., *22*:79, 1953.

151. de Gruchy, G. C., Santamaria, J. N., Parson, I. C., and Crawford, H.: Nonspherocytic congeni-tal hemolytic anemia. Blood, *16*:1371, 1960.

152. Dern, R. J., Beutler, E., and Alving, A. S.: The hemolytic effect of primaquine. II. The natural course of the hemolytic anemia and the mechanism of its self-limited character. J. Lab. Clin. Med., *44*:171, 1954.

153. Dern, R. J., Weinstein, I. M., LeRoy, G. V., Talmage, D. W., and Alving, A. S.: The hemolytic effect of primaquine. I. The localization of the drug-induced hemolytic defect in prima-quine-sensitive individuals. J. Lab. Clin. Med., *43*:303, 1954.

154. Earle, D. P., Jr., Bigelow, F. S., Zubrod, C. G., and Kane, C. A.: Studies on the chemotherapy of the human malarias. IX. Effect of primaquine on the blood cells of man. J. Clin. Invest., *27*:121(suppl.), 1948.

155. Gant, F. L., and Winks, G. F., Jr.: Primaquine sensitive hemolytic anemia complicating diabetic acidosis. Clin. Res., *9*:27, 1961. Abstr.

156. Hanel, H. K., and Cohn, J.: Adenosine-triphosphatase deficiency in a family with non-spherocytic haemolytic anaemia. Scand. J. Haematol., *9*:28, 1972.

157. Harkness, D. R.: A new erythrocytic enzyme defect with hemolytic anemia: glyceraldehyde-3-phosphate dehydrogenase deficiency. J. Lab. Clin. Med., *68*:879, 1966.

158. Harvald, B., Hanel, K. H., Squires, R., and Trap-Jensen, J.: Adenosine-triphosphatase de-ficiency in patients with nonspherocytic haemolytic anaemia. Lancet, *2*:18, 1964.

159. Hockwald, R. S., Arnold, J., Clayman, C. B., and Alving, A. S.: Status of primaquine. IV. Toxicity of primaquine in Negroes, J.A.M.A., *149*:1568, 1952.

160. Hsu, T. H. J., Robinson, A. R., and Zuelzer, W. W.: Genetic polymorphism of hemolytic anemia associated with erythrocyte pyruvic kinase deficiency. Blood, *28*:977, 1966 Abstr.

161. Jacob, H. S., and Jandl, J. H.: Screening test for glucose-6-phosphate dehydrogenase de-ficiency. N. Engl. J. Med., *274*:1162, 1966.

162. Jaffé, E. R.: Clinical profile: hereditary hemolytic disorders and enzymatic deficiencies of human erythrocytes. Blood, *35*:116, 1970.

163. Kattamis, C. A., Kyriazakou, M., and Chaidas, S.: Favism. Clinical and biochemical data. J. Med. Genet., *6*:34, 1969.

164. Keitt, A. S.: Pyruvate kinase deficiency and related disorders of red cell glycolysis. Am. J. Med., *41*:762, 1966.

165. Keitt, A. S.: Hemolytic anemia with impaired hexokinase activity. J. Clin. Invest., *48*:1997, 1969.
166. Kellermeyer, R. W.: Drugs and G-6-PD Deficiency of Red Cells. *In* Dimitrov, N. V., and Nodine, J. H. (eds.): Drugs and Hematologic Reactions. Grune and Stratton, 1974.
167. Kirkman, H. N., Kidson, C., and Kennedy, M.: Variants of human glucose-6-phosphate dehydrogenase. Studies of Samples from New Guinea. *In* Beutler, E. (ed.): Hereditary Disorders of Erythrocyte Metabolism. Grune & Stratton, New York, 1968.
168. Konrad, P. N., Richards, F. II, Valentine, W. N., and Paglia, D. E.: α-glutamyl-cysteine synthetase deficiency: a cause of hereditary hemolytic anemia. N. Engl. J. Med., *286*:557, 1972.
169. Kraus, A. P., Langston, M. F., Jr., and Lynch, B. L.: Red cell phosphoglycerate kinase deficiency. A new cause of non-spherocytic hemolytic anemia. Biochem. Biophys. Res. Commun., *30*:173, 1968.
170. Luzzatto, L.: Inherited haemolytic states: glucose-6-phosphate dehydrogenase deficiency. Clin. Haematol., *4*:83, 1975.
171. Luzzatto, K., Usanga, E. A., and Reddy, S.: Glucose-6-phosphate dehydrogenase deficient red cells: resistance to infection by malarial parasites. Science, *164*:839, 1969.
172. Mentzer, W. C., Jr., Baehner, R. L., Schmidt-Schonbein, H., Robinson, S. H., and Nathan, D. G.: Selective reticulocyte destruction in erythrocyte pyruvate kinase deficiency. J. Clin. Invest., *50*:688, 1971.
173. Mohler, D. N., and Crockett, C. L., Jr.: Hereditary hemolytic disease secondary to glucose-6-phosphate dehydrogenase deficiency: report of three cases with special emphasis on ATP metabolism. Blood, *23*:427, 1964.
174. Mohler, D. N., Majerus, P. W., Minnich, V., Hess, C. E., and Garrick, M. D.: Glutathione synthetase deficiency as a cause of hereditary hemolytic disease. N. Engl. J. Med., *283*:1253, 1970.
175. Necheles, T. F., Rai, U. S., and Cameron, D.: Congenital non-spherocytic hemolytic anemia associated with unusual erythrocyte hexokinase abnormality. J. Lab. Clin. Med., *76*:593, 1970.
176. Oski, F. A., Nathan, D. G., Sidel, V. W., and Diamond, L. K.: Extreme hemolysis and red-cell distortion in erythrocyte pyruvate kinase deficiency. N. Engl. J. Med., *270*:1023, 1964.
177. Oski, F. A., and Whaun, J. M.: Hemolytic anemia and red cell glyceraldehyde-3-phosphate dehydrogenase deficiency. Clin. Res., *17*:601, 1969. Abstr.
178. Paglia, D. E., Holland, P., Baughan, M. A., and Valentine, W. N.: Occurrence of defective hexosephosphate isomerization in human erythrocytes and leukocytes. N. Engl. J. Med., *280*:66, 1969.
179. Phillips, S. M., and Silvers, N. P.: Glucose-6-phosphate dehydrogenase deficiency, infectious hepatitis, acute hemolysis, and renal failure. Ann. Intern. Med., *70*:99, 1969.
180. Prins, H. K., Oort, M., Looms, J. A., Zürcher, C., and Beckers, T.: Congenital nonspherocytic hemolytic anemia associated with glutathione deficiency of the erythrocytes. Hematologic, biochemical and genetic studies. Blood, *27*:145, 1966.
181. Ramot, B., Fisher, S., Szeinberg, A., Adam, A., Sheba, C., and Gafni, D.: A study of subjects with erythrocyte glucose-6-phosphate dehydrogenase deficiency. II Investigation of leukocyte enzymes. J. Clin. Invest., *38*:2234, 1959.
182. Ramot, B., Szeinberg, A., Adam, A., Sheba, C., and Gafni, D.: A study of subjects with erythrocyte glucose-6-phosphate dehydrogenase deficiency. Investigation of platelet enzymes. J. Clin. Invest., *38*:1659, 1959.
183. Salen, G., Goldstein, F., Haurani, F., and Werts, C. W.: Acute hemolytic anemia complicating viral hepatitis in patients with glucose-6-phosphate dehydrogenase deficiency. Ann. Intern. Med., *65*:1210, 1966.
184. Salvidio, E., Pannacciulli, I., Tizianello, A., and Ajmar, F.: Nature of hemolytic crises and the fate of G6PD deficient drug-damaged erythrocytes in Sardinians. N. Engl. J. Med., *276*:1339, 1967.
185. Schneider, A. S., Valentine, W. N., Baughan, M. A., Paglia, D. E., Shore, N. A., and Heins, H. L., Jr.: Triosephosphate Isomerase Deficiency. A Multisystem Inherited Enzyme Disorder. Clinical and Genetic Aspects. *In* Beutler, E. (ed.): Hereditary Disorders of Erythrocyte Metabolism. Grune & Stratton, New York, 1968.
186. Schneider, A. S., Valentine, W. N., Hattori, M., and Heins, H. L., Jr.: Hereditary hemolytic anemia with triosephosphate isomerase deficiency. N. Engl. J. Med., *272*:299, 1965.
187. Selwyn, J. G., and Dacie, J. V.: Autohemolysis and other changes resulting from the incubation in vitro of red cells from patients with congenital hemolytic anemia. Blood, *9*:414, 1954.
188. Sparkes, R. S., Carrel, R. E., and Paglia, D. E.: Probable localization of a triosephosphate isomerase gene to the short arm of the number 5 human chromosome. Nature, *224*:367, 1969.

189. Stefanini, M.: Chronic hemolytic anemia associated with erythrocyte enolase deficiency exacerbated by ingestion of nitrofurantoin. Am. J. Clin. Pathol., *58*:408, 1972.
190. Szeinberg, A., Kahawa, D., Gavendo, S., Zaidman, J., and Ben-Ezzer, J.: Hereditary deficiency of adenylate kinase in red blood cells. Acta Haematol., *42*:111, 1969.
191. Tanaka, K. R., and Paglia, D. E.: Pyruvate kinase deficiency. Semin. Hematol., *8*:367, 1971.
192. Tanaka, K. R., and Valentine, W. N.: Pyruvate Kinase Deficiency. *In* Beutler, E. (ed.): Hereditary Disorders of Erythrocyte Metabolism. Grune & Stratton, New York, 1968.
193. Tanaka, K. R., Valentine, W. N., and Miwa, S.: Pyruvate kinase (PK) deficiency hereditary nonspherocytic hemolytic anemia. Blood, *19*:267, 1962.
194. Tarlov, A. R., Brewer, G. J., Carson, P. E., and Alving, A. S.: Primaquine sensitivity. Arch. Intern. Med., *109*:209, 1962.
195. Tarui, S., Kono, N., Nasu, T., and Nishikawa, M.: Enzymatic basis for the coexistence of myopathy and hemolytic disease in inherited muscle phosphofructose kinase deficiency. Biochem. Biophys. Res. Commun., *34*:77, 1969.
196. Twomey, J. J., O'Neal, F. B., Alfrey, C. P., and Moser, R. H.: ATP metabolism in pyruvate kinase deficient erythrocytes. Blood, *30*:576, 1967.
197. Valentine, W. N.: Deficiencies associated with Embden-Meyerhof pathway and other metabolic pathways. Semin. Hematol., *8*:348, 1971.
198. Valentine, W. N., Bennett, J. M., Krivit, W., Konrad, P. N., Lowman, J. T., Paglia, D. E., and Wakem, C. J.: Hereditary hemolytic anemia with increased red cell adenine nucleotides, glutathione and basophilic stippling and ribosphosphate pyrophosphokinase (RPK) deficiency: studies on two new kindreds. Br. J. Haematol., *24*:157, 1973.
199. Valentine, W. N., Hsieh, H. S., Paglia, D. E., Anderson, H. M., Baughan, M. A., Jaffé, E. R., and Garson, O. M.: Hereditary hemolytic anemia associated with phosphoglycerate kinase deficiency in erythrocytes and leukocytes. A probable x-chromosome-linked syndrome. N. Engl. J. Med., *280*:528, 1969.
200. Valentine, W. N., and Kurschner, K. K.: Studies on human erythrocyte nucleotide metabolism. Blood, *39*:666, 1972.
201. Valentine, W. N., Oski, F. A., Paglia, D. E., Baughan, M. A., Schneider, A. S., and Nauman, J. L.: Hereditary hemolytic anemia with hexokinase deficiency. Role of hexokinase in erythrocyte aging. N. Engl. J. Med., *276*:1, 1967.
202. Valentine, W. N., and Tanaka, K. R.: Pyruvate Kinase Deficiency Hereditary Hemolytic Anemia. *In* Stanbury, J. B. et al. (eds.): The Metabolic Basis of Inherited Disease. 3rd Ed. McGraw-Hill, Inc., New York, 1972.
203. Valentine, W. N., Tanaka, K. R., and Miwa, S.: A specific erythrocyte glycolytic enzyme defect (pyruvate kinase) in three subjects with congenital non-spherocytic hemolytic anemia. Tr. Assoc. Am. Physicians, *74*:100, 1961.
204. Waller, H. D.: Glutathione Reductase Deficiency. *In* Beutler, E. (ed.): Hereditary Disorders of Erythrocyte Metabolism. Grune & Stratton, New York, 1968.
205. Waterbury, L., and Frenkel, E. P.: Hereditary nonspherocytic hemolysis with erythrocyte phosphofructokinase deficiency. Blood, *39*:415, 1972.
206. Yoshida, A.: The Structure of Normal and Variant Human Glucose-6-phosphate Dehydrogenase. *In* Beutler, E. (ed.): Hereditary Disorders of Erythrocyte Metabolism. Grune & Stratton, New York, 1968.
207. Yoshida, A.: Hemolytic anemia and glucose-6-phosphate dehydrogenase deficiency. Science, *179*:532, 1973.
208. Yoshida, A., Beutler, E., and Motulsky, A.: Table of human glucose-6-phosphate dehydrogenase variants. Bull. W. H. O., 1971.
209. Zuelzer, W. W., Robinson, A. R., and Hsu, T. H. J.: Erythrocyte pyruvate kinase deficiency in nonspherocytic hemolytic anemia: a system of multiple genetic markers? Blood, *32*:33, 1968.

SICKLE CELL ANEMIA

210. Allen, T. D.: Sickle cell disease and hematuria: a report of cases. J. Urol., *91*:177, 1964.
211. Barnes, P. M.: Hendrickse, R. G., and Watson-Williams, E. J.: Low molecular weight dextran in treatment of bone pain crises in sickle cell disease—a double-blind trial. Lancet, *2*:1271, 1965.
212. Barreras, L., Diggs, L. W., and Bell, A.: Erythrocyte morphology in patients with sickle cell anemia and pulmonary emboli. J.A.M.A., *203*:569, 1968.
213. Barrett-Connor, E.: Cholelithiasis in sickle cell anemia. Am. J. Med., *45*:889, 1968.
214. Bell, W. R., and Pitney, W. R.: Management of priapism by therapeutic defibrination. N. Engl. J. Med., *280*:649, 1969.

215. Bernstein, J., and Whitten, C. F.: A histologic appraisal of the kidney in sickle cell anemia. Arch. Pathol., *70*:407, 1960.
216. Brody, J. I., Goldsmith, M. H., Parks, S. K., and Soltys, H. D.: Symptomatic crises of sickle cell anemia treated by limited exchange transfusion. Ann. Intern. Med., *72*:327, 1970.
217. Callender, S. T. E., and Nickel, J. F.: Survival of transfused sickle cells in normal subjects and of normal red blood cells in patients with sickle cell anemia. J. Lab. Clin. Med., *32*:1397, 1947.
218. Callender, S. T. E., Nickel, J. F., Moore, C. V., and Powell, E. O.: Sickle cell disease: studied by measuring the survival of transfused red blood cells. J. Lab. Clin. Med., *34*:90, 1949.
219. Cerami, A., and Manning, J. M.: Potassium cyanate as an inhibitor of the sickling of erythrocytes in vitro. Proc. Natl. Acad. Sci., U.S.A., *68*:1180, 1971.
220. Charache, S., and Page, D. L.: Infarction of bone marrow in the sickle-cell disorders. Ann. Intern. Med., *67*:1195, 1967.
221. Charache, S., and Richardson, S. N.: Prolonged survival of a patient with sickle cell anemia. Arch. Intern. Med., *113*:844, 1964.
222. Clinicopathologic conference, a patient with sickle cell anemia surviving forty-eight years. Am. J. Med., *48*:226, 1970.
223. Cooperative urea trial group: Clinical trials of therapy for sickle cell vasoocclusive crises. J.A.M.A., *228*:1120, 1974.
224. Cooperative urea trial group: Treatment of sickle cell crises with urea in invert sugar. J.A.M.A., *228*:1125, 1974.
225. Diggs, L. W.: The sickle cell phenomenon. The rate of sickling in moist preparations. J. Lab. Clin. Med., *17*:913, 1932.
226. Diggs, L. W., and Bibb, J.: The erythrocyte in sickle cell anemia; morphology, size, hemoglobin content, fragility and sedimentation rate. J.A.M.A., *112*:695, 1939.
227. Diggs, L. W., and Ching, R. E.: The pathology of sickle cell anemia. South. Med. J., *27*:839, 1934.
228. Diggs, L. W., Pulliam, H. N., and King, J. C.: The bone changes in sickle cell anemia. South. Med. J., *30*:249, 1937.
229. Donegan, C. C., MacIlwaine, W. P., and Leavell, B. S.: Hematologic studies in patients with sickle cell anemia following multiple transfusions. Am. J. Med., *17*:29, 1954.
230. Emmel, V. E.: A study of the erythrocytes in a case of severe anemia with elongated and sickle-shaped red blood corpuscles. Arch. Intern. Med., *20*:586, 1917.
231. Fink, A. I., Funahansi, T., Robinson, M., and Watson, R. J.: Conjunctival blood flow in sickle cell disease. Arch. Ophthalmol., *66*:82, 1961.
232. Gill, F. A., Kaye, D., and Hook, E. W.: The influence of erythrophagocytosis on the interaction of macrophages and *Salmonella* in vitro. J. Exp. Med., *124*:173, 1966.
233. Gillette, P. N., Manning, J. M., and Cerami, A.: Increased survival of sickle cell erythrocytes after treatment in vitro with sodium cyanate. Proc. Natl. Acad. Sci. U.S.A., *68*:2791, 1971.
234. Greenberg, S. R., Atwater, J., and Israel, H. L.: Frequency of hemoglobinopathies in sarcoidosis. Ann. Intern. Med., *62*:125, 1965.
235. Greenberg, N. S., Kass, E. H., and Castle, W. B.: Studies on the destruction of red blood cells. XII. Factors influencing the role of S hemoglobin in the pathologic physiology of sickle cell anemia and related disorders. J. Clin. Invest., *36*:833, 1957.
236. Hahn, E. V., and Gillespie, E. B.: Sickle cell anemia: report of a case greatly improved by splenectomy. Experimental study of sickle cell formation. Arch. Intern. Med., *39*:233, 1927.
237. Harris, J. W., Brewster, H. H., Ham, T. H., and Castle, W. B.: Studies on destruction of the red blood cells. X. The biophysics and biology of sickle cell disease. Arch. Intern. Med., *97*:145, 1956.
238. Harrow, B. R., Sloane, J. A., and Liebman, N. C.: Roentgenologic demonstration of renal papillary necrosis in sickle cell trait. N. Engl. J. Med., *268*:969, 1963.
239. Hatch, F. E., and Diggs, L. W.: Fluid balance in sickle cell disease. Arch. Intern. Med., *116*:10, 1965.
240. Henderson, A. B.: Sickle cell anemia. Clinical study of fifty-four cases with autopsy. Am. J. Med., *9*:757, 1950.
241. Herrick, J. B.: Peculiar elongated and sickle-shaped red blood corpuscles in a case of severe anemia. Arch. Intern. Med., *6*:517, 1910.
242. Hill, F. S., Hughes, J. G., and Davis, B. C.: Electroencephalographic findings in sickle cell anemia. Pediatrics, *6*:277, 1950.
243. Hill, R. J., Konigsberg, W., Guidotti, G., and Craig, L. C.: Structure of human hemoglobin: I. The separation of the $\alpha-$ and $\beta-$chains and their amino acid composition. J. Biol. Chem., *237*:1549, 1962.
244. Hirschman, R. J., and Johns, C. J.: Hemoglobin studies in sarcoidosis. Ann. Intern. Med., *62*:129, 1965.

245. Hook, E. W., Campbell, C. G., Weens, H. S., and Cooper, G. R.: *Salmonella* osteomyelitis in patients with sickle-cell anemia. N. Engl. J. Med., *257*:403, 1957.
246. Huck, J. G.: Sickle cell anemia. Johns Hopkins Med. J., *34*:335, 1923.
247. Hughes, J. G., Diggs, L. W., and Gillespie, C. E.: The involvement of the nervous system in sickle cell anemia. J. Pediatr., *17*:66, 1940.
248. Ingram, V. M.: A specific chemical difference between the globins of normal human and sickle cell anaemia haemoglobin. Nature, *178*:792, 1956. Conference on Hemoglobin. Natl. Acad. Sci., 1958, Pub. 557, p. 233.
249. James, G. W. III, and Abbott, L. D., Jr.: Erythrocyte destruction in sickle-cell anemia: simultaneous N^{15}-hemin and N^{15} stercobilin studies. Proc. Soc. Exp. Biol. Med., *88*:398, 1955.
250. Jenkins, M. E., Scott, R. B., and Baird, R. C.: Studies in sickle cell anemia. XVI. Sudden death during sickle cell crisis. J. Pediatr., *56*:30, 1960.
251. Jones, S. R., Binder, R. A., and Donowho, E. M., Jr.: Sudden death in sickle cell trait. N. Engl. J. Med., *282*:323, 1970.
252. Kabins, S. A., and Lerner, C.: Fulminant pneumococcemia in sickle cell anemia. J.A.M.A., *211*:467, 1970.
253. Kaye, D., Gill, F. A., and Hook, E. W.: Factors influencing host resistance to *Salmonella* infections: the effects of hemolysis and erythrophagocytosis. Am. J. Med. Sci., *254*:101, 1967.
254. Kimmelstiel, P.: Vascular occlusion and ischemic infarction in sickle cell disease. Am. J. Med. Sci., *216*:11, 1948.
255. Knochel, J. P.: Hematuria in sickle cell trait. Arch. Intern. Med., *123*:160, 1969.
256. Leavell, B. S., and MacIlwaine, W. A.: Sickle Cell Anemia. *In* Bean, W. B. (ed.): Monographs in Medicine. Series 1. William & Wilkins Co., Baltimore, 1952.
257. Lieb, W. A., Geeracts, W. J., and Guerry, D. III: Sickle-cell retinopathy. Ocular and systemic manifestations of sickle cell disease. Acta Ophthalmol. (Kbh.)(Suppl.), *58*:1, 1959.
258. Macht, S. H., and Roman, P. W.: The radiologic changes in sickle cell anemia. Radiology, *51*:697, 1948.
259. Mahmood, A.: A double-blind trial of a phenothiazine compound in the treatment of clinical crisis of sickle cell anaemia. Br. J. Haematol., *16*:181, 1969.
260. Margolis, M. P.: Sickle cell anemia. A composite study and survey. Medicine, *30*:357, 1951.
261. Murayama, M.: Molecular mechanism of red cell sickling. Science, *153*:145, 1966.
262. Murayama, M.: Tertiary structure of sickle cell hemoglobin and its functional significance. J. Cell Physiol., *67*:211, 1966.
263. Neel, J. V.: The inheritance of the sickling phenomenon with particular reference to sickle cell disease. Blood, *6*:389, 1951.
264. Neel, J. V.: Genetic aspects of abnormal hemoglobins. Conference on hemoglobin. Natl. Acad. Sci., Pub. 557, 1958, p. 253.
265. Paton, D.: The conjunctival sign of sickle-cell disease. Arch. Ophthalmol., *68*:627, 1962.
266. Pauling, L., Itano, H. A., Singer, S. J., and Wells, I. C.: Sickle cell anemia, a molecular disease. Science, *110*:543, 1949.
267. Pauling, L., Itano, H. A., Wells, I. C., Schroeder, W. A., Kay, L. M., Singer, S. J., and Corey, R. B.: Sickle anemia hemoglobin. Science, *111*:459, 1950.
268. Pearson, H. A., Cornelius, E. A., Schwartz, A. D., Zelson, J. H., Wolfson, S. L., and Spencer, R. P.: Transfusion-reversible functional asplenia in young children with sickle-cell anemia. N. Engl. J. Med., *283*:334, 1970.
269. Pearson, H. A., and Diamond, L. K.: The critically ill child: sickle cell disease crises and their management. Pediatrics, *48*:629, 1971.
270. Pearson, H. A., Spencer, R. P., and Cornelius, E. A.: Functional asplenia in sickle cell anemia. N. Engl. J. Med., *281*:923, 1969.
271. Perillie, P. E., and Epstein, F. H.: Sickling phenomena produced by hypertonic solutions; a possible explanation for the hyposthenuria of sickle cell anemia. J. Clin. Invest., *42*:570, 1963.
272. Perutz, M. F., and Mitchison, J. M.: State of haemoglobin in sickle cell anaemia. Nature, *166*:677, 1950.
273. Ponder, E.: Red cell cytochemistry and architecture. Ann. N.Y. Acad. Sci., *48*:579, 1947.
274. Porter, F. S., and Thurman, W. G.: Studies in sickle cell disease. Am. J. Dis. Child., *106*:35, 1963.
275. Ricks, P.: Further experiences with exchange transfusion in sickle cell anemia and pregnancy. Am. J. Obstet. Gynecol., *100*:1087, 1968.
276. Ryerson, C. S., and Terplan, K. L.: Sickle cell anemia. Two unusual cases with autopsy. Folia Haematol., *53*:353, 1935.
277. Scott, R. B.: Health care priority and sickle cell anemia. J.A.M.A., *214*:731, 1970.
278. Shotton, D., Crockett, C. L., Jr., and Leavell, B. S.: Splenectomy in sickle cell anemia: report of a case and review of the literature. Blood, *6*:365, 1951.

279. Singer, K., Motulsky, A. G., and Wile, S. A.: Aplastic crisis in sickle cell anemia. A study of its mechanism and its relationship to other types of hemolytic crises. J. Lab. Clin. Med., 35:721, 1950.
280. Statius van Eps, L. W., Pinedo-Veels, C., DeVries, G. H., and DeKong, J.: Nature of concentrating defect in sickle-cell nephropathy. Lancet, 1:450, 1970.
281. Symposium on hemoglobinopathies in pregnancy. Clin. Obstet. Gynecol., 12:13, 1969.
282. Winkelstein, J. A., and Drachman, R. H.: Deficiency of pneumococcal serum opsonizing activity in sickle cell disease. N. Engl. J. Med., 279:459, 1968.
283. Winsor, T., and Burch, G. E.: The electrocardiogram and cardiac state in active sickle cell anemia. Am. Heart J., 29:685, 1945.
284. Wintrobe, M. M.: The cardiovascular system in anemia: with a note on the particular abnormalities in sickle cell anemia. Blood, 1:121, 1946.

THALASSEMIA

285. Atwater, J., Schwartz, I. R., Erslev, A. J., Montgomery, T. L., and Tocantins, L. M.: Sickling of erythrocytes in patients with thalassemia–hemoglobin-I disease. N. Engl. J. Med., 263:1215, 1960.
286. Baglioni, C.: Fusion of two polypeptide chains in hemoglobin Lepore and its interpretation as genetic deletion. Proc. Natl. Acad. Sci., 48:1880, 1962.
287. Bank, A., and Marks, P. A.: Excess α chain synthesis relative to β chain synthesis in thalassemia major and minor. Nature, 212:1198, 1966.
288. Beard, M. E., Necheles, T. F., and Allen, D. M.: Clinical experience with intensive transfusion therapy in Cooley's anemia. Ann. N.Y. Acad. Sci., 165:415, 1969.
289. Benesch, R., and Benesch, R. E.: Properties of haemoglobin H and their significance in relation to function of haemoglobin. Nature, 202:773, 1964.
290. Benz, E. J., Jr., and Forget, B. G.: The biosynthesis of hemoglobin. Semin. Hematol., 11:463, 1974.
291. Cooley, T. B., and Lee, P.: Series of cases of splenomegaly in children with anemia and peculiar bone changes. Tr. Am. Pediatr. Soc., 47:29, 1925.
292. Dormandy, K. M., Lock, S. P., and Lehmann, H.: Haemoglobin Q-alpha-thalassemia. Br. Med. J., 1:1582, 1961.
293. Fessas, P., and Mastrohalos, N.: Demonstration of small components in red cell haemolysates by starch-gel electrophoresis. Nature, 183:30, 1959.
294. Fessas, P., and Stamatoyannopoulos, G.: Absence of haemoglobin A$_2$ in an adult. Nature, 195:1215, 1962.
295. Fessas, P., Stamatoyannopoulas, G., and Karaklis, A.: Hemoglobin "Pylos": study of a hemoglobinopathy resembling thalassemia in the heterozygous homozygous and double heterozygous state. Blood, 19:1, 1962.
296. Gabuzda, T. G.: Analytic review, Hemoglobin H and the red cell. Blood, 27:568, 1966.
297. Harton, B. F., Thompson, R. B., Dozy, A. M., Nechtman, C. M., Nichols, E., and Huisman, T. H. J.: Inhomogeneity of hemoglobin VI. The minor hemoglobin components of cord blood. Blood, 20:302, 1962.
298. Hollan, S. R., Szelenyi, J. S., Bremhall, B., Duerst, M., Jones, R. T., Koler, R. D., and Stocklen, Z.: Multiple alpha chain loci for human haemoglobins. Hb. J-Buda and Hb. G-Pest. Nature, 235:47, 1972.
299. Ingram, V. M.: The Hemoglobins in Genetics and Evolution. Columbia University Press, New York, 1963.
300. Kan, Y. W., Schwartz, E., and Nathan, D. G.: Globin chain synthesis in the alpha thalassemia syndromes. J. Clin. Invest., 45:2515, 1968.
301. Lehmann, H.: Inheritance of human haemoglobin. Br. Med. Bull., 15:40, 1959.
302. Marks, P. A.: Thalassemia syndromes: biochemical, genetic and clinical aspects. N. Engl. J. Med., 275:1363, 1966.
303. Minnich, V., Na-Nakorn, S., Chongchareonsuk, S., and Kochaseni, S.: Mediterranean anemia. A study of 32 cases in Thailand. Blood, 9:1, 1954.
304. Nathan, D. G., and Gunn, R. B.: Thalassemia: the consequence of unbalanced hemoglobin synthesis. Am. J. Med., 41:819, 1966.
305. Nathan, D. G., Stossel, T. B., Gunn, R. B., Zarkowsky, H. S., and Laforet, M. T.: Influence of hemoglobin precipitation on erythrocyte metabolism in alpha and beta thalassemia. J. Clin. Invest., 48:33, 1969.
306. Neel, J. V., and Valentine, W. N.: The frequency of thalassemia. Am. J. Med. Sci., 209:568, 1945.
307. Ottolenghi, S., Lanyon, W. G., Paul, J., Williamson, R., Weatherall, D. J., Clegg, J. B., Pritchard,

J., Poortrakul, S., and Boon, W. H.: The severe form of thalassaemia is caused by a hemo-globin gene deletion. Nature, *251*:388, 1974.

308. Pearson, H. A., Gerald, P. S., and Diamond, L. K.: Thalassemia intermedia due to interaction of Lepore trait with thalassemia trait: report of three cases. J. Dis. Child., *97*:464, 1959.

309. Piomelli, S., Danoff, S. J., Becker, M. H., Lipera, M. J., and Travis, S. F.: Prevention of bone malformation and cardiomegaly in Cooley's anemia by early hypertransfusion regimen. Ann. N.Y. Acad. Sci., *165*:427, 1969.

310. Rigas, D. A., Koler, R. D., and Osgood, E. E.: New hemoglobin possessing a higher electro-phoretic mobility than normal adult hemoglobin. Science, *121*:372, 1955.

311. Singer, K.: Hereditary hemolytic disorders associated with abnormal hemoglobins. Am. J. Med., *18*:633, 1955.

312. Slater, L. M., Muir, W. A., and Weed, R. I.: Influence of splenectomy on insoluble hemoglobin inclusion bodies in β thalassemic erythrocytes. Blood, *31*:766, 1968.

313. Smith, C. H., Erlandson, M. E., Stern, G., and Schulman, I.: The role of splenectomy in the management of thalassemia. Blood, *15*:197, 1960.

314. Taylor, J. M., Dozy, A., Kan, Y. W., Varmus, H. E., Lie-Injo, L. E., Ganesan, J., and Todd, D.: Genetic lesion in homozygous thalassaemia (hydrops fetalis). Nature, *251*:392, 1974.

315. Valentine, W. N., and Neel, J. V.: Hematologic and genetic study of the transmission of thalassemia. Arch. Intern. Med., *74*:185, 1944.

316. Weatherall, D. J., and Clegg, J. B.: The Thalassemia Syndromes. 2nd Ed. Blackwell Scientific Publications, Oxford, 1972.

317. Wintrobe, M. M., Matthews, E., Pollack, R., and Dobyns, B. M.: A familial hemopoietic dis-order in Italian adolescents and adults. J.A.M.A., *114*:1530, 1940.

318. Wolff, J. A., and Lukem, K. H.: Management of thalassemia: a comparative program. Ann. N.Y. Acad. Sci., *165*:423, 1969.

319. Wolman, I. J.: Transfusion therapy in Cooley's anemia: growth and health as related to long-range hemoglobin levels, a progress report. Ann. N.Y. Acad. Sci., *119*:736, 1964.

320. Wolman, I. J., and Ortolani, M.: Some clinical features of Cooley's anemia patients as related to transfusion schedules. Ann. N.Y. Acad. Sci., *165*:407, 1969.

321. Zaino, E. C.: Paleontologic thalassemia. Ann. N.Y. Acad. Sci., *119*:402, 1964.

OTHER HEMOGLOBINOPATHIES

322. Bookchin, R. M., Davis, R. P., and Ranney, H. M.: Clinical features of hemoglobin C Harlem, a new sickling hemoglobin variant. Ann. Intern. Med., *68*:8, 1968.

323. Carrell, R. W., and Lehmann, H.: The unstable haemoglobin haemolytic anaemias. Semin. Hematol., *6*:116, 1969.

324. Cawein, M. J., Lappat, E. J., Brangle, R. W., and Farley, Z. H.: Hemoglobin S-D disease. Ann. Intern. Med., *64*:62, 1966.

325. Charache, S., Conley, L. L., Waugh, D. F., Ugoretz, R. J., and Spurrell, R.: Pathogenesis of hemolytic anemia in homozygous hemoglobin C disease. J. Clin. Invest., *40*:1795, 1967.

326. Chernoff, A. I.: Studies on hemoglobin E. J. Lab. Clin. Med., *44*:780, 1954.

327. Chernoff, A. I.: On the prevalence of hemoglobin D in the American Negro. Blood, *11*:907, 1956.

328. Chernoff, A. I., Smith, G., and Steinkamp, R.: Homozygous hemoglobin D disease. J. Lab. Clin. Med., *48*:795, 1956.

329. Conley, J. C. L., and Charache, S.: Inherited hemoglobinopathies. Hosp. Pract., *4*:35, 1969.

330. Diggs, L. W., and Bell, A.: Intraerythrocytic hemoglobin crystals in sickle cell–hemoglobin C disease. Blood, *25*:218, 1965.

331. Diggs, L. W., Kraus, A. P., Morrison, D. B., and Rudnicki, R. P. T.: Intraerythrocytic crystals in a white patient with hemoglobin C in the absence of other types of hemoglobin. Blood, *9*:1172, 1954.

332. Fairbanks, V. F., Opfell, R. W., and Burgert, E. O., Jr.: Three families with unstable hemo-globinopathies (Köln, Olmsted and Santa Ana) causing hemolytic anemia with inclusion bodies and pigmenturia. Am. J. Med., *46*:344, 1969.

333. Gerald, P. S., and Path, C. E.: Hemoglobin C Georgetown; first abnormal hemoglobin due to two different mutations in the same gene. J. Clin. Invest., *45*:1012, 1966.

334. Heller, P.: Hemoglobinopathic dysfunction of the red cell. Am. J. Med., *41*:799, 1968.

335. Huehns, E. R.: Diseases due to abnormalities of hemoglobin structure. Ann. Rev. Med., *21*:157, 1970.

336. Itano, H. A.: A third abnormal hemoglobin associated with hereditary hemolytic anemia. Proc. Natl. Acad. Sci., *37*:775, 1951.

337. Itano, H. A., and Neel, J. V.: A new inherited abnormality of human hemoglobin. Proc. Natl. Acad. Sci., *36*:613, 1950.

338. Jacob, H. S.: Mechanisms of Heinz body formation and attachment to red cell membrane. Semin. Hematol., *7*:341, 1970.

339. Kaplan, E., Zuelzer, W., and Neel, J. V.: A new inherited abnormality of hemoglobin and its interaction with sickle cell hemoglobin. Blood, *6*:1240, 1951.

340. Kraus, A. P., Miyaji, T., Iuchi, I., and Kraus, L. M.: A new variety of sickle cell anemia with clinically mild symptoms due to an α chain variant of hemoglobin ($\alpha^{23\ Glu\ NH_2}$). J. Lab. Clin. Med., *66*:886, 1965.

341. Kraus, L. M., Miyaji, T., Iuchi, I., and Kraus, A. P.: Characterization of $\alpha^{23\ Glu\ NH_2}$ in hemoglobin Memphis. Hemoglobin Memphis S, a new variant of molecular disease. Biochemistry, *5*:3701, 1966.

342. Lessin, L. S., Jensen, W. N., and Porter, E.: Molecular mechanism of hemolytic anemia in homozygous hemoglobin C disease. J. Exp. Med., *130*:443, 1969.

343. Pierce, L. E., Path, L. E., and McCoy, K.: A new hemoglobin variant with sickling properties. N. Engl. J. Med., *268*:862, 1963.

344. Powell, W. N., Rodarte, J. G., and Neel, J. V.: The occurrence in a family of Sicilian ancestry of the traits for both sickling and thalassemia. Blood, *5*:887, 1950.

345. Ranney, H. M.: Clinically important variants of human hemoglobin. N. Engl. J. Med., *282*:144, 1970.

346. Rieder, R. F.: Human hemoglobin stability and instability: molecular mechanisms and some clinical correlations. Semin. Hematol., *11*:423, 1974.

347. Silvestroni, E., and Bianco, I.: Singulare associazone de "anemia microcitica" constituzionale con "depranocitiro-anemia" in sogetto di razza bianca. Policlinico [Prat.], *53*:265, 1946.

348. Singer, K., Chapman, A. Z., Goldberg, S. R., Rubinstein, H. M., and Rosenblum, S. A.: Studies on abnormal hemoglobins. IX. Pure (homozygous) hemoglobin C disease. Blood, *9*:1023, 1954.

349. Singer, K., Kraus, A. P., Singer, L., Rubinstein, H. M., and Goldberg, S. R.: Studies on abnormal hemoglobins X. A new syndrome: hemoglobin C–thalassemia disease. Blood, *9*:1032, 1954.

350. Smith, E. W., and Conley, C. L.: Filter paper electrophoresis of human hemoglobins with special reference to the incidence and clinical significance of hemoglobin C. Johns Hopkins Med. J., *93*:94, 1953.

351. Smith, E. W., and Conley, C. L.: Clinical features of the genetic variants of sickle cell disease. Johns Hopkins Med. J., *94*:289, 1954.

352. Smith, E. W., and Conley, C. L.: Sickle cell–hemoglobin D disease. Ann. Intern. Med., *50*:94, 1959.

353. Spaet, T. H., Alway, R. H., and Ward, G.: Homozygous type C hemoglobin. Pediatrics, *12*:483, 1954.

354. Tanaka, K. R., and Clifford, G. O.: Homozygous hemoglobin C disease: report of three cases. Ann. Intern. Med., *49*:30, 1958.

355. Wheby, M. S., Thorup, O. A., and Leavell, B. S.: Homozygous hemoglobin C disease in siblings; further comment on intraerythrocytic crystals. Blood, *11*:266, 1956.

356. Zuelzer, W., and Kaplan, E.: Thalassemia–hemoglobin C disease. A new syndrome presumably due to the combination of the genes for thalassemia and hemoglobin C. Blood, *9*:1047, 1954.

357. Zuelzer, W. W., Neel, J. V., and Robinson, A. R.: Abnormal hemoglobins, Progr. Hematol., *1*:91, 1956.

ERYTHROBLASTOSIS FETALIS

358. Allen, F. H., Jr., and Diamond, L. K.: Erythroblastosis fetalis. N. Engl. J. Med., *257*:659, 1957; *257*:705, 1957; *257*:761, 1957.

359. Allen, F. H., Jr., Diamond, L. K., and Vaughan, V. C.: Erythroblastosis fetalis. Prevention of kernicterus. Am. J. Dis. Child., *80*:779, 1950.

360. Behrman, R. E.: Preliminary report of the committee on phototherapy in the newborn infant. J. Pediatr., *84*:135, 1974.

361. Bowman, J. M., Friesen, R. F., Bowman, W. D., McInnis, A. L., Barnes, P. H., and Grewar, D.: Fetal transfusion in severe Rh isoimmunization. J.A.M.A., *207*:1101, 1969.

362. Brown, A. K., and Zuelzer, W. W.: Studies on the neonatal development of the glucuronide conjugating system. J. Clin. Invest., *37*:332, 1958.

363. Brown, A. K., Zuelzer, W. W., and Robinson, A. R.: Studies in hyperbilirubinemia. II. Clearance of bilirubin from plasma and extravascular space in newborn infants during exchange transfusion. Am. J. Dis. Child., *93*:274, 1957.

364. Clarke, C. A.: Prevention of rhesus iso-immunization. Semin. Hematol., *6*:201, 1969.

365. Cohen, F., Zuelzer, W. W., Gustafsan, D. C., and Evans, M. M.: Mechanisms of isoimmunization. I. The transplacental passage of fetal erythrocytes in homospecific pregnancies.
Blood, 23:621, 1964.
366. Cunningham, M. D., Mace, J. W., and Peters, E. R.: Clinical experience with phenobarbital in
icterus neonatorum. Lancet, 1:550, 1969.
367. Diamond, L. K., Blackfan, K. D., and Baty, J. M.: Erythroblastosis fetalis and its association
with universal edema of the fetus, icterus gravis neonatorum and anemia of the newborn.
J. Pediatr., 1:269, 1932.
368. Finn, R., Clarke, C. A., Donohoe, W. T. A., Sheppard, P. M., Lebane, D., and Kulke, W.: Experimental studies on the prevention of Rh haemolytic disease. Br. Med. J., 1:1486, 1961.
369. Hsia, D. Y., Allen, F. H., Jr., Gellis, S. S., and Diamond, L. K.: Erythroblastosis fetalis, VIII.
Studies of serum bilirubin in relation to kernicterus. N. Engl. J. Med., 247:668, 1952.
370. Kelsall, G. A., Vos, G. H., Kirk, R. L., and Shield, J. W.: The evaluation of cord blood hemoglobin, reticulocyte percentage and maternal antiglobulin titer in the prognosis of hemolytic disease of the newborn. Pediatrics, 20:221, 1957.
371. Landsteiner, K., and Wiener, A. S.: An agglutinable factor in human blood recognizable by
immune sera for Rhesus blood. Proc. Soc. Exp. Biol., 13:223, 1940.
372. Leading Article: Massive pulmonary haemorrhage in the newborn. Br. Med. J., 3:553, 1973.
373. Leading Article: Management of neonatal jaundice. Br. Med. J., 1:469, 1974.
374. Levine, P., Katzin, E. M., and Burnham, L.: Isoimmunization in pregnancy. J.A.M.A., 116:825,
1941.
375. Levine, P., and Stetson, R. E.: Unusual cases of intragroup agglutination. J.A.M.A., 113:126,
1939.
376. Levine, P., Vogel, P., Katzin, E. M., and Burnham, L.: Pathogenesis of erythroblastosis fetalis:
statistical evidence. Science, 94:371, 1941.
377. Lilley, A. W.: Intrauterine transfusion of fetus in hemolytic disease. Br. Med. J., 2:1107, 1963.
378. Lilley, A. W.: Errors in the assessment of hemolytic disease from amniotic fluid. Am. J. Obstet.
Gynecol., 86:485, 1963.
379. Little, B., McCutcheon, E., and Desforges, J. F.: Amniocentesis and intrauterine transfusion
in Rh-sensitized pregnancy. N. Engl. J. Med., 27:332, 1966.
380. Mollison, P. L.: Survival of transfused erythrocytes in hemolytic disease of the newborn.
Arch. Dis. Child., 18:161, 1943.
381. Mollison, P. L.: Blood Transfusion in Clinical Medicine. 5th Ed. Blackwell Scientific Publications, Oxford, 1972.
382. Nevanlinna, H. R., and Vaino, T.: The influence of mother-child ABO incompatibility on Rh
immunization. Vox Sang., 1:26, 1956.
383. Odell, G. B.: Studies in kernicterus. I. The protein binding of bilirubin. J. Clin. Invest., 38:823,
1959.
384. Oski, F. A., and Nauman, J. L.: Hematologic problems in the newborn. Erythroblastosis fetalis.
Major Problems in Clin. Pediatr., 4:176, 1972.
385. Pollack, W., Gorman, J. G., and Freda, V. J.: Prevention of Rh hemolytic disease. Progr.
Hematol., 6:121, 1969.
386. Voak, D., and Williams, M. A.: An explanation of the failure of the direct antiglobulin test to
detect erythrocyte sensitization in ABO hemolytic disease of the newborn and observations on pinocytosis of IgG anti-A antibodies by infant (cord) red cells. Br. J. Haematol.,
29:9, 1971.
387. Walker, W.: Haemolytic anaemia in the newborn infant. Clin. Haematol., 4:145, 1975.
388. Wallerstein, H.: Treatment of severe erythroblastosis by simultaneous removal and replacement of blood of the newborn infant. Science, 103:583, 1946.
389. Wilson, J. T.: Phenobarbital in the neonatal period. Pediatrics, 43:324, 1969.
390. Woodrow, J. C.: Rh immunization and its prevention. Series Haematol., 3:3, 1970.
391. Zipursky, A.: The universal prevention of Rh immunization. Clin. Obstet. Gynecol., 14:869,
1971.
392. Zuelzer, W. W., and Cohen, F.: ABO hemolytic disease and heterospecific pregnancy. Pediatr.
Clin. North Am., 4:405, 1957.

DRUG-INDUCED AND AUTOIMMUNE HEMOLYTIC ANEMIA

393. Allgood, J. W., and Chaplin, H., Jr.: Idiopathic acquired auto-immune hemolytic anemia.
A review of forty-seven cases treated from 1955 through 1965. Am. J. Med., 43:254, 1967.
394. Atkinson, J. P., and Frank, M. M.: Complement-independent clearance of Ig-G sensitized
erythrocytes: inhibition by cortisone. Blood, 44:629, 1974.
395. Bakemeier, R. F., and Leddy, J. P.: Heavy chain:light chain relationships among erythrocyte
autoantibodies. J. Clin. Invest., 46:1033, 1967.

396. Bakemeier, R. F., and Leddy, J. P.: Erythrocyte autoantibody associated with alpha-methyl-dopa: heterogeneity of structure and specificity. Blood, *32*:1, 1968.
397. Bell, C. A., Zwicker, H., and Sacks, H. J.: Autoimmune hemolytic anemia: routine serologic evaluation in a general hospital population. Am. J. Clin. Pathol., *60*:903, 1973.
398. Bird, G. W. G., Eeles, G. H., Litchfield, J. A., Rahman, N., and Wingham, J.: Haemolytic anaemia associated with antibodies to tolbutamide and phenacetin. Br. Med. J., *1*:728, 1972.
399. Bolton, F. G., and Dameshek, W.: Thrombocytopenic purpura due to quinidine. I. Clinical studies. Blood, *11*:527, 1956.
400. Bourne, H. R., Lichtenstein, L. M., Melmon, K. L., Kenney, C. S., Weinstein, Y., and Shearer, G. M.: Modulation of inflammation and immunity by cyclic AMP. Science, *189*:19, 1974.
401. Brouillard, R. F., and Barret, O., Jr.: Methyldopa associated hepatitis, J.A.M.A., *224*:904, 1973.
402. Carstairs, K. L., Breckenridge, A., Dollery, C. T., and Worlledge, S. M.: Incidence of a positive direct Coombs test in patients on methyldopa. Lancet, *2*:133, 1966.
403. Chaplin, H.: Clinical usefulness of specific antiglobulin reagents in autoimmune hemolytic anemia. Progr. Hematol., *8*:25, 1973.
404. Coombs, R. R. A., Mourant, A. E., and Race, R. R.: A new test for the detection of weak and "incomplete" Rh agglutinins. Br. J. Exp. Pathol., *26*:255, 1945.
405. Corley, L. E., Lessner, H. E., and Larsen, W. E.: Azathioprine therapy of "autoimmune" diseases. Am. J. Med., *41*:404, 1966.
406. Costea, N., Yakulis, V. J., and Heller, P.: Inhibition of cold agglutinins (anti-I) by M. pneumoniae antigen. Proc. Soc. Exp. Biol. Med., *139*:476, 1972.
407. Croft, J. D., Jr., Swisher, S. N., Jr., Gilliland, B. C., Bakemeier, R. F., Leddy, J. P., and Weed, R. I.: Coombs-test positivity induced by drugs: mechanisms of immunologic reactions and red cell destruction. Ann. Intern. Med., *68*:176, 1968.
408. Dacie, J. V.: The Auto-immune Haemolytic Anemias. Part II in The Haemolytic Anaemias, Congenital and Acquired. 2nd Ed. Grune & Stratton, New York, 1962.
409. Dacie, J. V.: Drug-induced Hemolytic Anaemias, Paroxysmal Nocturnal Haemoglobinuria, Haemolytic Disease of the Newborn. Part IV in The Haemolytic Anaemias, Congenital and Acquired. 2nd Ed. Grune & Stratton, New York, 1967.
410. Dacie, J. V., and Worlledge, S. M.: Auto-immune hemolytic anemias. Progr. Hematol., *6*:82, 1969.
411. Dameshek, W., and Schwartz, S. O.: Acute hemolytic anemia (acquired hemolytic icterus, acute type). Medicine, *19*:231, 1940.
412. de Gruchy, G. C.: The diagnosis and management of acquired haemolytic anaemia. Australia. Ann. Med., *3*:106, 1954.
413. DeTorregrosa, M. V. V., Rosada, A. L. R., and Montella, E.: Hemolytic anemia secondary to stibophen therapy. J.A.M.A., *186*:598, 1963.
414. Donath, J., and Landsteiner, R.: Über paroxysmalen Hämoglobinurie. Münch. Med. Wochnschr., *51*:1590, 1904.
415. Evans, R. S., Takahashi, K., Duane, R. T., Payne, R., and Lui, C. K.: Primary thrombocytopenic purpura and acquired hemolytic anemia. Evidence for a common etiology. Arch. Intern. Med., *87*:48, 1951.
416. Eyster, M. E.: Melphalan (Alkeran®) erythrocyte agglutinin and hemolytic anemia. Ann. Intern. Med., *66*:573, 1967.
417. Eyster, M. E., and Jenkins, D. E., Jr.: Erythrocyte coating substances in patients with positive direct antiglobulin reactions. Correlation of γ G globulin and complement coating with underlying diseases, overt hemolysis and response to therapy. Am. J. Med., *46*:360, 1969.
418. Eyster, M. E., Nachman, R. L., Christenson, W. N., and Engel, R. L., Jr.: Structural characteristics of red cell auto-antibodies. J. Immunol., *96*:107, 1966.
419. Faulk, W. P., Tomsovie, E. J., and Fudenberg, H. H.: Insulin resistance in juvenile diabetes mellitus. Immunologic studies. Am. J. Med., *49*:133, 1970.
420. Feltkamp, T. E., Mees, E. J. D., and Nieuwenhuis, M. G.: Autoantibodies related to treatment with chlorthalidone and α-methyldopa. Acta Med. Scand., *187*:219, 1970.
421. Freedman, A. L., Barr, R. S., and Brody, E. A.: Hemolytic anemia due to quinidine: observations on its mechanism. Am. J. Med., *20*:806, 1956.
422. Gabor, E. P., and Goldberg, L. S.: Levodopa induced Coombs positive haemolytic anaemia. Scand. J. Haematol., *11*:201, 1973.
423. Garratty, G., and Petz, L. D.: Drug-induced immune hemolytic anemia. Am. J. Med., *58*:398, 1975.
424. Gilliland, B. C., Baxter, E., and Evans, R. S.: Red cell antibodies in acquired hemolytic anemia with negative antiglobulin serum tests. N. Engl. J. Med., *285*:252, 1971.
425. Gottlieb, A. J., and Wurzel, H. A.: Protein-quinone interaction: in vitro induction of indirect antiglobulin reactions with methyldopa. Blood, *43*:85, 1974.

426. Gralnick, H. R., Wright, L. D., Jr., and McGinniss, M. D.: Coombs positive reactions associated with sodium cephalothin therapy. J.A.M.A., *199*:725, 1967.
427. Ham, T. H.: Hemoglobinuria. Am. J. Med., *18*:990, 1955.
428. Harris, J. W.: Studies on the mechanism of a drug-induced hemolytic anemia. J. Lab. Clin. Med., *44*:809, 1954.
429. Hinz, C. F.: Serologic and physicochemical characterization of Donath-Landsteiner antibodies from six patients. Blood, *22*:600, 1963.
430. Hippe, E., Jensen, K. B., Olesen, H., Lind, K., and Thomsen, P. E. B.: Chlorambucil treatment of patients with cold agglutinin syndrome. Blood, *35*:68, 1970.
431. Huber, H., Polley, M. J., Linscott, W. D., Fudenberg, H. H., and Muller-Eberhard, H. J.: Human monocytes: distinct receptor sites for the third component of complement and for immunoglobulin G. Science, *162*:1281, 1968.
432. Jandl, J. H., Greenberg, M. S., Yonemoto, R. H., and Castle, W. B.: Clinical determination of the sites of red cell sequestration in hemolytic anemia. J. Clin. Invest., *35*:842, 1956.
433. Jandl, J. H., Richardson-Jones, A., and Castle, W. B.: Destruction of red cells by antibodies in man. I. Observations of the sequestration and lysis of red cells altered by immune mechanisms. J. Clin. Invest., *36*:1428, 1957.
434. Kerr, R. O., Cardamone, J., Dalmasso, A. P., and Kaplan, M. E.: Mechanisms of erythrocyte destruction in penicillin-induced hemolysis. N. Engl. J. Med., *287*:1322, 1972.
435. Lakshminarayan, S., Sahn, S. A., and Hudson, L. D.: Massive hemolysis caused by rifampicin. Br. Med. J., *2*:282, 1973.
436. Lay, W. H.: Drug-induced hemolytic reaction due to antibodies against the erythrocyte-dipyrone complex. Vox Sang., *11*:601, 1966.
437. Levine, B. B., and Redmond, A. P.: Immune mechanisms of penicillin-induced Coombs' positivity in man. J. Clin. Invest., *46*:1085, 1967. Abstr.
438. Lindberg, L. G., and Nordin, A.: Severe hemolytic reaction due to chlorpromazine. Acta Med. Scand., *170*:195, 1961.
439. LoBuglio, A. F., Cotran, R. J., and Jandl, J. H.: Red cells coated with immunoglobin G: binding and sphering by mononuclear cells in man. Science, *158*:1582, 1967.
440. LoBuglio, A. F., and Jandl, J. H.: The nature of the alpha-methyldopa red-cell antibody. N. Engl. J. Med., *276*:658, 1967.
441. LoBuglio, A. F., and King, G. W.: α-Methyldopa and Red Blood Cells. *In* Dimitrov, N. V., and Nodine, J. H. (eds.): Drugs and Hematologic Reactions. Grune & Stratton, 1974.
442. Logue, G. L., Boyd, A. E., III, and Rosse, W. F.: Chlorpropamide-induced immune hemolytic anemia. N. Engl. J. Med., *283*:900, 1970.
443. Mac Gibbon, B. H., Loughridge, C., Hourihane, W., O'B. D., and Boyd, D. W.: Autoimmune haemolytic anemia with acute renal failure due to phenacetin and p-amino-salicylic acid. Lancet, *1*:7, 1960.
444. Maddrey, W. C., and Boitnott, J. K.: Severe hepatitis from methyldopa. Gastroenterology, *68*:361, 1975.
445. Mohler, D. N., Farris, B. L., and Pearre, A. A.: Paroxysmal cold hemoglobinuria with acute renal failure. Arch. Intern. Med., *112*:36, 1963.
446. Mohler, D. N., Husband, R. A., and Boothe, P. E.: Methyldopa (MD)-induced increase of lymphocyte cAMP. In abstracts of Seventeenth Annual Meeting of the Am. Soc. Hematol., 1974.
447. Mollison, P. L.: The effect of isoantibodies on red-cell survival. Ann. N.Y. Acad. Sci., *169*:199, 1970.
448. Moltlan, L., Reidenberg, M. M., and Eichman, M. F.: Positive direct Coombs' test due to cephalothin. N. Engl. J. Med., *277*:123, 1967.
449. Monohitharajah, S. M., Jenkins, W. J., Roberts, P. D., and Clarke, R. C.: Methyldopa and associated thrombocytopena. Br. Med. J., *1*:494, 1971.
450. Muirhead, E. E., Halden, E. R., and Groves, M.: Drug-dependent Coombs (antiglobulin test) and anemia: observations on quinine and acetophenetidin (Phenacetin). Arch. Intern. Med., *101*:87, 1958.
451. Nesmith, L. W., and Davis, J. W.: Hemolytic anemia caused by penicillin. J.A.M.A., *203*:27, 1968.
452. Perry, H. M., Chaplin, H., Carmody, S., Haynes, C., and Frei, C.: Immunologic findings in patients receiving methyldopa: a prospective study. J. Lab. Clin. Med., *78*:905, 1971.
453. Petz, L. D., and Fudenberg, H. H.: Coombs-positive hemolytic anemia caused by penicillin administration. N. Engl. J. Med., *274*:171, 1966.
454. Petz, L. D., and Garratty, G.: Drug-induced haemolytic anaemia. Clin. Haematol., *4*:181, 1975.
455. Pirofsky, B.: Immune haemolytic disease: the autoimmune haemolytic anaemias. Clin. Haematol., *4*:167, 1975.
456. Poole, G., Stradling, P., and Worlledge, S.: Potentially serious side effects of high-dose twice-weekly rifampicin. Br. Med. J., *3*:343, 1971.

457. Ries, C. A., Garratty, G., Petz, L. D., and Fudenberg, H. H.: Paroxymal cold hemoglobinuria: report of a case with an exceptionally high thermal range Donath-Landsteiner antibody. Blood, *38*:491, 1971.
458. Ries, C. A., Rosenbaum, T. J., Garratty, G., Petz, L. D., and Fudenberg, H. H.: Penicillin-induced immune hemolytic anemia. Occurrence of massive intravascular hemolysis. J.A.M.A. *233*:432, 1975.
459. Robertson, J. H., Kennedy, C. C., and Hill, C. M.: Haemolytic anaemia associated with mefenamic acid. Ir. J. Med. Sci., *140*:226, 1971.
460. Robinson, M. G., and Foadi, M.: Hemolytic anemia with positive Coombs test. Association with isoniazid therapy. J.A.M.A., *208*:656, 1969.
461. Rosenthal, M. C., Pisciotta, A. V., Kominos, Z. D., Goldberg, H., and Dameshek, W.: The auto-immune hemolytic anemia of malignant lymphocytic disease. Blood, *10*:197, 1955.
462. Ross, J. F.: Hemoglobinemia and the hemoglobinurias. N. Engl. J. Med., *233*:691, 732, 1945.
463. Rosse, W. F.: Quantitative immunology of immune hemolytic anemia. I. The fixation of C1 by auto-immune antibody and heterologous anti-IgG antibody. II. The relationship of cell-bound antibody to hemolysis and the effect of treatment. J. Clin. Invest., *50*:727, 734, 1971.
464. Rosse, W. F.: Correlation of in vivo and in vitro measurements of hemolysis in hemolytic anemia due to immune reactions. Progr. Hematol., *8*:51, 1973.
465. Rosse, W. F., and Logue, G. L.: Immune hemolytic anemias. Mod. Treat., *8*:379, 1971.
466. Schubothe, H.: The cold hemagglutinin disease. Semin. Hematol., *33*:27, 1966.
467. Schwartz, R. S., and Costea, N.: Autoimmune hemolytic anemia: clinical correlations and biological implications. Semin. Hematol., *3*:2, 1966.
468. Schwartz, R., and Dameshek, W.: The treatment of autoimmune hemolytic anemia with 6-mercaptopurine and thioguanine. Blood, *19*:483, 1962.
469. Scott, G. L., Myles, A. B., and Bacon, P. A.: Autoimmune haemolytic anaemia and mefenamic acid therapy. Br. Med. J., *3*:534, 1968.
470. Shinton, N. K., and Wilson, L.: Autoimmune haemolytic anaemia due to phenacetin and p-aminosalicylic acid. Lancet, *1*:226, 1960.
471. Shulman, N. R.: A mechanism of cell destruction in individuals sensitized to foreign antigens and its implications in autoimmunity. Ann. Intern. Med., *60*:506, 1964.
472. Slugg, P. H., and Kunkel, R. S.: Complications of methysergide therapy, retroperitoneal fibrosis, mitral regurgitation, edema and hemolytic anemia. J.A.M.A., *213*:297, 1970.
473. Snapper, I., Marks, D., Schwartz, L., and Hollander, L.: Hemolytic anemia secondary to mesantoin. Ann. Intern. Med., *37*:619, 1953.
474. Spath, P., Garratty, G., and Petz, L.: Studies on the immune response to penicillin and cephalothin in humans. II. Immunohematologic reactions to cephalothin administration. J. Immunol., *107*:860, 1971.
475. Swanson, M. A., Chanmougan, D., and Schwartz, R. S.: Immunohemolytic anemia due to antipenicillin antibodies. Report of a case. N. Engl. J. Med., *274*:178, 1966.
476. Territo, M. C., Peters, R. W., and Tanaka, K. P.: Autoimmune hemolytic anemia due to levodopa therapy. J.A.M.A., *226*:1347, 1973.
477. Weiner, W.: To be or not to be an antibody: the "agent" in auto-immune hemolytic anemia. Blood, *14*:1057, 1959.
478. Weiner, W., and Vos, G. H.: Serology of acquired hemolytic anemias. Blood, *22*:606, 1963.
479. Weiss, H. J., Berger, R. E., and Tice, E. D.: Fatal disseminated intravascular coagulation and hemolytic anemia following stibophen therapy; a study of basic mechanisms. Am. J. Med. Sci., *264*:375, 1972.
480. White, J. M., Brown, D. L., Hepner, G. W., and Worlledge, S. M.: Penicillin-induced haemolytic anaemia. Br. Med. J., *3*:26, 1968.
481. Worlledge, S. M.: Immune drug-induced hemolytic anemias. Semin. Hematol., *10*:327, 1973.
482. Worlledge, S. M.: Immune Drug-induced Haemolytic Anaemias. *In* Girdwood, R. H. (ed.): Blood Disorders Due to Drugs and Other Agents. Excerpta Medica, Amsterdam, 1973.
483. Worlledge, S. M., Carstairs, K. C., and Dacie, J. V.: Autoimmune haemolytic anaemia associated with α-methyldopa therapy. Lancet, *2*:135, 1966.
484. Worlledge, S. M., and Rousso, C.: Studies on the serology of paroxysmal cold haemoglobinuria (P.C.H.), with special reference to its relationship with the P blood group system. Vox Sang., *10*:293, 1965.
485. Young, L. E., Miller, G., and Christian, R. M.: Clinical and laboratory observations on auto-immune hemolytic disease. Ann. Intern. Med., *35*:507, 1951.

Paroxysmal Nocturnal Hemoglobinuria

486. Aster, R. H., and Enright, S. E.: A platelet and granulocyte membrane defect in paroxysmal nocturnal hemoglobinuria: usefulness for the detection of platelet antibodies. J. Clin. Invest., *48*:1199, 1969.

487. Beal, R. W., Kronenberg, H., and Firkin, B. G.: The syndrome of paroxysmal nocturnal hemoglobinuria. Am. J. Med., 37:899, 1964.
488. Brubaker, L. H., Schaberg, D. R., Jefferson, D. H., and Mengel, C. E.: A potential rapid screening test for paroxysmal nocturnal hemoglobinuria. N. Engl. J. Med., 288:1059, 1973.
489. Carmel, R., Cotman, C. A., Jr., Yatteau, R. F., and Costanzi, J. J.: Association of paroxysmal nocturnal hemoglobinuria with erythroleukemia. N. Engl. J. Med., 283:1329, 1970.
490. Cartwright, G. E.: Diagnostic Laboratory Hematology. 4th Ed. Grune & Stratton, New York, 1968.
491. Charache, S.: Prolonged survival in paroxysmal nocturnal hemoglobinuria. Blood, 33:877, 1969.
492. Crookston, J. H., Crookston, M. C., Burnie, K. L., Francombe, W. H., Dace, J. V., Davis, J. A., and Lewis, S. M.: Hereditary erythroblastic multinuclearity associated with a positive acidified-serum test: a type of congenital dyserythropoietic anaemia. Br. J. Haematol., 17:11, 1969.
493. Dacie, J. V., and Gilpin, A.: Refractory anaemia (Fanconi type). Its incidence in three members of one family, with one case a relationship to chronic haemolytic anemia with nocturnal haemoglobinuria (Marchiafava-Micheli disease or "nocturnal haemoglobinuria"). Arch. Dis. Child., 19:155, 1944.
494. Dacie, J. V., and Lewis, S. M.: Paroxysmal nocturnal haemoglobinuria: Clinical manifestations, haematology, and nature of the disease. Ser. Haematol., 5:3, 1972.
495. Firkin, F., Goldberg, H., and Firkin, B. G.: Glucocorticoid management of paroxysmal nocturnal haemoglobinuria. Australas. Ann. Med., 17:127, 1968.
496. Gaither, J. C.: Paroxysmal nocturnal hemoglobinuria. N. Engl. J. Med., 265:421, 1961.
497. Gotze, O., and Muller-Eberhard, H. J.: Paroxysmal noctural hemoglobinuria. Hemolysis initiated by the C3 activator system. N. Engl. J. Med., 286:180, 1972.
498. Hansen, N. E., and Killmann, S. A.: Paroxysmal nocturnal hemoglobinuria in myelofibrosis. Blood, 36:428, 1970.
499. Hartmann, R. C., Auditore, J. V., and Holland, W. C.: Erythrocyte acetylcholinesterase defect in paroxysmal nocturnal hemoglobinuria. J. Clin. Invest., 37:900, 1958.
500. Hartmann, R. C., and Jenkins, D. E., Jr.: Paroxysmal nocturnal hemoglobinuria: current concepts of certain pathophysiologic features. Blood, 25:850, 1965.
501. Hartmann, R. C., and Jenkins, D. E., Jr.: The "sugar-water" test for paroxysmal nocturnal hemoglobinuria. N. Engl. J. Med., 275:155, 1966.
502. Hartmann, R. C., Jenkins, D. E., Jr., and Arnold, A. B.: Diagnostic specificity of sucrose hemolysis test for paroxysmal nocturnal hemoglobinuria. Blood, 35:462, 1970.
503. Hartmann, R. C., and Kolhouse, J. F.: Viewpoints on the management of paroxysmal nocturnal hemoglobinuria (PNH). Ser. Haematol., 5:42, 1972.
504. Holden, D., and Lichtman, H.: Paroxysmal nocturnal hemoglobinuria with acute leukemia. Blood, 33:283, 1969.
505. Jenkins, D. E., Jr., and Hartmann, R. C.: Paroxysmal nocturnal hemoglobinuria terminating in acute myeloblastic leukemia. Blood, 33:274, 1969.
506. Johns, R. J.: Familial reduction in red-cell cholinesterase. N. Engl. J. Med., 267:1344, 1962.
507. Kan, S. Y., and Gardner, F. H.: Life span of reticulocytes in paroxysmal nocturnal hemoglobinuria. Blood, 25:759, 1965.
508. Kaufman, R. W., Schecter, G. P., and McFarland, W.: Paroxysmal nocturnal hemoglobinuria terminating in acute granulocytic leukemia. Blood, 33:287, 1969.
509. Kuo, C., Van Voolen, A., and Morrison, A. N.: Primary and secondary myelofibrosis: its relationship to "PNH-like defect." Blood, 40:875, 1972.
510. Lewis, S. M., and Dacie, J. V.: The aplastic anemia-paroxysmal nocturnal hemoglobinuria syndrome. Br. J. Haematol., 13:236, 1967.
511. Metz, J., Stevens, K., van Rensburg, N. J., and Hart, D.: Failure of in-vivo inhibition of acetylcholinesterase to affect erythrocyte life-span: the significance of the enzyme defect in paroxysmal nocturnal haemoglobinuria. Br. J. Haematol., 7:458, 1961.
512. Quagliana, J. M., Cartwright, G. E., and Wintrobe, M. M.: Paroxysmal nocturnal hemoglobinuria following drug-induced aplastic anemia. Ann. Intern. Med., 61:1045, 1964.
513. Rosse, W. F.: The complement sensitivity of PNH cells. Ser. Haematol., 5:101, 1972.
514. Rosse, W. F., and Dacie, J. V.: Immune lysis of normal human and paroxysmal nocturnal hemoglobinuria red blood cells. II. The role of complement components in the increased sensitivity of PNH red cells to immune lysis. J. Clin. Invest., 45:749, 1966.
515. Rosse, W. F., and Gutterman, L. A.: The effect of iron therapy in paroxysmal nocturnal hemoglobinuria. Blood, 36:559, 1970.
516. Sirchia, G., and Lewis, S. M.: Paroxysmal nocturnal haemoglobinuria. Clin. Haematol., 4:199, 1975.
517. Storb, R., Evans, R. S., Thomas, E. D., Buckner, C. D., Clift, R. A., Fefer, A., Neiman, P., and

Wright, S. E.: Paroxysmal nocturnal haemaglobinuria and refractory marrow failure treated by marrow transplantation. Br. J. Haematol., *24*:743, 1973.

518. Yachnin, S., and Ruthenberg, J. M.: The initiation and enhancement of human red cell lysis by activators of the first component of complement and by first component esterase, studies using normal red cells and red cells from patients with paroxysmal nocturnal hemoglobinuria. J. Clin. Invest., *44*:518, 1965.

MECHANICAL HEMOLYSIS

519. Brain, M. C.: Microangiopathic hemolytic anemia. N. Engl. J. Med., *281*:833, 1969.
520. Brain, M. C.: The hemolytic-uremic syndrome. Semin. Hematol., *6*:162, 1969.
521. Brain, M. C.: Microangiopathic hemolytic anemia. Br. J. Haematol., *23*(Suppl):45, 1972.
522. Brain, M. C., Dacie, J. V., and Hourihane, D. O'B.: Microangiopathic haemolytic anemia: the possible role of vascular lesions in pathogenesis. Br. J. Haematol., *8*:358, 1962.
523. Bull, B. S., and Kuhn, I. N.: The production of schistocytes by fibrin strands (a scanning electron microscope study). Blood, *35*:104, 1970.
524. Chaplin, H., Perkoff, G. T., Frisbie, J. H., Tateishi, S., and Haynes, C. R.: March hemoglobinuria. J.A.M.A., *208*:1700, 1969.
525. Dacie, J. V.: Secondary or Symptomatic Haemolytic Anaemias. Part III in The Hemolytic Anaemias, Congenital and Acquired. 2nd Ed. Grune & Stratton, New York, 1967.
526. Davidson, R. J. L.: Exertional haemoglobinuria: a report on three cases with studies on the haemolytic mechanism. J. Clin. Pathol., *17*:536, 1964.
527. Davidson, R. J. L.: March or exertional haemoglobinuria. Semin. Hematol., *6*:150, 1969.
528. Ducrou, W., Harding, P. E., Kimber, R. J., and Kutkaite, D.: Traumatic haemolysis after heart valve replacement: a comparison of haematological investigations. Aust. N.Z. J. Med., *2*:118, 1972.
529. Ellman, L., and Knock-Macauley, H.: Traumatic hemolysis with rupture of aneurysm of sinus of Valsalva. Arch. Intern. Med., *126*:1019, 1970.
530. Eyster, E., Mayer, K., and McKenzie, S.: Traumatic hemolysis with iron deficiency anemia in patients with aortic valve lesions. Ann. Intern. Med., *68*:995, 1968.
531. Gilligan, D. R., Altschule, M. D., and Katersky, E. M.: Physiologic intravascular hemolysis of exercise. Hemoglobinemia and hemoglobinuria following cross-country runs. J. Clin. Invest., *22*:859, 1943.
532. Hollingsworth, J. H., and Mohler, D. N.: Microangiopathic hemolytic anemia caused by purpura fulminans. Ann. Intern. Med., *68*:1310, 1968.
533. Kaden, W. S.: Traumatic haemoglobinuria in conga-drum players. Lancet, *1*:1341, 1970.
534. Marsh, G. W., and Lewis, S. M.: Cardiac haemolytic anaemia. Semin. Hematol., *6*:133, 1969.
535. Nevaril, C. G., Lynch, E. C., Alfrey, C. P., and Hellums, J. D.: Erythrocyte damage and destruction induced by shearing stress. J. Lab. Clin. Med., *71*:784, 1968.
536. Pirofsky, B.: Hemolysis in valvular heart disease. Ann. Intern. Med., *65*:373, 1966.
537. Rubenberg, M. L., Regoeczi, E., Bull, B. S., Dacie, J. V., and Brain, M. C.: Microangiopathic haemolytic anemia: the experimental production of haemolysis and red cell fragmentation by defibrination in vivo. Br. J. Haematol., *14*:627, 1968.
538. Spicer, A. J.: Studies on march hemoglobinuria. Br. Med. J., *1*:155, 1970.
539. Streeton, J. A.: Traumatic hemoglobinuria caused by karate exercises. Lancet, *2*:191, 1967.
540. Stuard, I. D., Heusinkveld, R. S., and Moss, A. J.: Microangiopathic hemolytic anemia, thrombocytopenia and pulmonary hypertension. N. Engl. J. Med., *287*:869, 1972.
541. Venkatachalam, M. A., Jones, D. B., and Nelson, D. A.: Microangiopathic hemolytic anemia in rats with malignant hypertension. Blood, *32*:278, 1968.
542. Walinsky, P., Spitzer, S., Brodsky, I., Kasparian, H., and Mason, D.: Hemolytic anemia with a Cross-Jones prosthesis. Am. J. Med. Sci., *254*:831, 1967.
543. Ziperovich, S., and Paley, H. W.: Severe mechanical hemolytic anemia due to valvular heart disease without prosthesis. Ann. Intern. Med., *65*:342, 1966.

INFECTIONS, CHEMICAL AGENTS, PHYSICAL AGENTS, HYPOPHOSPHATEMIA

544. Adner, M. M., Alstatt, L. B., and Conrad, M. E.: Coombs positive hemolytic disease in malaria. Ann. Intern. Med., *68*:33, 1968.
545. Banwell, J. G., and Kibukamusoke, J. W.: Haemolytic anemia and relapsing fever. East Afr. Med. J., *40*:124, 1963.
546. Bennett, J. M., and Healey, P. J. M.: Spherocytic hemolytic anemia and acute cholecystitis caused by Clostridium welchii. N. Engl. J. Med., *268*:1070, 1963.

547. Caulfield, L. J.: Renal and hematologic complications of acute falciparum malaria in Vietnam. Bull. N.Y. Acad. Med., *45*:1043, 1969.
548. De, S. E., Sengupta, K. P., and Chandra, N. N.: Intravascular haemolysis in cholera. Lancet, *1*:807, 1954.
549. Deiss, A., Lee, G. R., and Cartwright, G. E.: Hemolytic anemia in Wilson's disease. Ann. Intern. Med., *74*:413, 1970.
550. Easton, J. W., Koplin, D. F., Swofford, H. S., Kellstrand, C. M., and Jacob, H. S.: Chlorinated urban water: a cause of dialysis-induced hemolytic anemia. Science, *181*:463, 1973.
551. Fairbanks, V. F.: Copper sulphate-induced hemolytic anemia. Arch. Intern. Med., *120*:429, 1967.
552. Fowler, B. A., and Weiseberg, J. B.: Arsine poisoning. N. Engl. J. Med., *291*:1171, 1974.
553. Jacob, H. S., and Amsden, T.: Acute hemolytic anemia with rigid red cells in hypophosphatemia. N. Engl. J. Med., *285*:1446, 1971.
554. Jenkins, G. C.: Arsine poisoning. Br. Med. J., *2*:78, 1965.
555. Kalderon, A. E., Kikkawa, Y., and Bernstein, J.: Chronic toxoplasmosis associated with severe hemolytic anemia. Arch. Intern. Med., *114*:95, 1964.
556. Kimber, R. J., and Lander, H.: The effect of heart on human red cell morphology, fragility and subsequent survival in vivo. J. Lab. Clin. Med., *64*:922, 1964.
557. Klein, W. J., Metz, E. N., and Price, A. R.: Acute copper intoxication: a hazard of hemodialysis. Arch. Intern. Med., *129*:578, 1972.
558. Klock, J. C., and Mentzer, W. C.: Hemolytic anemia and somatic cell dysfunction in severe hypophosphatemia. Arch. Intern. Med., *134*:360, 1974.
559. Manzler, A. D., and Schreiner, A. W.: Copper-induced hemolytic anemia. A new complication of hemodialysis. Ann. Intern. Med., *73*:409, 1970.
560. Retief, F. P., and Hofmeyer, N. G.: Acute hemolytic anemia as a complication of typhoid fever. S. Afr. Med. J., *39*:96, 1965.
561. Reynafarje, C., and Ramos, J.: The hemolytic anemia of human bartonellosis. Blood, *17*:562, 1961.
562. Shen, S. C., and Ham, T. H.: Studies on the destruction of red blood cells. III. Mechanism and complication of hemoglobinuria in patients with thermal burns, spherocytosis and increased osmotic fragility or red blood cells. N. Engl. J. Med., *229*:701, 1943.

CHAPTER **8**

ANEMIA ASSOCIATED
WITH OTHER CONDITIONS

CHRONIC DISEASE

Anemia, generally without neutropenia or thrombocytopenia, often develops in patients with chronic disease, particularly infections, neoplasms, chronic renal disease, rheumatoid arthritis, connective tissue disorders, fractures, and severe tissue injuries.[1-6] It is the commonest type of anemia seen in hospitalized patients, but it usually does not become apparent until the patient has been ill for a month or more.

The anemia is mild, and only rarely is the hemoglobin less than 9 gm. per 100 ml. and the hematocrit less than 27 per cent; lower figures indicate the probable presence of some other factor. The anemia is usually normocytic and normochromic, less often normocytic and hypochromic, and rarely microcytic and hypochromic.

Studies of patients with this type of anemia have indicated that several mechanisms are faulty. The survival time of the erythrocytes is modestly shortened because of an extracorpuscular factor. This shortening would not be of any consequence were it not for impaired bone marrow response which, in some patients, not all, may be the result of diminished erythropoietin production. In addition, iron metabolism[4] is disordered; there is diminished flow of iron from the storage cells to the erythropoietic cells in the bone marrow, a situation which causes the accumulation of iron in the storage cells and a reduction in the number of sideroblasts. Apparently the available iron which reaches the normoblasts is handled in a normal manner.

The defective mechanisms that have been found in this type of anemia produce a characteristic picture which consists of the following: (1) reduced plasma iron (10 to 70 micrograms per 100 ml.); (2) decreased iron-binding capacity (100 to 300 micrograms per 100 ml.); (3) reduced saturation of the plasma transferrin (10 to 25 per cent); (4) decreased numbers of bone marrow sideroblasts (reduction from 40 per cent to less than 20 per cent); (5) normal or

289

increased storage iron. Erythropoiesis is normoblastic in type unless there is some associated deficiency of folate or vitamin B_{12}.

Factors which are responsible for the subnormal erythropoietin response to the anemia, and those concerned in the trapping of the iron in the reticulo-endothelial cells, which produces an unusual functional type of iron deficiency, are poorly understood. It has been suggested that the decreased levels of plasma albumin, transferrin, and erythropoietin seen in chronic disease are a reflection of impaired protein synthesis that occurs in these disorders.[4] The anemia usually improves when the underlying disease improves. Androgens, which stimulate the production of the erythropoietin, are rarely used because of the possible occurrence of undesirable side-effects. The anemia is seldom severe enough to warrant blood transfusion, the only really effective treatment available at the present time, but some older patients with vascular disease and circulatory insufficiency require transfusions when the hemoglobin level is no lower than 9 or 10 gm. per 100 ml.

MYXEDEMA

The occurrence of anemia in myxedema was first noted by Charcot in 1881,[10] and in 1883 Kocher reported that anemia appeared gradually following surgical removal of the thyroid gland.[14] Since that time anemia has been recognized as a frequent development in patients with spontaneous myxedema and also in those who develop thyroid deficiency following surgery. The incidence of anemia was reported as 52 per cent in one series of patients,[17] and was 43 per cent in a series of 100 patients seen at the University of Virginia Hospital.

MECHANISM OF THE ANEMIA

Several different types of anemia occur singly or in combination in patients with myxedema. They are: the uncomplicated anemia of hypothyroidism; anemia caused by vitamin B_{12} deficiency; and anemia of iron deficiency.

The uncomplicated anemia of hypothyroidism, which is normochromic and normocytic or slightly macrocytic, is rarely if ever severe; usually the red count is over 3.0 mil. per cu.mm. and the hematocrit is over 30 per cent. The weight of evidence supports the concept advanced by Wälchli[24] and Bomford[8] that the anemia in myxedema is an adaptation to a condition of relative oxygen surfeit in the tissues, rather than the consequence of an illness associated with partial failure of bone marrow function that is the result of the lack of thyroid factor. Clinical observation has shown that patients with myxedema and anemia associated with a deficiency of vitamin B_{12} or iron can respond at least partially to vitamin B_{12} or iron without treatment with thyroid hormone. Experiments have demonstrated that the hematopoietic response of hypothyroid rats subjected to bleeding or exposure to low pressure chambers is the same as that of normal rats.[13, 20] Clinical investigations in patients with myxedema and anemia have revealed that erythropoiesis is stimulated by phlebotomy and by dinitrophenol, a preparation which increases oxygen consumption without increasing

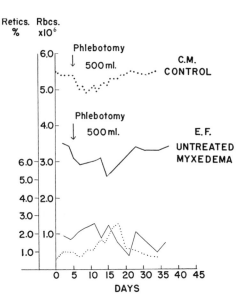

Figure 8–1 Response to bleeding of a normal patient and a patient with untreated myxedema. The restoration of the erythrocyte count to the pre-phlebotomy level within the normal period of time indicates that the bone marrow of patients with untreated myxedema is capable of responding to a stimulus for erythropoiesis. (From Leavell, Thorup, and McClellan: Tr. Am. Clin. Climatol. A., vol. 68, 1956.)

thyroid function (Fig. 8–1).[15, 22] These clinical and experimental observations demonstrate that the marrow in the hypothyroid state is able to respond to an appropriate stimulus without the administration of thyroxin, and they support the concept that the anemia is the result of an adaptation to the hypometabolic state.

Pernicious anemia and myxedema may coexist in the same patient, and the incidence of this association, variously estimated as being from 1 to 12 per cent, appears to be increased.[9] The cause of the increased frequency of vitamin B_{12} deficiency in myxedema is not apparent. Although there may be occasional instances of an effect of the thyroid hormone on the absorption of vitamin B_{12},[16] this absorption is normal in most patients with myxedema, and the administration of thyroid preparation does not lead to an increase in the absorption or in the serum level of vitamin B_{12} in hypothyroid patients with vitamin B_{12} deficiency.[22, 23] The increased incidence of antibodies to thyroglobulin, 25 to 50 per cent, that has been found in patients with pernicious anemia suggests that autoimmunity may be a mechanism in the production of myxedema and pernicious anemia in the same patient.[11, 12]

Iron deficiency occurs in some patients with myxedema. Although the possible importance of a reported defective absorption of dietary iron[21] has not been determined, it is likely that in most patients with myxedema the causes of iron deficiency are the same as in other individuals. One possible difference is an increased frequency of excessive menstrual flow in premenopausal women with hypothyroidism.[9]

CLINICAL MANIFESTATIONS

The onset of the symptoms in myxedema is often insidious, with increasing weakness, muscular aches, lack of energy, and increased tolerance to heat and intolerance to cold. Severe constipation is often a troublesome symptom. Puffiness of the eyelids and swelling of the face and extremities are often apparent to the patient. Contrary to the popular lay opinion, weight gain is by no means a universal symptom in thyroid deficiency.

When the patient is examined the diagnosis may be suggested by the appearance of the patient's face, which is often pale, dull, and expressionless. The trunk and extremities frequently appear edematous, but the edema does not pit on pressure. Much of the hair normally present on the head and body may be lost, and that which remains is coarse in texture. In severe cases the skin is dry and scaly and has a pale yellow tinge. The voice is usually hoarse and deep, and speech is slow and deliberate. In many patients the tongue is enlarged. The recovery phase of the deep tendon reflexes is sluggish. In addition to the signs characteristic of myxedema, the patient may have the signs of associated cardiovascular disturbance such as edema, ascites, and pericardial effusion.

LABORATORY EXAMINATIONS

The anemia is not severe in the uncomplicated case of myxedema. The lowest erythrocyte count observed in the authors' series was 3.0 mil. per cu.mm. The MCV ranged from 81 to 110 cu. μ and was over 94 cu. μ in 60 per cent. The blood smears showed little or no poikilocytosis or anisocytosis. There was no instance of hypochromic microcytic anemia in this group, but the serum iron level was found reduced in four of ten patients in whom it was measured. The values ranged from 32 to 99 micrograms per 100 ml. (normal 60 to 150). Three of the patients with low serum iron levels were women who had mild normocytic anemia, and the fourth was a man with a hematocrit of 40 per cent in whom no chronic blood loss could be demonstrated. Whether these values indicate undetected blood loss or the poor absorption of food iron that has been reported to occur in myxedema is uncertain. Leukocyte counts varied from 3400 to 13,000 per cu.mm., but were usually normal. The platelet counts were also normal. Although bone marrow hypoplasia has been reported to be a feature of myxedema,[7] bone marrow aspiration in this series revealed the cellularity of the marrow to be within normal limits in slightly more than one-half the patients, and hypocellular in the remainder. Erythropoiesis was normoblastic in every instance.

The results of the other laboratory tests are those usually found in any patient with myxedema.

DIAGNOSIS AND PROGNOSIS

If myxedema is considered in the differential diagnosis, its presence can usually be established or excluded without difficulty by a consideration of the clinical features and by means of appropriate laboratory tests. Myxedema is sometimes mistaken for pernicious anemia because the pallor and yellowish tint of the skin of patients with myxedema suggest it, as does the macrocytosis.

An incorrect diagnosis of aplastic anemia is also made at times because of the failure of the anemia to respond to treatment with iron, vitamin B_{12}, and other preparations.

The anemia of myxedema generally responds to the administration of thyroid substance in the usual dosage (desiccated thyroid 0.03 to 0.1 gm. per day) by a gradual rise in the hemoglobin and erythrocytes to normal levels in from three to nine months. The prognosis is excellent as long as the patient continues treatment. If there is an associated deficiency of iron or vitamin B_{12} the appropriate preparation must be given in addition to desiccated thyroid in order to restore the blood to normal.

ACUTE BLOOD LOSS

Anemia that is caused by the sudden loss of a large volume of blood may occur in a variety of circumstances. Among these are trauma, postoperative hemorrhage, ruptured ectopic pregnancy, ruptured aneurysm, ruptured esophageal varices, esophageal tears (Mallory-Weiss syndrome) from vomiting (especially if a hemorrhagic tendency is present), and ulcerative lesions of the gastrointestinal tract. Massive bleeding occurs spontaneously or after minor trauma in patients with the various hemorrhagic disorders. The clinical picture that the patient presents depends on the amount, location, and acuteness of the bleeding, as well as the nature of the underlying disorder and the previous condition of the patient. The usual symptoms of an acute hemorrhage are sudden weakness, dizziness, pallor, thirst and sweating. The marked variability in the manifestations is shown by the fact that in some patients syncope is the initial symptom, whereas in others the passage of bloody or tarry stools may be the only indication that a hemorrhage has occurred.

The changes in the peripheral blood depend on the time that has elapsed since the hemorrhage, the size and location of the hemorrhage, and the nature of the underlying disease. The amount of blood lost can be measured better by a determination of the blood volume than by the hematocrit reading, because the latter may not reach its lowest point until 48 or 72 hours after the hemorrhage.[25] Unless preceding iron deficiency or a brisk reticulocytosis is present, the anemia is usually of the normocytic type. Thrombocytosis and leukocytosis, accompanied by an increase in the younger forms, occur after a few hours. Reticulocytosis begins in two or three days and reaches a peak in from four to seven days.[26] Reticulocyte counts as high as 12 or 14 per cent often follow an acute hemorrhage severe enough to reduce the red blood count to about 3.0 mil. per cu.mm. (Fig. 8–2). Hemorrhage into the tissues or body cavities may be followed by rises in both reticulocytes and serum bilirubin. If bleeding has ceased, an increase in the erythrocyte count becomes evident by the time the reticulocytosis reaches its maximum; the count continues to rise, even without treatment, until the normal level is reached, usually in from four to six weeks. The erythrocyte count is reported to return to a level of 4.5 mil. per cu.mm. within about 33 days after an acute episode irrespective of the size of the hemorrhage.[27]

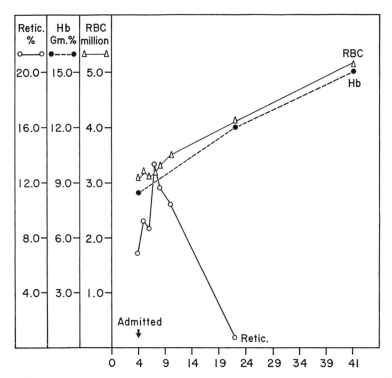

Figure 8–2 Chart showing hematologic response to acute hemorrhage. The peak reticulocyte response of 13 per cent occurred on the seventh day. The hemoglobin level and erythrocyte counts returned to normal during the fifth week.

There are two important aspects in the diagnosis of the patient with an acute hemorrhage. These are the recognition of acute blood loss as the cause of anemia, and the determination of the cause of the bleeding. Recognition of the hemorrhage usually presents no difficulties, but at times its severity may not be appreciated unless it is remembered that the hematocrit reading may give little or no indication of the amount of blood that has been lost. If the stool has not been examined for occult blood, an elevated reticulocyte count associated with a normocytic anemia or an elevation of the blood urea level may be the first clue to a recent hemorrhage. In order to determine the cause of the hemorrhage, roentgenographic study of the gastrointestinal tract, gastroscopy, celiac angiograms, liver function tests, special studies for blood dyscrasias, and even surgical exploration may be necessary.

Treatment of acute hemorrhage is often the treatment of shock by means of intravenous fluids, vasopressor agents, and blood transfusions. Other treatment is directed toward the underlying disease. Unless the patient's iron stores have become depleted because of previous bleeding or some other factor, the hemoglobin and red cell count will return to normal levels after a moderate-sized hemorrhage without therapy with iron.

PREGNANCY

During normal pregnancy reductions in the hematocrit, hemoglobin, and erythrocyte count are found. The maximal decrease occurs during the last trimester when the reduction may amount to 15 or 25 per cent.[29, 31, 35] These changes are due at least in part to hemodilution, since the plasma volume increases by 800 to 1300 ml. (around 1000 ml.), whereas the red cell volume increases by only about 300 ml.[28] These values return to normal a few weeks after delivery.[37] Because of these disproportionate changes, decreases in hematocrit, erythrocytes, and hemoglobin levels can be considered to be physiologic to a certain extent.

Not all changes that occur in the blood during pregnancy can be explained by hemodilution, because the level of the serum iron falls while the values for the free erythrocyte protoporphyrin and the latent iron-binding capacity rise.[31, 33, 34] In nonpregnant patients elevations of the free erythrocyte protoporphyrin and latent iron-binding capacity are most often seen in iron deficiency. More direct evidence of the frequent development of actual iron deficiency during pregnancy is the observation that the serum iron level fell in about 80 per cent of a group of patients who received no supplemental iron during pregnancy, but remained normal in 80 per cent of those who received iron salts orally.[35, 36]

The mother loses iron to the fetus and also with bleeding during delivery. The iron requirements for the fetus, which will be met at the expense of the mother, amount to about 400 mg. As the absence of menstruation during pregnancy allows the mother to conserve 325 mg. of iron that would ordinarily be lost through menstruation, the net added requirement of pregnancy is about 75 mg. However, the loss of iron in the placenta and in bleeding at the time of parturition has been estimated to average about 325 mg. Calculations from these figures therefore indicate that the net additional iron necessary for pregnancy is 400 mg. or 500 mg.[40]

There is disagreement concerning the normal range of the blood values during pregnancy. The following values have been said to represent the lower normal limits of hemoglobin and erythrocytes during pregnancy: hemoglobin 10 gm. per 100 ml.; erythrocytes, 3.5 mil. per cu.mm.;[39] hemoglobin 11.3 to 11.5 gm. per 100 ml.; red cells 3.7 mil. per cu.mm.; hematocrit 35 per cent.[29, 34] The W.H.O. places the lower limit of normal hemoglobin in pregnant females at 11.0 gm. per 100 ml.[37] The reported frequency of anemia in pregnancy varies from 30 per cent to 80 per cent.[35, 39]

TYPES OF ANEMIA

Iron deficiency is the commonest cause of anemia during pregnancy. It occurred in about 75 per cent of one series of patients.[35] In many instances some degree of iron deficiency antedates the pregnancy.[29, 35, 39] Severe iron deficiency is evidenced by the occurrence of a hypochromic microcytic type of anemia, but a milder degree of iron deficiency may be associated with only minor changes in the indices and in the appearance of the erythrocytes. When iron deficiency is present, the serum iron level is reduced to less than 60 micrograms per 100 ml., and the latent iron-binding capacity is increased; erythropoiesis is normoblastic in type.

Other types of anemia are much less common than that due to iron deficiency. Macrocytic anemia, attributed to dietary deficiency, was observed in 8.4 to 25.7 per cent of the patients in one series.[30] The higher incidence of this type of anemia occurred in a group of 70 patients of a low economic status. Anemia associated with a megaloblastic type of erythropoiesis sometimes occurs during pregnancy or the puerperium. In one series of 45 patients with megaloblastic erythropoiesis indistinguishable from that seen in pernicious anemia, the mean corpuscular volume was greater than 100 cu. μ in only one-half the patients. The changes in the blood smears were similar to those seen in pernicious anemia but were less marked. Free hydrochloric acid was present in the gastric secretion in three-quarters of the patients.

The megaloblastic anemia of pregnancy is nearly always the result of folate deficiency. Megaloblastic maturation in the bone marrow, hypersegmented granulocytes in the peripheral blood, thrombocytopenia, and low serum folate levels occur. Multiple factors, such as increased need during pregnancy, inadequate intake, and malabsorption may be responsible. Evidence of intestinal malabsorption, as measured by xylose absorption, serum carotene levels, and fecal excretion of fat, is found in some pregnant patients.[41] The thrombocytopenia which occurs in folate deficiency may be responsible for serious vaginal bleeding during or after delivery.[38] A relationship between folate deficiency and toxemia, infection, and premature delivery has been suspected but not established. Serum vitamin B_{12} levels have been variously reported as normal or slightly reduced in pregnancy, but vitamin B_{12} deficiency rarely is responsible for the megaloblastic anemia of pregnancy, probably because large reserve stores of the vitamins are normally present.

The development of aplastic anemia during pregnancy is serious but fortunately rare. Of the more than 30 cases reported, three-quarters died during pregnancy; nearly all the survivors recovered within a few weeks after delivery.[32]

Recognition of the factors responsible for anemia during pregnancy is not always easy, because iron deficiency occurs in association with normal indices and megaloblastic anemia occurs with normal indices or even with microcytosis. Determination of the serum iron level, which is reduced in iron deficiency and normal or elevated in other types of anemia, measurement of the serum folate level, and a study of the bone marrow usually enable the diagnosis to be established. Even with the benefit of the bone marrow examination, recognition of the type of anemia may be difficult if the patient has taken multivitamin tablets. These often contain amounts of folic acid that may be sufficient to convert a megaloblastic type of erythropoiesis to the normoblastic type, and yet be inadequate to correct the anemia.

When the patient with anemia is seen for the first time during pregnancy, the possibility that the anemia may be the result of some coexisting disease rather than the pregnancy must be considered. Leukemia, diseases of the lymphoma group, renal disease, or almost any other cause of anemia may be recognized for the first time during pregnancy. The occurrence of pregnancy in a patient with one of the hemoglobinopathies may be serious because of the high incidence of complications in the mother or the child. When one of the hemoglobinopathies is considered in the diagnosis, it is important to differentiate the benign combination of a trait condition and an anemia of pregnancy from the more serious homozygous or doubly heterozygous abnormalities.

TREATMENT AND PROGNOSIS

The best therapy for the anemia of pregnancy is preventive. In most patients, iron deficiency anemia can be prevented by the ingestion of an adequate diet or by supplementation with 0.3 gm. of ferrous sulfate three times a day. A single 0.3 gm. tablet taken at bedtime is also effective. Most macrocytic anemias can be prevented by a liberal daily diet which contains one quart of milk, one-quarter pound of lean meat, and one egg a day, or by supplementing the diet with 5 mg. of folic acid.[39] When multivitamin preparations are used to supplement the diet of pregnant patients, it is important to be sure that the multivitamin preparation includes at least 400 micrograms of folic acid.[38] If an iron deficiency anemia has developed it can generally be corrected by the administration of 0.3 gm. of ferrous sulfate three times a day. In the occasional patient, who does not tolerate oral iron because of gastrointestinal symptoms, parenteral iron may be required. Most patients with megaloblastic anemia do not respond to vitamin B_{12}, but usually respond to folic acid in a dose of from 5 to 20 mg. a day. The unusual occurrence of a response to the combination of vitamin B_{12} and ascorbic acid after the failure of each preparation singly has been reported.[33] As is true in other circumstances, the pregnant patient who is seriously ill with a severe degree of anemia may need blood transfusions before the diagnosis of the type of anemia can be established. Even in this situation it is rare that the necessary hematologic studies cannot be initiated or the necessary specimens obtained before the therapy is started.

The prognosis of the patients who develop anemia during pregnancy is excellent when proper treatment is given, if no serious complicating disorders are present. If iron deficiency develops, therapy with iron may be necessary for some months after the pregnancy in order to replenish the iron stores. Megaloblastic anemia rarely relapses after adequate therapy, but may recur in subsequent pregnancies.

CHRONIC RENAL DISEASE

The majority of patients with chronic renal insufficiency develop anemia. In patients with severe renal disease, the hematocrit is usually in the range of 15 to 30 vol. per cent. Numerous studies have shown that the anemia is a result of one or more of the following factors: diminished erythropoiesis, hyperhemolysis, or bleeding. At times a deficiency of iron or folate is important.[42, 46, 53]

The anemia associated with chronic renal disease is nearly always normochromic and normocytic in type, but a macrocytic anemia occurs occasionally. In one series of patients with uremia secondary to various types of renal disease, the hemoglobin levels ranged from 5.6 to 8.4 gm. per 100 ml. and the erythrocyte counts ranged from 1.5 to 3.5 ml. per cu.mm.[53] In the same series varying degrees of reticulocytosis, 2.4 to 22.5 per cent, occurred irregularly. The leukocyte and platelet counts are usually normal. Examination of the bone marrow reveals erythrocytic hypoplasia, normal cellularity, or erythrocytic hyperplasia. The serum iron level and the unsaturated iron-binding capacity are usually normal or slightly decreased unless significant blood loss has occurred. The antiglobulin (Coombs) test, hypotonic saline fragility test, mechanical fragility test, and serum bilirubin levels are usually normal. The fecal urobilinogen excretion is increased when hyperhemolysis is present.

For many years the anemia of uremia was ascribed to an accumulation in the blood of poisons secondary to defective renal function. It was noted that, whatever the nature of these "poisons" might be, the action on the marrow appeared to be selective because erythrocyte precursors seemed to be depressed, although activity was normal or increased in the other marrow elements. Histologic evidence of hypoplasia of the erythroid series was found on examination of the marrow only when the nonprotein nitrogen level of the blood was above 150 mg. per 100 ml. Complete aplasia was not found, and it was suggested that a defect in the delivery of red blood cells to the peripheral blood from the bone marrow might be a factor in the anemia.

The diminished erythropoiesis in uremia has been demonstrated in several ways. It has been reported that in patients with uremia there is a decreased rate of utilization of radioactive iron[48, 53] and an increased storage of iron in the liver and spleen.[51] In vitro studies of bone marrow cells suspended in culture media containing uremic serum have revealed a decrease in the rate of maturation of erythrocyte precursors[54] and a diminished rate of removal of iron from the culture media.[56] The depression of erythropoiesis is probably due mainly to faulty erythropoietin production by the diseased kidneys. The presence of an additional factor, an impaired response of the bone marrow to appropriate stimulation, is shown by observations made on patients being treated by chronic dialysis;[42] with this treatment erythropoiesis improved and erythropoietin levels rose, the latter probably coming from extrarenal sources.

In 1949 Emerson and Burroughs[45] published the first of a series of reports indicating that hyperhemolysis, manifested by a rapid fall in the hematocrit, difficulty in maintaining a hematocrit level of 15 vol. per cent, and an absolute rise in reticulocyte count, contributes to the production of anemia in uremia in some circumstances. When the survival time of erythrocytes was measured by the Ashby technique of differential agglutination, it was found that normal donor cells were destroyed in the recipient uremic patient at one-and-a-half to three times the normal rate. Erythrocytes from uremic patients survived normally in the normal recipient. It was concluded that some extracorpuscular factor present in the plasma of uremic patients was responsible for the premature destruction of red blood cells. Other investigators demonstrated that this hemolytic activity was not found in all patients and was not constant in the same patient.[52] The occurrence of hemolysis appeared to coincide with the periods of rapid progression of the underlying renal disease. Nevertheless, hyperhemolysis is not the only mechanism concerned in the anemia of uremia. Even during periods of increased hemolytic activity, the decrease in the life span of the red blood cells is not sufficient to produce anemia if the marrow responds normally.[43] Thus, although hemolysis contributes to the anemia in certain patients, it appears that depression of erythropoiesis is the most important and most common factor.

Another aspect of this complex problem has been indicated by the studies of Rees et al., which suggest that a disorganization of metabolism occurs in red blood cells that are suspended in uremic serum.[55] The transfer of iron into the developing erythrocyte seems to be energy-dependent, and it is possible that a metabolic dysfunction which alters energy output interferes with iron uptake in vivo and in vitro.

Patients being treated by chronic dialysis sometimes develop other hematologic complications. Some develop folate depletion, which may result in a megoblastic anemia, and others develop iron deficiency anemia, probably the result of loss of red cells in the dialyzer. In some patients undergoing hemodialysis, an oxidant Heinz-body type of hemolytic anemia has developed as a result of the action of chloramines present in the water that was used.[42] Iron overload from repeated transfusions of patients treated with chronic dialysis has not proved to be the problem that it was expected to be.

Renal transplant patients who are being treated with immunosuppressive agents develop varying degrees of bone marrow depression with resultant anemia, granulocytopenia, or thrombocytopenia. In some, study of the bone marrow discloses striking dyserythropoiesis with morphologic abnormalities in the red cell precursors similar to those seen in the Di Guglielmo syndrome.

Unless renal function improves, treatment of the anemia usually produces

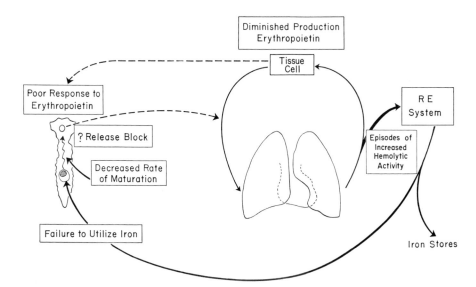

Figure 8–3   Schematic representation of the factors thought to be concerned in the production of anemia in chronic renal disease. Despite the presence of anemia and the reduced oxygen-carrying capacity of the blood there is a failure of the factors which normally operate to compensate for this deficiency.

only temporary or modest benefit. For a prompt increase in hematocrit, red cell transfusions are necessary. Androgens, which act mainly by stimulating erythropoietin production, may produce significant elevations of the hematocrit after three to six months of treatment in patients who still have renal tissue; anephric patients respond poorly, if at all, to these preparations.[47, 49]

Figure 8–3 summarizes the various factors thought to play a role in the production of anemia in decompensated renal disease.

CHRONIC LIVER DISEASE

Anemia occurs often in patients with chronic liver disease. The morphologic characteristics of the anemia, which may be macrocytic, normocytic, or hypochromic microcytic, depend on the mechanisms responsible for the anemia. Blood loss, increased hemolysis, or deficient erythropoiesis may be the most important factor in a particular individual.

Hypochromic microcytic anemia may indicate iron deficiency or chronic blood loss from the gastrointestinal tract. It may be the result of repeated severe hemorrhages from ruptured esophageal varices or mild chronic blood loss from irritation of the gastrointestinal tract. Increased pressure in the portal circulation and a defect in blood coagulation may be contributing factors.

In chronic liver disease the anemia is usually macrocytic, but is sometimes normocytic. The mean corpuscular volume is usually between 100 and 120.[64] The marked anisocytosis and poikilocytosis which are usually seen in pernicious anemia are often absent in chronic liver disease, but target cells are often numerous; nucleated red cells rarely appear in the peripheral circulation. Although significant poikilocytosis is rarely seen in the peripheral blood smear, a severe deformity, "burr poikilocytosis," and a severe hemolytic anemia occur occasionally. In addition, examination of wet preparations of peripheral blood reveals a higher incidence of acanthoid cells. All these are reversible morphologic abnormalities that appear to be related to a serum factor.[60] Erythropoiesis is normoblastic in type unless acute alcoholism, vitamin B_{12} deficiency, or folate deficiency are also present, and the reticulocytes are often slightly increased. Leukocyte and platelet counts are usually normal but they may be greatly reduced if "hypersplenism" or folate deficiency is present.

The mechanisms responsible for the macrocytic anemia of cirrhosis of the liver have been clarified by the studies of Jandl.[64] Sixteen of 20 patients with cirrhosis and anemia who were studied were found to have a definite hemolytic anemia, evidenced by the triad of elevated excretion of fecal urobilinogen, persistent reticulocytosis, and increased concentration of the erythrocyte precursors in the bone marrow. The extracorpuscular nature of the hemolytic process was shown by the survival times of transfused normal cells that were determined by the Ashby differential agglutination method. The exponential type of survival curve that was found suggested a random destruction of the red cells in a local site, such as the liver or spleen. Additional studies that utilized erythrocytes tagged with Cr^{51} indicated that the spleen is the major site of destruction. A correlation was found between the rate of red cell destruction and the degree of anemia.

Zieve syndrome, first reported in 20 patients, consists of hemolytic anemia, hyperlipemia, and liver disease;[67] the patients are usually alcoholic and often have pancreatitis. The hyperhemolysis was originally attributed to hyperlipemia, particularly lysolecithin, but later studies have failed to confirm that the hyperlipemia is responsible for the hyperhemolysis.[58]

Although demonstration of the hemolytic nature of the anemia in cirrhosis of the liver affords the best explanation of the anemia in the majority of patients who have a macrocytic anemia associated with a normoblastic marrow, factors other than hyperhemolysis are important in patients with macrocytic anemia and the megaloblastic type of bone marrow.[64, 66] The anemia in most of these patients has been more severe than that usually seen in cirrhosis. The erythrocyte count has been in the neighborhood of 1.0 mil. per cu.mm. in most patients and less than 2.0 mil. per cu.mm. in nearly all; the mean corpuscular volume usually has been over 130 cu. μ. In such patients hematologic recovery has followed the administration of folic acid,[64] vitamin B_{12},[66] liver extract, and ascorbic acid. The possibility of a coexisting pernicious anemia can be excluded if the gastric analysis and determinations of the serum vitamin B_{12} level are normal. Patients with cirrhosis often have grossly deficient diets for long periods. In the majority of patients with chronic alcoholism and liver disease, macrocytosis is related to a deficiency in folic acid; borderline or low serum folate concentration has been found in 80 per cent of a group of patients of this type.[62, 65] Herbert has shown that in normal conditions the storage of folate represents about a month's reserve supply.[61] Ingestion of alcohol, folate deficiency, and hypersplenism all may be important in the anemia, thrombocytopenia, or leukopenia that occurs in some patients with chronic liver disease.

Increased plasma volume and hemodilution may be responsible for reduction in the hematocrit and other blood values in some patients with chronic liver disease and splenomegaly.

DISORDERS OF THE SPLEEN

ANATOMY

The anatomy of the spleen resembles that of a lymph node, but certain important peculiarities of the circulation in the spleen make it unique (Fig. 8–4). Lymphatic tissue, the so-called "white pulp," forms a sheath about the arteries; the stroma, composed of reticular fibers and fixed macrophages, is filled with free lymphocytes of various sizes. The tissue forms a nodule which is denser in the periphery than in the center. The "red pulp" consists of the venous sinuses and the tissue in the spaces between them, termed "splenic cords" or "Billroth's cords." The reticulum fibers from the white pulp continue into the red pulp which contains lymphocytes, free macrophages, and other cells of the blood; fixed macrophages and free monocytes are present in great numbers. The spleen is unusual in that it has two circulations, one fast and one slow (Fig. 8–5).

In the "fast" circulation, blood from some of the arterial branches flows directly into the venous sinuses which promptly empty into the veins. In the "slow" circulation, branches of the arteries end in the cords of Billroth; the slow progress of the cells through the red pulp provides an opportunity for incubation and for a sort of filtration in which the macrophages remove certain cells. Those that are not phagocytized still must pass through small openings in the capillary wall in order to enter the venous sinuses and continue to the connecting veins. The slow circulation through the phagocyte-rich cords of Billroth is important in one of the main functions of the spleen in adult life, the removal of all types of damaged cells from the circulating blood.

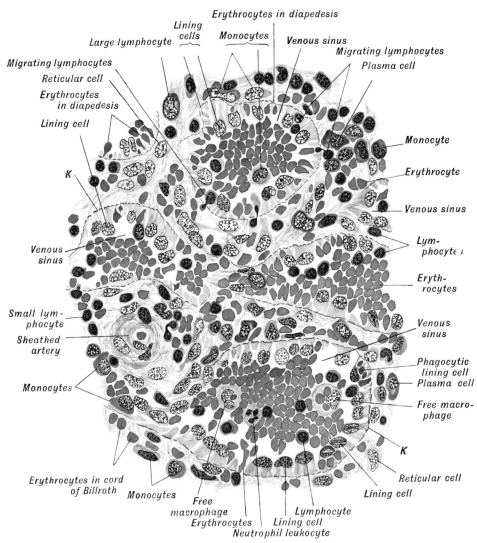

Figure 8–4   Red pulp of the human spleen. (From Bloom and Fawcett: A Textbook of Histology. Philadelphia, W. B. Saunders Co., 1968.)

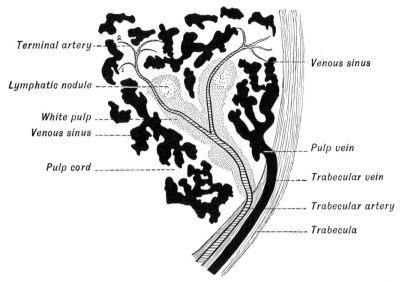

Terminal artery

Lymphatic nodule

White pulp
Venous sinus

Pulp cord

Venous sinus

Pulp vein

Trabecular vein

Trabecular artery

Trabecula

Figure 8–5 Diagram to show closed (*1*) and open (*2*) circulation through the spleen. (From Bloom and Fawcett: A Textbook of Histology. Philadelphia, W. B. Saunders Co., 1975.)

FUNCTION

The spleen has varied functions. In the embryo it is an organ of hematopoiesis. This function does not continue after birth in a normal baby, but in later life hematopoiesis may reappear in the spleen in certain disease states, such as myelofibrosis, that are accompanied by extramedullary hematopoiesis. Experiments in animals have also demonstrated that the cells from the adult spleen can repopulate the marrow and restore hematopoiesis after the marrow cells have been severely damaged by irradiation.

The spleen is a major site of immunoglobulin production, and thus an important factor in the body's resistance to infection. It is also a major factor in certain disease syndromes characterized by excessive immunoglobulin production, particularly autoimmune antibodies; autoimmune hemolytic anemia and thrombocytopenic purpura may arise in this manner.

The spleen, with its numerous macrophages in the reticuloendothelial system, is an important organ of cellular defense against infection. Young children who have had the spleen removed, and those who have a "packed" reticuloendothelial system as a result of hemolytic anemia, are unusually susceptible to some infections, particularly those caused by the pneumococcus; such infections may be sudden, overwhelming, and fatal in a matter of hours. Although not as susceptible as children, some adults may be similarly affected by splenectomy.

Probably the function of the spleen that is most important in hematologic disorders is the destruction of circulating blood cells. Although this function is shared by the phagocytic cells of the bone marrow and liver, the spleen is normally the major site for the destruction of senescent normal cells and also for a variety of abnormal cells of all types. Destruction of the erythrocytes in vivo involves three stages: (1) injury to the red cell; (2) sequestration in the spleen; and (3) cell destruction, usually by macrophages of the reticuloendothelial system. The slow circulation in the spleen allows for sequestration and incubation of the cells in the cords of Billroth, a situation in which some cellular defects are magnified. The stasis in the cords also provides an unusually favorable situation for cells which are coated with antibodies to become attached to specific receptor sites on the macrophages, a prelude to phagocytosis and destruction. The erythrocytes in most hemolytic states have membranes that are more rigid than normal, a defect that renders them susceptible to fragmentation in the general circulation and in the spleen, particularly when passing through the walls that separate the cords from the venous sinuses; the macrophages engulf many red cell fragments, schistocytes, produced in this way. The enlargement of the spleen that is seen in nearly all hemolytic anemias probably develops as a result of the increasing back pressure and dilatation in the cords, and the accompanying hyperplasia of the phagocytic cells.

CAUSES OF SPLENOMEGALY

Most diseases of the spleen, with the notable exceptions of idiopathic thrombocytopenic purpura and disorders associated with the splenic infarction such as sickle cell anemia, are associated with splenomegaly. The most common causes are listed in Table 8–1. As the classification indicates, splenomegaly nearly always is only one aspect of an underlying disease that is not confined to the spleen.

Hypersplenism is the term often used to denote a syndrome characterized by the following: splenomegaly; anemia; leukopenia; thrombocytopenia singly or in combination; a marrow with cellularity that is normal or increased; and correction of the blood picture by splenectomy. The syndrome may occur with splenomegaly of sufficient degree from virtually any cause.

Various mechanisms have been suggested to explain the changes that occur in the peripheral blood of patients with large spleens. One of the earlier explanations offered, the existence of an inhibiting effect on the marrow exerted by the enlarged spleen, has not been proved. Sequestration of cellular elements in the spleen without destruction produces cytopenias in some patients. Up to 90 per cent of the platelets and as much as 1000 ml. of red cells and 800 ml. of plasma may be removed from the circulation by this mechanism.[73] Destruction of cells, particularly erythrocytes and platelets, produces cytopenias in some patients; the anatomy of the slow circulation in the spleen and the abundance of macrophages are important mechanisms that increase as the spleen enlarges. Still another mechanism that produces cytopenias, hemodilution, has been recognized in recent years. An increase in plasma volume of a degree sufficient to affect the values in the peripheral circulation occurs in many patients with greatly enlarged spleens, those that weigh 1000 gm. or more and extend to the umbilicus.

Table 8–1   *Causes of Splenomegaly*

1. Congestive splenomegaly
      (Intrahepatic or extrahepatic; obstruction of portal or splenic vein)

2. Myeloproliferative disorders
      (Leukemia, myelofibrosis, polycythemia vera, idiopathic thrombocythemia)

3. Lymphoproliferative disorders
      (Leukemia, malignant lymphoma, including Hodgkin's disease)

4. Hemolytic anemia
      (Usual in virtually all varieties, congenital or acquired, with extravascular
         hemolysis; rare in SS disease in adults)

5. Infections
      (Viral, bacterial, protozoan or fungal; infectious mononucleosis, tuberculosis, sub-
         acute bacterial endocarditis, splenic abscess, malaria, syphilis, brucellosis, kala-
         azar, histoplasmosis, and others)

6. Storage disorders
      (Gaucher's, Niemann-Pick, Schüller-Christian, Letterer-Siwe, Sky-blue histiocytic)

7. Connective tissue disorders
      (Felty's syndrome, systemic lupus erythematosus, polyarteritis, and others)

8. Primary splenic disease
      (Neoplasms, cysts,? "idiopathic splenomegaly," hamartomas)

9. Others
      (Sarcoidosis, chronic iron deficiency, amyloidosis, tropical splenomegaly)

DIAGNOSIS OF THE PATIENT WITH SPLENOMEGALY

The physical examination usually suffices to determine whether a mass in the left upper quadrant is spleen or something else. A palpable spleen is almost invariably an enlarged one; usually the spleen is at least twice the normal size before it is palpable, but on occasion a spleen that weighs 800 gm. is not palpable because of abdominal fluid, splenic adhesions, or displacement or paralysis of the diaphragm. The enlarged spleen is usually associated with percussion dullness low in the left axilla. The edge is usually palpable, and if the spleen is considerably enlarged a notch or two may be felt on the medial or upper medial border. On respiration the spleen moves diagonally downward from the left upper quadrant to the right lower quadrant. At times it may be palpable only when the patient lies on the right side and breathes deeply with maximum use of the diaphragm. Sometimes a greatly enlarged spleen fills almost the entire abdomen. The anterior surface of the spleen is nearly always smooth; palpation of a mass with an irregular anterior surface in the left upper quadrant should make one suspicious of a tumor, pancreatic, renal, mesenteric, retroperitoneal, or bowel, or something other than the spleen. A benign tumor arising from the stomach wall may be very difficult to distinguish from the spleen because its surface is smooth and the gastrointestinal x-rays may be normal. When the spleen is considerably enlarged and reaches to the umbilicus or below, there is nearly always some associated disturbance in the peripheral blood counts, either an increase or decrease in the red cells, leukocytes, or platelets. Indeed, if the patient has a mass which seems to be a spleen extending below the umbilicus, and there is no abnormality in the peripheral blood, a neoplasm rather than an enlarged spleen, should be suspected.

If the physical examination leaves doubt whether a mass is spleen, other studies usually settle the question. Flat x-rays of the abdomen, an intravenous pyelogram, or barium study of the gastrointestinal tract may suffice. More definitive measures are the scans with radioactive materials, celiac angiograms, and splenoportograms.

Establishing the cause of the splenomegaly may be easy or difficult. If congestive splenomegaly is suspected, a detailed history for possible liver disease, and careful search for hepatomegaly, palmar erythema, or spider angiomata may be helpful. Liver function tests, measurement of the bilirubin, and a search for varices either by barium study or by gastroscopy may be necessary. Percutaneous liver biopsy is sometimes helpful. In some patients with congestive splenomegaly secondary to splenic vein thrombosis caused by trauma, malignancy, or changes in the blood viscosity, all of the above tests may be normal and the diagnosis is established only by celiac angiogram or splenoportogram.

If a myeloproliferative disorder is responsible for splenomegaly, its presence can usually be determined by bone marrow aspiration, bone marrow biopsy, or careful study of the peripheral blood. Determination of the total red cell mass and plasma volume may be necessary to establish the presence of polycythemia vera on occasions.

Lymphoproliferative disorders are one of the commonest causes of splenomegaly. If biopsy of the bone marrow or an accessible lymph node does not provide the diagnosis, x-ray study of the gastrointestinal tract, percutaneous liver biopsy, and lymphangiograms may be rewarding. Although lymphoma of the spleen is usually accompanied by evidence of disease elsewhere, sometimes the diagnosis is established only after operation and careful study of the removed spleen and lymph nodes. Whether the diagnostic search should be pursued to the point of laparotomy, in preference to a longer period of observation, must be decided in each individual case.

If the presence of hemolytic anemia is suggested by the association of anemia, splenomegaly, reticulocytosis, and mild elevation of the serum bilirubin, further diagnostic measures discussed in Chapters 3 and 7 are necessary for a more precise diagnosis. A careful study of the morphology both of the red cells and the leukocytes on the peripheral blood smear, and a determination of the Coombs test, are two simple procedures that make good starting points.

Numerous infections cause splenomegaly of varying degree. Cultures of the blood, sputum, lymph nodes, bone marrow, lungs, liver, and other tissues, or special staining of biopsy material, may provide a definite diagnosis. Serial complement fixation tests and agglutination tests may help to establish a definite diagnosis in some infections when cultures fail.

The occurrence of acute hemolytic anemia in the course of systemic infections, viral and bacterial, has been reported;[72] splenic sequestration of red cells and splenomegaly were present. The hypothesis was advanced that splenomegaly was a consequence of pyrogen excess, and that this led to stasis, damage, and destruction in the spleen.

Storage disorders are usually diagnosed by biopsy of the bone marrow, lymph node, or liver; electron microscopy may be especially valuable. Clinical features of the different syndromes and skeletal x-rays are helpful at times.

Connective tissue disorders are generally suggested by the history and other clinical features of the case, but additional measures such as skin or muscle biopsy, determination of the serum complement level, tests for antinuclear factor, cryoglobulin and rheumatoid factors, serum protein electrophoresis, or immunoelectrophoresis usually are necessary to establish the diagnosis.

Primary splenic diseases are rare and are usually diagnosed only after splenectomy.

BIG SPLEEN DISEASE (TROPICAL SPLENOMEGALY)

"Big spleen disease" has been studied extensively in Uganda,[70, 74] where most of these patients have pancytopenia. Study has revealed that the anemia is due in part to hyperhemolysis, but in larger part to an expanded plasma volume with hemodilution; sequestration of red cells in the spleen appears to be of minor importance. This disorder is characterized by hyperplasia of the Kupffer's cells in the liver accompanied by varying degrees of lymphocytic infiltration of the liver; considerable hyperplasia of the lymphoid tissue is evident in the spleen and sometimes in the marrow. Although repeated studies for malarial parasites in these patients have been negative, the presence of antibodies to quartan malaria and the distribution of the cases in Uganda suggest that the disorder is related to quartan malaria infection. Splenectomy is usually followed by a decrease in the plasma volume, which is not accounted for by removal of the plasma contained in the spleen, and improvement in the hematologic values. In some patients, long-term antimalarial therapy, particularly with Paludrine, has been followed by a decrease in the size of the spleen and improvement in the hematologic values.

The clinical manifestations of patients with "nontropical idiopathic splenomegaly" are similar to those seen in the tropics. In a group of such patients, splen megaly, leukopenia, and neutropenia of a severe degree, moderate thrombocytopenia, and slight-to-moderate reticulocytosis were present: all the patients who were studied were "anemic," although in only two was the total red cell volume subnormal.[68] Splenectomy produced a sustained and striking hematologic improvement in most patients. Two patients later died with illnesses unconnected with splenomegaly, and one died of lymphosarcoma and autoimmune hemolytic anemia.

Whether these patients have: (1) an unusual response to some infection, which appears to be the case when tropical splenomegaly occurs in certain patients with malaria; (2) an autoimmune disorder of uncertain origin, the main feature being exaggerated lymphoreticular cell proliferation; or (3) some atypical or "premalignant" early form of lymphoma is uncertain. It is possible that the presence of lymphoma is a late manifestation of, or a response to, one of the other disorders.

The studies of Hess and associates confirm that an expanded plasma volume is responsible for the cytopenias found in a number of patients with massive splenomegaly from a variety of causes[71] (leukemia, myelofibrosis, sarcoidosis, lymphoma, and congestive splenomegaly). In some patients who had only one-half the normal venous hematocrit, the red cell mass was normal whereas the plasma volume was twice the normal; in many patients both splenic sequestration and cellular destruction were also factors. Various studies before, during, and after splenectomy disclosed the presence of portal hypertension, which has been shown to correlate with an expanded plasma volume in several studies. An increased portal blood flow was suggested as a possible explanation; studies of arteriovenous oxygen differences and distribution of Cardio-Green dye apparently failed to demonstrate any significant arteriovenous shunting in the spleen. Other factors operative in the expanded plasma volume include a decrease in resistance in the cutaneous circulation and stimulation of the renin–angiotensin–aldosterone system with salt and water retention. The plasma volume and venous hematocrit may not return to normal until several months after splenectomy.

INDICATIONS FOR SPLENECTOMY

A decision regarding the advisability of splenectomy can be made only after careful consideration of the individual patient. In some disorders, such as hereditary spherocytosis, splenectomy is indicated in nearly every patient because the operation restores the blood picture to normal by removing the organ of the red cell destruction, although the inherited defect in the red cells persists. Likewise the indications for splenectomy in other hemolytic disorders and thrombocytopenia purpura are fairly well defined. On the other hand, in many splenomegalic disorders, such as the lymphomas and myeloid metaplasia, the indications for splenectomy are not clear-cut because of the operative risks and the unknown chances of success.

Splenectomy relieves only one aspect of the underlying disorder, and rarely if ever effects a cure of the primary disease. One must also consider that even a successful splenectomy may carry some risk. Splenectomy in very young children, particularly those with a reticuloendothelial system loaded from hyperhemolysis or other causes, may be followed by a lowered resistance to infection, especially to those caused by the pneumococcus; similarly, splenectomy in children or adults may seriously impair the body's reaction to malaria. If the underlying disease responsible for the splenomegaly is amenable to more definitive treatment, splenectomy probably is not necessary because the hypersplenism syndrome usually disappears after appropriate therapy. When the nature and course of the underlying disease are such that an early fatal outcome is expected, splenectomy is rarely justified even if hypersplenism is fairly severe. If the underlying process cannot be diagnosed, or if it is identified as one for which no satisfactory therapy is available, splenectomy is often performed if anemia, neutropenia, or thrombocytopenia is disabling or hazardous to the patient. An increase in the plasma volume of 50 per cent also has been considered an indication for splenectomy, particularly if combined with evidence of red cell pooling, which can occur without increased destruction.[73] In such circumstances gratifying results occur often, but not invariably. Clinical improvement in the patient may continue even though a partial hematologic relapse may develop some months later.

Rupture of the spleen is a clear-cut indication for splenectomy, which is usually a life-saving measure. Symptoms of rupture usually are manifest soon after trauma, but may be delayed and become apparent only after from two to ten days. Occasionally rupture may not occur for weeks or even months after an injury. Abdominal pain, particularly in the left upper quadrant, a left upper quadrant mass, a falling hematocrit, and other evidences of an acute abdomen lead to the recognition of the difficulty. When a spleen is diseased and enlarged, as in leukemia or infectious mononucleosis, rupture may occur spontaneously or after an event no more traumatic than a physical examination. A subcapsular hemorrhage usually is the initial lesion.

FELTY'S SYNDROME

Felty's syndrome, characterized by the triad of arthritis, splenomegaly, and neutropenia, was described first in 1924.[76] The syndrome is more likely to occur in middle-aged or older persons who have had arthritis, which may or may not be disabling, for 15 years or more. Enlargement of the superficial lymph nodes and nodular lymphoid proliferation in some areas of the marrow are common. Some patients with the syndrome have repeated bacterial infections and chronic leg ulcers, attributable at least in part to the neutropenia.

The mechanisms responsible for the neutropenia are not understood. A recent study of 17 patients using diisopropylfluorophosphate ($DF^{32}P$) led to the conclusion that the principal mechanism responsible for the neutropenia is excessive margination of the cells. Subnormal granulocyte production was also found in about one-third, but excessive destruction was rare.[79]

In a series of 15 patients aged 43 to 67 seen by one of us and treated by splenectomy, the spleen size varied from 265 to 880 gm.; spleens as large as 2420 gm. have been reported.[77] Presplenectomy total leukocyte counts ranged from 900 to 3300 per cu. mm., and granulocytes from 64 to 2100 per cu. mm. In 12 of the 15 patients the leukocyte count returned to normal within 48 hours after splenectomy, and in ten it remained normal from one to thirteen years. Rheumatoid and antinuclear factors were present in 13 of the 14 patients studied. Twelve of the 15 patients were anemic, and three had thrombocytopenia. Normoblastic erythroid and myeloid hyperplasia were seen in virtually all of the marrow biopsies; lymphocytosis occurred in three.

The effect of splenectomy on infections in patients with Felty's syndrome is more difficult to evaluate. Nine of the patients in the above-mentioned series had repeated infections during the year before splenectomy, and in five there was a marked decrease in frequency during the year after splenectomy. Nevertheless, two patients with normal neutrophil counts died within two months of splenectomy, probably from septicemia, and two who did not have significant improvement in the leukocyte counts have continued to have recurrent infections. In view of the unpredictable effect on the blood counts and the undetermined influence on the body defense mechanism, splenectomy is warranted only in those patients with marked neutropenia who have severe trouble or invalidism because of infection.

HEMATOLOGIC DISORDERS OF ALCOHOLISM

Patients who are chronic alcoholics may suffer from a variety of hematologic disorders (Table 8–2). The hematologic abnormalities, which may involve the red cells, granulocytes, or platelets, are the result of many factors, including the pharmacologic effect of excessive alcohol ingestion, the presence of acute or chronic liver disease, dietary insufficiency, and bleeding. These changes have been the subject of recent reviews.[83, 86] In one study of 65 patients, 75 per cent had a disorder of red cell production, 20 per cent had thrombocytopenia, and 6 per cent had leukopenia.

The anemia seen in chronic alcoholics evolves through several stages. The first is one of negative vitamin balance when alcohol replaces other food substances in the diet; the equivalent of 300 ml. of absolute ethanol a day can produce folate deficiency within a few weeks. The second stage, which may appear as early as a week after heavy drinking and poor diet, is evidenced by megaloblastic changes in the bone marrow. Later, in some patients, ringed sideroblasts appear in the marrow. In one series, megaloblastic erythropoiesis secondary to

---

Table 8–2   *Effects of Alcohol on Circulating Blood Cells and Precursors*

I Erythrocytic Series
   A. Bone Marrow
      (1) Megaloblasts
      (2) Vacuolization of red cell precursors
      (3) Sideroblasts
   B. Erythrocytes
      (1) Acanthocytosis
      (2) Stomatocytosis
      (3) Zieve syndrome

II Platelets
   A. Thrombocytopenia
      (1) Decreased production
      (2) Increased destruction
   B. Platelet dysfunction

III Leukocytes
   A. Granulocytopenia
   B. Granulocyte dysfunction

folate deficiency occurred in 40 per cent of the patients, and sideroblastic changes in 30 per cent.[83]

Several different types of hemolytic anemia occur in chronic alcoholics. The anemia seen in patients with chronic portal cirrhosis is often hemolytic, the result of splenic sequestration of erythrocytes. Another type of hemolytic anemia characterized by transient stomatocytosis has been reported;[82] the anemia, which was associated with shortened red cell survival in the absence of acanthocytosis or hyperlipemia, disappeared with abstinence from alcohol, only to recur with the resumption of heavy drinking. Hemolytic anemia associated with "spur cells" has been reported, most often in patients with alcoholic hepatic cirrhosis, jaundice, hepatomegaly, and splenomegaly. The characteristic features of the cells are a striking increase in cholesterol and cholesterol–phospholipid ratio.[81] The cell membrane with its spurlike projections lacks plasticity and the cells are destroyed in the spleen. Severe liver disease seems to be more important than alcoholism per se in producing "spur cell" anemia. Spur cells are similar morphologically, but different chemically, from the acanthocytes seen in abetalipoproteinemia.[81] The syndrome reported by Zieve in 1958, characterized by transient hemolytic anemia, jaundice, hyperlipemia or hypercholesterolemia, and alcoholic liver disease, is poorly understood.[67] Its status is uncertain; hyperlipemia has been excluded as a cause of the hemolysis, and even the existence of hyperhemolysis has been questioned.

Thrombocytopenia that occurs in some chronic alcoholics may be caused by splenomegaly, dietary folate deficiency, or the direct toxic effect of alcohol on the marrow. An incidence of 14 per cent (counts 68,000 to 138,000 cu. mm.) was found in one study.[88] It was first shown in 1964 that alcohol can produce thrombocytopenia in the absence of folate deficiency by a direct effect on the marrow.[92] The disappearance of the megakaryocytes and a fall in platelet count were not prevented in alcoholic subjects who were given 75 micrograms of folic acid a day while ingesting alcohol, which apparently also depressed the platelet production by megakaryocytes that were present. Alcohol per se is likely to produce only mild thrombocytopenia, 60,000 to 130,000 per cu. mm. More severe thrombocytopenia usually means that additional factors, such as folate deficiency or hypersplenism, are present, but exceptions occur.[89]

Leukopenia may be important in alcoholics if they contract bacterial infection, particularly pneumonia. In some such patients seen by the authors, the total leukocyte count has been less than 1,000 cu. mm., with a virtual absence of granulocytes associated with a marrow almost totally devoid of granulocyte precursors older than myelocytes. Severe, often fatal, septicemia is common. The abnormalities are the result of the direct effect of alcohol on cell maturation, folate deficiency, and, less frequently, the presence of an overactive spleen. Granulocyte counts that ranged from 900 to 1900 cu. mm. were found on nine occasions in six alcoholics without infection or splenomegaly;[89] the leukopenia was accompanied by thrombocytopenia and anemia in eight, and low serum folate in five. In addition to the quantitative effect on the granulocytes, other studies have indicated that granulocyte mobilization may be diminished within a few hours after the administration of alcohol; the effect lasts only a few hours,[80] and its clinical importance has not been determined.

The megaloblastic changes seen in the bone marrow are nearly always the result of folate deficiency; serum folate levels are usually low, whereas vitamin B_{12} levels are normal. The alcoholic's diet is generally deficient in folate, and folate stores are low. Alcoholic patients on a low folate diet developed megalo-blastosis within one to three weeks when alcohol was administered; without alcohol, they developed deficiency within five to ten weeks compared to the 19-week-interval required in the normal patient. Ethanol has a direct effect on folate metabolism: it may induce malabsorption of folate and also block the action of physiologic doses of folate. The morphologic manifestation of the direct effect of alcohol is the presence of vacuoles in the erythrocyte precursors produced by endocytosis. The associated physiologic inhibition is shown by the improved iron metabolism and reticulocytosis that occur after abstinence from alcohol, even without any change in diet.

Reversible sideroblastic abnormalities in patients with severe alcoholism accompanied by dimorphic peripheral smears, low folate levels in the serum and red cells, megaloblastic red cell precursors, elevated serum iron levels, and numerous ring sideroblasts have been described. Such changes were seen in one-half of the group of 20 anemic patients admitted to one hospital.[85, 86] The marrows became normal within one to three weeks after abstinence from alcohol. Alcohol apparently produces sideroblasts by interfering with the con-version of pyridoxine to pyridoxal phosphate, because the defect was corrected by parenteral pyridoxal phosphate but not by pharmacologic amounts of folic acid or pyridoxine.[86] Such a block to ALA synthesis would cause a diminution in heme synthesis and an increase in iron in the mitochondria.

LEAD POISONING

Chronic lead poisoning can produce encephalopathy, nephropathy, peri-pheral neuropathy, and anemia. The review by Aub, Reznikoff, et al. is still a classic.[94] The most common symptoms are fatigue, constipation colic, nausea, vomiting, headache, anorexia, and irritability; in more seriously ill patients there may be focal or generalized seizures, coma, and even death. The physical examination may show evidence of neuropathy or encephalopathy; a lead line in the gums has been found in 43 per cent of patients.

Lead poisoning from industrial sources has become virtually unknown in the United States. Although lead poisoning has been traced to water pipes, glazed pottery, and certain glass washed in a dishwasher,[96] the most common cause at present in adults is illicit "moonshine" whiskey. In children the com-monest sources are pica and the consumption of lead-containing paint and inhalation of smoke from burning batteries containing lead. The diet of the nor-mal healthy adult is said to contain from 0.3 to 0.5 mg. of lead. The normal level of lead in the blood, almost exclusively confined to the erythrocytes, is between 20 and 30 micrograms per 100 ml. of blood;[93] the bone marrow con-tains 50 times as much as the peripheral blood. Both levels are elevated con-siderably in heavy wine-drinkers.

The hematologic effects of lead are confined to the red cell series. Anemia, generally normocytic or slightly hypochromic, is a late sign; the hematocrit is usually between 20 and 30 per cent and ranges from 18 to 39 per cent.[98] Reticulocytosis and basophilic stippling are constant findings; the half-life of erythrocytes labeled with the Cr^{51} techniques is two-thirds normal.[96] This modest reduction in the life span of the cells, apparently the consequence of membrane damage, is accompanied by marked hyperplasia of the erythroid precursors in the marrow. This marrow cellularity reflects dyserythropoiesis rather than a simple compensatory reaction; the sideroblasts are increased and the incorporation of iron into red cells is reduced.[96]

Lead has several effects on the erythrocytes and normoblasts. It damages the mitochondria and causes disturbances in porphyrin metabolism and hemoglobin synthesis. This is apparent in the increased sideroblasts visible by light microscopy. The increase in reticulocytes and stippled erythrocytes may reflect lead damage to the cytoplasmic ribosomes and/or soluble RNA.

The simplest screening test for lead poisoning is a study of the peripheral blood smears for basophilic stippling; normal persons have 3 or 4×10^5 red cells per cu.mm., and more than 50×10^5 red cells per cu.mm. is strongly suggestive of increased lead absorption.[96] Determination of urinary lead excretion before and after the administration of CaEDTA (Calcium versenate) was considered the most reliable diagnostic test in one study.[98] In another, the finding of more than 60 micrograms of lead per 100 ml. of blood was considered evidence of lead poisoning.[96]

The most important aspect of treatment, of course, is removal from the source of the poisoning. Calcium versenate (CaEDTA) is the treatment for elimination of lead from the body preferred by some,[98] but a daily dose of no more than 0.5 to 1.0 gm. has also been advised in order to avoid increased toxicity when lead is mobilized.[96]

ARSENIC POISONING

When the organic arsenic compounds arsphenamine and neoarsphenamine were used in the treatment of syphilis, thrombocytopenia, leukopenia, and aplastic anemia were well-recognized reactions. The neutropenia-producing effect of inorganic arsenic was also well-known. Fowler's solution was one of the first chemotherapeutic agents used in the treatment of chronic granulocytic leukemia, and as late as the 1930s it was being used in patients with chronic granulocytic leukemia who had pulmonary tuberculosis, which was thought to be a contraindication to radiotherapy.

Chronic poisoning with inorganic arsenic produces anemia which is very similar to that seen in lead poisoning;[99] in addition, neutropenia occurs regularly and thrombocytopenia frequently.

The symptoms of chronic arsenic poisoning are nausea, vomiting, diarrhea, weakness, and some ataxia. Physical examination often discloses brownish pigmentation of the skin, which with the symptoms may suggest Addison's disease, hyperkeratosis of the palms and soles, splenomegaly, and signs of peripheral neuropathy. The nails may be yellowish in color, and if the exposure to arsenic was also acute a defined line of demarcation may be apparent.

Anemia, usually moderately severe with red cell counts between 2.0 and 4.0 mil./cu.mm.,[99] is an almost constant feature; it is generally normocytic but mild hypochromia has been noted. Anisopoikilocytosis and basophilic stippling are present. The reticulocyte count in the reported cases has been from 1.5 to 15 per cent. Neutropenia occurs in almost all patients, and in reported cases the total leukocyte count has been between 1000 and 2400 per cu.mm. Platelet counts have ranged from 36,000 to 210,000 per cu.mm. and were thrombocytopenic in one-half.

The bone marrow is hypercellular. There is a striking increase in the red cell precursors; these are predominantly normoblastic, but "megaloblastoid" or even megaloblastic changes with normal serum levels of vitamin B_{12} and folate have been reported.[100] Karyorrhexis, binuclearity, and mitotic abnormalities are prominent. In the granulocytic series some increases in myelocytes, with a diminution of older cells and occasional giant metamyelocytes are found.

Arsenic poisoning usually indicates an attempt at homicide. With present-day restrictions on its purchase, accidental arsenic poisoning because of agricultural use or careless housekeeping (such as keeping arsenic and baking powder on the same shelf in the kitchen) has become a rarity.

The diagnosis is usually made by testing the urine for arsenic; more than 0.2 mg./per liter is definitely abnormal and strongly suggestive of chronic poisoning. Arsenic accumulates in the hair and nails, and persists for months; these tissues often offer the best material to examine for suspected poisoning. The hematologic abnormalities generally disappear within two or three months after ingestion of arsenic ceases.

COPPER DEFICIENCY

Copper deficiency, known to produce anemia in animals, is rare in humans. It has been reported in malnourished infants, and also in adults following extensive bowel resection.[101] Anemia, leukopenia, mild macrocytosis, and hypochromia were found when copper stores were depleted after long-term hyperalimentation; the abnormalities were corrected by the administration of copper. The presence of megaloblastoid erythropoiesis with sideroblastosis in the bone marrow during copper deficiency suggested abnormalities in RNA/DNA metabolism and mitochondrial activity.

KWASHIORKOR

Kwashiorkor is seen only occasionally in the United States and other Western countries, but unfortunately is not rare in Africa and other parts of the world. The disorder is caused by a severe protein deficiency associated with an adequate or nearly adequate intake of calories in the form of carbohydrate. Anemia, hypoalbuminemia, and edema occur in nearly all patients, and some develop hepatomegaly and ascites. In some, particularly in East Africa, the reddish color of the hair and skin combined with a prominent abdomen suggest the diagnosis at a distance. The disease is essentially one of young children, often occurring in next to the youngest who is no longer breast-fed; growth retardation may be evident. Anemia usually is not severe unless the protein deficiency is associated with other causes of anemia, such as infection or iron or folate deficiency. The disorder is a serious one with a mortality rate of over 10 per cent. Treatment is directed toward the fluid excess, a search for infection, and correction of any dietary deficiencies that are present.

ANEMIA OF PREMATURITY

The fall in hemoglobin that occurs after birth is more marked in prematures than in full-term infants. The so-called anemia of prematurity that occurs during the first six to 12 weeks of life and does not respond to hematinics appears to be a physiologic adjustment;[102] important factors are an expanding plasma volume, accompanied by diminished erythropoiesis that is probably the result of improved tissue oxygenation. In full-term infants the hemoglobin may fall to 11.4 gm./100 ml. The fall is greater in premature infants, to 9.6 gm./100 ml. in infants weighing 1200 to 2350 g, and 7.8 gm./100 ml. in those weighing less than 1200 g.[102]

References

ANEMIA ASSOCIATED WITH CHRONIC DISEASE

1. Barrett-Connor, E.: Anemia and infection. Am. J. Med., 52:242, 1972.
2. Cartwright, G. E.: The anemia of chronic disorders. Semin. Hematol., 3:351, 1966.
3. Cartwright, G. E., and Lee, G. R.: Annotation: the anaemia of chronic disorders. Br. J. Haematol., 21:147, 1971.
4. Douglas, S. W., and Adamson, J. W.: The anemia of chronic disorders: studies of marrow regulation and iron metabolism. Blood, 45:55, 1975.
5. Kurnick, J. E., Ward, H. P., and Pickett, J. C.: Mechanism of the anemia of chronic disorders. Arch. Intern. Med., 130:323, 1972.
6. Ward, P., Gordon, B., and Pickett, J. C.: Serum levels of erythropoietin in rheumatoid arthritis. J. Lab. Clin. Med., 74:93, 1969.

ANEMIA ASSOCIATED WITH MYXEDEMA

7. Axelrod, A. R., and Berman, L.: The bone marrow in hyperthyroidism and hypothyroidism. Blood, 6:436, 1951.
8. Bomford, R.: Anaemia in myxoedema and the role of the thyroid gland in erythropoiesis. Q. J. Med., 7:495, 1938.
9. Carpenter, J. T., Mohler, D. N., Thorup, O. A., and Leavell, B. S.: Anemia in Myxedema. In Crispell, K. R. (Ed.): Current Concepts in Hypothyroidism. Pergamon Press, New York, 1963.
10. Charcot, M.: Myxoedème, cachexie pachydermique ou état crétinoïde. La Lancette française Gazette des Hôpitaux. January 25, 1881.

11. Doniach, D., Roitt, I. M., and Taylor, K. B.: Autoimmune phenomena in pernicious anaemia. Serologic overlap with thyroiditis, thyrotoxicosis and systemic lupus erythematosus. Brit. M. J., *1*:1374, 1963.
12. Fisher, J. M., and Taylor, K. B.: A comparison of autoimmune phenomena in pernicious anemia and chronic atrophic gastritis. N. Engl. J. Med., *272*:499, 1965.
13. Gordon, A. S., Kadow, P. C., Finkelstein, G., and Charipper, H. A.: The thyroid and blood regeneration in the rat. Am. J. Med. Sci., *212*:385, 1946.
14. Kocher, T.: Über Kropf Extirpation and ihre Folgen. Arch. Chir., *29*:254, 1883.
15. Leavell, B. S., Thorup, O. A., and McClellan, J. E.: Observations on the anemia in myxedema. Tr. Am. Clin. Climatol. Assoc., *68*:137, 1956.
16. Leithhold, S. L., David, D., and Best, W. R.: Hypothyroidism with anemia demonstrating abnormal vitamin B_{12} absorption. Am. J. Med., *24*:535, 1958.
17. Lerman, J., and Means, J. H.: Treatment of the anemia of myxedema. Endocrinology, *16*:553, 1932.
18. McClellan, J. E., Donegan, C., Thorup, O. A., and Leavell, B. S.: Survival time of the erythrocyte in myxedema and hyperthyroidism. J. Lab. Clin. Med., *51*:91, 1958.
19. Muldowney, F. P., Crooks, J., and Wayne, E. J.: The total red cell mass in thyrotoxicosis and myxedema. Clin. Sci., *16*:309, 1957.
20. Myer, O. O., Thewlis, E. W., and Rusch, H. P.: The hypophysis and hemopoiesis. Endocrinology, *27*:932, 1940.
21. Pirzio-Biroli, G., Bothwell, T. H., and Finch, C. A.: Iron absorption. II. The absorption of radioiron administered with a standard meal in man. J. Lab. Clin. Med., *51*:37, 1958.
22. Tudhope, G. R., and Wilson, G. M.: Anemia in hypothyroidism. Q. J. Med., *29*:513, 1960.
23. Tudhope, G. R., and Wilson, G. M.: Deficiency of vitamin B_{12} in hypothyroidism. Lancet, *1*:703, 1962.
24. Walchli, E.: Hypo- und athyreosis und blutbild. Folia Haematol., *27*:135, 1922.

ANEMIA ASSOCIATED WITH ACUTE BLOOD LOSS

25. Ebert, R. V., Stead, E. A., Jr., and Gibson, J. G., II: Response of normal subjects to acute blood loss. Arch. Intern. Med., *68*:578, 1941.
26. Gordon, A. S.: Quantitative nature of the red cell response to a single bleeding. Proc. Soc. Exp. Biol. Med., *31*:563, 1934.
27. Schiødt, E.: Observations on blood regeneration in man. I. The rise in erythrocytes in patients with hematemesis or melena from peptic ulcer. Am. J. Med. Sci., *193*:313, 1937.

ANEMIA ASSOCIATED WITH PREGNANCY

28. Berlin, N. I., Goetsch, C., Hyde, G. M., and Parsons, R. J.: The blood volume in pregnancy as determined by P-32 labeled red blood cells. Surg. Gynecol. Obstet., *97*:173, 1953.
29. Bethell, F. H.: The blood changes in normal pregnancy and their relation to the iron and protein supplied by the diet. J.A.M.A., *107*:564, 1936.
30. Bethel, F. H., and Blecha, E.: Diet in pregnancy. Clinics, *1*:346, 1936.
31. Fay, J., Cartwright, G. E., and Wintrobe, M. M.: Studies on free erythrocyte protoporphyrin, serum iron, serum iron-binding capacity and plasma copper during normal pregnancy. J. Clin. Invest., *28*:487, 1949.
32. Goldstein, I. M., and Coller, B. S.: Aplastic anemia in pregnancy: recovery after normal spontaneous delivery. Ann. Intern. Med., *82*:537, 1975.
33. Holly, R. G.: Megaloblastic anemia in pregnancy. Remission following combined therapy with ascorbic acid and vitamin B_{12}. Proc. Soc. Exp. Biol. Med., *78*:238, 1951.
34. Holly, R. G.: The iron and iron-binding capacity of serum and the erythrocyte protoporphyrin in pregnancy. Obstet. Gynecol., *2*:119, 1953.
35. Holly, R. G.: The value of iron therapy in pregnancy. Journal-Lancet, *74*:211, 1954.
36. Holly, R. G.: Anemia in pregnancy. Obstet. Gynecol., *5*:562, 1955.
37. Lange, R. D., and Dynesius, R.: Blood volume changes during normal pregnancy. Clin. Haematol., *2*:453, 1973.
38. Lawrence, C., and Klipstein, F. A.: Megaloblastic anemia of pregnancy in New York City. Ann. Intern. Med., *66*:25, 1967.
39. Sturgis, C. C.: Hematology. Charles C Thomas, Springfield, Ill., 1948.
40. Wallerstein, R. O.: Iron metabolism and iron deficiency during pregnancy. Clin. Haematol., *2*:453, 1973.
41. Whitfield, C. R., and Love, A. H. G.: Intestinal malabsorption in megaloblastic pregnancy anemia. J. Obstet. Gynaecol. Br. Commonw., *75*:844, 1968.

Anemia Associated with Chronic Renal Disease

42. Adamson, J. W., Eschbach, J., and Finch, C. A.: The kidney and erythropoiesis. Am. J. Med., *44*:725, 1968.
43. Chaplin, H., and Mollison, P. L.: Red cell life-span in nephritis and in hepatic cirrhosis. Clin. Sci., *12*:351, 1953.
44. Eaton, D. W., Koplin, C. F., Swofford, H. S., Kjellstrand, C. M., and Jacob, J. S.: Chlorinated urban water: a cause of dialysis-induced hemolytic anemia. Science, *181*:463, 1973.
45. Emerson, C. P., Jr., and Burroughs, B. A.: The mechanism of anemia and its influence on renal function in chronic uremia. J. Clin. Invest., *28*:779, 1949.
46. Erslev, A. J.: Anemia of chronic renal disease. Arch. Intern. Med., *126*:774, 1970.
47. Eschbach, J. W., and Adamson, J. W.: Improvement in the anemia of chronic renal failure with fluoxymesterone. Ann. Intern. Med., *78*:527, 1973.
48. Finch, C. A., Gibson, J. G., III, Peacock, W. C., and Fluharty, R. G.: Iron metabolism, utilization of intravenous radioactive iron. Blood, *4*:905, 1949.
49. Fried, W., Jonasson, O., Lang, G., and Schwartz, F.: The hematologic effect of androgen in uremic patients. Ann. Intern. Med., *79*:823, 1973.
50. Jacobson, L. O., Goldwasser, E., Fried, W., and Plzak, L.: Role of the kidney in erythropoiesis. Nature, *179*:633, 1957.
51. Kaye, M.: The anemia associated with renal disease. J. Lab. Clin. Med., *52*:83, 1958.
52. Loge, J. P., Lange, R. D., and Moore, C. V.: Characterization of the anemia of chronic renal insufficiency. J. Clin. Invest., *29*:830, 1950.
53. Loge, J. P., Lange, R. D., and Moore, C. V.: Characterization of the anemia associated with chronic renal insufficiency. Am. J. Med., *24*:4, 1958.
54. Markson, J. L., and Rennie, J. B.: The anaemia of chronic renal insufficiency. Scott. Med. J., *1*:320, 1956.
55. Rees, S. B., et al.: Effect of dialysis and purine ribosides upon the anemia of uremia. J. Clin. Invest., *36*:923, 1957.
56. Thorup, O. A., Jr., Strole, W. E., and Leavell, B. S.: The rate of removal of iron from culture medium by human bone marrow suspension. J. Lab. Clin. Med., *52*:266, 1958.
57. Yawata, Y., Howe, R., and Jacob, H. S.: Abnormal red cell metabolism causing hemolysis in uremia. Ann. Intern. Med., *79*:362, 1973.

Anemia Associated with Chronic Liver Disease

58. Blass, J. P., and Dean, H. M.: The relation of hyperlipemia to hemolytic anemia in an alcoholic patient. Am. J. Med., *40*:283, 1966.
59. Brown, A.: Megaloblastic anemia associated with adult scurvy: report of a case which responded to synthetic ascorbic acid alone. Br. J. Haematol., *1*:345, 1955.
60. Grahn, E. P., Dietz, A. A., Stefani, S. S., and Donnelly, W. J.: Burr cells, hemolytic anemia and cirrhosis. Am. J. Med., *45*:78, 1968.
61. Herbert, V.: Minimum daily adult folate requirement. Arch. Intern. Med., *110*:649, 1962.
62. Herbert, V., Zalusky, R., and Davidson, C. S.: Correlation of folate deficiency with alcoholism and associated macrocytosis, anemia, and liver disease. Ann. Intern. Med., *58*:977, 1963.
63. Hines, J. D.: Reversible megaloblastic and sideroblastic marrow abnormalities in alcoholic patients. Br. J. Haematol., *16*:87, 1969.
64. Jandl, J. H.: The anemia of liver disease: observations on its mechanism. J. Clin. Invest., *34*:390, 1955.
65. Klipstein, F. A., and Lindenbaum, J.: Folate deficiency in chronic liver disease. Blood, *25*:443, 1965.
66. Movitt, E. R.: Megaloblastic erythropoiesis in patients with cirrhosis of the liver. Blood, *5*:468, 1950.
67. Zieve, L.: Jaundice hyperlipemia and hemolytic anemia: A heretofore unrecognized syndrome associated with alcoholic fatty liver and cirrhosis. Ann. Intern. Med., *48*:471, 1958.

Disorders of the Spleen

68. Dacie, J. V., Brain, M. C., Harrison, C. V., Lewis, S. M., and Worlledge, S. M.: Non-tropical idiopathic splenomegaly ("primary hypersplenism"): a review of ten cases and their relationship to malignant lymphomas. Br. J. Haematol., *17*:317, 1969.
69. Eraklis, A. J., Kevy, S. V., Diamond, L. K., and Gross, R. E.: Hazard of overwhelming infection after splenectomy in childhood. N. Engl. J. Med., *276*:1225, 1967.
70. Hamilton, P. J. S., Richmond, J., Donaldson, G. W. K., Williams, R., Hutt, M. S. R., and Lugumba, V.: Splenectomy in "big spleen disease." Br. Med. J., *3*:823, 1967.

71. Hess, C. E., Ayers, C. R., Wetzel, R. A., Mohler, D. N., and Sandusky, W. R.: Dilutional anemia in splenomegaly: an indication for splenectomy. Ann. Surg., *173*:693, 1971.
72. Jandl, J. H., Jacob, H. S., and Daland, G. P.: Hypersplenism due to infection. N. Engl. J. Med., *264*:1063, 1961.
73. Prankerd, T. A. J.: The spleen and anaemia. Br. Med. J., *2*:517, 1963.
74. Richmond, J., Donaldson, G. W. K., Williams, R., Hamilton, P. J. S., and Hutt, M. S. R.: Hematologic effect of idiopathic splenomegaly seen in Uganda. Br. J. Haematol., *13*:348, 1967.
75. Sandusky, W. R., Leavell, B. S., and Benjamin, B. I.: Splenectomy: indications and results in hematologic disorders. Ann. Surg., *159*:695, 1964.

FELTY'S SYNDROME

76. Felty, A. R.: Chronic arthritis in the adult associated with splenomegaly and leukopenia. Johns Hopkins Med. J., *36*:16, 1924.
77. Moore, R. A., Brunner, C. M., Sandusky, W. R., and Leavell, B. S.: Felty's syndrome: long-term follow-up after splenectomy. Ann. Intern. Med., *75*:381, 1971.
78. Sandusky, W. R., Rudolf, L. E., and Leavell, B. S.: Splenectomy for control of neutropenia in Felty's syndrome. Ann. Surg., *167*:744, 1968.
79. Vincent, P. C., Levi, J. A., and MacQueen, A.: The mechanism of neutropenia in Felty's syndrome. Br. J. Haematol., *27*:463, 1974.

HEMATOLOGIC DISORDERS OF ALCOHOLISM

80. Brayton, R. G., Stokes, P. E., Schwartz, M. S., and Louria, D. B.: Effect of alcohol and various diseases on leukocyte mobilization phagocytosis and intracellular bacterial killing. N. Engl. J. Med., *282*:123, 1970.
81. Cooper, R. A.: Anemia with spur cells: a red cell defect acquired in serum and modified in the circulation. J. Clin. Invest., *48*:1820, 1969.
82. Douglas, C. C., and Twomey, J. J.: Transient stomatocytosis with hemolysis: a previously unrecognized complication of alcoholism. Ann. Intern. Med., *72*:159, 1970.
83. Eichner, E. R.: The hematologic disorders of alcoholism. Am. Jour. Med., *54*:621, 1973.
84. Eichner, E. R., and Hillman, R. S.: The evolution of anemia in alcoholic patients. Am. J. Med., *50*:218, 1971.
85. Hines, J. D.: Reversible megaloblastic and sideroblastic marrow abnormalities in alcoholic patients. Br. J. Haematol., *16*:87, 1969.
86. Hines, J. D., and Cowan, D. H.: Studies on the pathogenesis of alcohol-induced sideroblastic bone marrow abnormalities. N. Engl. J. Med., *283*:441, 1970.
87. Hines, J. D., and Cowan, D. H.: Anemia in Alcoholism. *In*: Dimitrov, N. V., and Nodine, J. H. (eds.): Drugs and Hematologic Reactions. Grune & Stratton, N.Y., 1974.
88. Lindenbaum, J., and Hargrove, R. L.: Thrombocytopenia in alcoholics. Ann. Intern. Med., *68*:526, 1968.
89. Liu, Y. K.: Leukopenia in alcoholics. Am. J. Med., *54*:605, 1973.
90. McCurdy, P. R., Pierce, L. E., and Rath, C. E.: Abnormal bone-marrow morphology in acute alcoholism. N. Engl. J. Med., *266*:505, 1962.
91. Straus, D. J.: Hematologic aspects of alcoholism. Semin. Hematol., *10*:183, 1973.
92. Sullivan, L. W., and Herbert, V.: Suppression of hematopoiesis by ethanol. J. Clin. Invest., *43*:2048, 1964.

LEAD POISONING

93. Albahary, C.: Lead and hematopoiesis. Am. J. Med., *52*:367, 1972.
94. Aub, J. C., Fairhill, L. T., Minot, A. S., and Reznikoff, P.: Lead Poisoning. Medicine, *4*:1, 1925.
95. Boyett, J. D., and Butterworth, C. E., Jr.: Lead poisoning and hemoglobin synthesis. Report of 15 patients with chronic lead intoxication. Am. J. Med., *32*:884, 1962.
96. Dickinson, L., Reichert, E. L., Reginald, C. S. H., Rivers, J. B., and Kominami, N.: Lead poisoning in a family due to cocktail glasses. Am. J. Med., *52*:391, 1972.
97. Waldron, H. A.: The anemia of lead poisoning—a review. Br. J. Ind. Med., *23*:83, 1966.
98. Whitfield, C. L., Ch'ien, L. T., and Whitehead, J. D.: Lead encephalopathy in adults. Am. J. Med., *52*:289, 1972.

ARSENIC POISONING

99. Kyle, R. A., and Pease, D. C.: Hematologic aspects of arsenic intoxication. N. Engl. J. Med., *273*:18, 1965.
100. Westhoff, D. D., Sahaha, R. J., and Barnes, A. J.: Arsenic intoxication as a cause of megalo-blastic anemia. Blood, *45*:241, 1975.

COPPER DEFICIENCY

101. Dunlap, W. M., James, G. W., III, and Hume, D. M.: Anemia and neutropenia caused by copper deficiency. Ann. Intern. Med., *80*:470, 1974.

ANEMIA OF PREMATURITY

102. Stockman, J. A., III: Anemia of prematurity. Semin. Hematol., *12*:163, 1975.

CHAPTER **9**

GRANULOCYTES AND MONOCYTES

Credit for distinguishing between the red and white corpuscles in the circulating blood has been given to William Hewson.[34] The term "leukocytosis" was introduced by Virchow to indicate a temporary increase in the number of circulating leukocytes; he recognized that increases occurred in a variety of normal and disease states. The association of leukocytosis with infectious processes attracted considerable attention and stimulated numerous investigations. Over 50 years ago the authors of one book on hematology wrote, "The problem of leukocytosis has been subjected to as much discussion as any question of modern medicine. An exhaustive recital of the work devoted to it, of its methods, and of the results of this work would fill a whole volume and would be out of place in a treatise on blood diseases."[22] Since that time other investigations of the origin and function of the leukocytes, and the variations therein, have added to our knowledge, but many important details remain to be clarified.

The origin and morphology of the leukocytes are discussed in Chapter 1. The present chapter deals with cellular kinetics, the functions these cells perform, the numbers of the different types of leukocytes that are found in normal circumstances, the variations that occur under different physiologic and pathologic conditions, and the mechanisms that are considered important in producing these changes.

The phagocytic cells, granulocytes and mononuclear macrophages, are essential for the body's defense against bacterial infection. Without these cells, even with antibiotics, an individual can survive for only a short period; if the cells are significantly reduced in number, infections are frequent, often severe, and difficult to control. The phagocytic function of the macrophage is also important in the body's immune mechanism, the antigen–antibody and graft–versus–host reactions. (Chap. 14).

320

GRANULOCYTES

THE ORIGIN OF GRANULOCYTES

All hematologic cells, including granulocytes and monocytes, plasma cells, lymphocytes, and marrow fibroblasts are thought to arise in the bone marrow from a common precursor cell termed the pluripotent stem cell.[29] This cell is considered able to replicate in order to maintain a pool of stem cells, or to differentiate into a specific hematopoietic cell series. The evidence for this concept comes from a murine cell culture system. When lethally irradiated mice are transfused with bone marrow elements from nonirradiated mice[70] the spleen develops discrete colonies containing erythrocytes, granulocytes, and megakaryocytes.[70] Chromosomal analyses show distinctive chromosomal markers within each colony, which indicates that each colony is a clone.[5, 81] In this murine spleen culture system, cells with the capacity to form colonies are called "colony-forming units" (CFU). The stem cell that forms these spleen colonies has been partially separated from the other donor marrow cells, and strongly resembles the small lymphocyte when examined with the light microscope; this cell, however, is said to have a distinctive intracellular architecture and can be distinguished from the small lymphocyte by electron microscopy.[18, 72]

The pluripotential stem cell is considered able to differentiate into committed stem cells, which have different capacities for further differentiation into specific hematopoietic cell lines. Thus a committed stem cell may be unipotent and able to produce a single cell line such as erythrocytes, megakaryocytes, or granulocytes; it may be multipotent, able to produce more than one cell line, such as granulocytes and macrophages.[14] Experimentally, a committed granulocyte–monocyte stem cell (GMS stem cell) can be assayed in man by the growth of mixed granulocyte and monocyte colonies on soft agar, through a modification of the method devised by Bradley and Metcalf;[10] this committed granulocyte–monocyte stem cell does not have the ability to produce megakaryocytes or erythrocytes.

The stem cell committed to the granulocytic series gives rise to the myeloblast, which develops into a promyelocyte, the common precursor of the neutrophilic, eosinophilic, and basophilic granulocytes. As the myeloblasts mature into promyelocytes, proteins are synthesized and packed into granules in the Golgi apparatus in the cytoplasm. These primary or nonspecific granules persist in the mature neutrophil. They are azurophilic with Wright's stain and contain a number of enzymes including the hemoprotein myeloperoxidase, which has peroxidase activity; these granules probably also contain other low molecular weight proteins with bactericidal activity.[68] As the promyelocyte differentiates into a myelocyte, the secondary or specific granules are formed in the Golgi apparatus; they are small, and stain poorly with Wright's stain as compared to the primary granules. These secondary granules contain no peroxidase or digestive enzymes, but they do contain alkaline phosphatase and the microbicidal protein lactoferrin.[68] In maturing from the myeloblast to the myelocyte the neutrophil converts from primary aerobic to anaerobic metabolism, losing many mitochondria and gaining glycogen, which becomes the source of energy for its metabolism.

GRANULOPOIESIS-KINETICS

The granulocytes constitute a tissue of considerable size. Only a small part of this tissue is contained in the circulating blood, where the number of granulocytes normally ranges from 2000 to 6000 cells per cu. mm. Osgood estimated that 60 per cent of the total number of granulocytes are in the bone marrow, with 0.7 per cent of the total in the circulating blood and 40 per cent in the tissues exclusive of the blood and blood-forming organs.[55] The quantity and distribution of the granulocytes can be appreciated by considering the total mass of cells. It is estimated that the weight of granulocytes in the marrow is 900 gm., in the circulating blood 10 gm., and in the other tissues 600 gm., compared to the normal adult liver of 1500 gm. and spleen of 150 gm.

It is customary to consider the existence in the marrow of different pools or compartments; these are the stem cell pool, the mitotic pool in which cell division and maturation occur, the nonmitotic pool in which only maturation occurs, and the mature granulocyte pool which serves as a reservoir for future systemic release.[62] Mature granulocytes are released from the bone marrow into the peripheral blood, where one-half of the total granulocyte pool (TBGP) forms the circulating granulocyte pool (CGP) and the other half is sequestered in the capillaries as the marginal granulocyte pool (MGP).[8] Mature granulocytes migrate from the intravascular space through capillary walls into the tissues, where they perform their phagocytic functions and finally die or are excreted. Experimental evidence indicates that once the granulocytes leave the intravascular compartment they are unable to return in significant numbers. The location and function of the extravascular granulocytes is an intriguing problem; the lungs, liver, and spleen are known sites of extravascular accumulation.[6, 32]

Donohue and others, employing a radioiron technique, calculated that the average number of total marrow granulocyte forms in man is 11.4×10^9 cells per kg., or 79.8×10^{10} for a 70 kg. man; of this total 61.6×10^{10} are metamyelocytes, bands, and segmented forms, cells that can be released from the marrow quickly. The same authors placed the CGP at 2.1×10^{10} in a 70 kg. man;[20] an equal number of cells, 2.1×10^{10}, is sequestered in the capillaries of the body as the MGP.[2] The total daily production of neutrophils in a 70 kg. man has been placed at 1.2×10^{11} neutrophils per day.[14]

Granulopoiesis begins with the pluripotential stem cell; most of the stem cells are in a resting phase, and only a small proportion divide or differentiate into committed stem cells and myeloblasts.[14] The fact that most stem cells are not dividing has important implications in the treatment of acute leukemia because most chemotherapeutic agents are cycle-active drugs that mainly affect the rapidly-dividing committed granulocyte precursors. Thus, the stem cell would be relatively unaffected by these agents and could constitute a reservoir for either normal or leukemic stem cells. The major granulocyte production pool is composed of myeloblasts, promyelocytes, and myelocytes. The number of cell divisions between myeloblast and myelocyte has been estimated at between three and seven.[62] Cells older than myelocytes do not divide; the mature neutrophil remains in the marrow reserve pool, possibly for days. The time necessary for a myelocyte to progress to a mature neutrophil has been variously estimated to be between six and 14 days.[62] Both the tritiated thymidine (^{3}HT) method to label cells synthesizing DNA and the radioactive diisopropylfluorophosphate (DF^{32}P) method to label cells with neutrophilic granules indicate that the marrow granulocyte reserve pool is at least 13 times the size of the total blood granulocyte pool.[8, 9]

After release into the blood the mature granulocytes are distributed almost equally between the CGP and MGP. The half-life of granulocytes in the blood is approximately six to seven hours;[62] the cells do not leave the circulation because of senescence as red blood cells do, but appear to exit randomly. After entering the tissue the granulocytes survive for an average of four to five days.[62] The survival time in the tissue depends on many factors and varies from minutes to several days.[62] The main sites of extravascular accumulation are the lungs, liver, spleen, gastrointestinal tract, bone marrow, striated muscle, and kidney. Studies that employed catheterization of various vessels have revealed that the lungs remove large numbers of leukocytes from the circulation.[6] The fate of cells trapped in the pulmonary circulation is uncertain, but several possibilities have been suggested: (1) transient trapping with later entry into the general circulation; (2) migration and excretion through the sputum and gastrointestinal tract; (3) re-entry into the general circulation by way of the lymphatics and thoracic duct; (4) disintegration in the lung. A failure of the removal mechanism has been suggested as a cause of leukocytosis in certain diseases, especially leukemia.

Colony-stimulating activity (CSA) can be demonstrated in serum, or feeder layers of peripheral white blood cells placed under the agar bed of transplanted granulocyte–monocyte stem cells.[14, 62] The most potent sources of CSA in humans are the peripheral blood monocytes.[29] One potent stimulus for the release of CSA by macrophages is endotoxin from gram-negative bacteria; thus the macrophages may be the key to the activation of the body defenses in the presence of infection. Studies of human serum and urine have shown that most of the CSA resides in a glucoprotein with a molecular weight of 45,000 that migrates electrophoretically as an alpha globulin.[14, 29] Whether this colony-stimulating glycoprotein is a granulopoietin that acts on the appropriate stem cell in a fashion analogous to erythropoietin remains undecided at the present time.

Although there is strong evidence for the existence of a granulopoietin that stimulates granulocyte production, there is only minor evidence to support the existence of an inhibitor to complete the negative feedback mechanism. Chalones are defined as tissue specific, species nonspecific regulator substances which are produced within the tissue on which they act to inhibit cell proliferation in a reversible manner. Such a substance active in vitro and in vivo has been isolated from neutrophils; an action on the proliferation of the committed granulocyte–monocyte stem cell has been postulated, but a physiologic role for this granulocyte chalone has not been established.[65]

REGULATION OF CELL PRODUCTION

The factors that control the level of the granulocytes in the circulation in normal and abnormal conditions have not been defined precisely. In Ehrlich's and Lazarus's textbook of 1910, chemotaxis was accepted as the explanation of the migration of leukocytes into areas of infection, and it was postulated that the marrow cells were stimulated by a chemical that led to increased proliferation and output of these cells.[22] The importance of the reactive ability of the marrow was recognized, for it was known that an injection of oil of turpentine produced leukocytosis in normal individuals, but failed to do so in patients with typhoid fever and leukopenia until after the fever and leukopenia had disappeared. More recent studies have provided a better understanding of the factors regulating granulocyte levels in the blood.

Alteration in the peripheral blood granulocyte count, either leukocytosis or leukopenia, could be the result of diminished production, an increase in destruction, or a shift in granulocytes from one pool to another. The rate of release of neutrophils from the marrow appears to be influenced by a humoral factor. Several experimental models in which animals have been rendered leukopenic by chemotherapy,[8] leukapheresis,[20] or antiserum and irradiation[30] have demonstrated the presence of a plasma "granulocyte releasing factor" which mobilizes cells from the marrow granulocyte storage pool to the circulating blood pool. These experiments indicate that the marrow granulocyte storage pool serves as the major immediate source of new blood granulocytes during acute bacterial infection, when large numbers of circulating granulocytes migrate to the site of infection. How these plasma factors produce granulocyte mobilization is still unclear.

Hormones and bacterial products can stimulate mobilization of granulocytes from the bone marrow. Both ACTH and hydrocortisone produce an increase in circulating neutrophils and a decrease in circulating eosinophils.[21] Intravenous hydrocortisone exerts its earliest effect through release of granulocytes from the marrow storage pool.[62] Hydrocortisone also inhibits the movement of neutrophils from the vascular compartment. Ethiocholanolone, typhoid vaccine, and a Salmonella endotoxin also induce the release of marrow granulocytes, but so far none of these agents has proved very useful clinically in assessing the marrow reserve of leukopenic patients.[62, 63]

Changes in the peripheral granulocyte count may also be the result of shifts between the MGP and the CGP; the leukocytosis that follows strenuous physical exertion or the intravenous injection of epinephrine is the result of such a shift. Although the leukocyte-releasing factors produce peripheral leukocytosis, they do not function as a granulopoietin to stimulate the production of new granulocytes, which is essential if leukocytosis is to be sustained during periods of infection.

The existence of both a stimulatory factor and an inhibiting factor that operate by a negative feedback system, a common phenomenon in biology, appears a likely mechanism to explain the control of bone marrow function. The development of satisfactory methods for studying bone marrow culture in vitro[8, 10] has stimulated research in this field.[8] Inoculation of human bone marrow into specially-prepared soft agar will result in the growth of colonies of granulocytes and monocytes varying from 40 to 2000 cells; each colony originates from a single committed stem cell.[29, 62] Growth in this system does not occur spontaneously unless a colony stimulating factor (CSF) or CSA is present to initiate and sustain growth.[62]

MONOCYTES AND MACROPHAGES

Studies of the effect of radiation on the marrow in various animals have shown that the monocytes are formed in the bone marrow.[67] Migration of macrophages in rats and their labeling by tritiated thymidine were suppressed by radiation, but not if the bone marrow was shielded; in addition, labeled cells present in the bone marrow suspension that were injected intravenously appeared as labeled macrophages in the exudate, but cells from the thoracic duct, lymph nodes, and thymus prepared in the same way and injected intravenously did not produce the labeled macrophages. The promonocytes develop from the GMS stem cell in the bone marrow. During maturation complex changes in morphology and function occur; the cells appear to ingest proteins, which in some way leads to an increase in the lysosomal enzymes. Like the granulocytes, monocytes contain two types of cytoplasmic granule; one, the "primary," contains peroxidase and lysosome enzymes; the contents of the "secondary" granule are not known. When the monocyte becomes transformed into the macrophage the peroxidase-containing granules disappear, but lysomal enzymes continue to be synthesized.[68]

Monocytes or mononuclear macrophages are found normally in the circulating blood, bone marrow, lymph nodes, spleen, and loose connective tissue. They constitute from 3 to 7 per cent of the circulating leukocytes, the total number in the circulation being approximately 0.5×10^{11}. The ratio of those in the tissues to those in the circulating blood has been estimated to be 400:1.[55]

Data concerning the circulation of the monocytes in the peripheral blood are not as complete as those for granulocytes. Recent studies using autotransfused cells labeled with (^{3}H-DFP) indicate that the circulating monocyte pool constitutes only about one-quarter of the monocytes in the circulation, the others belonging to a marginal monocyte pool. T $\frac{1}{2}$ times in the circulation in normal subjects was found to be 8.4 hours, but was as high as 15 hours in some patients with monocytosis. The turnover was estimated at 6×10^8 monocytes per hour, 7×10^6 per hour per kilogram of body weight.[48]

When the monocyte leaves the circulation it develops into a macrophage in the lung, peritoneum, liver (Kupfer's cells), or in an area of inflammation. The macrophages undergo adaptation at the new tissue sites, and pulmonary macrophages behave differently from macrophages found in the peritoneum. Although the main source of macrophages is the circulating monocytes, under special conditions macrophages may reproduce themselves, a process seen particularly in the liver and lung. Formerly the macrophages were considered to be a part of a "reticuloendothelial" system. The endothelial cells, fibroblasts, reticular cells, and dendritic cells are now considered by some to belong to a different system, because these cells do not have the morphologic characteristics of mononuclear phagocytes, cannot be shown to be derived from the peripheral blood monocyte, and are not highly phagocytic.[73] Monocytes and both the fixed and mobile macrophages are characterized by their highly-developed capacity for phagocytosis.

The mechanism that recognizes an antigen that gains access to the body as "foreign" or "not self," and brings it into contact with the immunological system, is not completely understood. Chemotaxis of macrophages has been difficult to demonstrate, possibly because of their slow movement. Recently sensitized lymphocytes have been demonstrated to elaborate a chemotactic factor for mononuclear cells, as well as a migration inhibitory factor (MIF) which inhibits random migration of normal macrophages in vitro. These factors may play a major role in the accumulation of macrophages at sites of infection or allergic reactions. The specificity of the immunologic activity of the macrophage seems to be increased by globulin components of the serum known as cytophilic antibodies.[53] These bind to the macrophage in such a way that the cell is subsequently able to adsorb antigen. There is evidence that the cytophilic antibodies may occur "naturally" without known prior immunization.[52]

Structural units which consist of macrophages surrounded by lymphocytic cells have been observed in lymph nodes of immunized animals. Such clones suggest a physical means of transfer between cells, and actual physical joining between the cytoplasm of macrophages and lymphocytes has been reported.[66] In addition, it has been demonstrated that labeled RNA, which had been produced in macrophages incubated with tritiated cytidin and then extracted, was incorporated into lymph node cells after incubation.[24]

Antigen appears to be unable to stimulate antibody production by antibody-producing cells directly on first exposure or possibly even on subsequent exposures, but the evidence is not conclusive. Apparently the antigen must first be engulfed and processed by the macrophage before the message can be transferred to the antibody-producing cells. Antigen is initially localized in macrophages and later in the reticulum cells in lymphoid follicles. Once in the macrophage, antigen becomes associated with large granules, probably lysosomes. Later macrophage RNA, with or without antigen fragments, is passed to the lymphocytes which cluster about the macrophage.[26] Soon thereafter, new antibody-forming cells appear in the spleen and lymph nodes. Significant titers of antibody do not appear for three to four days after stimulation, although minute quantities may be detected in the first 24 hours. Stimulation or depression of macrophage activity in vivo is accompanied by stimulation or depression of antibody production.

THE EOSINOPHIL

The eosinophil is a granulocyte with a high content of peroxidase that differs from the neutrophil in many respects.[15, 44, 76] After maturation in the bone marrow it spends less than a day, perhaps only three or four hours, in the circulation before it migrates to tissue sites, where it may survive morphologically intact for from eight to 12 days. Several eosinophil chemotactic factors responsible for its migration into an area of inflammation have been demonstrated. One related to complement is produced by the reaction of antigen with IgG, and a second is elaborated by antigen-stimulated leukocytes. Another, important in allergic disorders, apparently results from the action of antigen and antibody of the IgE class on the surface of the mast cell or basophil. Other reactions that activate complement, such as those associated with endotoxins and tissue injury, can produce eosinophil chemotactic factors. Recent work has demonstrated that some malignant cells produce a chemotactic factor and eosinophilia, perhaps in a manner analogous to the production of erythropoietin and parathormone by certain neoplasms.

The eosinophil lacks some of the proteolytic enzymes, cathepsin and phagocytin, found in neutrophils, but it can phagocytize antigen-antibody complexes and certain microorganisms; it is less effective in killing bacteria. There is no evidence that the cell causes tissue damage, such as tissue necrosis, per se.

The function of the eosinophil remains unclear, although eosinophilia occurs in many conditions including bronchial asthma, parasitic infestations, dermatoses, drug reactions, "hypereosinophilic syndromes," Löffler's pulmonary syndrome, Löffler's endocarditis, periarteritis nodosa, diffuse eosinophilic collagen vascular disease, and eosinophilic leukemia. An eosinophilic reaction may be seen in patients with carcinoma or Hodgkins disease. Adrenal steroids produce eosinopenia in man, but the mechanism remains a mystery.

THE BASOPHIL

The basophil and its tissue counterpart, the mast cell, are concerned in allergic reactions. Basophils contain over one-half, possibly 85 per cent, of the histamine found in the blood, probably in the cytoplasmic granules.

Radioautograph studies have shown IgE on or in basophils of atopic patients and some normal individuals, but not on other leukocytes. The IgE-anti-IgE reaction causes degranulation of the basophils and release of histamine;[23, 39, 78] serum components are not necessary.

The basophils in the blood, normally 28 to 44 per cu. mm. of blood, are often increased in chronic granulocytic leukemia and other myeloproliferative disorders; elevations also occur in some patients with hypothyroidism. ACTH produces a fall in basophils and eosinophils in the circulating blood. The tissue basophils are increased in delayed hypersensitivity reactions, but not in nonspecific exudates or immediate types of hypersensitivity reaction.

PHAGOCYTOSIS

The importance of phagocytosis as one of the main defense mechanisms of the body was suggested by Metchnikoff in 1882 after he had observed the accumulation of mobile cells at a thorn placed under the skin of a starfish larva.[80] Numerous studies since that time have confirmed Metchnikoff's concept. The serious infections with a high mortality rate that occur in most patients with agranulocytosis from any cause amply substantiate it. Granulocytes and monocytes are also the main sources of pyrogens responsible for the febrile response seen in most infections and in tissue necrosis. Phagocytosis is a complex process that involves the following phases: (1) chemotaxis, both humoral and cellular; (2) recog-

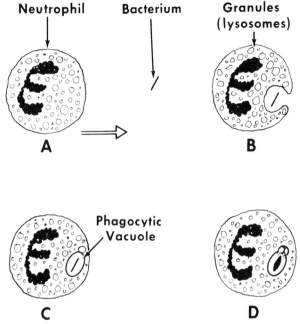

Figure 9–1 Phagocytosis of a bacterium by a neutrophil leukocyte. *A,* Chemotaxis. *B,* Engulfment. *C,* Formation of a phagocytic vacuole. *D,* Fusion of lysosomes and phagocytic vacuole.

nition of the foreign body; (3) engulfment; and (4) killing of the ingested organisms (Fig. 9–1).

CHEMOTAXIS

Different processes related to inflammation can influence chemotaxis, the movement of the granulocytes or monocytes into the proximity of the offending particle. The reaction between the microorganism and the host tissue may produce humoral chemotactic factors in several ways. In one, an active chemotactic factor is released by some bacteria in the body. A second and more important active process is generated by the action of bacteria on serum complement.[68] The antigen–antibody reaction on the surface of the organism activates the hemolytic component of complement C-1, C-4, and C-2. The complex of antigen–antibody C-1, 4, 2 reacts with C-3 and C-5 to split off C-3a and C-5a, low molecular weight peptides with chemotactic activity. C-3a and C-5a, the chemotactic factors in complement, are also produced in the absence of specific antibodies by action of nonspecific proteases on C-3, C-5; in addition, some microorganisms cause the necessary changes in C-3, C-5 by acting through the properdin system.[68] Still other factors are chemotactic to a certain extent. Among these are the Hageman factor activation which liberates kallikrein and plasminogen. Chemotactic substances are also released by neutrophils that have phagocytosed certain particles.

Lymphokines released from lymphocytes that have been stimulated by antigens are also chemotactic.

The response of the cell to the chemotactic stimulus is a necessary part of the reaction. Neutrophils move more rapidly to areas of inflammation than do monocytes, apparently in response to the same chemotactic stimulus; after the monocytes have reached a certain concentration in the area of inflammation, the migration of neutrophils to the area ceases. The factors which mediate this change in the cell population are not understood. Although the details of the cell's motile response in chemotaxis, presumably initiated by the action of the chemotactic agent on the plasma membrane of the cell, are unknown, contractile proteins beneath the cell membranes, ATPase activity, and the microtubules are thought to be involved.[68] Hirsch and Cohn have employed cinemicrophotography to study phagocytosis.[35, 36] They observed that a polymorphonuclear leukocyte moved in a random fashion until the cell came within 10 to 20 μ of a particle or a bacillus; at this range chemotaxis became evident and the cell moved in a straight line to the particle. The rapid motion of the granules in the neutrophil during movement gives the impression that the granulocyte is streaming rapidly towards the object to be engulfed: the motile behavior of the mononuclear phagocyte is similar but less rapid, and the edges of the membrane are more likely to project in a number of different directions.[68]

RECOGNITION AND ENGULFMENT

Recognition of the object to be phagocytosed is essential if phagocytosis is to be beneficial. Particles exposed to fresh serum or coated with specific antibody are engulfed readily and rapidly. This coating of the particles is termed opsonization. Heat-resistant serum IgG antibodies are strong opsonins, but such antibodies are present in significant amounts only in hyperimmune sera. The heat labile opsonins found in normal serum are fragments of C-3 produced by the action of bacteria on C-1, C-4, and C-2; this fragment is the only known opsonically-active complement protein. Without opsonins phagocytosis proceeds slowly, particularly in a liquid medium where some entrapment between two cells or against a surface, such as the wall of an alveolus, is necessary. Apparently the opsonin portion of the particle–opsonin–complex attaches to specific binding sites on the plasma membrane of the cells prior to ingestion. Human monocytes contain receptor sites for immunoglobulin-G and for complement; the latter facilitates the attachment of cells or particles after the reaction of IgG or IgM with the complement components.[4, 37] The attached particle thus becomes firmly adherent to the cell membrane. When this has occurred rapid phagocytosis, complete within 30 seconds to 2 minutes, is accomplished as the cytoplasm of the cell flows around the particle; the cell membrane invaginates until it fuses to close the ingested particle in a ring of cell membrane that has become detached. The ingestion of particles is energy-dependent and ATP generating processes are activated.

Various factors influence phagocytosis. It is enhanced by opsonization of the particle and also by increased temperature. The properties of the particle to be engulfed affect it. Many bacteria produce antiphagocytic substances which are toxic for the phagocytic cell, such as the somatic "O" antigen on the surface of many gram-negative species, exotoxins, and leukocidins. The growing type III pneumococcus resists phagocytosis by producing a polysaccharide "slime" layer composed of long chain carbohydrate polymers of glucose and glucuronic acid, which protects the organism from phagocytosis and contributes to its virulence. The stickiness of certain bacteria, such as type I gonococci, may contribute to their resistance; many become attached to the surface of the granulocyte and escape ingestion.[19]

KILLING OF THE ORGANISMS

The vital step of killing the ingested organisms is accomplished by the fusion of the leukocyte granules in the neutrophils and monocytes (lysomes) with the phagocytic vacuole, followed by the discharge of digestive enzymes into the vacuoles. During phagocytosis glycolysis is accelerated and acid production is increased; the slight change in pH may suffice to release the bactericidal substance from the granules. Corticosteroids, antimalarial drugs, mycobacterium tuberculosis, Toxoplasma gondii, and other agents apparently sometimes interfere with degranulation in some manner.[68]

Several different systems important in the bactericidal activity of granulocytes have been identified: among these are antibacterial proteins, low intracellular pH, production of hydrogen peroxide, and production of superoxide. The pH of the phagocytic vacuole in neutrophils, 3.5 to 4.0, may be low enough to inhibit or kill some organisms. Lysozyme has some antimicrobial activity alone or in combination with ascorbic acid and hydrogen peroxide. The phagosome also contains lactoferrin, an iron-binding protein that inhibits the growth of microorganisms, as well as hydrolytic enzymes.[41, 68]

The most potent microbicidal agent in the granulocytes is hydrogen peroxide; by itself it is active against bacteria, fungi, and viruses, a function that is greatly augmented by the presence of myeloperoxidase in the presence of the halide ions, iodine or chloride, which probably enter the phagocytic vacuole by diffusion. The serious disorder, chronic granulomatous disease, is characterized by a defect in this mechanism. Peroxide production in granulocytes, monocytes, and some macrophages is rapid after phagocytosis has commenced. This enzymatic conversion of oxygen to H_2O_2 is not inhibited by cyanide, which indicates that the enzyme is not a heme protein. Whether this is accomplished by NADH or NADPH is uncertain; the observation that neutrophils totally lacking G6PD, which generates NADPH from NADP, are unable to produce H_2O_2 has been interpreted as favoring either concept.[46, 68]

Mechanisms which reduce or destroy the hydrogen peroxide generated in the cell may function in the virulence of the organism; the staphylococcal catalase of Staphylococcus aureus is an example.[45] Low pO_2 interferes with the bactericidal function of granulocytes, and may be a factor in the persistence of infections in abscesses.[33]

The mechanisms for killing in monocytes are similar to those described in the neutrophil, except that these cells do not contain lactoferrin or bactericidal cationic proteins and have less myeloperoxidase.[68]

Table 9-1 *Total and Differential Leukocyte Counts in Normal Adults According to Various Authors*

AUTHOR	TOTAL (PER) (CU.MM.)	NEUTRO. (%)	EOSIN. (%)	BASO. (%)	LYMPH. (%)	MONO. (%)
Osgood et al	4,000–11,000	33–75	0–6	0–2	15–60	0–9
Sturgis and Bethell[69]	6,000– 7,400	55–67	2–3	0.5–0.7	23–38	4–6
Schilling[67]	5,000– 8,000	51–67	2–4	0–1	21–35	4–8
Wintrobe	5,000–10,000	54–62	1–3	0–0.75	25–33	3–7

NORMAL VALUES

The normal values for the total and differential leukocyte counts in adults according to various authors are shown in Table 9–1. Both the total count and the percentages of the different cells vary with the age of the individual. In the newborn, total counts varying from 3600 to 45,000 per cu.mm. have been reported, but the great majority are in the range of 10,000 to 25,000 per cu.mm.;[27, 69] at this time the neutrophils constitute about 60 per cent of the cells. From the second week through the second year, when the total count ranges from 8000 to 13,000 per cu.mm., the lymphocytes predominate and make up from 50 to 69 per cent of the total. During childhood the total count is usually around 8000 per cu.mm. and the range is 4000 to 13,000 per cu.mm.; during the same period the percentage of lymphocytes decreases to a range of 25 to 48 per cent by the 12th year. At about the 15th year the adult values are reached and these are maintained throughout the remainder of the individual's life.

Wintrobe found the following values (mean/cu.mm. and 95 per cent confidence limits) in 105 male medical students; neutrophils, 4300, 1800 to 6700; lymphocytes, 2700, 1500 to 3900; monocytes, 500, 100 to 900; eosinophils, 200, 0 to 600; basophils 40, 0 to 120.[77]

In one report of counts on 663 whites and 123 blacks, the granulocyte counts were lower in blacks (white males, 4463; black males, 3722; white females, 4440; black females, 4098).[12, 13] There were no differences in the levels in hemoglobin, hematocrit, or lymphocytes. A drop in the leukocyte count from 7800 per cu.mm. to 3500 per cu. mm., due mainly to a decrease in neutrophils, has been observed in healthy men in isolation at the South Polar Plateau.[51]

VARIATIONS

PHYSIOLOGIC VARIATIONS

In addition to the variations in leukocytes that are found at different ages, changes occur as a result of other physiologic processes, probably because of the shifting of granulocytes from the marginal pool along the vessel walls into the circulating granulocyte pool. These variations, which since the time of Virchow have been recognized to occur independently of disease, have been the subject of several detailed reviews.[27, 69]

Spontaneous fluctuations in the leukocyte count occur during the day. These appear to be inconstant, irregular, and unrelated to the ingestion of food; the changes have been interpreted as indicative of a redistribution of leukocytes within the body rather than an increased production of new cells, because these fluctuations are not associated with an increase in immature cells. An hourly rhythm of the leukocytes and an afternoon increase regardless of food ingestion have been reported, but not confirmed.

Strenuous exercise produces a marked leukocytosis. Total counts as high as 27,000 per cu.mm. have been found in marathon runners and football players. Leukocytosis that develops within 11 seconds has also been found after a 100-yard dash. After exercise the count returns to normal within several hours. Although pregnancy is associated with only a slight increase in leukocytes and neutrophils, at the onset of labor there is a marked increase, sometimes with the appearance of myelocytes, that may reach levels of 17,000 to 34,000 per cu.mm.[27, 42, 69]

Other causes of leukocytosis are paroxysmal tachycardia (13,000 to 20,000 per cu.mm.) and convulsions (37,000 to 43,000 per cu.mm.). Emotional states may be associated with changes in the leukocyte counts; the count has been noted to rise from 8000 to 18,000 per cu.mm. with the development of a panic reaction, and to decrease 6000 to 12,000 per cu.mm. in 1 hour when amobarbital administered intravenously induced a change in the emotional status.[49]

VARIATIONS DUE TO DISEASE

Changes that occur in the leukocytes in the peripheral blood in disease are often helpful in considering both the diagnosis and prognosis. In general, the changes in the peripheral blood reflect the type of injury, the extent of the process, and the body's reaction to the injury. Significant alterations may occur in the total number of leukocytes, in the proportion of the various cells present, and in the morphologic appearance of the individual cells. After removal of the spleen for any cause there is an increase in the neutrophil count, which returns to normal or near normal levels after several weeks or months. At this time the number of circulating lymphocytes and monocytes rises and apparently remains elevated.

Although no unconditional statements can be made concerning the reaction of the body to infection, certain generalizations can be stated. A leukocytosis is more likely to occur in acute infections than in chronic disorders. Blacks, who have lower granulocyte counts than whites, have a lower neutrophil count response to acute appendicitis than whites.[38] A mild infection most often is associated with no change in the leukocytes, or with a slight increase to 11,000 or 15,000 per cu.mm. In infectious or destructive processes a marked neutrophilic leukocytosis, accompanied by an increase in the younger forms, indicates a severe injury and a brisk reaction of the body's defense mechanism. A low or normal total leukocyte count associated with a marked increase in younger forms in

Table 9-2 *Causes of Neutrophilic Leukocytosis*

1. Infections: especially with pyogenic bacteria; either localized, as appendiceal abscess, or generalized, as septicemia.
2. Other disorders associated with acute inflammation or cellular necrosis: infarction, collagen disease, acute hemolysis.
3. Neoplasms: leukemia, carcinoma, lymphomas, especially with areas of tissue necrosis and widespread metastases.
4. Intoxications: drugs, chemicals; especially in poisonings with liver damage.
5. Acute hemorrhage.

the presence of infection indicates either an early stage of the infectious process or a subnormal response to a severe infection. Severe infection and extensive tissue destruction are also manifested by morphologic changes in the granulocytes such as cytoplasmic basophilia, vacuolation of the cytoplasm, and toxic granulation. Bacterial infections, particularly those due to cocci, are apt to be accompanied by an increase in the total leukocyte count and the neutrophilic granulocytes; viral infections are likely to be associated with a low or normal total leukocyte count and a relative or absolute lymphocytosis. Neoplastic disease, leukemia excepted, is usually associated with a normal leukocyte count unless the process is extensive and tissue necrosis has occurred; in this circumstance neutrophilic leukocytosis of marked degree is often present.

Neutrophilia has been defined as more than 7500 neutrophils per cu.mm. and neutropenia as less than 1500 per cu.mm. in the venous blood.[56] Both familial[126] and apparently acquired[152] chronic neutrophilic leukocytoses have been described. Both conditions appear to be benign and none of the reported individuals developed leukemia.

The most common causes of increases in neutrophilic granulocytes, lymphocytes, monocytes, and eosinophilic granulocytes are presented in Tables 9-2 to 9-5.

A decrease in the number of circulating leukocytes, which is generally due to a decrease in the granulocytes, is found in a variety of clinical conditions. The most frequent causes of neutropenia are listed in Table 9-6. Although the factors that may produce neutropenia are not as well understood as those that produce anemia, the possible mechanisms can be classified in a similar fashion: (1) diminished production; (2) increased destruction; and (3) the "loss" of leukocytes from the circulation, by sequestration in the various organs or tissues. In the majority of clinical conditions with neutropenia, diminished production appears to be the important mechanism.

Table 9-3 *Causes of Lymphocytosis*

1. Infections	(a) Acute: infectious mononucleosis, pertussis; infectious lymphocytosis; other viral and bacillary infections.
	(b) Convalescence: especially viral infections.
	(c) Chronic: tuberculosis, brucellosis, syphilis.
2. Neoplasms	Lymphocytic leukemia, lymphosarcoma.
3. Metabolic disease	Hyperthyroidism.

Table 9–4   *Causes of Monocytosis*

1. Infections	(a) Bacterial: tuberculosis, subacute bacterial endocarditis, brucellosis, typhoid fever.
	(b) Protozoal: malaria, kala-azar.
	(c) Rickettsial: Rocky Mountain spotted fever.
2. Neoplasms	Monocytic leukemia, Hodgkin's disease, reticuloendotheliosis.
3. During recovery from infections and marrow depression	Drugs; radiotherapy.
4. Other causes	Polycythemia vera; connective tissue disorder.

Diminished production may be due to a deficiency of essential substances, such as vitamin B_{12} and folic acid, or to the presence of metabolic antagonists, such as aminopterin and 6-mercaptopurine. Diminished granulocytopoiesis may also be the result of damage to the precursor cells in the marrow by irradiation, chemicals, marrow replacement, drug idiosyncrasy, and other unknown causes.

The importance of leukocyte antibodies as a mechanism responsible for the production of neutropenia is uncertain. The occurrence of nonspecific transfusion reactions characterized by chills, fever, and leukopenia associated with the presence in the recipient's blood of agglutinins against the donor leukocytes has been reported.[11] In another study it was found that leukoagglutinins were demonstrable in 38 of 350 patients with hematologic disorders. However, 64 per cent of the patients with leukoagglutinins had no leukopenia, and only one of 22 patients with leukopenia had leukoagglutinins. Ninety per cent of the patients with leukoagglutinins had received transfusions, and the likelihood of a positive test was greater after multiple transfusions. Because of this observation and the failure to demonstrate any agglutination of autologous leukocytes, it was concluded that at least the majority of leukoagglutinins are isoagglutinins.[57] A different experience is reported by Tullis, who employed a different technique.[71] He found positive tests for leukocyte antibodies in 59 of 132 sera from patients with leukopenia, and in only 11 of 102 sera from patients with hematologic and hepatic disorders without leukopenia. Antibodies were demonstrated in patients with primary agranulocytosis, primary hypersplenism, secondary hypersplenism, myelophthisic anemia, leukemia, and drug sensitivity. The antileukocyte antibody activity, which appeared to be made up of two components, decreased as clinical improvement occurred, and the granulocyte counts rose after treatment with steroids or splenectomy. Autoimmune leukopenia has been reported in lymphomas, Felty's syndrome, infectious mononucleosis, systemic lupus erythematosus, periarteritis nodosa, and chronic hepatitis.[109]

Table 9–5   *Causes of Eosinophilia*

1. Allergic reactions	Bronchial asthma, drug reactions, allergic dermatitis, hay fever, angioneurotic edema.
2. Parasitic infestation	Intestinal (hookworm, tapeworm, ascaris, Taenia echinococcus); especially with muscle invasion by trichina.
3. Skin diseases	Exfoliative dermatitis, pemphigus, dermatitis herpetiformis.
4. Neoplasms	Metastatic carcinoma, myelocytic leukemia, Hodgkin's disease.
5. Other diseases	Periarteritis nodosa, eosinophilic granuloma, Löffler's syndrome, Löffler's endocarditis, hypereosinophilic syndrome

Table 9–6   *Causes of Neutropenia*

1. Infections: acute viral (rubeola, infectious hepatitis); bacterial (brucellosis, typhoid fever); protozoal (malaria, kala-azar); and overwhelming infections (septicemia).
2. Bone marrow damage: aplastic anemia or neutropenia due to unknown cause; irradiation, toxic drugs, and chemicals (benzol, mustard drugs, antimetabolic agents); drug idiosyncrasy (amidopyrine, sulfonamides, and others).
3. Disorders associated with splenomegaly: congestive splenomegaly, diseases of the reticuloendothelial system (parasitic diseases, chronic infections, neoplasms), Felty's syndrome.
4. Other disorders: disseminated lupus erythematosus, anaphylaxis, "aleukemic" leukemia.
5. Nutritional deficiency: vitamin B_{12}, folic acid.
6. Neutropenia: chronic idiopathic, familial benign, cyclic.

Splenomegaly from diverse causes, such as portal hypertension, tuberculosis, kala-azar, and involvement by diseases of the lymphoma group, may be associated with a neutropenia that is relieved by splenectomy. Splenectomy may remove an organ of leukocyte destruction, a site of the production of leukocyte antibodies, or a "depressive influence" on the bone marrow; correction of a large plasma volume may be important in some patients.

The neutropenia that occurs in anaphylactic shock and after the administration of histamine and nicotinic acid is thought to be due to a loss of the leukocytes from the circulation as a result of sequestration in the tissues of the body, particularly the splanchnic circulation, liver, spleen, and lungs. Excessive margination of granulocytes may be an important factor in the neutropenia of Felty's syndrome.[151]

In some patients with fatal bacterial infections, particularly pneumonia or septicemia, severe leukopenia develops in the absence of medication. The authors have seen several such patients with total leukocyte counts of less than 1000 per cu.mm. and no more than a few hundred granulocytes. Examination of the bone marrow revealed an absence of cells older than myelocytes and an increased number of myelocytes and promyelocytes, nearly all of which stained poorly, contained many vacuoles, and appeared to be degenerating; no evidence of leukemia was found in the autopsies. Whether the severe leukopenia developed acutely or the infections developed in someone with unrecognized chronic neutropenia is uncertain. The occurrence of infection further reduces the level of the neutrophils in patients who have granulocytopenia, particularly when this is a consequence of treatment with cytotoxic drugs.

Leukemoid Reactions

A leukemoid reaction is defined as a leukocyte response in the peripheral blood that simulates a form of leukemia in its magnitude or in the morphology of the cells involved. High leukocyte counts (up to 100,000 per cu.mm.) involving the neutrophils occur in some patients who have bacterial pneumonia, ulcerative colitis, and other severe infections. The smear usually manifests an orderly increase in the immature cells rather than the "leukemic hiatus;" in the latter conditions young cells such as myeloblasts and promyelocytes or young myelocytes may be increased more than the older myelocytes and metamyelocytes. A leukocyte count of 15,000 to 25,000 or more occurs in patients with polycythemia vera, and may mimic leukemia after hemorrhage which has produced anemia. In myeloid metaplasia, Hodgkin's disease, and advanced carcinoma a very marked leukocytic reaction is sometimes encountered. High eosinophil counts which may exceed 75,000 sometimes occur in Hodgkin's disease, other lymphomas, periarteritis, Loeffler's syndrome, and other disorders. Leukemoid reactions characterized by the presence of blast cells and promyelocytes, often with leukopenia, sometimes occur in patients with disseminated tuberculosis and fungus infection. In such patients the marrow is not usually packed with cells, as is often the case in acute leukemia.

Leukemoid reactions characterized by a great increase in the lymphocytes are seen most often in infectious mononucleosis and whooping cough, but occasionally they occur in tuberculosis and during convalescence from various diseases.

The monocytic type of leukemoid reaction is most likely to occur in tuberculosis, Hodgkin's disease, or histiocytic lymphoma.

Usually the examination of the bone marrow, special tests of the peripheral blood such as the heterophil agglutination test, leukocyte alkaline phosphatase, and other examinations such as x-rays of the chest and possibly biopsies suffice for the recognition of the leukemoid reaction. Sometimes, however, the answer only becomes apparent after the patient has been observed for some weeks or months.

DISORDERS ASSOCIATED WITH QUANTITATIVE DEFECTS IN GRANULOCYTES

AGRANULOCYTOSIS (GRANULOCYTOPENIA)

Introduction

Although isolated cases of this disease had been seen prior to that time, it was Schultz's report in 1922 that established agranulocytosis as an entity.[103] This report described five fatal cases that occurred in women whose illness was characterized by necrotic ulceration of the oropharynx accompanied by marked leukopenia and granulocytopenia. After this description additional instances of the same disorder, which was thought to be the result of some infectious agent, were soon recognized. Soon afterward, Roberts and Kracke established that the sepsis which occurred in nearly all patients with the disorder followed the agranulocytosis and was not a causative factor.[102] A further advance in the knowledge of the disease came when Kracke noted that the disease occurred largely in Germany and the United States, particularly in middle-aged women who gave a history of treatment with drugs. He also noted that the coal tar derivatives had come into wide usage in these countries following World War I. The fact that benzene is a leukocyte depressant led him to suspect that benzene or its products should be seriously considered as the cause of the condition, a belief that was strengthened when he was able to produce the hematologic and clinical features of agranulocytosis in rabbits by the subcutaneous injection of benzene and its oxidation products.[90, 91]

Madison and Squier,[93] Plum,[100] and others[92] established that drugs containing amidopyrine were responsible for most cases of agranulocytosis at that time. In 1935 Kracke and Parker noted that, of 172 cases that had been reported in the literature, 153 had occurred after the administration of amidopyrine.[92] In the same report they listed 46 American proprietary compounds that contained amidopyrine. Because the number of reported instances of agranulocytosis was small in comparison to the large number of persons who took amidopyrine in one compound or another, an idiosyncrasy was suspected. This was demonstrated conclusively by Madison and Squier in 1934[93] and by Plum in 1935.[100] It was recognized that agranulocytosis could be caused by other drugs, and in 1938 Fitz-Hugh listed 14 drugs thought to be responsible.[88] This list was compiled at the beginning of the sulfonamide era and since then the list has lengthened steadily. More recently, nearly 90 per cent of all episodes of agranulocytosis have been attributed to the use of therapeutic drugs.[97]

Mechanism of the Disease

Agranulocytosis was considered to be an infectious disease until it was demonstrated that the primary factor was the reduction of the granulocytes in the peripheral blood, which lowered resistance and led to bacterial invasion. The drugs that were the most common offenders contained a known leukocyte depressant in the form of the benzene ring, and it was known that the marrow of some fatal cases was almost completely devoid of cells of the granulocytic series. Because of these observations it was thought that the responsible drugs or their breakdown products acted by direct suppression of granulocytopoiesis in the marrow.[90, 92, 102] The greater likelihood of a different mechanism was shown by Madison and Squier.[93] They administered small doses of amidopyrine to two patients who had recovered from agranulocytosis caused by amidopyrine; symptoms developed in two or three hours and the circulating granulocytes diminished greatly or disappeared completely by the 12th hour; recovery occurred in four days. These observations, which were confirmed by others,[85, 100] indicated that some mechanism other than depression of granulocytopoiesis must have acted to produce so profound a change in such a short time.

A possible explanation of the rapid disappearance of the circulating granulocytes in these circumstances was provided by the experiments of Moeschlin and Wagner.[95] Blood was obtained from a Pyramidon-sensitive patient three hours after the administration of 0.3 gm. Pyramidon. When 300 ml. of this blood was given to two normal recipients, severe granulocytpoenia developed in from 20 to 40 minutes and persisted for three or four hours. The same workers also demonstrated that, at the height of the Pyramidon agranulocytosis, the plasma and serum contained a substance that caused agglutination of both homologous and heterologous leukocytes. It was suggested that leukocytes agglutinated in this manner were removed from the circulation and destroyed mainly in the lungs. The existence of such a mechanism was demonstrated in guinea pigs which were injected with the antileukocyte serum produced by the injection of guinea pig leukocytes into rabbits.[94]

Although the presence of leukocyte antibodies may explain the occurrence of agranulocytosis in certain hypersensitive patients, it appears that this mechanism is not the only one concerned in all instances of agranulocytosis that occur as a result of drug idiosyncrasy. Amidopyrine appears to produce agranulocytosis by means of a true immunologic reaction that may follow the administration of only a very small amount of the drug. However, the agranulocytosis that sometimes follows the administration of sulfonamide compounds probably is the result of another mechanism, because agranulocytosis is rarely seen during therapy with these drugs unless a fairly large amount of the drug has been administered.

The role that the bone marrow plays in the production of agranulocytosis has not been clearly defined. It is probably an important one in the development of the clinical syndrome. The depletion of the granulocytic series of the marrow that is seen at autopsy, and the delay in the development of agranulocytosis until one or two weeks after the last dose of offending drug that is seen in some patients, appear to be explained best by the action of the responsible mechanism on all members of granulocytic series in the marrow. The normal and hyperplastic marrows that have been found in some patients with the disorder have been interpreted by some as evidence of partial recovery from previous damage[84, 102] and by others as a maturation arrest.[89] Still another interpretation has been offered, namely that the hyperplasia of the granulocytic elements in the marrow is an effort to compensate for the destruction of leukocytes in the circulation; according to this concept, the picture of marrow depletion develops only when the bone marrow has become exhausted.[94, 95] This interpretation appears unlikely in view of the results that have been obtained with leukapheresis experiments which indicate that the normal marrow is almost inexhaustible.

A recent study of agranulocytosis produced by phenothiazine derivatives, a group of drugs frequently implicated in this disease, showed that the dyscrasia did not occur until after more than ten days of treatment, usually after more than 20 days, and did not occur if it had not appeared within 90 days.[98] Bone marrow aplasia was demonstrated during the disease, and recovery usually occurred within two weeks of discontinuation of the drug. Studies of cultures of human bone marrow cells by means of H^3-thymidine or H^3-uridine suggested that chlorpromazine inhibited cell division in both sensitive and nonsensitive patients. Further investigation disclosed that, even in the absence of chlorpromazine, cells from sensitive patients had a lower labeling index than the "normal" group, suggesting an inherent defect, possibly of an enzyme concerned with DNA synthesis. When patients with sensitive marrows, as determined by culture studies, were given varying amounts of chlorpromazine, some developed leukopenia, but others adapted to the drug and showed no clinical evidence of toxicity.

The drugs that are most likely to produce a decrease in one or more of the types of cells in the blood because of an idiosyncrasy are listed in Table 9–7; usu-

Table 9-7   *Drugs That Sometimes Produce Hematologic Abnormalities (Classification and Estimated Risk)*

1. Anticonvulsants	methylphenylethylhydantoin – high; trimethadione – moderate.
2. Antihistaminics	phenothiazine type – moderate; ethylenediamine type – low.
3. Antimicrobial Agents	arsenobenzol – high; chloramphenicol – high; sulfonamides – moderate; thiosemicarbazone – moderate; streptomycin – low; oxytetracycline, chlortetracycline – low.
4. Antithyroid Agents	thiouracils – high; methimazole – moderate.
5. Sedatives	(2-isopropyl-4-pentenoyl) urea – high; amidopyrine – high; phenacemide – moderate; pyrithyldione – low; chlorpromazine – moderate.
6. Spasmolytics	phenothiazine – moderate; procaine amide – low.
7. Unclassified	gold preparations – high; phenylbutazone – high; nitrophenols – high; mercurial diuretics – low; quinidine – low; quinacrine hydrochloride – low; mercury, amphetamine – low.

ally the association of the drug and leukopenia is known, but a causal relationship often has not been established. Although the frequency of reactions is unknown, the following drugs can be considered "high risk;" methylphenylethylhydantoin; arsenobenzol; chloramphenicol; thiouracils; amidopyrine; gold preparations; phenylbutazone; nitrophenols. The following can be classed as "moderate risk:" trimethadione; phenothiazines; sulfonamides; methimazole; phenacemide; chlorpromazine.[96, 105] The drugs shown in Table 9–8 have been called the most common offenders.[104]

Clinical Manifestations

Agranulocytosis occurs in both sexes and may develop at any age. Prodomal symptoms such as fatigue, headache, weakness, insomnia, and restlessness usually occur. Most patients complain of a sore throat. This often progesses rapidly as chills, increasing fever, and dysphagia develop. Unless improvement occurs the temperature rises to 105° F or more, and the patient becomes mentally confused, irrational, prostrated, or stuporous.

Physical examination early in the disease may reveal nothing more than a few small areas of necrosis in the tonsillar areas. Later the areas of necrotic ulceration enlarge as edema and slight reddening of the mucous membranes develop. The cervical lymph nodes become enlarged and slightly tender, and in some patients the soft tissue of the neck becomes swollen. At times vaginal and rectal ulceration occur as the result of local infection.

Table 9-8   *The More Common Drugs Reported to Cause Agranulocytosis*

Amidopyrine	Phenylbutazone
Chloramphenicol	Propylthiouracil
Gold Salts	Sulphonamides
Phenothiazine	Methimazole (Tapazole)

Laboratory Examination

The most significant feature is the occurrence in the peripheral blood of severe leukopenia and granulocytopenia unaccompanied by anemia or thrombocytopenia. Many patients develop lymphocytopenia as well as granulocytopenia, and the total leukocyte count falls to levels as low as 100 to 2000 per cu.mm. Granulocytes often constitute less than 10 per cent of the total cells, and may be entirely absent. Those that are present often show extreme degrees of toxic granulation. Monocytes often make up an appreciable percentage of the cells, especially during recovery, and a total monocyte count of over 100 per cu.mm. is considered a sign of good prognosis.[101]

The appearance of the bone marrow varies with the stage of the disease. In most of the severe cases at the height of the disease the cells of the granulocytic series are greatly reduced or absent and the percentages of lymphocytes, plasma cells, and reticuloendothelial cells are increased. In other patients, particularly when recovery is taking place, examination of the marrow reveals hyperplasia of the granulocytic series; in such circumstances toxic granulation is evident in many of the younger cells.

In severe cases blood cultures often establish the presence of septicemia. Smears made from the ulcerated lesions or sputum often show masses of bacteria accompanied by but few cells.

Differential Diagnosis

The most important consideration in the differential diagnosis is acute leukemia. The distinction usually is not difficult because leukemia is generally associated with anemia, thrombocytopenia, and hemorrhagic manifestations, which are not a part of agranulocytosis. Examination of the bone marrow and study of smears made from the buffy coat of the peripheral blood nearly always reveal the presence of blasts and other young cells when leukemia is present. A carefully-taken history regarding recent exposure to drugs or chemical agents is often helpful.

The presence of agranulocytosis may be suspected in some patients with infectious mononucleosis who have ulcerative pharyngeal lesions and a marked reduction in the granulocytes in the peripheral blood. The degree and distribution of the adenopathy, the presence of pathologic lymphocytes in the blood smear, and the positive heterophil agglutination test usually lead to the recognition of infectious mononucleosis; in doubtful cases a few days of observation generally resolve the difficulty, because leukopenia rarely persists for more than a few days in infectious mononucleosis.

Other diseases are less likely to be confused with agranulocytosis. Sepsis is rarely responsible for a leukocyte count of less than 3000 per cu.mm. or a depression of the granulocytes to less than 30 per cent of the total. Other diseases such as those of the lymphoma group, tuberculosis, and subacute bacterial endocarditis are sometimes associated with severe leukopenia. In such patients the underlying disease is usually easily recognized because of splenomegaly or other features that lead to the correct diagnosis.

Prognosis and Treatment

Before antibiotics became available agranulocytosis was a serious disease, with a mortality rate in the well-developed cases that varied from 50 to 90 per cent. The mortality rate was nearly 100 per cent in patients whose leukocyte counts fell to less than 1000 per cu.mm. and in persons over 60 years of age. The general condition of the patient and the amount of drug that had been administered also appeared to influence the outcome.[84]

In the pre-antibiotic era many forms of treatment were employed in an effort to produce an increase in granulocytes. These included x-ray therapy, blood transfusion, injections of pentose nucleotide, leukocyte concentrates, extracts of liver or bone marrow. The early reports on each method were hopeful but subsequent experience was disappointing. The first real advance in treatment came when Dameshek and Wolfson administered sulfathiazole, a drug known to be capable of producing agranulocytosis, to two moribund patients whose disease was due to some other drug; the therapy appeared to bring the infection under control and the patients recovered.[86]

The most important aspects of treatment are the withdrawal of the offending drug and the administration of an antimicrobial agent to combat infection.

Illustrative Case

This 62-year-old white widow was in good health until six weeks prior to admission, when she developed hematuria, frequency of urination, dysuria, and suprapubic pain. A diagnosis of urinary tract infection was made and she was treated with a sulfonamide 0.5 gm. three times a day. The urinary symptoms improved and the medication was continued for about five weeks. At this time the patient complained of fatigue, lassitude, and chilliness. She was admitted to her community hospital, where she was found to have a leukocyte count of 600 per cu.mm. and a temperature of 101° F. She was treated with penicillin, transfusions, and cortisone. Four days later the leukocyte count had risen to 2000 per cu.mm., but granulocytes were still absent from the peripheral blood and she was referred for further treatment.

Physical examination. Temperature 103, pulse 84, respirations 22. There was no ulceration of the nasopharynx or vagina, and the liver, spleen, and lymph nodes were not enlarged. The remainder of the examination was non-contributory.

Laboratory examination. Blood studies on admission: Hct. 55 per cent; W.B.C. 2000 per cu.mm.; differential count (per cent), juveniles 1, bands 6, segmented 9, lymphocytes 70, monocytes 12, basophils, 2; reticulocytes 1.3 per cent; platelet count normal. Bone marrow obtained by aspiration five days after the agranulocytosis was recognized was cellular, erythropoiesis was normoblastic in type, and the megakaryocytes were normal. The cells of the granulocytic series were increased. Differential count of the marrow leukocytes (per cent): promyelocytes 0.5, myelocytes 16, juveniles 14, bands 46, segmented cells 18, lymphocytes 5, eosinophils 1. The patient was treated with penicillin, 500,000 units per day. Her temperature returned to normal by the third day and remained normal thereafter. The leukocyte count rose rapidly. On the day after admission it was 3500, the third day 10,000, the sixth day 18,000, the 14th day 21,000. One month after discharge from the hospital and about seven weeks after onset of symptoms of agranulocytosis her hematocrit was 47 per cent, hemoglobin 15 gm. per 100 ml., leukocyte count 5000 per cu.mm., platelets 230,000 per cu.mm. The differential count was normal.

Comment. This elderly patient had agranulocytosis manifested by severe leukopenia associated with normal red cell and platelet counts. The bone marrow specimen, examined after recovery had begun, appeared hyperplastic. That obtained at another hospital a week earlier was either "aplastic or dilute." The extremely low leukocyte count in this patient would have augured a poor prognosis in the days before antibiotics. On treatment with penicillin and supportive measures she made an uneventful recovery. When agranulocytosis is caused by a sulfonamide drug, which was suspected but not proved in this case, the fall in granulocytes usually does not occur until after the patient has been taking the drug for several weeks. The patient was warned against future use of the suspected drug.

NEUTROPENIA

Cyclic Neutropenia

Cyclic neutropenia is a well-established but poorly-understood entity that was first described by Leale in 1910.[136] Other reviewers have found 30 cases reported in the literature.[121, 143] This rare disorder, which may occur at any age, is characterized by the regular diminution or disappearance of the circulating neutrophilic granulocytes at approximately 21-day intervals. During the neutropenic phase fever, malaise, and oral pharyngeal ulceration usually appear and are often accompanied by arthralgia, headache, sore throat, and lymph node enlargement. Relatively minor intercurrent infections occur commonly but severe infections are unusual.

By serial bone marrow studies, Page and Good showed that the recurrent neutropenia is due to the cyclic arrest of production of the entire neutrophilic series.[143] Neither a neutropenia-producing factor nor leukoagglutinins could be demonstrated in the blood of the patient. The patient's serum exerted no demonstrable influence on the motility function of normal neutrophils. Although the influence of a hormonal factor could not be excluded, none was demonstrated. The occurrence of neutropenia bore no relationship to menstruation or to the urinary excretion of FSH or 17-ketosteroids.

Studies by Wolff, Guerry, Dale and associates on human beings and gray collie dogs with cyclic neutropenia have produced the best understanding of the disorder.[115, 116, 124, 131] The cyclic neutropenia is a reflection of a cyclic depression of hematopoiesis which involves all cell lines and occurs approximately every 21 days. Because of the short life-span of the circulating granulocytes, neutropenia with its sequellae is the most prominent clinical manifestation. Nevertheless, monocytes, lymphocytes, platelets, and reticulocytes also cycle with strict periodicity. Periodic failure of marrow production, rather than peripheral destruction, has been established as the responsible mechanism. Apparently marrow production is turned on during neutropenia and switched off after the peripheral neutrophil counts return to normal. Investigation of patients with the disorder has shown that the levels of colony stimulating factor (CSF) and erythropoietic-stimulating factor (ESF) in the urine increased during the neutropenic phase concomitant with the maximum peripheral monocytosis; the increases in ESF and CSF before the occurrence of reticulocytosis and the increase in the neutrophils suggest a negative feedback regulation system. The successful transplantation of normal marrow cells to a gray collie dog with the disease with production of normal hematopoiesis indicates that the cyclic changes occur because the hematopoietic stem cells are defective in the subjects with the disorder.[116] Conversely, successful transplantation of the marrow from a collie dog with cyclic neutropenia into an irradiated normal collie produced the disease in the recipient with cyclic rises and falls of the granulocytes, platelets, and reticulocytes. Erythropoietic peaks were noted at 11- to 12-day intervals in the donor collie and at similar intervals in the recipient after engraftment.[131]

Other observations on these subjects indicate that the marrow transit time of reticulocytes is four to five days, neutrophils nine to 11 days, and monocytes six to eight days; it was thought that monocytes arise from the same stem cell as the granulocytes but do not reside in marrow storage pool for any appreciable time. In dogs, the platelets were the first elements to increase.

Cyclic neutropenia is at times familial.[141] In a study of 20 patients with the familial disorder, the clinical course was similar to that in patients previously reported. It was noted that patients whose minimal neutrophil counts were less than 200 per cu.mm. were most severely affected; none of the "symptom-free" patients had minimal neutrophil counts of less than 500 per cu.mm.

Antibiotics are important in the treatment of infections during the neutropenic phases but their long-term prophylactic use is not recommended.

Familial Benign Chronic Neutropenia

This disorder, characterized by constant neutropenia and relatively mild recurring infections, has been reported in several generations of the same family; it is thought to be transmitted on a non-sex-linked dominant.[114] In the reported cases the total leukocyte counts were in the neighborhood of 4000 per cu.mm., but the neutrophil granulocytes were only 300 to 500 per cu.mm. The eosinophils were 300 to 700 per cu.mm.; lymphocytes and monocytes were increased in the peripheral blood and marrow. In the marrow there was a reduction in the number of cells older than myelocytes.

A defect in proliferation and differentiation presumably beyond the specific granule stage of the myelocyte has been demonstrated in vivo and vitro in two children with the congenital disorder; the presence of functioning myelocytes and eosinophils is probably important in the survival of these patients.[156]

A study of Yemenite Jews with genetic neutropenia who had absolute neutropenia (300 to 1200 granulocytes per cu.mm.) and no special tendency to infection indicated that there was no deficiency of granulocyte colony-forming cells. This disorder differs from the one discussed earlier in that the bone marrow appeared normal, having neither a lack of mature granulocytes nor degeneration of mature granulocytes; a defect in the release mechanism was suggested.[140]

Chronic Idiopathic Neutropenia

Chronic idiopathic neutropenia is a serious disorder.[137, 148] The reported patients have had moderate to severe leukopenia and severe granulocytopenia, and sometimes virtual absence of the granulocytes from the circulating blood. The severity of the disease is reflected in the paucity or lack of granulocytic cells in the areas of infection. In the bone marrow, cells of the granulocytic series are reduced and cells beyond the myelocyte or metamyelocyte stage are absent; nucleated red cells and lymphocytes predominate. Three-quarters of the reported cases have been in women more than 40 years of age. Many have died with pneumonia, septicemia, or abscess formation. Although some patients appeared to respond favorably to corticosteroids, treatment with corticosteroids, immunosuppressive agents, and splenectomy has usually been ineffective.

Other patients who appear to have had the same disease pursue a milder course and are not plagued by infections, even though the circulating granulocyte count may be zero.[113, 134] In one group of 15 patients with chronic idiopathic neutropenia, observed from one to 19 years, neutrophil counts varied between 0 and 152 per cu.mm. in the patient with the lowest counts, and between 546 and 823 per cu.mm. in the patient with the highest counts. The frequency of infection was not increased above normal and no serious diseases developed. Bone marrow examinations were made in all the patients, and in each the cellularity was normal or increased; there were normal numbers of band cells and younger forms but segmented cells were virtually absent. Treatment with corticosteroids and splenectomy did not change the blood counts.

Studies made in a patient with chronic benign neutropenia of childhood during stress and after large doses of corticosteroid led to the conclusion that the neutropenia most probably resulted from a failure to release cells from the marrow in nonstressful conditions.[87] Study of the bone marrow in patients with the disorder disclosed normocellularity or hypercellularity with granulocyte maturation to the band forms at least.

DISORDERS ASSOCIATED WITH QUALITATIVE DEFECTS IN GRANULOCYTES

The clinical syndromes associated with qualitative leukocyte abnormalities have been classified as: (1) a defect in neutrophil chemotaxis; (2) defects in the ingestion phase of phagocytosis; or (3) defects in intracellular killing of organisms.[119] A number of qualitative defects in granulocytes have been described.[144] With a better understanding of the steps involved in phagocytosis and other aspects of cellular defense and the availability of more refined techniques of study, it may be anticipated that an increasing number of disorders characterized by qualitative defects of the leukocytes will be described. Also (as has occurred in the coagulation field) recognition of these abnormalities, even though rare, may be expected to provide a better comprehension of the various processes involved in normal function.

CHRONIC GRANULOMATOUS DISEASE

Chronic granulomatous disease in childhood was reported first in 1957.[107, 135] The first six cases reported were in males. Symptoms developed within the first few years of life and the children died within two or three years. The disease is characterized by suppurative lymphadenitis, particularly in the neck and groin, eczematoid dermatitis about the eyes, nose, and mouth, pulmonary infiltrations, hepatosplenomegaly, lymphadenopathy, recurrent suppurative infections, and granuloma formation. Early observations did not reveal the nature of the disorder, but it was noted that the patients developed leukocytosis in response to infection and had normal or increased gamma globulins. Many of the infections were the result of staphylococci, and others were apparently due to *Klebsiella*, *Serratia marcescens*, and other organisms that ordinarily do not manifest great virulence. This hereditary disorder is transmitted as a sex-linked recessive, and the heterozygous state has been demonstrated in some asymptomatic mothers.[123, 129]

A better understanding of this disorder was provided by the demonstration that, although there was no defect in phagocytosis by the leukocytes, cultures disclosed that organisms phagocytized by cells from patients with the disorder survived much better than they did when exposed to normal cells.[123, 129] The defect in killing phagocytized organisms was related to a lack of release of bactericidal factors rather than to their absence because normal quantities of acid phosphatase, glucuronidase, lysozyme, and phagocytin were present in the lysosomes. A failure of lysosomes to degranulate because of lack of fusion of the lysosome with the phagocytic vacuole was postulated, but normal degranulation has been found subsequently in some patients.[46, 120] Other leukocyte abnormalities in these patients have been demonstrated, including a defect in the hexosemonophosphate shunt, defective hydrogen peroxide production after phagocytosis, and a deficiency in reducing nitroblue tetrazolium; this test has shown that mothers of some patients with chronic granulomatous disease have two populations of granulocytes, one normal and one defective.

Hydrogen peroxide is essential for normal intracellular killing of bacteria, and the defect in its production, probably the result of absence of a glucose oxidase enzyme, is the likely explanation of the failure of these cells to kill bacteria which do not themselves produce significant amounts of H_2O_2.[138] Some bacteria, such as streptococci or pneumococci, are killed by the combination of their own H_2O_2 production, peroxidase, and appropriate ions, such as chloride or iodide; other bacteria, such as *S. aureus* and *S. marcescens*, survive and multiply in cells with deficient H_2O_2 production. The importance of hydrogen peroxide was shown by the improved killing of *S. aureus* and *S. marcescens* that followed the in vitro introduction of glucose oxidase absorbed on latex particles into leukocytes of patients with chronic granulomatous disease; phagocytosis of these particles corrected an enzyme defect and promoted peroxide generation.[130] It has been reported that chronic granulomatous disease in females differs from that in males, in that, in the former, leukocyte glutathione peroxidase activity is significantly reduced.[128]

Job's syndrome, a disorder of young red-headed girls characterized by a life-long history of recurrent colds, abscesses, purulent sinusitis, ear disease, skin lesions, and pulmonary disease, first reported in 1966,[177] may be a variant of chronic granulomatous disease.[120] It appears likely that numerous other enzymatic defects, congenital or acquired, will be found with continued study.

CHEDIAK-HIGASHI SYNDROME

Chediak in 1952 and Higashi in 1954 independently reported instances of the syndrome now known as the "Chediak-Higashi Syndrome."[110, 127] This unusual disorder, apparently inherited as an autosomal recessive, is mainly a disease of childhood, but it also occurs in young adults, and a mild form (heterozygote) occurs in middle age. The most characteristic feature is the great enlargement of the granules in the leukocytes, which at times resemble Döhle bodies, and the presence of red-staining bodies in the cytoplasm of the lymphocytes (Fig. 9–2). The abnormalities which are present in nearly all the band and segmented cells appear in the myelocytes and metamyelocytes in the bone marrow as well; the granules are peroxidase positive. The large granules and inclusions that are characteristic of the cells have been shown to be giant abnormal lysosomes. An abnormality in the limiting membranes of the large lysosomes has been postulated on the basis of histochemical supravital staining.[132]

Among the clinical features of this disorder is semialbinism, which gives a peculiar grayish-brown color to the hair.[154] Upon transillumination of the globe of the eyes, a red light can be readily visualized through the pale blue irides. The optic fundi are pale and nystagmus is usually present. There is an increased incidence of pyogenic infections which may be severe and incapacitating. A tendency to excessive sweating in some patients and hyperpigmentation of the areas of skin exposed to sunlight are common. In some patients, at least terminally, lymphadenopathy, splenomegaly, and hepatomegaly develop and suggest the presence of a lymphoma.

The increased susceptibility of these patients to pyogenic infections is probably related to dysfunction of the granulocytes. The disease occurs in man, the Aleutian mink, and other animals. Studies in affected men and minks have demonstrated several defects.[111, 122, 144, 155] Chemotaxis of the granulocytes was subnormal, apparently the result of a cellular defect. Phagocytosis was normal but intracellular killing of ingested bacteria was defective, probably because of the failure of postphagocytic degranulation and delivery of the lysosomal contents to the phagocytic vacuole.

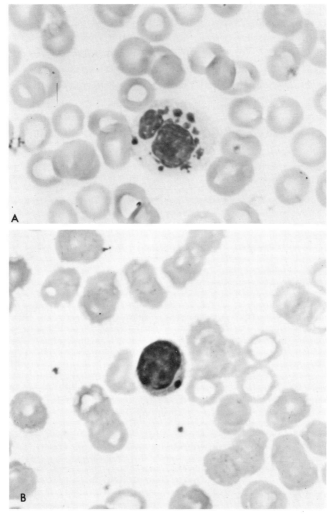

Figure 9-2   Leukocytes in Chediak-Higashi syndrome. *A,* Neutrophil. *B,* Lymphocyte.

A markedly increased rate of granulocyte turnover reflected by elevation of muramidase is the result of intramedullary cellular destruction.[108]

OTHER DISORDERS

Hereditary myeloperoxidase deficiency in neutrophils and monocytes has been associated with systemic infection with *Candida* and impaired killing of *Candida* and bacteria in vitro.[146] Recurrent infections with impaired bactericidal function occurred in a boy with morphologic abnormalities in the nuclei and granules in the granulocytes; granules were not seen with Wright-Giemsa stain, and alkaline phosphatase activity was absent.[149]

A familial disorder characterized by susceptibility to infection and deficient phagocytosis has been reported. The defect in phagocytosis was the result of dysfunction of a plasma-mediated factor (opsonin); plasma from normal persons corrected the defect, possibly by adding a labile activator of complement.[139] Defective phagocytosis and bacterial killing by neutrophils has been found in a 65-year-old man.[150]

Defective chemotaxis has been reported in a number of disorders including diabetes mellitus.[142] The occurrence of frequent prolonged infections with *Klebsiella* and *E. coli* associated with impaired neutrophil leukotaxis has been reported in a 4-year-old child.[153] The defect was due, at least in part, to an inhibitor in the patient's serum; normal serum largely restored the leukotactic function. A serum inhibitor has also been described in patients with hepatic cirrhosis.[118] Defective chemotaxis related to an intrinsic defect in the phagocytes has been reported in neutrophils[112] and monocytes.[147]

INFECTIOUS MONONUCLEOSIS
Synonym: Glandular Fever

INTRODUCTION

Credit for the first description of this disease has often been given to Pfeiffer for his report on "Drusenfieber" which appeared in 1889.[193] Pfeiffer described an illness occurring in children five to eight years of age which was characterized by fever of one to ten days' duration, sore throat, adenopathy, splenomegaly, and hepatomegaly. The disorder was considered to be an infectious and epidemic disease. Following this account, reports of unusual cases of adenitis that were associated with marked lymphocytosis and resembled lymphocytic leukemia appeared in the literature, but the report of Sprunt and Evans in 1920 provided the first clear description of the disease to which they gave the name "infectious mononucleosis."[202] They studied six young adults whose illness was characterized by fever, enlargement of the cervical, axillary, and inguinal lymph nodes, splenomegaly, and leukocytosis. The differential count was unusual because of an increase in mononuclear elements, chiefly "large lymphocytes;" even more important was the observation that "all types of pathological lymphocytes, some resembling Türk's irritation forms, were to be seen." Study of lymph nodes removed from three patients disclosed definite hyperplasia, distinct from Hodgkin's disease, tuberculosis, and lymphosarcoma, that could not be distinguished from lymphocytic leukemia. It was concluded that the cases constituted a clinical syndrome that had a good prognosis. Although at one time it was thought that the "glandular fever" reported by Pfeiffer before microscopic study of the blood was available and the "infectious mononucleosis" of Sprunt and Evans were the same disorder, more recent authors have concluded that they are not and that priority for describing the disease should go to Sprunt and Evans.[169, 174]

The abnormal mononuclear cells that had been noted were studied carefully by Downey and McKinlay in 1923.[165] Their observations have been confirmed many times but little has been added to their description. In a study of nine cases, they recognized three types of abnormal lymphocytes in the blood and concluded that there was "no danger of confusing the blood picture with leukemia, if well studied."

An important contribution that facilitated the recognition of the disease was made by Paul and Bunnell in 1932.[192] These investigators utilized a sheep cell agglutination test to study the presence of heterophil antibodies in patients with rheumatic fever, and in a group of individuals who served as controls. In their report they stated: "Quite by accident it was discovered that heterophil antibodies were present in a specimen of serum from a patient ill with infectious mononucleosis in much higher concentration than has been described in serum disease or any other clinical condition that we studied." They obtained similar results in three other patients with infectious mononucleosis and, apart from serum sickness and one other exception, failed to find high titers of heterophil antibodies in a large number of other conditions. Since that time the heterophil agglutination test has proved helpful in diagnosing infectious mononucleosis. However, an increasing number of positive tests have since been found in conditions other than infectious mononucleosis, and for this reason Davidsohn's differential test has proved valuable.[164]

A number of monographs on infectious mononucleosis are available.[159, 169, 174, 183]

ETIOLOGY AND PATHOLOGY

Ever since infectious mononucleosis was described and epidemics reported, the disease has been considered to be a viral infection, but numerous attempts to isolate an etiologic agent have failed. The degree of infectivity seemed to be low, and the incubation period seemed to vary from one day[159] to eight weeks.[173]

In recent years, the studies of Henle and others[168, 170–172] on the association of the Epstein-Barr virus (EB virus) and infectious mononucleosis have attracted considerable interest. They have demonstrated the absence of antibodies to EB virus before the development of the disease and their appearance during the acute stage of the disease; in contrast to heterophil antibodies which rise and fall rapidly, those induced by EB virus persist for years. The demonstration that a leukocyte-transforming factor which appeared to be the EB virus was present in throat-washings of patients with infectious mononucleosis for months after resolution of the clinical symptoms, and absent in normal controls, also strongly suggests that the EB virus is the causative agent in this disease.[189] The occurrence of EB virus in culture of cells obtained from patients with Burkitt's lymphoma has stimulated considerable speculation concerning the role of the EB virus in these two diseases and the relationship of the diseases to each other.[166] Three possibilities have been considered: (1) that EB virus is the etiologic agent of infectious mononucleosis; (2) that it is a superinfection; or (3) that it acts as a latent and poorly immunogenic virus which is activated nonspecifically in subsequent lymphoreticular proliferation. Furthermore, it has been suggested that the different clinical diseases, and even the lack of disease associated with EB virus, may be a reflection of the lymphoreticular response of the patient. When antibodies to the EB virus are present, the patient is immune to infectious mononucleosis; when absent, the patient is susceptible.[169] It is likely that many young children become immunized by infection with EB virus that is mild or asymptomatic; clinical infectious mononucleosis may reflect infection at an older age—in young adults particularly.

Recent studies have shown that the EB virus infects only B-lymphocytes whereas the majority of atypical lymphocytes seen in infectious mononucleosis are T-lymphocytes;[191] the relationship suggests that the T-cells are part of the immune response to the virus.

Most of the clinical manifestations of the disease are explained by the pathologic findings. The most complete report is that of Custer and Smith.[163] In a study of nine autopsies they found that the lymph nodes were usually enlarged as a result of an increase in the size of the lymph follicles. Enlargement of the lymph nodes was not invariable and in some cases the architecture of the nodes wal blurred and the follicles were inconspicuous. Splenic enlargement occurred in every instance and was associated with lymphocytic infiltration of the trabeculae and capsule. Varying degrees of lymphocytic infiltration were also found in the tissue of the central nervous system, meninges, myocardium, and in the periportal areas of the liver. In this series the bone marrows were normal or hyperplastic. In another study of 23 bone marrow biopsies granulomatous lesions were found in nine.[177]

CLINICAL MANIFESTATIONS

Infectious mononucleosis occurs in both sexes and is predominantly a disease of children and young adults. The disease has been reported in a 4-month-old infant and in an adult 70 years of age. About 80 per cent of the cases occur between the ages of 15 and 30 and the disease is rarely seen in persons over 40. At one time it was considered rare in blacks, but a more recent report indicates that the incidence in blacks is about the same as that in whites.[210]

Although infectious mononucleosis varies a great deal in its manner of onset, severity, and clinical manifestations, most patients have a similar clinical picture. They usually complain of malaise, sore throat, headache, and weakness of several days' duration. Anorexia and cough are not unusual. Fever of less than 102° F is usually present, and the pulse is generally normal or slow in proportion to the temperature. Examination of the pharynx usually reveals diffuse infection of the mucous membranes or follicular tonsillitis. Palpable enlargement of the cervical lymph nodes is usually evident when the patient is first seen, or develops within a few days. Involvement of the nodes in the cervical region, which is gen-

---

Figure 9–3 Acute leukemia.

Figure 9–4 Infectious mononucleosis.

From Heilmeyer, L., and Begemann, H.: Atlas der klinischen Hämatologie und Cytologie. Berlin-Göttingen-Heidelberg, Springer, 1955.

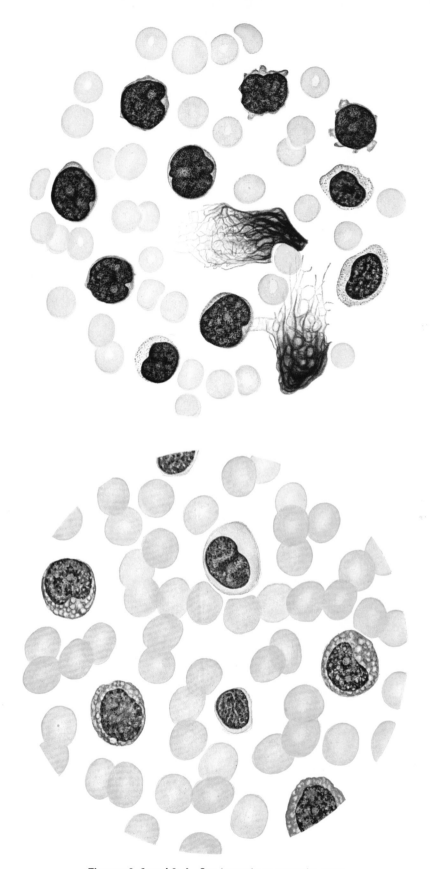

Figures 9–3 and 9–4 See legends on opposite page.

erally bilateral, is soon followed by the appearance of enlargement of the axillary and inguinal nodes. The spleen and liver are often palpable. Usually both the characteristic findings in the blood, a lymphocytosis associated with "pathologic lymphocytes" and the positive heterophil agglutination test, are present when the patient is first seen, or develop during the first week or ten days thereafter. As a rule, the fever subsides by lysis within the first or second week, and the symptoms disappear during the second or third week. Convalescence is rapid in most patients. The glandular enlargement often improves within a few days, but some residual enlargement may persist for months. In three-quarters of the patients the blood picture returns to normal in two months and the heterophil agglutination becomes negative in less than four months.

The "usual" clinical picture is not seen in a number of patients with infectious mononucleosis. Some patients are essentially asymptomatic, and the presence of the disease is manifested only by painless adenopathy and the characteristic laboratory findings. Others become acutely ill with high fever and present the appearance of a severe overwhelming infection. In still others, the clinical features are dominated by the presence of the disease in a particular organ; in such patients the presenting complaints are abdominal pain, jaundice, hematuria, or disease of the central nervous system.

The characteristic features of infectious mononucleosis are fever, glandular enlargement, faucial infection, and lymphocytosis. The incidence of symptoms and signs varies in different series.[164, 173, 175, 206, 207, 210] The extremes are shown in Table 9–9.

Skin Lesions

Various types of cutaneous eruptions occur and an incidence of 18 per cent was found in one series. The rash usually makes its appearance between the fourth and seventh days, but may appear as late as the 20th day. The commonest type is a fine macular or maculopapular rash, pink or pinkish-brown in color, that involves mainly the trunk. The rash is often virtually indistinguishable from that seen in rubella; it may consist of only eight or ten lesions, and usually appears in a single crop that lasts from three to seven days. Other types of lesions that have been seen less often are erythematous, urticarial, morbilliform, and

Table 9–9   *The Incidence of Various Symptoms and Signs in Infectious Mononucleosis as Reported by Different Authors*

SYMPTOMS	PER CENT	PHYSICAL SIGNS	PER CENT
Sore throat	50–80	Fever	70–100
Malaise	25–63	Enlarged nodes	76–100
Headache	35–67	Pharyngitis	68–82
Weakness	13–54	Splenomegaly	26–70
Anorexia	17–41	Hepatomegaly	6–37
Abdominal pain or disease	14–22	Rashes	0–18
Ocular symptoms	6–15	Jaundice	5–8
		Hematuria	1–7

vesicular. Lesions like those seen in erythema multiforme and erythema nodosum also occur.

Two independent reports appeared in 1967 showing that a rash occurred in virtually 100 per cent of patients with infectious mononucleosis who were treated with ampicillin.[190, 194] Copper-colored macules and papules appeared first on the trunk and quickly spread to involve the entire body; pruritus was almost invariably present. The rash usually appeared from seven to ten days after the patient began taking ampicillin, and cleared up a week after the drug was stopped; neither antihistaminics nor corticosteroids exerted any effect on the course. These authors noted a rash in less than 15 per cent of patients with infectious mononucleosis who received no antibacterial drugs, and in less than 20 per cent of the general population who took ampicillin. The incidence of rash in patients taking tetracycline and penicillin was about the same as that in untreated patients.

Liver Damage

Although jaundice occurs in only about 6 per cent of patients with infectious mononucleosis, it is probable that some impairment of liver function occurs in a high percentage of patients with the disease. Study of liver tissue obtained by biopsy and at autopsy indicates that the jaundice is due to a form of hepatitis and is not the result of extrahepatic obstruction from enlarged nodes.[163] The lesion consists mainly of periportal infiltration with mononuclear cells; there are minimal changes in the hepatic cells which are not accompanied by necrosis or alteration of the hepatic architecture. A good correlation between the severity of the infiltrative process and the frequency of abnormal liver function tests (BSP, SGPT, and alkaline phosphatase) has been reported.[180] A high incidence of abnormal liver function tests has been found in patients with infectious mononucleosis without jaundice. Hepatitis is a feature of nearly all cases. Although abnormal liver function tests may persist for long periods (up to 22 months in one report),[206] the prognosis for complete recovery is excellent, even in the patients with jaundice. Cirrhosis of the liver has been reported only once and this patient had an alcoholic history.[184]

Central Nervous System Involvement

Involvement of the central nervous system, first reported in 1931,[167, 178] was found in 5.5 per cent of 144 patients who were hospitalized for infectious mononucleosis.[200] Other estimates place the incidence at less than 1 per cent of all patients with infectious mononucleosis.[160] Although unusual, in some patients the nervous system involvement provides the only clinical manifestations that are recognized; in others it is the presenting or major manifestation. At least 64 cases have been reported.[202] Involvement of the central nervous system has been manifested by headache, nuchal rigidity, drowsiness, stupor, coma, paralysis, convulsions, and changes in the spinal fluid such as pleocytosis, increased protein, and increased pressure. The types of central nervous system involvement were classified by Bernstein and Wolff as follows: (1) serous meningitis; (2)

meningitis; (3) encephalitis; (4) meningoencephalitis; (5) meningitis or meningo-encephalitis with acute polyneuritis; (6) peripheral neuropathy.[160] Meningitis, encephalitis, and meningitis or meningoencephalitis with polyneuritis (Guillain-Barré syndrome) make up about three quarters of the reported cases. Cerebral involvement with diplopia, nystagmus, papilledema, or an abnormal Babinski sign occurs in some patients without associated abnormalities in the cerebrospinal fluid. When death occurs it is usually the result of respiratory paralysis. Despite a course that is frequently stormy, the prognosis is good in patients with central nervous system involvement; 85 per cent recover within a period that varies from a few days to several months after the onset of the complication.

Cardiac Involvement

The occurrence of cardiac involvement has been reviewed.[176] There is rarely any clinical evidence of cardiac involvement, but pericarditis which was diagnosed by the occurrence of chest pain, pericardial friction rub, electrocardiographic abnormalities, and changes in heart size has been reported nine times. Most of the reported cardiac abnormalities are not obvious and consist of electrocardiographic changes in the T wave, PR interval, or cardiac rhythm. Routine electrocardiograms have revealed abnormalities in from 5 to 50 per cent of patients. Postmortem studies have revealed focal interstitial infiltration of abnormal lymphocytes in the myocardium that appears to offer an explanation for the electrocardiographic findings.[163] Pericarditis has not been present in the autopsied cases. Although the electrocardiographic changes persist for months in some patients, there is little or no evidence that chronic heart disease occurs in patients with infectious mononucleosis.

Rupture of the Spleen

This is a serious complication that has been seen in at least 21 patients with infectious mononucleosis, it has a mortality rate of about 33 per cent in the reported cases and is one of the most frequent causes of death.[163] Rupture of the spleen occurs as a consequence of splenic enlargement associated with capsular infiltration and subcapsular hemorrhage. The rupture rarely occurs before the third week of the disease, but has been reported as early as the end of the second week, and as late as 30 days after onset. The presence of this complication is generally manifested by severe pain in the upper abdomen or left upper quadrant followed by circulatory collapse. In some patients the occurrence of this complication has not been recognized because the diagnosis of infectious mononucleosis had not been made prior to the rupture, and was not suspected then because the intraperitoneal hemorrhage was associated with polymorphonuclear leukocytosis.[201] Although rupture of the spleen in infectious mononucleosis is usually termed "spontaneous," the importance of slight trauma associated with a trivial blow or the performance of the physical examination has been emphasized.

Hematologic Complications

The most important hematologic complications that occur in infectious mononucleosis are hemolytic anemia and thrombocytopenic purpura. Both complications are rare but each has been reported at least 16 times.[202] In the reported cases the hemoglobin levels have ranged from 4.3 to 9.8 gm. per 100 ml., the reticulocyte count from 7.0 to 37.5 per cent, and the level of indirect-reacting bilirubin in the serum from 1.6 to 6.0 mg. per 100 ml.[208] The antiglobulin (Coombs) test has been positive in most of the patients with hemolytic anemia when it has been performed, which suggests that the hyperhemolysis is due to autoimmune antibodies. Normally the i antigen disappears from the red cell in postnatal life and is replaced by the I antigen. In infectious mononucleosis the i antigen appears to be unmasked, and antibodies against the i antigen have been found in 20 to 80 per cent of patients; high titers are found in some but not all of the patients who develop hemolytic anemia. Both the anemia and the thrombocytopenia disappear spontaneously or with appropriate treatment, and no deaths have been reported from these complications. Thrombocytopenia (which is not rare, unlike clinical purpura) may persist for six months or more, but at least partial recovery usually occurs in from two to four weeks.

Hematuria

Hematuria occurs in from 1 to 7 per cent of patients and may be the presenting complaint. It presumably results from lymphocytic infiltration in the kidney. Chronic renal disease secondary to infectious mononucleosis has not been reported.

LABORATORY MANIFESTATIONS

The most characteristic abnormalities in the peripheral blood in infectious mononucleosis are leukocytosis, absolute lymphocytosis, and the presence of abnormal lymphocytes. Leukocyte counts of 3000 per cu.mm. or less may occur early in the disease, but the total count is usually elevated by the second week. Counts over 40,000 per cu.mm. are rare. The most constant feature in infectious mononucleosis is the presence of the "pathologic lymphocytes" first described by Sprunt and Evans[204] and classified into three types of Downey and McKinlay.[165] The type I cell is a highly differentiated mature lymphocyte with a nucleus that has a cloudy appearance owing to the presence of a coarse network of chromatin strands or masses that is not sharply separated from the parachromatin. The nucleus is often indented. The cytoplasm is very basophilic and somewhat mottled in appearance. The type II cell has a nucleus with a course chromatin structure somewhat similar to that of the plasma cell. The cytoplasm is less basophilic than the type I cell and contains fewer vacuoles. The type III cell, which more closely resembles leukemic cells, has a less differentiated nucleus that contains nucleoli. In Downey and McKinlay's report the type III cells were un-

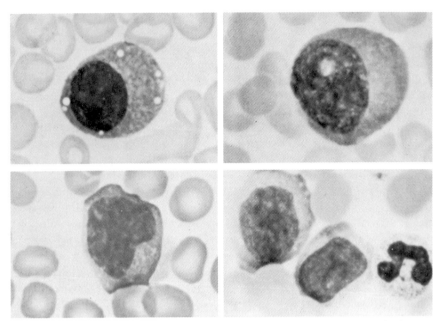

Figure 9-5 Various forms of pathologic lymphocytes seen in patients with infectious mononucleosis.

common, being seen in small numbers in only one of nine cases; the types I and II cells were numerous in all nine cases that were studied.

Other abnormalities, such as nuclear indentation, cytoplasmic vacuolation, and nuclear fenestration, may be seen in lymphocytes of all sizes. In patients who are diagnosed as having infectious mononucleosis, mononuclear cells almost invariably constitute over 50 per cent of the leukocytes at some stage of the disease, and counts as high as 96 per cent have been observed. Abnormal lymphocytes probably occur in all patients with infectious mononucleosis, but are not pathognomonic of the disease. Apparently identical cells, for which the name "virocyte" has been suggested, have been observed in the following conditions: infectious hepatitis, virus pneumonia, herpetic infections, rubella, rubeola, roseola infantum, undulant fever, rickettsialpox, and allergic states. In these disorders the percentage of abnormal lymphocytes is generally less than in infectious mononucleosis, and elevated total leukocyte counts are unusual. Although absolute lymphocytosis nearly always occurs in infectious mononucleosis, it is not a constant finding. An increase in polymorphonuclear cells sometimes occurs in the prodromal phase and early in the disease.

Eosinophilia, which is more likely to develop during convalescence, has been found in 14 per cent of one series[198] and in 10 per cent of another.[210] The eosinophils are usually less than 15 per cent but counts as high as 21 per cent occur. Except in rare instances complicated by hemolytic anemia and thrombocytopenia, the hemoglobin, red cell count, and platelet counts are normal.

Although the heterophil agglutination (Paul-Bunnell) test is nonspecific, it is a very helpful procedure in the diagnosis of infectious mononucleosis.[192] Titers of 1:56,[198] 1:160,[163] and 1:224[164] have been considered confirmatory of infectious mononucleosis if the clinical and hematologic findings are suggestive of the disease. The differential adsorption test of Davidsohn is more specific because agglutinins for sheep cells sometimes occur in normal persons and in patients with serum sickness and other diseases.[164] Davidsohn found that the heterophil antibodies in infectious mononucleosis are not completely removed from the serum by adsorption with guinea pig kidney, but are removed completely when adsorbed with beef red cells. The heterophil antibodies found in normal individuals and in patients with serum sickness and other diseases are different in that they are removed from the serum when adsorbed with guinea pig kidney. The test is useful in excluding patients with high titers that are not due to infectious mononucleosis and in establishing the diagnosis of infectious mononucleosis in patients with low titers. The test has been particularly helpful in patients with monocytic leukemia and acute leukemia; titers as high as 1:896 have been seen in these diseases, but they could be distinguished from infectious mononucleosis by the guinea pig absorption test.[161, 203] The incidence of positive heterophil agglutination tests in infectious mononucleosis has been reported to be from 50 per cent to 100 per cent. The frequency of positive tests depends on the criteria used for establishing the diagnosis of infectious mononucleosis, the stage of the disease, and the number of the tests performed. The test is usually positive when the patient is first seen, but the time of development of a positive test varies from 1 to 89 days.[175] In the vast majority of patients the test will be positive, if at all, in the first two weeks of the disease. The heterophil agglutination test may remain positive from nine days to 63 weeks,[175] but generally it becomes negative in from two to four months.[159] In one series the test became negative in 75 per cent of the patients within four months.[175]

The thymol turbidity, BSP excretion, and cephalin flocculation tests and the serum alkaline phosphatase level have been found to be abnormal in a high percentage of patients with infectious mononucleosis. A significant increase in α 2-globulin has been reported in 81 of 85 patients in one series.[197] There was no correlation with the heterophil antibody level, liver function, or lymphocytosis. The elevated level was readily reversed by corticosteroid therapy, and it was inferred that the hypergammaglobulinemia was a manifestation of a response of the reticuloendothelial system, a delayed hypersensitivity reaction, possibly to a virus.

The occurrence of false positive Wassermann and Kahn tests in infectious mononucleosis is well known. Incidences of 2 per cent,[206] 3 per cent,[210] 10 per cent,[173] and 18 per cent,[159] have been reported. The test usually becomes positive during the second week and reverts to negative by the eighth week, but the duration of positivity varies from a few days to more than three months. The finding of a positive routine serologic test for syphilis in a young adult may be the first intimation that the patient may have infectious mononucleosis.

False positive agglutination tests for Br. melitensis, S. typhosa, S. paratyphii A and B, and Proteus X-19 have been reported.[181] In some patients several agglutination tests may be positive at the same time. When repeated titrations have been done, it has been noted that the titers rose abruptly, sometimes to as high as 1:1280, but fell quickly.

Transient urinary abnormalities in the form of red blood cells, white blood cells, albuminuria, and casts have been reported in 3 per cent and 6 per cent of patients.[202]

DIAGNOSIS

The possibility of infectious mononucleosis is suggested by the occurrence of sore throat, fever, enlarged lymph nodes, or lymphocytosis in children and young adults. The presence of more than 50 per cent lymphocytes and more than 10 per cent pathologic lymphocytes is even stronger evidence. It is probable that almost all physicians now require some serologic confirmation before making a diagnosis of infectious mononucleosis, even if the clinical and hematologic picture seems characteristic, because the cytomegalic virus and probably others can produce a clinical picture similar to that seen in this disease.

The Monospot test developed by Lee and associates is the slide test most often used as a screening test for infectious mononucleosis.[182] In the test, either finely-ground guinea pig kidney or beef red cell stroma is added to serum on the slide, followed by a drop of horse red cells. The test is positive if agglutination occurs in the presence of the guinea pig kidney, but not with the beef red cell stroma; the guinea pig kidney absorbs Forssman antibody but not the heterophile antibody. The heterophile agglutination test, which in a sense is a presumptive test, is considered adequate to establish the diagnosis if the titer is 1:224 or higher and the clinical picture and hematologic findings suggest the disease. It has been recommended that the differential adsorption test be used if the titer is less than 1:224 and the findings suggest infectious mononucleosis, and also in circumstances when the titer is over 1:224 but is associated with no evidence of the disease.[164] If the titer is reduced more than 75 per cent by adsorption with guinea pig kidney, the antibody is probably not of the infectious mononucleosis type.

The diagnosis of infectious mononucleosis may be difficult if the patient is seen before the characteristic hematologic and serologic findings appear, especially when the clinical features are those more often associated with other diseases. When jaundice, hematuria, a septic type of fever, adenopathy, or evidence of central nervous system involvement is the presenting complaint, the diagnosis may not be considered in sporadic cases when the patient is first seen. When the diagnosis of infectious mononucleosis is considered, repeated examination of the peripheral blood, repeated agglutination tests, and a period of observation may be necessary before the question can be settled.

The "postperfusion syndrome" closely resembles infectious mononucleosis.[195] This syndrome occurs from one to eight weeks (usually two to five weeks) after open-heart surgery, and lasts from one to four weeks. It is characterized by fever (100° to 103° F), splenomegaly, and abnormal lymphocytes in the circulating blood; liver function tests are often abnormal and at times the liver is enlarged. The total leukocyte count is almost invariably normal; lymphocytes constitute 21 to 79 per cent of the cells and atypical cells have ranged from 3 to 60 per cent. In one series of 11 patients who had heterophil tests, three were negative; five had a titer of 1:7 or 1:14, two a titer of 1:28, and one a titer of 1:112. Both EB virus and cytomegalic virus infection have been incriminated, apparently from exposure to blood containing the live viruses.

A clinical illness similar to infectious mononucleosis has been reported in patients with proved cytomegalovirus infection. It was characterized by mild sore throat, cervical adenopathy in most, and splenomegaly in a minority. Myalgia, fever, and chills were present. The leukocyte count was mildly elevated, and lymphocytes constituted 60 to 75 per cent of the total; 15 to 34 per cent of the lymphocytes were abnormal forms. The heterophile agglutination test was negative in all. Most of the reported cases have been in young women but it has also occurred in men; the disease is not confined to patients who have had open-heart surgery. Thus, a patient with the clinical and peripheral blood picture of infectious mononucleosis and a negative heterophile agglutination test should be studied for cytomegalovirus disease with throat culture and urine culture, as well as for EB virus.[196]

The report of a patient with infectious mononucleosis who had a mass in the anterior mediastinum that regressed spontaneously is yet another example of the protean manifestations of this disease, and the difficulty one may encounter in making a diagnosis.[209] The rare occurrence of a positive heterophil test in patients with lymphoma is sometimes puzzling but of uncertain significance, especially in view of the recent studies on Burkitt's tumor. Although it usually is not difficult to distinguish between infectious mononucleosis and Hodgkin's disease, the occurrence of "Reed-Sternberg-like" cells in biopsy material from the tonsil and cervical lymph nodes in some patients with proven infectious mononucleosis may cause difficulty.[157, 187]

COURSE AND PROGNOSIS

Infectious mononucleosis usually runs an acute course characterized by fever for ten days or less, followed by prompt recovery. A recrudescence of fever and symptoms is not unusual after the temperature has returned to normal for several days. In some patients the manifestations of the disease are so mild that its presence is recognized only by the laboratory tests. In other patients malaise and weakness may persist for months before complete recovery occurs. Nearly all patients recover completely, but deaths have occurred. In one report of 30 fatal cases, the causes of death were as follows: spontaneous splenic rupture, 13; Guillain-Barré syndrome, 6; hemorrhage from nasopharyngeal or gastrointestinal tract, 4; miscellaneous, mainly secondary infections, 7.[186] True recurrences of the disease, with serologic confirmation of the diagnosis, must be extremely rare if they occur at all.

TREATMENT

The treatment of infectious mononucleosis is largely symptomatic and supportive. Parenteral fluids may be necessary if the throat is much involved. Prolonged bed rest is not necessary in patients with abnormal liver function tests or abnormal electrocardiograms. Treatment with sulfonamides, penicillin, chlortetracycline, and chloramphenicol has not been found to shorten significantly the duration of symptoms or fever, or to reduce the incidence of complications.

In certain circumstances corticosteroid drugs appear to be of benefit.[199] A favorable effect with the corticosteroid drugs in those patients (approximately 10 per cent) who had the severe form of disease has been reported.[158] Shortening of the period of fever together with striking improvement in the pharyngeal inflammation, malaise, lethargy, and anorexia was noted; no adverse effect from the treatment was observed.

Illustrative Case

A 17-year-old white male student was in excellent health until two weeks prior to admission, when he first noticed malaise. Ten days prior to admission transient chilly sensations occurred. Five days before admission severe headache appeared, and was accompanied by sore throat and enlargement of the cervical lymph nodes. The sore throat became progressively worse and on the day of admission the patient was unable to swallow liquids.

Physical examination. The oral temperature on admission was 100° F. The tonsillar areas were covered with a white, thick, pseudomembranous type of exudate. There was bilateral enlargement of the cervical and axillary lymph nodes which measured 1 to 3 cm. in diameter. A soft spleen edge was palpable 1 cm. below the left costal margin. The neurologic examination and the remainder of the routine examination were within normal limits.

Laboratory examination. Admission blood studies: Hct. 50 per cent; W.B.C. 14,000 per cu.mm., differential count (per cent), granulocytes 28, lymphocytes 64, monocytes 8. Many of the lymphocytes appeared abnormal: they were large and had an opaque basophilic cytoplasm. The nuclei of many of the smaller cells were indented or fenestrated. Other examinations showed the following: serum bilirubin level 0.7 mg. per 100 ml.; alkaline phosphatase 6.3 (B.U.); thymol turbidity 9-6 units; cephalin flocculation 4 plus in 48 hours; spinal fluid normal. The heterophil agglutination test was positive in dilutions of 1:3564 before adsorption, and positive in a dilution of 1:792 after differential adsorption.

A diagnosis of infectious mononucleosis was made. The patient responded well to symptomatic measures and was essentially asymptomatic when discharged from the hospital eight days later. One month after discharge nodes that measured 1 × 1 cm. were still palpable in the cervical area and in the left axilla. The leukocyte count was 7000 per cu. mm., and the differential count was (per cent): bands 1, segmented 47, lymphocytes 40, monocytes 9, eosinophils 2, basophils 1. A few atypical lymphocytes persisted. The heterophil test was still positive in dilutions of 1:24 after adsorption.

Comment. This patient illustrates most of the typical features of infectious mononucleosis. The majority of patients are young adults who complain of fever, malaise, sore throat, and cervical adenopathy. As often happens, the heterophil agglutination test was positive and the blood smear was typical of infectious mononucleosis when the patient was first seen. The patient is typical of many with the disease in that he had neither clinical jaundice nor elevation of the serum bilirubin, but did exhibit evidence of liver dysfunction in the various tests. Because of his severe headache the complication of a meningoencephalitis was considered, but was discarded when the neurologic examination and cerebrospinal fluid proved to be normal.

References

LEUKOCYTES AND LEUKOPOIESIS

1. Alper, C. A., Abramson, N., Johnston, R. B., Jr., Jandl, J. H., and Rosen, F. S.: Increased susceptibility to infection associated with abnormalities of complement-mediated functions and of the third component of complement (C3). N. Engl. J. Med., 282:349, 1970.
2. Athens, J. W., Mauer, A. M., Raab, S. O., Haab, O. P., and Cartwright, G. E.: Studies of granulocytic kinetics. J. Clin. Invest., 39:969, 1960.
3. Athens, J. W., Raab, S. O., Haab, O. P., Boggs, D. R., Ashenbrucker, H., Cartwright, G. E., and Wintrobe, M. M.: Leukokinetic studies. X. Blood granulocyte kinetics in chronic myelocytic leukemia. J. Clin. Invest., 44:765, 1965.
4. Atkinson, J. P., and Frank, M. M.: Complement-independent clearance of IgG-sensitized erythrocytes: inhibition by cortisone. Blood, 44:629, 1974.
5. Becker, A. J., McCulloch, E. A., and Till, J. E.: Cytological demonstration of the clonal nature of spleen colonies derived from transplanted mouse marrow cells. Nature, 197:452, 1963.
6. Bierman, H. R., Kelly, K. H., and Cordes, F. L.: The sequestration and visceral circulation of leukocytes in man. Ann. N.Y. Acad. Sci., 59:850, 1955.
7. Bloom, B. R., and Bennett, B.: Macrophages and delayed-type hypersensitivity. Semin. Hematol., 7:215, 1970.
8. Boggs, D. R.: The kinetics of neutrophilic leukocytes in health and disease. Semin. Hematol., 4:359, 1967.
9. Boggs, D. R., Athens, J. W., Cartwright, G. E., and Wintrobe, M. M.: Leukokinetic studies. IX. Experimental evaluation of a model of granulopoiesis. J. Clin. Invest., 44:643, 1965.
10. Bradley, T. R., and Metcalf, D.: The growth of mouse bone marrow cells in vitro. Aust. J. Exp. Biol. Med. Sci., 44:287, 1966.
11. Brittingham, T. E., and Chaplin, H., Jr.: Sensitivity to buffy coat a cause of "nonspecific" transfusion reactions. J. Clin. Invest., 36:877, 1957.
12. Broun, G. O., Herbig, F. K., and Hamilton, J. R.: Leukopenia in Negroes. N. Engl. J. Med., 275:1410, 1966.
13. Broun, G. O., Herbig, F. K., and Hamilton, J. R.: Leukopenia in Negroes. N. Engl. J. Med., 277:899, 1967.
14. Cline, M. J., Craddock, C. G., Gale, R. P., Golde, D. W., and Lehrer, R. I.: Granulocytes in human disease. Ann. Intern. Med., 81:801, 1974.
15. Cohen, S. G.: The eosinophil and eosinophilia. N. Engl. J. Med., 290:457, 1974.
16. Craddock, C. G.: The production, utilization and destruction of white blood cells. Progr. Hematol., 3:92, 1962.
17. Craddock, C. G., Jr., Perry, S., and Lawrence, J. S.: The dynamics of leukopoiesis and leukocytosis, as studied by leukopheresis and isotopic techniques. J. Clin. Invest., 35:285, 1956.
18. Dicke, K. A., van Noord, M. J., Maat, B., Shaefer, V. W., and van Bekkum, D. W.: Identification of cells in primate bone marrow resembling the hematopoietic stem cell in the mouse. Blood, 42:195, 1973.
19. Dilworth, J. A., Hendley, J. O., and Mandell, G. L.: Attachment and ingestion of gonococci by human neutrophils. Infection and Immunity, 11:512, 1975.
20. Donohue, D. M., Reiff, R. H., Hanson, M. C., Betson, Y., and Finch, C. A.: Quantitative measurements of erythrocytic and granulocytic cells of the marrow and blood. J. Clin. Invest., 37:1571, 1958.
21. Dougherty, T. F., and White, A.: Influence of hormones on lymphoid tissue structure and function. The role of the pituitary adrenotrophic hormone in the regulation of the lymphocytes and other cellular elements of the blood. Endocrinology, 35:1, 1944.
22. Ehrlich, P., and Lazarus, A.: Anemia. Rebman, Ltd., London, 1910.
23. Fernex, M.: The Mast Cell System. Wm. Wilkins Co., Baltimore, USA, 1968.
24. Fishman, M., Hammerstram, R. A., and Bond, V. P.: In vitro transfer of macrophage RNA to lymph node cells. Nature, 198:549, 1963.
25. Ford, W. L., and Gowans, J. L.: The traffic of lymphocytes. Semin. Hematol., 6:67, 1969.
26. Friedman, H. P., Stavitsky, A. B., and Solomon, J. M.: Induction in vitro of antibodies to phage T2: antigens in the RNA extract employed. Science, 149:1106, 1965.
27. Garrey, W. E., and Bryan, W. R.: Variations in white blood cell counts. Physiol. Rev., 15:597, 1935.
28. Golde, D. W., and Cline, M. J.: Identification of the colony stimulating cell in human peripheral blood. J. Clin. Invest., 51:2981, 1972.
29. Golde, D. W., and Cline, M. J.: Regulation of granulopoiesis. N. Engl. J. Med., 29:1388, 1974.

30. Gordon, A. S.: Some aspects of hormonal influences upon the leukocytes. Ann. N.Y. Acad. Sci., 59:907, 1955.
31. Gordon, A. S., Handler, E. S., Siegel, C. D., Dornfest, B. S., and Lo Bue, J.: Plasma factors influencing leukocyte release in rats. Ann. N.Y. Acad. Sci., 113:766, 1964.
32. Gowans, J. L.: Life-history of lymphocytes. Br. Med. Bull., 15:50, 1959.
33. Hays, R. C., and Mandell, G. L.: pO₂ pH, and redox potential of experimental abscesses (38275). Proc. Soc. Exp. Biol. Med., 147:29, 1974.
34. Hewson, W.: The Works of William Hewson. Printed for the Sydenham Society. London, 1846.
35. Hirsch, J. G.: Cinemicrophotographic observations on granule lysis in polymorphonuclear leukocyte during phagocytosis. J. Exp. Med., 116:827, 1962.
36. Hirsch, J. G., and Cohn, Z. A.: Degranulation of polymorphonuclear leukocytes following phagocytosis of microorganisms. J. Exp. Med., 112:1005, 1960.
37. Huber, H., Polley, M. J., Linscott, W. D., Fudenberg, H. H., and Muller-Eberhard, H. J.: Human monocyte: distinct receptor sites for the third component of complement and for immunoglobulin G. Science, 162:1281, 1968.
38. Hyman, P., and Westring, D. W.: Leukocytosis in acute appendicitis. J.A.M.A.,229:1630, 1974.
39. Ishizaka, T., Tomioka, H., and Isizaka, K.: Degranulation of human basophil leukocytes by anti IgE antibody. J. Immunol., 106:705, 1971.
40. Kindred, J. E.: A quantitative study of the hemopoietic organs of young adult albino rats. Am. J. Anat., 71:207, 1942.
41. Klebanoff, S. J.: Antimicrobial mechanisms in neutrophilic polymorphonuclear leukocytes. Semin. Hematol., 12:117, 1975.
42. Kuvin, S. F., and Brecher, G.: Differential neutrophil counts in pregnancy. N. Engl. J. Med., 266:877, 1962.
43. Mackaness, G. B.: The monocyte in cellular immunity. Semin. Hematol., 7:172, 1970.
44. Mahmoud, A. A. F., Kellermeyer, R. W., and Warren, K. S.: Production of monospecific rabbit antihuman eosinophil serums and demonstration of blocking phenomenon. N. Engl. J. Med., 290:417, 1974.
45. Mandell, G.: Catalase, superoxide dismutase, and virulence of Staphylococcus aureus. J. Clin. Invest., 55:561, 1975.
46. Mandell, G. L., and Hook, E. W.: Leukocyte function in chronic granulomatous disease of childhood. Am. J. Med., 47:473, 1969.
47. McCredie, K. B., Hersh, E. M., and Freireich, E. J.: Cells capable of colony formation in the peripheral blood of man. Science, 171:293, 1971.
48. Meuret, G., Bammert, J., and Hoffman, G.: Kinetics of human monocytopoiesis. Blood, 44: 801, 1974.
49. Milhorat, A. T., Small, S. M., and Diethelm, O.: Leukocytosis during various emotional states. Arch. Neurol. Psychiatr., 47:779, 1942.
50. Morley, A., and Stohlman, F., Jr: Studies on the regulation of granulopoiesis. I. The response to neutropenia. Blood, 35:312, 1970.
51. Muchmore, H. G., Blackburn, A. B., Shurley, J. T., Pierce, C. M., and McKown, B. A.: Neutropenia in healthy men at the South Polar Plateau. Arch. Intern. Med., 125:646, 1970.
52. Nelson, D. S.: In Neuberger, A., and Tatum, F. I. (eds.): Frontiers Biology Macrophages and Immunity, Vol. 2. John Wiley and Sons, Inc., New York, 1969.
53. Nelson, D. S., and Boyden, S. V.: Macrophage cytophilic antibodies and delayed hypersensitivity. Br. Med. Bull., 23:15, 1967.
54. North. R. J.: Endocytosis. Semin. Hematol., 7:161, 1970.
55. Osgood, E. E.: Number and distribution of human hemic cells. Blood, 9:1141, 1954.
56. Osgood, E. E., Brownlee, I. E., Osgood, M. W., Ellis, D. M., and Cohen, W.: Total differential and absolute leukocyte counts and sedimentation rates. Arch. Intern. Med., 64:105, 1939.
57. Payne, Rose: Leukocyte agglutinins in human sera. Arch. Intern. Med., 99:587, 1957.
58. Perry, S., Goodwin, H. A., and Zimmerman, T. S.: Physiology of the granulocyte. J.A.M.A., 203:937, 1025, 1968.
59. Perry, S., Weinstein, I. M., Craddock, C. G., Jr., and Lawrence, J. S.: The combined use of typhoid vaccine and P³² labeling to assess myelopoiesis. Blood, 12:549, 1957.
60. Pluznik, D. H., and Sachs, L.: The cloning of normal "mast" cells in tissue culture. J. Cell Physiol., 66:319, 1965.
61. Quittner, H. N., Wald, N., Sussman, L. N., and Antopol, W.: The effect of massive doses of cortisone on the peripheral blood and bone marrow of the mouse. Blood, 6:513, 1951.
62. Robinson, W. A., and Mangalik, A.: The kinetics and regulation of granulopoiesis. Semin. Hematol., 12:7, 1975.

63. Robinson, W. A., and Pike, B. L.: Leukopoietic activity in human urine. N. Engl. J. Med., *282*: 1291, 1970.

64. Rothstein, G.: The regulation of granulocyte production. N. Engl. J. Med., *286*:262, 1972.

65. Rytomaa, T.: Role of chalone in granulopoiesis. Br. J. Haematol., *24*:141, 1973.

66. Schoenberg, M. D., Mumaw, V. R., Moore, R. D., and Weisberger, A. S.: Cytoplasmic interaction between macrophages and lymphocytic cells in antibody synthesis. Science, *143*: 964, 1964.

67. Schilling, V.: The Blood Picture. C. V. Mosby Co., St. Louis, 1929.

68. Stossel, T. P.: Phagocytosis. N. Engl. J. Med., *290*:717, 774, 833, 1974.

69. Sturgis, C. C., and Bethell, F. H.: Quantitative and qualitative variations in normal leukocytes. Physiol. Rev., *23*:279, 1943.

70. Till, J. E., and McCulloch, E. A.: A direct measurement of the radiation sensitivity of normal mouse bone marrow cells. Radiat. Res., *14*:213, 1961.

71. Tullis, J. L.: Prevalence, nature and identification of leukocyte antibodies. N. Engl. J. Med., *258*:569, 1958.

72. vanBekkum, D. W., van Noord, M. J., and Dicks, K. A.: Attempts at identification of hemapoietic stem cell in mouse. Blood, *38*:347, 1971.

73. Van Furth, R.: Origins and kinetics of monocytes and macrophages. Semin. Hematol., *7*:125, 1970.

74. Van Furth, R., and Cohn, Z. A.: The origin and kinetics of mononuclear phagocytes. J. Exp. Med., *128*:415, 1968.

75. Volkman, A., and Gowans, J. L.: The origin of macrophages from bone marrow in the rat. Br. J. Exp. Pathol., *46*:62, 1965.

76. Wasserman, S. I., Goetzl, E. J., Ellman, L., and Austin, K. F.: Tumor-associated eosinophilotactic factor. N. Engl. J. Med., *290*:420, 1974.

77. Wintrobe, M. M.: Clinical Hematology. 6th Ed. Lea & Febiger, Philadelphia, 1967.

78. Wolf-Jurgensen, P.: The basophilic leukocyte. Ser. Haematol., 1, *4*:45, 1968.

79. Wood, W. B., Jr., and Smith, M. R.: The nature and biological significance of the capsular slime layer of pneumococcus Type III. Tr. Assoc. Am. Physicians, *62*:90, 1949.

80. Wright, C. S., and Dodd, M. C.: Phagocytosis. Ann. N.Y. Acad. Sci., *59*:945, 1955.

81. Wu, A. M., Till, J. E., Siminovitch, L., and McCulloch, E. A.: A cytological study of the capacity for differentiation of normal hemopoietic colony-forming cells. J. Cell. Physiol., *69*:177, 1967.

82. Yoffey, J. M.: The quantitative study of the leukocytes. Ann. N.Y. Acad. Sci., *59*:928, 1955.

83. Zarafonetis, C., Harmon, D. R., and Clark, P. F.: The influence of temperature upon opsonization and phagocytosis. J. Bacteriol., *53*:343, 1947.

AGRANULOCYTOSIS

84. Dameshek, W.: Leukopenia and Agranulocytosis. Oxford University Press, New York, 1944.

85. Dameshek, W., and Colmes, A.: The effect of drugs in the production of agranulocytosis with particular reference to amidopyrine hypersensitivity. J. Clin. Invest., *15*:85, 1936.

86. Dameshek, W., and Wolfson, L. E.: A preliminary report on the treatment of agranulocytosis with sulfathiazole. Am. J. Med. Sci., *203*:819, 1942.

87. Deinard, A. S., and Page, A. R.: A study of steroid-induced granulocytosis in a patient with chronic benign neutropenia of childhood. Br. J. Haematol., *28*:333, 1974.

88. Fitz-Hugh, T., Jr.: Sensitivity reactions of the blood and bone marrow to certain drugs. J.A.M.A., *111*:1643, 1938.

89. Fitz-Hugh, T., Jr., and Krumbhaar, E. B.: Myeloid cell hyperplasia of the bone marrow in agranulocytic angina. Am. J. Med. Sci., *183*:104, 1932.

90. Kracke, R. R.: Recurrent agranulocytosis: report of an unusual case. Am. J. Clin. Pathol., *1*:385, 1931.

91. Kracke, R. R.: The experimental production of agranulocytosis. Am. J. Clin. Pathol., *2*:11, 1932.

92. Kracke, R. R., and Parker, F. P.: The relationship of drug therapy to agranulocytosis. J.A.M.A., *105*:960, 1935.

93. Madison, F. W., and Squier, T. L.: The etiology of primary granulocytopenia (agranulocytic angina). J.A.M.A., *102*:755, 1934.

94. Moeschlin, S., Meyer, H., Israels, L. G., and Tarr-Gloor, E.: Experimental agranulocytosis. Its production through leukocytic agglutination by antileukocytic serum. Acta Haematol., *11*:73, 1954.

95. Moeschlin, S., and Wagner, K.: Agranulocytosis due to the occurrence of leukocyte-agglutinins (Pyramidon and cold agglutinins). Acta Haematol., 8:29, 1952.
96. Osgood, E. E.: Hypoplastic anemias and related syndromes caused by drug idiosyncrasy. J.A.M.A., 152:816, 1953.
97. Palva, I. P., and Mustalo, O. O.: Drug agranulocytosis with special reference to aminophenazone. Acta Med. Scand., 187:109, 1970.
98. Pisciotta, A. V.: Agranulocytosis induced by certain phenothiazine derivatives. J.A.M.A., 203: 1862, 1969.
99. Pisciotta, A. V.: Immune and toxic mechanisms in drug-induced agranulocytosis. Semin. Hematol., 10:279, 1973.
100. Plum, P.: Agranulocytosis due to amidopyrine. An experimental and clinical study of seven new cases. Lancet, 1:14, 1935.
101. Reznikoff, P.: The etiologic importance of fatigue and the prognostic significance of monocytosis in neutropenia (agranulocytosis). Am. J. Med. Sci., 195:627, 1938.
102. Roberts, S. R., and Kracke, R. R.: Agranulocytosis: report of a case. J.A.M.A., 95:780, 1930.
103. Schultz, W.: Über eigenartige Halserkrankungen (a) Monozytenangina; (b) Gangränezierende Prozesse und Defekt des Granulozytensystems. Dtsch. Med. Wochenschr., 48: 1495, 1922.
104. Stohlman, F., Jr.: Drug-related haematological problems during pregnancy. Clin. Haematol., 2:525, 1973.
105. Welch, H., Lewis, C. N., and Kerlan, I.: Blood dyscrasias. A nationwide survey. Antibiot. Chemother., 4:607, 1954.

CYCLIC NEUTROPENIA AND OTHER DISORDERS OF NEUTROPHILS

106. Baehner, R. L., and Nathan, D. G.: Quantitative nitroblue tetrazolium test in chronic granulomatous disease. N. Engl. J. Med., 278:971, 1968.
107. Berendes, H., Bridges, R. A., and Good, R. A.: Fatal granulomatous disease in childhood: clinical study of new syndrome. Minn. Med., 40:309, 1957.
108. Blume, R. S., Bennett, J. M., Yankee, R. A., and Wolff, S. M.: Defective granulocyte regulation in the Chediak-Higashi syndrome. N. Engl. J. Med., 279:1009, 1968.
109. Boxer, L. A., Yokoyama, M., and Wiebe, R. A.: Autoimmune neutropenia associated with chronic hepatitis., Am. J. Med., 52:279, 1972.
110. Chediak, M.: Nouvelle anomalie leucocytaire de la charactère constitutionnel et familial. Rev. Hematol., 7:362, 1962.
111. Clark, R. A., Kimball, H. R., and Padgett, G. A.: Granulocyte chemotaxis in the Chediak-Higashi syndrome of mink. Blood, 39:644, 1972.
112. Clark, R. A., Root, R. K., Kimball, H. R., and Kirkpatrick, C. H.: Defective neutrophil chemotaxis and cellular immunity in a child with recurrent infections. Ann. Intern. Med., 78:515, 1973.
113. Crosby, W. H.: How many "polys" are enough? Arch. Intern. Med., 123:722, 1969.
114. Cutting, H. O., and Lang, J. E.: Familial benign chronic neutropenia. Ann. Intern. Med., 61: 876, 1964.
115. Dale, D. C., Alling, D. W., and Wolff, S. M.: Cyclic hematopoiesis: the mechanism of cyclic neutropenia in gray collie dogs. J. Clin. Invest., 51:2197, 1972.
116. Dale, D. C., and Graw, R. G., Jr.: Transplantation of allogeneic bone marrow in canine cyclic neutropenia. Science, 183:83, 1974.
117. Davis, S. D., Schaller, J., and Wedgwood, R. J.: Job's syndrome. Recurrent "cold" staphylococcal abscesses. Lancet, 1:1013, 1966.
118. DeMeo, A. N., and Anderson, B. R.: Defective chemotaxis associated with a serum inhibitor in cirrhotic patients. N. Engl. J. Med., 286:735, 1972.
119. Douglas, S. D.: Analytic review: disorders of phagocyte function. Blood, 35:851, 1970.
120. Douglas, S. D., Davis, W. C., and Fudenberg, H. H.: Granulocytopathies: pleomorphism of neutrophil dysfunction. Am. J. Med., 46:901, 1969.
121. Duane, G. W.: Periodic neutropenia. Arch. Intern. Med., 102:462, 1958.
122. Gallin, J. I., Bujak, J. S., Patten, E., and Wolff, S. M.: Granulocyte function in the Chediak-Higashi syndrome of mice. Blood, 43:201, 1974.
123. Good, R. A., Quie, P. G., Windhorst, D. B., Page, A. R., Rodey, G. E., White, J., Wolfson, J. J., and Holmes, B. H.: Fatal (chronic) granulomatous disease of childhood: a hereditary defect of leukocyte function. Semin. Hematol., 5:215, 1968.
124. Guerry, D., IV, Adamson, J. W., Dale, D. C., and Wolff, S. M.: Human cyclic neutropenia: urinary colony-stimulation factor and erythropoietin levels. Blood, 44:257, 1974.

125. Guerry, D., IV, Dale, D. C., Omine, M., Perry, S., and Wolff, S. M.: Periodic hematopoiesis in human cyclic neutropenia. J. Clin. Invest., 52:3220, 1973.

126. Herring, W. B., Smith, L. G., Walker, R. I., and Herion, J. C.: Hereditary neutrophilia. Am. J. Med., 56:729, 1974.

127. Higashi, O.: Congenital gigantism of peroxidase granules. Tohoku J. Exp. Med., 59:315, 1954.

128. Holmes, B., Park, B. H., Malawista, S. E., Quie, P. G., Nelson, D. L., and Good, R. A.: Chronic granulomatous disease in females. N. Engl. J. Med., 283:217, 1970.

129. Holmes, B., Quie, P. G., Windhorst, D. B., and Good, R. A.: A fatal granulomatous disease of childhood: inborn abnormality of phagocytic function. Lancet, 1:1225, 1966.

130. Johnson, R. B., Jr., and Baehner, R. L.: Improvement of leukocyte bactericidal activity in chronic granulomatous disease. Blood, 35:350, 1970.

131. Jones, J. B., Lange, R. D., Yant, T. J., Vodopick, H., and Jones, E. S.: Canine cyclic neutropenia: erythropoietin and platelet cycles after bone marrow transplantation. Blood, 45:213, 1975.

132. Kanfer, J. N., Blume, R. S., Yankee, R. A., and Wolff, S. M.: Alteration of sphingolipid metabolism in leukocytes from patients with the Chediak-Higashi syndrome. N. Engl. J. Med., 279:410, 1968.

133. Klebanoff, S. J., and White, L. R.: Iodination defect in leukocytes of chronic granulomatous disease. N. Engl. J. Med., 280:460, 1969.

134. Kyle, R. A., and Linman, J. W.: Chronic idiopathic neutropenia. N. Engl. J. Med., 279:1015, 1968.

135. Landing, B. H., and Shirkey, H. S.: Syndrome of recurrent infection and infiltration of viscera by pigmented lipid histiocytes. Pediatrics, 20:431, 1957.

136. Leale, M.: Recurrent furunculosis in an infant showing an unusual blood picture. J.A.M.A., 54:1854, 1910.

137. Lipton, A.: Chronic idiopathic neutropenia. Arch. Intern. Med., 123:694, 1969.

138. Mandell, G. L., and Hook, E. W.: Leukocyte bactericidal activity in chronic granulomatous disease: correlation of bacterial hydrogen peroxide production and susceptibility to intracellular killing. J. Bacteriol., 100:531, 1969.

139. Miller, M. E., Seals, J., Kaye, R., and Levitsky, L. C.: Familial plasma-associated defect of phagocytosis: new cause of recurrent bacterial infections. Lancet, 2:60, 1968.

140. Mintz, U., and Sachs, L.: Granulocyte colony forming cells in the bone marrow of Yemenite Jews with genetic neutropenia. Blood, 41:745, 1973.

141. Morley, A. A., Carew, J. P., and Baikie, A. G.: Familial cyclical neutropenia. Br. J. Haematol., 13:719, 1967.

142. Mowat, A. G., and Baum, J.: Chemotaxis of polymorphonuclear leukocytes from patients with diabetes mellitus. N. Engl. J. Med., 284:621, 1971.

143. Page, A. R., and Good, R. A.: Studies on cyclic neutropenia. Am. J. Dis. Child., 94:623, 1957.

144. Quie, P. G.: Pathology of bactericidal power of neutrophils. Semin. Hematol., 12:143, 1975.

145. Quie, P. G., Kaplan, E. L., Page, A. R., Gruskay, F. L., and Malawista, S. E.: Defective polymorphonuclear-leukocyte function and chronic granulomatous disease in two female children. N. Engl. J. Med., 278:976, 1968.

146. Salmon, S. E., Cline, M. J., Schultz, J., and Lehrer, R. I.: Myeloperoxidase deficiency. N. Engl. J. Med., 282:250, 1970.

147. Sniderman, R., Altman, L. C., Frankel, A., and Blaese, R. M.: Defective mononuclear leukocyte chemotaxis: a previously unrecognized immune dysfunction. Ann. Intern. Med., 78:509, 1973.

148. Spaet, T. H., and Dameshek, W.: Chronic hypoplastic neutropenia. Am. J. Med., 13:35, 1952.

149. Strauss, R. G., Bove, K. E., Jones, J. F., Mauer, A. M., and Fulginiti, V. A.: Anomaly of neutrophil morphology with impaired function. N. Engl. J. Med., 290:478, 1974.

150. Tan, J. S., Strauss, R. G., Akabutu, J., Kauffman, C. A., Mauer, A. M., and Phar, J. P.: Persistent neutrophil dysfunction in an adult. Am. J. Med., 57:251, 1974.

151. Vincent, P. C., Levi, J. A., and MacQueen, A.: The mechanism of neutropenia in Felty's syndrome. Br. J. Haematol., 27:463, 1974.

152. Ward, H. N., and Reinhard, E. H.: Chronic idiopathic leukocytosis. Ann. Intern. Med., 75:193, 1971.

153. Ward, P. A., and Schlegel, R. J.: Impaired leucotactic responsiveness in a child with recurrent infections. Lancet, 2:344, 1969.

154. Weary, P. E., and Bender, A. S.: Chediak-Higashi syndrome with severe cutaneous involvement. Arch. Intern. Med., 119:381, 1967.

155. Wolff, S. W., Dale, D. C., Clark, R. A., Root, R. K., and Kimball, H. R.: The Chediak-Higashi syndrome: studies of host defenses. Ann. Intern. Med., 76:293, 1972.

156. Wriedt, K., Kauder, E., and Mauer, A. M.: Defective myelopoiesis in congenital neutropenia. N. Engl. J. Med., 283:1072, 1970.

Infectious Mononucleosis

157. Agliozzo, C. M., and Reingold, I. M.: Infectious mononucleosis simulating Hodgkin's disease. Am. J. Clin. Pathol., 56:730, 1971.
158. Bender, C. E.: The value of corticosteroids in the treatment of infectious mononucleosis. J.A.M.A., 199:529, 1967.
159. Bernstein, A.: Infectious mononucleosis. Medicine, 19:85, 1940.
160. Bernstein, T. C., and Wolff, H. G.: Involvement of the nervous system in infectious mononucleosis. Ann. Intern. Med., 33:1120, 1950.
161. Carpenter, G., Kahler, J., and Reilly, E. B.: Elevated titers of serum heterophil antibodies in three instances of monocytic leukemia. Am. J. Med. Sci., 220:195, 1950.
162. Chang, R. S., Lewis, J. P., and Abildgaard, C. F.: Prevalence of oropharyngeal excretors of leukocyte-transforming agents among a human population. N. Engl. J. Med., 289:1325, 1973.
163. Custer, R. P., and Smith, E. B.: The pathology of infectious mononucleosis. Blood, 3:830, 1948.
164. Davidsohn, I., Stern, K., and Kashiwagi, C.: The differential test for infectious mononucleosis. Am. J. Clin. Pathol., 21:1101, 1951.
165. Downey, H., and McKinlay, C. A.: Acute lymphadenosis compared with acute lymphatic leukemia. Arch. Intern. Med., 32:82, 1923.
166. E.B. virus, infectious mononucleosis and Burkitt's lymphoma. Lancet, 2:887, 1969.
167. Epstein, S. H., and Dameshek, W.: Involvement of the central nervous system in a case of glandular fever. N. Engl. J. Med., 205:1238, 1931.
168. Gerber, P., Hamre, D., Moy, R. A., and Rosenblum, E. N.: Infectious mononucleosis: complement-fixing antibodies to herpes-like virus associated with Burkitt lymphoma. Science, 161: 173, 1968.
169. Glade, P. R.: Infectious mononucleosis. J. B. Lippincott, Philadelphia, 1973.
170. Henle, G., Henle, W., and Volker, D.: Relation of Burkitt's tumor-associated type virus in infectious mononucleosis. Proc. Natl. Acad. Sci. U.S.A., 59:94, 1968.
171. Henle, G., and Henle, W.: EB virus in the etiology of infectious mononucleosis. Hosp. Pract., 5:33, 1970.
172. Hirshaut, Y., Glade, P., Moses, H., Manaker, R., and Chessin, L.: Association of herpes-like virus infection with infectious mononucleosis. Am. J. Med., 47:520, 1969.
173. Hoagland, R. J.: Infectious mononucleosis. Am. J. Med., 13:158, 1952.
174. Hoagland, R. J.: Infectious Mononucleosis. Grune & Stratton, New York & London, 1967.
175. Hobson, F. G., Lawson, B., and Wigfield, M.: Glandular fever: A field study. Br. Med. J., 1: 845, 1958.
176. Houck, G. H.: Involvement of the heart in infectious mononucleosis. Am. J. Med., 14:261, 1953.
177. Hovde, R. F., and Sundberg, R. D.: Granulomatous lesions in the bone marrow in infectious mononucleosis. Blood, 5:209, 1950.
178. Johansen, A. H.: Serous meningitis and infectious mononucleosis. Acta Med. Scand., 76:269, 1931.
179. Jordan, M. C., Rousseau, W. E., Stewart, J. A., Noble, G. R., and Chin, T. D. Y.: Spontaneous cytomegalovirus mononucleosis. Ann. Intern. Med., 79:153, 1973.
180. Kilpatrick, Z. M.: Structural and functional abnormalities of liver in infectious mononucleosis. Arch. Intern. Med., 117:47, 1966.
181. Leavell, B. S., and McNeel, J. O.: Infectious mononucleosis: unusual manifestations. Va. Med. Mon., 69:180, 1942.
182. Lee, C. L., Davidsohn, I., and Panczyszyn, O.: The spot test. Am. J. Clin. Pathol., 49:12, 1968.
183. Leibowitz, S.: Infectious Mononucleosis. Modern Medical Monographs. Grune and Stratton, New York, 1953.
184. Leibowitz, S., and Brody, H.: Cirrhosis of the liver following infectious mononucleosis. Am. J. Med., 8:675, 1950.
185. Longcope, W. T.: Infectious mononucleosis (glandular fever) with a report of ten cases. Am. J. Med., Sci., 164:781, 1922.
186. Lukes, R. J., and Cox, F. H.: Clinical and morphologic findings in 30 fatal cases of infectious mononucleosis. Am. J. Pathol., 34:586, 1958.
187. Lukes, R. J., Tindle, B. H., and Parker, J. W.: Reed-Sternberg-like cells in infectious mononucleosis. Lancet, 2:1003, 1969.
188. MacKinney, A. A., and Cline, W. S.: Infectious mononucleosis. Br. J. Haematol., 27:367, 1974.
189. Miller, G., Niederman, J. C., and Andrews, L.: Prolonged oropharyngeal excretion of Epstein-Barr virus after infectious mononucleosis. N. Engl. J. Med., 288:229, 1973.
190. Patel, B. M.: Skin rash with infectious mononucleosis and ampicillin. Pediatrics, 40:910, 1967.

191. Pattengale, P. K., Smith, R. W., and Perlin, E.: T and B cell markers. Atypical lymphocytes in acute infectious mononucleosis. N. Engl. J. Med., *291*:1145, 1974.

192. Paul, J. R., and Bunnell, W. W.: The presence of heterophile antibodies in infectious mononucleosis. Am. J. Med., Sci., *183*:90, 1932.

193. Pfeiffer, S.: "Drusenfieber." Jahrb. f. Kinderh., *29*:257, 1889.

194. Pullen, H., Wright, N., Murdoch, J. McC.: Hypersensitivity reactions to antibacterial drugs in infectious mononucleosis. Lancet, *2*:1176, 1967.

195. Reyman, T. A.: Postperfusion syndrome: a review and report of 21 cases. Am. Heart J., *72*:116, 1966.

196. Rifkind, D.: Cytomegalic mononucleosis. Ann. Intern. Med., *69*:842, 1968.

197. Rose, K. D.: Serum proteins in infectious mononucleosis. Ann. Intern. Med., *64*:826, 1966.

198. Schultz, A. L., and Hall, W. H.: Clinical observations in 100 cases of infectious mononucleosis and the results of treatment with penicillin and Aureomycin. Ann. Intern. Med., *36*:1498, 1952.

199. Schumacher, H. R., Jacobson, W. A., and Bemiller, C. R.: Treatment of infectious mononucleosis. Ann. Intern. Med., *58*:217, 1963.

200. Silverstein, A., Strinberg, G., and Nathanson, M.: Nervous system involvement in infectious mononucleosis. Arch. Neurol., *26*:353, 1972.

201. Smith, E. B., and Custer, R. P.: Rupture of the spleen in infectious mononucleosis. A clinicopathologic report of seven cases. Blood, *1*:317, 1946.

202. Smith, J. N., Jr.: Complications of infectious mononucleosis. Ann. Intern. Med., *44*:861, 1956.

203. Southam, C. M., Goldsmith, Y., and Burchenal, J. H.: Heterophile antibodies and antigens in neoplastic diseases. Cancer, *4*:1036, 1951.

204. Sprunt, T. P., and Evans, F. A.: Mononuclear leukocytosis in reaction to acute infections (infectious mononucleosis). Johns Hopkins Med. J., *31*:410, 1920.

205. Stevens, D. A.: Editorial: Infectious mononucleosis and malignant lymphoproliferative diseases. J.A.M.A., *219*:897, 1972.

206. Stevens, J. E.: Infectious mononucleosis: a clinical analysis of 210 sporadic cases. Va. Med. Mon., *79*:74, 1952.

207. Templeton, H. J., and Sutherland, R. T.: The exanthem of acute mononucleosis. J.A.M.A., *113*:1215, 1939.

208. Thurm, R. H., and Bassen, F.: Infectious mononucleosis and acute hemolytic anemia. Blood, *10*:841, 1955.

209. Waterhouse, B. E., and Lapidus, P. H.: Infectious mononucleosis associated with a mass in the anterior mediastinum. N. Engl. J. Med., *227*:1137, 1967.

210. Wechsler, H. F., Rosenblum, A. H., and Sills, C. T.: Infectious mononucleosis: report of an epidemic in an army post. Ann. Intern. Med., *25*:113, 1946.

CHAPTER 10

MYELOPROLIFERATIVE DISORDERS

In 1951 Dameshek introduced the term "myeloproliferative syndrome" to indicate a group of diseases or syndromes thought to be the result of some primary bone marrow disturbance.[7] He included the following: chronic granulocytic leukemia; polycythemia vera; idiopathic or agnogenic myeloid metaplasia; megakaryocytic leukemia; and erythroleukemia (including the di Guglielmo syndrome). He suggested that the fibrosis of the marrow, which is a frequent finding in these disorders, is a manifestation of active proliferation of fibroblasts and reticulum cells. At present the term "myeloproliferative disorder" has a broader connotation which usually includes the disorders listed in Table 10-1. Paroxysmal nocturnal hemoglobinuria would be included by some authors. The term remains a useful one for several reasons. At times the clinical and laboratory observations in a patient may indicate a definite disturbance of the bone marrow elements which is not well enough defined to warrant a more precise diagnosis; in such circumstances, further observation in the ensuing months usually serves to clarify the diagnosis. The term also implies some relationship among the disorders, particularly when the typical findings of one disorder are replaced by those of another of the group (Table 10-2).

Chronic granulocytic leukemia is discussed in Chapter 12. It is usually manifested by anemia, leukocytosis, splenomegaly, and proliferation of the granulocytic cells in the bone marrow; often the megakaryocytes are increased, and

Table 10-1 *Classification of Myeloproliferative Disorders*

1. Chronic granulocytic leukemia (CGL)
2. Acute granulocytic leukemia (AGL)
3. Polycythemia vera (PV)
4. Agnogenic myeloid metaplasia (AMM)
5. Idiopathic thrombocythemia (hemorrhagic thrombocythemia) (HT)
6. Erythroleukemia (di Guglielmo's) (EL)
7. Acquired sideroblastic anemia (refractory normoblastic anemia) (ASA)
8. Preleukemia

Table 10–2 *Hematologic Characteristics of the Myeloproliferative Disorders*

	WBC	RBC	Pl	Spl	Ph Cr	LAP
CGL	+++	N –	+ N	+	+	–
PV	+	++	+	+	0	+
AMM	+ N –	N –	+ N –	+	0	N
HT	+	N –	+++	+	0	N
EL	+ N –	–	–	+ N	0	N
ASA	+ N –	–	– N	+ N	0	N

Legends
CGL = chronic granulocytic leukemia
PV   = polycythemia vera
AMM = agnogenic myeloid metaplasia
HT   = hemorrhagic thrombocythemia
EL   = erythroleukemia
ASA = acquired sideroblastic anemia
+ = increased;   N = normal;   – = decreased;   0 = absent

sometimes thrombocytosis is striking. It appears that there may be two types of chronic granulocytic leukemia with similar clinical findings. In one, the Philadelphia chromosome is present and the score of the leukocyte alkaline phosphatase test is very low; in the other, the Philadelphia chromosome is absent and the leukocyte alkaline phosphatase reaction is low, normal, or even increased. In both groups the leukemia terminates as acute myeloblastic leukemia in a high percentage of patients.

Acute granulocytic or *myeloblastic leukemia,* discussed in Chapter 12, occurs most frequently in adults and is manifested by anemia, thrombocytopenia, and mild splenomegaly; the leukocyte count is usually elevated, but leukopenia may be present. The characteristic finding is a definite pathologic increase in myeloblasts and promyelocytes in the marrow; at times these cells fill the marrow cavity. Auer bodies are seen in the blast cells, particularly in the peripheral blood, of some patients. The disease does not transform into other members of the group. "Smoldering leukemia" is a term sometimes used to indicate a syndrome of anemia, leukopenia, and a bone marrow which contains a pathologically increased number of myeloblasts.[26,35] This picture differs from the usual one seen in acute myeloblastic leukemia in that thrombocytopenia is not as common, leukocytosis is absent, the anemia usually is not marked, and the course of the disease appears to be milder and somewhat slower. Nevertheless, patients with this syndrome have acute myeloblastic or myelomonoblastic leukemia.

Polycythemia vera, discussed in Chapter 11, is characterized by increases in the red cell mass, hematocrit, and red cell counts, leukocytosis (in three-quarters of the patients), splenomegaly (in three-quarters of the patients), and a normal or increased platelet count; at times, platelet counts reach levels of 5 to 10 million per cu. mm. Examination of the bone marrow usually shows hyperplasia of all the hematopoietic elements, but at times some areas of fibrosis are apparent. The Philadelphia chromosome is absent, and the leukocyte alkaline phosphatase reaction is normal or increased. The abnormalities in the circulating blood reflect the proliferation of all the cell lines in the bone marrow. The erythropoietin level in the blood is not increased as it is in patients with erythrocytosis or "secondary polycythemia."

The earliest form of treatment for polycythemia vera was phlebotomy. Later, many patients were treated with some form of radiation, particularly x-ray or radioactive phosphorus. The median survival time in patients with polycythemia vera treated with radioactive phosphorus was reported to be 13.2 years, compared to 6.7 years in those treated with other methods. The validity of this comparison has, however, been questioned.[30] In addition, there has been increasing concern over the influence of radiation (and possibly drugs) on the frequency of the later development of myelofibrosis or acute leukemia; some authors question whether acute leukemia has developed in patients with polycythemia vera who have not received prior therapy of this sort.

In myeloproliferative disorders, lymphomas, and leukemia, when one disease or syndrome seems to follow another in the same patient, it is sometimes difficult to know if it is part of the natural history of the disease, an unwanted result of therapy, or a reflection of some defect in the patient, immunologic or otherwise.

MYELOID METAPLASIA

Synonyms. One review lists 25 different names that have been suggested for this syndrome.[18] Those used most commonly are: agnogenic myeloid metaplasia, chronic nonleukemic myelosis, aleukemic myelosis, leukanemia, leukoerythroblastic anemia, myelosclerosis, and myelofibrosis.

This syndrome is characterized by splenomegaly, anemia, the presence of nucleated red blood cells and immature granulocytes in the circulating blood, and the occurrence of extramedullary hematopoiesis in the liver and spleen. There is considerable variation in the histologic appearance of the bone marrow in the reported cases. Credit for the first report of a case of this type is usually given to Heuck, who in 1879 reported two cases that were considered to show the chance association of myelogenous leukemia and osteosclerosis.[20] Ever since that time there has been considerable confusion and controversy concerning terminology, classification, and causation of the syndrome. Several comprehensive reviews of the clinical or pathologic aspects of the problem have appeared that also contain extensive bibliographies.[4,16,19,22,23,28,31,32,41] Although some authors differ as to what should be classified as "primary" and "secondary" types of this syndrome, some such grouping is desirable for a better understanding of the problem.

Secondary Myeloid Metaplasia; Leukoerythroblastic Anemia

The syndrome is characterized by anemia associated with myelocytes or younger cells of the granulocytic series and nucleated red cells in the peripheral blood; splenomegaly, anisopoikilocytosis of the circulating erythrocytes, and extramedullary hematopoiesis are usually present and mild reticulocytosis is frequent. The leukocyte and platelet counts are usually normal, or nearly so. The syndrome is thought to be the result of encroachment on the hematopoietic tissue of the marrow by space-consuming lesions.

Carcinomatosis, with bone marrow metastases, is probably the commonest cause of this syndrome: it has also been reported in patients with disseminated tuberculosis, multiple myeloma, Hodgkin's disease, septicemia, neurofibromatosis, leukemia, and polycythemia vera.[10,21,31] Immature cells of the granulocytic and erythrocytic series also appear in the circulating blood of patients who are seriously ill with infections and many other disorders, often as an agonal event.

The simple occurrence of nucleated red cells in the peripheral blood, without other evidence of extramedullary hematopoiesis, is not sufficient for the diagnosis of this syndrome. Nucleated red cells have been found in the circulating blood in a number of disorders. They are seen most often in association with hemorrhage, pernicious anemia, hemolytic anemia, leukemia, and carcinoma, but also occur in other disorders such as heart failure, severe infection, and cerebrovascular accidents.[37]

Primary or Agnogenic Myeloid Metaplasia (Nonleukemic Myelosis, Myelofibrosis)

Most of the controversy regarding patients in this category has centered around the nature of the underlying process. It has been considered to be: (1) leukemic in nature; (2) a proliferative or neoplastic disorder closely related to, but different from, myelocytic leukemia and polycythemia; (3) a response of the marrow and reticuloendothelial tissue to injury of some sort.

The evidence for the leukemic nature of the process has been reviewed by Heller; Lewison, and Palin.[49] These authors studied the material obtained at autopsy of two patients. The bone marrow of both showed intense myeloid hyperplasia, and only one showed small, widely scattered areas of fibrosis, but the authors emphasized that they considered their comments applicable to cases reported in the literature under the 25 other names as well as to the term "aleukemic myelosis," which they used. The authors, who concluded that the syndrome is a form of myelogenous leukemia, considered that the presence of fibrosis in the marrow and osteosclerosis in the bones, the absence of leukemic invasion in the organs, and the appearance of the spleen were not adequate grounds for excluding leukemia.

Wyatt and Sommers[44] studied 30 patients, 20 of whom were autopsied, and concluded that the disorder was nonleukemic in nature. It was thought that the primary lesion was a necrobiosis of the maturing hematopoietic cells, which was followed by overgrowth of the marrow reticulum, ossification, and extramedullary hematopoiesis. The study of the histories and a retrospective analysis for possible causative agents in these cases revealed a list of possible factors similar to those considered important in aplastic anemia. This suggested that prolonged marrow exposure to certain substances might be an important factor. A similar conclusion is suggested by another report of six patients with "agnogenic myeloid metaplasia." It was noted that two patients gave histories of heavy exposure to benzol, two had daily exposure to "paint removers," one worked with carbon tetrachloride, and one washed auto parts with "high-test gasoline."[34] The increased incidence of myelofibrosis found in survivors of the atomic bomb explosion in Hiroshima, a pattern similar to that found for leukemia, is evidence that ionizing radiation is the causative agent in some patients with the disorder.

The development of aplastic anemia after radiation and certain toxic agents is well recognized. Leukemia develops in some patients who have or have had aplastic anemia, and the development of myeloid metaplasia may be an analogous sequence. The development of massive enlargement of the spleen and liver with myeloid metaplasia, seen in many patients, is different from an effort to compensate for a bone marrow rendered functionless by fibrosis. The postmortem examination in some patients discloses evidence of myeloid metaplasia (the proliferation of normoblasts, granulocytes, and megakaryocytes) that is so widespread, involving the myocardium, lungs, pleura, and other tissues, as well as the liver, spleen, and lymph nodes, that it has every appearance of an invasive process which involves several cell lines rather than one, as is seen characteristically in leukemia. The extramedullary hematopoiesis, which is usually of little clinical significance, occasionally becomes more aggressive and forms tumors large enough to cause intestinal obstruction, pleural and ascitic effusions, spinal cord compression, portal hypertension, and partial obliteration of a kidney and ureter.[15]

An unusual type of myeloproliferative disease has been reported in nine children.[33] The disorder became manifest between 5 months and 4 years of age and was characterized in most by chronic illness, anemia, and massive splenomegaly; there was a leukocytosis of between 2700 and 128,000 per cu.mm., accompanied in nearly all by young cells of the granulocytic series in the peripheral blood. The bone marrow was hyperplastic. The leukocyte alkaline phosphatase was low in the four patients in whom it was measured, and the Philadelphia chromosome was not found in four patients who were examined for it. The course of the disease was variable, ranging from early death through improvement after splenectomy to apparently spontaneous complete recovery after 10 or 12 years of illness. It closely resembled chronic granulocytic leukemia, but its familial distribution, the absence of the Philadelphia chromosome, and the apparent recovery in some patients suggest that it is a different disorder.

Although it is probable that the controversy as to the nature and causation of this syndrome will continue, the concept of this syndrome as a myeloproliferative disorder, which does not exclude a reaction to toxic agents, affords the best working hypothesis at the present time.

CLINICAL MANIFESTATIONS

This rather uncommon disorder occurs in either sex, but is rare in blacks. Symptoms generally appear first after the age of 50, but sometimes begin before the age of 40. Onset is usually gradual, and the patients complain of weakness and easy fatigue, or of upper abdominal discomfort caused by enlargement of the spleen and liver. Weight loss of 15 to 20 pounds is common. Aching and severe pain in the extremities, leg cramps, and peripheral edema sometimes occur. Cutaneous hemorrhages, either petechiae or ecchymoses, are not unusual, and serious gastrointestinal hemorrhage is not rare. Night sweats and fever occur in an appreciable number of patients. Occasionally, ascites and esophageal varices develop late in the course of the disease. The architecture of the liver is usually little altered, and a greatly augmented portal flow is considered the most likely explanation of the elevated portal venous pressure. Attacks of gout or gouty arthritis are a troublesome feature in some patients with high levels of uric acid in the blood.

The most significant feature of the physical examination is the splenomegaly. Palpable enlargement of the spleen is almost invariably present, and is sometimes so extreme that the firm spleen fills the entire left side of the abdomen and extends into the right lower quadrant. Some authors report that the degree of splenomegaly correlates roughly with the duration of the disease. Hepatomegaly generally occurs, but usually is less prominent than the splenomegaly. In some patients, after the spleen is removed, the liver becomes enormous and virtually fills the abdominal cavity. Significant enlargement of the superficial lymph nodes is exceedingly rare. Not infrequently, a bleeding tendency is manifested by ecchymoses and petechiae or retinal hemorrhages. Pallor of the skin and mucous membranes is usually evident, and jaundice of mild degree is sometimes apparent in the skin and sclerae. The other abnormalities found on the physical examination are those that occur commonly in older persons with a chronic disease associated with anemia, such as loss of weight, cardiac enlargement, and precordial systolic murmurs.

Anemia in this disorder is often the result of multiple factors, which include the degree of cellularity of the marrow, the effectiveness of the medullary erythropoiesis, hemolysis, bleeding, and expanded plasma volume with hemodilution: the effectiveness of the extramedullary hematopoiesis and even folate deficiency are important factors. Studies with radioactive iron and chromium have shown that the spleen plays a significant role in hyperhemolysis in only about one-quarter of the patients. Such studies also indicate that extramedullary erythropoiesis is largely ineffectual. Hyperhemolysis associated with paroxysmal nocturnal hemoglobinuria has developed in some patients.

LABORATORY EXAMINATION

The most significant hematologic feature of this disorder is an anemia characterized by marked anisocytosis and poikilocytosis associated with the occurrence of nucleated red cells and myelocytes or myeloblasts in the peripheral blood. The degree of anemia, the levels of leukocytes and platelets, and the numbers of immature erythrocytes and granulocytes vary within a wide range. Patients with normal or elevated blood levels sometimes are also included as examples of this syndrome if immature cells are present in the circulating blood.

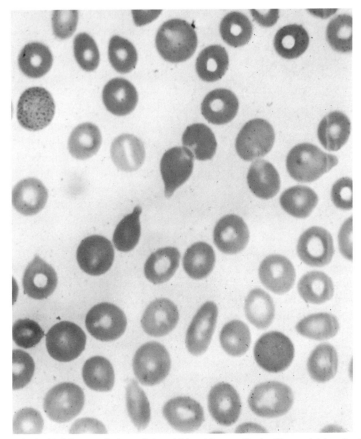

Figure 10–1 Poikilocytosis in peripheral blood in a patient with myeloid metaplasia.

In the reported series, which includes observations on more than 150 patients, the hemoglobin ranged from 5.0 to 14.0 gm. per 100 ml., and was less than 9.0 gm. per 100 ml. in 21 patients. The mean corpuscular volume varied from 71 to 103 cu.μ, and was normal in 60 per cent of subjects. The mean corpuscular hemoglobin was normal in 60 per cent, and low in the remainder. Examination of the blood smear often suggests the diagnosis because of the presence of a marked degree of poikilocytosis—particularly "teardrop forms" and elongated cells—anisocytosis, and the presence of nucleated red cells (Fig. 10–1). The changes in the peripheral blood are not diagnostic. The nucleated red cells are usually few in number, less than 5 per 100 leukocytes, but occasionally they outnumber the leukocytes. Most often these cells are late normoblasts, but basophilic and polychromatophilic normoblasts and cells that resemble megaloblasts are sometimes seen. The reticulocyte count is often normal, but mild or moderate reticulocytosis of 3 to 5 per cent is common.

The leukocyte count is usually elevated, but the range in the reported cases is from 1200 to 92,000 per cu.mm.; in one series the initial leukocyte counts in over 80 per cent of patients were less than 20,000 per cubic mm., and the reverse was true in a series of patients with chronic granulocytic leukemia.

Myeloblasts, promyelocytes, and myelocytes are usually found in the peripheral blood. It has been noted that the number and identity of the immature granulocytes in the peripheral blood represent a "shift to the left" rather than a "leukemic hiatus." The authors have seen marked diminution and even disappearance of the immature leukocytes follow a series of transfusions in several patients with this disorder, but such a change has not been found in patients with leukemia who have been treated similarly. Eosinophilia, monocytosis, and basophilia sometimes occur in myelofibrosis. The leukocyte alkaline phosphatase stain in patients with myelofibrosis gives variable results; low, normal, and high values have been found. Although a differentiation between leukemia and myelofibrosis cannot be made by this reaction, a high value favors myelofibrosis. The Philadelphia chromosome, which occurs in a high percentage of patients with chronic myelocytic leukemia, is rarely found in those with myelofibrosis.

The platelets are often large and the total count varies widely in different patients. Neither a marked reduction to less than 100,000 per cu.mm. nor a marked increase to over a million per cu. mm. is uncommon, but a normal or slightly increased count is usual.

Specimens of bone marrow obtained by aspiration are usually very hypocellular, but normal cellularity or even hyperplasia of some or all elements is found in some patients. Biopsy specimens obtained by operation or needle and postmortem marrows show increased fibrosis as well as hypocellularity, although some marrows contain areas of hyperplasia. Hickling has studied the bone marrow histology in 68 patients with the disorder.[22] He concluded that the marrow undergoes a transition ranging from general hyperplasia involving all of the normal hematopoietic cells, followed by megakaryocytic hyperplasia, to varying degrees of fibrosis and eventual bony replacement of nearly all the marrow. Between these extremes he recognized seven categories. Splenic aspiration and hepatic puncture usually reveal extramedullary hematopoiesis in the form of nucleated red cells, young granulocytes, and megakaryocytes.

Other laboratory tests frequently are abnormal in patients with this disorder. Uric acid levels in the blood are elevated in more than one-half of the patients and in many of these the levels are twice the normal value. The liver function tests often are mildly abnormal. Serum bilirubin and fecal urobilinogen excretion are usually increased in patients who have significant hyperhemolysis. The Coombs test is occasionally positive. Abnormalities of coagulation in the form of defective platelet function or an abnormality in a plasma coagulation factor have been found in some patients. The level of vitamin B_{12} in the serum is sometimes elevated, but usually is normal; the level probably depends more on the leukocyte count than on anything else.

Roentgenograms of the bones, particularly of the long bones, may show a decreased density of the inner surface of the central area of bone and patchy irregular densities in the spongiosa.[42] The changes may be indistinguishable from those sometimes found in leukemia. Increased bone density was demonstrated on roentgenograms in one-quarter of the patients in one series.[28] Osteosclerosis, particularly in the axial skeleton, vertebrae, ribs, and the metaphyses of the femur and humerus, has been reported in from 30 to 70 per cent of patients with the disorder.[43] So frequent is the occurrence of osteosclerosis that its presence associated with splenomegaly in a person middle-aged or older strongly suggests the diagnosis of myeloid metaplasia.

DIFFERENTIAL DIAGNOSIS

When a patient presents with splenomegaly and anemia associated with nucleated red cells and immature granulocytes in the peripheral blood, the important differential diagnosis is between chronic myelocytic leukemia and the myeloid metaplasia syndrome. The appearance of marked poikilocytosis in the smear is suggestive but not diagnostic of myeloid metaplasia. Failure to obtain a specimen that is consistent with leukemia by marrow aspiration strongly suggests that leukemia is not present; nevertheless the diagnosis of leukemia cannot be discarded in this circumstance, because hypocellular samples and "dry taps" are sometimes obtained in patients with leukemia even when the marrow is packed with cells. The distinction between leukemia and myeloid metaplasia sometimes cannot be made until after a surgical biopsy of the bone marrow or a needle aspiration of the liver. A splenic aspiration biopsy which reveals young granulocytes, normoblasts, and megakaryocytes is strong evidence of myeloid metaplasia, but the risks of the procedure have restricted its use in most institutions. Although a diagnosis of myelofibrosis with myeloid metaplasia is not justified without a biopsy of the bone marrow that demonstrates fibrosis, it must be remembered that fibrosis in the bone marrow occurs in other conditions, particularly in leukemia. Sometimes even after these studies the evidence is inconclusive, and the distinction between these two disorders cannot be made with assurance until after a longer period of observation.

A search for the Philadelphia chromosome and determination of the leukocyte alkaline phosphatase help to distinguish chronic myelocytic leukemia from myeloid metaplasia. The Philadelphia chromosome is present in from 90 to 95 per cent of patients with chronic myelocytic leukemia, and is present rarely, if at all, in patients with myeloid metaplasia. Nearly all the latter have a normal or increased score with the leukocyte alkaline phosphatase determination, whereas patients with chronic myelocytic leukemia have subnormal values; this is not diagnostic of chronic granulocytic leukemia, but an elevated value is strong evidence against the diagnosis.

If leukemia appears to be excluded, further study for possible causes of the secondary type of extramedullary hematopoiesis, such as carcinomatosis, tuberculosis, and other disorders, is indicated. If these appear to be excluded and the appearance of the bone marrow biopsy is consistent, a diagnosis of myelofibrosis or agnogenic myeloid metaplasia is made. A history of preceding polycythemia vera favors this diagnosis.

TREATMENT AND COURSE

The disorder is a chronic one that usually continues over a period of years. In some patients, at least early in the disease, the main symptoms are those referable to the anemia or enlarged spleen. Night sweats, weight loss, and fever usually appear later in the course. Gastrointestinal hemorrhages are not infrequent and may be serious; poorly-understood severe pains in the extremities and abdomen are very troublesome in some patients. Phlebothrombosis, pulmonary embolism, and infarction may occur and present as an acute emergency or as respiratory distress, cor pulmonale, and right-sided heart failure.

There is no specific treatment for this disorder. Neither iron nor vitamin B_{12} is of any value in the uncomplicated case. Most patients require blood transfusions which are given as often as symptoms warrant. Several other forms of treatment, including splenectomy and radiotherapy, have been tried with inconsistent results; the drugs used most often are androgens, corticosteroids, and busulfan.

For many years splenectomy was thought to be contraindicated because of the high operative mortality rate and because it appeared that the operation removed a needed area of hematopoiesis. A different opinion was expressed by Green, Conley, Ashburn, and Peters,[16] who reported that, in a series of 24 patients, splenectomy was rarely harmful and sometimes produced beneficial effects. Others too have reported favorable results.[6, 12] In one study of 35 patients treated with splenectomy, 14 responded well and survived for up to eight years. Splenectomy is most likely to be helpful in patients with hemolytic anemia who require many transfusions, and in those with associated thrombocytopenia. Patients with dilution anemia are often benefitted, although several months may be required for the large plasma volume to return to normal. Pronounced discomfort in the splenic area and severe hypermetabolism manifested by sweats and weight loss have also been considered indications for splenectomy. The dangers and ineffectiveness of the operation in some patients are apparent from published reports. Of 28 patients who had splenectomy, 12 died at operation or in the the immediate, postoperative period, and seven others died within one year.[32] Excellent results were obtained in a small number of patients. Since there is appreciable risk associated with the operation in patients with this disorder, splenectomy is not indicated in those who can be managed adequately by other forms of treatment. In elderly patients, and those with very high platelet counts, splenectomy is contraindicated because of the risk of operation and the chance of postoperative complications such as thrombosis and hemorrhage secondary to thrombocytosis.

Although splenic irradiation has been used sporadically over a period of years, its value or danger is still uncertain, possibly because some patients so treated have differed from others in unrecognized but important details.

Androgens, first reported by Gardner and Pringle, have proved to be very effective in some patients; from one-half to three-quarters experience either complete remission or distinct improvement.[13, 25] Results appear to be better in women, in patients who have had polycythemia vera, in those who have had splenectomy, and in those whose spleens are not massively enlarged. The response is also much better in patients with adequate radioiron uptake in the marrow and peripheral blood. Testosterone enanthate, 6 mg. kg. of body weight I.M. once a week, Dianabol (methandrostenolone) orally 5 mg. 4 times per day, and oxymetholone 40 to 200 mg. per day may be effective. Gardner emphasizes that androgens, which have their major effect on the committed red cell compartment, should be tried for at least three months; if there has been no response in this period, a trial with another androgen is recommended. Undesirable sequelae of treatment with androgens are the virilizing effects in women and the occasional occurrence of jaundice associated with hepatic damage, which may be severe and even fatal. Androgen therapy should be discontinued if jaundice develops.

Corticosteroids benefit some patients with hyperhemolysis or thrombocytopenia and bleeding. Busulfan, 6 mg. per day, helps some, probably by reducing hyperhemolysis, but a variety of effects have occurred; hematologic improvement unaccompanied by a diminution in the size of the spleen occurs in some patients, and in others splenomegaly diminishes without any improvement in the peripheral blood. Busulfan may produce an adverse effect on the remaining marrow elements, and its use should be discontinued if thrombocytopenia develops. The authors have seen severe pulmonary fibrosis and bone marrow aplasia in a patient treated continuously for over two years. Intermittent therapy should be used if possible. Busulfan is a useful agent, however, in treating thrombocytosis that is sometimes present and an apparent factor in both phlebothrombosis and bleeding.

The prognosis for patients with myeloid metaplasia is better than for those with chronic leukemia. Although the survival time varies from a few weeks to more than 20 years, the median survival time in one group of 143 patients was about four years.[28] The mortality rate was greatest during the first year. The three-year survival rate in the disease is about 30 per cent, five-year survival about 20 per cent, and 10-year survival about 10 per cent. In one series of 45 patients, half were alive five years after diagnosis and ten years after symptoms first appeared.[43] Death is most often the result of infection, thrombosis, or hemorrhage. Other patients die with heart failure, and a few develop chronic myelocytic leukemia or acute myeloblastic leukemia as a terminal event. An acute form of myeloid metaplasia that has a course of less than a year has been described.[3a]

Illustrative Case

A 40-year-old white librarian was largely asymptomatic when an "abdominal tumor" was found on routine physical examination in October 1945. At that time the erythrocyte count was 6.6 million per cu.mm. and the hematocrit 62 per cent. A diagnosis of polycythemia vera was made, and during the next four years she received a total of 3250 R of x-radiation to the spleen and a total of 460 R over the long bones. Phlebotomies were performed at frequent intervals. Following treatment with radiophosphorus in 1950 she had a good symptomatic remission, and in 1953 the blood values were: Hct. 49 per cent, Hb. 12.7 gm. per 100 ml., R.B.C. 6 million per cu. mm., W.B.C. 13,000 per cu.mm., platelets 516,000 per cu.mm. During the late spring and summer of 1954 the patient noticed progressive weakness, easy fatigue, slight dyspnea on exertion, easy bruising, and recurrent left upper quadrant pain. Because of these symptoms she was admitted to the hospital on August 2, 1954.

Physical examination. Loud systolic murmurs were heard in the aortic area and in the mitral region. The liver was palpable three fingerbreadths below the right costal margin; the spleen filled the entire left side of the abdomen. The remainder of the physical examination was noncontributory.

Laboratory examination. Admission blood studies disclosed: Hct. 28 per cent, R.B.C. 2.8 million per cu.mm., Hb. 8.4 gm. per 100 ml., retics. 0.7 per cent, W.B.C. 7400 per cu. mm.; differential count (per cent), myelocytes 2, juveniles 2, bands 7, segs. 68, lymphs. 18, monocytes 1, eosinophils 1, basophils 1. There were 5 nucleated red cells per 100 white cells. The serum bilirubin was 0.54 mg. per 100 ml. Bone marrow obtained by aspiration and also surgical biopsy of the iliac crest revealed marked hypoplasia.

Treatment and course. The patient responded moderately well to steroid therapy, but in the fall of 1955 her symptoms and anemia increased. A hemolytic factor was demonstrated, and splenectomy was performed in September 1956. The spleen weighed 1975 gms. Microscopic study of the spleen revealed the presence of many islands of myeloid tissue associated with evidence of erythropoiesis and an increased number of megakaryocytes. The findings were considered to be characteristic of myeloid metaplasia.

The patient improved, but in the fall of 1957 the symptoms changed, and from then on heart failure was a problem. She became increasingly refractory to treatment, and died in April 1958 after an episode of abdominal pain.

At autopsy the usual manifestations of congestive heart failure were present. In addition there was marked coronary arteriosclerosis, as well as calcific aortic valvulitis and calcification of the annulus fibrosus of the mitral valve. Of particular interest was the presence of generalized fibrosis of the bone marrow associated with areas of hypercellularity and evidence of extramedullary hematopoiesis in the liver.

Comment. This patient's course is similar to that seen in many with myelofibrosis. At one time she had well-developed polycythemia vera which was treated with phlebotomies, x-radiation, and radiophosphorus. About eight years after the polycythemia was first recognized she developed anemia. This was associated with fibrosis in the bone marrow, marked splenomegaly, the presence of immature leukocytes and red cells in the peripheral blood, and evidence of hematopoiesis in the spleen. Splenectomy produced only moderate temporary benefit, and the patient succumbed to recurrence of the anemia and heart failure several years later. The relationship of the myelofibrosis to the preceding polycythemia vera and to the radiation therapy is interesting, but difficult to interpret.

IDIOPATHIC THROMBOCYTHEMIA (HEMORRHAGIC THROMBOCYTHEMIA)

Idiopathic or hemorrhagic thrombocythemia occurs almost exclusively in middle-aged or older persons. The clinical features are splenomegaly, anemia, abnormal bleeding (usually from the nose or gastrointestinal tract), and thrombocytosis. An abnormal tendency to thrombosis, particularly of the veins of the legs or spleen, is sometimes manifest.[18]

Platelet counts range from 1.0 to 5.0 mil. per cu.mm. or even more; large clumps of platelets and giant platelets frequently are present on the smear of the peripheral blood. The severity of the anemia is related to the amount of bleeding; it usually is normocytic, but may be hypochromic and microcytic if repeated bleeding has occurred. In nearly all the reported patients the leukocyte count has been slightly elevated; counts have ranged from 10,000 to 60,000 per cu. mm. Examination of the bone marrow discloses striking hyperplasia of the megakaryocytes, many of which appear young or bizarre. Erythroid and granulocytic hyperplasia are often evident.

Whether or not this syndrome constitutes a separate clinical entity is debatable. Unquestionably some patients with myeloid metaplasia, polycythemia vera, or chronic granulocytic leukemia develop all features of the syndrome during the course of their illness. Others, however, have the fully-developed syndrome when they first consult their physician. In addition to the other myeloproliferative disorders, other causes of thrombocytosis such as carcinomatosis, Hodgkin's disease, and iron deficiency must be considered in the differential diagnosis, particularly in patients without detectable splenomegaly. Abnormal bleeding is not a prominent feature of these other forms of thrombocytosis. It is the result of the excessive number of platelets and their poor function; both bleeding and thrombocytosis are often controlled by treatment with busulfan, radioactive phosphorus or melphalan.

ERYTHROLEUKEMIA

Synonyms: Di Guglielmo syndrome; erythremic myelosis

Di Guglielmo first described this disorder as one characterized by malignant proliferation of the erythrocytic cells in the bone marrow.[9] He later recognized the occurrence of mixed forms involving both the erythrocytes and the granulocytes, "erythroleukemia." Practically all the patients seen clinically fit into the "mixed" forms of disturbance involving both red cells and granulocytes, and for this reason the syndrome is now considered to be one of the myeloproliferative disorders.[8, 9, 38] Some authors consider that the disorder passes through three stages, namely predominant erythroblastic proliferation, mixed erythroblastic and myeloblastic growth, and preponderant myeloblastic proliferation. Others are unable to recognize these stages, and consider the disorder to be one with variable proliferation of both the erythroid and myeloid cells, or erythroleukemia at all stages.[38] Dameshek considered that some, if not all, instances of refractory normoblastic anemia and acquired sideroblastic anemia are variants of the Di Guglielmo syndrome.[8] The high percentage of patients with the "refractory normoblastic anemia" or "acquired sideroblastic anemia" who develop acute myeloblastic leukemia terminally supports the concept of a relationship.

The disorder has been reported in patients from 11 to 85 years of age, but it occurs most frequently at 40 years of age or older. Males have outnumbered females 2:1 in the reported cases. Presenting symptoms usually are weakness, easy fatigue, dyspnea on exertion, and weight loss. Less often, bleeding in the skin and mucous membranes or from the gastrointestinal tract occurs. Severe pains of an unusual character occur commonly in the trunk, epigastrium, back, or extremities. Examination usually discloses pallor and evidence of weight loss. Hemorrhages into the skin, mucous membranes, or fundi are not unusual. Splenomegaly and hepatomegaly have been reported in about one-third of the patients.

Laboratory examinations reveal severe or moderate anemia that is normochromic and normocytic or slightly macrocytic. Leukopenia is common, and normal counts are not unusual, but leukocytosis is rare. The platelet count is normal or reduced. The reticulocytic count is often from 2 to 4 per cent. Study of the peripheral blood smear usually shows nucleated red cells and myeloblasts in addition to anisocytosis and poikilocytosis of the erythrocytes.

The bone marrow is usually hypercellular, mainly because of a striking increase in the erythrocytic precursors. Many of the cells are large, basophilic, multinucleated, immature pronormoblasts, and others are megaloblasts; nuclear maturation is abnormal in nearly all. Morphologically-similar erythrocyte precursors develop in some patients receiving antileukemic chemotherapy or immunosuppressive drugs. Auer bodies are sometimes present in young cells of the myeloid series.

Studies of anemia in patients with this disease have disclosed that the serum vitamin B_{12} level is unusually high, vitamin B_{12} absorption is normal, and the anemia fails to respond to either vitamin B_{12} or folic acid. The hemolytic character of the anemia is shown by the increased fecal urobilinogen excretion and the decreased cell survival measured with chromium-tagged cells. Failure of erythropoiesis has been demonstrated by studies with radioactive iron which disclose an increased clearance from the plasma associated with decreased utilization and incorporation into the circulating red cells, the prototype of "ineffective" erythropoiesis. Hypertransfusion reduces the bizarre erythroid hyperplasia seen in the disease, but qualitative abnormalities persist.[1]

The anemia is usually refractory to treatment other than transfusions. Steroids, vitamin B_{12}, folic acid, and splenectomy are ineffective. One report of multiple drug chemotherpay, daunorubicin — prednisone, is encouraging; of nine patients so treated, four had complete remissions, median duration six months, and three had partial remissions.[5]

The prognosis is very poor. Most patients develop frank acute myeloblastic leukemia within a year after the appearance of the first symptoms. A chronic form with survivals for ten years or more has been reported, however. As the disease pursues its relentless course, the myeloblasts in the marrow increase and almost always become the predominant cells before death occurs.

ACQUIRED SIDEROBLASTIC ANEMIA (REFRACTORY NORMOBLASTIC ANEMIA)

Acquired sideroblastic anemia, which is discussed in Chapter 5, is a poorly-understood disorder. The "sideroblastic" anemias are those associated with significant numbers of ringed sideroblasts in the marrow. The ringed appearance of the cells is caused by the location of the stainable iron in the mitochondria, a circumstance which indicates a defect in iron and heme metabolism.

Some of the acquired cases have been "idiopathic", and others have been associated with certain drugs or diseases. Nearly all reported instances of the idiopathic acquired type have been in patients over 40 years of age, usually much older. In most instances of the acquired type the erythropoiesis is ineffective and the anemia has been refractory to treatment with pyridoxine, folate, and androgen, but apparent responses occasionally have been observed. It appears likely that many, if not all, patients diagnosed as having "refactory normoblastic anemia" also belong to this syndrome.

The anemia is usually normocytic or macrocytic. A population of hypochromic erythrocytes was found in all patients in one group of the idiopathic variety. Reticulocytes are normal (or slightly increased), and platelet and leukocyte counts are normal or slightly reduced. Usually, but not invariably, the serum iron level and transferrin saturation are increased. More often than not the serum iron is above 175 micrograms, per 100 ml. and the transferrin saturation is 75 per cent or more. Stores of marrow iron and the number of ringed sideroblasts are markedly increased, and erythropoiesis is normoblastic and hyperplastic. Although many physicians have seen patients with this disorder develop frank leukemia months or years after coming under observation, one report emphasizes the mild nature of the disorder in some patients with survivals of ten years or more. In this group of the acquired idiopathic variety, a leukemic termination was found in only 7 per cent of 61 cases.[27] It is possible that this transformation occurs more often in patients with malignant disease and in those who have been treated with radiation or chemotherapy.

PRELEUKEMIA

Preleukemia is a term introduced to designate patients with various clinical manifestations, listed in Table 10–3, who eventually develop definite leukemia.[11,17] The initial symptoms usually are weakness, recurrent infections, or fever. Pallor and splenomegaly occur frequently, and petechiae and ecchymoses are not unusual. In many instances the only symptoms are those related to the anemia.

Pancytopenia or varying combinations of anemia, thrombocytopenia, and

Table 10–3   *Hematologic Abnormalities Reported Most Frequently in "Preleukemia"*

PERIPHERAL BLOOD	BONE MARROW
Pancytopenia	Hypercellularity
Anemia, granulocytopenia, or thrombocytopenia	Dyserythropoiesis
Anisocytosis and poikilocytosis	Megaloblastoid forms
Oval macrocytes	Increase in young cells of granulocytic series
Basophilic stippling	Maturation defect in granulocytes
Nucleated red cells	Storage iron increased
Monocytosis	Chromosomal abnormalities
Pelger-Huët anomaly	

granulocytopenia occur. Anemia, which is almost invariably present, usually is accompanied by striking abnormalities in the peripheral blood smear including aniso- and poikilocytosis, polychromatophilic cells, oval macrocytes, teardrop forms, shistocytes, and nucleated red cells. Monocytosis and an increase in basophiles occur frequently. An acquired Pelger-Huët-like abnormality and other defects in nuclear or cytoplasmic development may be apparent in the granulocytes. The platelets are often abnormally large.

The bone marrow is usually hypercellular, particularly the red cell series which in the vast majority of instances will manifest some "megaloblastoid" features. Chromosomal abnormalities have been found in 50 to 60 per cent of patients; the abnormalities usually have been in the C group, but no consistent defects have been observed. Patients with preleukemia have a defect in the granulocytic colony stimulating capacity similar to that seen in those with acute myeloblastic leukemia.[17] The iron stores in the marrow are usually increased.

Nearly all patients with the recognized syndrome have developed definite acute myeloblastic or myelomonoblastic leukemia within three to 24 months, but occasionally only after as long as nine years. The survival time after the appearance of definite leukemia is usually very short.

Some have objected to the term preleukemia because they feel it is valid only in retrospect. The clinical features of this syndrome are similar to those seen in sideroblastic anemia, refractory normoblastic anemia, aplastic anemia with cellular marrow and ineffective erythropoiesis. Nevertheless, many of the features described in this syndrome occur in patients with lymphoma or other malignancies who have been treated with radiation or chemotherapeutic drugs during what appears to be a transitional phase that is followed by definite leukemia. Despite the objections that have been raised, the term and the concept it implies seem apt in some clinical situations.

TRANSITIONS IN MYELOPROLIFERATIVE DISORDERS

The frequency of transition of one of the myeloproliferative syndromes to another member of the group is of considerable importance. In his original communication on the subject in 1951, Dameshek considered the occurrence of "transition forms" to be common and thought that the diagnostic label assigned to a patient, whether "chronic granulocytic leukemia" or "agnogenic myeloid metaplasia" for example, was sometimes simply a matter of taste.[8] In the succeeding decade, the occurrence of transitions between the disorders was generally accepted and was not considered rare. More recently, with the benefit of greater knowledge and better diagnostic methods of distinguishing the diseases or syndromes, the concept has been re-examined.

In one series of 110 patients diagnosed as having agnogenic myeloid metaplasia, 20 per cent developed terminal leukemia.[6] In another series of 194 patients with myeloid metaplasia, 165 were classified as idiopathic and 29 as post-polycythemia vera; eight patients of the 165 with the idiopathic type died with acute leukemia, as did five who had the disorder following polycythemia vera. Most, but not all, who developed acute leukemia had been treated with radiotherapy or chemotherapeutic agents. In another series of 45 patients with agnogenic myeloid metaplasia, none developed acute leukemia.[43] In a report which emphasized the infrequency of transition among the myeloproliferative disorders, the incidence of development of acute leukemia was found to be as follows: polycythemia vera 7 per cent; agnogenic myeloid metaplasia 7 per cent; chronic granulocytic leukemia 39 per cent. The therapy which had been employed was considered responsible for the development of acute leukemia in the first two groups.[14] In one group of 207 patients diagnosed as having polycythemia vera, agnogenic myeloid metaplasia developed in 29; this transition occurred more frequently in those who were treated with radiotherapy or chemotherapy, in 25 out of 130.[40]

Ward and Block proposed that these disorders constitute two distinct groups, with little overlapping but with changes occurring within the groups.[43] Figure 10–2 is a modification of theirs. One group, called "the myeloleukemia syndrome," is viewed as characterized by a neoplastic proliferation of a single cell line that invades and destroys the normal architecture of organs. Transition to acute leukemia is expected in all patients with chronic granulocytic leukemia or erythroleukemia who live long enough. The second group, called "the myeloproliferative syndrome," is considered to be a benign proliferation of a trilineage of hematopoietic cells in organs that were previously hematopoietic, a process different from leukemic transformation or invasion.

The concept is attractive, but apparent crossovers between these groups

Myeloleukemic Syndrome

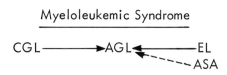

Myeloproliferative Syndrome

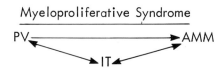

Figure 10–2 Transitions in myeloproliferative disorders. (After Ward and Block.[43])

occur, for example, from polycythemia vera and agnogenic myeloid metaplasia to acute myeloblastic leukemia. One possible explanation for the apparent exceptions to the concept is that the original diagnosis was incorrect, and that the proper one should have been chronic granulocytic leukemia rather than myeloid metaplasia or polycythemia vera; such diagnostic dilemmas will persist until there are more precise diagnostic methods. The criteria used for the diagnosis of the different disorders probably vary, and the diagnosis made sometimes remains a matter of judgment. Other possible explanations implicate the effect of therapy given for the primary disease; apparently the development of leukemia can be triggered by radiation and chemotherapeutic drugs, but whether by androgens or pre-existing anemia is uncertain. Another unmeasurable, but probably important, element is the host's resistance to malignancy, immunologic or otherwise; the occurrence of secondary primary malignancies in patients who have not received any anti-cancer therapy is well known.

References

1. Adamson, J. W., and Finch, C. A.: Erythropoietin and regulation of erythropoiesis in the Di Guglielmo's syndrome. 36:590, 1970.
2. Anderson, R. E., Hoshino, T., and Yamamoto, T: Myelofibrosis with myeloid metaplasia in survivors of atomic bomb in Hiroshima. Ann. Intern Med., 60:1, 1964.
3. Bensinger, T. A., Logue, G. L., and Rundles, R. W.: Hemorrhagic thrombocythemia: control of postoperative thrombocytosis with melphalan. Blood, 36:61, 1970.
3a. Bergsman, K. L., and Van Slyck, E. J.: An accelerated variant of agnogenic myeloid metaplasia. Ann. Intern. Med., 74:232, 1971.
4. Block, M., and Jacobson, I. O.: Myeloid metaplasia. J.A.M.A., 143:1390, 1950.
5. Bloomfield, C. D., Brunning, R. D., and Kennedy, B. J.: Daunorubicin—prednisone treatment of erythroleukemia. Ann. Intern. Med., 81:746, 1974.
6. Bouroncle, B. A., and Doan, C. A.: Myelofibrosis: clinical, hematologic and pathologic study of 110 patients. Am. J. Med. Sci., 243:697, 1962.
7. Dameshek, W.: Some speculations on the myeloproliferative syndromes. Blood, 6:372, 1951.
8. Dameshek, W., and Baldini, M.: The Di Guglielmo syndrome. Blood, 13:192, 1958.
9. Di Guglielmo, G.: Acute Erythemic Disease. In Proc. 6th Congr. Int. Soc. Hematol. Grune and Stratton, New York, 1958.
10. Erf, L. A., and Herbut, P. A.: Primary and secondary myelofibrosis (a clinical and pathological study of thirteen cases of fibrosis of the bone marrow). Ann. Intern Med., 21:863, 1944.
11. Fisher, W. B., Armentroutm S. A., Weisman, R., Jr., and Graham, R. C., Jr.: "Preleukemia." Arch. Intern. Med., 132:226, 1973.
12. Fishman, N., and Ballinger, W. F.: Splenectomy for agnogenic myeloid metaplasia and myelofibrosis. Arch. Surg., 90:940, 1965.
13. Gardner, F. H., and Pringle, J. C., Jr.: Androgens and erythropoiesis. II. Treatment of myeloid metaplasia. N. Engl. J. Med., 264:103, 1961.
14. Glaser, R. M., and Walker, R. I.: Transitions among the myeloproliferative disorders. Ann. Intern. Med., 71:285, 1969.
15. Glew, R. H., Jaese, W. H., and McIntyre, P. A.: Myeloid metaplasia with myelofibrosis: clinical spectrum of extramedullary hemopoiesis and tumor formation. Johns Hopkins Med. J., 132:253, 1973.
16. Green, T. W., Conley, C. L., Ashburn, L. L., and Peters, H. R.: Splenectomy for myeloid metaplasia of the spleen. N. Engl. J. Med., 248:211, 1953.
17. Greenberg, P. L., Nichols, W. C., and Schrier, S. L.: Granulopoiesis in acute myeloid leukemia and preleukemia. N. Engl. J. Med., 284:1225, 1971.
18. Gunz, F. W.: Hemorrhagic thrombocythemia: a critical review. Blood, 15:706, 1960.
19. Heller, E. L., Lewisohn, M. G., and Palin, W. E.: Aleukemic myelosis. Chronic non-leukemic myelosis, agnogenic myeloid metaplasia, osteosclerosis, leukoerythroblastic anemia and synonymous designations. Am. J. Pathol., 23:327, 1947.
20. Heuck, G.: Zwei Fälle von Leukämie mit eigenthümlichen Blut-resp. Knochenmarksbefund. Virchows Arch., 78:475, 1879.

21. Hickling, R. A.: Chronic non-leukemic myelosis. Q. J. Med., *6*:253, 1937.
22. Hickling, R. A.: The natural history of chronic non-leukemic myeloses. Q. J. Med., *37*:267, 1968.
23. Hutt, M. S. R., Pinninger, J. L., and Wetherley-Mein, G.: The myeloproliferative disorders. With special reference to myelofibrosis. Blood, *8*:295, 1953.
24. Jackson, H., Jr., Parker, F., Jr., and Lemon, H. M.: Agnogenic myeloid metaplasia of the spleen. A syndrome simulating other more definite hematologic disorders. N. Engl. J. Med., *222*:985, 1940.
25. Kennedy, B. J.: Effect of androgenic hormone in myelofibrosis. J.A.M.A., *182*:116, 1962.
26. Knospe, W. H., and Gregory, S. A.: Smoldering acute leukemia. Arch. Intern. Med., *127*:910, 1971.
27. Kushner, J. P., Lee, G. R., Wintrobe, M. N., and Cartwright, G. E.: Idiopathic refractory sideroblastic anemia. Clinical and laboratory investigation of 17 patients and review of the literature. Medicine, *50*:139, 1971.
28. Linman, J. W., and Bethell, F. H.: Agnogenic meyloid metaplasia. Its natural history and present day management. Am. J. Med., *22*:107, 1957.
29. Milner, G. R., Geary, C. G., Wadsworth, L. D., and Doss, A.: Erythrokinetic studies as a guide to the value of splenectomy in primary meyloid metaplasia. Br. J. Haematol., *25*:467, 1973.
30. Modan, B., and Lillienfeld, A. M.: Polycythemia vera and leukemia — the role of radiation treatment; a study of 1222 patients. Medicine, *44*:305, 1965.
31. Nakai, G. S., Graddock, C. G., and Figueroa, W. C.: Agnogenic myeloid metaplasia. Ann. Intern. Med., *57*:419, 1962.
32. Pitcock, J. A., Reinhard, E. H., Justus, B. W., and Mendelsohn, R. S.: A clinical and pathological study of seventy cases of myelofibrosis. Ann. Intern. Med., *57*:73, 1962.
33. Randall, D. L., Reiquam, C. W., Githens, J. H., and Robinson, A.: Familial myeloproliferative disease: new syndrome closely simulating myelogenous leukemia in childhood. Am. J. Dis. Child., *110*:479, 1965.
34. Rawson, R., Parker, F., Jr., and Jackson, H., Jr.: Industrial solvents as possible etiologic agents in myeloid metaplasia. Science, *93*:541, 1941.
35. Rheingold, J. J.: Acute leukemia. Its smoldering phase. J.A.M.A., *230*:985, 1974.
36. Saarni, M. I., and Linman, J. W.: Preleukemia. Am. J. Med., *55*:38, 1973.
37. Schwartz, S. O., and Stansbury, F.: Significance of nucleated red blood cells in peripheral blood. J.A.M.A., *154*:1339, 1954.
38. Sheets, R. F., Drevets, C. C., and Hamilton, H. E.: Erythroleukemia (Di Guglielmo's syndrome). Arch. Intern. Med., *111*:295, 1963.
39. Silverstein, M. N.: Postpolycythemia myeloid metaplasia. Arch. Intern. Med., *134*:113, 1974.
40. Silverstein, M. N., Brown, A. J., Jr., and Linman, J. W.: Idiopathic myeloid metaplasia. Arch. Intern. Med., *132*:709, 1973.
41. Silverstein, M. N., Gomes, M. R., Re-Mine, W. H., and Elveback, L. R.: Agnogenic myeloid metaplasia, natural history and treatment. Arch. Intern. Med., *120*:546, 1967.
42. Vaughan, J. M., and Harrison, C. V.: Leuco-erythroblastic anaemia and myelosclerosis. J. Pathol., Bacteriol., *48*:339, 1939.
43. Ward, H. P., and Block, M. H.: The natural history of agnogenic myeloid metaplasia (AMM) and a critical evaluation of its relationship with the myeloproliferative syndrome. Medicine, *50*:357, 1971.
44. Wyatt, J. P., and Sommers, S. C.: Chronic marrow failure, myelosclerosis and extramedullary hematopoiesis. Blood, *5*:329, 1950.

CHAPTER 11

POLYCYTHEMIA

Strictly speaking, the term polycythemia (polys, many; kytos, cell; haima, blood) refers to an increase of all the cellular elements in a known volume of blood, and erythrocythemia (erythros, red; kytos, cell; haima, blood) to an increase in red blood cells alone. By common usage, and in this text, polycythemia refers to an increase in red blood cells, and is modified by the terms leukocytosis or thrombocytosis if those elements are also increased.

RELATIVE POLYCYTHEMIA

An increase in red blood cell count above normal may be *relative* or *absolute*. If the volume of fluid in which the red blood cells are suspended is reduced, an increase in their concentration results. The number of cells per unit volume of whole blood is increased, and this increase is reflected in the red blood cell count and the hematocrit. The total body red cell mass remains unchanged. Such a condition of *relative* polycythemia exists in any situation in which the plasma volume is reduced without a concomitant reduction in red cell mass. *Acute relative polycythemia* is most frequently associated with a shift or loss of body water, and in such circumstances the red cell count and hematocrit determination are valuable aids in the recognition and quantification of such changes. A careful history will generally lead to a correct interpretation of the laboratory findings. Changes in plasma osmolality will influence the volume of the red cell. Ingress or egress of water from the red cell in response to altered osmotic forces outside the cell may be sufficient to affect the hematocrit. *Chronic relative polycythemia* is believed to be secondary to an abnormally low plasma volume. This condition has been referred to as Gaisböck's disease,[117] stress polycythemia,[117] and spurious (relative) polycythemia.[28] The cause of the low plasma volume is not understood, but it has been attributed to a variety of causes including emotional stress,[117] alcoholism,[166] heavy smoking,[158a] chronic anxiety,[117] a position at the extreme of a normal frequency distribution curve,[28, 57] and systemic hypertension.[51] Most patients are white males in early middle age of somewhat stocky build and moderately overweight. Leukocytosis, thrombocytosis, and spleno-

Table 11–1 *Classification of Polycythemia*

I. Relative Polycythemia: an acute or chronic decrease in plasma volume with no change in red cell mass.
II. Polycythemia vera: a proliferative disorder involving all elements of the bone marrow.
III. Secondary polycythemia: an increase in red cell mass with no involvement of other marrow elements.
   A. Associated with known hypoxic stimulus.
      1. Cardiovascular disease with right to left shunt.
      2. Pulmonary disease with decreased arterial oxygen saturation.
      3. Low barometric pressure.
      4. Abnormal hemoglobin.
   B. Associated with inappropriate erythropoietin production.
   C. Associated with excess adrenocortical steroids or androgens.
IV. Benign familial polycythemia: a familial disorder of unknown etiology manifested by an increase in red cell mass.

---

megaly are absent. Many have been reported to be tense and anxious.[99, 117] Further studies are needed to establish the specificity of the condition.

ABSOLUTE POLYCYTHEMIA

An *absolute* increase in red blood cell mass may occur either as the result of a physiologic response to tissue hypoxia, or in the pathologic state known as polycythemia vera. In the first instance, the polycythemia is secondary to some recognized inciting cause; in the second, the polycythemia is classified as "primary" since no inciting cause has been identified.[8, 162]

The various conditions which cause an increase in red cell mass are classified in Table 11–1.

POLYCYTHEMIA VERA

Synonyms: Primary Polycythemia, Vaquez' Disease, Osler's Disease, Polycythemia Rubra Vera, Erythremia

Vaquez in 1892 gave the first description of polycythemia that was not associated with pulmonary or cardiac disease.[140] The second description of such a patient was published by Cabot in 1899.[33] In 1903 Osler collected eight cases, four from the literature and four of his own, and pointed out many features of the disease.[140] In 1908 he clearly defined the disorder, and discussed the course and prognosis as well as the therapeutic use of bleeding, oxygen, and irradiation of the spleen.[141] Excellent comprehensive reviews of the disease have been written by Harrop,[75] Lawrence, Berlin, and Huff[118] Pike,[147] Modan,[132] and Jepson.[94]

PATHOGENESIS

The etiology of polycythemia vera is unknown. Because of the proliferation of all the cell lines in the bone marrow and the frequent transformation of polycythemia vera into leukemia, myelofibrosis, and other related syndromes, polycythemia vera has been considered to be a myeloproliferative disorder[33, 44, 107, 123, 183] (Chapter 10).

Owing to the known development of polycythemia in response to hypoxia, numerous attempts have been made to explain polycythemia vera as a marrow hypoxia mechanism of some sort, but none has been satisfactory.[18, 160] The greater frequency of leukocytosis and thrombocytosis, and the finding of normal arterial oxygen saturation, in polycythemia vera serve to differentiate it from hypoxic polycythemia.[58]

The increased red cell mass in polycythemia vera is due to increased production, rather than an increased life span, of cells. Studies with radioactive iron showed that the plasma iron turnover in this disease is five times normal.[148] Studies on life span of cells have shown that it is normal,[125] or that there is a dual population of cells, one with a normal life span, and another with very short life span.[20] The stimulus for the increased erythropoiesis in this disease has not been identified. Extracts of plasma from patients with polycythemia vera have been reported by some to stimulate erythropoiesis when injected into test animals;[42, 123] others have been unable to confirm these results.[47, 100, 143] These conflicting data indicate the need for a more sensitive technique by which to assay plasma erythropoietin. There is no evidence that the marrow cells of patients with polycythemia are hypersensitive to erythropoietin or consume more erythropoietin than normal. The defect appears to reside in the stem cell.[111]

Most of the clinical manifestations of polycythemia vera can be explained by alterations in the peripheral blood. The total blood volume is increased two or three times due almost entirely to an increase in the total mass of circulating red cells. Associated with this increase in erythrocytes, there is an increase in blood viscosity that may be five to eight times normal.[75, 128] The increased blood volume and the slowed circulation in the congested capillaries are responsible for the plethoric appearance of the patient and the ruddy cyanosis which appears when the level of the nonoxygenated hemoglobin in the capillaries rises above 5 gm. per 100 ml.[8, 162] The increased blood volume and viscosity place a load on the heart which may result in cardiac decompensation, and may lead to thrombosis of pulmonary vessels.[32] The consistently increased stroke volume with a normal or elevated cardiac output is thought to result from increased central blood volume and increased diastolic filling.[40] Recent studies have shown that the increase in cardiac output more than compensates for the increased viscosity, and that oxygen transport is actually increased.[35] These patients frequently have vascular disease, however, and the vessels are unable to carry an increased flow of blood. For this reason, the effect of viscosity may not be offset and local tissue ischemia may occur. This often improves markedly when the underlying disease is treated effectively. The frequent occurrence of thrombosis in this disorder appears to be related to the presence of the vascular disease in association with increased blood viscosity, decreased blood flow, and an increased number of blood platelets. A recent report suggests the presence of fibrinolytic inhibitors in the platelets of patients with polycythemia vera.[112]

One of the puzzling features of polycythemia, a disease characterized by thrombosis, is the frequent occurrence of abnormal bleeding. The distention of the blood vessels has been considered a possible explanation.[118] In addition, abnormalities in the quality of the blood clot and in clot retraction have been demonstrated. It has also been shown that the presence of very large numbers of platelets interferes with the early stages of blood coagulation.[106] Several qualitative platelet defects have been studied.[106,137,178] The reported decrease in platelet factor III availability is not corrected by sonication of the platelets. Still another factor that may be important is the occurrence of increased fibrinolysis that has been demonstrated in polycythemia vera, but not in secondary polycythemia.[22, 178]

CLINICAL MANIFESTATIONS

Polycythemia vera occurs more often in males than in females, the ratio being about 1.3:1 or 2:1.[38, 107, 118, 145, 183] The disease appears to be more common in whites than in blacks; in a series of 50 patients with polycythemia vera seen at the University of Virginia Hospital, the ratio of whites to blacks was 24:1, although in the total hospital admissions the ratio of whites to blacks was 4.5:1.[145] Clinical manifestations of the disease appear most often between the ages of 40 and 60, though the disease has been reported in children.[46,118] In the authors' series the age at onset ranged from 21 to 88 years, but only 10 per cent were below the age of 40.[145]

Most of the symptoms of polycythemia vera are related to the increased red cell mass, the associated vascular disease, and the tendency to hemorrhage and thrombosis.

Onset is usually insidious and the manifestations variable. Weakness, easy fatigue, irritability, and dizziness are common early complaints. At other times onset is abrupt, and the first indication of the presence of the disease is the occurrence of a catastrophe such as a gastrointestinal hemorrhage, myocardial infarction, thrombosis of a retinal vessel, or the development of hemiplegia.

The most common clinical manifestations relate to the cardiovascular system. Complaints such as dyspnea on exertion, ankle edema, angina pectoris, palpitation, headache, dizziness, and intermittent claudication are present in about two-thirds of the patients when first seen.[145]

In about one-third of the patients, gastrointestinal symptoms such as epigastric pain, nausea, bloating, vomiting, and constipation are prominent. The incidence of duodenal ulcer demonstrable by x-ray is reported to be 10 to 19 per cent.[118, 145, 147] Both hematemesis and melena occur not infrequently, and either may be the first manifestation of the disease. On occasion the patient's history of severe bleeding may be doubted because of the failure of the laboratory tests to demonstrate the degree of anemia suggested by the history.

Other symptoms occur much less often in polycythemia vera, but are recognized as part of the disease. In some patients severe pruritus, particularly after a hot bath, and night sweats constitute the main complaints. Patients are sometimes treated for "conjunctivitis" for a time before the underlying disease is recognized.[11] Hyperuricemia is a common finding, and clinical gout occurs in approximately 10 per cent.[184] Other less common complaints relate to the genitourinary system, such as hematuria, dysuria, and urinary frequency.

Often the most striking feature of the physical examination is the appearance of the patient—a ruddy and florid face, telangiectasia of the cheeks and nose, and purplish cyanosis of the lips and ears. The appearance frequently suggests the diagnosis, but the countenance of the middle-aged man who has spent most of his life out-of-doors and indulged freely in alcohol may be virtually indistinguishable. Marked reddening is often evident in the palms, conjunctivae, pharynx, and vaginal mucous membranes. Examination of the fundus frequently reveals retinal veins that are distended and dark purple in color. Hypertension is present in about one-half of the patients. The spleen is enlarged in about three-quarters of the patients; it is usually firm, and rarely extends as low as the umbilicus unless the disease has been present for some years;[175] late in the course of the disease, especially when leukemia or myelofibrosis has developed, the spleen may become greatly enlarged and fill most of the abdominal cavity. Hepatomegaly occurs in about one-third to one-half of the patients.

LABORATORY FINDINGS

The laboratory data in patients with polycythemia vera illustrate the involvement of the granulocytic and megakaryocytic series, and not the red cells alone.[45,118,155] The untreated patient typically has an erythrocyte count in the range of 6 to 10 million, a hemoglobin between 18 and 24 gm. per 100 ml., and a hematocrit that ranges from 55 to 80 per cent.[147] The total red cell mass is increased, but the plasma volume may be normal, slightly elevated, or even decreased.[1,19] (Normal values: R.B.C. vol., ml./kg., men 28.27 ± 4.11, women 24.24 ± 2.59; plasma vol., ml./kg., men 33.45 ± 5.18, women 34.77 ± 3.24[88]) Equations using combined height-weight, surface area, height-weight-skinfold thickness, or lean body mass have been used.[153a] The leukocyte count is usually elevated. In our series of 50 patients a range of 5400 to 88,000 per cu. mm. was found; 70 per cent had counts higher than 10,000 per cu. mm.,[145] a figure comparable to that of 74 per cent found in a much larger series.[118] The total blood granulocytic pool in patients with polycythemia vera has been shown by studies of granulocytic kinetics to be increased.[129]

The leukocyte alkaline phosphatase score is usually high when there is leukocytosis; rarely, it will be elevated when the leukocyte count is in the normal range.[10] Myelocytes and metamyelocytes are often present on the blood smear, and nucleated red blood cells occur not infrequently. Platelet counts range from 100,000 to 1.5 mil. per cu.mm.[145] In one series, 50 per cent of the platelet counts were above 400,000 per cu.mm., and in another, 65 per cent were over 300,000 per cu.mm.[118]

The serum concentration of vitamin B_{12} has been reported to be elevated in 36 per cent of patients with untreated polycythemia vera. The capacity of the serum proteins to bind vitamin B_{12} was increased in 70 per cent of patients in the same study. These findings are similar to those in other myeloproliferative disorders, but may help to differentiate between polycythemia vera and secondary polycythemia.[65]

Study of fixed sections of bone marrow is reported to show a characteristic pattern consisting of clumps of stem cells and early normoblasts in about 85 per

Table 11–2 *Diagnostic Criteria*

CATEGORY A

    A1. Increased red cell mass, measured with Cr^{51} labeled red cells (male $\geq$ 36 ml./kg., female $\geq$ 32 ml./kg.).

    A2. Normal arterial oxygen saturation $\geq$ 92%.

    A3. Splenomegaly.

CATEGORY B

    B1. Thrombocytosis (platelets $>$ 400,000/mm.^{3}).

    B2. Leukocytosis (white count $>$ 12,000/mm.^{3} in absence of fever or infection).

    B3. Elevated leukocyte alkaline phosphatase score. ($>$ 100 in absence of fever or infection).

    B4. Elevated serum Vitamin B_{12} or unbound B_{12} binding capacity ($B_{12} >$ 900 pg./ml., $USB_{12}C >$ 2200 pg./ml.).

The diagnosis of polycythemia vera is acceptable if (a) all three from Category A are present, or (b) the combination A1 and A2 is present plus any two from Category B.

Adapted from Wasserman, L. R.: The management of polycythaemia vera. Brit. J. Haematol., *21*:371, 1971.

cent of patients.[14,23] Study of smears made from material obtained by aspirations was rarely helpful in our series, since about one-half of the marrows appeared to be normal and the remainder showed varying degrees of hyperplasia;[145] a stain for iron usually indicates that storage iron is greatly reduced or absent.

Ferrokinetic studies indicate that, as the disease progresses, an uncompensated shortening of the red cell life span occurs and produces progressive decrease in red cell mass. This happens regardless of therapy, and appears to be part of the natural history of the disease.[148] Associated with this are increases in erythrocyte glutamic oxaloacetic transaminase, glucose-6-phosphate dehydrogenase, and hexokinase, which reflect a young red cell population.[15] Splenic sequestration of the red cells increases as the red cell survival decreases.

Other laboratory features of the disease are an increased basal metabolic rate, an increased level of uric acid,[126,160] increased plasma iron turnover,[87] and normal arterial oxygen saturation.[58]

The National Polycythemia Vera Study Group in 1968 set up rigid criteria for documenting the presence of polycythemia vera for purposes of their studies (Table 11–2).[184]

COURSE AND PROGNOSIS

It has been pointed out that the natural history of polycythemia vera is virtually unknown, since some form of therapy has always been available.[147] Developments such as thrombosis, hemorrhage, and the occurrence of other myeloproliferative syndromes are so frequent that it is difficult to decide whether they should be considered as complications of the disorder or as incidents in its natural history.

A high incidence of vascular thrombosis is to be expected in a disease characterized by an increased red cell mass, increased viscosity of the blood, and elevated numbers of platelets when the disease occurs in an age-group in which vascular disease is common. The incidence of thrombosis is reported to be 22 per cent,[183] 28 per cent,[177] and as high as 40 per cent in our own series.[145] Thrombosis probably occurs in any of the vessels, but appears to

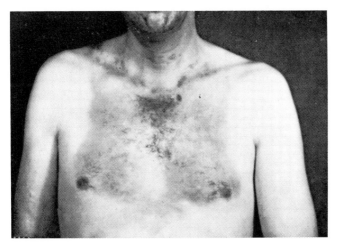

Figure 11–1 Extensive subcutaneous hemorrhage following dental extraction in a patient with polycythemia vera.

be most common in the coronary, cerebral, mesenteric, pulmonary, retinal, and peripheral arteries, and in the leg, retinal, and portal veins.[39,41] The episodes of thrombosis are seen more often when there is inadequate control of the red cell mass and platelet level by therapy.

Hemorrhage is a frequent occurrence in polycythemia vera. An incidence of 16 per cent,[183] 59 per cent,[177] and 30 per cent[145] has been observed. In our experience the most serious hemorrhages have been intracranial, gastrointestinal, and those occurring after various surgical procedures, but extensive ecchymoses, hemarthroses, epistaxis, bleeding after dental extractions, and bleeding after minor technical procedures have also proved extremely troublesome (Fig. 11–1).[39,154,187]

Peptic ulcer is not uncommon in this disease, and the incidence has been found to be from 10 to 14 per cent,[147] 12 per cent,[145] and 19 per cent.[116] The incidence of gastrointestinal symptoms is higher, from 17 per cent[145] to 25 per cent,[118] and severe gastrointestinal hemorrhage occurs not infrequently. The rare association of polycythemia vera and pregnancy has been noted.[83,157] The platelets, leukocytes, and hemoglobin fell progressively during the first two trimesters, followed by a sharp rise in these elements in the seventh month. Fetal salvage was low.[16, 36, 74]

The median survival time in polycythemia vera has been reported[118] to be 13.2 years in patients treated with radiophosphorus and 6.7 years in those treated with various methods other than P^{32}. Survival times in individual patients vary from a few months to 25 years.[52] The commonest causes of death are thrombosis, hemorrhage, leukemia, and other myeloproliferative states. In Lawrence's series, the causes of death in 57 patients treated with P^{32} were as follows: chronic myelogenous leukemia, 11 (6 were acute terminally); cerebral hemorrhage, 7; coronary thrombosis, 8; congestive heart failure, 9; carcinoma, 8; postoperative deaths, 5; miscellaneous, 4; unknown, 5.[118] In our own series of 24 patients who died, 12 had received no form of radiation therapy and 12 had received treatment with P^{32} or x-ray. The causes of death in the 12 who had received no irradiation were: heart failure or cerebrovascular accident, 8; postoperative hemorrhage, 1; carcinoma, 1; miscellaneous (peritonitis, multiple sclerosis, renal insufficiency), 3. The causes of death in 12 who had received P^{32} or x-ray were: heart failure or thromboses, 3; myelogenous leukemia (acute), 3; myeloid metaplasia, 2; miscellaneous (hepatic cirrhosis, unknown), 3.[145]

Although the complications of thrombosis and hemorrhage are the most common serious developments in most patients with polycythemia vera, it is definitely established that leukemia, myelofibrosis, or some other myeloproliferative disorder develops in an appreciable number, perhaps 20 to 30 per cent. These complications are more likely to develop in patients with long survival times. If the incidence of these disorders is higher in patients treated with P^{32}, it is possible that this is related to the longer survival of the patients so treated, and/or to their exposure to some form of radiation.

DIAGNOSIS

In most patients with polycythemia vera the diagnosis is made without difficulty. The clinical findings of plethora and splenomegaly, in association with laboratory values indicating an absolute increase in red cell mass, leukocytosis, and thrombocytosis, are characteristic. Occasionally it is difficult to decide if polycythemia is present in plethoric-appearing middle-aged hypertensive men with borderline blood counts, and it is not easy to determine whether a well-established polycythemia is primary or secondary. Another problem arises when the leukocyte values are such that the distinction from chronic myelocytic leukemia is not easily made.

If the hematocrit is 55 per cent and the erythrocyte count is elevated to 5.8 to 6.0 mil. per cu.mm., the possibility of an early polycythemia vera cannot be excluded merely because splenomegaly, leukocytosis and thrombocytosis are absent. While splenomegaly, leukocytosis, and thrombocytosis do not occur in secondary polycythemia, they need not be present in early polycythemia vera. Once it has been established that the apparent increase in red cell mass is absolute and not secondary to a reduced plasma volume, polycythemia secondary to reduced arterial oxygen saturation must be ruled out. A negative family history and normal studies of hemoglobin structure and function will exclude hemoglobinopathy as a cause. Elevated erythropoietin levels must be considered inappropriate in a patient with normal arterial oxygen saturation and hemoglobin function who has not received androgens or cobaltous chloride. Careful studies must then be undertaken to rule out lesions of the kidney, liver, adrenal, brain, or uterus which may elaborate erythropoietin and produce an increase in red cell mass.

Although the presence of frank myelocytic leukemia, either acute or chronic, is easily recognized, a decision as to when polycythemia vera with a markedly elevated leukocyte count becomes transformed into chronic myelocytic leukemia or myelofibrosis may be virtually impossible without special techniques, since young cells of the myelocytic series appear in the peripheral blood in each circumstance. Metabolic differences are demonstrable between the leukocytes in chronic myelocytic leukemia and those seen in polycythemia vera.[176]

These consist of differences in alkaline phosphatase activity, myeloid leukocyte glycogen, and blood histamine. The Philadelphia chromosome (Ph[1]), formerly thought to be diagnostic of chronic myelocytic leukemia, has now been reported in preparations from a small percentage of patients with polycythemia vera, myelofibrosis, granulocytic leukemia, with high leukocyte alkaline phosphatase, and acute myelocytic leukemia.[159] Further studies of the Ph[1] chromosome and its significance in these disorders are needed.[121] Nevertheless, the finding of the Ph[1] chromosome almost invariably means that the patient has chronic myelocytic leukemia.[55]

TREATMENT

At present there is no cure for polycythemia vera. Therapy is directed toward reducing the increased blood volume, increased viscosity, and increased platelet counts. Since it has been recognized for many years that these abnormalities are responsible for the clinical manifestations of the disease, numerous methods of treatment have been introduced. One author lists 24 methods or agents that have been tried.[52] Among these are many that were once considered to be the treatment of choice, such as benzol, Fowler's solution, phenylhydrazine, spray roentgen radiation, roentgen irradiation of the spleen and bones, phlebotomy, and a low iron diet. Some forms of therapy such as splenectomy, thyroidectomy, and oxygen inhalation never enjoyed much popularity because they were impractical, ineffective, and even dangerous. Numerous chemotherapeutic agents have been tried in polycythemia, and some, such as nitrogen mustard, TEM, demecolcin, pyrimethamine, and 6-mercaptopurine, have been found to be inferior to radiophosphorus. Bleeding, radioactive phosphorus, and chemotherapeutic agents are the therapeutic methods used most widely at the present time.

Venesection

Venesection is the oldest form of therapy for polycythemia vera. It is a means of reducing the blood volume promptly, and it often provides prompt symptomatic relief. Because of the development of undesirable symptoms when the blood volume is reduced too rapidly in middle-aged and elderly patients, it is desirable to remove only 500 ml. of blood once or twice a week if the blood volume is to be reduced to normal by this method. If the hematocrit is very high and more frequent bleedings are necessary, the use of plasma expanders[35] or the reinfusion of the patient's separated plasma reduces side-effects and decreases viscosity. Although phlebotomy is an effective means of reducing the red cell mass in these patients, it is not a satisfactory method of treatment when used alone if high platelet levels must be reduced; also, symptoms resulting from a state of chronic iron deficiency may develop.[47]

Radioactive Phosphorus

Radioactive phosphorus, P[32] was introduced as a method of treatment for polycythemia vera by Lawrence in 1938[114] and has many advantages for therapy.

It can be administered orally or intravenously. It has a half-life of 14.3 days, and emits only beta rays which travel less than 0.7 cm. in tissue.[52] It is concentrated in tissues that have a high rate of phosphorus turnover, particularly the bone marrow, liver, spleen, and lymph nodes. In these tissues it produces ionization within the cells and halts cell division. Radioactive phosphorus depresses erythropoiesis, granulocytopoiesis, and platelet production, which results in a reduction of these elements in the circulating blood. Since radioactive phosphorus does not cause any significant increase in the destruction of mature erythrocytes, a significant decrease in the red cell count does not occur for two or three months.

The effectiveness of this form of therapy is indicated by reports of the reduction in the incidence of thromboses in several large series from 14.8 to 27.4 per cent in patients treated with conventional means exclusive of radiation to 2.7 to 4.2 per cent in patients with P^{32}.[189] In another series the incidence of thromboses was 50 per cent in 32 patients treated with other forms of therapy, and less than 5 per cent in 148 patients treated with P^{32}.[172] Comparison of the life expectancy revealed an increase from seven years in patients treated with drugs, phlebotomy, and roentgen ray to 13.3 years in those treated with P^{32}.[116] Splenomegaly and hepatomegaly often respond in a gratifying manner to the latter form of therapy.

Radioactive phosphorus is administered either intravenously or orally.[52] In about one-half of the patients a satisfactory remission follows the initial dose, but 40 per cent require a second treatment and 10 per cent a third.[1, 147, 151] In one series the duration of remissions averaged about 2.5 years, but sometimes they lasted as long as ten years.[52] In another report, the average interval between courses was about 15 months; however, the greatest number of re-treatments occurred in the first six to ten months. After the patient had a satisfactory remission, the interval between treatments increased to about 33 months.[118]

It has been strongly suspected that therapy with P^{32} and other forms of radiation is associated with an increased incidence of leukemia, particularly the acute variety, and other myeloproliferative disorders.[39,133,139,151,161] The evaluation of survival data of retrospective case-control studies of patients with polycythemia vera has been challenged recently. Studies of the effects of P^{32} therapy in this disorder are being carried out.[71,73,120,131,184,185,186]

Chemotherapy

Nitrogen mustard (HN_2), triethylenemelamine (TEM), demecolcin, and pyrimethamine have been used in the treatment of polycythemia vera.[50,52,90] All have a suppressive effect on the marrow, but the short duration of the remissions that occur and the difficulty in avoiding undesired toxic effects on the marrow have prevented their gaining an important place in therapy.

The recent concern over the use of P^{32} has prompted the use of the alkylating agents chlorambucil, cyclophosphamide, and busulfan. All are effective in about 80 per cent of patients, but there is a long latent period during which the patient must be controlled with phlebotomy. Although chlorambucil and cyclophosphamide may be given in maintenance doses, busulfan should be used intermittently, because long-term therapy has been associated with pulmonary fibrosis and other complications.[103,179,185]

Plan of Treatment

In the treatment of polycythemia vera it is important that the patient be kept ambulatory if possible. If the disease is even moderately severe, bed rest is dangerous because of the increased likelihood of thrombosis. For this reason, patients should be treated without hospitalization whenever possible. Because of the tendency both to hemorrhage and thrombosis that exists in polycythemia vera, surgical procedures should be performed only if absolutely necessary. Prior treatment of the polycythemia reduces the likelihood of these complications, but does not prevent them in all cases.[154,187]

A divergence of opinion regarding the preferred therapy of polycythemia vera is evident in a review of the literature and has been emphasized in a symposium on this subject.[60,105] Because of the lack of more definite data concerning the late complications of treatment with radioactive phosphorus, many hematologists treat patients with phlebotomy, or a combination of phlebotomy and busulfan; radioactive phosphorus is employed if satisfactory control is not obtained with other methods. The value of treatment with cytotoxic agents, which may have the same hazards as radioactivity, has not been established.

The National Polycythemia Vera Study Group was organized under the auspices of the National Cancer Institute to determine optimum therapy in polycythemia vera and related disorders such as myelofibrosis and myeloid metaplasia. Only preliminary results have appeared thus far,[105] but these suggest that myelosuppressive agents supplemented by phlebotomy appear to be the treatment of choice for most patients with polycythemia vera. Simple phlebotomy may be most effective for women of childbearing age and those with an inactive form of the disorder without symptoms. If there is any doubt as to the nature of the underlying disorder, neither chemotherapy nor radioactive phosphorus should be used. The results of this very important national study will be awaited with great interest.

The aim of treatment in our clinic is to keep the hematocrit below 50 per cent and the platelet count below 500,000 per cu.mm. Patients are treated initially by phlebotomy, 500 ml. once or twice a week. If the platelet count is over 700,000, if thromboses occur, or if bleeding occurs in association with thrombocythemia, busulfan is used as found necessary to control the platelet count; this often requires three weeks or more, and anticoagulants are used if thrombosis is a problem. When control is established, treatment by phlebotomy or busulfan is given when necessary.

If control is not obtained by the method outlined above, the patient is considered for treatment with radioactive phosphorus. The patient is observed at monthly intervals, and if the hematocrit rises appreciably during this interval a phlebotomy is performed. After remission has been produced, the patient is followed at regular intervals and treatment repeated as necessary.

Should it be established conclusively that radiotherapy does not significantly increase the incidence of leukemia and myelofibrosis, even in younger patients, or that risk of these disorders is small compared to other benefits of the therapy, treatment with radioactive phosphorus would be employed more widely.

The complication of hyperuricemia and high urate excretion secondary to increased nucleoprotein turnover may be effectively treated with the xanthine oxidase inhibitor, allopurinol, while myelosuppression is being effected.

SECONDARY POLYCYTHEMIA
(Erythrocytosis, Erythrocythemia)

A remarkable increase in total red cell mass may occur in any situation which results in tissue hypoxia. Oxygen deprivation leads to an increase in the level of erythropoietin, a humoral substance believed to be primarily responsible for the regulation of erythropoiesis.[54,67,68,152] Although not the sole source, the kidney is the chief site of production or activation of erythropoietin. Erythropoietin appears to mediate the response of the bone marrow to hypoxia by increasing the number of pluri-potential stem cells which become erythroblasts, and by increasing the rate at which they develop their full complement of hemoglobin.[4, 64, 86, 144] (See Chapter 2.)

The increase in red cell mass found in polycythemia vera is not accompanied by any increase in erythropoietin that can be detected by techniques currently available, whereas high levels are found in that which is secondary to hypoxia. In addition, there are forms of erythrocytosis associated with high levels of erythropoietin unrelated to hypoxia or other known stimuli. In secondary polycythemia, the increase in the red cell mass is often accompanied by a decrease in plasma volume; in primary polycythemia vera, the plasma volume is usually normal.[20,70] Excessive elevations of the red blood cell mass may produce sufficient alterations of the viscosity of the blood to cause circulatory embarrassment and increase the danger of thrombosis.[128]

Associated with Known Hypoxic Stimulus

CARDIAC AND VASCULAR MALFORMATIONS

Any cardiac or vascular lesion which results in a high grade venoarterial shunt may produce polycythemia. As the result of the mixing of venous and arterial blood, inadequately oxygenated arterial blood reaches the peripheral tissues. An increase in erythropoietin is thought to occur and to stimulate erythropoiesis. The subsequent polycythemia increases the oxygen-carrying capacity of the blood and affords a measure of relief to the patient.

PULMONARY DISORDERS

Polycythemia occurs in some chronic pulmonary disorders in which it appears to be physiologic response to the decreased arterial oxygen saturation. The commonest pulmonary abnormalities that lead to hypoxemia are:
1. Perfusion of nonaerated or poorly-aerated alveoli;
2. Altered alveolar membrane characteristics interfering with gaseous exchange;
3. Direct pulmonary arteriovenous fistulas.

One end-result of each of these conditions is decreased arterial oxygen saturation which may occur for only a few hours during sleep.[162] In the first instance, the blood flow is through poorly-aerated or nonaerated segments and there is inadequate exposure of the blood to oxygen. In the second instance, the pulmonary segments are well-aerated, but the alveolar membranes have been so altered as to interfere with gaseous exchange between the alveoli and the capillaries. Direct pulmonary arteriovenous fistulas cause anoxia because the blood by-passes vessels in which gaseous exchange takes place.[31] A large reduction in the red cell mass of patients with polycythemia secondary to hypoxic lung disease was achieved by continuous oxygen administration. The effects lasted from six to 15 months.[37]

LOW BAROMETRIC PRESSURE

Persons who reside at high altitude with lowered barometric pressure have a decreased alveolar oxygen tension which leads to incomplete arterial oxygen saturation. The polycythemia which occurs in response to the hypoxia appears to bear a direct relationship to the severity of the oxygen deficit.[89] If an individual is already compromised by lowered barometric pressure, the occurrence of any chronic pulmonary disorder may be catastrophic. Marked polycythemia, severe cyanosis, pulmonary hypertension, and right heart strain may result.[130] Some degree of improvement usually follows removal to sea level.[31,135,162]

ABNORMAL HEMOGLOBINS: METHEMOGLOBINEMIA

A variety of abnormalities in hemoglobin structure or red cell enzyme function result in the persistence of the ferric (Fe^{+++}) state of iron in the hemoglobin molecule. This form of hemoglobin is known as methemoglobin, and is incapable of oxygen transport since it cannot bind oxygen. Methemoglobinemia may occur as an acquired or inherited disorder. The acquired form is the result of exposure to some oxidant which overwhelms the normal intracellular reducing mechanisms and leaves iron in the oxidized state.

Hereditary methemoglobinmeia may arise as the result of autosomal recessive transmission of deficient or abnormal intracellular reducing enzymes, or the occurrence of one of the hemoglobin variants known collectively as *hemoglobin M*. These hemoglobin variants are transmitted as an autosomal dominant and have specific amino acid substitutions in the alpha or beta chain near the site of attachment of the heme group, which facilitates electron transfer and results in persistence of iron in the ferric state.[61, 77]

Polycythemia has been noted in conjunction with methemoglobinemia, but it is inconsistent and not as marked as might be expected from the level of the abnormal pigment.[79,91,98]

Carboxyhemoglobin levels sufficient to cause clinically significant erythrocytosis have been noted in heavy smokers. The condition was reversible with cessation of smoking.[158a]

Table 11–3 *Stable Hemoglobins with Increased Oxygen Affinity*
Associated with Erythrocytosis

HEMOGLOBIN	SUBSTITUTION	REFERENCE
Chesapeake	α 92 Arg → Leu	38
J Capetown	α 92 Arg → Gln	122
*Olympia	β 20 Val → Met	171
*Malmo	β 97 His → Gln	17, 56
Yakima	β 99 Asp → His	97
Kempsey	β 99 Asp → Asn	150
Ypsilanti	β 99 Asp → Tyr	63
*Brigham	β 100 Pro → Leu	124
Rainier	β 145 Tyr → Cys	5, 76
Bethesda	β 145 Tyr → His	29
Hiroshima	β 146 His → Asp	72
*Heathrow	β 103 Phen → Leu	188
*San Diego	β 109 Val → Met	138

*Electrophoretically silent
(Adapted from Lokich, J. J., et al.: Electrophoretically silent. J. Clin. Invest. 52:2060, 1973.)

ABNORMAL OXYGEN DISSOCIATION CURVE

The structural differences between the oxy- and deoxy-confirmation of hemoglobin have been extensively studied by x-ray crystallography.[146] These studies indicate the deoxyhemoglobin A subunits are stabilized by inter- and intra-subunit salt bonds which include residues responsible for the binding of 2-3–DPG and Bohr protons. The hemoglobin subunits change their tertiary structure in response to the binding of oxygen with a step-by-step release of constraints on the unreactive quarternary structure which causes the equilibrium to shift in favor of the reactive oxyhemoglobin form. Each step in the process of change in subunit constraint diminishes the work required to change the teritary structure of the next subunit.[146]

A number of abnormal stable hemoglobins with increased oxygen affinity associated with varying levels of erythrocytosis have been reported. Since several of these hemoglobins are electrophoretically silent, the determination of the oxygen dissociation curve is a necessary part of the study of a patient with secondary polycythemia of obscure origin (Table 11–3).

The variant substitutions in these abnormal hemoglobins are believed to interfere with subunit and ligand interaction and to shift conformational stability in favor of the oxy- form. This could occur as the result of an increase in the stability of the oxy- form, as in the case of hemoglobin San Diego,[9, 138] or a reduction in the stability of the deoxy-form, as in the case of hemoglobin Bethesda.[29] The shift of the dissociation curve to the left results in a reduction of tissue oxygen tension, a hypoxic stimulus, and erythrocytosis.[38, 63]

Associated with Inappropriate Erythropoietin Production

The preceding forms of secondary polycythemia appear to be the result of decreased delivery of oxygen to the tissues, which results in the release of a humoral substance capable of stimulating erythropoiesis. Secondary polycythemia may also occur in conditions in which delivery of oxygen to the tissues is normal and the mechanism is unexplained. Among these are hypernephroma,[59, 82] Wilms' tumor,[163, 174] polycystic kidney disease,[110] hydronephrosis,[43,93,119] renal tuberculosis,[172] cerebellar hemangioblastoma,[40,84] hydrocephalus,[149] ovarian tumors,[66] uterine myomata,[80,85,169,173] pheochromocytoma,[25,180] renal adnoma,[49] hepatic carcinoma,[34,100] and Bartter's syndrome.[53]

Fluid obtained from renal cysts,[156] uterine fibromyomata,[81, 142] a cystic cerebellar hemangioblastoma,[181] and extracts of hypernephroma, Wilms' tumor,[163] and pheochromocytoma tissue[82, 180] have been demonstrated to have erythropoietin activity. However, the erythropoietin activity could not always be correlated with elevated plasma or urine erythropoietin levels, and was not consistently associated with a secondary polycythemia.[156]

The mechanisms by which these lesions may stimulate erythrocytes remain unclear, and their direct association with secondary polycythemia must rest on a return to normal hematologic values following their removal.

Associated with Excess Adrenocortical Steroids or Androgens

Secondary polycythemia may be seen in patients with Cushing's syndrome if they have androgen as well as corticosteroid production. Both androgens and corticosteroids have been used successfully in the treatment of bone marrow failure. The exact mechanism of action of these steroid compounds is unknown, but androgens do exert an effect on renal mass,[127] and an increase in the production of renal erythropoietic factor has been reported.[153] There is an increase in the plasma levels of erythropoietin in experimental animals and in the urinary concentration in humans after administration of androgens.[60, 65, 101] Although there is little evidence to indicate that androgens act directly on the marrow, several metabolites of androgenic steroids have been shown to effect erythroid precursor cells.[136]

BENIGN FAMILIAL POLYCYTHEMIA

Recently the rare syndrome known as benign familial polycythemia or primary erythrocytosis has received further attention. In patients with this syndrome, mostly children, there is an increase in total red cell mass without leukocytosis or thrombocytosis. There may be slight splenomegaly. Reports have emphasized the familial nature of the disorder and its persistence into adult life. Both autosomal dominant and recessive forms have been described.

One dominant form is associated with a functionally abnormal hemoglobin with increased oxygen affinity.[171] A second results from disturbed red cell glycolysis leading to inappropriate 2–3 DPG levels which affect the oxygen affinity of the normal hemoglobin. There remain other dominant forms of familial erythrocytosis with normal oxygen affinity and hemoglobin for which no cause has been detected.[30, 48, 63]

Patients with the recessive form have a markedly elevated hematocrit. The disorder has been found in sibs only, and consanguinity has been noted in some of the reported families.[170] Recent studies of members of two families have revealed excessive erythropoietin production which was independent of the oxygen-carrying capacity of the blood.[6] A defect in the intracellular mechanism of erythropoietin production, rather than the oxygen sensor, was suggested. Others have suggested that abnormal intrarenal blood flow distribution could result in an hypoxic stimulus and elevated erythropoietin levels.[104]

The pathophysiology of this condition has not been clearly defined, and careful studies of these families are indicated.[170]

Despite the usual benign course,[168] some have noted an increased incidence of thromboembolic events. These patients should be followed carefully, and phlebotomy carried out as indicated.[2, 12, 70, 108, 134]

Illustrative Cases

CASE 1

This 53-year-old white housewife enjoyed good health until 12 months prior to admission, when she had a single profuse nosebleed. Six months later she had a fall, and in examining herself to ascertain its effects noted a nontender mass in the left upper quadrant of her abdomen. One month prior to admission she developed dyspnea and ankle edema. Examination by her family physician revealed splenomegaly, and the patient was referred for investigation.

Physical examination. The spleen extended almost to the level of the umbilicus and was moderately firm. The liver was palpable two finger-breadths below the right costal margin. The remainder of the physical examination was noncontributory.

Laboratory studies. Erythrocyte count 5.2 million per cu.mm., hematocrit 47 per cent, leukocyte count 15,000 per cu.mm., reticulocytes 0.2 per cent. Differential count (per cent): myelocytes 1, juvenile 1, bands 10, segmented 79, lymphocytes 4, monocytes 1, eosinophils 3, basophils 1. Platelet count was 426,000 per cu.mm. Bone marrow examination revealed the marrow to be hypercellular with hyperplasia of all cell lines.

It was thought that this patient had either an early polycythemia vera or chronic myelocytic leukemia. Treatment was withheld pending further periodic examinations.

Treatment and course. Six months later the diagnosis of polycythemia vera was evident. She had a very florid complexion; the spleen and liver were unchanged. The hematocrit was 59 per cent, leukocyte count 14,000 per cu.mm., platelets 580,000 per cu.mm. The hematocrit was reduced to 55 per cent after three phlebotomies over the next eight days, and she was given 4.0 millicuries of P[32] orally.

Four months later the hematocrit had risen to 65 per cent, erythrocyte count was 7.3 mil. per cu.mm., and platelets 772,000 per cu.mm. Five hundred ml. of blood was removed by phlebotomy on two occasions to reduce the red cell count, and the patient was given an additional 6.0 millicuries of P^{32} by the oral route. For the next 18 months the hematocrit remained between 48 and 50 per cent, platelets less than 500,000 per cu.mm., and leukocyte count between 9000 and 13,000 per cu.mm., and the spleen edge was at the costal margin. At the end of that period, however, it was found that the hematocrit had risen, and the spleen edge reached the level of the umbilicus. The patient was given another 4 millicuries of P^{32} by the oral route, and four months later the hematocrit was 51 per cent and platelet count 500,000 per cu.mm.

Two and one-half years after the third dose of P^{32} the hematocrit had risen to 58, erythrocyte count had risen to 7.4 mil. per cu.mm., platelets were 1,200,000 per cu.mm., and the spleen had once again increased in size. At this juncture it was decided to institute therapy with busulfan. Phlebotomy once again reduced the hematocrit, and the administration of busulfan 2 mg. twice a day was initiated. The levels of the cellular elements in the peripheral blood were followed at weekly intervals and were satisfactory. After 50 days the busulfan was stopped, and three months later the hematocrit was 46 per cent, platelet count 300,000, and leukocyte count 9800 per cu.mm. The spleen was still at the level of the umbilicus.

Comments. As is true of the majority of patients with polycythemia vera, this patient's initial symptoms appeared in middle age. The evidence of increased red blood cell mass, the presence of a markedly enlarged spleen, and generalized marrow hyperplasia suggested the possibility of chronic myelogenous leukemia or polycythemia vera. The diagnosis could not be made with certainty on the initial visit. The first remission required 10 millicuries of P^{32} and lasted 18 months. Following the administration of an additional 4 millicuries of P^{32}, the hematocrit returned to normal levels, and the patient remained free of symptoms for 36 months longer despite the fact that her platelet count was not adequately controlled. When the hematocrit values once again rose to abnormal levels, it was decided to use the chemotherapeutic agent busulfan in an attempt to obtain a satisfactory reduction of erythrocytes, leukocytes, and platelets. This was successful. This patient's course has now extended over 12 years, during which time she has had no complications and has lived a normal life.

CASE 2

A 69-year-old white housewife with known diabetes mellitus of 15 years' duration was admitted with a history of passing tarry stools for four days. The most significant abnormalities on physical examination were splenomegaly and hepatomegaly. On this admission the hemoglobin was 7.5 gm. per 100 ml., erythrocyte count was 2.8 million per cu.mm., and the leukocyte count was 22,000 per cu.mm. Differential count (per cent): myelocytes 1, juvenile 1, bands 3, segmented 58, lymphocytes 15, monocytes 21, eosinophils 1. No nucleated red cells were seen. Occult blood was present in the stool, but barium studies of the entire gastrointestinal tract revealed no intrinsic lesion. The sternal marrow was markedly hypercellular and the myeloid-erythroid ratio was 3:1.

It was thought that the patient probably had chronic myelocytic leukemia with gastrointestinal hemorrhage. She was treated with blood transfusions and had a satisfactory response. Follow-up examinations for several months revealed normal hemoglobin and red count values, leukocyte counts of about 17,000 per cu.mm., and a differential count similar to that noted in the hospital. Six months later the patient again had a severe gastrointestinal hemorrhage with melena and hematemesis. Following this episode the hemoglobin was 10.5 gm. per 100 ml., red count 3.3 million per cu.mm., and leukocyte count 36,000 per cu.mm.

After recovery from this hemorrhage the red count rose to 6.3 million and hemoglobin to 17 to 18 gm., and it was apparent that the diagnosis of polycythemia vera was the correct one. Her leukocyte count varied from 12,000 to 36,000 per cu.mm. Because of the discomfort from the size of the spleen, she received several courses of roentgen therapy over the spleen which resulted in a reduction of the splenic size as well as reduction in the leukocytes, hematocrit, and red cell count.

When she was 73 years of age, she had angina pectoris and intermittent claudication. During the next five years the erythrocyte cell count rose to 7.7 mil. per cu.mm. on several occasions, and phlebotomies were performed as indicated. She fell and suffered an intertrochanteric fracture of the hip. During the operation to pin the fracture there was considerable bleeding; two days later a cerebral vascular accident occurred. The patient improved slowly and returned home. Six months later the patient's hematocrit was 45 per cent, and erythrocyte count 4.7 mil. per cu.mm., but the leukocyte count had risen to 102,000 per cu.mm. Differential count (per cent): myelocytes 5, juveniles 8, bands 7, segmented 70, monocytes 8, eosinophils 1. It was the clinical impression that the patient had developed leukemia. Three weeks later the patient was admitted to the hospital after an episode of mental confusion followed by unconsciousness. She remained unconscious and died a few hours after admission. Death was attributed to an intracranial hemorrhage.

Autopsy showed extensive intracranial hemorrhage. There was evidence of old infarction of the myocardium and generalized arteriosclerosis. Marked splenomegaly and hepatomegaly were present. Microscopic examination of the liver, spleen, and bone marrow disclosed chronic myelocytic leukemia.

Comment.   The patient died at the age of 78, some ten years after the onset of her symptoms. Earlier in her illness she was thought to have myelocytic leukemia, rather than polycythemia vera, because the hematologic values were obtained after a massive gastrointestinal hemorrhage. Later in her course the diagnosis of polycythemia vera appeared to be well-established. Subsequently the patient had many complications of this disease, such as angina pectoris, intermittent claudication, cerebral thrombosis, and postoperative bleeding. Her final episode was an intracranial hemorrhage. As is often the case, it was difficult to determine whether these episodes were due to her blood dyscrasia or to the diabetes mellitus and arteriosclerosis which were present. It appeared likely, however, that the blood dyscrasia was a factor. The incidence of complications of this type has been reduced by treatment with radioactive phosphorus, and had this agent been used the course of her illness might have been altered. Late in her course this patient also developed chronic myelocytic leukemia which was evident at autopsy. This development illustrates the unsettled problem of the relationship between polycythemia vera and myelocytic leukemia, and the important question as to whether there is any relationship between radiation therapy of polycythemia and the development of the leukemia.

References

1. Abbatt, J. D., Chaplin, H., Darte, J. M. M., and Pitney, W. R.: Treatment of polycythaemia vera with radiophosphorus: haemological studies and preliminary clinical assessment. Q. J. Med., 23:91, 1954.

2. Abildgaard, C. F., Cornet, J. A., and Schulman, I.: Primary erythrocytosis. J. Pediatr., 63: 1072, 1964.

3. Abraham, J. P., Ulutin, O. N., Johnson, S. A., and Caldwell, M. J.: A study of the defects in the blood coagulation mechanisms in polycythemia vera. Am. J. Clin. Pathol., 36:7, 1961.

4. Adamson, J. W., and Finch, C. A.: Erythropoietin and the polycythemias. Ann. N.Y. Acad. Sci., 149:560, 1968.

5. Adamson, J. W., Parer, J. T., and Stamatoyannopoulos, G.: Erythrocytosis associated with hemoglobin Rainier: oxygen equilibria and marrow regulation. J. Clin. Invest., 48:1376, 1969.

6. Adamson, J. W., Stamatoyannopoulos, G., Kontras, S., and Lascari, A.: Recessive familial erythrocytosis: aspects of marrow regulation in two families. Blood, 41:641, 1973.

7. Alexanian, R.: Erythropoietin and erythropoiesis in anemic man following androgens. Blood, 33:564, 1969.

8. Altschule, M. D., Volk, M. C., and Henstell, H.: Cardiac and respiratory function at rest in patients with uncomplicated polycythemia vera. Am. J. Med. Sci., 200:478, 1940.

9. Anderson, N. L.: Hemoglobin San Diego (B109[G11]Val→Met) crystal structure of the deoxy form. J. Clin. Invest., 53:329, 1974.

10. Anstey, L., Kemp, N. H., Stafford, J. L., and Tanner, R. K.: Leukocyte alkaline-phosphatase activity in polycythaemia rubra vera. Br. J. Haematol., 9:91, 1963.

11. Ascher, K. W.: Eye manifestation in polycythemia. J.A.M.A., 215:295, 1971.

12. Auerback, M. L., Wolff, J. A., and Mettier, S. R.: Benign familial polycythemia in childhood. Pediatrics., 21:54, 1958.

13. Bader, R. A., Bader, M. E., and Duberstein, J. L.: Polycythemia vera and arterial oxygen saturation. Am. J. Med., 34:435, 1963.

14. Barabas, A. P., Offen, D. N., and Meinhard, E. A.: The arterial complications of polycythemia vera. Br. J. Surg., 60:183, 1973.

15. Bartos, H. R., and Desforges, J. F.: Erythrocyte enzymes in polycythemia vera. Blood, 29:916, 1967.

16. Baxandall, J. D.: Primary erythrocytosis and pregnancy. J. Obstet. Gynaecol. Br. Commonw., 80:996, 1973.

17. Berglund, S.: The oxygen dissociation curve of whole blood containing hemoglobin Malmö. Scand. J. Haematol., 9:377, 1972.

18. Berk, L., Burchenal, J. H., Wood, T., and Castle, W. B.: Oxygen saturation of sternal marrow blood with special reference to the pathogenesis of polycythemia vera. Proc. Soc. Exp. Biol. Med., 69:316, 1948.

19. Berlin, N. L., Lawrence, J. H., and Gartland, J.: Blood volume in polycythemia as determined by P^{32} labeled red blood cells. Am. J. Med., 9:747, 1950.

20. Berlin, N. I., Lawrence, J. H., and Lee, H. C.: The life span of the red blood cell in chronic leukemia and polycythemia. Science, 114:385, 1951.

21. Beutler, E., Lang, A., and Lehmann, H.: Hemoglobin Duarte: ($\alpha_2\beta_2^{62(E6) Ala \rightarrow Pro}$): a new unstable hemoglobin with increased oxygen affinity. Blood, 43:527, 1974.

22. Bjorkman, S. E., Laurell, C-B., and Nilsson, I. M.: Serum proteins and fibrinolysis in polycythemia vera. Scand. J. Clin. Lab. Invest., 8:304, 1956.

23. Block, M., and Bethard, W. F.: Bone marrow studies in polycythemia. J. Clin. Invest., 31:618, 1952.

24. Blum, A. S., and Zbar, M. J.: Relative polycythemia. Arch. Intern. Med., 104:385, 1959.

25. Bradley, J. E., Young, J. D., Jr., and Lentz, G.: Polycythemia secondary to pheochromocytoma. J. Urol., 86:1, 1961.

26. Brodsky, I.: The use of ferrokinetics in the evaluation of busulphan therapy in polycythemia vera. Br. J. Haematol., 10:291, 1964.

27. Brodsky, I., Kahn, S. B., and Brady, L. W.: Polycythemia vera: differential diagnosis by ferrokinetic studies and treatment with busulphan (Myleran). Br. J. Haematol., 14:351, 1968.

28. Brown, S. M., Gilbert, H. S., Krauss, S., and Wasserman, L. R.: Spurious (relative) polycythemia: a non-existent disease. Am. J. Med., 50:200, 1971.

29. Bunn, H. F., Bradley, T. B., Davis, W. E., Drysdale, J. W., Burke, J. F., Beck, W. S., and Laver, M. D.: Structural and functional studies on hemoglobin bethesda ($\alpha_2\beta_2^{145His}$), a variant associated with compensatory erythrocytosis. J. Clin. Invest., 51:2299, 1972.

30. Bunn, H. F., and Jandl, J. H.: Control of hemoglobin function within the red cell. N. Engl. J. Med., *282*:1414, 1970.
31. Burchell, H. B., and Clagett, O. T.: The clinical syndrome associated with pulmonary arteriovenous fistulas, including a case report of a surgical cure. Am. Heart J., *34*:151, 1947.
32. Burgess, J. H., and Bishop, J. M.: Pulmonary diffusing capacity and its subdivisions in polycythemia vera. J. Clin. Invest., *42*:997, 1963.
33. Cabot, R. C.: A case of chronic cyanosis without discoverable cause ending in cerebral hemorrhage. Boston Med. Surg. J., *141*:574, 1899.
34. Cannon, P., and Penington, D. C.: Erythropoietin and hepatoma. Lancet, *2*:1276, 1967.
35. Castle, W. B., and Jandl, J. H.: Blood viscosity and blood volume: opposing influence upon oxygen transport in polycythemia. Semin. Hematol., *3*:193, 1966.
36. Centrone, A. L., Freda, R. N., and McGowan, L.: Polycythemia rubra vera in pregnancy. Obstet. Gynecol., *30*:657, 1967.
37. Chamberlain, D. A., and Millard, F. J. C.: The treatment of polycythemia secondary to hypoxic lung disease by continuous oxygen administration. Q. J. Med., *32*:341, 1963.
38. Charache, S., Weatherall, D. J., and Clegg, J. B.: Polycythemia associated with a hemoglobinopathy. J. Clin. Invest., *45*:813, 1966.
39. Chievitz, E., and Thiede, T.: Complications and causes of death in polycythemia vera. Acta Med. Scand., *172*:513, 1962.
40. Clinicopathologic Conference: Polycythemia and neoplastic disease. Am. J. Med., *33*:942, 1962.
41. Cobb, L. A., Kramer, R. J., and Finch, C. A.: Circulatory effects of chronic hypervolemia in polycythemia vera. J. Clin. Invest., *39*:1722, 1960.
42. Contopoulos, A. N., McCombs, R., Lawrence, J. H., and Simpson, M. E.: Erythropoietic activity in the plasma of patients with polycythemia vera and secondary polycythemia. Blood, *12*:614, 1957.
43. Cooper, W. M., and Tuttle, W. B.: Polycythemia associated with a benign kidney lesion: report of a case of erythrocytosis with hydronephrosis with remission of polycythemia following nephrectomy. Ann. Intern. Med., *47*:1008, 1957.
44. Dameshek, W.: Some observations on polycythemia vera. Bull. N. Engl. Med. Center., *16*:53, 1954.
45. Dameshek, W., and Henstell, H. H.: The diagnosis of polycythemia. Ann. Intern. Med., *13*:1360, 1940.
46. Damon, A., and Holub, D. A.: Host factors in polycythemia vera. Ann. Intern. Med., *49*:43, 1958.
47. DeGowin, R. L., and Gurney, C. W.: Hemopoiesis in polycythemia vera after phlebotomy and iron therapy. Arch. Intern. Med., *114*:424, 1964.
48. Delivoria-Papadopoulos, M., Oski, F. A., and Gottlieb, A. J.: Oxygen-Hemoglobulin dissociation curves: effect of inherited enzyme defects of the red cell. Science, *165*:601, 1969.
49. DeMarsh, Q. B., and Warmington, W. J.: Polycythemia associated with a renal tumor. N. W. Med., *54*:976, 1955.
50. Ellison, R. R., Ginsberg, V., and Watson, J.: Triethylene melamine in polycythemia vera. Cancer, *6*:327, 1953.
51. Emery, A. C., Jr., Whitcomb, W. H., and Frohlich, E. D.: "Stress" polycythemia and hypertension. J.A.M.A., *229*:159, 1974.
52. Erf, L. A.: Radioactive Phosphorus in the Treatment of Primary Polycythemia (Vera). *In* Tocantins, L. M.: Progress in Hematology. Vol. 1. Grune & Stratton, New York, 1956, p. 153.
53. Erkelens, D. W., and Van Eps, L. W.: Bartter's syndrome and erythrocytosis. Am. J. Med., *55*:711, 1973.
54. Erslev, A.: Humoral regulation of red cell production. Blood, *8*:349, 1953.
55. Ezdinli, E. Z., Sokal, J. E., Crosswhite, L., and Sandberg, A. A.: Philadelphia chromosome—positive and negative—chronic myelocytic leukemia. Ann. Intern. Med., *72*:175, 1970.
56. Fairbanks, V. F., Maldanado, J. E., Charache, S., and Boyer, S. H.: Familial erythrocytosis due to electrophoretically undetectable hemoglobin with impaired oxygen dissociation (hemoglobin Malmö $\alpha_2\beta_2$ 97Gln). Mayo Clin. Proc., *46*:721, 1971.
57. Fessell, W. J.: Odd men out. Arch. Intern. Med., *115*:736, 1965.
58. Fisher, J. M., Bedell, G. N., and Seebohm, P. M.: Differentiation of polycythemia vera and secondary polycythemia by arterial oxygen saturation and pulmonary function tests. J. Lab. Clin. Med., *50*:455, 1957.
59. Forssell, J.: Polycythemia and hypernephroma. Acta Med. Scand., *150*:155, 1954.
60. Gardner, F. H.: Polycythemia (conclusion). Semin. Hematol., *3*:232, 1966.
61. Gerald, P. S., and Efron, M. L.: Chemical studies of several varieties of Hb. M. Proc. Natl. Acad. Sci. U.S.A., *47*:1758, 1961.
62. Gilbert, H. S., Krauss, S., Pasternack, B., Herbert, V., and Wasserman, L. R.: Serum vit. B_{12}

content and unsaturated vit. B_{12}-binding capacity in myeloproliferative disease. Ann. Intern. Med., *71*:719, 1969.

63. Glynn, K. P., Penner, J. A., Smith, J. R., and Rucknagel, D. L.: Familial erythrocytosis: a description of three families, one with hemoglobin Ypsilanti. Ann. Intern. Med., *69*:769, 1968.

64. Gordon, A. S., Cooper, G. W., and Zanjani, E. D.: The kidney and erythropoiesis. Semin. Hematol., *4*:337, 1967.

65. Gordon, A. S., Mirand, E. A., Weinig, J., Katz, R., and Zanjani, E. D.: Androgen actions on erythropoiesis. Ann. N.Y. Acad. Sci., *149*:318, 1968.

66. Gottschalk, R. G., and Furth, J.: Polyerythemia with features of Cushing's syndrome produced by luteomas. Acta Haematol., *5*:100, 1951.

67. Grant, W. C., and Root, W. S.: Fundamental stimulus for erythropoiesis. Physiol. Rev., *32*:449, 1952.

68. Gurney, C. W., Goldwasser, E., and Pan, C.: Studies on erythropoiesis. VI. Erythropoietin in human plasma. J. Lab. Clin. Med., *50*:534, 1957.

69. Hall, C. A.: Gaisböch's disease. Redefinition of an old syndrome. Arch. Intern. Med., *116*: 4, 1965.

70. Hallock, P.: Polycythemia of morbus caeruleus (cyanotic type of congenital heart disease). Proc. Soc. Exp. Biol. Med., *44*:11, 1940.

71. Halnan, K. E., and Russell, M. H.: Polycythemia vera. Comparison of survival and causes of death in patients managed with and without radiotherapy. Lancet, 2:760, 1965.

72. Hamilton, H. B., Iuchi, I., Miyaji, T., and Shibata, S.: Hemoglobin Hiroshima (β143 Histidine $\rightarrow$ aspartic acid): a newly identified fast-moving beta chain variant associated with increased oxygen affinity and compensatory erythremia. J. Clin. Invest., *48*:525, 1969.

73. Harman, J. B., Ledlie, E. M.: Survival of polycythemia vera patients treated with radioactive phosphorus. Br. Med. J., 2:146, 1967.

74. Harris, R. E., and Conrad, F. G.: Polycythemia vera in the childbearing age. Arch. Intern. Med., *120*:697, 1967.

75. Harrop, G. A., Jr.: Polycythemia. Medicine, 7:291, 1928.

76. Hayashi, A., Stamatoyannopoulos, G., Yoshida, A., and Adamson, J.: Haemoglobin Rainier: β145 (HC2) tyrosine $\rightarrow$ cysteine and haemoglobin Bethesda: β145 (HC2) tyrosine $\rightarrow$ histidine. Nature. New Biol., *230*:264, 1971.

77. Heller, P.: Hemoglobinopathic dysfunction of the red cell. Am. J. Med., *41*:799, 1966.

78. Heller, P., Coleman, R. D., and Yakulis, V.: Hemoglobin M Hyde Park: a new variant of abnormal methemoglobin. J. Clin. Invest., *45*:1021, 1966.

79. Heller, P., Weinstein, H. G., Yakulis, V. J., and Rosenthal, I. M.: Hemoglobin M. Kankakee: a new variant of hemoglobin M. Blood, *20*:287, 1962.

80. Hertko, E. J.: Polycythemia (erythrocytosis), associated uterine fibroids and apparent surgical cure. Am. J. Med., *34*:288, 1963.

81. Hertko, E. J.: Polycythemia (erythrocytosis) associated with uterine fibroids: a case report with erythropoietic activity demonstrated in the tumor. Ann. Intern. Med., *68*:1169, 1968. (Abstr.)

82. Hewlett, J. S., Hoffman, G. C., Senhauser, D. A., and Battle, J. D., Jr.: Hypernephroma with erythrocythemia. Report of a case and assay of the tumor for an erythropoietic-stimulating substance. N. Engl. J. Med., *262*:1058, 1960.

83. Hochman, A., and Stein, J. A.: Polycythemia and pregnancy. Report of a case. Obstet. Gynecol., *18*:230, 1958.

84. Holmes, C. R., Kredel, F. E., and Hanna, C. B.: Polycythemia secondary to brain tumor. South. Med. J., *45*:967, 1952.

85. Horwitz, A., and McKelway, W. P.: Polycythemia associated with uterine myomas. J.A.M.A., *158*:1360, 1955.

86. Huff, R. L., Elmlinger, P. J., Garcia, J. F., Oda, J. M., Cockrell, M. C., and Lawrence, J. H.: Ferrokinetics in normal persons and in patients having various erythropoietic disorders. J. Clin. Invest., *30*:1512, 1951.

87. Huff, R. L., Hennessy, T. G., Austin, R. E., Garcia, J. F., Roberts, B. M. and Lawrence, J. H.: Plasma and red cell iron turnover in normal subjects and in patients having various hematopoietic disorders. J. Clin. Invest., *29*:1041, 1950.

88. Huff, R. L., and Feller, D. D.: Relation of circulating red cell volume to body density and obesity. J. Clin. Invest., *35*:1, 1956.

89. Hurtado, A., Merino, C., and Delgado, E.: Influence of anoxemia on the hematopoietic activity. Arch. Intern. Med., *75*:284, 1945.

90. Isaacs, R.: Treatment of polycythemia vera with Daraprim. J.A.M.A., *156*:1491, 1954.

91. Jaffe, E. R.: Hereditary methemoglobinemias associated with abnormalities in the metabolism of erythrocytes. Am. J. Med., *41*:786, 1966.

92. Jandl, J. H., Davidson, C. S., Abelmann, W. H., and MacDonald, R. A.: Hemochromatosis terminating in polycythemia and hepatoma with observations on the natural history of hemochromatosis. N. Engl. J. Med., 269:1054, 1963.
93. Jaworski, Z. F., and Wolan, C. T.: Hydronephrosis and polycythemia. A case of erythrocytosis relieved by decompression of unilateral hydronephrosis and cured by nephrectomy. Am. J. Med., 34:523, 1963.
94. Jepson, J. H.: Polycythemia: diagnosis pathophysiology and therapy. Can. Med. Assoc. J., 100:271, 327, 1969.
95. Jones, N. F., Payne, R. W., Hyde, R. D., and Price, T. M. L.: Renal polycythemia. Lancet, 1:299, 1960.
96. Jones, R. T., Brimhall, B., Huisman, T. H. J., Kleihauer, E., and Betke, K.: Hemoglobin Freiburg: abnormal hemoglobin due to deletion of a single amino acid residue. Science, 154:1024, 1966.
97. Jones, R. T., Osgood, E. E., Brimhall, B., and Koler, R. D.: Hemoglobin Yakima. I. Clinical and biochemical studies. J. Clin. Invest., 46:1840, 1967.
98. Josephson, A. M., Weinstein, H. G., Yakulis, V. J., Singer, L., and Heller, P.: A new variant of hemoglobin M disease: hemoglobin M Chicago. J. Lab. Clin. Med., 59:918, 1962.
99. Kaung, D. T., and Peterson, R. E.: "Relative polycythemia" or "pseudopolycythemia." Arch. Intern. Med., 110:456, 1962.
100. Keighley, G., Hammond, D., and Lowy, P. H.: The sustained action of erythropoietin injected repeatedly into rats and mice. Blood, 23:99, 1964.
101. Kennedy, B. J., and Gilbertsen, A. S.: Increased erythropoiesis induced by androgenic-hormone therayp. N. Engl. J. Med., 256:719, 1957.
102. Kiely, J. M., Stroebel, C. F., Hanlon, D. G., and Owen, C. A., Jr.: Clinical value of plasma iron turnover rate in diagnosis and management of polycythemia. J. Nucl. Med., 2:1, 1961.
103. Killmann, S. A., and Cronkite, E. P.: Treatment of polycythemia vera with Myleran. Am. J. Med. Sci., 241:218, 1961.
104. Kisker, C. T., and Kleinman, L. I.: Primary benign erythrocytosis and abnormal renal perfusion. Lancet, 1:1162, 1972.
105. Klein, H., and Wasserman, L. R. (eds.): Polycythemia Theory and Management. Charles C Thomas, Springfield, Ill. 1973. Pub. #872 p. 238. Epilogue.
106. Klein, F., Farber, S., Freeman, G., and Fiorentino, R.: The effects of varying concentrations of human platelets and their stored derivatives on the recalcification time of plasma. Blood, 11:910, 1956.
107. Klemperer, P.: Reticuloentheliosis. Bull. N.Y. Acad. Med., 30:526, 1954.
108. Knock, H. L., and Githens, J. H.: Primary erythrocytosis of childhood. Am. J. Dis. Child., 100: 189, 1960.
109. Kurnick, J. E., Ward, H. P., and Block, M. H.: Bone marrow sections in the differential diagnosis of polycythemia. Arch. Pathol., 94:489, 1972.
110. Kurrle, G. R.: A case of Gaisböck's disease (polycythaemia hypertonica). M. J. Aust., 1:777, 1954.
111. Krantz, S. B.: Application of the in vitro erythropoietin system to the study of human bone marrow disease: polycythemia vera. Ann. N.Y. Acad. Sci., 149:430, 1968.
112. Kwaan, H. C., and Suwanwela, N.: Inhibitors of fibrinolysis in platelets in polycythaemia vera and thrombocytosis. Br. J. Haematol., 21:313, 1971.
113. Labie, D., Lerous, J.-P., Najman, A., and Reyrolle, C.: Familial Diphophoglycerate mutase deficiency. Influence on the oxygen affinity curves of hemoglobin. FEBS, letters, 9:37, 1970.
114. Lawrence, J. H.: Nuclear physics and therapy: preliminary report on a new method for the treatment of leukemia and polycythemia. Radiology, 35:51, 1940.
115. Lawrence, J. H.: The control of polycythemia by marrow inhibition. J.A.M.A., 141:13, 1949.
116. Lawrence, J. H.: Polycythemia: physiology, diagnosis, and treatment based on 303 cases. Grune & Stratton, New York, 1955.
117. Lawrence, J. H., and Berlin, N. I.: Relative polycythemia—polycythemia of stress. Yale J. Biol. Med., 24:498, 1952.
118. Lawrence, J. H., Berlin, N. I., and Huff, R. L.: The nature and treatment of polycythemia vera. Medicine, 32:323, 1953.
119. Lawrence, J. H., and Donald, W. G., Jr.: Polycythemia and hydronephrosis or renal tumors. Ann. Intern. Med., 50:959, 1959.
120. Lawrence, J. H., Winchell, H. S., and Donald, W. G.: Leukemia in polycythemia vera. Ann. Intern. Med., 70:763, 1969.
121. Levin, W. C., Houston, E. W., and Ritzmann, S. E.: Polycythemia vera with Ph[1] chromosomes in two brothers. Blood, 30:503, 1967.
122. Lines, J. G., and McIntosh, R.: Oxygen binding by hemoglobin J. Capetown ($\alpha_2$92 Arg $\rightarrow$ Gln). Nature, 215:297, 1967.

123. Linman, J. W., Bethell, F. H., and Long, M. J.: Studies on the nature of the plasma erythropoietic factor(s). J. Lab. Clin. Med., *51*:8, 1958.
124. Lokich, J. J., Moloney, W. C., Bunn, H. F., Bruckheimer, S. M., and Ranney, H. M.: Hemoglobin Brigham ($\alpha_2{}^A\beta_2{}^{100\text{Pro}\to\text{Leu}}$). J. Clin. Invest., *52*:2060, 1973.
125. London, I. M., Shemin, D., West, R., and Rittenberg, D.: Heme synthesis and red blood cell dynamics in normal humans and in subjects with polycythemia vera, sickle cell anemia and pernicious anemia. J. Biol. Chem., *179*:463, 1949.
126. Lynch, E. C.: Uric acid metabolism in proliferative diseases of the marrow. Arch. Intern. Med., *109*:639, 1962.
127. Mann, D. L., Donati, R. M., and Gallagher, N. L.: Relationship of Renal Mass to Erythropoietin Production. Lab. Invest., *19*:406, 1968.
128. Martin, W. J., and Bayrd, E. D.: Erythroleukemia, with special emphasis on the acute or incomplete variety. Blood, *9*:321, 1954.
129. Mauer, A. M., and Jarrold, T.: Granulocyte kinetic studies in patients with proliferative disorders of the bone marrow. Blood, *22*:125, 1963.
130. Mendlowitz, M.: The effect of anemia and polycythemia on digital intravascular blood viscosity. J. Clin. Invest., *27*:565, 1948.
131. Modan, B.: Computing survival in long-term disease. J.A.M.A., *192*:609, 1965.
132. Modan, B.: Polycythemia: a review of epidemiological and clinical aspects. J. Chron. Dis., *18*:605, 1965.
133. Modan, B., and Lilienfeld, A. M.: Leukemogenic effect of ionising-irradiation treatment in polycythemia. Lancet, *2*:439, 1964.
134. Modan, B., and Modan, M.: Benign erythrocytosis. Br. J. Haematol., *14*:375, 1968.
135. Monge, C.: High altitude disease. Arch. Intern. Med., *59*:32, 1937.
136. Necheles, T. F., and Rai, U. S.: Studies on the control of hemoglobin synthesis: the in vitro stimulating effect of a 5-β-H steroid metabolite on heme formation in human bone marrow cells. Blood, *34*:380, 1969.
137. Niewiarowski, S., Zywicka, H., and Latallo, Z.: Coagulation disorders in thrombocythaemia; a study of seven cases. Thromb. Diath. Haemorrh., *7*:114, 1962.
138. Nute, P. E., Stamatoyannopoulos, G., Hermodson, M. A., and Roth, D.: Hemoglobinopathic erythrocytosis due to a new electrophoretically silent variant hemoglobin San Diego (beta 109 [G11] val $\to$ met). J. Clin. Invest., *53*:320, 1974.
139. Osgood, E. E.: Contrasting incidence of acute monocytic and granulocytic leukemias in P^{32} treated patients with polycythemia vera and chronic lymphocytic leukemia. J. Lab. Clin. Med., *64*:560, 1964.
140. Osler, W.: Chronic cyanosis, with polycythemia and enlarged spleen: a new clinical entity. Am. J. Med. Sci., *126*:187, 1903.
141. Osler, W.: A clinical lecture on erythraemia. Lancet, *1*:143, 1908.
142. Ossias, A. L., Zanjani, E. D., Zalusky, R., Solomon, E., and Wasserman, L. R.: Case report: studies on the mechanism of erythrocytosis associated with a uterine fibromyoma. Br. J. Haematol., *25*:179, 1973.
143. Penington, D. G.: Red-cell regulators. Letter to editor. Lancet, *1*:975, 1960.
144. Penington, D. G.: The relation of erythropoietin to polycythemia. Proc. Roy. Soc. Med., *59*:1091, 1966.
145. Personal observation.
146. Perutz, M. F.: Stereochemistry of cooperative effects in haemoglobin. Nature, *228*:726, 1970.
147. Pike, G. M.: Polycythemia vera. N. Engl. J. Med., *258*:1250, 1297, 1958.
148. Pollycove, M., Winchell, H. S., and Lawrence, J. H.: Classification and evolution of patterns of erythropoiesis in polycythemia vera as studied by iron kinetics. Blood, *28*:807, 1966.
149. Primrose, D. A.: Polycythemia in association with hydrocephalus. Lancet, *2*:1111, 1952.
150. Reed, C. S., Hampson, R., Gordon, S., Jones, R. T., Novy, M. J., Brimhall, B., Edwards, M. J., and Koler, R. D.: Erythrocytosis secondary to increased oxygen affinity of a mutant hemoglobin, hemoglobin Kempsey. Blood, *31*:623, 1968.
151. Reinhard, E. H., and Hahneman, B.: The treatment of polycythemia vera. J. Chron. Dis., *6*:332, 1957.
152. Reissmann, K. R.: Studies on the mechanism of erythropoietic stimulation in parabiotic rats during hypoxia. Blood, *5*:372, 1950.
153. Rencricca, H. J., Solomon, J., Fimian, W. J., Jr., Howard, D., Rizzoli, V., and Stohlman, F., Jr.: The effect of testosterone on erythropoiesis. Scand. J. Haematol., *6*:431, 1969.
153a. Retzlaff, J. A., Tauxe, N., Kiely, J. M., and Strobel, C. F.: Erythrocyte volume, plasma volume, and lean body mass in adult men and women. Blood, *33*:649, 1969.
154. Rigby, P. G., and Leavell, B. S.: Polycythemia vera. A review of fifty cases with emphasis on the risk of surgery. Arch. Intern. Med., *106*:622, 1960.
155. Rosenthal, N., and Bassen, F. A.: Course of polycythemia. Arch. Intern. Med., *62*:903, 1938.

156. Rosse, W. F., Waldmann, T. A., and Cohen, P.: Renal cysts, erythropoietin and polycythemia. Am. J. Med., 34:76, 1963.
157. Ruch, W. A., and Klein, R. L.: Polycythemia and pregnancy. Obstet. Gynecol., 23:107, 1964.
158. Russel, R. P., and Conley, C. L.: Benign polycythemia: Gaisböck's syndrome. Arch. Intern. Med., 114:734, 1964.
158a. Sagone, A. L., Jr., and Balcerzak, S. P.: Smoking as a cause of erythrocytosis. Ann. Intern. Med., 82:512, 1975.
159. Sandberg, A. A., Ishihara, T., Crosswhite, L. H., and Hauschka, T. S.: Comparison of chromosome constitution in chronic myelocytic leukemia and other myeloproliferative disorders. Blood, 20:393, 1962.
160. Schwartz, B. M., and Stats, D.: Oxygen saturation of sternal marrow blood in polycythemia vera. J. Clin. Invest., 28:736, 1949.
161. Schwartz, S. O., and Ehrlich, L.: The relationship of polycythemia vera to leukemia; a critical review. Acta Haematol., 4:129, 1950.
162. Selzer, A.: Chronic cyanosis. Am. J. Med., 10:334, 1951.
163. Shalet, M.F., Holder, T. M., and Walters, T. R.: Erythropoietin-producing Wilms' Tumor. J. Pediatr., 70:615, 1967.
164. Shullenberger, C. C.: Long-range treatment of polycythemia vera with 6-mercaptopurine. Cancer Chemother. Rep., 16:251, 1962.
165. Silverstein, A., Gilbert, H., and Wasserman, L. R.: Neurologic complications of polycythemia. Ann. Intern. Med., 57:909, 1962.
166. Smith, J. F. B., and Lucie, N. P.: Alcohol—a cause of stress erythrocytosis? Lancet, 1:637, 1973.
167. Smith, J. R., and Kay, N. E.: Polycythemia-1973. Laboratory and clinical evaluation. Postgrad. Med., 54:141, 1973.
168. Smith, L. F., Jr., and Battle, J. D., Jr.: Benign familial erythrocytosis. A 24-year study. Clin. Res., 14:436, 1966.
169. Spurlin, G. W., Van Nagell, J. R., Jr., Parker, J. C., Jr., and Roddick, J. W., Jr.: Uterine myomas and erythrocytosis. Obstet. Gynecol., 40:646, 1972.
170. Stamatoyannopoulos, G.: Familial Erythrocytosis. Blood. Birth Defects. Orignial Article Series, 8:39, 1972.
171. Stamatoyannopoulos, G., Nute, P. E., Adamson, J. W., Bellingham, A. J., and Funk, D.: Hemoglobin Olympia (B20 Valine → Methionine): an electrophoretically silent variant associated with high oxygen affinity and erythrocytosis. J. Clin. Invest., 52:342, 1973.
172. Stroebel, C. F., Hall, B. E., and Pease, G. L.: Evaluation of radiophosphorus therapy in primary polycythemia, J.A.M.A., 146:1301, 1951.
173. Thompson, A. P., and Marson, F. G. W.: Polycythaemia with fibroids. Lancet, 2:759, 1953.
174. Thurman, W. G., Grabstald, H., and Lieberman, P. H.: Elevation of erythropoietin levels in association with Wilms' tumor. Arch. Intern. Med., 117:280, 1966.
175. Tinney, W. D., Hall, B. E., and Griffin, H. Z.: The liver and spleen in polycythemia vera. Proc. Staff Meet. Mayo Clin., 18:46, 1943.
176. Valentine, W. N., Beck, W. S., Follette, J. H., Mills, H., and Lawrence, J. S.: Biochemical studies in chronic myclocytic leukemia, polycythemia vera and other idiopathic myeloproliferative disorders. Blood, 7:959, 1952.
177. Videback, A.: Polycythemia vera: course and prognosis. Acta Med. Scand., 138:179, 1950.
178. Vries, S. L. de, Braat-Van Straaten, M. A. J., Müller, E., and Wettermark, M.: Antiplasmin deficiency in polycythaemia: a form of thrombopathy. Thromb. Diath. Haemorrh., 6:445, 1961.
179. Wald, N., Hoshino, T., and Sears, M. E.: Therapy of polycythemia vera with Myleran. Blood. 13:757, 1958.
180. Waldman, T. A., and Bradley, J. E.: Polycythemia secondary to a pheochromocytoma with production of an erythropoiesis stimulating factor by the tumor. Proc. Soc. Exp. Biol. Med., 108:425, 1961.
181. Waldman, T. A., Levin, E. H., and Baldwin, M.: The association of polycythemia with cerebellar hemangioblastoma. The production of an erythropoiesis stimulating factor by the tumor. Am. J. Med., 31:318, 1961.
182. Ward, H. P., Bigelow, D. B., and Petty, T. L.: Postural hypoxemia and erythrocytosis. Am. J. Med., 45:880, 1968.
183. Wasserman, L. R.: Polycythemia vera—its course and treatment; relation to myeloid metaplasia and leukemia. Bull. N. Y. Acad. Med., 30:343, 1954.
184. Wasserman, L. R.: Annotation. The management of polycythemia vera. Br. J. Haematol., 21:371, 1971.
185. Wasserman, L. R., and Gilbert, H. S.: The treatment of polycythemia vera. Med. Clin. North Am., 50:1501, 1966.

186. Watkins, P. J., Fairley, G. H., and Bodley-Scott, R.: Treatment of polycythemia vera. Br. Med. J., 2:664, 1967.
187. Wasserman, L. R., and Gilbert, N. S.: Surgery in polycythemia vera. N. Engl. J. Med., 269: 1226, 1963.
188. White, J. M., Szur, L., Gillies, I. D. S., Lorkin, P. A., and Lehmann, H.: Familial polycythemia caused by a new haemoglobin variant: hb Hearthrow, beta 103 (G5) phenylalanine → leucine. Br. Med. J., 3:665, 1973.
189. Wiseman, B. K., Rohn, R. J., Bouroncle, B. A., and Myers, W. G.: The treatment of polycythemia vera with radioactive phosphorus. Ann. Intern. Med., 34:311, 1951.
190. Yamaoka, K.: Hemoglobin Hirose: $\alpha_2 B_2 37(C3)$ tryptophan yielding serine. Blood, 38:730, 1971.

CHAPTER **12**

LEUKEMIA

HISTORIC ASPECTS

In 1845 Bennett,[6] Craigie,[30] and Virchow[177] independently reported patients with undoubted leukemia. Bennett and Craigie attributed the remarkable numbers of white blood cells to the presence of "purulent matter in the blood." In 1846 Virchow, who introduced the term "leukemia," did not agree that the changes in the blood were the result of the invasion of the blood stream by a suppurative process, and considered that the hematologic changes were part of a definite pathologic process that involved certain organs in the body. The conflicting claims regarding the priority of discovery of leukemia were reviewed by Osler,[122] who concluded that Virchow deserved priority because he was the first to realize that the increase in white blood cells was an essential feature of the disease to which he gave the name "leukemia." Two forms of leukemia were recognized by Virchow. In one, the small forms of white cells predominated and enlargement of the lymph nodes was common; in the second, the large white cells were increased in number and marked splenomegaly occurred. Acute leukemia was first described by Friedrich in 1857,[35, 50] and in 1913 the first case of monocytic leukemia was reported by Reschad and Schilling-Torgau.[134]

CLASSIFICATION

A classification of leukemia is given in Table 12–1. "Myelo" in the term "myelogenous" refers to bone marrow. The terms "acute" and "chronic" originally were accurate in describing the course of the illness. Now, with present modes of treatment, children with acute lymphoblastic leukemia show a longer median survival than children and adults with chronic granulocytic leukemia. Thus the term "acute leukemia" better describes the situation in which there is little or no differentiation of the involved cell line. Leukemias exhibiting a well-differentiated cell line are referred to as "chronic leukemias." On the basis of morphologic and cytochemical findings, "acute monocytic leukemia" is included with "acute myelomonocytic leukemia."[71]

412

Table 12–1 *Classification of Leukemia*

LEUKEMIA	PREDOMINANT CELL
1. Myelogenous	
A. Acute	
1. Myeloblastic	Myeloblast, promyelocyte
2. Myelomonocytic	Myeloblast, and monocytes
3. Erythroleukemia	Myeloblast, abnormal erythroblasts
B. Chronic	
1. Granulocytic	Granulocytic series
2. Eosinophilic	Eosinophil and precursors
3. Basophilic	Basophil and precursors
4. Myelomonocytic	Granulocytic series and monocytes
2. Lymphocytic	
A. Acute lymphoblastic	Lymphoblast
B. Chronic	
1. Lymphocytic	Lymphocyte
3. Others	
A. Leukemic reticulo-endotheliosis ("Hairy" cell)	"Hairy" cell (lymphocyte or histiocyte)
B. Plasma cell	Plasma cell
C. Mast cell	Mast cell

THE INCIDENCE OF LEUKEMIA

It is reported that in the last 50 years there has been a three- to sixfold increase in leukemia, the greatest that has occurred in any disease except coronary thrombosis and carcinoma.[84] In England and Wales the incidence of leukemia has increased from 1.7 per 100,000 in 1900 to 5 per 100,000 in 1955;[151] in the United States comparable studies indicate an increase from 1 per 100,000 in 1900 to 6.3 per 100,000 in 1952. In the period 1943 to 1952 the incidence of leukemia in males was 7.3 per 100,000, and that for females 5.77 per 100,000.[58, 96, 139] Such factors as improved diagnosis, more frequent hospitalization, improved treatment, and the increased number of older persons in the general population may help to explain the apparent increase. In the last few decades the rise has been almost entirely in those over 50 years of age, and the only consistent increase in the last 20 years has been in those over 65; in the last 15 years the rate in those under 65 in New Zealand and the U. S. A. has been declining. On the basis of a detailed review of the statistics, Gunz and Baikie concluded that no decisive evidence now exists to prove that an actual, rather than an apparent, rise in the incidence of leukemia has occurred in past decades.[66] With regard to ethnic groups and race, the disease is more common in Jews than in non-Jews, and is less common in blacks than in whites.[97] The incidence in whites and blacks is about the same if the Jewish population is excluded.

Approximately 60 per cent of patients with leukemia have the chronic form of the disease. Age and sex distribution is shown in Figure 12–1, and is virtually identical to that described 45 years earlier.[178] Chronic lymphocytic leukemia is

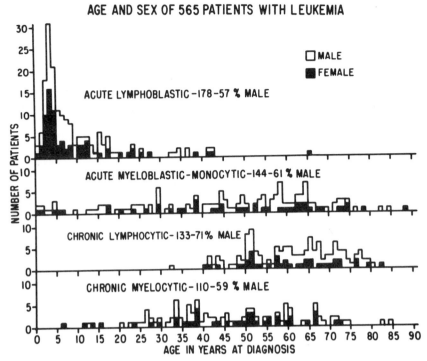

AGE AND SEX OF 565 PATIENTS WITH LEUKEMIA

Figure 12–1   From Boggs, Wintrobe and Cartwright: Medicine 41:163, 1962 with permission of the authors and publishers.

slightly more common than chronic granulocytic leukemia.[92] Eosinophilic leukemia is very rare, and in some of the reported patients the diagnosis has been questioned.[171] Basophilic leukemia and mast cell leukemia are even rarer, but have been reported.[35] Plasma cell leukemia is also quite rare,[130] and may be seen before the underlying multiple myeloma is diagnosed.[89] Acute leukemia occurs most commonly in children and young adults, but an increasing incidence in older persons has been reported.[28, 68]

ETIOLOGY AND PATHOGENESIS

In 1894 Osler wrote of leukemia, "Notwithstanding most careful clinical study and thorough histological and bacteriological investigation, the secret of the causative factor of this disease is as profound as it was half a century ago."[122] Although the cause of leukemia is unknown, there is considerable evidence to support the view that it is a neoplasm.[53,66,84] The progressive, ultimately fatal course of the leukemias together with accumulation of the involved cell line, usually in abnormal locations, fits the clinical pattern of a neoplastic disease. The essential alteration is thought to reside in the leukemic cell and to be responsible for its failure to respond to the forces which ordinarily control its reproduction and maturation. Metcalf presented an alternative view based on work with cultures of leukemic cells. He held that disturbed levels of factors regulating granulopoiesis may be necessary for the development and progression of acute and chronic granulocytic leukemia.[103] Whether a single factor or multiple factors are responsible for the essential alteration of the cell is unknown. Because of ignorance on this point, the question arises whether all the clinically-recognized forms of acute and chronic leukemia are the same disease. Different types of leukemia differ considerably in age distribution, clinical manifestations, survival time, and response to various types of therapy; these differences could be explained by a varied host response as well as by multiple causative factors.

Although our knowledge of many essentials of the leukemic process remains inadequate, a considerable body of information has accumulated relative to the production of leukemia by external agents and the genetic predisposition to leukemia. Much of this evidence has been derived from the study of laboratory animals, but important deductions have also been drawn from consideration of the occurrence of the disease in man.

Miller has tabulated certain high risk groups, those in whom the risk of developing leukemia within 10 to 15 years is greater than 1 in 100. These groups are: (1) identical twin of patient with leukemia, 1 in 5; (2) patients with radiation-treated polycythemia vera, 1 in 6; (3) those with Bloom's syndrome and Fanconi's aplastic anemia, 1 in 8 up to 30 years old; (4) atomic bomb survivors within 1000 meters of the hypocenter (Hiroshima and Nagasaki), 1 in 60; and (5) children with Down's syndrome, 1 in 95 under 10 years of age.[106] Other high risk groups include: (1) radiation-treated patients with ankylosing spondylitis, 1 in 270; (2) sibs of leukemic children, 1 in 720; and (3) U.S. Caucasian children less than 15 years of age, 1 in 2880.[106]

Ionizing Radiation

Evidence from a number of sources indicates that ionizing radiation can be a leukemogenic agent in man as well as in mice. The incidence of leukemia in physicians is twice that of the general population. In 1950 the incidence in radiologists was reported to be from eight to nine times that in physicians in general; a decade later the incidence was reported as 3.05 per cent in radiologists and 0.51 in physicians who were not radiologists.[99] An increased incidence of chronic granulocytic and acute lymphoblastic leukemia appears to be well established in survivors of atomic bombings in a frequency directly related to the severity of the exposure to radiation.[49, 90, 111] The peak incidence occurred between four and eight years after the irradiation, and the first cases were seen as early as one to two years after exposure.[175] The therapeutic use of x-ray for spondylitis in adults[29] and for thymic enlargement in children[160] has been reported to be responsible for leukemia. In British spondylitic patients the peak occurred four to five years after radiation, but the incidence remained elevated for up to 15 years; in children exposed to radiation before birth, the increased incidence reached its peak between the third and fifth years of life and was not increased after the age of 7. It is suspected but not proved that the incidence of leukemia, particularly acute leukemia, is higher in patients with polycythemia vera who have been treated with x-ray or radioactive phosphorus than in those treated by other means.[109,148] There appears to be an increasing incidence of acute leukemia in patients with Hodgkin's disease, perhaps related to more aggressive use of radiation treatment and longer survival.[140] Even the use of diagnostic x-ray during pregnancy has been suspected as a factor in the development of leukemia in childhood.[67,167] Myelogenous leukemia, acute or chronic, is the type usually induced in man by radiation.

Drugs and Chemicals

The evidence that exposure to benzol (benzene) may produce leukemia is circumstantial, but a number of suspicious instances have been reported.[2,78] The individual response to this chemical appears to vary, and both the concentration and length of exposure are probably important. The incidence of leukemia in patients with aplastic anemia may be increased, but a leukemogenic action of the drugs involved has not been proved.[27,51] Leukemia may develop if an abnormal clone of cells develops in a hypoplastic marrow. The development of acute leukemia after prolonged treatment with cytotoxic chemotherapy has been reported.[62,86,89a] Although the leukemogenic effect of these drugs in man is not yet established unequivocally, it should be kept in mind when considering their use for treatment of nonmalignant disorders.

Infection

Severe infections of various types usher in some 50 per cent of cases of acute leukemia in childhood.[84] Some authors have suspected that infection may cause leukemia, but most workers have concluded that such infections occur as a consequence of the pre-existent leukemia.[53] Although the early concept of leukemia as an infectious disease is no longer tenable, the relationship of viruses to leukemogenesis is currently stimulating much interest and investigation.

Viruses

Studies of the role of viruses in leukemia have been carried out largely in mice and fowl, and the relationship of the leukemia that occurs in these species to that of man is still uncertain.[82,147] Gross[63] has shown that leukemia may be transmitted to mice by the injection of a suspension of cells or cell-free extracts. He suggested that a causative virus might be transmitted from parent to offspring and remain dormant for some time. Cell-free extracts of liver, spleen, or lymphatic tumors of AKR* mice have produced leukemia and epitheliomas when injected into newborn mice of the C_3H† strain less than 16 hours old.[64] This observation suggests a relationship between leukemia and other malignancy in mice, a relationship that is well recognized in man.[110] Other reports

---

*AKR strain — mice having a high incidence of spontaneous leukemia.
†C_3H strain — mice having a low incidence of spontaneous leukemia.

have indicated that injections of cell-free extracts of brain from mice or human beings with leukemia cause the development of leukemia in a strain of mice not ordinarily susceptible to the disease.[145, 149] These and other studies demonstrate that leukemia can be produced in both mammals and fowl by the injection of cell-free filtrates.[98] Studies with mice indicate that leukemia and lymphomas can be induced by radiation and chemicals, including methylcholanthrene and urethan. The presence of murine leukemia virus (MuLV) in a majority of those developing active disease supported the concept that a latent leukemogenic virus had been activated, but did not exclude the possibility that it was only a passenger virus.[81] Viruses are known to cause leukemia in mice and chickens and probably cause the disease in a number of animals.[41,82] The leukemogenic viruses in these animals are RNA type C viruses. Studies of the disease in these species suggest that the disease complex is the same in all, and probably similar to that in man.

In the last few years, studies in animal leukemia have revealed a complex type C virus–cell relationship quite unlike the usual relationship. It is now known that cells may be infected with these viruses and yet show little or no evidence of that infection. The virus is assembled at, and buds from, the cell membrane. Although complete virus is not found in the cytoplasm, viral RNA and RNA-dependent DNA polymerase, reverse transcriptase,[142] enter the cell cytoplasm. DNA is transcribed from the RNA and presumably becomes part of the host cell genome, as provirus. Virus replication occurs only when the cell synthesizes DNA. This finding, plus the rarity of horizontal transmission of virus (i.e., spread between contacts) in most animal models, has led to the oncogene hypothesis.[173] This states that vertical transmission to the zygote results in a viral genome (oncogene) being present in every somatic cell. Ordinarily this genome is repressed. Derepression brings about production of infectious virus (virogene), resulting in leukemia. Factors such as radiation, chemicals, or even other viruses could trigger derepression.

With regard to RNA type C viruses, no unequivocal example of human leukemia has been proved to be caused by these agents. Nevertheless, the similarity to animal leukemia, and accumulating evidence, strongly favor the possibility. Of great importance is the recent demonstration that peripheral blood leukocytes from a patient with acute myelocytic leukemia released particles containing viral RNA and reverse transcriptase closely related to a primate cancer virus.[54]

In man, virus-like particles have been demonstrated in the plasma of patients with acute or chronic lymphocytic or granulocytic leukemia; these particles, which resemble the murine leukemia virus on electron microscopic examination, were not found in control plasmas,[20] but their morphology is not sufficiently unique to warrant the designation of virus on the basis of ultrastructure alone.[34]

Genetic Considerations

To what extent genetic factors influence the development of leukemia is still unknown. In certain highly inbred strains of mice, leukemia develops spontaneously in nearly all the animals. Although this suggests strongly the importance of genetic factors, the previously-discussed role of viruses in mouse leukemia complicates the interpretation.

Some constitutional susceptibility to leukemia in man was suggested by the studies of Videbaek,[176] but later reports have not confirmed his conclusions.[65] Reports of the occurrence of several instances of leukemia in the same family suggest a genetic influence, but are not conclusive, because some unrecognized factor in the family environment may be responsible. Observations on the occurrence of leukemia in identical twins do not afford definite evidence of the existence of a hereditary factor.[66] In the rare instances of congenital leukemia that have been reported, the disease has not been demonstrated in the mother.[132] One report described the occurrence of leukemia in a nine-month-old child born of a leukemic mother.[31] In all other reported instances of children born of leukemic mothers, the offspring have remained free of the disease.[10] The great majority of instances of familial leukemia have been of the chronic lymphocytic variety, but not more than 100 of these have been reported.[35]

Better evidence supporting a genetic background for some forms of leukemia is the relationship between leukemia and conditions characterized by chromosomal abnormalities.[141] Acute leukemia, myeloblastic or lymphoblastic, occurs at least 15 times the normal rate in mongolism (Down's syndrome), which is characterized by an extra chromosome (trisomy 21).[66] In addition, subjects with Fanconi's and Bloom's syndromes show unusual fragility of cultured lymphocyte chromosomes and an increased incidence of acute leukemia.[66]

Aneuploidy is found in 50 per cent of patients with acute lymphoblastic and acute myeloblastic leukemia.[141] Although one-half of the patients have no visible karyotypic abnormalities, sub-microscopic alterations might be present. Even so, the fact that the visible abnormalities are so different from case to case suggests that no consistent chromosomal changes contribute to the etiology of acute leukemia.

Although not involved with inheritance, the most consistent chromosomal abnormality associated with leukemia is the Philadelphia (Ph[1]) chromosome[117,118] found in 80 to 90 per cent of patients with typical chronic granulocytic leukemia. This is a G-group chromosome, number 22,[121] which has lost a portion of its long arms by translocation to chromosome number 9.[138]

In marrow and peripheral blood, leukemic cells capable of division show the chromosomal abnormality, although skin fibroblasts and lymphocytes do not.[80] The Ph[1] chromosome is an acquired rather than an inherited abnormality, and is not eradicated by treatment of the leukemia. When blastic transformation occurs in chronic granulocytic leukemia, other chromosomal abnormalities, usually aneuploidy, may develop, but the Ph[1] persists.[141] A majority of marrow cells, including megakaryocytes and erythroid cells, show the Ph[1] chromosome, indicating that the involved cell is a progenitor of all these cell lines. Apparently the granulocytic progeny of this stem cell acquire a selective growth advantage over adjacent normal cells.[116] This evidence, combined with studies of cellular enzymes, strongly indicates a clonal origin of chronic granulocytic leukemia.[66] Subjects heterozygous for the A and B isozymes of glucose–6–phosphate dehydrogenase normally show a mixture of these enzyme types in groups of their cells. In such heterozygous patients with chronic granulocytic leukemia, skin fibroblasts showed a mixture of A and B isozymes, but only one enzyme type was found in collections of red and white cells, indicating a clonal origin of the leukemia.[46]

ACUTE LEUKEMIA

Acute leukemia, both lymphoblastic and myeloblastic, is a much more severe disease than any of the chronic leukemias. The illness usually begins as acute leukemia, but blastic transformation may develop as the terminal event in a patient who has had chronic granulocytic leukemia for months or years. The presence of acute leukemia is characterized by the occurrence of appreciable numbers of young cells, particularly blast forms, in the circulating blood and bone marrow. The different types of acute leukemia cannot be distinguished from one another with certainty on clinical grounds alone, and, because of the extreme immaturity of the cells, it may be difficult to identify the cell type even after careful hematologic study. Hayhoe et al. correlated cytologic, cytochemical, and clinical findings in 140 consecutive cases of acute leukemia.[71] Their data provided evidence for the classification shown in Table 12–1. Acute monocytic leukemia was not distinguishable as a separate entity, and is included with acute myelomonocytic leukemia. Erythroleukemia is discussed in Chapter 10. Lymphoblastic leukemia clearly differs in nature from the others. Those cases showing cytologic and cytochemical features of lymphoblastic leukemia had a different age distribution, the incidence being very low after the age of 30. In addition, duration of survival was usually greater, and the preponderance of males found in other acute leukemias was less marked. Myeloblastic leukemia is rare in children. In another series of 226 patients over 14 years of age with acute leukemia, 11.5 per cent had lymphoblastic leukemia; in those over 30 years of age, the incidence was 8 per cent.[9] Other authors report that the myeloblastic type is fairly evenly divided among the different age-groups; it is generally agreed that the myelomonocytic type occurs most often in the middle and older age-groups.[56,68,151]

CLINICAL MANIFESTATIONS

The clinical characteristics of acute leukemia vary from case to case and depend mainly on the organ systems involved in the disease and the extent to which normal blood elements are lacking. Thus, pallor or symptoms referable to anemia are common presenting complaints. Bleeding, such as epistaxis, bleeding gums, petechiae, or ecchymoses, occurs some time in the course of the illness in nearly all patients with acute leukemia, and may be the presenting symptom. In one series of 580 patients with acute leukemia, the presenting symptoms were related to anemia in 61 per cent and to bleeding in 15 per cent.[136] Bleeding is usually on the basis of thrombocytopenia, but a severe hemorrhagic disorder associated with intravascular coagulation and/or fibrinolytic activity occurs in some patients with acute leukemia, particularly those in whom the promyelocyte is the predominating cell.[66]

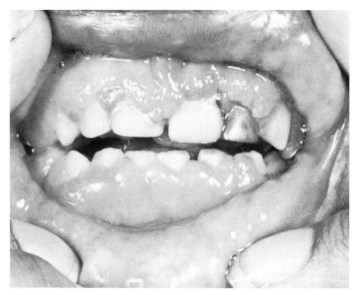

Figure 12–2   Hypertrophied gums in a patient with acute myelomonocytic leukemia.

Often the initial symptoms may give no hint of the seriousness of the under-lying disease. In children, especially, the onset may be characterized by the development of listlessness, fretfulness, poor appetite, and pallor. In some, aching and pains in the extremities lead to an initial diagnosis of rheumatic fever. The onset of the disease often resembles that of an acute respiratory in-fection with fever, malaise, fatigue, and sore throat, or may mimic a severe infection with high fever, headache, sweats, and severe prostration. Such episodes often occur as a result of infections that develop because of the lowered resis-tance of these patients, but they also arise in the absence of demonstrable infection. Physical examination generally reveals marked pallor of the skin and mucous membranes. Petechial hemorrhages and ecchymoses of different sizes occur commonly in all parts of the skin and mucous membranes. Leukemic infiltration of the skin, which has a characteristic purplish color, occurs occasion-ally, but is less common than in chronic leukemia. Not infrequently the gums appear hypertrophic, swollen, and ulcerated, a condition seen more often in myelomonocytic leukemia than in other types (Figure 12–2). One explanation for this occurrence is that the immature leukemic cells with monocytic features have sufficient cytoplasmic development of those qualities which normally enable the monocyte to enter tissues.[94]

In acute leukemia, enlargement of the liver is inconstant, and hepatic tenderness is unusual. A soft spleen edge is usually, but not invariably, palpable a few centimeters below the left costal margin. Splenomegaly and lymph node enlargement are more likely to occur in acute lymphoblastic leukemia, and are therefore found more often in children than in adults. In adults, the observation that the spleen edge is very firm and extends as far down as the umbilicus sug-gests that the patient had chronic granulocytic leukemia before onset of the acute phase. Mild or moderate (0.5 to 1.5 cm.) enlargement of the superficial lymph nodes is usually present, but it may be so slight as to escape detection. In children the node enlargement may become massive, particularly in the thorax. Tenderness on light pressure over the bones, particularly the lower portion of the sternum, is commonly demonstrable in acute leukemia.

Occasionally an extramedullary mass of leukemic tissue will be found on physical examination. Breast masses have been reported[57] although involvement of periosteal and perineural structures is more frequent.[120] These, usually granulocytic sarcomas[131] consisting of myeloblasts, are called chloromas if they possess myeloperoxidase, which imparts a green color seen on sectioning the tumor.

LABORATORY MANIFESTATIONS

Anemia, which may result from blood loss, decreased blood production, increased hemolysis, or a combination of these factors, occurs in almost every patient with acute leukemia. The anemia is often severe and hemoglobin levels as low as 2 to 3 gm. per 100 ml. sometimes are seen. The erythrocyte count and hematocrit are reduced proportionally, and the anemia is generally of the normocytic, normochromic variety.

The most important abnormality in acute leukemia involves the leukocytes. The total leukocyte count varies from subnormal levels of a few hundred to several hundred thousand per cu.mm. Characteristically, very immature cells occur in significant numbers. Often in routinely stained blood smears classification of the immature cells is difficult, if not impossible, unless some maturation occurs or a characteristic finding is present, such as an Auer rod (see below and (Fig. 12–3). When the total leukocyte count is low, examination of smears made from a concentrate of the leukocyte fraction after centrifugation of the peripheral blood (buffy coat smear) is often useful in demonstrating the presence of immature cells. In cases of pancytopenia, study of the peripheral blood in this manner often makes it possible to distinguish between leukemia and aplastic anemia, and is also helpful in identifying the type of leukemia prior to examination of bone marrow smears. Nucleated red cells are seen commonly in the peripheral blood in all types of acute leukemia.

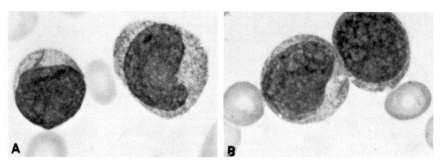

Figure 12–3 Blast cells with Auer bodies. *A:* Monoblasts from patient with acute myelomonocytic leukemia. *B:* Myeloblasts from patient with acute myeloblastic leukemia.

Thrombocytopenia occurs sooner or later in nearly all types of acute leukemia. Usually the platelets are markedly reduced when the patient is first seen.

Examination of the bone marrow, even when there may be little or equivocal evidence in the peripheral blood, reveals infiltration by the immature leukemic cells responsible for the disease. On occasion, only very immature atypical blast cells are found, and even with special stains the type of leukemia cannot be identified with assurance; such unusual cases are classified as undifferentiated or "stem cell" leukemia.

Classification of the acute leukemias on the basis of Romanowsky stains is fraught with difficulty and is being supplemented by other methods. These include the peroxidase reaction, the periodic acid–Schiff (PAS) reaction for glycogen, Sudan black B stain for intracellular lipids, and other cytochemical techniques which help to differentiate the acute leukemias,[71] e.g., immature cells showing a negative reaction to Sudan black and peroxidase, but coarse granules on PAS stain are most likely to be lymphoblasts.[71] The presence of Auer rods excludes lymphoblastic leukemia and indicates myeloblastic or myelomonocytic leukemia (Fig. 12–3). On the basis of ultrastructural and cytochemical studies, these rods, or bodies, appear to be lysosomal in nature and composed of fused azurophilic granules.[71] In addition, elevated levels of plasma and urine lysozyme (muramidase) and plasma vitamin B_{12} binding capacity favor the diagnosis of myeloblastic or myelomonocytic leukemia.[4] When the predominant immature cell in the marrow is a promyelocyte, some hematologists use the term "acute promyelocytic leukemia." Perhaps further studies of cellular products, cell culture, and the use of electron microscopy will allow better classification of acute leukemias.

DIAGNOSIS

The diagnosis of acute leukemia is generally made without difficulty when there is marked increase in immature leukocytes in the peripheral blood and bone marrow, associated with anemia and thrombocytopenia. On occasion, acute leukemia must be distinguished from infectious mononucleosis. The absence of anemia and thrombocytopenia, the absence of blast cells in the peripheral blood, the varied morphologic appearance of the cells in the peripheral blood, and the positive reaction with the heterophil agglutination test, usually serve to distinguish infectious mononucleosis without much difficulty (see Chapter 9). Aplastic anemia is more difficult because anemia, leukopenia, thrombocytopenia, fever, and abnormal bleeding may occur in both diseases. The presence of lymphadenopathy and splenomegaly, and the appearance of the bone marrow, nearly always permit a correct diagnosis, but occasionally a prior period of observation is necessary.

Whenever there is doubt about the diagnosis of acute leukemia a re-evaluation of the situation becomes necessary. Good quality blood smears and marrow preparations, including bone marrow biopsy (see chapter 3), must be obtained. A period of observation to allow clarification will usually benefit the patient more than early treatment based on an uncertain diagnosis.

Leukemoid reactions secondary to infections usually cause no difficulty because the proportion of very immature cells in acute leukemia is generally out of all proportion to that seen in severe infections in which there is a more orderly increase in the intermediate and immature forms. Disseminated tuberculosis is an exception: a leukemoid reaction, usually of the myeloblastic type, sometimes develops and so mimics leukemia that the true nature of the primary disease may be discovered only at autopsy.[174] Similar leukemoid reactions have been reported in patients with disseminated histoplasmosis.[11] On occasion, the presence of immature granulocytes and nucleated red cells in the peripheral blood (leukoerythroblastic smear) may lead to an initial impression of leukemia in a patient who has metastatic bone marrow involvement; further examinations, including a study of the bone marrow, nearly always indicate the correct diagnosis.

CLINICAL COURSE AND COMPLICATIONS

With rare exceptions,[19] acute leukemia is a fatal disease that usually runs a short course. Before the widespread use of transfusions, antibiotics, and chemotherapeutic agents, survival time was from six days to six weeks. The use of chemotherapy has resulted in significant improvement in the outlook for patients with lymphoblastic leukemia, particularly children, but these preparations are not as effective in other types of acute leukemia. The prognosis is worse in children under one year of age, and better in patients with low or normal leukocyte counts. Other factors, such as the duration of disease before treatment or the initial appearance of the bone marrow, are not related to prognosis. In adults the prognosis has not improved greatly with newer methods of treatment;[4] patients with lymphoblastic leukemia often survive more than a year, but those with the other types seldom have a remission lasting more than six or eight months, and usually do not live as long as a year. With current aggressive therapy, an increasing number of children, perhaps 50 per cent of those with lymphoblastic leukemia, are surviving free of demonstrable leukemia for as long as five years.[159]

The complications of acute leukemia occur as a result of bone marrow failure or tissue infiltration by the leukemic cells. Infection and hemorrhage are the most frequent causes of death and will be discussed later under supportive care.

Central nervous system involvement is a prominent complication of acute leukemias. Hemorrhage or leukemic infiltrations in the brain and other parts of the central nervous system occur frequently. The incidence of objective signs of neurologic involvement (other than retinal changes) was reported to be 20 per cent in one series of 334 cases.[146] In 163 patients with leukemia of all types, the incidence of central nervous system involvement was 35 per cent.[127] Lesions occurred most often in acute myeloblastic leukemia, in which intracranial hemorrhage was the commonest manifestation; the frequency of this serious event appeared to be related more to an elevated leukocyte count (over 50,000 per cu.mm.) than to thrombocytopenia.

In another series of 117 cases, intracranial hemorrhage was the cause of death in 20 per cent of patients.[112] Most of the fatal intracerebral hemorrhages occurred in those with preterminal leukocyte counts over 100,000 per cu.mm.

At autopsy these patients were found to have leukostasis in small intracerebral vessels, an occurrence which may be related to the relative rigidity of blast cells.[95] Proliferation of leukemic cells seemed to result in destruction of the vessel wall and the formation of leukemic nodules which coalesced to form larger lesions. In contrast to intracerebral hemorrhage, fatal subarachnoid hemorrhage was not related to the leukocyte count, but to thrombocytopenia.[112] In this series, meningeal infiltration was seen most often in lymphocytic leukemia, especially in males less than 20 years of age. The frequency of CNS involvement in lymphoblastic and myeloblastic leukemia in children, when expressed per month at risk, is not greatly different.[42] Thus, the greater frequency of CNS involvement in lymphoblastic leukemia may be related to the longer duration of survival. Meningeal leukemia is usually manifested by vomiting, headache, and other signs of increased intracranial pressure, but it may occur with a normal cerebrospinal fluid examination; the complication may develop when the disease is apparently in complete remission. Convulsions, sensory disturbances, papilledema, cranial nerve palsies, and signs of pyramidal tract involvement are not uncommon.

Demonstration of leukemic cells in the spinal fluid is the most reliable test to establish the diagnosis of CNS leukemia. Use of the cytocentrifuge,[39] which concentrates any cells present onto a glass slide, is essential, permitting identification of blast cells when the total cell count is normal and when there are no signs or symptoms of CNS involvement. Sugar and protein content of spinal fluid are not reliable tests for determining the presence of meningeal leukemia.[18]

Other complications of leukemia are numerous, and include infiltration in various sites such as the bladder and kidney, producing pain and hematuria; severe joint and bone pain as a result of involvement of synovial membranes or subperiosteal infiltration or hemorrhage; and perianal and anorectal problems such as abscess formation.[154]

TREATMENT

The treatment of acute leukemia involves the use both of supportive measures and specific therapy. Included in the former are blood transfusions for anemia, fresh blood and platelet concentrates for thrombocytopenia and bleeding, granulocyte transfusions and antibiotics for associated infection, and analgesics for pain. One of the most important supportive measures is the attitude of the physician toward the patient and his family. The "human interest" stories in the press have made leukemia a tragic story known to nearly all. The physician's support of members of the family, his sympathetic understanding of their anxieties, and his willingness to take time to talk with them all contribute greatly to their comfort. It is important that the parents of children with leukemia be urged to treat them during periods of remission as they would a normal child. The children should be allowed to return to school and play, and normal discipline should be enforced. In this way the over-all emotional impact of the disease on the family may be reduced.

Current chemotherapeutic approaches to treatment of human acute leukemia are based largely on experimental mouse leukemia.[162] Simply stated, these studies show that the fractional kill of leukemic cells is the same for a given amount of treatment, regardless of the actual number of cells present. In addition, they show that one leukemic cell leads ultimately to death from leukemia; thus, correctly or not, treatment of human acute leukemia has moved toward the concept of "total cell kill." This approach utilizes combinations of drugs in schedules that attempt to achieve additive antileukemic effects without combining toxic side-effects. Initial treatment aimed at returning the blood and marrow to normal is referred to as *induction*. Even when induction is successful with return of blood and marrow to normal (complete hematologic remission), leukemic cells remain in the kidney, liver, and other organs.[100, 114] This finding led to what is called *consolidation* treatment. In this stage, either the drugs used during induction or additional drugs are given in an attempt to kill remaining leukemic cells. Following this phase, *maintenance* therapy is used to prevent recurrence of leukemia. Many elaborate combinations and schedules have been, and are being, tried by various leukemia study groups. In such a situation, views on the best, or even most acceptable treatment may vary from one year to the next. Nevertheless, changes and constant investigations are necessary in a disease such as acute leukemia, the treatment of which leaves so much to be desired despite the definite progress made.

Lymphoblastic Leukemia

At present, combination chemotherapy results in complete remission in about 90 per cent of children[165] and adults[126] with lymphoblastic leukemia. Table 12–2 lists the drugs used. Currently preferred induction treatment consists of daily oral prednisone, 40 to 100 mg. per M^2 body surface, together with intravenous vincristine 1 to 2 mg. per M^2 each week. In general, four to six weeks are required to achieve bone marrow remission. This highly effective combination is lethal to leukemic cells and spares normal cells, so that production of severe marrow hypoplasia is not necessary to achieve complete remission, as appears to be the case in acute myeloblastic leukemia. Unless maintenance therapy is given, the median duration of remission tends to be short-lived, approximately eight weeks,[165] but it can be extended significantly with further treatment. Improved methods of maintenance are now being investigated, and these include alternating various drugs such as methotrexate and 6–mercaptopurine,[186] periodic reinduction with prednisone, daunomycin, and vincristine, use of immunotherapy,[101] and prophylactic treatment of the central nervous system in children.[159] The latter approach has resulted in improved survival in children, the most optimistic report showing 51 per cent five-year leukemia-free survival.[159] Various methods have been used for CNS prophylaxis including intrathecal methotrexate, alone or combined with cranial radiation, and craniospinal radiation alone.[159] As expected, along with improving survival, these vigorous approaches to treatment have also resulted in serious toxicity, including fatal opportunistic infection despite control of leukemia[159] and CNS toxicity related to cranial radiation followed by systemic administration of methotrexate.[128] It is not known whether CNS prophylactic treatment is of benefit in adults with lymphoblastic

Table 12–2   *Drugs used for Remission Induction in Children with Lymphoblastic Leukemia*[165]

Drug	Number of Patients	% Complete Remission	Mode of Action	Toxicity
Cyclophosphamide	44	18	Alkylating agent	Myelosuppression, Alopecia
Methotrexate	48	21	Folate antagonist	Myelosuppresion, oral and gastro-intestinal ulcerations
Cytosine Arabinoside	10	30	Pyrimidine antagonist	Myelosuppression
Daunorubicin	32	33	Interferes with RNA transcription	Myelosuppression Cardiac toxicity Alopecia
L-Asparaginase	21	43	Deprives leukemic cells of asparagine	Anaphylaxis Hepatitis Pancreatitis
Vincristine	119	55	Interferes with mitotic spindles	Peripheral neuropathy Alopecia
Prednisone	72	57	Unknown	Cushingoid manifestations
Drug Combinations				
Prednisone + Mercaptopurine	154	82		
Prednisone + Vincristine	63	84		
Prednisone + Vincristine + Methotrexate + Mercaptopurine	35	94		
Prednisone + Vincristine + Daunomycin	33	97		

leukemia but with the same chemotherapy used for children, excluding CNS prophylaxis, median survival is approximately 11 months.[72]

When meningeal (CNS) leukemia occurs, treatment consists of intrathecal methotrexate 7.5 mg. per M^2 given every three to four days until the spinal fluid cell mononuclear count is less than $10/mm^3$ and no leukemic cells are found on cytocentrifuge of the spinal fluid. Treatment thereafter is given monthly. Cytosine arabinoside is also effective when given intrathecally.[165]

Myeloblastic Leukemia (Includes Myelomonocytic)

Progress in the treatment of AML has been slow in developing. Prior to the introduction of cytosine arabinoside and daunomycin, induction of complete remissions occurred in about 10 per cent of patients, and median survival was four months.[36]

Table 12–3   *Drugs Used for Remission Induction in Acute Myeloblastic Leukemia*

DRUG	NUMBER OF PATIENTS	% COMPLETE REMISSION	REFERENCE
Methotrexate	34	3	52
6-Mercaptopurine	31	10	52
Cytosine Arabinoside	57	32*	12
Daunomycin	22	50	179
Drug Combinations			
Mercaptopurine + Vincristine + Methotrexate + Prednisone	21	29	179
Cytosine Arabinoside + Daunomycin + Vincristine	23	48	137
Cytosine Arabinoside + Cyclophosphamide + Vincristine + Prednisone	66	48**	12
Cytosine Arabinoside + Daunomycin	30	53	59
Cytosine Arabinoside + Thioguanine	43	65***	26

*54% ⎫
**74% ⎬ excluding those dying in
***87% ⎭   first 6 weeks

At present, various drug combinations produce complete remission in approximately 50 per cent of patients. Duration of survival is definitely prolonged for those patients achieving complete remission. Drugs used for this purpose are shown in Table 12–3.

To achieve complete remission, most of the leukemic cells must be eliminated. Since the drugs which are reliably lethal to leukemic myeloblasts are also very toxic to normal marrow cells, remission induction is very hazardous owing to the resulting severe marrow hypoplasia. Thus, intensive supportive therapy is essential for good results. Many induction attempts are complicated by sepsis, bleeding, and side-effects such as anorexia, nausea, vomiting, and oral mucosal lesions. The patients are usually very sick and their discomfort is increased by the frequent examinations, cultures, transfusions, and radiologic and other studies required in their management. In view of this, Crosby questioned whether all patients with acute myeloblastic leukemia (AML) should be treated with the toxic drugs that are employed.[32] He identified six types of AML which he considered to be refractory to treatment: (1) blast crisis of CML; (2) smoldering leukemia; (3) AML with megaloblastosis; (4) myelomonocytic leukemia; (5) promyelocytic leukemia; and (6) AML in middle age (those over 50). He thought that patients in these groups differ from children and younger adults with the disease. He suggested that, if the physician feels he must treat patients in one of the other groups, milder measures are probably better than aggressive therapy. Our current approach is to decide in each individual case how aggressive an approach to pursue, aided by discussions with the patient and family. As a result, almost all our patients enter a program for an attempt at complete remission. Exceptions include patients with smoldering acute leukemia,[135] and those with such serious additional disease that more than a few months' survival is unlikely despite the leukemia (e.g., acute leukemia in a patient with widespread metastatic carcinoma). Patients in relatively good health with "smoldering" acute leukemia, in whom the rate of progression of the disease, as judged by history, appears slow, should be observed to see how rapidly the disease is in fact progressing. Sometimes such a patient does well for months, with only transfusions for anemia, before requiring specific chemotherapy. Although advanced age lessens the chance of complete remission,[4] treatment decision is based not on age but on the patient's general condition.

In our experience,[115] after administration of mainly cytosine arabinoside alone,[164] combined with thioguanine,[26] or with cyclophosphamide, vincristine, and prednisone,[12] 31 per cent of all patients obtained complete remission defined as follows: (1) bone marrow normocellular and containing less than 5 per cent blast forms; (2) peripheral blood granulocyte count greater than $1000/mm^3$; (3) peripheral platelet count greater than $100,000/mm^3$; (4) no blast forms demonstrated in the peripheral blood after recovery from hematologic toxicity of the induction chemotherapy; and (5) absence of physical findings suggestive of leukemic infiltration of the spleen, liver, lymph nodes, or other organs. Maintenance treatment consisted of monthly five-day infusions of cytosine arabinoside, or weekly cytosine arabinoside combined with oral thioguanine three to five days per week. Median duration of complete remission was 8.2 months. Median survival was 17 months for those with complete remission, 6.5 months for those with only partial remission, and only 2.8 months for treatment failures. Patients not treated with chemotherapy had a median survival of 2.1 months. The efficacy of consolidation and maintenance therapy is less clear in AML than in ALL. Nevertheless, once complete remission is obtained, most hematologists give maintenance drugs. Different approaches to maintenance are being studied, including immunotherapy.[4, 101]

Supportive Treatment

As previously discussed, hemorrhage and infection account for most of the deaths in acute leukemia. Particularly in AML, these complications may occur during induction chemotherapy before an adequate attempt to bring about remission has been accomplished. Since thrombocytopenia is the major risk factor for bleeding, platelet transfusions, 6 or more units, should be given to an adult with a platelet count below 50,000 per mm^3 in the presence of bleeding. This may need to be repeated every other day. Serious bleeding is more likely to occur when the platelet count is below 10,000 per mm³, so in that situation prophylactic use of platelet transfusion is advocated by some, particularly during induction chemotherapy, or when the patient is febrile, or if mucosal ulceration is present.[23] Platelets from ABO, HL-A compatible donors represent ideal therapy,[182] but this usually is not practical. Granulocytopenia from incompatible platelets has been noted,[74] and could be very dangerous in patients with already reduced levels of granulocytes.

Transfusion of packed red cells may be required to control anemia. Although there is no definite critical level of hemoglobin concentration, less than 7 gm./100 ml. is undesirable, since hemorrhage may be more likely to occur in the severely anemic patient.

Infection remains the most serious threat to the leukemic patient in relapse. Many infections are due to organisms acquired from the hospital environment which colonize the patient, particularly the gastrointestinal tract, and cause infection when host resistance is impaired by severe granulocytopenia. Attempts to prevent this sequence of events include use of laminar air flow room reverse isolation combined with oral, nonabsorbable antibiotic prophylaxis.[144] Although this combination was reported to produce a significant reduction in severe infections in those patients able to tolerate it, no dramatic effect on remission rate was noted owing to resistance of the leukemia to chemotherapy.

Detection of fever in the leukopenic patient (less than 1000 granulocytes per mm³) should necessitate an immediate search for infection, by means of chest x-ray and collection of culture material: blood, urine, sputum if available, and a swab from any skin lesion. Following this, antibiotic therapy must be begun at once with a combination of drugs designed to give very broad coverage, with particular emphasis on gram-negative bacteria. As new antibiotics are developed the most effective drug combinations will change, but at present we institute therapy of the febrile, leukopenic patient with intravenous carbenicillin (5 gm. every four hours) and cephalothin (2 gm. every four hours). On the basis of subsequent results of cultures, the antibiotics are changed appropriately. Many times cultures are negative, but defervescence occurs. In this case, the original antibiotics are continued until the patient is afebrile for at least three consecutive days. If cultures and other studies are negative, but the fever persists despite use of antibiotics for four to seven days, the antibiotics should be discontinued and further search should be made for the cause of fever.[93]

Leukocyte transfusion may replace granulocytes sufficiently to aid antibiotic treatment of severe infections.[16,37,76,143] Granulocytes obtained by filtration leukapheresis or continuous centrifugation can be used safely and are effective. Leukocyte transfusions are available for clinical use in some centers, and in the near future will almost certainly become as routine as the use of other blood components.

Other measures important in the treatment of acute leukemia include an adequate fluid intake, plus the use of allopurinol to prevent urate nephropathy during cytotoxic therapy. In addition, hypokalemia is often noted before or during induction therapy of acute leukemia, particularly the myelomonocytic variety.[129] Use of carbenicillin[169] may also produce hypokalemia, which should be corrected.

Illustrative Cases

CASE 1

This 65-year-old man noted easy fatigue eight months before admission to another hospital for a minor surgical procedure. At that time he was found to have a leukopenia. He was not anemic, and platelets were adequate. Shortly after this he became weaker, and developed swelling of the gums. He also noted pallor, and was then admitted to the hospital.

Physical examination. Pallor, hypertrophy of the gums, and evidence of a perirectal abscess were noted. There was no adenopathy and the liver and spleen were not palpable.

Laboratory examination. Hematocrit 20%, WBC 3,000 cells/cu.mm. Blood smear showed myeloblasts, promyelocytes, myelocytes, nucleated red cells, and an increased number of monocytes. Platelet count was 70,000/cu. mm. Bone marrow specimen was hyperplastic with myeloblasts predominating. Some promyelocytes and monocytes were present, and the diagnosis of acute myelomonocytic leukemia was made.

Course. On the day of admission the patient began an eight-day course of intravenous cytosine arabinoside and oral 6–thioguanine, each given every 12 hours. A severe pancytopenia ensued. During the 30-day hospitalization complications were numerous, including recurrent spiking fever, anocutaneous fistula, Pseudomonas urinary tract infection, enterococcal bacteremia, and acute gastrointestinal hemorrhage. He required repeated red cell and platelet transfusions, and frequent courses of antibiotics including carbenicillin, cephalothin, gentamicin, and penicillin. On the 21st hospital day platelet count began to rise, followed by a rise in mature granulocytes and general improvement without subsequent infection. Repeat bone marrow showed normal granulocytic maturation. He was discharged on the 30th hospital day with hematocrit of 39%, WBC 2100/cu.mm. with 64% neutrophils, 20% lymphocytes, 12% bands, 2 myelocytes, and 2 promyelocytes. Platelet count was 75,000/cu.mm.

Since discharge he has continued to do well and has received maintenance therapy with cytosine arabinoside, one injection weekly, and 6–thioguanine given orally four days a week. He has returned to full-time work and the blood counts remain normal. He has now been in complete clinical and hematologic remission for two years and six months.

Comment. This relatively elderly man nearly died as a result of his disease and the induction therapy. Vigorous treatment of complications and use of combination chemotherapy for induction brought about a complete remission. He illustrates very well the hazardous induction period usually encountered in the treatment of acute myeloblastic leukemia. The cost of hospitalization was $6,300, but he is living an enjoyable and productive life which would not have been possible without chemotherapy.

CASE 2

This 3-year-old white girl was in excellent health until two months prior to her first visit, when increasing pallor, bruises, and fatigue were noticed. Two months before admission her family physician found her hemoglobin to be 10.7 gm. per 100 ml. and her leukocyte count 14,500 per cu.mm. with "a normal differential." She was treated with penicillin for tonsillitis, but weakness, pallor, and a tendency to bruise continued until admission.

Physical examination. Temperature 102° F; pulse 108; height 39½ inches; and weight 34 pounds. Multiple 1 by 1 cm. nodes were palpated in the anterior and posterior cervical areas, both the axillary regions, and the inguinal areas. A systolic murmur was heard over the precordium. On inspiration the liver edge was felt 6 cm. below the right costal margin and the spleen 5 cm. below the left. The remainder of the examination was normal except that she was very pale.

Laboratory examination. Hemoglobin, 5.7 gm.%; hematocrit, 16.5%; white count, 15,000 per cu.mm.; and platelets, 5000 per cu.mm. Reticulocytes were 0.2%. Differential count: lymphoblasts, 39%; lymphocytes, 55% (many immature); and segmented cells, 6%. Uric acid was 5.4 mg. per 100 ml.

Course. The patient was treated with platelet concentrates and packed red cells, after which bone marrow aspiration was performed. The cellularity was greatly increased, and 95% of the cells were considered to be lymphoblasts; megakaryocytes, myelocytes, erythroid cells, and myeloid cells were significantly diminished.

A diagnosis of acute lymphoblastic leukemia was made, and the following treatment given: prednisone, 10 mg. every six hours; 1.7 mg. of vincristine sulfate intravenously each week; and allopurinol, 50 mg. three times a day.

In the third week of treatment the hemoglobin was 8.8 gm. per 100 ml.; hematocrit, 27%; white count, 2400 per cu.mm.; platelets, 400,000 per cu.mm.; and reticulocytes, 0.7%; bone marrow examination disclosed remission in the leukemia. After five weeks the treatment was discontinued. Two weeks later the splenomegaly and hematomegaly had disappeared. The hemoglobin was 11 gm. per 100 ml., hematocrit was 34%, platelets were 470,000 per cu.mm., and white count was 3300 per cu.mm. Differential count showed segmented cells to be 63%, lymphocytes 34%, and monocytes 3%.

The patient was placed on 6–mercaptopurine for maintenance therapy, and continued free of symptoms and with bone marrow remission for six months, when slight cervical adenopathy reappeared, blasts became evident in the peripheral blood, and bone marrow examination disclosed relapse with a large infiltration of lymphoblasts. She was again treated with 35 mg. of prednisone q.i.d. and 1.7 mg. of vincristine intravenously at weekly intervals. One month later she was asymptomatic except for developing alopecia; peripheral blood was essentially normal except for mild anemia with leukopenia, but bone marrow examination showed continued relapse with 13% blasts. Vincristine at weekly intervals was continued for two more weeks, and the patient became asymptomatic with bone marrow remission. Prednisone dosage was tapered, then discontinued, and she was given methotrexate 25 mg. per M² (17.5 mg.) twice a week.

The patient continued in clinical and hematologic remission for six more months, when she developed diarrhea accompanied by moderate lymphadenopathy. Hematocrit was 38%, hemoglobin 12.6 gm. per 100 ml., and white count 12,000 per cu.mm.; bone marrow examination disclosed 35% lymphoblasts. Because of the relapse, the patient was treated with daunomycin, 25 mg. per M² per day for three days, repeated after a four-day interval, with vincristine, 1.5 mg. per M² per week for four doses, and with prednisone, 10 mg. four times a day for 28 days.

For the next eight months relapses occurred with increasing frequency, becoming more resistant to all forms of therapy, and she died during an episode of infection almost three years from onset of leukemia.

   Comment.   This child had acute lymphoblastic leukemia for three years. She had numerous relapses, which responded to different forms of treatment, but ultimately became refractory to treatment.

CHRONIC LYMPHOCYTIC LEUKEMIA

   In 1924 Minot and Isaacs[108] presented data on 97 patients with chronic lymphocytic leukemia. They noted that the disorder occurred most commonly between 45 and 55 years of age, a decade later than the peak incidence of chronic myelogenous leukemia. The disease occurred in males more than three times as often as in women. Scott[152] in 1957 reviewed a series of 227 patients and found the greatest number of cases occurring between the ages of 60 and 70 years. He noted that there seemed to be a growing number of women with chronic lymphatic leukemia. In 1929[125] a small series revealed a male:female ratio of 4:1; in Scott's series the ratio was more nearly 2:1.

CLINICAL MANIFESTATIONS

   Chronic lymphocytic leukemia may make its appearance in a variety of ways. The onset is sometimes so insidious that the diagnosis is made before symptoms appear, when an individual undergoes a routine examination or consults his physician for some unrelated complaint. In such circumstances the usual manifestations are previously unrecognized enlargement of the superficial lymph nodes and/or a moderate increase in the leukocyte count, accompanied by an absolute increase in the small lymphocytes. Probably the most common complaint that leads the patient to seek medical advice is the accidental discovery of enlarged superficial nodes. Any group of nodes may be involved, but enlargement of the cervical nodes is most often noted. At times the initial complaint is that of involvement of the lacrimal and salivary glands — Mikulicz's syndrome. Enlargement of intra-abdominal lymph nodes may produce gastrointestinal or abdominal complaints; involvement of the mediastinal nodes may result in cough, hoarseness, or dyspnea.

   Abnormalities in peripheral blood are responsible for the initial symptoms in some patients. If anemia is severe, easy fatigue, exertional dyspnea, and weakness occur. Thrombocytopenia may cause bleeding gums, easy bruising, petechiae, or gastrointestinal bleeding. Fever rarely occurs in the absence of infection.

   A variety of skin lesions occur in about 10 per cent of patients some time during the course of the disease. Nonspecific lesions such as pruritus, areas of hyperpigmentation, macular and papular eruptions, exfoliative dermatitis, and herpes zoster occur without actual leukemic infiltration of the skin. Specific lesions, the result of actual infiltration of the skin by leukemic cells, are usually discrete and bright red or purple in color. These lesions, which vary greatly in number, usually measure a few mm. in diameter. Generalized leukemic involvement of the skin—leukemia cutis universalis—generally produces intense itching. In some patients the disease assumes the form of mycosis fungoides.

Rarer manifestations of chronic lymphocytic leukemia are massive gastro-intestinal hemorrhage, visual disturbances, and complaints referable to the skeletal system. Skeletal lesions, such as rarefaction of the bones, pathologic fracture, and collapse of vertebrae with cord compression, occur in 5 per cent of patients with this disease.[158]

On physical examination, the most constant abnormality is enlargement of the superficial lymph nodes (Fig. 12–4). In practically every patient some enlargement occurs of at least a few of the superficial lymph nodes. In most patients the individual nodes are moderately enlarged and measure from 2 to 3 cm. in diameter. The nodes are moderately firm, freely movable, and nontender. Clusters of nodes may measure 10 cm. or more in diameter. Splenomegaly occurs in nearly all patients with chronic lymphocytic leukemia; usually the spleen is moderately firm and extends several centimeters below the left costal margin, but occasionally it fills the entire left side of the abdomen. Hepatomegaly is also an almost constant finding. Retinal hemorrhages may occur without other evidence of abnormal bleeding or in association with ecchymoses, petechiae, and bleeding from the mucous membranes. Leukemic infiltration of the tonsil occurs in a small percentage of patients, and can usually be recognized by its reddish purple color. The leukemic infiltrations of the skin are usually recog-

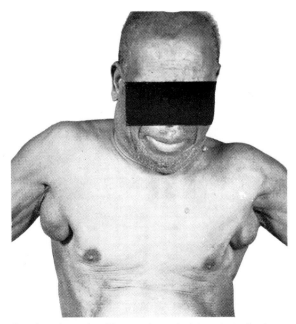

Figure 12–4 Greatly enlarged axillary and cervical lymph nodes in a patient with chronic lymphocytic leukemia.

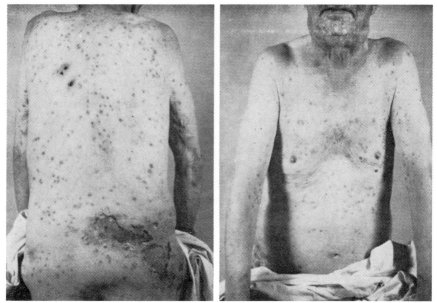

Figure 12–5   Leukemia cutis and herpes zoster in a patient with chronic lymphocytic leukemia.

nized by the reddish purple color and discrete nature of the lesions; if severe pruritus and excoriation are present, the underlying nature of the skin lesions may not be apparent (Fig. 12–5).

LABORATORY MANIFESTATIONS

The most characteristic features of chronic lymphocytic leukemia are increases in the total leukocyte count and the absolute number of small lymphocytes (>4500 mm³). Leukopenia rarely occurs. The leukocyte count is nearly always above 15,000 per cu.mm., and often reaches levels of from 200,000 to 400,000 per cu.mm. Most of the cells in the peripheral blood are small well-differentiated lymphocytes (Fig. 12–6). These constitute 65 to 75 per cent of the cells in the early stage of the disease, and usually amount to 95 to 98 per cent in the more advanced stages. A small number of larger lymphocytes, some less well-differentiated, occur at times, but blast forms are not seen. Smears of peripheral blood often show many "smudge" and "basket cells" which are apparently leukemic lymphocytes disrupted in the process of preparing the smear.

Bone marrow involvement by the leukemic process varies. In smears of marrow aspirates, lymphocytes nearly always constitute more than 40 per cent of the cells. Bone marrow biopsy sections show diffuse infiltration with lymphocytes, and at times the marrow is almost replaced by them.

Anemia is sometimes absent at first, but it develops in nearly every patient at some time during the course of the disease; it may be the result of leukemic infiltration of the bone marrow with underproduction of erythrocytes, hemorrhage, hyperhemolysis, or a combination of these factors. In some patients with splenomegaly, an apparent anemia with a low hematocrit is actually hemo-dilution, i.e., total red cell mass is normal and plasma volume increased. Unless there has been chronic blood loss the anemia is usually normocytic and normochromic in type. Severe anemia with hemoglobin as low as 3 or 5 gm. per 100 ml. is sometimes seen, but more often the hemoglobin is above 7.5 gm. per 100 ml. If a hemolytic anemia is present, it is usually associated with reticulocytosis, polychromatophilia, mild macrocytosis, and the presence of nucleated red cells in the peripheral blood. The degree of hyperhemolysis may be so mild that it is detectable only by cell survival studies, or it may be so severe that it threatens the life of the patient. In the latter situation it is usually of the autoimmune type, and the Coombs test is positive (See Chapter 7). Although platelet count is often normal, thrombocytopenia usually develops in the course of the disease.

Serum globulin abnormalities occur in most patients with chronic lympho-cytic leukemia. In one study, 67 per cent developed hypogammaglobulinemia.[44] Quantitative measurement of immunoglobulins showed severe reductions of IgA and IgM levels in the majority of one group of 57 patients.[47] A few patients show protein abnormalities resembling those seen in multiple myeloma or macroglobulinemia, i.e., a monoclonal increase in IgG or IgM levels.[47]

Another abnormality is elevation of the basal metabolic rate to plus 20 to 40 per cent, which may occur when the leukemic process is active, and at times results in symptoms of hypermetabolism.

DIAGNOSIS

The diagnosis of chronic lymphocytic leukemia is made without difficulty in most patients because generalized lymphadenopathy and lymphocytosis are usually present. Not infrequently, the disease is diagnosed in an asymptomatic stage when the patient has a general examination or enters the hospital for an operation such as herniorrhaphy. The total leukocyte count is often 10,000 to 12,000 per cu.mm.; from 50 to 70 per cent of the leukocytes in the peripheral blood are small lymphocytes. Bone marrow examination is not essential for diag-nosis, but if one is performed an increased number of lymphocytes may be found. Lymphocytic leukemoid reactions are unusual, particularly in adults, but at times it may be difficult to distinguish between lymphocytosis due to leu-kemia and that due to some other cause. Infectious mononucleosis is rare in persons over 40 years of age, whereas lymphocytic leukemia is seen most fre-quently in older people. Abnormal-appearing lymphocytes of various sizes, particularly large cells, are characteristic of infectious mononucleosis and other viral illnesses, whereas in chronic lymphocytic leukemia the blood smear con-tains mainly small lymphocytes or smudge forms. The heterophil agglutination test helps in this differentiation, since it is negative in leukemia and positive with mononucleosis.

At times the differential diagnosis between lymphocytic lymphoma and the early stage of chronic lymphocytic leukemia may be difficult. If lymphocytosis in the peripheral blood is inconstant and involvement of the bone marrow is not diffuse, lymphocytic lymphoma should be suspected. The diseases cannot always be distinguished even after biopsy of a lymph node.

Many patients have clinical pictures that appear to be transitional between leukemia and lymphoma. One group of patients exemplifies the difficulty in distinguishing between these closely-related disorders. This problem may or may not be merely a matter of semantics. There are patients with splenomegaly and pancytopenia without an absolute lymphocytosis in the peripheral blood. Aspirate of the marrow often produces only a dilute, hypocellular specimen, whereas on biopsy a packed marrow diffusely infiltrated with mononuclear cells is found; most of the cells are small, well-differentiated lymphocytes, but some are larger and more immature. Such patients may improve with corticosteroid treatment or after splenectomy; at operation there may or may not be involvement of the intra-abdominal and retroperitoneal nodes. It is uncertain whether the disorder in these patients should be classified as an atypical aleukemic form of chronic lymphocytic leukemia, or as lymphocytic lymphoma largely confined to the spleen and bone marrow. Another disorder which may present an almost identical clinical picture and be difficult to distinguish is leukemic reticuloendotheliosis (see below). Care should be taken to detect the characteristic cellular morphology and cytochemistry of the "hairy" cell which separates this entity from aleukemic chronic lymphocytic leukemia.[25]

The term "lymphosarcoma cell leukemia" has been applied to patients with clinical findings typical of chronic lymphocytic leukemia, but whose blood and bone marrow contain lymphocytes which are more variable in size, are more immature, and which tend to have an oval or notched nucleus.[183] A small number of such cells may be found in many patients with chronic lymphocytic leukemia, so that most hematologists do not separate these patients from those with classical lymphocytic leukemia. Since patients with the more immature lymphocytes have a shorter survival than those with classic lymphocytic leukemia, 40 per cent and 56 per cent five-year survival respectively,[183] separation may be worthwhile. Preferably, a term should be used for this variant of lymphocytic leukemia which does not connote a different disease process, but only indicates less differentiation of the leukemic cell. Thus, we favor the term chronic lymphocytic leukemia, prolymphocytic variety, or chronic prolymphocytic leukemia.

CLINICAL COURSE AND PROGNOSIS

Studies of lymphocyte kinetics have shown that, except for a small pool of rapidly dividing lymphocytes, most are nonproliferating and long-lived, recirculating for months or years (see Chapter 14). In chronic lymphocytic leukemia,

---

Figure 12–6 Chronic lymphocytic leukemia.

Figure 12–8 Chronic granulocytic leukemia.

From Heilmeyer, L., and Begemann, H.: Atlas der klinischen Hämatologie und Cytologie. Berlin-Göttingen-Heidelberg, Springer, 1955.

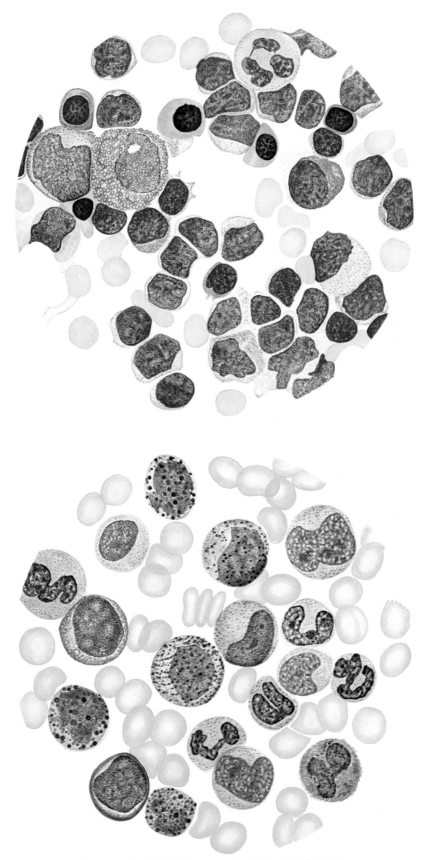

Figures 12–6 and 12–8 *See legends on opposite page*

studies indicate that long-lived lymphocytes predominate,[184] and, as the disease progresses, long-lived and apparently functionally inert lymphocytes accumulate in massive amounts in the sites through which they usually circulate, viz., lymph nodes, spleen, blood, and bone marrow. Thus, the course of the disease is characterized by: (1) progressive enlargement of the lymph nodes and spleen; (2) progressive marrow replacement with leukemic lymphocytes with resulting decrease in normal blood elements and an increased number of lymphocytes; (3) a state of altered immunity characterized by deficient levels of immunoglobulins and an increased propensity for infection and autoimmune disorders. The latter may be explained by the finding that the leukemic cells have characteristics of B lymphocytes. Cellular immunity, a T lymphocyte function, remains intact (Chapter 14).

All of these features influence survival. The survival time in chronic lymphocytic leukemia as reported by different authors varies considerably. Median survival time has ranged from 1.5 to 7.7 years, as shown in Table 12–4. Many factors, such as the sex of the patients, the dating of onset of disease, the selection of patients to be included, and the source of the material, may be responsible for the differences.

Boggs and colleagues studied the factors influencing survival in 130 patients with chronic lymphocytic leukemia whom they saw between 1945 and 1964.[13] The median survival of the entire group was six years. The survival period was nine years if those who died with other diseases were excluded, and a ten-year life-span from the time of onset of disease was suggested. Patients who had the poorer prognosis, a survival time of less than five years, manifested more clinical or laboratory evidence of disease at the time of diagnosis, were older, and were more likely to have symptoms; these features suggested that the disease probably had been present and asymptomatic for a longer period. Patients treated infrequently survived as long as did those treated regularly; this observation, and the known added hazards of bleeding and infection

Table 12–4   *Survival in Chronic Lymphocytic Leukemia*
(after onset of symptoms)

Author	Date	No. of Patients	Avg. Survival Time (Yrs.)	Median (Yrs.)	Treatment
1. Minot et al.[108]	1924	30	3.5		None
		50	3.5		X-ray
2. Leavell[92]	1938	49	3.6	3.0	X-ray
3. Wintrobe and Hasenbush[180]	1939	152	3.3		X-ray
4. Bethell[9]	1942	68	4.9		
5. Tivey[172]*	1954	685		2.8	
6. Osgood et al.[124]	1955	100		4.8	[32]P
7. Reinhard et al.[133]	1959	77†	3.5		[32]P
		25‡	6.5		
8. Feinleib and MacMahon[45]	1960	359		1.5	Various
9. Steinkamp et al.[166]	1963	119†	5.3	5.4	[32]P
		42‡	8.9		
10. Hill et al.[77]	1964	97		7.7	[32]P
11. Boggs et al.[13]	1966	130†		6.0	Various

*Series collected from literature
†Survival from diagnosis until death
‡Survival since diagnosis (patients living at time of report)

that follow treatment with radiation, cytotoxic drugs, and corticosteroids, led these authors to question whether leukemia-directed therapy prolonged survival. This study and a more recent report[185] afford strong support for the practice of individualizing treatment in each patient.

Many patients with chronic lymphocytic leukemia lead practically normal lives over a course of many years, and about one-third die of causes unrelated to leukemia. Generally, however, the disease progresses; the lymph nodes, liver, and spleen increase in size, and other manifestations of the disease, such as weakness, loss of weight, anemia, and bleeding, appear. The appearance of anemia and thrombocytopenia is associated with a relatively poor prognosis. A shortening of the length of remission after treatment, failure of the nodes and spleen to regress with therapy, the appearance of skin lesions, and the occurrence of serious bleeding are also signs of more rapid progression of the disease.

Infection eventually becomes a major problem. Deficient immunoglobulin levels combined with neutropenia secondary to marrow infiltration and chemotherapy lead particularly to bacterial infections. As a result of repeated bouts of pneumonia, sinusitis, and other infections, the patients lose weight, become weaker, and eventually die. Fatal hemorrhage may occur in the thrombocytopenic patient. In contrast to chronic granulocytic leukemia, blastic transformation does not seem to occur in chronic lymphocytic leukemia, and although acute leukemia has developed in some patients the incidence is not greater than in the general population.[66] Interestingly, the acute leukemias reported have often not been lymphoblastic.[66]

The occurrence of autoimmune hemolytic anemia is a serious development. When the anemia is severe, weakness, palpitation, fatigue, and obvious jaundice may be present. The hemolytic anemia usually responds to adrenal corticosteroid therapy, but in some patients the serum agglutinin is so reactive that crossmatching with donors is extremely difficult or even impossible. This situation is even more hazardous if the patient needs an urgent operation. It is uncertain whether this type of anemia occurs more frequently in patients treated with radiation therapy. An incidence of 26 per cent was noted in one series.[123]

When patients with chronic lymphocytic leukemia develop either gastrointestinal bleeding associated with a gastric lesion apparent on a roentgenographic study, or a mass in some part of the body, the question arises whether the lesion is a leukemic tumor or some other neoplasm. Often only a biopsy will give the answer. We have seen a variety of neoplasms, including carcinoma of the breast, pancreas, colon, prostate, and lung in patients with lymphocytic leukemia. Six reports from the literature, covering 1261 patients with chronic lymphocytic leukemia, revealed a combined incidence of various sorts of malignancies of 8 per cent.[35]

THERAPY

As in any serious disease which is incurable, the attitude of the physician is of great importance in the care of the patient. Continuing interest, periodic unhurried examinations, a certain amount of optimism, and a degree of enthusiasm for the treatment employed all help the patient to adjust to his disease.

Measures other than the "specific" therapeutic agents have contributed to the improvement in the treatment of leukemia in recent decades. Better antibiotics for the treatment of infections and the greater use of transfusions for anemia have saved lives that would have been lost in earlier years. Adrenal corticosteroids are valuable in the treatment of hemolytic anemia and thrombocytopenia when these develop. Splenectomy is occasionally employed in the treatment of the hemolytic anemia and thrombocytopenia, but the result is unpredictable and, when good, is often of short duration.

The most widely-used forms of therapy at present are irradiation, alkylating agents, and adrenal corticosteroids. There is at present no clear-cut evidence that treatment increases longevity. In addition, all forms of treatment now used may result in undesirable toxic side-effects, including decreased production of normal blood cells and immunoglobulins. Thus, in patients with chronic lymphocytic leukemia who are asymptomatic and who have only mild enlargement of the superficial lymph nodes accompanied by a mild lymphocytosis, it is advisable to defer specific treatment until progression of the disease occurs. Some patients in this category survive 10, 20, or 30 years, or even longer, and lead entirely normal lives without treatment. More often, the disease progresses and some form of therapy becomes necessary. No rigid criteria, only general guidelines, can be given regarding when to begin treatment. The leukocyte count is not a reliable guide since marked spontaneous fluctuations may occur. Most hematologists would agree that progressive adenopathy and splenomegaly, particularly if associated with weight loss and other systemic symptoms, are indications for treatment. There is, however, no general agreement about methods of treatment.

Therapeutic Agents

Radiation.   Roentgen ray therapy has been used in chronic lymphocytic leukemia for many years. Therapy may consist of whole-body radiation[83] or localized treatment for symptoms producing enlarged nodes or spleen. Radiation in the form of radioactive phosphorus (^{32}P) is considered by some to be the treatment of choice,[77, 124, 133] particularly when administered in regular doses "titrated" to maintain optimum status.[124] ^{32}P may also be used at irregular intervals as indicated by changes in the patient's condition.[77] Both forms of whole-body radiation, χ-radiation and ^{32}P, are effective in lowering the lymphocyte count and decreasing the adenopathy and splenomegaly. Neither has been shown to increase duration of survival and, in one comparative study,[79] patients treated with ^{32}P showed a shorter survival than those treated with alkylating agents.

Alkylating Agents.   The nitrogen mustard derivatives chlorambucil and cyclophosphamide are the drugs most widely used now, and they have an equally satisfactory antileukemic effect.[157] Both are marrow-suppressive but, in addition, cyclophosphamide may produce hemorrhagic cystitis. These agents may be used alone or combined with prednisone. In one controlled study, a combination of chlorambucil, 6 mg. daily, and prednisone, 30 mg. daily, for six weeks was found to be superior to chlorambucil alone, judged by tumor regression and effect on normal blood cells.[69]

Chlorambucil, 0.1 to 0.2 mg./kg. (usually 6 to 12 mg.) a day by mouth, or cyclophosphamide, 100 to 200 mg. daily, also orally, is effective. Treatment may be given continuously on a daily basis after adjustment of the dose, or intermittently. With the latter method the drug is discontinued when a satisfactory response occurs, and recommenced when indicated. Complete remission is unusual in this disease, and usually is not the aim of treatment. Studies comparing these methods show no difference in survival.[79,157] Continuous therapy is more likely to result in depression of normal blood elements, so we prefer the intermittent method. With either method, blood counts must be checked regularly to avoid serious marrow depression. There are, as yet, no good studies evaluating short (four- to five-day) courses of larger amounts of chemotherapeutic agents given intermittently to increase the antileukemic effects while allowing time for recovery of normal blood cells between courses, as used in treatment of lymphocytic lymphoma.[3]

Adrenal Corticosteroids. As discussed above, prednisone may be given together with alkylating agents, or may be used for three to four weeks prior to use of an alkylating agent. Given in 0.5 to 1 mg. per kg. amounts, dramatic reduction in the size of lymph nodes often occurs, accompanied by a sharp increase in peripheral lymphocyte count which may persist for a month or more. Lessening of symptoms and a feeling of well-being also occur. Lack of bone marrow toxicity is a definite advantage of prednisone. Nevertheless, other side-effects, including an increase of the patient's susceptibility to infection, limit its usefulness as an antileukemic agent.

Large doses of prednisone, 60 to 145 mg. daily, may improve patients with advanced disease who either are refractory to alkylating agents or, owing to marrow depression, cannot tolerate more of these drugs.[157] Because of the undesirable sequelae of steroid treatment, the dose should be reduced and the drug discontinued as soon as possible. Intermittent maintenance therapy, such as administration of the drug two or three days a week, may reduce the incidence of complications.

Other Forms of Treatment. A number of other methods have been used to decrease the lymphocyte mass in chronic lymphocytic leukemia. These include antilymphocyte serum,[66] leukapheresis,[33] and extracorporeal irradiation of the blood.[48] None of these is preferable to the combined use of prednisone and an alkylating agent once the decision is made to treat.

Use of androgens[87] may be of benefit when anemia is severe and studies indicate decreased production of erythrocytes. In this situation, bone marrow biopsy usually shows massive infiltration with lymphocytes. Combining use of alkylating agents to decrease the marrow infiltration, and a less virilizing androgen such as oxymetholone to stimulate erythropoiesis, may be successful when either agent fails on its own.

Unfortunately, none of the present methods of treatment improves the serious and life-shortening immunoglobulin deficiency. When infections occur repeatedly, prophylactic use of gamma globulin and antibiotics may be helpful.[105] It should be stressed, however, that no controlled clinical trials have been conducted to study the efficacy of antibiotics or gamma globulin in preventing infection in chronic lymphocytic leukemia.

Illustrative Case

This 54-year-old white male noticed the onset of fatigue and weight loss in the summer of 1964. He was found to have an elevated white count with a predominance of lymphocytes, and he was referred for consideration of treatment.

Physical Examination. There was generalized lymphadenopathy, and the spleen was palpable 4 cm. below the left costal margin.

Laboratory Examination. WBC 42,000 per mm³ with 86% small lymphocytes, 12% segmented neutrophils, 1 eosinophil, and 1 basophil. Hematocrit 46%, platelet count 91,500 per mm³.

Course. A diagnosis of chronic lymphocytic leukemia was made and no treatment given. Over the next year the patient continued to feel below par, began to have some night sweats, and enlarging lymph nodes were noted together with slight increase of size of spleen. In August, 1966 treatment with cyclophosphamide, 150 mg. a day, was begun. After six weeks the WBC had decreased to 25,000 per mm³ with 83% lymphocytes, and the treatment was stopped. The lymph nodes became smaller, the spleen decreased somewhat in size, and the symptoms improved. Over the next two years he remained relatively stable but in April, 1968 the hematocrit had decreased to 34% associated with a reticulocyte count of 1.2% and a negative Coombs test. Platelet count had decreased to 54,000 per mm³, and the white count had risen to 281,000 with 98% lymphocytes. Over the next six months the spleen continued to enlarge and was palpable at the pelvic brim. Radioactive isotope studies showed a remarkably expanded plasma volume and a normal red cell mass. For this reason, a splenectomy was performed in November, 1968. Four months later the hematocrit had risen to 34% with return of the plasma volume to normal. Over the next six months anemia slowly progressed in severity and in June, 1969 a bone marrow biopsy revealed almost complete replacement of the marrow with small well-differentiated lymphocytes. The anemia was thought to be primarily related to inadequate production of erythrocytes secondary to marrow replacement with lymphocytes. Prednisone, 60 mg. a day, was begun together with methandrostenolone, 30 mg. a day. After a month prednisone was decreased to 10 mg. a day, and after three months the hematocrit had risen to 41%. When, despite this treatment, the anemia recurred with an hematocrit of 21% in March, 1970, cyclophosphamide was restarted at 100 mg. a day, and oxymetholone, 80 mg. a day, was substituted for the methandrostenolone. From March to June, 1970 there was progressive improvement in the hematocrit up to 50%, a decrease in the white count from 327,000 to 37,000 and a rise in platelets from 89,000 to 197,000.

The patient felt better and continued to improve for approximately two years, but in December, 1972 the liver had enlarged markedly to a span of 20 cm., the generalized adenopathy had increased, the hematocrit had decreased to 35%, and the white count had risen to 210,000 with a platelet count of 62,000. His energy had decreased and he did not feel well. Combination chemotherapy was begun consisting of cyclophosphamide, 300 mg. a day for five days, prednisone, 400 mg. a day for five days, and an injection of vincristine, 2 mg. This was repeated every four weeks for nine courses and produced remarkable improvement. The patient felt stronger, the liver decreased to a span of 9 cm., the hematocrit rose to 47%, the white count fell to 13,000 with 68% lymphocytes, and the platelets rose to 305,000. He then did well with no treatment from July, 1973 until October, 1974, when an apparent cholecystitis developed associated with obstructive jaundice, and he was hospitalized. At exploratory laparotomy, multiple enlarged lymph nodes partially occluding the common bile duct were seen. Lymph nodes removed from around the common duct showed changes typical of chronic lymphocytic leukemia.

Following operation he has made good progress, with complete clearing of jaundice. He continues to have generalized small lymphadenopathy, a liver span of 13.5 cm., hematocrit of 42%, and a white count of 20,500 with 20% segs and 77% lymphocytes. He is not on any treatment at present.

Comment. This patient illustrates a number of features of chronic lymphocytic leukemia. He shows the prolonged course that can occur, sometimes extending for several years without treatment. The massive splenomegaly resulted in expansion of the plasma volume with dilutional anemia which responded in part to removal of the spleen. Anemia related to replacement of the marrow with lymphocytes and inadequate production of red cells responded completely to a combination of cytotoxic therapy and androgens. Another feature was the excellent response to intermittent high dose chemotherapy as used for lymphocytic lymphomas. Obstructive jaundice caused by enlarged lymph nodes around the common bile duct was relieved by removal of the nodes. This case also illustrates the fact that such patients usually do well as long as their immunologic status does not predispose them to infection.

LEUKEMIC RETICULOENDOTHELIOSIS

Several terms have been proposed for this group of patients who have, in the peripheral blood and bone marrow, abnormal cells that display features of both lymphocytes and histiocytes. Most of the terms used were based on morphologic interpretation of the characteristic cell, and include chronic reticulolymphocytic leukemia, "hairy-cell" leukemia, and reticulum cell leukemia.[25] Recent functional studies suggest that the abnormal cell is of lymphocytic origin,[24] whereas others suggest that the cells are histiocytes.[88a] This disorder may make up 2 per cent of all leukemias.[17]

Typically, adults are affected, the majority being over 50 years of age, with a four-to-one male predominance. Onset is characteristically slow and insidious. Infection may be the presenting finding. The outstanding physical finding is splenomegaly, which is present in almost every case and often reaches a massive size. Lymphadenopathy is infrequent, but moderate enlargement of the liver occurs in about one-half of the cases. Pancytopenia is present in almost all patients. Leukopenia, particularly neutropenia, is a striking finding. The characteristic abnormal cells are present in the blood in most patients, although a buffy coat smear may be required to locate them.

The diagnosis is established by discovery of the characteristic cells in the blood and bone marrow. A varying percentage of the cells which resemble lymphocytes has an irregular cytoplasmic border. The nuclear chromatin pattern is quite fine and differs from the more smudged nuclear chromatin pattern of the lymphocyte. A specific cytochemical reaction is a tartrate-resistant acid phosphatase.[181] Bone marrow biopsy sections show extensive infiltration with the abnormal cell, usually with an associated dense reticulin network.

The disease runs a chronic steadily progressive course. Median survival has been reported to be between three and five years. Since there is no known cure, treatment usually consists of observation only, unless leukopenia leads to problems of infection, or anemia leads to symptoms. In this situation splenectomy is the treatment of choice, and patients progress well thereafter for a time, but anemia usually recurs and may respond to androgens. Sometimes adrenal corticosteroids plus vincristine may bring about clinical improvement. Use of cytotoxic drugs usually is not helpful, and may indeed be harmful.

Illustrative Case

On admission to another hospital in 1972 for vaginal bleeding, this 61-year-old woman was found to have leukopenia of approximately 2500 cells/cu.mm. She had a history of easy bruising for $1\frac{1}{2}$ years. She was not anemic, but platelets were slightly decreased at 100,000/cu.mm. Blood smear showed 50% lymphocytes, 2 myelocytes, and 48% band and segmented granulocytes. Bone marrow aspirate was hypocellular, and she was thought to have marrow depression related to drug toxicity. Following this she had no complaints until she injured her thumb in February, 1974. Cellulitis developed at the site of injury and progressed to involve the hand, and at the same time a necrotizing skin infection developed along the right side of the neck. She became febrile. During this time the white cell count was approximately 2000, with 60% segmented neutrophils. Blood cultures revealed a group A beta-hemolytic streptococcus for which penicillin was prescribed. There was no improvement, and she was referred to the University of Virginia in March, 1974.

Physical Examination. There was no adenopathy, but the spleen was palpable 4 cm. below the left costal margin. There was cellulitis of the right arm from the midhumerus to the wrist. An area of cellulitis was also present on the right leg, in addition to a necrotic area of skin infection on the right side of the neck.

Laboratory Examination. Hematocrit 27%, reticulocytes 2%, WBC 1600 with 47% segs, 51% lymphocytes, 1% monocytes, and 1% eosinophils. Platelet count 143,000 per mm³. Bone marrow biopsy sections revealed a very hyperplastic marrow with an increase in reticulin fibers. Touch preparation of the marrow aspirate revealed many "hairy" cells diagnostic of leukemic reticuloendotheliosis.

Hospital Course. The patient required intensive antibiotic treatment and débridement of the neck. She had a stormy hospital course complicated by bilateral pneumonia and middle ear effusions, and was febrile for the first 26 hospital days. During this time anemia became more severe, blood transfusions were required.

After she was afebrile for approximately ten days and the general condition had improved, splenectomy was performed. Sections of the spleen revealed intense leukemic infiltrate. Touch preparations of the spleen revealed complete replacement with "hairy" cells. Two days after splenectomy the white count had risen to the range of 7000 per cu.mm., with the percentage of segmented neutrophils ranging from 29 to 45%. The platelet count rose to 300,000 per mm³ and the hematocrit remained stable at the transfused level of 39%. Postoperatively good progress was made, and the patient was discharged from the hospital a week after splenectomy.

Since discharge she has remained well with no further infections. When seen one year after surgery she was doing well and had a white blood cell count of 11,600 with 30% neutrophils, 40% hairy cells, and 30% lymphocytes. Hematocrit was 39%.

Comment. This patient exemplifies the slowly-developing, insidious onset of leukemic reticuloendotheliosis. She had a two-year period with mild cytopenias without serious difficulty. As is often the case, diagnosis was not made until serious infection developed and a bone marrow study revealed the typical "hairy" cells. The patient had a difficult time clearing the infections, but once splenectomy was performed the neutrophil number became adequate and she had no further infections for a year postsplenectomy. This case illustrates the good progress made by many patients after splenectomy.

CHRONIC GRANULOCYTIC LEUKEMIA

INCIDENCE

Chronic granulocytic (myelocytic) leukemia is found in all races and in both sexes, and is primarily a disease of middle age. In 1924 Minot, Buckman, and Isaacs[107] presented data on 130 patients with chronic granulocytic leukemia. In this series the commonest age of onset was from 35 to 45 years. Fifty-six per cent of patients were males. In 1951 Shimkin, Mettier, and Bierman[156] reviewed the incidence and distribution of chronic myelogenous leukemia, compared their data with those of Minot, Buckman, and Isaacs, and noted an increased incidence of the disease, particularly in women, and an increased age at onset.

CLINICAL MANIFESTATIONS

The onset of chronic granulocytic leukemia is usually gradual; occasionally its presence is discovered during a routine examination. The period between the appearance of symptoms and the time the patient seeks medical advice is usually from eight to nine months. The most common initial symptoms are the presence of discomfort in the left upper quadrant or the upper abdomen, or the accidental finding of a mass in this area. The patient often complains of a sensation of fullness and gaseous eructations after eating. Not infrequently, signs of active disease such as loss of weight, fever, and night sweats are present.

Usually the persistence and progression of these relatively mild symptoms lead the patient to consult his physician.

Less often the disease makes itself known more abruptly. Massive gastro-intestinal hemorrhage manifested by either hematemesis or melena may be the first definite indication of disease. Others seek medical advice because of aching in the back and extremities, or because of a pleuritic type of pain in the left upper quadrant and lower portion of the left chest which radiates to the left shoulder, evidence of splenic infarction. The occurrence of hemorrhages or infiltrative lesions in the skin may be the first evidence of the disease. Visual disturbance from retinal hemorrhages is at times the initial complaint. In some patients, the initial symptoms are those of anemia—dyspnea on exertion, dizziness, palpitation, easy fatigue, and weakness.

Fever from the leukemia per se is a late manifestation of the disease, and when it occurs it often continues until the death of the patient. Priapism develops in chronic granulocytic leukemia more often than in other types of leukemia, but is very rare.

The most striking abnormality on physical examination is splenomegaly, present in nearly all patients at the time of initial examination. In one series of patients the lower border of the spleen extended below the umbilicus at the time of the initial visit in 70 per cent.[153] As the disease progresses, the splenomegaly

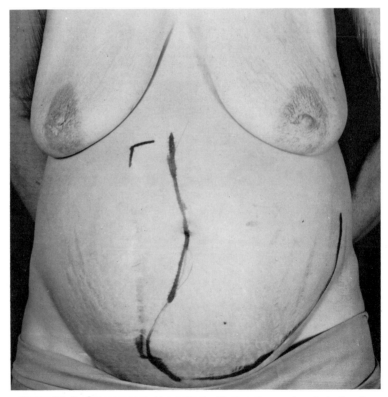

Figure 12–7 Splenomegaly in a patient with chronic granulocytic leukemia.

responds less to treatment and sometimes steadily increases in size until it eventually fills the entire left half of the abdomen and occasionally the right lower abdomen as well (Fig. 12–7). The sudden appearance of hernia or uterine prolapse has been noted in some patients with massive splenomegaly. In most patients the splenomegaly is associated with considerable enlargement of the liver, which is usually firm and nontender. Mild degrees of enlargement of the superficial lymph nodes may be seen in patients with chronic leukemia, but the enlargement does not reach the degree seen in those with lymphocytic leukemia; frequently, no significant lymphadenopathy is present. Retinal lesions, such as engorgement of the veins and white-centered areas of hemorrhage, are seen in a high percentage of the patients with chronic leukemia. At times leukemic infiltration along the peripheral portion of the distended veins and blurring of the disc margin are present. The skin and mucous membranes are often pale, and petechial lesions and ecchymoses are not unusual. Light or moderate pressure on the lower portion of the sternum produces pain in many patients; this tenderness is present during the active phase of the disease, and often subsides as the disease responds to treatment.

LABORATORY MANIFESTATIONS

Anemia occurs at some time in practically all patients with chronic granulocytic leukemia, but is not invariably present when the patient is first seen. The anemia tends to increase as the disease progresses and improve as the disease regresses in response to treatment. It is usually normocytic and normochromic. On blood smear, erythrocyte morphology is usually normal, but an occasional nucleated red cell may be seen. The hemoglobin may be as low as 4 or 5 gm. per 100 ml., but is more often in the range of 7 to 9 gm. per 100 ml. on first examination. The reticulocyte count is usually normal or slightly elevated. Anemia may be the result either of bleeding, diminished erythropoiesis secondary to the encroachment on the erythropoietic tissue of the marrow by the leukemic cells, or hemodilution in patients with massive splenomegaly. In some patients with this disease hyperhemolysis is present.

The most striking abnormality in granulocytic leukemia is found in the leukocytes. The total leukocyte count is increased, and although it may exceed 1 million per cu.mm., it is commonly between 100,000 and 300,000 per cu.mm. Such high values are the result of an increase in segmented neutrophils, band cells, juveniles, and myelocytes; a few myeloblasts and promyelocytes may be seen, but they do not constitute a large percentage of the cells in chronic granulocytic leukemia. The eosinophils and basophils are usually increased (Fig. 12–8).

At the time of diagnosis the platelet count is increased in over one-half of the patients, with counts over 1 million per cu.mm. sometimes seen. Thrombocytopenia is often present later in the disease.

Examination of bone marrow usually reveals a marked increase in cellularity due chiefly to an increase in cells of the granulocytic series. The M:E ratio (Chapter 3) is very high. Often the percentage of the younger cells in this series is increased, but at times the differential count of the marrow falls within normal limits. Thus, except for cytogenetic study and as baseline information useful for comparison later in the course, marrow aspirate is not of much help diagnostically. Erythropoiesis is normoblastic in type, and megakaryocytes usually are present in normal or increased numbers. Biopsy of the marrow shows marked hyperplasia of granulocytic elements. In addition, fibrosis may be demonstrable, particularly later in the disease.[60]

Cytogenetic study of the bone marrow reveals the Philadelphia (Ph[1]) chromosome in 70 to 95 per cent of patients with chronic granulocytic leukemia.[43, 116, 117, 118] The Ph[1] chromosome is a G-group chromosome, number 22,[121] which has lost a portion of its long arms by translocation to chromosome number 9.[138] When present, with rare exceptions,[168] it is found in all metaphases seen in direct preparations of marrow. The exceptions may represent residual nonleukemic cells. Patients with apparent chronic granulocytic leukemia who do not show the Ph[1] chromosome differ from the classic Ph[1] (+) group, as discussed below.

Cytochemical determination of the peripheral blood neutrophil (leukocyte) alkaline phosphatase activity reveals a value lower than normal in 90 per cent of patients with chronic granulocytic leukemia.[43]

Serum vitamin B_{12} and B_{12} binding capacity are both greatly elevated in this disease.[73] These findings reflect the increased mass of granulocytes which apparently synthesize the vitamin B_{12} binding proteins, transcobalamin I and III.[150]

Other abnormalities include an increased serum uric acid and an elevated basal metabolic rate not related to thyroid function. Roentgenologic examination may reveal osseous lesions in various parts of the skeleton. Subperiosteal new bone formation, osteolytic lesions, and transverse bands of diminished density at the ends of the long bones are the commonest abnormalities.[35,113,158] Osteosclerotic lesions are less common.

DIAGNOSIS

Many infectious, inflammatory, and malignant disorders may simulate chronic granulocytic leukemia by producing a granulocytic leukemoid reaction. With these conditions, the leukocyte count usually does not exceed 50,000 per cu.mm., but the whole array of granulocytic precursors may be seen in the blood smear. Often the clinical setting permits the differential diagnosis to be made, but at times this is difficult. It is helpful in establishing the diagnosis if the findings usually associated with granulocytic leukemia are present, i.e., eosinophilia, basophilia, thrombocytosis, and splenomegaly. Fortunately most of the conditions resulting in a reactive granulocytosis are also associated with elevated leukocyte alkaline phosphatase activity, in distinct contrast to the abnormally low values usually found in chronic granulocytic leukemia. Demonstration of the Ph[1] chromosome by karyotypic analysis of marrow cells confirms the diagnosis of chronic granulocytic leukemia.

Distinguishing this condition from other myeloproliferative conditions (see Chapter 10) may be extremely difficult since many of their features overlap. Again, the leukocyte alkaline phosphatase is usually elevated in these disorders, and the Ph[1] chromosome is rarely, if ever, found in conditions other than chronic granulocytic leukemia.[66]

CLINICAL COURSE AND PROGNOSIS

Reported survival times vary considerably (Table 12–5). With most forms of treatment, the median survival time from onset of symptoms is probably between three and four years; the prognosis is better for females than for males by about six to twelve months. The five-year survival rate is probably between 15 and 25 per cent, but a few patients live for 15 or 20 years. The initial course of treatment may be followed by an excellent clinical remission, but relapse inevitably occurs. The leukocyte count usually rises during relapse, but clinical relapse does not invariably follow an increase in the leukocyte count. In fact, marked cyclical oscillation of the leukocyte count has been noted suggesting persistence of some marrow regulatory mechanism in chronic granulocytic leukemia.[168] If the leukocyte count continues to rise over a period of several months, a relapse is likely.

Subsequent courses of therapy generally bring remissions of shorter duration, and the response of the spleen and blood usually is not nearly so satisfactory as in the first remission. As the disease progresses, splenomegaly and anemia become more constant features. The course of this disorder is sometimes accompanied by severe attacks of left upper quadrant pain and fever which are the result of splenic infarction or perisplenitis.

Transformation into acute leukemia (blastic transformation) occurs in 70 per cent of patients, and usually leads to death in a few weeks or months.[170] Most of the remaining patients enter an accelerated phase[85] characterized by cachexia, fever, night sweats, persistent anemia, and the occurrence of hemorrhage. This phase leads to death within a few months, with hemorrhage or infection as the terminal event.

Some unfavorable signs occur in the course which predict the imminent onset of blastic transformation or the accelerated phase.[170] These include: (1) peripheral blood basophilia in excess of 20 per cent; (2) an unexplained increase

Table 12–5 *Survival in Chronic Granulocytic Leukemia*
(after onset of symptoms)

AUTHOR	DATE	NO. OF PATIENTS	MEDIAN SURVIVAL (YRS.)	TREATMENT
1. Minot et al.[107]	1924	52	2.6	None
		78		X-ray
2. Leavell[92]	1938	87	2.5	X-ray
3. Tivey[172]*	1954	1090	2.7	
4. Osgood et al.[124]†	1956	100	4.8	^{32}P
5. Reinhard et al.[133]	1959	118	2.6	^{32}P
6. Haut et al.[70]	1961	30	3.6	Busulfan
7. M.R.C.[102]	1968	48	3.6	Busulfan
		54	3.0	X-ray
8. Kennedy[88]	1972	10	4.2**	Hydroxyurea
9. Canellos et al.[22]	1975	20	3.7**	Dibromomannitol

*Series collected from literature
**After diagnosis
†Chronic lymphocytic leukemia and chronic granulocytic leukemia — same survival

in the leukocyte alkaline phosphatase activity; (3) development of marrow fibrosis;[60] (4) cytogenetic demonstration of multiple Philadelphia chromosomes, or chromosomal aneuploidy; (5) fever without infection; (6) shortening of the time required for the immature circulating granulocytes to double in number.[168]

At time of diagnosis an unfavorable prognosis is suggested by myelofibrosis[60] and by absence of the Ph[1] chromosome.[43] Compared to Ph[1] (+) patients, those without the Ph[1] chromosome had lower leukocyte and platelet counts, did not respond as well to antileukemic therapy, and developed blastic transformation earlier. Median survival of Ph[1] (−) patients was eight months compared to 40 months in the Ph[1] (+) group.[43]

TREATMENT

Although chronic granulocytic leukemia may be discovered on a routine examination when the patient is asymptomatic, it is unusual if more than a few months elapse before the patient develops symptoms and needs treatment. Both supportive and more specific measures are employed in the treatment of this disease.

The most important supportive measures are transfusions and antibiotics. Anemia is treated by transfusion only if it is severe, or if it fails to respond as the disease improves with specific therapy. Antibiotics are used when infections are present. Any patient who presents with what appears to be a febrile relapse of leukemia should be studied carefully for infection that may be treated successfully.

The specific measures available for treatment include radiation and chemotherapy. At the present time the available treatment is palliative, its aim to reduce the granulocytic mass toward normal, thereby decreasing the splenomegaly, improving marrow function, and abolishing symptoms. Even when complete clinical and hematologic remission occur, the Ph[1] chromosome remains, indicating persistence of the disease. In addition, although available therapy has definitely improved the quality of life, survival has been extended only slightly and no treatment method has prevented blastic transformation. In view of this, vigorous attempts to eradicate the disease are being evaluated and will be discussed later.

Radiation Therapy

For many years splenic irradiation was used extensively for treatment of chronic granulocytic leukemia. It has been largely abandoned since the report of better results with busulfan in a randomized controlled clinical trial comparing the two methods (Table 12–5).[102]

Radiation in the form of radioactive phosphorus (^{32}P) is effective in the treatment of this disease.[91, 123] Osgood et al. advocated the use of regularly spaced titrated amounts of ^{32}P to maintain the patient in "optimum" status.[123] They reported a somewhat longer median duration of survival than other centers either using ^{32}P in a different schedule[133] or using chemotherapeutic agents (Table 12–5). Whether this method of treatment is superior, or the results are related to patient selection or other factors, is not certain.

Chemotherapy

Busulfan is currently the agent of choice for treating chronic granulocytic leukemia based on efficacy, availability, and ease of treatment.[70,102,168] Busulfan is an alkylating agent whose main toxicity is bone marrow depression. The daily dose is more important in terms of toxicity than the total dose. The initial daily dose for an adult is 4 to 6 mg. orally. Since the rate at which the leukocyte count decreases is dose-related, the decrease will be slow with this relatively low dose. As a result, weekly leukocyte and platelet counts are sufficient to regulate the dose and prevent serious marrow depression. If the platelet count goes below normal limits during treatment, the dose must be decreased and the patient followed carefully since irreversible thrombocytopenia and marrow depression may result. The leukocyte count may not begin to decrease for two weeks, but when it does it may continue for three to four weeks after the drug is discontinued. Thus, busulfan should be stopped when the leukocyte count is around 15,000 per cu.mm. This level is achieved by over three-quarters of the patients in three months or less. At this time, the blood smear usually appears normal and the spleen is no longer palpable. About one-half of the patients who respond have remissions that last over six months, occasionally more than two years. The longer remissions are more likely to follow if treatment is continued until the leukocyte count is in the normal range, but this is associated with increased risks. When relapse occurs, the course of treatment is repeated. Subsequent remissions are usually of shorter duration than the first. We prefer intermittent treatment to continuous treatment with small doses. However, if relapse occurs within one to two months, maintenance therapy of 2 mg. per day, or 2 mg. two or three times per week, may be employed. Maintenance therapy is preferred by some, but no controlled study has finally settled this question.

Although adverse effects aside from those on the bone marrow are not common, busulfan has produced a variety of toxic reactions.[168] These include generalized skin pigmentation, amenorrhea, gynecomastia, impotence, sterility, alopecia, pulmonary fibrosis, and renal damage with hyperuricemia. Nausea, vomiting, diarrhea, cheilosis, and glossitis are not common, but may occur.

Other chemotherapeutic agents effective in chronic granulocytic leukemia include dibromomannitol[22,168] and hydroxyurea (See Table 12–5).[88,168]

Dibromomannitol (DBM) is a brominated sugar alcohol which is cytotoxic. Compared to busulfan, the myelosuppressive effect of DBM is more predictable, but duration of induced remission is not as long.[22] DBM may be effective in patients who no longer respond to busulfan, if blastic transformation has not occurred.

Hydroxyurea is a specific inhibitor of DNA synthesis. It results in rapid lowering of the elevated leukocyte count,[88] but it is not preferable to busulfan in chronic granulocytic leukemia. Like DBM, hydroxyurea may be effective in patients refractory to busulfan.[88]

Other therapeutic methods being investigated include extracorporeal irradiation of the blood, leukapheresis, and immunotherapy.[168] Splenectomy[168] may be beneficial in a few patients who are not in the blastic phase but who have chemotherapy-resistant massive splenomegaly associated with any or all of the following: (1) symptoms of gastric compression; (2) repeated splenic infarctions; (3) marked thrombocytopenia; or (4) severe dilutional anemia.[75]

Blastic Transformation

This catastrophic occurrence is the major threat to survival in chronic granulocytic leukemia. It occurs in 70 per cent of patients, is usually resistant to treatment, and leads to death within a few weeks or months.[170] The blood and marrow findings usually are similar to those seen in acute myeloblastic leukemia, with at least 20 per cent blast cells in the marrow. Anemia, thrombocytopenia, splenomegaly, and a deteriorating clinical state are usually present. In some patients the immature cells have morphologic[14] and enzymatic[55] features of lymphoblasts. This has led to speculation that chronic granulocytic leukemia is a disease of a pluripotential stem cell capable of undergoing myeloblastic or lymphoblastic differentiation.[14,55]

Treatment of blastic transformation is like that described for acute myeloblastic leukemia (page 426), but the results are worse. In view of the report showing 30 per cent remission with prednisone and vincristine,[21] and the possibility that some of the transformations may be lymphoblastic, a drug combination[12] may be preferable that includes agents active against both myeloblastic and lymphoblastic leukemia, e.g., cyclophosphamide, cytosine arabinoside, prednisone, and vincristine.

Aggressive Approach to Treatment

A prospective study has been started in an attempt to determine if intensive treatment will eliminate the leukemic cells, prevent blastic transformation, and improve survival.[38] The experimental treatment consists of splenic irradiation followed first by splenectomy and then by multiple drug chemotherapy. This approach is based on several observations: (1) presence of the Ph[1] chromosome in patients brought into otherwise complete remission with busulfan indicates persistence of leukemic cells; (2) this cell line undergoes blastic transformation as suggested by the finding of the Ph[1] chromosome in blast metaphases analyzed during the stage of blastic transformation; (3) there is good evidence that chronic granulocytic leukemia is of clonal origin (page 418),[66] and that suppression of the Ph[1] (+) leukemic clone may result in appearance of Ph[1] (−) presumably nonleukemic cells.[168] More time is needed before the results of this aggressive approach can be evaluated.

Illustrative Case

This 60-year-old woman was well until she developed nausea and vomiting in May, 1972.

Physical Examination. No adenopathy was present, but the liver was slightly enlarged and the spleen was palpable 7 cm. below the left costal margin.

Laboratory Examination. Hematocrit 29%. Red cell indices showed a normocytic normochromic anemia; reticulocyte count 3%. Leukocyte count 310,000/cu.mm. with 2% myeloblasts, 3% promyelocytes, 10% metamyelocytes, 28% band forms, 40% segmented forms, 8% basophils, 5% eosinophils, and 4% lymphocytes. Platelet count 438,000/mm³ (elevated). The leukocyte alkaline phosphatase score was 1 (normal = 14-120). Bone marrow examination revealed marked granulocytic hyperplasia, and the Philadelphia chromosome was present.

Course. The patient was treated with intermittent busulfan to keep her white count under 30,000/mm³, and she did well for 16 months.

In September, 1973 she developed fatigue, jaundice, and fever without infection. On admission to the hospital her WBC count was 6,700/mm,³ with an occasional blast seen on blood smear. Platelet count was 26,000/mm³ and hematocrit 30%. Bone marrow aspirate was hypercellular with many blasts morphologically resembling lymphoblasts. She was treated intensively with cytosine arabinoside, vincristine, and prednisone. After two courses of therapy the patient had a complete clinical and hematologic remission which was maintained with weekly cytosine arabinoside and 6–thioguanine, and intermittent vincristine.

She did well for four months, but then developed weakness of the legs followed by severe bitemporal headaches and confusion. Her peripheral WBC count and differential were normal at this time. She was admitted to the hospital where lumbar puncture revealed an elevated opening pressure and approximately 1000 cells/mm³. On slides prepared by cyto-centrifugation these cells appeared to be lymphoblasts exhibiting the characteristic large PAS-positive cytoplasmic granules and a negative peroxidase reaction. Treatment was begun with intrathecal methotrexate, 15 mg. weekly, and the patient had marked symptomatic improvement with partial return of strength in her legs. She did not want further intrathecal treatment, and approximately six weeks later developed fever and pancytopenia. Bone marrow aspiration again revealed large numbers of immature cells resembling lymphoblasts. The patient died before further therapy could be given.

Comment. This patient had classic chronic granulocytopenia leukemia with diagnostic clinical features, plus abnormally low leukocyte alkaline phosphatase and the Ph¹ chromosome on cytogenetic study of the marrow. Busulfan controlled the disease until the abrupt onset of blastic transformation. Interestingly, the blasts appeared morphologically and cytochemically to be lymphoblasts, and complete remission was achieved with combination chemotherapy which included prednisone and vincristine. Extramyeloid blastic disease developed in the CNS which responded to intrathecal treatment. Nevertheless, she died 34 months after diagnosis and 18 months after onset of blastic transformation.

EOSINOPHILIC LEUKEMIA

Although the existence of eosinophilic leukemia is questioned by some authors and is considered a variant of chronic granulocytic leukemia by others, a number of cases, including 43 with autopsy, have been reported.[7,8] The following criteria have been proposed for the diagnosis of eosinophilic leukemia: hepatosplenomegaly, lymphadenopathy, and marked persistent eosinophilia, usually accompanied by anemia and thrombocytopenia. Some of the autopsied patients had chloromas; those with evidence of other diseases which might have caused eosinophilia were excluded. The leukocyte counts ranged between 50,000 and 200,000 per cu.mm. Over 60 per cent were eosinophilic granulocytes; blast cells were observed in the peripheral blood of 27 patients, and in one patient constituted 80 per cent of the cells. Features of the disease different from those usually seen in chronic granulocytic leukemia were the high incidence of involvement of the central nervous system (20 per cent) without association of bleeding or thrombocytopenia, and intractable heart failure which occurred in several patients; at autopsy, cardiac fibrosis and eosinophilic infiltration of the myocardium were found. The Philadelphia chromosome was not found in the two patients in whom it was sought. Response to treatment was poor.

CHRONIC MYELOMONOCYTIC LEUKEMIA

A variant of myelomonocytic leukemia[104,155,161] has been described which differs in several important ways from the usual acute variety. Patients with this variant often have a prodromal illness characterized by fever and fatigue which lasts for four to six months. At diagnosis, severe anemia is common and thrombocytopenia is often present. An absolute monocytosis is found in the blood. The bone marrow is hyperplastic and shows a monocytosis, but less than 20 per cent myeloblasts are present. The predominant cell is an atypical myelocyte.[104] Developmental abnormalities in both the myeloid and erythroid precursors are common. Survival, without treatment, of more than 12 months is common and one patient survived for 11 years.[161] On occasion the white blood cell count will rise to more than 50,000/mm^3 (more than 50 per cent of these cells being monocytes), but the consistent elevation of white blood cell count seen in chronic granulocytic leukemia is not common. Transformation into acute leukemia, usually of the myelomonocytic variety, is the most frequent terminal event, but patients may die of infection or bleeding without such transformation. Infection is frequent during the course.

Experience with combination chemotherapy in this disorder has been disappointing, but few trials have been reported. Survival may be prolonged with supportive care alone.

SPECIAL THERAPEUTIC PROBLEMS IN THE LEUKEMIAS

Management of the pregnant patient with leukemia requires special consideration. Although there is no evidence that pregnancy has an adverse effect on the course of any type of leukemia, the hazards of pregnancy and delivery are greatly increased. Another problem is the effect that antileukemic therapy might have on the fetus.[163] Because of this possibility, an effort should be made to avoid any treatment during pregnancy; treatment should be given during the first three months only if absolutely essential. For the patient with chronic leukemia, usually granulocytic, therapy may be delayed until delivery, or at least past the first trimester when the potential mutagenic effect of chemotherapy is greatest. Busulfan has been used safely even in the first trimester.[40] It may not be possible to delay treatment of acute leukemia past this stage. The chemotherapeutic agents previously discussed are the agents of choice in this situation. One thorough review found no recorded instance of congenital abnormality attributable to the treatment of leukemia in pregnancy.[66] Intrauterine and neonatal death of the infant is a frequent occurrence even without chemotherapy. These and other aspects must be considered in early pregnancy when the question of therapeutic abortion arises. This can be decided only by discussion with the patient, her husband, and obstetrician.

At times, the advisability of surgical operation arises in some patients with leukemia. In acute leukemia in relapse the risk of surgery is so great and the prognosis usually so poor, particularly in adults, that only life saving operations are ever considered. In a patient with any type of leukemia, the decision for or against operation must be an individual one made only after an evaluation of all the aspects of the problem.

Not infrequently, patients with chronic leukemia need operations such as prostatic resection, cholecystectomy, hysterectomy, cataract extraction, or pinning of a fractured hip; at times more serious ones, such as resection of the colon for carcinoma, may be necessary. Although complications of bleeding and infection are not uncommon, the operative survival rate for patients with chronic lymphatic leukemia approaches that of other patients of the same age. Patients with chronic granulocytic leukemia have more complications and a more difficult time.[5]

For elective procedures in a patient with uncomplicated chronic lymphocytic leukemia, it may be necessary to correct the anemia. This should be done without treatment with cytotoxic drugs, because of the attendant risk of thrombocytopenia. Mild autoimmune hemolytic anemia is often controlled by corticosteroid drugs, but severe anemia of this type increases the risk and may lead to difficulty in cross-matching for blood transfusion. Before elective surgery, it is advisable to bring the patient with chronic granulocytic leukemia into good clinical and hematologic remission.

References

1. Aisenberg, A. C., Bloch, K. J., Long, J. C., and Colvin, R. B.: Reaction of normal human lymphocytes and chronic lymphocytic leukemia cells with an antithymocyte antiserum. Blood, *41*:417, 1973.

2. Aksoy, M., Dincol, K., Erdem, S., and Dincol, G.: Acute leukemia due to chronic exposure to benzene. Am. J. Med., *52*:160, 1972.
3. Bagley, C. M., Jr., DeVita, V. T., Jr., Berard, C. W., and Canellos, G. P.: Advanced lympho-sarcoma: intensive cyclical combination chemotherapy with cyclophosphamide, vincristine, and prednisone. Ann. Intern. Med., *76*:227, 1972.
4. Beard, M. E. J., and Fairley, G. H.: Acute leukemia in adults. Semin. Hematol., *2*:5, 1974.
5. Bender, A., and Leavell, B. S.: Surgical procedures in patients with chronic leukemia. Va. Med. Mon., *9*:753, 1967.
6. Bennett, J. H.: Case of hypertrophy of the spleen and liver in which death took place from suppuration of the blood. Edinburgh Med. Surg. J., *64*:413, 1845.
7. Bentley, H. P., Jr., Reardon, A. E., Knoedler, J. P., and Krivit, W. K.: Eosinophilic leukemia. Am. J. Med., *30*:340, 1961.
8. Benvenisti, D. S., and Ultmann, J. E.: Eosinophilic leukemia (report of five cases and review of literature). Ann. Intern. Med., *71*:731, 1969.
9. Bethell, F. H.: The relative frequency of the several types of chronic leukemia and their man-agement. J. Chron. Dis., *6*:403, 1957.
10. Bierman, H. R., Aggeler, P. M., Thelander, H., Kelly, K. H., and Cordes, H. I.: Leukemia and pregnancy. J.A.M.A., *161*:220, 1956.
11. Bird, R. M., and Marshall, R. A.: Unusual hematological manifestations in disseminated his-toplasmosis. Tr. Am. Clin. Climatol. Assoc., *79*:177, 1967.
12. Bodey, G. P., et al.: Chemotherapy of acute leukemia. Arch. Intern. Med., *133*:260, 1974.
13. Boggs, D. R., Sofferman, S. A., Wintrobe, M. M., and Cartwright, G. E.: Factors influencing the duration of survival of patients with chronic lymphocytic leukemia. Am. J. Med., *40*:243, 1966.
14. Boggs, D. R.: Hematopoietic stem cell theory in relation to possible lymphoblastic conversion of chronic myeloid leukemia. Blood, *44*:449, 1974.
15. Boggs, D. R., Wintrobe, M. M., and Cartwright, G. E.: The acute leukemias. Medicine, *41*:163, 1962.
16. Boggs, D. R.: Transfusion of neutrophils as prevention or treatment of infection in patients with neutropenia. N. Engl. J. Med., *290*:1055, 1974.
17. Bouroncle, B. A., Wiseman, B. K., and Doan, C. A.: Leukemic reticuloendotheliosis. Blood, *13*:609, 1958.
18. Broder, L. E., and Carter, S. K.: Meningeal Leukemia. Plenum Press, New York and London, 1972.
19. Burchenal, J. H.: Long-term survival in Burkitt's tumor and in acute leukemia. Cancer Res. *27*:2616, 1967.
20. Burger, C. I., Harris, W. W., Anderson, N. G., Bartlett, T. W., and Kniseley, R. M.: Virus-like particles in human leukemic plasma. Proc. Soc. Exp. Biol. Med., *115*:151, 1964.
21. Canellos, G. P., DeVita, V. T., Whang-Peng, J., and Carbone, P. P.: Hematologic and cyto-genetic remission of blastic transformation in chronic granulocytic leukemia. Blood, *38*:671, 1971.
22. Canellos, G. P., Young, R. C., Nieman, P. E., and DeVita, V. T., Jr.: Dibromomannitol in the treatment of chronic granulocytic leukemia: a prospective randomized comparison with busulfan. Blood, *45*:197, 1975.
23. Cash, J. D.: Platelet transfusion therapy. Clin. Haematol., *1*:395, 1972.
24. Catovsky, D., Pettit, J. E., Galetto, J., Okos, A., and Galton, D. A. G.: The B-lymphocyte nature of the hairy cell of leukemic reticuloendotheliosis. Br. J. Haematol., *26*:29, 1974.
25. Catovsky, D., Pettit, J. E., Galton, D. A. G., Spiers, A. S. D., and Harrison, C. V.: Leukemic reticuloendotheliosis ("hairy" cell leukemia): a distinct clinicopathological entity. Br. J. Haematol., *26*:9, 1964.
26. Clarkson, B.: Acute myelocytic leukemia in adults. Cancer, *30*:1572, 1972.
27. Cohen, T., and Creger, W. P.: Acute myeloid leukemia following seven years of aplastic anemia induced by chloramphenicol. Am. J. Med., *43*:762, 1967.
28. Cooke, J. V.: The occurrence of leukemia. Blood, *9*:340, 1954.
29. Court-Brown, W. M., and Abatt, J. D.: The incidence of leukemia in an infant born of a mother with leukemia. N. Engl. J. Med., *259*:727, 1958.
30. Craigie, D.: Case of disease of the spleen in which death took place in consequence of the pres-ence of purulent matter in the blood. Edinburgh Med. Surg. J., *64*:400, 1845.
31. Cramblett, H. G., Friedman, J. L., and Najjar, S.: Leukemia in an infant born of a mother with leukemia. N. Engl. J. Med., *259*:727, 1958.
32. Crosby, W. H.: To treat or not to treat acute granulocytic leukemia. Arch. Intern. Med., *122*:79, 1968.
33. Curtis, J. E., Hersh, E. M. and Freireich, E. J.: Leukapheresis therapy of chronic lymphocytic leukemia. Blood, *39*:163, 1972.

34. Dameshek, W.: The outlook for eventual control of leukemia. N. Engl. J. Med., *250*:131, 1954.
35. Dameshek, W., and Gunz, F.: Leukemia, Grune & Stratton, New York and London, 1964.
36. Dameshek, W., Necheles, T. F., and Finkel, H. E.: Survival in myeloblastic leukemia of adults. N. Engl. J. Med., *275*:700, 1966.
37. Djerassi, I.: Transfusions of filtered granulocytes. N. Engl. J. Med., *292*:802, 1975.
38. Dowling, M. D., Hopfan, S., Knapper, W. H., Vaartaja, T., Gee, T., Haghbin, M., and Clarkson, B. D.: Attempt to induce true remission in chronic myelogenous leukemia (C. M. L.). Proc. Am. Assoc. Cancer Res., *15*:189, 1974.
39. Drewinko, D., Sullivan, M. P., and Martin, T.: Use of the cytocentrifuge in the diagnosis of meningeal leukemia. Cancer, *31*:1331, 1973.
40. Dugdale, M., and Fort, A. T.: Busulfan treatment of leukemia during pregnancy. J.A.M.A., *199*:131, 1967.
41. Dutcher, R. M.: Viruses as Etiologic Factors in Leukemia. *In* Dameshek, W., and Dutcher, R. M. (eds.): Perspectives in Leukemia. Grune & Stratton. New York, 1968.
42. Evans, A. E., Gilbert, E. S., and Zandstra, R.: The increasing incidence of central nervous system leukemia in children. Cancer, *26*:404, 1970.
43. Ezdinli, E. Z., Sokal, J. E., Crosswhite, L., and Sandberg, A. A.: Philadelphia chromosome-positive and negative chronic myelocytic leukemia. Ann. Intern. Med., *72*:175, 1970.
44. Fairley, G. H., and Scott, R. B.: Hypogammaglobulinemia in chronic lymphocytic leukemia. Br. Med. J., *2*:920, 1961.
45. Feinleib, M., and MacMahon, B.: Variation in the duration of survival of patients with chronic leukemias. Blood, *15*:332, 1960.
46. Fialkow, P. J., Lisker, R., Giblett, E. R., Zavala, C., Cobo, A., and Detter, J.: Genetic markers in chronic myelocytic leukaemia: evidence opposing autosomal inactivation and favoring 6–PGD–Rh linkage. Ann. Hum. Genet., *35*:321, 1972.
47. Fiddes, P., Penny, R., Wells, J. V., and Rozenberg, M. C.: Clinical correlations with immunoglobulin levels in chronic lymphatic leukemia. Aust. N. Z. J. Med., *4*:346, 1972.
48. Field, E. O., Dawson, K. B., Pelkham, M. J., Hammersley, P. A., Cooling, C. L., Morgan, R. L., and Smithers, D. W.: The response of chronic lymphocytic leukemia to treatment by extracorporeal radiation of the blood. Assessed by isotope-labeling procedures. Blood, *36*:87, 1970.
49. Folley, J. H., Borges, W., and Yamawaki, T.: Incidence of leukemia in survivors of the atomic bomb in Hiroshima and Nagasaki, Japan. Am. J. Med., *13*:311, 1952.
50. Forkner, C. E.: Leukemia and Allied Disorders. Macmillan Co., New York, 1938.
51. Fraumeni, J. F., Jr.: Bone marrow depression induced by chloramphenicol or phenylbutazone: leukemia and other sequelae. J.A.M.A., *201*:828, 1967.
52. Frei, E., et al.: Studies of sequential and combination antimetabolite therapy in acute leukemia: 6–mercaptopurine and methotrexate. Blood, *18*:431, 1961.
53. Furth, J.: Recent studies on the etiology and nature of leukemia. Blood, *6*:964, 1951.
54. Gallagher, R. E., and Gallo, R. C.: Type C RNA tumor virus isolated from cultured human acute myelogenous leukemia cells. Science, *187*:350, 1975.
55. Gallo, R. C.: Terminal transferase and leukemia. N. Engl. J. Med., *292*:804, 1975.
56. Gauld, W. R., Innes, J., and Robson, H. N.: A survey of 647 cases of leukemia 1938–1951. Br. Med. J., *1*:585, 1953.
57. Geelhoed, G. W., Graff, K. S., Duttera, M. J., Jr., and Henderson, E. S.: Acute leukemia presenting as a breast mass. J.A.M.A., *223*:1488, 1973.
58. Gilliam, A. G.: Age, sex, and race selection at death from leukemia and the lymphomas. Blood, *8*:693, 1953.
59. Gluckman, E., Basch, A., and Dreyfus, B.: Combination chemotherapy with cytosine arabinoside and rubidomycin in 30 cases of acute granulocytic leukemia. Cancer, *31*:487, 1973.
60. Gralnick, H. R., Harbor, J., and Vogel, C.: Myelofibrosis in chronic granulocytic leukemia. Blood, *37*:152, 1971.
61. Graw, R. G., Jr., Herzig, G., Peery, S., and Henderson, E. S.: Normal granulocyte transfusion therapy. N. Engl. J. Med., *278*:367, 1972.
62. Greenspan, E. M., and Tung, B. G.: Acute myeloblastic leukemia after cure of ovarian cancer. J.A.M.A., *230*:418, 1974.
63. Gross, L.: Mouse leukemia. Ann. N.Y. Acad. Sci., *54*:1184, 1952.
64. Gross, L.: A filterable agent recovered from Ak leukemic extracts, causing salivary gland carcinomas in C3H mice. Proc. Soc. Exp. Biol. Med., *83*:414, 1953.
65. Guasch, J.: Hérédité des leucémies. Le Sang, *25*:384, 1954.
66. Gunz, F., and Baikie, A. G.: Leukemia. Grune and Stratton, New York, San Francisco, and London, 1974.
67. Gunz, F. W., Borthwick, R. A., and Rolleston, G. L.: Acute leukemia in an infant following excessive intrauterine irradiation. Lancet, *2*:190, 1958.

68. Gunz, F. W., and Hough, R. F.: Acute leukemia over the age of fifty. Blood, *11*:882, 1956.

69. Han, T., Ezdinli, E. Z., Shimaoka, K., and Desai, D. V.: Chlorambucil vs. combined chlorambucil–corticosteroid therapy in chronic lymphocytic leukemia. Cancer, *31*:502, 1973.

70. Haut, A., Abbott, W. S., Wintrobe, M. M., and Cartwright, G. E.: Busulfan in the treatment of chronic myelocytic leukemia. The effect of long-term intermittent therapy. Blood, *17*: 1, 1961.

71. Hayhoe, F. G. J., and Cawley, J. C.: Acute leukemia: cellular morphology, cytochemistry and fine structure. Clin. Haematol., *1*:49, 1972.

72. Henderson, E. A.: Treatment of acute leukemia. Ann. Intern. Med., *69*:628, 1968.

73. Herbert, V.: Diagnostic and prognostic values of measurement of serum vitamin B_{12}-binding proteins. Blood, *32*:305, 1968.

74. Herzig, R. H., Poplack, D. G., and Yankee, R. A.: Prolonged granulocytopenia from incompatible platelet transfusions. N. Engl. J. Med., *290*:1720, 1974.

75. Hess, C. E., Ayers, C. R., Wetzel, R. A., Mohler, D. N., and Sandusky, W. R.: Dilutional anemia of splenomegaly: an indication for splenectomy. Ann. Surg., *173*:693, 1971.

76. Higby, D. J., Yates, J. W., Henderson, E. S., and Holland, J. F.: Filtration leukapheresis for granulocyte transfusion therapy. N. Engl. J. Med., *292*:761, 1975.

77. Hill, J. M., Loeb, E., and Speer, R. J.: Colloidal zirconyl phosphate ^{32}P in chronic leukemia and lymphomas. J.A.M.A., *187*:106, 1964.

78. Hueper, W. C.: Occupational Tumors and Allied Diseases. Charles C Thomas, Springfield, Ill., 1942.

79. Huguley, C. M., Jr.: Survey of Current Therapy and Problems in Chronic Leukemia in Leukemia–Lymphoma. Chicago Year Book, Medical Publishers, 1970.

80. Hungerford, D. A.: The Philadelphia chromosome and some others. (Edit.) Ann. Intern. Med., *61*:789, 1964.

81. Igel, H. J., Huebner, R. J., Turner, H. C., Katin, P., and Falk, H. L.: Mouse leukemia virus activation by chemical carcinogens. Science, *166*:1624, 1969.

82. Jarrett, W. F. H.: Viruses and leukemia. Br. J. Haematol., *25*:287, 1973.

83. Johnson, R. E.: Total body irradiation of chronic lymphocytic leukemia: incidence and duration of remission. Cancer, *25*:523, 1970.

84. Kaplan, H. S.: On the etiology and pathogenesis of the leukemias: a review. Cancer Res., *14*: 535, 1954.

85. Karanas, A., and Silver, R. T.: Characteristics of the terminal phase of chronic granulocytic leukemia. Blood, *32*:445, 1968.

86. Kaslow, R. A., Wisch, N., and Glass, J. L.: Acute leukemia following cytotoxic chemotherapy. J.A.M.A., *219*:75, 1972.

87. Kennedy, B. J.: Androgenic hormone therapy in lymphatic leukemia. J.A.M.A., *190*:1130, 1964.

88. Kennedy, B. J.: Hydroxyurea therapy in chronic myelogenous leukemia. Cancer, *29*:1052, 1972.

88a. King, G. W., Hurtubise, P. E., Sagone, A. L., LoBuglio, A. F., and Metz, E. N.: Leukemic reticuloendotheliosis: study of the origin of the malignant cell. Am. J. Med. *59*:411, 1975.

89. Kyle, R. A., Maldonado, J. E., and Bayrd, E. D.: Plasma cell leukemia. Arch. Intern. Med., *133*:813, 1974.

89a. Kyle, R. A., Pierre, R. V., and Bayrd, E. D.: Multiple myeloma and acute myelomonocytic leukemia. N. Engl. J. Med., *283*:1121, 1970.

90. Lange, R. D., Moloney, W. C., and Yamawaki, T.: Leukemia in atomic bomb survivors. Blood, *9*:575. 1954.

91. Lawrence, J. H., Dobson, R. L., Low-Beer, B. V. A., and Brown, B. R.: Chronic myelogenous leukemia: a study of 129 cases in which treatment was with radioactive phosphorus. J.A.M.A. *136*:672, 1948.

92. Leavell, B. S.: Chronic leukemia. A study of the incidence and factors influencing the duration of life. Am. J. Med. Sci., *196*:329, 1938.

93. Levine, A. S., Schimpff, S. C., Graw, R. G., Jr., and Young, R. C.: Hematologic malignancies and other marrow failure states: progress in the management of complicating infections. Semin. Hematol., *11*:141, 1974.

94. Lichtman, M. A., and Weed, R. I.: Peripheral cytoplasmic characteristics of leukocytes in monocytic leukemia: relationship to clinical manifestations. Blood, *40*:52, 1972.

95. Lichtman, M. A.: Cellular deformability during maturation of the myeloblast. N. Engl. J. Med., *283*:943, 1970.

96. MacMahon, B., and Clark, D.: Incidence of the common forms of human leukemia. Blood, *11*:871, 1956.

97. MacMahon, B., and Koller, E. K.: Ethnic differences in the incidence of leukemia. Blood, *12*:1, 1957.

98. Maduros, B. P., and Schwartz, S. O.: Viral etiology of leukemia. Adv. Intern. Med., *11*:107, 1962.
99. March, H. C.: Leukemia in radiologists 10 years later; with review of pertinent evidence for radiation leukemia. Am. J. Med. Sci., *242*:137, 1961.
100. Mathe, G., Schwarzenberg, L., Mery, A. M., Cattan, A., Schneider, M., Amiel, J. L., Schlumberger, J. R., Poisson, J., and Wajcner, G.: Extensive histological and cytological survey of patients with acute leukemia in "complete remission." Br. Med. J., *1*:640,1966.
101. Mathe, G.: Immunological approaches to the treatment of acute leukemia. Clin. Haematol., *1*:165, 1972.
102. Medical Research Council's Working Party for Therapeutic Trials in Leukemia: Chronic granulocytic leukemia: comparison of radiotherapy and busulfan. Br. Med. J., *1*:201, 1968.
103. Metcalf, D.: Human leukaemia: recent tissue culture studies on the nature of myeloid leukaemia. Br. J. Cancer, *27*:191, 1973.
104. Miescher, P. A., and Farquet, J. J.: Chronic myelomonocytic leukemia in adults. Semin. Hematol., *11*:129, 1974.
105. Miller, D. G., Budinger, J. M., and Karnofsky, D. A.: A clinical and pathological study of resistance to infection in chronic lymphocytic leukemia. Cancer, *15*:307, 1962.
106. Miller, R. W.: Persons with exceptionally high risk of leukemia. Cancer Res., *27*:2420, 1967.
107. Minot, G. R., Buckman, T. E., and Isaacs, R.: Chronic myelogenous leukemia. J.A.M.A., *82*:1489, 1924.
108. Minot, G. R., and Isaacs, R.: Lymphatic leukemia: age, incidence, duration and benefit derived from irradiation. Boston Med. Surg. J., *191*:1, 1924.
109. Modan, B., and Lilienfeld, A. M.: Polycythemia vera and leukemia. The role of radiation treatment. Medicine, *44*:305, 1965.
110. Moertel, C. G., and Hagedorn, A. B.: Leukemia or lymphoma and coexistent primary malignant lesions: a review of the literature and a study of 120 cases. Blood, *12*:788, 1957.
111. Moloney, W. C., and Kastenbaum, M. A.: Leukemogenic effects of ionizing radiation on atomic bomb survivors in Hiroshima City. Science, *121*:308, 1955.
112. Moore, E. W., Thomas, L. B., Shaw, R. K., and Freireich, E. J.: The central nervous system in acute leukemia. Arch. Intern. Med., *105*:451, 1960.
113. Nesbitt, J., III, and Roth, R. E.: Solitary lytic bone lesion in an adult with chronic myelogenous leukemia. Radiology, *64*:724, 1955.
114. Nies, B. A., Bodey, G. P., Thomas, L. B., Brecher, G., and Freireich, E. J.: The persistence of extramedullary leukemia infiltrates during bone marrow remission of acute leukemia. Blood, *26*:133, 1965.
115. Noon, M. A., and Hess, C. E.: Acute Leukemia in Adults. To be published.
116. Nowell, P. C.: Chromosome abnormalities in human leukemia and lymphoma. Proc. International Conference on Leukemia-Lymphoma. Zarafonetis, C. J. D. (ed.). Lea & Febiger, Philadelphia, 1968.
117. Nowell, P. C., and Hungerford, D. A.: Chromosome studies on normal and leukemic human leukocytes. J. Natl. Cancer Inst., *25*:85, 1960.
118. Nowell, P. C., and Hungerford, D. A.: Chromosome studies in human leukemia. II. Chronic granulocytic leukemia. J. Natl. Cancer Inst., *27*:1013, 1961.
119. Nowinski, R. C., Old, L. J., Sarkar, N. H., and Moore, D. H.: Common properties of the oncogenic RNA viruses (oncornaviruses). Virology, *42*:1152, 1970.
120. Nuss, H. B., and Moloney, W. C.: Chloroma and other myeloblastic tumors. Blood, *42*:721, 1973.
121. O'Riordan, M. L., Robinson, J. A., Buckton, K. E., and Evans, H. J.: Distinguishing between the chromosomes involved in Down's syndrome (trisomy 21) and chronic myeloid leukemia (Ph¹) by fluorescence. Nature, *230*:167, 1971.
122. Osler, W.: *In* Pepper, W. A. (ed.): System of Practical Medicine by American Authors. Vol. 11, Philadelphia, 1894.
123. Osgood, E. E., and Seaman, A. J.: Treatment of chronic leukemias. Results of therapy by titrated regularly spaced total body radioactive phosphorus or roentgen irradiation. J.A.M.A., *150*:1372, 1952.
124. Osgood, E. E., Seaman, A. J., and Koler, R. D.: Results of a 15 year program of treatment of chronic leukemia with titrated regularly spaced total body irradiation with ^{32}P or X-ray. *In* Proc. 6th Congr. Int. Soc. Hematol. Grune & Stratton, New York, 1956.
125. Panton, P. N., and Valentine, F. C. O.: Chronic lymphoid leukemia. Lancet, *216*:914, 1929.
126. Pavlovsky, S., Penalver, J., Eppenger-Helft, M., Sackmann, M. F., Bergna, L., Suarez, A., Vilaseca, G., and Pavlovsky, A.: Induction and maintenance of remission in acute leukemia. Cancer, *31*:273, 1973.
127. Phair, J. P., Anderson, R. E., and Namiki, H.: The central nervous system in leukemia. Ann. Intern. Med., *61*:863, 1964.

128. Price, R. A., and Jamieson, P. A.: The central nervous system in childhood leukemia. II. Subacute leukoencephalopathy. Cancer, *35*:306, 1975.
129. Pruzanski, W., and Platts, M. E.: Serum and urinary proteins, lysozyme (muramidase) and renal dysfunction in mono- and myelomonocytic leukemia. J. Clin. Invest., *49*:1694, 1970.
130. Pruzanski, W., Platts, M. E., and Ogryzlo, M. A.: Leukemic form of immunocytic dyscrasia (plasma cell leukemia). Am. J. Med., *47*:60, 1969.
131. Rappaport, H.: Atlas of Tumor Pathology. Sec. III. Fascicle 8, Armed Forces Institute of Pathology. Washington, D. C., 1966.
132. Reimann, D. L., Clemmens, R. L., and Pillsbury, W. A.: Congenital acute leukemia. J. Pediatr., *46*:415, 1955.
133. Reinhard, E. H., Neely, C. L., and Samples, D. M.: Radioactive phosphorus in the treatment of chronic leukemias. Long-term results over a period of 15 years. Ann. Intern. Med., *50*: 942, 1959.
134. Reschad, H., and Schilling-Torgau, V.: Über ein neue Leukämie durch echte Übergansformen (Splenzytenleukämie) und ihre Bedeutung für die Selbständigkeit dieser Zellen. München Med. Wochenschr., *60*:1981, 1913.
135. Rheingold, J. J., Kaufman, R., Adelson, E., and Lear, A.: Smoldering acute leukemia. N. Engl. J. Med., *268*:812, 1963.
136. Roath, S., Israels, M. C. G., and Wilkinson, J. F.: The acute leukemias: a study of 580 patients. Q. J. Med., *32*:257, 1964.
137. Rosenthal, D. S., and Moloney, W. C.: The treatment of acute granulocytic leukemia in adults. N. Engl. J. Med., *286*:1176, 1972.
138. Rowley, J. D.: A new consistent chromosomal abnormality in chronic myelogenous leukemia identified by quinacrine fluorescence and Giemsa staining. Nature, *243*:290, 1973.
139. Sacks, M. S., and Seeman, I.: A statistical study of mortality from leukemia. Blood, 2:1, 1947.
140. Sahaxian, G. J., Al-Mondhiry, H., Lacher, M. J., and Connolly, C. E.: Acute leukemia in Hodgkin's disease. Cancer, *33*:1369, 1974.
141. Sandberg, A. A., and Hossfeld, D. K.: Chromosomal abnormalities in human neoplasia. Annu. Rev. Med., *21*:379, 1970.
142. Sarngadharan, M. G., Sarin, P. S., Reitz, M. S., and Gallo, R. C.: Reverse transcriptase activity of human acute leukemic cells: purification of the enzyme, response to AMV 70S RNA, and characterization of the DNA Product. Nature [New Biol.] *24*:67, 1972.
143. Schiffer, C. A., Buchholz, D. H., Alsner, J., Betts, S. W., and Wiernik, P. H.: Clinical experience with transfusion of granulocytes obtained by continuous flow filtration leukapheresis. Am. J. Med., *58*:373, 1975.
144. Schimpff, S. C., Greene, W. H., Young, V. M., Fortner, C. L., Jepsen, L., Cusack, N., Block, J. B., and Wiernik, P. H.: Infection prevention in acute nonlymphocytic leukemia. Ann. Intern. Med., *82*:351, 1975.
145. Schoolman, H. M., Spurrier, W., Schwartz, S. O., and Szanto, P. B.: The induction of leukemia in Swiss mice by means of cell free filtrates of leukemic mouse brain. Blood, *12*:694, 1957.
146. Schwab, R. S., and Weiss, S.: Neurologic aspects of leukemia. Am. J. Med. Sci., *189*:766, 1935.
147. Schwartz, S. O.: Etiology of leukemia: a case for the virus theory. Blood, *11*:1045, 1956.
148. Schwartz, S. O., and Ehrlich, L.: The relationship of polycythemia vera to leukemia: a critical review. Acta Haematol., *4*:129, 1950.
149. Schwartz, S. O., Schoolman, H. M., and Szanto, P. B.: The acceleration of the development of AKR lymphoma by means of cell-free filtrates. Cancer Res., *16*:559, 1956.
150. Scott, J. M., Bloomfield, F. J., Stebbins, R., and Herbert, V.: Studies on derivation of transcobalamin III from granulocytes. J. Clin. Invest., *53*:228, 1974.
151. Scott, R. B.: Leukaemia. Lancet, *1*:1053, 1957.
152. Scott, R. B.: Leukaemia. Lancet, *1*:1162, 1957.
153. Scott, R. B.: Leukaemia. Lancet, *1*:1099, 1957.
154. Sehden, M. K., Dowling, M. D., Jr., Seal, S. H., and Stearns, M. W., Jr.: Perianal and anorectal complications in leukemia. Cancer, *31*:149, 1973.
155. Sexauer, J., Kass, L., and Schnitzer, B.: Subacute myelomonocytic leukemia. Am. J. Med., *57*:853, 1974.
156. Shimkin, M. B., Mettier, S. R., and Bierman, H. R.: Myelocytic leukemia: an analysis of incidence, distribution, and fatality. Ann. Intern. Med., *35*:194, 1951.
157. Silver, R. T.: The treatment of chronic lymphocytic leukemia. Semin. Hematol., *6*:344, 1969.
158. Silverman, F. N.: The skeletal lesions in leukemia. Am. J. Roentgenol., *59*:819, 1948.
159. Simone, J.: Acute lymphocytic leukemia in childhood. Semin. Hematol., *11*:25, 1974.
160. Simpson, C. L., Hempelmann, L. H., and Fuller, L. M.: Neoplasia in children treated with x-rays in infancy for thymic enlargement. Radiology, *64*:840, 1955.

161. Sinn, C. M., and Dick, F. W.: Monocytic leukemia. Am. J. Med., *20*:588, 1956.
162. Skipper, H. E., Schabel, F. M., Jr., and Wilcox, W. S.: Experimental evaluation of potential anticancer agents. XII. On the criteria and kinetics associated with "curability" of experimental leukemia. Cancer Chemother. Rep., *35*:1, 1964.
163. Sokal, J. E., and Lessmann, E. M.: Effects of cancer chemotherapeutic agents on the human fetus. J.A.M.A., *172*:1765, 1960.
164. Southwest Oncology Group. Cytarabine for acute leukemia in adults. Arch. Intern. Med., *133*: 251, 1974.
165. Spiers, A.S.D.: Chemotherapy of acute leukemia. Clin. Haematol., *1*:127, 1972.
166. Steinkamp, R. C., Lawrence, J. H., and Born, J. L.: Long-term experience with the use of ^{32}P in the treatment of chronic lymphocytic leukemia. J. Nucl. Med., *4*:92, 1963.
167. Stewart, A., Webb, J., Giles, D., and Hewitt, D.: Malignant disease in childhood and diagnostic irradiation in utero. Lancet, *2*:447, 1956.
168. Strychmans, P. A.: Current concepts in chronic myelogenous leukemia. Semin. Hematol., *11*:101, 1974.
169. Tattersall, M. H. N., Battersby, G., and Spiers, A. S. D.: Antibiotics and hypokalemia. Lancet, *1*:630, 1972.
170. Theologides, A.: Unfavorable signs in patients with chronic myelocytic leukemia. Ann. Intern. Med., *76*:95, 1972.
171. Thomas, J. R.: Eosinophilic leukemia presenting with erythrocytosis. Blood, *22*:639, 1963.
172. Tivey, H.: Prognosis for survival in chronic granulocytic and lymphocytic leukemia. Am. J. Roentgenol., *72*:68, 1954.
173. Todaro, G. J., and Huebner, R. J.: The viral oncogene hypothesis: new evidence. Proc. Natl. Acad. Sci. U.S.A., *69*:1009, 1972.
174. Twomey, J. J., and Leavell, B. S.: Leukemoid reactions to tuberculosis. Arch. Intern. Med., *116*:21, 1965.
175. Upton, A. C.: The role of radiation in the etiology of leukemia. Proc. Int. Conference Leukemia-Lymphoma. Zarafonetis, C. J. D. (ed.) Lea & Febiger, Philadelphia, 1968.
176. Videbaek, A.: Heredity in Human Leukemia. H. K. Lewis & Co., London, 1947.
177. Virchow, R.: Weisses Blut und Milztumoren. Med. Ztg., *15*:157, 163, 1846.
178. Ward, G.: The infective theory of acute leukemia. Br. J. Child. Dis., *14*:10, 1017.
179. Wiernik, P. H., and Serpick, A. A.: A randomized clinical trial of daunorubicin and a combination of prednisone, vincristine, 6–mercaptopurine, and methotrexate in adult acute nonlymphocytic leukemia. Cancer Res., *32*:2023, 1972.
180. Wintrobe, M. M., and Hasenbush, L. L.: Chronic leukemia. Arch. Intern. Med., *64*:701, 1939.
181. Yam, L. T., Li, C. Y., and Lam, K. W.: Tartrate-resistant acid phosphatase isoenzyme in the reticulum cells of leukemic reticuloendotheliosis. N. Engl. J. Med., *284*:357, 1971.
182. Yankee, R. A., Grumet, F. C., Rogentine, G. M.: Platelet transfusion therapy. The selection of compatible platelet donors for refractory patients by lymphocyte HL-A typing. N. Engl. J. Med., *281*:1208, 1969.
183. Zacharski, L. R., and Linman, J. W.: Chronic lymphocytic leukemia versus chronic lymphosarcoma cell leukemia. Am. J. Med., *47*:75, 1969.
184. Zimmerman, T. S., Godwin, H. A., and Perry, S.: Studies of leukocyte kinetics in chronic lymphocytic leukemia. Blood, *31*:277, 1968.
185. Zippin, C., Cutler, S. J., Reeves, W. J., Jr., and Lum, D.: Survival in chronic lymphocytic leukemia. Blood, *42*:367, 1973.

CHAPTER **13**

MALIGNANT LYMPHOMAS (LYMPHOMA, LYMPHOBLASTOMA)

DIAGNOSIS OF THE PATIENT WITH ENLARGED LYMPH NODES

The most accurate clinical diagnoses are made either by histologic study of diseased tissue or by demonstration of the presence of the agent responsible for the disease. In clinical practice the physician usually begins his diagnostic examination with the history and physical examination. With the recognition of some particular sign or symptom complex, such as lymphadenopathy, he proceeds with the differential diagnosis by an orderly consideration of the different diseases known to produce the manifestations that have been observed. The probability of the presence of one or more of the diseases under consideration increases as other evidence is found that supports those particular possibilities. This evidence is obtained by a systematic study of the patient that includes various laboratory tests and special procedures, such as a biopsy. The investigation is directed first toward the "probable" disease, and specific tests for "possible" but "improbable" disorders are deferred.

Enlarged lymph nodes, which provide the focal point of the diagnostic study in certain patients, occur in a number of different diseases. Probably the commonest causes are regional infections, such as infected wounds, dermatitis, pharyngitis, sinusitis, and abscessed teeth. Lymphadenopathy also occurs with relatively benign systemic infections, such as rubella, infectious mononucleosis, and viral hepatitis, and with more serious infections, such as tuberculosis, brucellosis, syphilis, fungal diseases, and tularemia. Enlargement of lymph nodes may be due to the presence of neoplastic disease, such as metastatic carcinoma, leukemia, lymphosarcoma, Hodgkin's disease, reticulum cell sarcoma, and giant follicular lymphosarcoma. Mild degrees of enlargement occur in

462

serum sickness and hyperthyroidism. Moderate enlargement occurs in disseminated lupus erythematosus and Boeck's sarcoid.

HISTORY

As is true for nearly all diagnostic problems, an accurate history is essential. Even the age of the patient is helpful information because the more benign systemic infections, such as rubella and infectious mononucleosis, are common in children and young adults but rare in middle-aged and older persons. Both the duration of the adenopathy and the presence or absence of various symptoms help in deciding which of the possible diagnoses are more probable. The recent development of adenopathy does not exclude a neoplasm from consideration, but the persistence of enlargement for some months makes an acute infection unlikely. Localizing symptoms, such as pain and tenderness in the gland, and evidence of associated inflammation, such as pharyngitis, favor infection. A history of weight loss, recurrent fever, night sweats, and pruritus suggests the presence of systemic disease, most often one of the lymphoma group.

PHYSICAL EXAMINATION

The physical examination, particularly the characteristics of the superficial nodes, generally gives helpful information. The distribution, size, consistency, and mobility of the nodes are important, as is the presence or absence of tenderness. Probably the most important observation is whether the adenopathy is generalized or localized. If the involvement is generalized, some systemic disease becomes the primary consideration and regional adenitis can be excluded. If the involvement appears to be localized, the presence of systemic disease is not excluded but the first consideration is given to a careful search for some associated disease, either infection or neoplasm, in the area drained by the enlarged lymph nodes. In any patient with enlarged nodes, the size is estimated carefully and is best recorded in centimeters rather than in less accurate terms, such as "pea-sized" and "egg-sized." An estimate of the size of the nodes gives some indication of the probability of the presence of certain diseases. The nodes in hyperthyroidism and serum sickness are rarely more than 0.5 or 1.0 cm. in diameter, and in disseminated lupus they seldom measure more than 1.0 to 3.0 cm. In the diseases of the lymphoma group the nodes are sometimes greatly enlarged. Careful estimations of the size of the nodes, and the constancy of size, are helpful in following the progress of the disease while the patient is under observation. The presence of tenderness in a node usually indicates infection, but marked tenderness also occurs in the nodes of some patients with other diseases, particularly Hodgkin's disease. Fixation of a node to the skin or deeper tissues indicates that the infection or neoplasm has involved the surrounding area. Sinus tracts or scars over an area of adenopathy suggest tuberculosis or fungal disease. A relatively small node that is stony hard in consistency suggests metastatic carcinoma, but extremely hard nodes that measure several centimeters in diameter also occur with calcification, in sarcoma, and in tuberculosis. In diseases of the lymphoma group characteristically the nodes are moderately firm, rubbery, and somewhat resilient, but there are many exceptions. The normal bean-shaped contour of the node is more apt to be maintained with infection than with neoplasm.

Other details of the physical examination are also important. The detection of a focus of infection in an area related anatomically to the adenopathy usually warrants a diagnosis of regional adenitis. The presence of splenomegaly and hepatomegaly suggests some generalized infectious process or a disease of the lymphoma group. If the spleen is firm and extends halfway to the level of the umbilicus or below, it is probable that the patient has some chronic disorder, such as a disease of the lymphoma group, rather than an acute infection, such as infectious mononucleosis or viral hepatitis.

LABORATORY EXAMINATION

Laboratory examinations sometimes establish the diagnosis in patients with large lymph nodes, and at other times permit the exclusion of certain diseases from further consideration. The routine studies of the blood, such as the hematocrit, leukocyte count, and differential count, are indicated. By such means leukemia usually can be detected if present, and the diagnosis of other diseases, such as infectious mononucleosis, can be provisionally established or excluded. An increase in the granulocytes favors bacterial infection or Hodgkin's disease, and an increase in "pathologic" lymphocytes favors infectious mono-nucleosis or a viral infection. Monocytosis suggests Hodgkin's disease, tuberculosis, or brucellosis. The presence of anemia indicates that the patient probably has more than a localized acute infection. More definitive information is provided by serologic tests such as the heterophile, tularemia, and other agglutination reactions, tests for anti-nuclear factor and "L.E." cells, and serial titers for toxoplasmosis and viral infections. Skin tests for tuberculosis and fungal diseases are sometimes helpful. In certain patients other studies, such as the electrophoretic study of the serum proteins and aspiration of bone marrow to obtain material for culture and cytologic study, are important.

ROENTGENOGRAPHIC EXAMINATION

Roentgenographic examinations often give valuable information about the nature of the process that is manifested by enlargement of the superficial nodes. A roentgenogram of the chest is usually necessary in order to detect disease in the lungs and determine the presence of involvement of the nodes in the hilar areas or mediastinum. The location, number, and appearance of the lesions in the lung may indicate the probability of tuberculosis, fungal disease, primary or metastatic carcinoma, or other disease. Details of the appearance and location of the involved nodes in the hilar areas and mediastinum may help to distinguish between Boeck's sarcoid and one of the lymphoma group, but are not diagnostic.

Examination of the gastrointestinal tract may reveal the presence of a primary carcinoma that was first suggested by the presence of Virchow's node behind the origin of the left sternocleidomastoid muscle. Radiologic evidence of diffuse infiltration of the stomach and hypertrophied rugal folds favors lymphosarcoma over Hodgkin's disease and other disorders that may present with superficial adenopathy. Evidence of skeletal involvement indicates that the adenopathy is part of a serious disorder, even though the roentgenographic appearance of the osseous lesion may not permit differentiation between the several possibilities.

LYMPH NODE BIOPSY

If the diagnosis is not made by other means, biopsy of a lymph node is often necessary, the decision being made after an evaluation of each patient individually. In one situation it may be apparent at the initial examination that a biopsy should be done promptly; in another, it may be decided that biopsy can be deferred for further observation and the performance of other tests. If an undiagnosed enlargement of the lymph node in an adult does not subside significantly within a few weeks, biopsy is nearly always indicated.

Although no fast rules can be made for the performance of the biopsy, the observance of some simple guides is helpful to both the pathologist and the clinician. Although the former bases his diagnosis on the histologic appearance of the specimen, it is helpful if pertinent clinical data are submitted along with the biopsy specimen. It is important that the pathologist receive representative tissue that is suitable for study. If more than one node is enlarged, the selection of the one to be biopsied is important. In general, cervical or supraclavicular nodes are preferable to axillary nodes; nodes from all of these sites are preferable to nodes from the femoral area, because the latter often have undergone alteration as a result of previous infection in the lower extremities. When the patient has a disease that involves the lymph nodes without significant enlargement of the superficial lymph nodes, the diagnosis frequently can be established by a supraclavicular biopsy or percutaneous liver biopsy; on occasion, thoracotomy or laparotomy may be necessary to establish a diagnosis. Mediastinoscopy and peritoneoscopy are valuable in experienced hands; these relatively minor operations may provide a tissue diagnosis and an assessment of the extent of certain tumors, information necessary for the decision regarding treatment, with less risk and morbidity than the usual thoracotomy or laparotomy. Although not as satisfactory for obtaining tissue as open thoracotomy, suction pleural or lung biopsy may be all that is necessary in some circumstances. The diagnosis should be established before the patient receives any specific therapy, because both radiation and chemotherapy can so change the appearance of the node that histologic diagnosis is difficult or impossible.

Careful handling of the node at the time of operation is important because trauma can distort the histologic appearance of the lesion. If an infectious etiology of the adenopathy is under consideration, part of the node should be sent for histologic examination and part for culture. Unless this is done, even tuberculosis or a fungal infection may pass unrecognized. If the patient has, or is thought to have, one of the lymphomas, particularly non-Hodgkin's lymphomas, study of a touch preparation of the sectioned node stained with Wright's and other stains can be very helpful, even essential, in determining the immaturity of the lymphocytes and histiocytes; whether the cells are well differentiated, poorly differentiated, or undifferentiated can be determined better with this method than by the usual H and E stained sections. If the biopsy of a node does not provide a definite diagnosis, a second biopsy[21] is indicated; if no suitable node is available at the time, periodic examination for the appearance of such a node is advisable.

FURTHER STUDY

If the biopsy establishes a diagnosis of Hodgkin's disease or some other lymphoma, further examinations to disclose the extent of the disease are necessary to determine the stage reached. These examinations include x-ray of the chest, possibly tomograms, and probably bone marrow biopsy and lymphangiograms. In some patients radiographic survey of the skeleton and gallium or other scans may be desirable. Staging laparotomy is necessary in some patients; the indications for this formidable diagnostic procedure currently vary from place to place, but it may be expected that with more experience these will be more clearly defined.

CLASSIFICATION

Malignant lymphoma is a term used to designate a group of diseases that have certain features in common. These diseases, which involve mainly the lymphoid structures of the body, cannot be distinguished from each other by their clinical manifestations. An accurate diagnosis is made only by microscopic study of a specimen of involved tissue, usually a lymph node. Although of unknown etiology, the diseases are generally considered to be neoplastic in nature.

The term "malignant lymphoma" is a convenient one for various reasons. In clinical practice it provides a designation for a provisional diagnosis until a more accurate one can be made. In addition, the histologic study of biopsy material sometimes makes it possible to place a disorder in this group of diseases even though a more precise diagnosis cannot be made with certainty. In this circumstance the patient often can be treated adequately without benefit of complete diagnosis, because the same principles of therapy and the same therapeutic agents are used in the management of the different diseases. It is convenient to group these diseases for the purpose of a clinical discussion because of the similarities in clinical manifestations, methods of diagnosis, treatment, and prognosis.

Hodgkin's disease is named after Thomas Hodgkin who first described the disorder in 1832.[68] In 1893 Kundrat recognized lymphosarcoma as a disease entity different from leukemia.[89] Giant follicular lymphoma, sometimes called "Brill-Symmers disease," was described by Brill, Baehr, and Rosenthal in 1925[22]

Table 13-1   *Classification of Lymphomas*

1. Hodgkin's Disease
   a. Lymphocyte predominant
   b. Nodular sclerosis
   c. Mixed cellularity
   d. Lymphocyte depletion

2. Non-Hodgkin's lymphoma

Cell Type	Nodular	Diffuse
a. Lymphocytic well differentiated	NLWD	DLWD
b. Lymphocytic poorly differentiated	NLPD	DLPD
c. Histiocytic	NH	DH
d. Mixed	NM	DM
e. Lymphocytic undifferentiated (stem cell)	NLU	DLU (Burkitt's lymphoma)

Mycosis fungoides
Histiocytic medullary reticulosis (? histiocytic, diffuse) (DH)

and by Symmers in 1927.[158] Roulet has been given credit for first clearly identifying reticulum cell sarcoma as a distinct type of tumor in 1930.[33]

Numerous classifications have been proposed for this group of diseases that involve the lymphoid tissue primarily. Two classifications are shown in Tables 13–1 and 13–2; that in Table 13–1 is the one most widely used at the present time. The term "lymphoma histiocytic diffuse" is replacing "reticulum cell sarcoma;" the newer terms, "lymphoma, nodular type, well differentiated lymphocytic" (or "poorly differentiated" or "undifferentiated") and "lymphoma, nodular type, histiocytic," are more precise than the older "giant follicular lymphoma." "Hodgkin's disease" as a diagnosis is incomplete unless one of the various types—lymphocyte predominant, nodular sclerosis, mixed cellularity, or lymphocyte depletion—is specified.

The newer diagnostic terms have already proved to be valuable both in estimating prognosis and in planning therapy. In fact most of the older literature on the frequency and prognosis of the various lymphomas has been rendered meaningless, or nearly so. Only a rough idea of the frequency of the disorders is provided even by the reliable report of 30 years ago that, of 618 cases of "lymphoma," 37 per cent were Hodgkin's disease, 35 per cent lymphosarcoma, 20 per cent reticulum cell sarcoma, and 8 per cent giant follicle lymphoma.[57]

Although a specific diagnosis can usually be made by histologic study of the involved tissue, at times the pathologist may have difficulty in identifying the disease from the material obtained by biopsy. Consultations with additional

Table 13-2   *Classification of Lymphomas*

1. Hodgkin's disease.
2. Lymphosarcoma.
3. Reticulum cell sarcoma.
4. Giant follicular lymphoma (Brill-Symmers disease, nodular lymphoblastoma).

pathologists, particularly hematopathologists, are utilized more often, as are the newer special techniques, staining and others, that help to identify the cells involved in the process. The reported instances of the finding of Hodgkin's disease, sarcoma, and giant follicle lymphoma[159] in a single lymph node, or the apparent transformation to other lymphomas often seen in nodes during the course of giant follicle lymphoma,[36, 159] and the variations from the original diagnoses found in later biopsies or autopsies in from 23 to 39 per cent of patients[36, 57] are difficult to interpret; the different diagnoses may reflect different diagnostic criteria of the pathologists, a tendency of the tumors to become less differentiated in appearance as they progress, or the occurrence of multiple tumors in a vulnerable host. There is little question, however, that cervical and para-aortic nodes at times seem to be involved by different types of Hodgkin's disease; in some patients, cervical biopsy shows the lymphocyte predominant picture and an intra-abdominal node or spleen of the mixed cellularity type. Although many pathologists consider that the histologic features of these diseases, with the exception of giant follicle lymphoma, remain relatively constant, the inconstancy noted in some cases has led to the suggestion that the whole lymphoma group is but a single neoplastic entity that has a number of variants.[36]

HODGKIN'S DISEASE

The extensive literature on Hodgkin's disease has been the subject of several excellent monographs.[85, 148] The clinical manifestations, histologic appearance, methods of diagnosis, and variable natural history of the disease are well established. Despite the numerous attempts that have been made to solve the problem, the cause (or causes) of Hodgkin's disease has not been determined. A recent review indicates that the data suggestive of a viral etiology are increasing. Although the occurrence of Hodgkin's disease in association with other diseases, notably tuberculosis and fungal infections, has suggested more than a chance association, all efforts to establish tuberculosis, the avian tubercle bacillus, diphtheroids, and other bacilli and fungi as causes of Hodgkin's disease have proved unsuccessful.

HISTOLOGIC CLASSIFICATION OF HODGKIN'S DISEASE

Lukes and Butler have proposed a histologic classification of Hodgkin's disease that offers certain advantages over that proposed by Jackson and Parker.[71] The modification of the former classification, which was adopted at the 1965 Conference on Hodgkin's Disease,[101] distinguishes four histologic types: (1) lymphocytic predominance; (2) nodular sclerosis; (3) mixed cellularity; and (4) lymphocytic depletion. The presence of Reed-Sternberg cells is a "sine qua non" for the diagnosis of Hodgkin's disease of any type.

Table 13-3 *Histologic Classification of Hodgkin's Disease*

JACKSON & PARKER		LUKES & BUTLER	
Type	*Incidence (%)*	*Type*	*Incidence (%)*
Paragranuloma	8	Lymphocytic predominance	15
Granuloma	91	Mixed	39
Sarcoma	1	Nodular sclerosis	40
		Lymphocytic depletion	6

A comparison of the two classifications of Hodgkin's disease based on Luke's review of 377 patients[101] is given in Table 13-3. In their original study of 301 patients, Jackson and Parker found the following distribution: paragranuloma, 12 per cent; granuloma, 80 per cent; and sarcoma, 8 per cent. Some difference in age distribution in the two series may be responsible for the discrepancies and the frequency of cases classed as sarcoma.

The Lukes classification has the advantage of providing a more definitive diagnosis for the type of disease which correlates better with prognosis and may reflect the status of the body's resistance to the disease. The nodular sclerosis picture occurs most often in the mediastinum, and many patients with this disease have a good prognosis, even if pulmonary tissue is involved.

CLINICAL MANIFESTATIONS

The varied clinical manifestations of Hodgkin's disease may appear at any age and in either sex. The disease occurred most frequently in the third decade in one series,[146] but in another study an even distribution was found in the first seven decades.[72] Males are affected more commonly than females, the ratio being about two to one.

The clinical manifestations of Hodgkin's disease are varied because virtually any organ in the body may be involved by the disease process. The incidence of lesions in various locations noted, either during life or at autopsy, in two series that totaled 485 patients[62, 71] are as follows: lungs, 33 per cent; mediastinum, 33 per cent; liver and spleen, 50 per cent and 70 per cent; skin, "common" and 38 per cent; bones, 20 per cent and 7 per cent. Involvement of the nervous system occurred in 12 per cent of another series.[151] Renal involvement was reported in 13 per cent. The disease is rarely found in the tonsils, but the salivary glands are involved in some patients.

Although nearly any sign or symptom may be the presenting one, the commonest initial symptom is painless enlargement of one or more lymph nodes (Fig. 13-1). An initial manifestation of this sort, usually in the cervical nodes, occurs in about 85 per cent of patients with Hodgkin's disease. The initial sites of involvement in one series were as follows: superficial lymph nodes in the cervical region, 60 to 80 per cent; axillary lymph nodes, 6 to 20 per cent; inguinal nodes, 6 to 12 per cent; mediastinal lymph nodes, 6 to 11 per cent. Enlargement of the retroperitoneal lymph nodes, liver, and spleen was seen less commonly

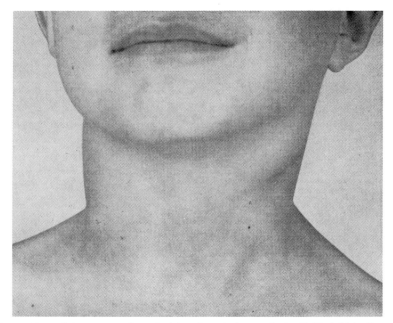

Figure 13-1 Enlargement of cervical lymph node in a patient with Hodgkin's disease.

in the early stages. Extranodal primary Hodgkin's disease is rare, even in the spleen, or the lymphoid tissues of the nasopharynx or the small intestine; nearly always what seems to be a primary lesion in some organ has been found on more extensive study to be associated with nodal disease.

The next most frequent symptoms are pain in the back, abdomen, or chest, weakness, loss of weight, and fever. Cough, dyspnea, and pruritus occur less often but are not rare. Severe pain in the abdomen, back, or chest after the ingestion of alcohol is a rare but striking symptom in some patients; the mechanism of the pain, which also occurs in other malignancies, is unknown. Pruritus is an unusual early symptom, but it develops in many during the course of the illness. This symptom, which is considered to be a sign of activity of underlying disease, may be extremely disagreeable and difficult to control unless the disease undergoes a remission.

Fever, which may be the chief and presenting symptom, occurs some time during the course of the disease in nearly every patient. It may be continuous, intermittent, or cyclic. An irregular type of fever that rises to 100° to 103° F at night occurs frequently and generally signifies that the disease is not confined to the superficial lymph nodes. The well known "Murchison" or "Pel-Ebstein" type of fever occurs in only a minority of patients. In this syndrome the temperature curve shows successive daily rises over a period of about a week until it reaches a peak of 103° to 105°, then subsides gradually to normal. After an interval of from ten days to two months, another febrile episode appears. The periods of remission gradually shorten unless the course of the disease is changed by therapy. This type of fever, particularly when accompanied by drenching night sweats, generally signifies mediastinal or intra-abdominal disease. A remittent type of fever similar to that seen in septicemia occurs in some patients with the acute fulminating type of Hodgkin's disease, even in the absence of demonstrable infection; shaking chills occur but are unusual. The urine of febrile patients with Hodgkin's disease contains a substance that acts like an endogenous pyrogen.[149] A pyrogen thought to be produced by mononuclear leukocytes has been extracted from the spleen and nodes of patients with Hodgkin's disease, but not from nonmalignant enlarged spleens.[20]

The immunologic status of many patients with Hodgkin's disease is abnormal.[117] Characteristically, there is impairment of the delayed hypersensitivity reaction, as measured by the response to tuberculin and other antigens, particularly those of fungal origin, and impairment of homograft rejection. Patients with localized disease may react normally to these tests; reactivity diminishes in those with more advanced stages of the disease. In advanced Hodgkin's disease, a state of "lymphocytic paralysis" develops; immunologic impairment has been correlated with the degree of lymphocyte reduction, either in the peripheral blood or in the lymph nodes. The impaired reactivity seen in patients with the active disease may improve, and even return to normal, when treatment induces a remission. Associated with the immunologic defect in Hodgkin's disease is an increased incidence of tuberculosis, cryptococcosis, histoplasmosis, nocardial infections, and various viral and bacterial infections, particularly in the late stages of the disease.

The variety of clinical manifestations that Hodgkin's disease may produce has been emphasized.[71, 105] Pruritus or exfoliative dermatitis may be the first manifestation. Disease in the intrathoracic region may present as an asymptomatic mediastinal tumor found on the roentgenogram or with evidence of the

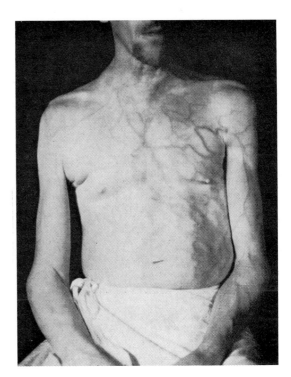

Figure 13–2 Infrared photograph demonstrating collateral circulation in a patient with Hodgkin's disease and superior vena caval obstruction.

superior mediastinal syndrome (Fig. 13–2). Intrathoracic disease may also be responsible for an unproductive cough, dyspnea, or pleural effusion. The first evidence of the disease sometimes appears in the abdominal region in the form of a retroperitoneal tumor, splenomegaly, or hepatomegaly. Skeletal involvement, which is most likely to occur in the vertebrae, is usually associated with pain that may be present for weeks before an osseous lesion is demonstrable in the roentgenograms. Hodgkin's disease is often found to be the cause of a persistent "fever of undetermined origin." In still other patients, splenomegaly, anemia, and other abnormalities in the peripheral blood are the principal manifestations.

Cutaneous Manifestations

Pruritus, localized or generalized, is a common, troublesome symptom in many patients with Hodgkin's disease; it indicates activity of the disease. Usually there are no apparent lesions in the skin to account for the pruritus. Symptomatic measures are often ineffective, but the symptom generally improves as the disease goes into remission.

Probably the most common dermatologic lesion in Hodgkin's disease is herpes zoster (Fig. 13–3). The reported incidence has varied from 15 to 25 per

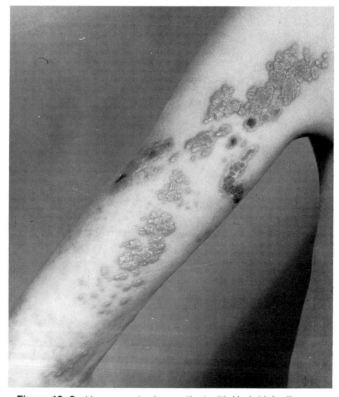

Figure 13–3   Herpes zoster in a patient with Hodgkin's disease.

cent, and in one series it occurred in 22 per cent of patients who had had splenectomy and in 13 per cent of those who had not.[60, 138, 142] At one institution over one-half of the patients who were treated with radiation, MOPP, and splenectomy later developed herpes zoster. A generalized herpetiform eruption occurred in nearly one-third of those with zoster; the recurrence rate was 8 per cent. These and other lesions probably reflect the lowered resistance to viral infection seen in Hodgkin's disease; one patient under our observation for years frequently had a remarkable spread of viral warts on his hands when the disease was active. Because of the extensive and severe reactions that have been reported, patients with Hodgkin's disease should not be vaccinated for smallpox.

Multiple brownish red elevated lesions of Hodgkin's tissue, which may or may not be pruritic, develop when the disease invades the skin. The disease at this stage is disseminated and may be very aggressive. We have observed some patients with lymphocyte depletion disease of the mediastinal nodes in whom the disease spread through the chest wall and skin, first producing ulceration and then tumor, despite high voltage irradiation of the area.

Exfoliative dermatitis and ichthyosis occur in some patients; when one of these is the main and presenting complaint, the correct diagnosis of the underlying disease may not be suspected.

Pulmonary Manifestations

A routine roentgenogram of the chest in an apparently healthy person sometimes brings the diagnosis of Hodgkin's disease into consideration for the first time when it discloses an unsuspected mediastinal tumor (Fig. 13–4). Involvement of the mediastinum and hilar nodes is common. Localized or scattered nodular lesions in the lungs also sometimes occur early in the course of the disease. When pericardial effusion is present, it usually is the result of direct invasion of the pericardium from disease in the mediastinal or hilar areas. At times the picture of constrictive pericarditis develops.

Pleural effusions, which may be serous or chylous, are more common than histologic evidence of pleural involvement by the primary disease; they are usually associated with disease of the mediastinal and hilar nodes. Hilar adenopathy often leads to invasion of the adjacent tissue by retrograde spread along the lymphatics.

Disseminated pulmonary lesions which have a nodular appearance suggest a hematogenous spread, either directly or via the thoracic duct to the pulmonary artery.[148] These lesions occur most commonly in patients with the lymphocyte depletion type of disease, but also occur in those with the nodular sclerosis and mixed cellularity types. Pulmonary lesions developed within several years in 14 per cent of a group of patients with Stage I and II disease treated with radiotherapy; approximately 80 per cent had involvement of the mediastinal or hilar nodes with the nodular sclerosing type of disease.[148] Tomograms are the most reliable examination for pulmonary lesions, which may not be apparent on the usual chest roentgenograms. It is often difficult to tell if the lesion seen on the radiograph is Hodgkin's disease, fibrosis secondary to previous treatment, or

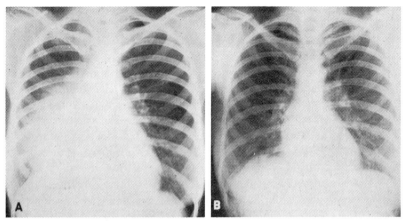

Figure 13–4 Chest roentgenograms of a patient with Hodgkin's disease. The diagnosis of the intrathoracic tumor (*A*) was established by biopsy. The patient responded unusually well to radiation and had no evidence of recurrence 12 years later (*B*). Although treated for recurrence of disease in the neck and elsewhere, she has no clinical evidence of disease 28 years after diagnosis. A review of her biopsy disclosed Hodgkin's disease, nodular sclerotic type.

a superimposed infection; not infrequently a biopsy is necessary to determine the precise diagnosis essential for proper management.

Neurologic Manifestations

The presence of disease in the nervous system most often becomes evident because of pressure on the spinal cord or the fifth, sixth, seventh, eighth, or ninth cranial nerve.[15] Involvement of the brain is generally associated with disease of the cranial bones, and the epidural tumor that causes cord compression is nearly always an extension from a lesion in a vertebra or from the adjacent mediastinal or retroperitoneal lymph nodes. Spinal cord compression by tumor is usually accompanied by pain; signs of compression such as constipation, urinary retention, and weakness or paralysis of the legs may develop rapidly. A myelogram should be made at the first suspicion of cord involvement.

As is now recognized in virtually all types of malignancy, almost any type of neuromyopathy can develop as a remote effect in patients with Hodgkin's disease, although the incidence is very low. Degenerative lesions have been described in all parts of the brain, the spinal cord, peripheral nerves, and muscles. Multifocal leukoencephalopathy, subacute cerebellar degeneration, and peripheral neuropathies are probably the commonest of these unusual lesions.[148] Acute paraplegia and massive necroses affecting both the gray and the white matter in the cord associated with a pathologic picture different from "progressive multifocal leukoencephalopathy" have been reported in patients with Hodgkin's sarcoma and nodular lymphoblastoma who had no invasion of the spinal cord by tumor. Peripheral neuritis in the lower extremities is a troublesome symptom in some patients; noninvasive peripheral neuropathy is unusual, but sometimes severe.

The attacks of herpes zoster, which are fairly common, are caused by involvement of the ganglia by the herpes virus rather than by Hodgkin's disease. The herpetic lesions disappear spontaneously without treatment (Fig. 13–3).

Gastrointestinal Tract

Hodgkin's disease involving the gastrointestinal tract is found in 20 to 50 per cent of autopsied patients, but primary involvement is rare, occurring in approximately 3 per cent.[47, 77] Approximately 50 patients with primary involvement of the small bowel have been reported.[46] In one series of 123 autopsied patients with Hodgkin's disease, 22 had lesions in the gastrointestinal tract, 16 in the stomach, two in the small intestines, and four in the colon. Nontumorous involvement of the gastrointestinal tract produced symptoms such as bleeding or obstruction more often than did actual involvement by tumor. Involvement of the gastrointestinal tract is a sign of poor prognosis. The survival time of patients who have had pain or a mass in the abdomen, vomiting, or bleeding is no more than one-half that of those without these manifestations; 75 per cent have been considered unsuitable for surgery, or have died shortly after surgical operation, and only a small number have survived for more than six months.

Jaundice occurs in from 3 to 8 per cent of patients with Hodgkin's disease.[95] Antemortem diagnosis of the cause of jaundice may be difficult. In autopsies on 57 jaundiced patients, the causes were: liver involvement with Hodgkin's disease, 70.2 per cent; no satisfactory explanation, 14 per cent; hemolytic anemia, 5.2 per cent; extrahepatic obstruction due to tumor, 3.5 per cent; hepatitis, 3.5 per cent; choledocholithiasis, 1.8 per cent; cirrhosis, 1.8 per cent. Although the jaundice may last from a few days to a year, its appearance is a preterminal event in more than 90 per cent of cases. Treatment is largely ineffective when icterus is caused by intrahepatic involvement.

Genitourinary Tract

Hodgkin's disease can affect the genitourinary tract in a number of ways. Perhaps the most common is obstruction of a ureter by intra-abdominal tumor. Although usually unilateral, the obstruction may be bilateral and may cause hydronephrosis with renal failure and uremia. Actual tumor involvement of one or both kidneys occurs much less commonly. The clinical manifestations of the nephrotic syndrome, massive proteinuria, hypercholesterolemia, low serum albumin, and paucity of red cells or casts in the urine are seen in some patients with Hodgkin's disease. It appears to be an immunologic reaction, because symptoms of the nephrosis develop without histologic evidence of Hodgkin's disease in the kidney, and generally subside following treatment with prednisone or immunosuppresive agents. The syndrome may appear when the Hodgkin's disease seems to be in remission or when active disease is apparent. A similar picture has occurred in some patients as the result of renal vein thrombosis or amyloidosis. If hematuria develops in a Hodgkin's disease patient who has been treated with Cytoxan, appropriate study is necessary, as in any other patient, to determine cause and source.

Bone Involvement

Various reviews place the incidence of bone involvement at between 10 and 15 per cent; current treatment may be reducing the frequency. The lesion may be sclerotic, lytic, or mixed. Involvement is seen most often in the vertebrae, but virtually any bone may be involved by direct extension from a diseased node or by hematogenous spread, and no histologic type of disease is exempt. Collapse of the diseased vertebra rarely occurs, but pain may be very troublesome.

PHYSICAL EXAMINATION

Abnormalities demonstrable by physical examination depend on the presence of the disease in various organs or systems in different parts of the body. Most commonly the lymph nodes, spleen, and liver are involved. The degree of lymphadenopathy, which is usually greatest in the cervical region, varies from slight to marked. The nodes are usually firm and rubbery in consistency, but may be either soft or stony hard. They are rarely tender and usually are not fixed to the skin or underlying structures. Occasionally the size of the nodes, especially in the cervical and submandibular areas, varies spontaneously from day to day. Palpable splenomegaly occurs in about 50 to 70 per cent of patients at some stage of the disease. The degree of enlargement found in different patients varies from a barely palpable spleen to one that nearly fills the entire left half of the abdominal cavity; usually the lower edge of the spleen is above the level of the umbilicus. Less commonly the examination reveals evidence of ascites, pleural effusion, pericardial effusion, superior vena caval obstruction, or neurologic involvement.

LABORATORY EXAMINATION

Laboratory examinations often disclose abnormalities, particularly in the peripheral blood. Normocytic anemia of some degree occurs in nearly all patients at some time during the course of the disease. Very rarely, pancytopenia is present when the patient is first seen. The anemia is usually the result of diminished erythropoiesis, but in some patients increased hemolysis is important. The total and differential leukocyte counts are often normal early in the disease, but a transitory increase in lymphocytes sometimes occurs. An increase in blood platelets and an absolute increase in monocytes have been reported to be constant throughout the disease.[24] In the more advanced stages of the disease leukocyte counts often rise to levels of 15,000 to 20,000 per cu.mm. or more. The leukocytosis is associated with an increase in cells of the granulocytic series and a decrease in lymphocytes. Often in the late stages, when lymphocytic paralysis develops, very few lymphocytes, 1000 cu.mm. or less, are found in the circulating blood. Eosinophilia of considerable degree occurs in some patients. Toxic granulation is often prominent and large bizarre platelets are often present. The erythrocyte sedimentation rate is usually elevated and the leukocyte alkaline phosphatase reaction increased when the disease is active. The electrophoretic pattern of the serum proteins may reveal a reduction in albumin associated with an increase in globulin in the moderately-advanced cases. Abnormalities in the proteins similar to those found commonly in multiple myeloma sometimes occur in Hodgkin's disease when there is an increase in plasma cells.[11] Reed-Sternberg cells can be found in bone marrow smears only rarely. Massive proteinuria is seen in some patients with Hodgkin's disease who develop amyloidosis.[30]

DIAGNOSIS AND STAGING

It is important to establish a histological diagnosis before treatment is started; unless the biopsy suffices to place the diagnosis, at least in this group of diseases, treatment is best deferred except in unusual circumstances. The decision regarding the type and amount of treatment must be based on a careful evaluation of the individual patient, and must take into consideration the condition of the patient as well as the type, extent, and location of disease. An evaluation of this sort is important because any treatment can prove deleterious or even fatal if given injudiciously.

Diagnosis of Hodgkin's disease involves two steps. First, a definite tissue diagnosis must be established by biopsy, and the histologic type determined, if possible; second, an attempt is made to define the extent of the disease by various staging procedures. Close collaboration between the internist, pathologist, surgeon, and radiotherapist is important when the patient first comes under observation and throughout the duration of the disease.

The histologic diagnosis of Hodgkin's disease in the excised node is not always easy. It is sometimes difficult to distinguish between Hodgkin's disease, non-Hodgkin's lymphoma, and lymphoid hyperplasia. The occurrence of Reed-Sternberg-like cells in biopsies from lymph nodes and tonsils of patients with proved infectious mononucleosis also presents difficulty, particularly in the younger age-group.

A more recently described disorder to be distinguished from Hodgkin's disease is *immunoblastic lymphadenopathy*, reported by Lukes and others in 1975.[102,140] The clinical manifestations are fever, sweats, weight loss, generalized lymphadenopathy, and occasional hepatosplenomegaly; hyperglobulinemia has been a consistent finding. This disorder has been considered to be a non-neoplastic hyperimmune proliferation of the B-lymphocytes with transformation of lymphocytes to immunoblasts and plasma cells. The disease is usually progressive, and in one group of 18 fatal cases the median survival was only 15 months. Complete remission, however, has followed the use of cytoxan, vincristine, and prednisone.

The staging classification recommended at the Ann Arbor Workshop in 1971[160] is the one in general use at present (Table 13–4). The recommendation

Table 13–4   *Staging of Hodgkin's Disease*

STAGE	SITE OF INVOLVEMENT
I	Single lymph node region
IE	Single extranodal site
II	Two or more lymph node regions on same side of diaphragm
IIE	Localized extranodal tissue plus one or more nodal regions on same side of diaphragm
III	Lymph node regions both sides of diaphragm
IIIS	Lymph node regions above and below diaphragm, plus spleen
IIIE	Localized extranodal tissue plus nodes on both sides of diaphragm
IIISE	Nodes, plus spleen, plus single extranodal site
IV	Diffuse or disseminated foci of one or more extralymphatic organs or tissues with or without associated nodal disease

"A" denotes absence and "B" presence of unexplained fever, night sweats, and/or unexplained loss of 10 per cent or more of body weight in preceding six months.

that the staging be further defined as "clinical" (based on usual examination and procedures), CS, or "pathologic" (based on the findings at laparotomy), PS, has not yet been widely accepted. The same is true for the more extensive and precise symbolism that has been recommended, N^+ or N^- for node biopsy, H^+ or H^- for liver biopsy, S^+ or S^- after study of the removed spleen, L^+ or L^- for lung biopsy, M^+ or M^- for marrow biopsy, P^+ or P^- for pleural biopsy or cytologic examination, O^+ or O^- for bone biopsy, and D^+ or D^- for cutaneous biopsy.

In order properly to classify a patient with histologically proved Hodgkin's disease according to stage, a systematic study is necessary. The studies which we employ differ slightly from those recommended by the Ann Arbor Conference on Staging;[130] our approach is shown in Table 13–5.

Lymphangiograms are made in patients who appear to have Stage I or

Table 13–5   *Staging of Patients with Hodgkin's Disease*

A. Required in virtually all patients
  1. History, with special attention to systemic symptoms
  2. Complete physical examination
  3. Laboratory tests: hematocrit, leukocyte count, differential count, platelet count, and sedimentation rate
  4. Bone marrow biopsy
  5. Radiograph of chest, PA and lateral
  6. Radiograph of lumbar spine and pelvis
B. Required in special circumstances
  1. Chest tomography: if pulmonary hilar, and/or mediastinal involvement is present or suspected
  2. Lymphangiograms: not necessary in Stage IV or III disease, unless of value in determining treatment to be given, or as an aid in laparotomy
  3. Staging laparotomy
  4. Peritoneoscopy
  5. Other radiographic examinations-I.V. pyelograms, inferior vena cavagram, myelogram, barium study of G.I. tract
C. Useful in certain circumstances
  1. Bone scans, gallium scan; scan of liver and spleen rarely of value
  2. Special studies of immunologic status; special blood chemistries

Stage II disease above or below the diaphragm. These studies usually are not indicated in patients with generalized disease, or in those with recognized disease below the diaphragm not confined to the groin areas, unless such studies are considered to be of special value in defining the field to be used in radiation treatment of a particular patient. Roentgenographic study of the gastrointestinal tract is made in patients who have symptoms suggesting involvement, but is not done routinely; x-rays of areas of the skeleton are taken when involvement is suspected.

In a group of 100 patients with Hodgkin's disease, abnormal lymphangiograms were found in 35 per cent of those thought to be Stage I, 51 per cent of those thought to be Stage II, and 89 per cent of those known already to be Stage III.[114] Similar results have been reported by others.[38] In a larger series of 192 patients, investigation disclosed that only two of 20 patients with cervical Stage I disease had abnormal lymphangiograms, whereas the same examination was abnormal in all six of those with Stage I disease in the groin. In the same study, lymphangiograms were abnormal in from 60 to 75 per cent of patients with lymphosarcoma and reticulum cell sarcoma who were thought to be in Stage I; the examination disclosed disease in over 80 per cent of those classed as Stage II and over 90 per cent of those in Stage III.[114] Interpretation of the lymphangiograms is often difficult. The level of error is probably at least 10 per cent, usually, but not always, due to a false negative reading, which may occur when a node does not fill because it is replaced by tumor or for some other reason. Some patients have more extensive disease, particularly below the diaphragm, than is disclosed by the studies. Nodes in the perisplenic, peripancreatic, celiac, and porta hepatis areas are not visualized by lymphangiograms.

Lymphangiography and vena cavography are not without risk. The complications of lymphangiography include oil embolism to the lung, kidney, brain, or liver, cellulitis at the site of the cutdown, and allergy to the injected dye. Transient pain, fever, hematoma, and pulmonary embolism also occur in some patients after vena cavography. Fatal reactions have been reported.[61, 112] Because of these complications, the following conditions are generally contraindications for lymphangiography: (1) pulmonary disease, symptomatic or asymptomatic; (2) history of allergy to iodine; and (3) known generalized Stage III disease, particularly with palpable involvement below the diaphragm.[92]

These shortcomings in lymphangiography and the other examinations led to the use of laparotomy and exploration to determine the extent of disease. The indications for staging laparotomy have varied widely, from a routine procedure at one extreme to "no laparotomy" in a series in which all patients were treated with radiation.

The use of the staging laparotomy in patients with Hodgkin's disease has provided much essential new knowledge about the behavior of the disease. The procedure usually involves the following: (1) abdominal operation; (2) splenectomy; (3) removal of obviously enlarged nodes for histologic study; (4) removal of apparently normal nodes if none appears diseased; and (5) two wedge and two needle biopsies of the liver. Splenectomy is performed because there seems to be little correlation between spleen size and histologic evidence of Hodgkin's disease, and large doses of radiation to the splenic region may damage the left kidney. Specimens of bone marrow (from two sites usually) are obtained.

The results of laparotomy in 100 consecutive untreated patients have proved valuable and interesting.[128] One-half of patients with splenomegaly did not have disease in the spleen (on the usual pathologic examination); one-third of the normal-sized spleens were diseased. Liver involvement was not found in the absence of splenic involvement; in addition, the larger the spleen, the greater was the likelihood of hepatic involvement. In 57 patients with "negative" lymphangiograms, only two were found to have para-aortic node involvement. Nodes were found in 17 of 23 patients with "positive" lymphangiograms, and in three of 20 patients with "equivocal" lymphangiograms. Other reports of the results of the laparotomy procedure have confirmed these findings, as has our personal experience with nearly 100 patients.

More data and more time will be necessary before the values and dangers of splenectomy as part of the staging laparotomy can be properly assessed.[40] The following benefits have been claimed: (1) certainty of diagnosis of the disease in the spleen; (2) more learned about the relationship to splenic involvement and hepatic involvement in Hodgkin's disease; (3) reduction of the field to be irradiated, with less danger to the left kidney; (4) possible increased tolerance to radiotherapy and chemotherapy; (5) an integral part of the knowledge necessary to evaluate results obtained with the different types of therapy.

The risk of septicemia with *Diplococcus pneumoniae* and *Hemophilus influenzae* in children less than 3 years of age following splenectomy for thalassemia or portal hypertension is well recognized; the incidence may be from 10 to 30 per cent of these patients, compared to 2 per cent when splenectomy is performed for other reasons, such as splenic rupture or thrombocytopenia.[40] Similar infections have occurred within a year of splenectomy in patients who have had staging laparotomy. Most of these have been young, 6 to 15 years of age. A review of 334 splenectomies in patients with Hodgkin's disease and 236 patients with lymphoma disclosed a morbidity rate of 1.4 per cent and mortality rate of 0.6 per cent; six of the 16 patients with infections were children. Similar infections also occur rarely following splenectomy performed for other reasons; because of the seriousness of this complication it must be considered in evaluating the staging laparotomy in Hodgkin's disease and other lymphomas.

In one study of 37 patients with Hodgkin's disease and 46 with non-Hodgkin's lymphoma, peritoneoscopy gave as much information about liver involvement as was obtained from staging laparotomy.[15] Neither the results of the liver function tests nor the size of the liver was of value in predicting the outcome of the examination. In this report, percutaneous liver biopsy gave a higher incidence of positive results than did peritoneoscopy in the patients with non-Hodgkin's lymphoma.

One review of the subject led to the conclusion that laparotomy should be used in only two situations: (1) to determine the frequency of node involvement in regions not visualized by lymphangiography (which would give some idea of the value or necessity of lymphangiography and para-aortic node biopsy); and (2) as part of a study to evaluate a treatment program. The authors took into consideration the rarity of unsuspected liver involvement, the high incidence of splenic involvement, the incidence of false negative lymphangiograms (10 per cent), the confirmation of positive results in 75 per cent, and the areas not visualized by lymphangiogram (porta hepatis; hilus of spleen; celiac, peripancreatic and periduodenal areas, and mesentery), as well as the risks involved in laparotomy.[7]

The authors of one report of the results of 100 consecutive staging laparotomies, which disclosed abdominal involvement in 44 patients, including 12 of 50 asymptomatic patients with negative lymphangiograms and 15 of 34 with symptoms and negative lymphangiograms, concluded that those with Stage I or II disease should either be explored or treated for intra-abdominal involvement. They considered that the need for laparotomy in patients with Stage III disease depends on the treatment plan.[4]

Although in our experience there have been no deaths, and only a rare major complication such as pneumonia or other postoperative infection, the procedure is a formidable one. Hospitalization is prolonged for ten days or two weeks, and therapy is delayed. We have recommended laparotomy in the following types of patients: (1) Stage IB and IIB with demonstrated disease above the diaphragm; (2) Stage IA and IIA disease above the diaphragm with equivocal lymphangiograms or vena cavograms; (4) Stage IIIA; and (5) Stage IA or IIA below the diaphragm. We have also explored patients with Stage IA disease in the left cervical region. It can be expected that the information gained from laparotomies, the longer follow-up period for evaluation of results obtained with different treatment regimes, and the increasing use of laparoscopy will better define the indications for laparotomy. In the meantime, the following comment made regarding the procedure at the Ann Arbor Conference on Staging of Hodgkin's Disease in 1971 warrants careful consideration:[160] "In view of the known and possible complications of exploratory laparotomy and splenectomy, the procedure should be considered required for diagnostic purposes if the therapeutic philosophy is to limit radiotherapy to only the known sites of the disease, or to patients of Stage I and II extent only. The procedure should be considered desirable but not required in attempting to exclude involvement of the liver in those patients who have the highest risk of liver involvement, those with apparent involvement of the para-aortic lymph nodes and spleen or those who have marked splenomegaly. In these circumstances, peritoneoscopy with liver biopsy is a suitable alternative procedure. Laparotomy is not considered required and is probably not justified if the risk for liver involvement is minimal *and* it is the therapeutic philosophy for an individual patient or, as a general rule, ... to treat the para-aortic lymph nodes and spleen with radiotherapy even in the absence of identified abdominal disease."

TREATMENT

Studies by Rosenberg and Kaplan, which included detailed clinical, laboratory, and radiologic evaluation as well as biopsy of equivocal areas, in 100 consecutive untreated patients with Hodgkin's disease indicated that the disease probably arises in a single focus and usually spreads along adjacent lymphoid channels. "Skipped" areas appeared in less than 25 per cent, and these were usually in the mediastinum. The good effects noted by Peters with "prophylactic" or "complementary" treatment of adjacent areas in patients with the disease point to the same conclusion, although she considers that there may be two types of Hodgkin's disease, one unifocal and the other multifocal in origin.[119] The latter is seen mainly in patients with Stage III disease. Both of these observations indicate that radiation treatment of the patient with Hodgkin's disease should be directed toward areas of probable involvement, and not limited to those actually demonstrated.

The most important therapy for patients with this disease is radiation. The role of chemotherapy is still being evaluated but is of increasing importance. Surgery, essential for diagnosis and staging, is employed in treatment in only a small percentage of patients, but in these it may be life-saving. Other details, including the treatment of infections, a sympathetic and understanding attitude toward the patient, and adequate time for discussions with the patient and family, are not specific but of great importance.

Radiotherapy

A good description and discussion of radiotherapy for Hodgkin's disease is given by Kaplan.[85] It is now generally accepted that high voltage radiotherapy which aims at cure is the treatment of choice for patients with localized disease. The five-year survival in patients treated with 3500 to 4000 rads is approximately double that of those treated with 2000 rads or less.[47] Kaplan has stated that intensive radiotherapy given with curative intent is "feasible and practical in all patients with Stage IA, IB, IIA, IIB, IIIA, IIIB and those with localized forms of disease in Rye Stage IV (Stanford stages IIE and IIIE)." He estimated that these groups comprise at least 90 per cent of untreated patients, and considered combination chemotherapy to be preferable for the other 10 per cent.[85]

In our institution, patients with stage IA, IB, IIA, IIB, and IIIA are treated with high voltage radiotherapy in large doses, 3500 to 4000 rads. On the assumption that Hodgkin's disease spreads to contiguous areas via the lymphatics, treatment is directed both at the involved areas and toward the adjacent drainage areas. The pattern of the area above the diaphragm to be radiated is "T"-shaped, a "mantle" that includes the cervical and supraclavicular areas on both sides, both axillary regions, and the mediastinum, front and back. Therapy below the diaphragm is directed in an "inverted Y" pattern with radiation to the para-aortic areas, the inguinal and femoral areas on both sides, and the splenic area. Radiation is directed away from normal tissue as much as possible.

If mediastinal disease is present, even though the patient is considered to have stage II disease, therapy is given to the para-aortic nodal area as well. "Total nodal" irradiation is aimed at all the nodal areas above and below the diaphragm, both the "mantle" and the "inverted Y" areas. The radiotherapy division at the University of Virginia Hospital alternates two weeks of radiation with two weeks of rest: this plan of interrupted therapy nearly always allows the desired amount of radiation to be given without interruption by side-effects. Radiotherapy is also used for patients with any stage of disease when the severity or magnitude of one area of disease is thought to warrant it.

Patients who are staged IIIB, IVA, and IVB are usually treated with chemotherapy initially, and the MOPP regimen is used unless there is some contraindication. Likewise, patients who have had radiotherapy with remission, but have relapsed, are usually treated with chemotherapy, as are patients who do not go into remission with radiotherapy. Occasionally, patients with extensive mediastinal disease are given chemotherapy for several months before radiotherapy in order to reduce the size of the field to be irradiated. We have not employed both chemotherapy and radiotherapy routinely in any type of patient.

Although there are not as many reports of Hodgkin's disease in children as there are in adults, several of the former indicate no unusual features.[52,139] Regional radiotherapy in stage I and II patients was associated with 80 per cent survival at 5 years and 60 per cent at 10 years, results comparable to those in adults. Nodular sclerosis is probably the commonest type of disease. Until the case for staging laparotomy has been defined more precisely, its use will probably be more restricted in children, particularly younger ones, because of the greater risk of postsplenectomy infection in this age-group.

Chemotherapy

Sulfur mustard, which was synthesized in 1854, was used with devastating effect as a chemical warfare agent in World War I. At that time, in addition to its vesicant action, serious systemic intoxication after exposure became apparent. Krumbhaar and Krumbhaar later reported a fatal case of a patient who had developed leukopenia and at autopsy was found to have aplasia of the bone marrow associated with necrotic changes in the lymphoid tissue and gastrointestinal tract.[88] In the decades that followed, various derivatives were prepared and tested against neoplasms of different types. One of the derivatives, mechlorethamine hydrochloride (nitrogen mustard), was shown to be effective in treating patients with Hodgkin's disease as well as those with myeloproliferative disorders in the mid-1940s; since that time it has remained one of the main chemotherapeutic agents used in Hodgkin's disease, first singly and then later in combination with other drugs.

The compounds that have been used most widely as single agents in treating Hodgkin's disease are: mechlorethamine hydrochloride, cyclophosphamide, vinblastine sulfate, vincristine sulfate, procarbazine hydrochloride, corticosteroids, methotrexate, and chlorambucil. The complete remission rate with these preparations varied from 17 to 37 per cent according to one report that combined the experience of several different groups.[156] When a complete remission was obtained with one of these preparations, it was usually of short duration (two or three months, rarely as many as six). The "improvement" reported in from 50 to 80 per cent of patients after use of these drugs usually represented only a partial remission (Table 13–6).

The demonstrated superiority of treatment of acute leukemia with several drugs led Devita and colleagues[42] to introduce quadruple therapy in patients with Hodgkin's disease in 1964. Their regimen, generally referred to as "MOPP," combined mechlorethamine hydrochloride, vincristine sulfate (Oncovin), procarbazine hydrochloride, and prednisone. These agents were selected because of their different modes of action and different limiting toxic effects. Their early results on 43 patients indicated that complete remission would occur in

Table 13–6 *Response in Hodgkin's Disease With Single Agent and Multiple Agent Chemotherapy**

	% of Patients With†		Median Duration of Response, Mo‡
	CR + PR	CR	
Single agents			
Mechlorethamine hydrochloride	63	...	2.5
Cyclophosphamide	54	22	2.5, 7.5
Vinblastine sulfate	65	33	3, 7.5
Vincristine sulfate	60	36	1
Procarbazine hydrochloride	69	37	4
Corticosteroids	54	...	<3
Methotrexate	...	17	...
Chlorambucil	80	...	4
NCI series§			
MOPP, little or no prior treatment	96	81	36‖
MOPP, extensive prior treatment	89	70	≥11
Present series§			
ALB	95	62	7
SEQ	90	53	7
MOPP, all patients	91	63	11
MOPP, little or no prior treatment	97	77	≥24
MOPP, extensive prior treatment	86	53	14

*(From Stutzman, et al.: J.A.M.A., *225*:1202, 1973. Copyright 1973, American Medical Association.)

81 per cent of those in Stage III and IV. Further, the median duration of remission was 36 months; 43 per cent of patients in remission remained disease-free without treatment for 5½ years or more. The protocol employed by these authors, and by nearly everyone since that time with but slight modification, is shown on page 487. The same group found no significant difference after remission was induced in patients who were given maintenance therapy with intermittent MOPP, and in those who received either no further therapy or intermittent therapy with BCNU.[175]

The encouraging early results obtained with MOPP therapy have been confirmed by others, although the results differ in some details.[54,109,113,156] The report from the S. W. Leukemia Chemotherapy Group (176 patients) showed that the complete remission rate in patients who had received major radiotherapy was 74 per cent, compared to 80 per cent in those who had no, or only minor, previous therapy; major chemotherapy or major radiotherapy plus chemotherapy reduced the remission rate to 35 or 40 per cent. Even in a group with stage IVB disease, the effect of previous chemotherapy and/or radiotherapy was apparent; in the group of 73 patients who had had no therapy or major radiotherapy the remission rate was approximately 70 per cent, compared to 30 per cent in 40 patients who had received previous chemotherapy and/or radiotherapy (Table 13–7).[54] This study showed that previous chemotherapy was a

Table 13–7 *Response in Hodgkin's*
Disease to Multiple Agent Chemotherapy

Pretreatment Characteristics	Patients		Complete Remission	
	Number	Percent	Number	Percent
Total patients	178	100	117	66
Age (years)				
Less than 20	26	15	17	65
20-39	94	53	60	64
40-59	47	26	34	72
Over 59	11	6	6	54
Sex				
Male	126	71	81	64
Female	52	29	36	69
Disease stage				
IIIA	9	5	7	78
IIIB	31	17	24	77
IVA	25	14	21	84
IVB	113	64	65	57
Prior therapy				
None or minor	93	52	74	80
Major radiotherapy	31	18	23	74
Major chemotherapy	25	14	10	40
Major radiotherapy and chemotherapy	29	16	10	35
Prior therapy by stage				
IIIA and B, IVA				
None or minor	39	22	34	87
Major radiotherapy	12	7	10	83
Major chemotherapy	8	4	5	62
Major radiotherapy and chemotherapy	6	3	3	50
IVB				
None or minor	54	30	40	74
Major radiotherapy	19	11	13	68
Major chemotherapy	17	10	5	29
Major radiotherapy and chemotherapy	23	13	7	30

(From Frei, et al.: Ann. Intern. Med., 79:376, 1973.)

significant limiting factor in treatment. In the entire series, 88 per cent of the calculated doses of the drugs were given to patients with little or no prior therapy and 80 per cent to patients with prior radiotherapy; in contrast, only 53 per cent could be given to those who had previously received major chemotherapy and 35 per cent to those who had previously received major chemotherapy plus radiotherapy.

The median time to complete remission in these patients was $3\frac{1}{2}$ months; it was estimated that this coincided with a 90 per cent decrease in tumor volume. The assumption that 10 per cent of active tumor remained was one of the factors governing the decision to give maintenance therapy for 18 additional months. The observation that there was a correlation between the initial site or sites of the largest masses of tumor before treatment, and the site of the initial recurrence, was consistent with the concept that relapses are manifestations of persisting tumor and not of reinduction of the disease. Although the report of the Southwestern Group indicated longer duration of the remission in patients who received maintenance therapy, the survival rate of four years was 70 to 80 per cent in both groups. The fact that those who had a shorter complete remission had the same survival time is probably a reflection of the success of MOPP therapy given when relapse occurred; 13 of 17 (77 per cent) of such patients responded, whereas those who relapsed after a while on maintenance therapy were no longer responsive to the MOPP.

The results obtained with the chemotherapy of this type will depend upon the composition of the group of patients, particularly the number with stage IVB disease with marrow involvement, the age of the patient, the number with systemic symptoms, and also the amount and type of previous therapy. The mortality rate in the reported series has varied from 20 per cent[109,113] to over 50 per cent;[54] in the authors' series it has been 45 per cent. The report from the NCI group of survival in a disease-free state for five to seven years by 15 of 35 patients who attained complete remission is most impressive, as is the survival curve which showed that all who were alive at 36 months were still alive and well at 66. Our experience, and that reported by Frei et al., is that approximately one-third of the patients who obtained complete remission have died within a few years.

The reported experience, which is in agreement with the results obtained by the authors in more than 50 patients, permits certain observations and conclusions:

1. The incidence of complete remission in previously untreated patients with stage IIIA, IIIB, IVA, and IVB disease has varied from 66 to 90 per cent.

2. The complete remission rate in patients with previous radiotherapy is approximately the same as that seen in the untreated group, but less than one-half of the patients who have received previous chemotherapy or chemotherapy plus radiotherapy attain a complete remission.

3. In the group treated at NCI and followed longer than the others, median duration of remission after entering remission was more than 36 months.

4. Relapse occurs in more than 50 per cent of those who have a complete remission, being most likely to occur within six to 12 months.

5. Maintenance therapy has not prolonged survival; whether it has prolonged the duration of remission is uncertain.

6. Patients with proved stage IVB disease are not as likely to obtain remission as are other patients, and their survival is less (50 per cent compared to 84 per cent stage IIIA, IIIB, and IVA).[54]

7. Sequential treatment with the agents used in the MOPP protocol is not as effective as their combined concurrent use.

8. The time required to obtain complete remission from the beginning of therapy may vary from three to 12 months, but is usually between three and six.

Both mechlorethamine and procarbazine produce bone marrow depression, which is the main toxic effect that causes revision of dosage or termination of the treatment in 80 to 90 per cent of patients. The major toxic effect of vincristine is on the peripheral nerves and may be manifested by paresthesias, muscular weakness, and absent knee and ankle jerks. Mild peripheral neuropathy occurs in the vast majority of patients during the six-months' course of MOPP, but is seldom severe enough to force cessation of the treatment. In a minority of patients, the undesirable effects which may develop in a short time are more serious: among these are weakness and atrophy in the muscles of the hands and arms, severe abdominal distention and obstipation, and even ortho-static hypotension. Alopecia, nausea, and vomiting are quite often troublesome but are rarely serious. Compazine and a sedative given one hour before the intravenous medication usually prevent nausea and vomiting.

The effect of sequential radiotherapy and chemotherapy in the treatment of Hodgkin's disease has been the subject of a prospective study.[108] One-hundred-and-two patients at stage IB through IIIB who had not received previous therapy were chosen at random and received total nodal irradiation, either alone or followed by six cycles of MOPP. In the former group there were ten relapses with two deaths from the disease, and in the latter group only one relapse. Mean duration of follow-up was 375 days. MOPP therapy was tolerated well. Although it significantly improved the probability of disease-free survival, actual survival was not significantly different for the two groups. All patients were thought to be in complete remission when MOPP therapy was started within two months after completion of total lymphoid radiation therapy. No problems with severe or prolonged leukopenia or thrombocytopenia were encountered in these patients who had had staging laparotomy with splenectomy earlier. Further studies of this type are necessary to determine the value of this combined sequential therapy.

"MOPP" THERAPY

The chemotherapy schedules that follow are those in most general use at the present time. One protocol for quadruple therapy of the MOPP regimen is the following:[42]

1. Nitrogen mustard   6 mg. per m^2 I.V.⎤ day 1 and day 8
                                                  ⎥ of each 28-day
2. Vincristine   1.4 mg. per m^2 I.V.⎥ period for 6
                                                  ⎦ cycles
3. Procarbazine   100 mg./m^2 per os day 1 through 14

4. Prednisone   (cycles 1 & 4 only)   40 mg./m^2 per os day 1 through 14

The dose of nitrogen mustard is reduced to one-half if the bone marrow is moderately impaired; if severe leukopenia or thrombocytopenia develops, the scheduled treatment is omitted. Patients with significant urea retention are not recommended for treatment in this manner. Dosage attenuation schedule for bone marrow depression is as follows:

If WBC count before starting new course was:	Then dosage was adjusted to:
>4,000	100% of all drugs
3999-3000	100% of vincristine, 50% nitrogen mustard and procarbazine
2999-2000	100% of vincristine, 25% nitrogen mustard and procarbazine
1999-1000	50% vincristine 25% nitrogen mustard
999-0	No drug

If platelet count before starting new course was:	The dosage was adjusted to:
>100,000	100% of all drugs
50,000-100,000	100% vincristine, 25% nitrogen mustard and procarbazine
< 50,000	No drug

We give prochlorperazine (Compazine), 10 mg., and sodium secobarbital (Seconal sodium), 100 mg., or similar medications one hour before the injection of nitrogen mustard, unless the patient is to drive home; the combination usually prevents nausea and vomiting. We do not give more than 2 mg. of vincristine in a treatment. If paresthesias are severe and the reflexes have disappeared, only one-half the calculated dose is given; if the neurologic toxicity progresses, the drug is discontinued. An attempt is made to give 6 cycles (6 two-week periods) of treatment. In some patients, particularly those who had prior treatment, more than six months is necessary to accomplish this; not infrequently, treatment is terminated before the full course of all the drugs can be given.

"COP" THERAPY[13]

Cyclophosphamide 400 mg./M² orally, days 1 through 5.
Vincristine 1.4 mg./M² I.V. day 1.
Prednisone 100 mg./M² orally day 1 through 5.

Repeat in 21 days for total of 6 cycles or until remission is obtained.

1. The daily amount of cyclophosphamide is preferably taken as a single morning dose.
2. Dose reduction schedule

WBC/cu.mm.	Platelets/cu.mm.	Dose
>4000	>100,000	100% of all drugs
3000–4000	50,000–100,000	75% cyclophosphamide, 100% others
2000–3000	50,000–100,000	50% cyclophosphamide, 100% others
1000–2000	<50,000	25% cyclophosphamide, 50% vincristine 100% prednisone
0–1000	<50,000	omit cyclophosphamide and vincristine, give 100% prednisone

When the patient becomes refractory to the "MOPP" treatment, or when marrow depression with cytopenia becomes a major limiting factor, other chemotherapy is generally used. Although the chance of a complete remission is small, and the duration short if it does occur, partial remission and some symptomatic improvement often follows. Most patients are better psychologically with some form of chemotherapy, even though it is not very effective, than with no treatment; it is rare that a patient with lymphoma requests that all treatment be stopped.

Drugs and combinations that we have found to be effective at times are: vinblastine 5 to 10 mg./week, monitored with the leukocyte count with or without prednisone; procarbazine 50 to 100 mg./day with or without prednisone;[39] chlorambucil 6 mg./day or o.d. with prednisone; Cytoxan 50 to 100 mg./day with or without prednisone.

When bone marrow depression is a limiting factor in therapy and there is no contraindication, vincristine, 1 to 2 mg. I.V. once a week, prednisone, 60 mg. on alternate days, and bleomycin, 10 to 20 mg./M^2 I.V. q 1 to 2 weeks to a total of 400 mg. may be used.[29] None of these drugs produces significant marrow toxicity. Bleomycin produces a short remission of from one to three months in between 40 and 50 per cent of patients with lymphoma. Toxic reactions include gastrointestinal upset, cutaneous reactions, alopecia and pulmonary complications, pneumonitis, dyspnea, and rales. Pulmonary toxicity, which occurs in 10 per cent of patients and may progress to pulmonary fibrosis, is the most serious toxic effect.

A combination treatment that has been effective in our experience in some patients with advanced Hodgkin's disease with marrow impairment who have become refractory to other forms of treatment is the following:

1. Adriamycin 30 mg./M^2 I.V. — once.
2. Bleomycin 15 units/M^2 I.M. — once.
3. Prednisone 60 mg./day orally for 10 days.

Repeat in 21 or 28 days if blood counts permit.

HAZARDS OF RADIOTHERAPY AND CHEMOTHERAPY

The hazards of radiotherapy may be delayed for months or even years, but the toxic effects of the chemotherapeutic agents usually appear promptly, within days or weeks; the main exception to this is the possible effect of the cytotoxic and immunosuppressive agents on the development of acute leukemia several years later, a development that has been reported in a few patients treated with radiation and chemotherapeutic agents.

The hazards of radiation to the skin and bone marrow elements have been known for many years. Radiation also usually produces transient but uncomfortable laryngitis and esophagitis, and gastrointestinal symptoms of anorexia, nausea, and diarrhea appear in some patients receiving radiation to the abdominal region. The use of high voltage therapy has meant a lessening of damage to the skin and administration of larger doses to the interior organs.

As a consequence of these higher doses, other sequelae, including pulmonary fibrosis, radiation damage to the spinal cord, and cardiac embarrassment from fibrosis of the pericardium, have been reported following such therapy.[47] These complications are serious and may be fatal. It may be the high voltage radiation rather than the recurrence of the lymphoma that is responsible for pericardial effusion, apparent cardiac enlargement, and constrictive pericarditis. Cardiac damage does not occur frequently enough to deter the physician from using this form of therapy when it is indicated, but such therapy should not be used unless there is a good chance of more than a palliative effect. In one report,[77] the most significant complication of high voltage large dose therapy was radiation pericarditis. This was noted in six out of 114 patients with clinical evidence of recurrence of Hodgkin's disease. Two were treated by aspiration and chemotherapy and eventually died of constrictive pericarditis. In the other four patients, pericardectomy was performed; Hodgkin's disease was found in one, but the other three have done well. In another series of 81 patients with stage I to III Hodgkin's disease treated with mantle radiotherapy, pericarditis developed in 30.8 per cent; 14 of the 25 effusions, often bloody, resolved spontaneously within two to seven months, and 11 were persistent; six patients required pericardectomy for symptoms of tamponade. There were no deaths. In 87 per cent of the cases the effusions occurred within one year of radiation therapy. Only four of the 25 patients had clinical evidence of acute pericarditis such as chest pain, fever, tachycardia, and pericardial friction rub.[142]

Long-term survival after radiation therapy may be followed in months or years by retroperitoneal fibrosis, interstitial fibrosis of the kidney, dilated lymphatics, telangiectasia, fibrosis, or stricture of the bowel which may be associated with malabsorption and perhaps chronic pancreatitis. As a result of the effect of radiation on the bone marrow, months may be required for hematologic recovery sufficient to permit the effective use of chemotherapy. When it is necessary to give chemotherapy after a shorter interval, the development of cytopenia of one sort or another often causes modification of the treatment regimen and limits its effectiveness.

Both radiation and chemotherapy can have adverse effects on testicular function in the male and ovarian function in the female. Aspermia and amenorrhea, temporary, partial, or permanent, have been reported.[137]

There appears to be a definite risk of second malignancies in patients treated with intensive radiation and intensive chemotherapy. In a group of 438 patients with Hodgkin's disease who received intensive radiation, the frequency of a second malignancy was 3.8 times that predicted; in those who received both intensive radiation and intensive chemotherapy, the incidence was 23 times that expected.[9]

Acute leukemia is being reported with increasing frequency in patients with Hodgkin's disease who have been treated with radiation and/or chemotherapy, and has been reported in over a hundred patients.[31, 32, 132, 135, 170] Only a small percentage of these have been diagnosed as having Reed-Sternberg cell leukemia; this type of leukemia has developed earlier in the course of the disease than the others, and may logically be considered as natural evolution of Hodgkin's disease. The vast majority of the patients, however, have had acute myeloblastic or acute myelomonoblastic leukemia. A smaller number have been diagnosed as having erythroleukemia, stem-cell, lymphoblastic, chronic lymphocytic, or chronic myelocytic leukemia. In over one-half of the patients, Hodgkin's disease has been present for more than five years, sometimes for eight or ten years. The late development and type of leukemia support the unproved interpretation that the leukemia probably developed as a result of therapy. Survival is usually short after this development. Although the frequency of leukemia seems to be increasing, it is still so rare that no-one has advocated withholding treatment which has proved so beneficial for the patient with Hodgkin's disease.

Nonleukemic pancytopenia has been reported as a late development in some patients with Hodgkin's disease treated with irradiation a year or two earlier. The development was associated with evidence of active Hodgkin's disease found at operation or autopsy.[78] The distinction between this type of reaction, preleukemia, and early acute leukemia is sometimes difficult to make.

The immediate toxic reactions to injections of nitrogen mustard are mainly nausea and vomiting, and occasionally diarrhea. The symptoms usually subside within eight to 24 hours and are usually prevented by administration of secobarbital, 100 to 300 mg., together with 10 mg. of Compazine. The most serious toxic effect is on the bone marrow, with resulting neutropenia and thrombocytopenia; the maximum effect on the marrow is apparent within ten days to two weeks after the injection, and in ordinary circumstances recovery ensues within a week or ten days. Local reactions, which may be severe, consist of tissue necrosis (if the preparation is injected into the tissues) and thrombophlebitis.

Cyclophosphamide (Cytoxan), an alkylating agent, which may be given orally or intravenously, produces toxic effects somewhat different from those seen with mechlorethamine hydrochloride. The effect on the bone marrow, although similar, is less pronounced, and alopecia is frequent. The most distinctive toxicity is hemorrhagic cystitis, which may be troublesome and serious. Chlorambucil (Leukeran) given orally produces toxic effects similar to the other alkylating agents, but they are less severe and develop gradually.

Vinblastine and vincristine are vinca alkaloids. The former is given intravenously in 5 to 10 mg. doses as a rule; the frequency and amount of injection are monitored by the leukocyte count. The maximum leukopenic effect is seen within seven to ten days, and recovery follows within another seven to 14 days. Disturbances in the peripheral nerves and autonomic nervous system develop in some patients. Vincristine, which is also given intravenously, has little toxic effect on the bone marrow. Its most striking toxic effects are on the nervous system, evidenced by paresthesias, loss of deep tendon reflexes, muscle weakness, footdrop, and weakness of the cranial nerves; a few patients develop severe constipation, abdominal distention, ileus, and postural hypotension. Alopecia occurs less frequently.

The dangers of treatment with high doses of prednisone for long periods are well-known. These include sodium and fluid retention, hypertension, diabetes mellitus, osteoporosis, myopathy, activation of pulmonary tuberculosis, and an increased susceptibility to infection. The manifestations of inflammation are usually suppressed, and body defenses against infections are often compromised. Purpura on the dorsum of the hands is common, particularly in the older patients, and superficial mucosal ulceration in the gastrointestinal tract may be a source of serious hemorrhage. A less common and less serious symptom is frequent nocturia. Because of these problems, antituberculous therapy is usually given to patients who have a positive tuberculin test, and antacid is often prescribed. The dose of prednisone is reduced as much as possible if long-term therapy is anticipated; the incidence of serious complications is reduced considerably if the daily dose is no more than 5 to 10 mg. Larger doses are well tolerated when given on an alternate-day basis; with this mode of administration, inflammatory responses are normal on the day the drug is not given.[37]

Procarbazine (Matulane) has been used in the treatment of lymphomas in doses of 3 to 4 mg./kg. of body weight q.d. (maximum daily dose 200 mg./M²), and in the MOPP program where the dose is 100 mg./M² daily for two weeks each month. The major toxicity is hematopoietic suppression in from one-half to two-thirds of the patients treated for a month. Nausea, vomiting, and neurotoxicity also occur.

Bleomycin has the merit of being virtually free of associated bone marrow toxicity. It does, however, produce gastrointestinal upsets, cutaneous reactions, and alopecia. The most serious toxic effects are pulmonary; dyspnea, rales, and pneumonitis occur in approximately 10 per cent of cases. In some patients this progresses to serious pulmonary fibrosis, which may be fatal.

Adriamycin[19] produces necrosis if it escapes into the tissues. Other toxic effects, usually transitory, are alopecia, which occurs in nearly all patients but is temporary; myelosuppression—particularly leukopenia, found in 10 per cent; gastrointestinal upset—nausea, vomiting, and mucositis; and cardiac disorder. The last is the most serious, and irreversible cardiac failure has developed in patients who received a total of 500 mg. of the drug, or even less. The drug is metabolized and excreted through the liver, and for this reason considerable dose reduction is necessary in patients with liver disease or jaundice.

PROGNOSIS

Statistics recorded in the literature regarding the prognosis of patients with Hodgkin's disease and the other lymphomas are of little value at present. Improved histologic diagnosis of the tumors, classification of patients by clinical stages, and improved methods of treatment with radiotherapy and chemotherapy, all make most earlier reports largely irrelevant to present-day management.

Despite advances in diagnosis and staging, it is virtually impossible to give an accurate prognosis in an individual patient with Hodgkin's disease; some patients with what appears to be localized disease have a rapid downhill course, probably because of undetected disease elsewhere, whereas others who appear to have generalized disease from the onset may respond well to treatment and survive for decades. Perhaps the most important factor in survival for patients with Hodgkin's disease, as for those with other malignancies, is their resistance to the tumor, the host-tumor relationship; at present there is no satisfactory way to evaluate this factor.

In one study of 1093 cases of Hodgkin's disease, 104 received no therapy at diagnosis; 68 per cent of these refused therapy and 32 per cent remained untreated because of initial doubt about the diagnosis; 80 patients remained untreated throughout. The mean age at diagnosis in the latter group was 56 years. The survival rate in those 80 untreated patients was 10 per cent at five years and 8 per cent at ten years. Twenty-four patients who received no therapy initially,

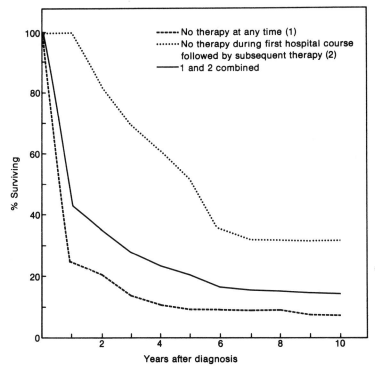

Figure 13–5   Survival in Hodgkin's disease. (From Greco, et al.: Arch. Intern. Med., *134*:1039, 1974, Copyright 1974, American Medical Association.)

but received various forms of therapy subsequently, had an average survival of 6.17 years, a five-year survival of 54 per cent, and a ten-year survival of 33 per cent (Fig. 13–5).[64]

As shown in Figures 13–6 and 13–7, the survival rate of patients with Hodgkin's disease stage IA and IIA treated with total nodal irradiation is probably over 90 per cent at seven years.[75] Kaplan's report indicates a five-year survival of approximately 90 per cent in stage I and IIA, and over 80 per cent in stage IIIA; patients in stage IIIB and IV had 40 per cent survival at five years; the five-year survival of patients in stage IIB was approximately 75 per cent, IIIB 60 per cent, and IV 40 per cent.[85] Factors other than the stage of the disease that influence the result of treatment are: "B" symptoms; age (prognosis being worse in elderly patients); and sex. Although it has long been felt that females survive better than males, recent studies indicate that this difference seems to be significant only in patients with stage III and IV disease, circumstances in which the outlook for females is appreciably better. The influences of histologic type and clinical stage on prognosis are not independent variables; patients with the lymphocyte predominant or the nodular sclerosis type of the disease have a better prognosis than others, but these types tend to be concentrated in the stage I and II cases, whereas the mixed cellularity and lymphocyte depletion types predominate in the more advanced cases and those with constitutional symptoms. The nodular sclerosis type involves the mediastinum and

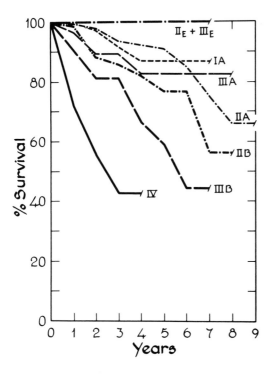

Figure 13-6 Survival in Hodgkin's disease after radiotherapy. (From Kaplan, H. S.: Hodgkin's Disease. Cambridge, Mass., Harvard University Press, 1972. © 1972 by the President and Fellows of Harvard College.)

supraclavicular nodes more than the other types, and tends to occur more frequently in females in the younger age-group.

The incidence of long-term survivors with Hodgkin's disease, ten years or more, has been placed at 14.2 per cent, 17 per cent, 9.8 per cent, 8 per cent, 5 per cent, and 35 per cent.[87, 155] These results were obtained with treatment much less aggressive than that used at present, and they should be compared with the 8 per cent survival in patients who had no treatment.[64] The vast majority of long-term survivors, 80 to 95 per cent, have either the nodular sclerosis type or the lymphocyte predominant type; a few have mixed cellularity, but lymphocyte depletion is exceedingly rare. In one study of 40 patients who survived for more than ten years, the cause of death was known in 21; 14 of these died of Hodgkin's disease, and in seven death was attributed to other causes. Of six autopsies in the latter group, four had evidence of active Hodgkin's disease which was not suspected clinically. These observations demonstrate that active disease can be present but not apparent clinically. They also suggest some equilibrium is reached between the patient and Hodgkin's disease which may permit a period of good general health, only later to break down with a further extension of the disease.

For a number of years many investigators have sought clues to the activity of disease or its prognosis in hematologic findings. As one would expect, these often reflect the stage of the disease. Thus, anemia is a manifestation of generalized disease, which would offer a poorer prognosis. An absolute lymphocyte count of less than 800 per cu. mm. indicates a worse prognosis than normal counts; a similar relationship has been noticed with the monocyte count. The

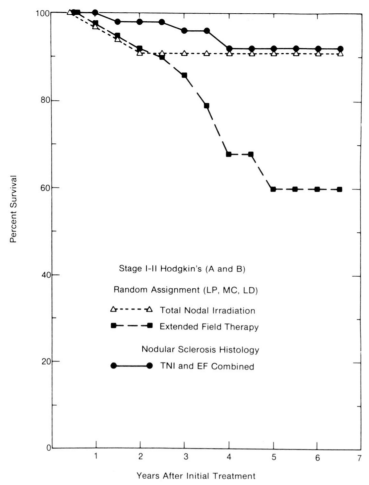

Figure 13-7 Survival in 125 patients with Hodgkin's disease following radiotherapy. (From Johnson, R.: J.A.M.A., 223:60, 1973. Copyright 1973, American Medical Association.)

erythrocyte sedimentation rate and the leukocyte alkaline phosphatase procedure are abnormal in most, but by no means all, patients with extensive and active Hodgkin's disease, and at times these suggest that relapse is impending; the sedimentation test, however, is often elevated for months after therapy.

The encouraging results of treatment in patients with these diseases, together with the realization that long-term survivors who were free of clinical disease eight or ten years after onset had as good a life expectancy as the general population of the same age-group, led Russell and Easson to introduce the concept of a cure in these diseases.[44] Their definition of a cure was "...of when in time—probably a decade or so after treatment—there remains a group of disease-free survivors whose progressive death rate from all causes is similar to that of a normal population of the same sex and age constitution." Such a definition, even though it may provoke some semantic difficulties, provides a stimulating and refreshing outlook for both the patient and the physician.

NON-HODGKIN'S LYMPHOMA

CLASSIFICATION

In recent years the term "non-Hodgkin's lymphoma" has found increasing favor. It has the virtue of providing a designation for a group of disorders in a field that is in transition. There are no well-defined guide lines for classification, diagnosis, treatment, necessary staging procedures, and prognosis because of lack of adequate information. A classification, shown in Table 13–1, and essentially that proposed by Rappaport, Winter, and Hicks in 1956, has come into the widest use in recent years.[122] Tumors are classified as "nodular" or "diffuse;" more specificity is gained in these two major groups by designating the nature of the cells involved, lymphocytes or histiocytes, and the degree of maturity of the cells. The more specific terms make evaluation of therapy and estimation of prognosis more precise and meaningful.

The frequencies of the different histologic types of non-Hodgkin's lymphoma vary in different reports (Table 13–8). It is interesting to note how infrequently the diagnosis of "well differentiated lymphocytic lymphoma," either "nodular" or "diffuse," was made in two of the series.

Although the classification proposed by Rappaport et al. has been a significant contribution and advance, it is probable that newer techniques of study, such as histochemical staining, electron microscopy, and staining for immunofluorescent antibodies, together with a broadened perspective, will provide greater accuracy and specificity in diagnosis that may require some revision in classification.

An example of the more precise information gained by newer techniques that promises to lead to a revision of the current classification of non-Hodgkin's lymphoma is the report by Jaffe et al.[73] Cells from six patients with nodular lymphomas were studied for characteristic binding sites and rosette formation in cell suspensions and frozen tissue sections with techniques that can distin-

Table 13–8   *Non-Hodgkin's Lymphoma, Frequency of Different Types*

NODULAR	(1) %	(2)	(3)	DIFFUSE	(1) %	(2)	(3)
NH	7.2		0	DH	28.7	20	32.5
NM	18.3		8.7	DM	10.5		5.0
NLPD	17.0		37.5	DLPD	10.8	20	11.5
NLWD	1.5		0	DLWD	2.5	35	5.0
				DU	3.5	15	
Total	44	10	46.2		56	90	53.8

NH = nodular histiocytic
NM = nodular mixed
NLPD = nodular lymphocytic poorly
 differentiated
NLWD = nodular lymphocytic well
 differentiated

DH = diffuse histiocytic
DM = diffuse mixed
DLPD = diffuse lymphocytic poorly
 differentiated
DLWD = diffuse lymphocytic well
 differentiated
DU = diffuse undifferentiated

(1) Jones, S. E., et al.: Cancer, *31*:806, 1973. (465 patients).
(2) Aisenberg, A. C.: N. Engl. J. Med., *288*:883, 1973.
(3) Schein, P. S., et al.: Blood, *43*:181, 1974 (80 patients).

guish between B lymphocytes (thymus-independent), T lymphocytes (thymus-dependent), and histiocytes. In all the tissues studied, cells from both the "poorly differentiated lymphocytic" and the "mixed lymphocytic histiocytic" types proved to be B lymphocytes; the studies also indicate that nodular lymphomas originate in lymphoid follicles, where the B-cell that bears the C-3 reactor is the predominant cell. If confirmed, these results indicate that diagnosis of "histiocytic" and "mixed" types of lymphoma will become less frequent.

Nearly all the lymphocytic lymphomas investigated have been found to be B cell proliferations, as identified by immunoglobulins on the cell surface.[3, 73, 94] Histiocytic lymphomas and mixed cell tumors have no demonstrable antibodies. The clonal character of the cell proliferation was established by demonstrating the presence of one predominant heavy chain and one predominant light chain. The studies strongly suggest the presence of at least two subtypes of neoplastic B lymphocyte. One, with the appearance of the adult small lymphocyte in the circulating blood, the cell involved in well differentiated lymphocytic lymphoma and chronic lymphocytic leukemia, had few immunoglobulins on the surface; another, which contained large amounts of immunoglobulins, was the cell seen in poorly differentiated lymphocytic lymphoma and lymphosarcoma cell leukemia.[3] The possibility was suggested that two lines of cells with abundant surface immunoglobulins could arise from the follicle, one producing nodular lymphoma, the other diffuse poorly differentiated lymphoma; the third B cell, with sparse immunoglobulin seen in well differentiated lymphomas, might arise in the mantle layer.[3]

T lymphocytes are characterized by the absence of surface immunoglobulins, the ability to form rosettes with sheep erythrocytes, and the reaction to antithymocyte globulin. This type of lymphocyte is the predominant one in normal nodes, inflammatory nodes, and nodes involved in Hodgkin's disease. Non-Hodgkin's lymphomas of T lymphocyte origin are unusual.[103]

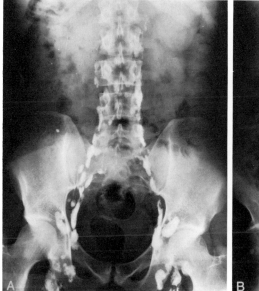 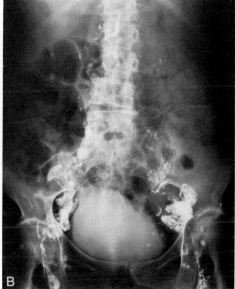

Figure 13–8 Lymphangiograms. *A*, Normal. *B*, Abnormal; Hodgkin's disease, Stage III A. (Courtesy of Dr. Anne Brower.)

CLINICAL MANIFESTATIONS OF DIFFUSE LYMPHOCYTIC LYMPHOMA AND DIFFUSE HISTIOCYTIC LYMPHOMA (LYMPHOSARCOMA AND RETICULUM CELL SARCOMA OR HISTIOCYTIC LYMPHOMA)

Lymphoma, Diffuse

The clinical manifestations of the diffuse lymphomas, lymphocytic (lymphosarcoma) and histiocytic (reticulum cell sarcoma), are very similar and are described together to avoid repetition.

These lymphomas occur at any age, but the highest incidence is found in the fifth and sixth decades. The incidence in males is approximately twice that in females.[57, 157]

The first evidence of disease is usually visible and palpable enlargement of superficial lymph nodes. In one series of 1269 patients, the disease made its appearance in this way in 65 per cent.[126] The cervical nodes were involved in 35 per cent, and the axillary, inguinal, and abdominal nodes were each involved in

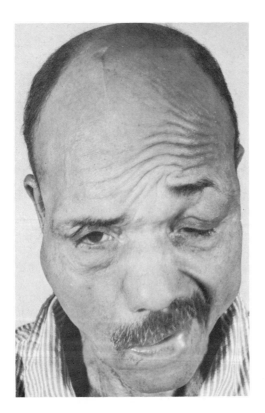

Figure 13–9 Lymphosarcoma involving the parotid gland with facial paralysis.

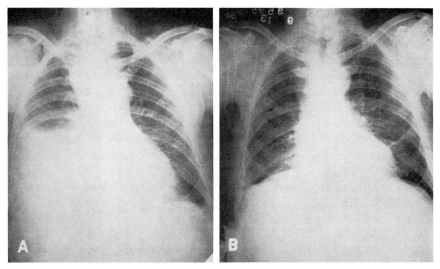

Figure 13-10   Chest roentgenograms in a patient with lymphosarcoma, showing mediastinal adenopathy and hydrothorax before therapy (*A*); appearance after irradiation (*B*).

about 12 per cent; mediastinal involvement was much less common. Intra-abdominal and mediastinal lymphosarcoma are causes of initial symptoms much more often in children than in adults. The involved nodes, which generally are moderately firm and resilient, are movable unless local invasion has occurred.

Although Hodgkin's disease cannot be distinguished from other lymphomas by the clinical manifestations in the individual patient, the diseases follow somewhat different patterns. Splenomegaly is less common and autoimmune hemolytic anemia is more common in other lymphomas than in Hodgkin's disease, fever occurs less often, and anemia develops later. The "Murchison-Pel-Ebstein" type of fever curve, which was observed during the course of the disease in 16 per cent of one group of patients with Hodgkin's disease, is rare in other members of the lymphoma group.[57] Almost any organ in the body can be involved by either of these diseases. Intrathoracic disease is the presenting symptom in only 5 per cent of patients, but about one-half of them develop clinical evidence of such involvement during the course of the disease; in 35 per cent it is mediastinal, in 30 per cent pleural, and in 20 per cent pulmonary. No part of the body is immune to involvement.

Lesions of the gastrointestinal tract occur more commonly than in Hodgkin's disease; the clinical incidence is reported to be 10 per cent and the frequency at autopsy 50 per cent.[68] The stomach, small intestine, or colon may be involved. In an autopsy series of 125 patients, 50 per cent had the disease in the gastrointestinal tract. The small intestine was involved most often, but lesions occurred frequently in the stomach and colon.[48] In 75 patients with "lymphosarcoma," involvement of the gastrointestinal tract, most often in the stomach or colon, occurred in 27 per cent. As in patients with Hodgkin's disease, involvement of the gastrointestinal tract with these diseases, except as the initial manifestation, was a sign of poor prognosis. Clinical symptoms such as bleeding, obstruction, and perforation occurred as often in patients without actual involvement of the gastrointestinal tract as in those with invasion; in the former group, ulceration, sometimes associated with prednisone and other therapy, was a frequent problem. The gastric lesion most often consists of a diffuse infiltration that may be recognized on the roentgenologic examination of the stomach because of the presence of exaggerated, stiffened rugae and diminished peristalsis. The most frequent site of disease in the small bowel is the terminal ileum, where the lesion may produce bleeding or intestinal obstruction.

Renal involvement, which often is not recognized clinically, occurs in about one-half of the patients. In one group, actual renal involvement occurred in 39 per cent of those with "lymphosarcoma" and in 46 per cent of those with "reticulum cell sarcoma." Various types of involvement occur.[86] The most common lesions are multiple nodules, cortical infiltration, possible evidence of the leukemic transformation, and invasion from a retroperitoneal tumor. More than one-half of the patients have some impairment of the renal function, most often from the disease outside the genitourinary tract, obstruction from tumors or retroperitoneal fibrosis, before the disease has run its course. The typical picture of the nephrotic syndrome occurs in some patients. At times renal vein thrombosis may be the responsible mechanism, but in other patients neither involvement by tumor nor vascular complications can be found; in these patients an abnormality in immunologic mechanism has been postulated. Other forms of renal disease that occur are amyloidosis and postradiation nephritis.

Involvement of the nasopharynx and tonsillar areas, rare in Hodgkin's disease, occurs more often in these lymphomas. Lesions of the nervous system and skeleton occur more frequently in histiocytic lymphoma (reticulum cell sarcoma) than in the others; when it involves the skeleton, the disease is usually widespread. In some patients, however, the disease appears to be primary in bone, and 50 per cent of these have been reported to survive five years after radiotherapy.[164]

Abnormalities occur in both the peripheral blood and bone marrow of many patients. Lymphocytosis of the peripheral blood, which is sometimes due partly to an increase in the large lymphocytes, is seen more often in these disorders than in Hodgkin's disease. Some patients who are diagnosed as having lymphocytic lymphoma (lymphosarcoma) later develop the peripheral blood picture of lymphocytic leukemia; this occurred in 7.3 per cent of adults and 13 per cent of children in one series. Acute leukemia was extremely rare except in children. Eosinophilia and polymorphonuclear leukocytosis sometimes occur but are less frequent than in Hodgkin's disease.[125]

At times patients with these lymphomas present with splenomegaly with or without evidence of hypersplenism. In some, the disease progresses slowly to involve the intra-abdominal lymph nodes and then the bone marrow. In this stage, when the total leukocyte count and the differential count are normal or nearly so, and the bone marrow is infiltrated with small lymphocytes, either as nodular, patchy, or diffuse involvement, it is difficult to know whether to make a diagnosis of "aleukemic lymphocytic leukemia" or "lymphosarcoma with involvement of the bone marrow." If the involvement is patchy, the situation is generally recognized as "Stage IV lymphoma." If it is diffuse, the proper terminology is "leukemia" of the recognized cell type. A biopsy, rather than an aspirate, is necessary to make this distinction, because an aspirate may be interpreted as diffuse if a nodule or localized area is aspirated. It is recognized that the diffuse picture in the marrow may evolve to some form of leukemia, but whether the patchy type of involvement ever becomes diffuse or transforms into leukemia is uncertain. Other patients with lymphoma, possibly those whose tumors contain the larger cell types, develop a picture of "leukosarcoma" characterized by the presence of cells resembling immature large lymphocytes; some cells have nucleoli and others have indented or folded nuclei. The "leukemoid" picture in these patients may persist or may be transient. Similar changes occur in some patients with histiocytic lymphoma; these are not as frequent but sometimes develop late in the disease, most often in the last few months.

Hemolytic anemia of the autoimmune type occurs in some patients, and at times is accompanied by thrombocytopenia. In one series of 515 patients with this type of tumor, the incidence of autoimmune hemolytic anemia and thrombocytopenic purpura was 2.1 per cent. In three of the four patients with idiopathic thrombocytopenic purpura, thrombocytopenia developed before there was any other evidence of the tumor. Both thrombocytopenia and hemolytic anemia usually respond to treatment with prednisone and/or splenectomy, but the ultimate prognosis in these patients is related to the type and extent of underlying disease.[79] The antiglobulin (Coombs) test is positive in at least one-half of the patients with malignant lymphoma who develop severe hemolytic anemia;[90] in some reports on the association of autoimmune hemolytic disease and lymphoma, only patients with positive tests are included.[131] Abnormalities in the serum protein, such as moderate decreases in albumin and gamma globulin and moderate increases in the alpha-1 and alpha-2 fractions, occur commonly; the occurrence of "myeloma-type" proteins is not rare.[11] IgG peaks in serum electrophoretic patterns were found in 4.5 per cent of patients with lymphocytic lymphoma of the diffuse type.[5]

Lymphoma, Nodular

This tumor (giant follicular lymphoma, nodular lymphoblastoma, Brill-Symmers disease) is about two and one-half times as common in males as in females, and occurs most often in the fifth or sixth decade.[57, 58] Less than 5 per cent of cases occur in individuals under 20 years of age. This disorder has a more benign course than the other members of the lymphoma group, but its tendency to undergo transformation is recognized.[12, 36, 50, 57, 58, 159]

Transformation into another type of lymphoma usually occurs after the disease has been present for five years. The most frequent transformation in one group of 64 patients was to "lymphosarcoma;"[52] other patients developed "reticulum cell sarcoma," chronic lymphocytic leukemia, and acute leukemia; in this series, transformation into Hodgkin's disease did not occur. The five-year survival was 72 per cent; ten-year, 60 per cent; and 15-year, 40 per cent. All the patients who died had lymphosarcoma or leukemia. According to Rappaport's concept, histiocytic lymphoma (reticulum cell sarcoma) develops only if the original nodular tumor was histiocytic or mixed cell in type; lymphocytic lymphoma rarely develops from the mixed type. The progression in the lymphocytic type is from nodular to diffuse, and in some patients the malignant cell seems to become less differentiated late in the disease. In 25 per cent of patients with nodular lymphoma, the disease was still nodular at autopsy.[122]

The present concept of this disorder may well need further modification in the future. In studies that utilized new and special techniques for identifying the tumor cell, the B lymphocyte (thymus-independent) was found in all cases; the same cell is the predominant one in follicles of the lymph nodes where these tumors apparently originate.[73, 94]

The most common initial manifestation is enlargement of the superficial lymph nodes or spleen. The involvement of the nodes is usually more or less generalized, but localized disease also occurs. In one report, the disease appeared to be localized at onset in one-half and generalized in one-third.[52] Twenty per cent developed lesions in the vertebrae or other parts of the skeleton; none had neurologic involvement. Enlargement of the mediastinal nodes may produce marked impairment of respiration. Enlargement of the retroperitoneal, mesenteric, and mediastinal nodes is common. The presence of the disease in these locations is often associated with ascites or hydrothorax, and the frequent occurrence of chylous ascites has been reported. The incidence of splenomegaly is reported to be 33 per cent.[58] Fever, cachexia, and other constitutional manifestations are rare. Although anemia is unusual until late in the disease, the frequent development of hemolytic anemia, thrombocytopenic purpura, and leukopenia in patients with splenomegaly has been reported.[50] Involvement of the skin, nervous system, and skeleton is rare.

Although radiotherapy has been reported to produce the best results in patients with this disease, even when the disorder is not localized,[52] some patients respond well to chemotherapeutic agents for a number of years.

Burkitt's Tumor

This disorder, now considered to be a lymphoma, was described first in 1958 by Burkitt, who observed the disease in 38 Ugandan children between the ages of 2 and 14.[25] Its most characteristic feature is rapidly growing osteolytic tumors that involve one or more quadrants of the jaw; tumors also occur in the salivary glands, kidneys, adrenals, liver, heart, retroperitoneum, and other sites. Central nervous system involvement, manifested by cranial nerve palsies and paraplegia from compression, is common, but usually responds well to treatment. The disease differs from the other types of lymphoma in that involvement of the superficial lymph nodes and the spleen is uncommon or minimal. This lymphoma is a disease of childhood, and in parts of Africa it comprises one-half of the tumors in children under 14 years of age. The distribution of the disease across Equatorial Africa has led to the suggestion that it is caused by an arthropod-borne virus.

The tumor is a malignant neoplasm of predominantly undifferentiated lymphoreticular cells which have a uniform and characteristic appearance in tissue sections and imprints.[27] The recommended classification is "malignant lymphoma, undifferentiated, Burkitt's type." It probably corresponds to the type designated "lymphoma, diffuse, stem cell" in some papers. The disease is not confined to the continent of Africa; a number of patients have been reported from the United States and other parts of the world. In American patients, the jaw is involved less often than in the Africans, but the ovary, the intra-abdominal organs, and the bone marrow are involved more often. Patients with the African form of the disease rarely have a terminal leukemic blood picture, but this has developed in about 30 per cent of the American series. In six patients with Burkitt's tumor and leukemia, special techniques indicated that the blast cells were of monoclonal B cell origin.[53]

Untreated Burkitt's lymphoma follows a rapidly fatal course, death usually occurring in less than six months, but the disease apparently responds well to treatment with cyclophosphamide (40 mg. per kg. I.V. × 6.)[10] About two-thirds of the patients, even some of those with Stage III and IV disease, obtain complete remission on such treatment. In nine patients treated with x-ray and a variety of chemotherapeutic agents, the mean survival time was only 2.5 months; in a group of 12 patients who received six or more injections of cyclophosphamide intravenously at intervals of three or four weeks, six patients survived from 52 to 112 weeks. Neurologic involvement which occurred in some patients responded well to intrathecal methotrexate, 10 mg. weekly for a minimum of four courses.[27] In one group of 101 patients in Uganda treated for longer than one week, 95 per cent had a complete remission; relapse occurred in 39 per cent of those with localized disease and in 70 per cent of those with generalized disease.[179] In 30 patients treated in the United States, the complete remission rate was 59 per cent;[10] relapse had occurred in only four of the 13 who experienced a complete remission. The value of therapy with multiple chemotherapeutic agents has not been determined.

The serologic aspects of Burkitt's tumor have created considerable interest. Although these have not been completely clarified, in every clinically confirmed case of African Burkitt's tumor the patient has had high levels of antibodies against a herpes-like virus; only 50 to 60 per cent of other Africans have similar titers. The virus (E–B virus) appears to be widely distributed in man. In young adults it is associated with infectious mononucleosis. The exact relationship of this virus to Burkitt's tumor and other diseases has not been defined.

Study of patients with Burkitt's lymphoma in Uganda has shown that many have delayed hypersensitivity responses to autologous tumor antigens; sustained remission was correlated with a positive reaction.[51]

Histiocytic Medullary Reticulosis

Histiocytic medullary reticulosis, first described by Scott and Robb-Smith in 1939,[141] is a rare disorder; 63 cases from virtually all parts of the world had been reported by 1968, the largest series being a group of 14 patients from Uganda.[143] Most of the reported patients were middle-aged or older, but some were under 20 years of age. The clinical manifestations of the disease are fever, wasting, lymphadenopathy, and hepatosplenomegaly; late in the disease abdominal pain, jaundice, hemolytic anemia, leukopenia, thrombocytopenia, and bleeding occur in a majority of patients. The disease is rapidly fatal; most patients have died within ten weeks of onset, and only an occasional patient has survived for from six to 15 months. Treatment with corticosteroids, 6-MP, alkylating agents, vincristine, and splenectomy has produced no more than short remissions.

The characteristic feature of the disease is a diffuse proliferation of the histiocytes and their precursors throughout the reticuloendothelial system. Erythrophagocytosis occurs frequently but is not specific for this disorder, since it also occurs in other lymphomas and various infections. The criteria suggested for a diagnosis are as follows: (1) sections that disclose proliferation of abnormal cells of the histiocytic series, not classified as Sternberg-Reed giant cells, with a tendency to erythrophagocytosis, must be found in at least two of the following organs: liver, lymph nodes, spleen, or bone marrow; and (2) there should be no evidence of local tumor formation in the liver, spleen, and marrow.[73] Sections of the liver and lymph nodes usually are better than those of the bone marrow for diagnosis.

Although many features described in this disorder seem to indicate a diagnosis of "lymphoma, histiocytic, diffuse," a recent review of 29 patients, aged 13 months to 71 years, concluded that the clinical and histologic findings warrant a separate classification. In this group, one-third achieved some remission with therapy, and median survival was six months, the range being from one month to eight years.[187]

Mycosis Fungoides

Mycosis fungoides is usually considered to be a form of malignant lymphoma of the skin.[18] The most common initial manifestation is some benign or nonspecific dermatitis, such as psoriasiform or neurodermatitis. After an interval that varies from months to decades, but which is usually several years, cutaneous tumors appear in all cases; in some patients the tumors are apparent at onset. Infection, especially staphylococcal septicemia or pneumonia (or some other disease), may lead to death at this stage of disease; in this circumstance, autopsy discloses no evidence of lymph node or visceral involvement by malignant lymphoma.

Clinical dissemination of the disease is generally manifested by fever, weight loss, generalized peripheral and hilar adenopathy, palpable hepatosplenomegaly, and often an increase in the circulating eosinophils. Histologic study of the nodes at this stage in 15 autopsied cases disclosed the pleomorphic mycosis fungoides cells mixed with inflammatory cells.[100] The authors concluded that dissemination is an ominous but distinct feature of the natural history of mycosis fungoides, and not an indication of the development of another form of lymphoma. Dissemination is not always easily recognized. In a group of 13 patients without known visceral involvement who had staging laparotomies, the abdominal lymph nodes were positive in three and the spleen was positive in four; the involvement was found on histologic study rather than by gross observation. The involved nodes and spleen were infiltrated with cells which had a deep nuclear indentation, but otherwise resembled lymphocytes with a nuclear size between that of the mature lymphocyte and histiocyte.

Prognosis depends on a number of factors. Patients with the localized cutaneous form of the disease sometimes remain well for decades and die from other causes. Patients under 51 years of age and those without cutaneous tumors, cutaneous ulcers, or palpable lymph node enlargement survive longer after diagnosis than the general group.[49] Average survival times of from 8 to 12.5 years after the onset of lesions have been reported; however, reported median survival times after tumor development are only 1.7 years and 2.3 years. At autopsy, widespread visceral lymphoma is usually found and infection is the commonest cause of death.[49]

Treatment with one of the chemotherapeutic agents used most often in other lymphomas and with radiotherapy has not been effective in the majority of patients with nonlocalized disease. The value of combined treatment such as the MOPP and COP regimens has not been determined, but they probably deserve a trial. A complete remission followed the use of bleomycin 10 mg./M^2 I.M. twice weekly in one patient who was not responsive to COP; when reported the remission had continued for almost a year on maintenance therapy with bleomycin 10 mg./wk., cyclophosphamide 200 mg./day orally for ten days each month, and prednisone 100 mg./day orally for five days q. two weeks.[152] Further trials of the newer agents are desirable. Although radiation and topical and systemic chemotherapy have not demonstrably lengthened the life of these patients, these treatments are often of considerable temporary symptomatic benefit.

Topical nitrogen mustard is the treatment of choice for treating skin plaques.[67] The regimen used at the University of Virginia utilizes a solution of 10 mg. of HN_2 in 20 ml. of distilled water. A physician or nurse wearing rubber gloves applies sterile 4×4 gauze flats soaked in the solution to the lesions for five minutes; in intertriginous areas the soaks are applied for only one minute. The treatment usually is given three times a week for one week. Advanced disease is treated by radiotherapy, intravenous nitrogen mustard, chlorambucil, or methotrexate. In the advanced stage, severe pruritus and widespread ulcerating infected lesions may present a distressing problem that taxes the ingenuity of the physician and the fortitude of the patient.

DIAGNOSIS

The diagnosis of non-Hodgkins lymphoma can be made only by tissue biopsy. The considerations discussed at the beginning of the chapter and in the section on Hodgkin's disease apply. Study of an imprint of the biopsied node with the benefit of special stains is always helpful and sometimes necessary in deciding the proper classification of the tumor cell. The possibility of one of the lymphoma group is suggested by enlargement of superficial lymph nodes, splenomegaly, prolonged fever, mediastinal tumors, hemolytic anemia, exfoliative dermatitis, and spinal cord compression. Infectious mononucleosis, tuberculosis, brucellosis, sarcoidosis, disseminated lupus erythematosus, and carcinomatosis often present problems in differential diagnosis. The difficulty can be resolved only by demonstrating the presence of one of the lymphoma group histologically or by satisfying the diagnostic criteria for the other disease under consideration. Whether the patient has lymphoma may remain uncertain even after biopsy if he has been taking anticonvulsant drugs.[70,150]

In most patients the distinction between lymphocytic lymphoma and lymphocytic leukemia is made without difficulty because of the increase in total leukocyte count and percentage of lymphocytes that are found in most cases of leukemia. However, in the occasional patient this differential diagnosis is not easy because there seems to be a close relationship or overlapping between the two diseases. The term "leukosarcoma" has been used to designate these transitional cases. In some such patients the classic features of leukemia develop later, but in others the abnormalities in the peripheral blood prove to be transient, and at necropsy months or years later there is no evidence of the widespread invasion of the various organs that usually occurs in leukemia. A leukocyte count of 30,000 per cu.mm. has been taken as the criterion of leukemia in some series when lymphocytes constitute more than one-half of the cells.[125]

At the present time diffuse bone marrow involvement with the lymphoid cell is considered diagnostic of leukemia, and patchy involvement as evidence of bone marrow involvement by lymphocytic lymphoma and not leukemia; a biopsy is necessary to make this distinction.

STAGING

The staging procedures to be employed in a patient with non-Hodgkin's lymphoma depend to a great extent on the physician's concept of the natural history of the disease, the prognosis, and the preferred method of treatment. At present, none of these is as well-defined as for the patient with Hodgkin's disease. The number of different diseases or types of disease that are recognized, the relative paucity of patients with any type, and the time, expense, morbidity, and risk involved in some diagnostic procedures, all contribute to the situation.

One important staging laparotomy study was made at Stanford University on 69 unselected patients with non-Hodgkin's lymphoma.[59] The procedure was similar to the staging procedure described for Hodgkin's disease. An interesting finding was that seven of the 69 patients had multiple histologic patterns in the same node, or in nodes from different areas. The staging procedure also gave a somewhat surprisingly even spread among the stages—stage I 20 per cent, stage II 24 per cent, stage III 23 per cent, and stage IV 30 per cent. Before laparotomy 37 patients were stage III and four stage IV; after laparotomy there were 16 stage III and 22 stage IV. Barium study of the gastrointestinal tract was of no value in patients without symptoms or other evidence of involvement. The report provided much interesting information, and the authors felt that laparotomy was valuable where clinical research is being carried out, although thus far it had not answered questions concerning its value in providing better management and improved survival.

The value of the bone marrow biopsy in staging patients with non-Hodgkin's lymphoma is firmly established, but reports differ regarding the frequency of positive results. In one report of 75 patients with lymph node proved lymphosarcoma (lymphoma, lymphocytic, nodular and diffuse, well differentiated and undifferentiated), marrow examination was positive in 47 (63 per cent); in over one-half of these the biopsy was positive when the aspirate was negative. In the study, 21 patients were considered to be stage I and II before the marrow examination; 13 of these were classed as stage IV after the examination. Thus, only approximately 10 per cent of the entire group of 75 patients remained stage I after bone marrow biopsy. In another report, however, the bone marrow biopsy was positive in none of nine patients called clinical stage I, in one of 19 in clinical stage II, and in 16 of 37 clinical stage III.[59] In another report[81] of the results of bone marrow examination in 218 untreated patients with non-Hodgkin's lymphoma, open marrow biopsy was positive more often than was needle biopsy, and both were superior to aspiration. The incidence of positive biopsy in the patients with different types of nodular disease and also in those with diffuse disease varied from 5 per cent of the histiocytic types to 30 per cent of the lymphocytic poorly differentiated types. In one report, bilateral trephine biopsies gave positive results in from 11 to 22 per cent more cases of lymphoma, Hodgkin's and non-Hodgkin's, than did a single posterior iliac spine biopsy.[23]

Primary extra nodal involvement with disease, rare in Hodgkin's disease, is not uncommon in non-Hodgkin's lymphoma. In one review of 12,447 cases of lymphoma, 2194 were considered to have originated in sites other than lymph nodes; only 90 of this group had Hodgkin's disease.[107] Extranodal involvement in the absence of disseminated disease was found in 24 per cent of patients with "reticulum cell sarcoma" (lymphoma, diffuse, histiocytic), in 15 per cent of those with "lymphosarcoma" (lymphoma, diffuse, lymphocytic), and in only 5 per cent of those with "giant follicular lymphoma" (nodular lymphoma). The stomach was involved in 346 patients, tonsils in 143, small bowel in 110, skin in 110, colon in 59, bone in 69, and salivary glands in 69.

Unless there is some contraindication, patients in our clinic have the following studies after diagnosis by tissue biopsy and study of imprints:
1. Hematocrit, leukocyte count, platelet count, differential count;
2. Roentgenogram of the chest;
3. Bone marrow biopsy;
4. If bone marrow is normal, percutaneous liver biopsy;
5. If marrow and hepatic biopsy are normal, lymphangiograms;
6. If cervical nodes are involved, otolaryngology consultation.

Staging laparotomy, various scanning techniques, barium study of the gastrointestinal tract, and radiologic bone survey are employed in selected patients as noted above.

TREATMENT AND PROGNOSIS

Treatment of the majority of patients with non-Hodgkin's lymphoma has been by radiotherapy, a single chemical agent, or combination chemotherapy. Knowledge of the histologic details of the tumor, such as cell type and nodularity, are essential for evaluation of results. In most patients the achievement of complete remission correlates best with the length of the disease-free interval and survival.

The results obtained with radiotherapy in 355 patients with non-Hodgkin's lymphomas classified according to the older system was reported by Molander in 1973.[107] In patients classified as stage I (31), the five-year survival was 84 per cent; in stage II (120), 74 per cent; in stage III (159), 43 per cent; stage IV (24), 46 per cent; extranodal (21), 71 per cent. The five-year survival statistics according to the histologic classification in use were: "giant follicular lymphoma," 83 per cent; "lymphosarcoma," 65 per cent; "reticulum cell sarcoma,"

56 per cent. The patients with localized disease, stage I and II, were treated with 4000 to 4500 rads to the involved and adjacent areas; those with stage III and IV received total nodal irradiation, 3000 to 3500 rads. In one group of 21 patients with extranodal lymphoma treated with surgery and radiotherapy, the survival was approximately that of stage II patients, a five-year survival of 71 per cent.

Johnson has reported his results at NCI obtained with primary radiotherapy in 27 previously untreated patients with stage III or stage IV (bone marrow) disease.[74] Twenty patients were classed as having the "lymphocytic poorly differentiated type" and 7 as "lymphocytic well differentiated;" 18 were nodular and nine diffuse. The patients were divided into three groups and treated with total body irradiation, total nodal irradiation, or a combination of the two. Complete remission occurred in 25 of the 27 (93 per cent), and lasted for a median duration of 26 months (three to 60 months); the three-year survival rate was 87 per cent (13 of 15); the five-year, 66 per cent (six of nine).

Jones et al. have reported their experience with single agent chemotherapy in 241 previously untreated patients with non-Hodgkin's lymphoma.[82] When the tumors were classed as "lymphosarcoma" or "reticulum cell sarcoma," the remission rate was from 10 to 20 per cent; in the "nodular" it was 28 to 48 per cent, and in the diffuse 5 to 22 per cent. Other results were histiocytic: nodular 28 per cent, diffuse 5 per cent; "mixed:" nodular 31 per cent, diffuse 13 per cent; poorly differentiated lymphocytic: nodular 48 per cent, diffuse 22 per cent.

The value of combination chemotherapy with different variations of the COP regimen in non-Hodgkin's lymphomas was reported by Hoogstraten et al.[69] and by Bagley et al.[13] In the former study, the combined chemotherapy proved to be superior to cyclophosphamide alone. In patients with "lymphosarcoma" the complete remission rate was approximately 33 per cent, and combined complete and partial, 90 to 100 per cent. In patients with "reticulum cell sarcoma" the incidence of complete remission was also approximately 33 per cent, the combined complete and partial, 54 to 85 per cent. The second report concerned 35 patients with advanced "lymphosarcoma," 32 without previous therapy. Twenty (70 per cent) complete and 12 (34 per cent) partial remissions were obtained. Eighty-nine per cent of the complete remissions lasted more than one year and 79 per cent of the entire group survived more than one year. The protocol employed in the study, probably the one in widest use today, is shown on page 488.

The value of the combination chemotherapy in patients with advanced disease and the important influence of the histologic diagnosis on the outcome has been confirmed.[136,147] The incidence of complete remission has been from 39 to 45 per cent. In one group of 30 patients with advanced lymphocytic lymphoma, 13 were classed as "nodular" and 17 as "diffuse;" ten (77 per cent) of the nodular group obtained complete remission compared to only two (12 per cent) of the diffuse. Median survival in the former group was 31 months, and eight were still alive for from 13 to 38 months; median survival in the diffuse group was only seven months. In another group of 80 patients treated with COP or MOPP, the complete remission rate varied from 22 to 71 per cent; 61 per cent of those who had a remission, and 28 per cent of the entire group were alive and free from disease for periods that varied from four months to over seven years, with a projected mean of remission of 3 ½ years.[136] Results varied in the different histologic categories; the subgroups with diffuse involvement had aggressive disease and did not fare as well as those with nodular patterns or well differentiated cells.

Currently, in our clinic, patients with localized non-Hodgkin's lymphomas are being treated in different ways. According to one plan, patients thought to be stage IA and IIA, and some with stage IIIA, are treated with radiotherapy, total nodal, or to the involved side of the diaphragm only. Another group receives radiotherapy to the involved area and adjacent regions, followed by the COP combination introduced by Bagley et al. for six courses.[13] If the disease is widespread, stage IV, or if systemic symptoms are prominent, chemotherapy (usually COP or MOPP) is given, and radiotherapy is used for problem areas of disease if necessary.

Single agent therapy or another combination of drugs is used less frequently, usually when other methods of treatment have failed. Prednisone alone in large doses, 60 to 100 mg. per day, often produces prompt and striking diminution in the size of tumor masses in patients with lymphocytic lymphoma. Suppression of the disease may continue for many months on maintenance therapy with a small daily dose of 5 to 20 mg., or a dose of 60 to 100 mg. on alternate days.

Some success has also been reported in lymphomas with adriamycin alone (30 to 56 per cent response rate) or combined with other agents.[29] In a study by the Southwest Oncology Group, complete response rates were obtained in from 62 to 67 per cent of 86 patients with non-Hodgkin's lymphomas with multiple therapy regimens used in cycles of two or three weeks. One, "CHOP" was:

Adriamycin (50 mg./M² I.V. day 1)
Cytoxan (750 mg./M² I.V. day 1)
Vincristine (1.4 mg./M² I.V. day 1)
Prednisone (100 mg./M² p.o. days 1 through 5)

The other, "HOP" was:

Adriamycin (80 mg./M² I.V. day 1)
Vincristine (1.4 mg./M² I.V. day 1)
Prednisone (100 mg./M² p.o. days 1 through 5)

SPECIAL PROBLEMS IN THERAPY OF HODGKIN'S DISEASE AND NON-HODGKIN'S LYMPHOMA

Certain clinical situations require special consideration in treatment. Patients with masses in the superior mediastinum, compression of the spinal cord, or involvement of the central nervous system are treated cautiously and kept under close supervision, because serious consequences may follow any increase in the mass. When a lesion of this type is irradiated, only a small dose is employed. A steroid drug is often given in this situation in an effort to reduce the size of the tumor mass quickly or to minimize the possibility of swelling secondary to radiation. The use of nitrogen mustard has been recommended in these situations because of the belief that the effects of these chemicals are different from those of x-rays and induce regression of the lesion without producing active congestion or edema.[172] However, we have seen one patient with Hodgkin's disease with signs of spinal cord compression who developed temporary paraplegia twice after courses of nitrogen mustard. A mediastinal mass often responds well to treatment and a long remission ensues. Close collaboration with a neurologist is often helpful in localizing the lesion to be treated and in the general management of the patient with neurologic involvement. Not infrequently, considerable damage to the spinal cord has occurred before the lesion is recognized, and varying degrees of paralysis outlast the regression of the tumor masses. Laminectomy is usually advisable in compression of the spinal cord.

Pleural effusion in lymphoma is usually, but not invariably, a sign of poor prognosis.[6,169] Obstruction to the lymph drainage of the lung and pleura by enlarged mediastinal nodes is the most common cause of pleural effusion in Hodgkin's disease and other lymphomas. Actual pleural involvement by the tumor occurs, but is rare, a situation different from that seen in metastatic carcinoma. Involvement of the lung on the affected side or chylous fluid does not alter the prognosis in these patients, but the presence of malignant cells indicates a worse prognosis. In the uncomplicated pleural effusion, irradiation of the mediastinum is probably the treatment of choice. If there is evidence of lung or pleural involvement, irradiation of the hemothorax is indicated. It has been recommended that, if active disease is present outside the thorax, chemotherapy should also be administered. For recurrent effusions, thoracentesis and a trial on closed tube drainage is recommended; if this fails, the instillation of nitrogen mustard or a radioactive isotope such as gold is advisable. These measures were successful in 37 per cent of patients for three months and in 29 per cent for six months.[6] After preliminary sedation, nitrogen mustard, 0.4 mg. per kg., is instilled in a single injection into the pleural cavity after about one-half of the fluid has been removed and a free flow of fluid is still present; after instillation, the position of the patient is changed every five to ten minutes over a period of one hour to insure more uniform distribution through the cavity.[171] Nitrogen mustard instillation has also been employed to treat recurrent ascites; chylous ascites often responds to corticosteroids.

Both the radiotherapy and the chemotherapy used in treating patients with lymphoma increase their vulnerability to a variety of infections. The commonest fungal infections seen in lymphoma are candidiasis, aspergillosis, cryptococcosis, mucormycosis, and histoplasmosis; amphotericin B is the treatment of choice for all.

Patients with Hodgkin's disease are prone to infection with *Cryptococcus neoformans* (Torula histolytica). Disseminated disease including meningitis formerly was considered uniformly fatal. When this infection is treated with amphotericin B, remission or even a cure of this complication is sometimes obtained. Pneumocystis carinii pneumonia, which has been diagnosed ante-mortem by needle biopsy of the lungs and successfully treated with pentamidine isethionate, occurs in some patients with long-standing Hodgkin's disease.[16] In one report, both tuberculosis and pyogenic infection were commoner than disseminated fungus disease in 137 patients with Hodgkin's disease.[97] Fever from Hodgkin's disease per se occurs twice as often as fever from infection; the latter was rarely seen except in advanced stages of the disease. The most frequent severe acute infections are caused by gram-negative bacteria (*Pseudomonas klebsiella, E. coli*); *S. aureus*, viral hepatitis, and varicella-zoster comprise most of the remainder. Candidiasis and aspergillosis are found with increasing frequency at autopsy.

Pregnancy may present a problem in patients with a lymphoma. There is no evidence that pregnancy causes any aggravation or acceleration of the condition. Because of danger to the fetus, either form of treatment, chemotherapy or radiation, is given before or after pregnancy, rather than during pregnancy, if possible. No area below the diaphragm is irradiated during the first three months of pregnancy, the most dangerous time for the fetus, if it can be avoided. Should it be necessary later, the fetus is protected as well as possible. In some circumstances, local irradiation and prednisone or an alkylating agent have been used successfully during the latter part of the pregnancy. Vinblastine sulfate has been administered orally, 5 mg. per day five days a week, throughout a pregnancy which ended with the birth of a normal thriving infant.[8] Women who develop lymphoma are advised against pregnancy for two years after diagnosis, the period when most relapses which require further therapy occur.

In some patients with lymphoma, fortunately a small percentage, persistent severe pain is a major problem. It is usually caused by pressure on or invasion of nerves, involvement of bone, obstruction of blood vessels or organs, or general pressure from the tumor mass. Treatment of the underlying disease by radiation or chemotherapy often brings relief. When it does not, analgesics in increasing strength are necessary and at times sedation is a helpful adjunct. Nerve block is effective in selected patients; chordotomy and lobotomy are almost "last resort" measures rarely employed.

In some patients, malignant lymphoma presents as splenomegaly without other apparent evidence of disease elsewhere; in others the splenomegaly is accompanied by fever, night sweats, and pancytopenia. Splenectomy produces prompt clinical remission in some patients,[154] but in many (eight in one group of 15) the disease became disseminated and fatal within two years;[99] two who lived more than three years developed lymphosarcoma cell leukemia. After evaluating the results of early splenectomy in 50 patients with lymphoproliferative disorders, early splenectomy for hypersplenism was recommended for those with chronic leukemia, well differentiated lymphocytic lymphoma, leukemic reticuloendotheliosis, and Hodgkin's disease; it was recommended "with caution" in histiocytic lymphoma and poorly differentiated lymphocytic lymphoma.[174] The results of splenectomy in patients with autoimmune hemolytic anemia are unpredictable, but are excellent in some after prednisone has failed.

Illustrative Cases

HODGKIN'S DISEASE

CASE 1

This 22-year-old white male was admitted to the University of Virginia Hospital in April, 1971 with a history of headache, malaise, night sweats, and fever for six weeks. He was referred because of pancytopenia and fever.

Physical examination. Pallor, marked enlargement of the spleen which extended to the iliac crest, moderate hepatomegaly, but no significant enlargement of the superficial lymph nodes. The temperature was 39° (C) and continued between 39° and 40° for the following week.

Laboratory examinations. Hematocrit, 30 per cent; leukocyte count, 1400 per cu.mm.; differential count (per cent), bands 44, segs 36, lymphocytes 16, monocytes 4; platelets were 155,000 per cu.mm., reticulocytes 2.1 per cent. Bone marrow obtained by aspiration was hypercellular with striking erythroid hyperplasia but no other significant abnormalities. Roentgenogram of the chest was normal.

Course. A lymphoma was suspected and percutaneous liver biopsy was obtained; this was reported as showing a granulomatous infiltrate "suggestive" of Hodgkin's disease but not diagnostic. A few days later a laparotomy was performed. The spleen was removed and the lymph nodes and liver were biopsied. The liver, spleen, and all the lymph nodes were positive for Hodgkin's disease, mixed cellularity type.

After the diagnosis was established as Hodgkin's disease, stage IVB, mixed cellularity type, the patient was treated according to the MOPP protocol. Treatment was started while the patient was in the hospital and he promptly became afebrile. He completed six months of MOPP therapy in October, 1971 with no untoward effect except mild peripheral neuropathy manifested mainly by absent ankle and knee jerks. Maintenance therapy was terminated in April, 1974. When last seen in October, 1975 he was in complete remission with normal x-rays of the chest, normal blood counts, and a sedimentation rate of 2 mm. He has been in complete remission since completing the six-month course of MOPP. He completed college work for a Bachelor's degree and was working full-time.

Comment. This case illustrates the good results obtained with MOPP therapy in 60 to 80 per cent of previously untreated patients in advanced Hodgkin's disease. Reports published since this patient was treated differ about the advisability of maintenance therapy such as this patient was given, since apparently it does not increase survival.

HODGKIN'S DISEASE

CASE 2

This 26-year-old white housewife was admitted to the University of Virginia Hospital in August, 1971 a few weeks after she noticed enlargement of a cervical lymph node. Biopsy of the node disclosed Hodgkin's disease, nodular sclerosis type. No other lymph node involvement was apparent. X-rays of the chest and lymphangiograms were reported as negative. At that time it was felt that there was involvement in the left cervical area, sometimes associated with "skipped" areas in the mediastinum, and staging laparotomy was performed. Histologic examination of the spleen, liver biopsies, and lymph nodes was entirely normal. Hodgkin's disease nodular sclerosis type, stage IA, was then diagnosed. The patient was treated with radiation to the mantle area and para-aortic area below the diaphragm. She appeared to be in complete remission at the completion of therapy of 4000 rads to the mantle area and 3500 to the para-aortic area.

Course. The patient was asymptomatic for the next two years, but in the autumn of 1973 developed an unproductive cough. X-ray at that time showed several circular densities in both lungs. Hodgkin's disease was strongly suspected and she was admitted to the hospital for open biopsy of one lung, which again disclosed Hodgkin's disease of nodular sclerosis type.

With the change from stage IA to IVA, the patient was started on MOPP therapy. At the end of six months, pulmonary lesions had cleared completely and the patient was asymptomatic. She was able to take only five cycles during this time; therapy was terminated because of pancytopenia, persistent nausea, vomiting, and peripheral neuritis. These symptoms all cleared within a few months, and when the patient was last seen in March, 1975, nine months after completing the MOPP and 3½ years after the original diagnosis, she appeared to be in complete remission.

Comment. This patient was thought to have stage IA disease and received radiotherapy to the mediastinum. In less than two years, lesions were present in the lungs. This has been reported to occur in 20 per cent of patients treated in this manner. The most likely explanation would appear to be the presence of small unrecognized foci of Hodgkin's disease in the lungs which were not included in the field of radiation when the mediastinum was treated. The foci increased in size and spread to the mediastinal nodes, which became enlarged. The patient had a good response to MOPP therapy although she was unable to complete the planned therapy. Previous radiotherapy such as this patient experienced has little influence on the response to the MOPP treatment; the incidence of complete remission is appreciably smaller in patients treated with MOPP after receiving previous chemotherapy.

LYMPHOMA, LYMPHOCYTIC

CASE 3

This 65-year-old white saleslady was well until December, 1955, when she noticed small purpuric lesions on the palms of the hands. During the next month the cutaneous lesions increased and became generalized. These lesions persisted, and during the following six weeks the patient noticed cramping pains and edema in the legs, mild anorexia, and weight loss of 10 pounds. She was admitted to the hospital in March, 1956.

Physical examination. Signs of hydrothorax were present bilaterally. The spleen was palpable three fingerbreadths below the left costal margin, and multiple orange-sized masses were palpable throughout the abdomen.

Pitting edema was present in both legs. The trunk, back, and upper arms were covered with maculopapular hemorrhagic rash. The remainder of the examination was essentially normal.

Laboratory examination. Hematocrit, white count, differential count, urinalysis, blood urea, stool examination, and prothrombin times were normal. Roentgenogram of the chest revealed small bilateral pleural effusions. Bone marrow examination disclosed the normoblastic type of erythropoiesis associated with a moderate increase in lymphocytes, a pattern that was thought to be consistent with lymphosarcoma or lymphocytic leukemia. Biopsy of an axillary lymph node was diagnosed as "lymphosarcoma."

Course. She was treated with a total of 12.5 mg. of TEM in three doses and was discharged from the hospital. She was readmitted three weeks after the last dose of TEM and four weeks after the first dose with a four-day history of fever, unproductive cough, pain in the left chest, and dyspnea. The intra-abdominal masses had become much smaller and the skin lesions had cleared almost completely. On admission the hematocrit was 35 per cent, white count 250 per cu.mm., and the platelet count 136,000 per cu.mm. Thoracentesis was performed on several occasions, and penicillin was administered because of the granulocytopenia and pneumonia. She improved promptly, and ten days after admission the white count had risen to 2200 per cu.mm. One month later, two months after the last dose of TEM, the hematocrit was 40 per cent, the white count was 4000 per cu.mm., and the differential count was normal.

The patient was largely asymptomatic and received no treatment for a year, when enlargement of the supraclavicular lymph nodes and intra-abdominal nodes recurred. The patient was given 5 mg. of TEM and developed nausea, vomiting, and diarrhea despite the fact that she had taken chlorpromazine before the TEM. The abdominal nodes decreased in size remarkably. The patient felt well for five months, at which time the superficial and intra-abdominal lymph nodes again increased in size. At this time a prolonged course of TEM consisting of a total of 57.5 mg. was administered over a six-month period. At the end of this time the axillary and supraclavicular nodes measured about 2 cm. in diameter, and the intra-abdominal masses remained, but the patient was largely asymptomatic and continued to work.

During the next two years the patient was treated on three occasions with TEM or chlorambucil for recurrent adenopathy. Four months after chlorambucil was started she appeared to be in complete remission. Remission continued for eight years without further treatment. Relapses occurred in September, 1965 and in June, 1969, but again complete remission followed treatment with chlorambucil.

In the spring of 1972 this patient, by then 81 years old, again relapsed and deteriorated rapidly. Huge masses appeared in the abdomen and neck and were completely unresponsive to treatment with radiation or various types of chemotherapy. She died in June, 1972.

Autopsy revealed that all the lymph nodes, the liver, and nearly all the organs were invaded by lymphosarcoma; in some nodes it was poorly differentiated. Both ureters were obstructed. Extensive pneumonia and bilateral pleural effusions were present.

A review of the original biopsy led to the diagnosis of lymphoma, lymphocytic, nodular, well differentiated type.

Comment. The course of the lymphoma in this patient is instructive.

From onset she had generalized disease. Fortunately, the disease was of the nodular type and the cells appeared to be well differentiated when studied in section. She responded well to different chemotherapeutic agents for over 17 years, and appeared to be in complete remissions without maintenance therapy for long periods, eight years at one point. Nevertheless, the disease eventually became very aggressive and completely refractory to further treatment.

References

1. Aisenberg, A. C.: Lymphocytopenia in Hodgkin's disease. Blood, *25*:1037, 1965.
2. Aisenberg, A. C.: Malignant lymphoma. N. Engl. J. Med., *288*:883 and 935, 1973.
3. Aisenberg, A. C., and Long, J. C.: Lymphocyte surface characteristics in malignant lymphoma. Am. J. Med., *58*:300, 1975.
4. Aisenberg, A. C., and Qazi, R.: Abdominal involvement at the onset of Hodgkin's disease. Am. J. Med., *57*:870, 1974.
5. Alexanian, R.: Monoclonal gammopathy in lymphoma. Arch. Intern. Med., *135*:62, 1975.
6. Anderson, C. B., Philpott, G. W., and Ferguson, T. B.: The treatment of malignant pleural effusions. Cancer, *33*:916, 1974.
7. Anderson, E., and Videbaek, A.: Diagnostic laparotomy in Hodgkin's disease. Scand. J. Haematol., *12*:5, 1974.
8. Armstrong, J. G., Dyke, R. W., Fouts, P. J., and Jansen, C. J.: Delivery of a normal infant during the course of oral vinblastine sulfate therapy for Hodgkin's disease. Ann. Intern. Med., *61*:106, 1964.
9. Arseneau, J. C., Sponzo, R. W., Levin, D. C., et al.: Nonlymphomatous malignant tumors complicating Hodgkin's disease. Possible association with intensive therapy. N. Engl. J. Med., *287*:1119, 1972.
10. Arseneau, J. C., Canellos, G. P., Banks, P. M., Berard, C. W., Gralnick, H. R., and DeVita, V. T., Jr.: American Burkitt's lymphoma, a clinicopathologic study of 30 cases. Am. J. Med. *58*:315, 1975.
11. Azar, H. A., Hill, W. T., and Osserman, E. F.: Malignant lymphoma and lymphatic leukemia associated with myeloma-type serum proteins. Am. J. Med., *23*:239, 1957.
12. Baehr, G.: The clinical and pathological picture of follicular lymphoblastoma. Tr. Assoc. Am. Physicians, *47*:330, 1932.
13. Bagley, C. M., Jr., DeVita, V. T., Jr., Bernard, C. W., and Canellos, G. P.: Advanced lymphosarcoma: intensive cyclical combination chemotherapy with cyclophosphamide, vincristine, and prednisone. Ann. Intern. Med., *76*:227, 1972.
14. Bagley, C. M., Jr., Roth, J. A., Thomas, L. B., and DeVita, V. T., Jr.: Liver biopsy in Hodgkin's disease. Ann. Intern. Med., *76*:219, 1972.
15. Bagley, C. M., Jr., Thomas, L. B., Johnson, R. C., Chretien, P. B., and DeVita, V. T., Jr.: Diagnosis of liver involvement by lymphoma. Result in 96 consecutive peritoneoscopies. Cancer, *31*:540, 1973.
16. Baker, W. H., and Castleman, B.: Cough and pulmonary infiltrates in a man with Hodgkin's disease of over four years' duration. N. Engl. J. Med., *277*:39, 1967.
17. Berkson, B. M., Lome, L. G., and Shapiro, I.: Severe cystitis induced by cyclophosphamide. J.A.M.A., *225*:605, 1973.
18. Block, J. B., Edgcomb, J., Eisen, A., and VanScott, E. J.: Mycosis fungoides. Am. J. Med., *34*:228, 1963.
19. Blum, R. H., and Carter, S. K.: Adriamycin. A new anticancer drug with significant clinical activity. Ann. Intern. Med., *80*:249, 1974.
20. Bodel, P.: Pyrogen release in vitro by lymphoid tissues from patients with Hodgkin's disease. Yale J. Biol. Med., *47*:101, 1974.
21. Bostick, W. L.: Evidence for the virus etiology of Hodgkin's disease. Ann. N.Y. Acad. Sci., *73*:307, 1958.
22. Brill, N. E., Baehr, G., and Rosenthal, N.: Generalized giant lymph follicle hyperplasia of lymph nodes and spleen. J.A.M.A., *84*:668, 1925.
23. Brunning, R. D., Bloomfield, C. D., McKenna, R. W., and Peterson, L.: Bilateral trephine bone marrow biopsies in lymphoma and other neoplastic diseases. Ann. Intern. Med., *82*:365, 1975.
24. Bunting, C. H.: Blood platelets and megalokaryocytes in Hodgkin's disease. Johns Hopkins Med. J., *22*:114, 1911.

25. Burkitt, D.: Sarcoma involving jaws in African children. Br. J. Surg., *46*:218, 1958–59.
26. Carbone, P. P.: Management of patients with non-Hodgkin's lymphoma. Arch. Intern. Med., *131*:455, 1973.
27. Carbone, P. P., Bernard, C. W., Bennett, J. M., Ziegler, J. L., Cohen, M. H., and Gerber, P.: NIH Clinical Staff Conference. Burkitt's tumor. Ann. Intern. Med., *70*:817, 1969.
28. Carey, R. M., Kimball, A. C., Armstrong, D., and Lieberman, P. H.: Toxoplasmosis. Am. J. Med., *54*:30, 1973.
29. Carter, S. K., and Blum, R. H.: New chemotherapeutic agents: bleomycin and adriamycin. Cancer J. Clin., *24*:322, 1974.
30. Case Records, Mass. Gen. Hosp.: Massive proteinuria in a patient with Hodgkin's disease. N. Engl. J. Med., *284*:95, 1971.
31. Castleman, B., Scully, R. E., and McNeely, B. U.: CPC. N. Engl. J. Med., *290*:1012, 1974.
32. Chan, B. W. B., and McBride, J. D.: Hodgkin's disease and leukemia. Can. Med. Assoc. J., *106*:558, 1972.
33. Chawla, P. L., Stutzman, L., DuBois, R. E., Kim, U., and Sokal, J. E.: Long survival in Hodgkin's disease. Am. J. Med., *48*:85, 1970.
34. Constable, W., and Leavell, B. S.: The management of Hodgkin's disease. Va. Med. Mon., *97*:381, 1970.
35. CPC. Hodgkin's disease complicated by thrombocytopenia and nephrotic syndrome. Am. J. Med., *51*:109, 1971.
36. Custer, R. P., and Bernhard, W. G.: The interrelationship of Hodgkin's disease and other lymphatic tumors. Am. J. Med. Sci., *216*:625, 1948.
37. Dale, D. C., Fauci, A. S., and Wolff, S. M.: Alternate day prednisone. Leukocyte kinetics and susceptibility to infections. N. Engl. J. Med., *291*:1154, 1974.
38. Davidson, J. W., and Clarke, E. A.: Influence of modern radiological techniques on clinical staging of malignant lymphomas. Can. Med. Assoc. J., *99*:1196, 1968.
39. DeConti, R. C.: Procarbazine in the management of late Hodgkin's disease. J.A.M.A., *215*:927, 1971.
40. Desser, R. K., and Ultmann, J. E.: Risk of severe infection in patients with Hodgkin's disease or lymphoma after diagnostic laparotomy and splenectomy. Ann. Intern. Med., *77*:143, 1972.
41. DeVita, V. T., Jr., Canellos, G. P., and Moxley, J. H., III: A decade of combination chemotherapy of advanced Hodgkin's disease. Cancer, *30*:1495, 1972.
42. DeVita, V. T., Jr., Serpick, A. A., and Carbone, P. P.: Combination chemotherapy in the treatment of advanced Hodgkin's disease. Ann. Intern. Med., *73*:881, 1970.
43. Donaldson, S. S., Moore, M. R., Rosenberg, S. A., and Vosti, K. L.: Characterization of postsplenectomy bacteremia among patients with and without lymphoma. N. Engl. J. Med., *287*:69, 1972.
44. Easson, E. C.: Long-term results of radical radiotherapy in Hodgkin's disease. Cancer Res., *26*:1244, 1966.
45. Easson, E. C., and Russell, M. H.: The cure of Hodgkin's Disease. Br. Med. J., *1*:1704, 1963.
46. Edwards, R. T.: Hodgkin's sarcoma of the small bowel. Va. Med. Mon., *96*:521, 1969.
47. Editorial. J.A.M.A., *206*:2309, 1968.
48. Ehrlich, A. N., Stalder, G., Geller, W., and Sherlock, P.: Gastrointestinal manifestations of malignant lymphoma. Gastroenterology, *54*:1115, 1968.
49. Epstein, E. H., Jr., Levin, D. L., Croft, J. D., Jr., and Lutzner, M. A.: Mycosis fungoides. Medicine, *51*:61, 1972.
50. Evans, T. S., and Doan, C. A.: Giant follicle hyperplasia: a study of its incidence, histopathologic variability, and the frequency of sarcoma and secondary hypersplenic complications. Ann. Intern. Med., *40*:851, 1954.
51. Fass, L., Herberman, R. B., and Ziegler, J.: Delayed cutaneous hypersensitivity reactions to autologous extracts of Burkitt-lymphoma cells. N. Engl. J. Med., *282*:776, 1970.
52. Firat, D., Stutzman, L., Studenski, E. R., and Pickren, J.: Giant follicular lymph node disease: clinical and pathological review of sixty-four cases. Am. J. Med., *39*:252, 1965.
53. Flandrin, G., Brouet, J. C., Daniel, M. T., and Preud'homme, J. L.: Acute leukemia with Burkitt's tumor cells: a study of six cases with special reference to lymphocyte surface markers. Blood, *45*:183, 1975.
54. Frei, E., III, Luce, J. K., Gamble, J. F., Coltman, C. A., Jr., Constanzi, J. J., Talley, R. W., Monto, R. W., Wilson, H. E., Hewlett, J. S., Delaney, F. C., and Gehan, E. A.: Combination chemotherapy in advanced Hodgkin's disease. Ann. Intern. Med., *79*:376, 1973.
55. Freman, C., Berg, J. W., and Cutler, S. J.: Occurrence and prognosis of extranodal lymphoma. Cancer, *29*:252, 1972.
56. Fuller, L. M., Sullivan, M., and Butler, J. J.: Results of regional radiotherapy in localized Hodgkin's disease in children. Cancer, *32*:640, 1973.

57. Gall, E. A., and Mallory, T. B.: Malignant lymphoma: a clinico-pathologic survey of 618 cases. Am. J. Pathol., *18*:381, 1942.

58. Gall, E. A., Morrison, H. R., and Scott, A. T.: The follicular type of malignant lymphoma. A survey of 63 cases. Ann. Intern. Med., *14*:2073, 1941.

59. Goffinet, D. R., Castellino, R. A., Kim, H., Dorfman, R. F., Fuks, Z., Rosenberg, S., Nelson, T., and Kaplan, H.: Staging laparotomies in unselected previously untreated patients with non-Hodgkin's lymphoma. Cancer, *32*:672, 1973.

60. Goffinet, D. R., Glatstein, E. J., and Merigan, T. C.: Herpes zoster-varicella infections and lymphoma. Arch. Intern. Med., *76*:235, 1972.

61. Gold, W. M., Youker, J., Anderson, S., and Nadel, J. A.: Pulmonary-function abnormalities after lymphangiography. N. Engl. J. Med., *273*:519, 1965.

62. Goldman, L. B.: Hodgkin's disease: an analysis of 212 cases. J.A.M.A., *114*:1611, 1940.

63. Goldsmith, M. A., and Carter, S. K.: Combination chemotherapy of advanced Hodgkin's disease: a review. Cancer, *33*:1, 1974.

64. Greco, R. S., Acheson, R. M., and Foote, F. M.: Hodgkin's disease in Connecticut from 1935 to 1963. Arch. Intern. Med., *134*:1039, 1974.

65. Greenberg, L. H., Wong, Y. S., Richardson, A. P., Jr., and Dollinger, M. R.: Combination chemotherapy of Hodgkin's disease in private practice. J.A.M.A., *221*:261, 1972.

66. Hanson, H. E., Skov, P. E., Askjaer, S. A., and Albertson, K.: Hodgkin's disease associated with nephrotic syndrome without kidney lesions. Acta Med. Scand., *191*:307, 1972.

67. Hayness, H. A., and VanScott, E. J.: Therapy of mycosis fungoides. Progr. Dermatol., *3*:1, 1968.

68. Hodgkin, T.: On some morbid appearances of the absorbent glands and spleen. Medico-Chirurg. Tr. London, *17*:68, 1832. Quoted from Major, R. H.: Classic Descriptions of Disease. Charles C Thomas, Springfield, Ill., 1955.

69. Hoogstraten, B., Owens, A. H., Lenhard, R. E., Gildewell, O. J., Leone, L. A., Olson, K. B., Harley, J. B., Townsend, S. R., Miller, S. P., and Spurr, C. L.: Combination chemotherapy in lymphosarcoma and reticulum cell sarcoma. Blood, *33*:370, 1969.

70. Hyman, G. A., and Sommers, S. C.: The development of Hodgkin's disease and lymphoma during anticonvulsant therapy. Blood, *28*:416, 1966.

71. Jackson, H., Jr., and Parker, F., Jr.: Hodgkin's disease. N. Engl. J. Med. I. General considerations, *230*:1, 1944; II. Pathology, *231*:35, 1944; III. Symptoms and course, *231*:639, 1944; IV. Involvement of certain organs, *232*:547, 1945; *233*:369, 1945.

72. Jackson, H., Jr., and Parker, F., Jr.: Hodgkin's Disease and Allied Disorders. Oxford University Press, New York, 1947.

73. Jaffe, E. S., Shevach, E. M., Frank, M. M., Berard, C. W., and Green, I: Nodular lymphoma—evidence for origin from follicular B lymphocytes. N. Engl. J. Med., *290*:813, 1974.

74. Johnson, R. E.: Remission induction and remission duration with primary radiotherapy in advanced lymphosarcoma. Cancer, *29*:1473, 1972.

75. Johnson, R. E.: Total nodal irradiation. J.A.M.A., *223*:59, 1973.

76. Johnson, R. E.: Total body irradiation (TBI) as primary therapy for advanced lymphosarcoma. Cancer, *35*:242, 1975.

77. Johnson, R. E., Kagan, A. R., Hafermann, M. D., and Keyes, J. W.: Patient tolerance to extended irradiation in Hodgkin's disease. Ann. Intern. Med., *70*:1, 1969.

78. Johnson, R. E., Kun, L. E., Belladonna, J. A., Johnson, S. K., Brereton, H. D., and Cohen, G. A.: Hematologic recovery and deterioration after "successful" radiotherapy for Hodgkin's disease. Ann. Intern. Med., *80*:213, 1974.

79. Jones, S. E.: Autoimmune disorders and malignant lymphoma. Cancer, *31*:1092, 1973.

80. Jones, S. E., Furs, Z., Bull, M., Kadin, M. E., Dorfman, R. F., Kaplan, H. S., Rosenberg, S. A., and Kim, H.: Non-Hodgkin's lymphomas. IV. Clincopathologic correlation in 465 cases. Cancer, *31*:806, 1973.

81. Jones, S. E., Rosenberg, S. A., Kaplan, H. S.: Non-Hodgkin's lymphomas. I. Bone marrow involvement. Cancer, *29*:954, 1972.

82. Jones, S. E., Rosenberg, S. A., Kaplan, H., Kadin, M. E., and Dorfman, R. L.: Non-Hodgkin's lymphoma. II. Single agent chemotherapy. Cancer, *30*:31, 1972.

83. Kadin, M. E., Glatstein, E., and Dorfman, R. F.: Clinicopathologic studies of 117 untreated patients subjected to laparotomy for the staging of Hodgkin's disease. Cancer, *27*:1277, 1971.

84. Kaplan, H. S.: Long-term results of palliative and radical radiotherapy of Hodgkin's disease. Cancer Res., *26*:1250, 1966.

85. Kaplan, H. S.: Hodgkin's Disease. Harvard University Press, Cambridge, Mass., 1972.

86. Kiely, J. M., Wagoner, R. D., and Holley, K. E.: Renal complications of lymphoma. Ann. Intern. Med., *71*:1159, 1969.

87. Korst, D. R., Meyer, O. O., and Jaeschke, W. H.: Survival in Hodgkin's disease. Arch. Intern. Med., *134*:1043, 1974.

88. Krumbhaar, E. B., and Krumbhaar, H. D.: Blood and bone marrow in mustard gas poisoning. J. Med. Res., 40:497, 1919.

89. Kundrat: Ueber lympho-sarkomatosis. Wien. Klin. Wochenschr., 6:211, 1893; 6:234, 1893.

90. Kyle, R. A., Kiely, J. M., and Stickney, J. M.: Acquired hemolytic anemia in chronic lymphocytic leukemia and the lymphomas. Arch. Intern. Med., 104:61, 1959.

91. LaMonte, C. S., and Lacher, M. J.: Lymphangiography in patients with pulmonary dysfunction. J.A.M.A., 132:365, 1973.

92. Lee, B. J.: Lymphangiography in Hodgkin's disease: indications and contraindications. Cancer Res., 26:1084, 1966.

93. Levin, W. C. (Editor): Symposium on Hodgkin's disease. Arch. Intern. Med., 131:331, 1973.

94. Levine, G. D., and Dorfman, R. F.: Nodular lymphoma: an ultrastructural study. Cancer, 35: 148, 1975.

95. Levitan, R., Diamond, H. D., and Craver, L. F.: Jaundice in Hodgkin's disease. Am. J. Med., 30:99, 1961.

96. Levy, R., and Kaplan, H.: Impaired lymphocytic function in untreated Hodgkin's disease. N. Engl. J. Med., 290:181, 1974.

97. Lobell, M., Boggs, D. R., and Wintrobe, M. M.: The clinical significance of fever in Hodgkin's disease. Arch. Intern. Med., 117:335, 1966.

98. Lokich, J. J., Galvanek, E. G., and Moloney, W. C.: Nephrosis of Hodgkin's disease. Arch. Intern. Med., 132:597, 1973.

99. Long, J. C., and Aisenberg, A. C.: Malignant lymphoma diagnosed at splenectomy and idiopathic splenomegaly. Cancer, 33:1054, 1974.

100. Long, J. C., and Minn, M. C.: Mycosis fungoides with extracutaneous dissemination: a distinct clinicopathologic entity. Cancer, 34:1745, 1974.

101. Lukes, R. J., and Butler, J. I.: Pathology and nomenclature of Hodgkin's disease. Cancer Res., 26:1063, 1966.

102. Lukes, R. J., and Tindle, B. H.: Immunoblastic lymphadenopathy. N. Engl. J. Med., 292:1, 1975.

103. Mann, R. B., Jaffe, E. S., Braylan, R. C., Eggleston, J. C., Ransom, L., Kaizer, H., and Berard, C. S.: Immunologic and morphologic studies of T cell lymphoma. Am. J. Med., 58:307, 1975.

104. McElwain, T. J.: Chemotherapy of the lymphomas. Semin. Hematol., 11:59, 1974.

105. Middleton, W. S.: Some clinical caprices of Hodgkin's disease. Ann. Intern. Med., 11:448, 1937.

106. Minot, G. R., and Isaacs, R.: Lymphoblastoma (malignant lymphoma): age and sex incidence, duration of disease, and the effect of roentgen-ray and radium irradiation and surgery. J.A.M.A., 86:1185, 1926.

107. Molander, G. W.: Lymphosarcoma, treatment and end results, 355 patients. Am. J. Roentgenol. Radium Ther. Nucl. Med., 117:54, 1973.

108. Moore, M. R., Bull, J. M., Jones, S. E., Rosenberg, S. A., and Kaplan, H. S.: Sequential radiotherapy and chemotherapy in the treatment of Hodgkin's disease. Ann. Intern. Med., 77:1, 1972.

109. Moore, M. R., Jones, S. E., Bull, J. M., William, L. A., and Rosenberg, S. A.: MOPP chemotherapy for advanced Hodgkin's disease. Cancer, 32:52, 1973.

110. Myers, C. E., Chabner, B. A., DeVita, V. T., Jr., and Gralnick, H. R.: Bone marrow involvement in Hodgkin's disease: pathology and response to MOPP chemotherapy. Blood, 44:197, 1974.

111. Neiman, R. S., Rosen, P. J., and Lukes, R. J.: Lymphocytic-depletion Hodgkin's disease. N. Engl. J. Med., 288:751, 1973.

112. Nelson, B., Rush, E. A., Takasugi, M., and Wittenberg, J.: Lipid embolism to the brain after lymphography. N. Engl. J. Med., 273:1132, 1965.

113. Nixon, D. W., and Aisenberg, A. C.: Combination chemotherapy in Hodgkin's disease. Cancer, 33:1499, 1974.

114. Owens, A. H., Jr., and Blazek, J. V.: Lymphography in the management of neoplastic disease. Johns Hopkins Med. J., 122:55, 1968.

115. Patchefsky, A. S., Brodovsky, H., Southard, M., Menduke, H., Gray, S., and Hoch, W. S.: Hodgkin's disease. A clinical and pathologic study of 235 patients. Cancer, 32:150, 1973.

116. Peckham, M. J.: Radiation therapy of the non-Hodgkin's lymphomas. Semin. Hematol. 11:41, 1974.

117. Perry, S., Thomas, L. B., Johnson, R. E., Carbone, P. P., and Haynes, H. A.: Hodgkin's disease (clincial staff conference). Ann. Intern. Med., 67:424, 1967.

118. Peters, M. V.: A study of survivals in Hodgkin's disease treated radiologically. Am. J. Roentgenol., 63:299, 1950.

119. Peters, M. V.: Prophylactic treatment of adjacent areas in Hodgkin's disease. Cancer Res., 26:1223, 1966.

120. Peters, M. V., and Middlemiss, K. C. H.: A study of Hodgkin's disease treated by irradiation. Am. J. Roentgenol., *79*:114, 1958.
121. Pettet, J. P., Pease, G. L., and Cooper, T.: An evaluation of paraffin sections of aspirated bone marrow in malignant lymphomas. Blood, *10*:820, 1955.
122. Rappaport, H., Winter, W. J., and Hicks, E. B.: Follicular lymphoma. A re-evaluation of its position in the scheme of malignant lymphoma. Based on a survey of 253 cases. (AFIP). Cancer, *9*:792, 1956.
123. Ravry, M., Maldonado, N., Velez-Garcia, E., Montalvo, J., and Santiago, P. J.: Serious infection after splenectomy for the staging of Hodgkin's disease. Ann. Intern. Med., 77:11, 1972.
124. Rosenberg, S. A.: Splenectomy in the management of Hodgkin's disease. Annotation. Br. J. Haemotol., *23*:271, 1972.
125. Rosenberg, S. A., Diamond, H. D., and Craver, L. F.: Lymphosarcoma: the effects of therapy and survival in 1269 patients in a review of 30 years' experience. Ann. Intern. Med., *53*:877, 1960.
126. Rosenberg, S. A., Diamond, H. D., Jaslowitz, B., and Craver, L. F.: Lymphosarcoma: a review of 1269 cases. Medicine, *40*:31, 1961.
127. Rosenberg, S. A., and Kaplan, H. S.: Evidence for an orderly progression in the spread of Hodgkin's disease. Cancer Res., *26*:1225, 1966.
128. Rosenberg, S. A., and Kaplan, H. S.: Hodgkin's disease and other malignant lymphomas. Calif. Med., *113*:23, 1970.
129. Rosenberg, S. A., and Kaplan, H.: The management of stage I, II and III Hodgkin's disease with combined radiotherapy and chemotherapy. Cancer, *35*:55, 1975.
130. Rosenberg, S. A., et al.: Report of the committee on Hodgkin's disease staging procedures. (Ann Arbor Symposium). Cancer Res., *3*:1862, 1971.
131. Rosenthal, M. C., Pisciotta, A. V., Komninos, Z. D., Goldenberg, H., and Dameshek, W.: The auto-immune hemolytic anemia of malignant lymphocytic disease. Blood, *10*:197, 1955.
132. Rosner, F., and Grunwald, H.: Hodgkin's disease and acute leukemia. Am. J. Med., *58*:339, 1975.
133. Roulet, F.: Das primäre Retothelsarkim der Lymphknoten. Virchows Arch. [Pathol. Anat.], *277*:15, 1930.
134. Rubin, P. (Editor): Updated Hodgkin's disease.
    A. Introduction. J.A.M.A., *222*:1292, 1972.
    B. Curability of Localized Disease. J.A.M.A., *223*:49, 1973.
    C. Advanced Disease and Special Problems. J.A.M.A., *223*:164, 1973.
135. Sahakian, G. J., Al-Mondhiry, H., Lacher, M. J., and Connolly, C. E.: Acute leukemia in Hodgkin's disease. Cancer, *33*:1369, 1974.
136. Schein, P. S., Chabner, B. A., Canellos, G. P., Young, R. C., Berard, C., and DeVita, V. T., Jr.: Potential for prolonged disease-free survival following combination chemotherapy of non-Hodgkin's lymphoma. Blood, *43*:181, 1974.
137. Schein, P. S., and Winokur, S. H.: Immunosuppressive and cytotoxic chemotherapy: long-term complications. Ann. Intern. Med., *82*:84, 1975.
138. Schimpff, S., Serpick, A., Stoler, B., Rumback, B., Mellin, H., Joseph, J. M., and Block, J. B.: Varicella-Zoster infection in patients with cancer. Arch. Intern. Med., *76*:241, 1972.
139. Schnitzer, B., Nishiyama, R. H., Heidelberger, K. P., and Weaver, D. K.: Hodgkin's disease in children. Cancer, *31*:560, 1973.
140. Schultz, D. R., and Yunis, A. A.: Immunoblastic lymphadenopathy with mixed cryoglobulinemia. N. Engl. J. Med., *292*:8, 1975.
141. Scott, R. B., and Robb-Smith, A. H. T.: Histiocytic medullary reticulosis. Lancet, *237*:194, 1939.
142. Scully, R. E., and McNeely, B. U.: Presentation of case. N. Engl. J. Med., *291*:1297, 1974.
143. Serck-Hanssen, A., and Purohit, G. P.: Histiocytic medullary reticulosis (report of 14 cases from Uganda). Br. J. Cancer, *22*:506, 1968.
144. Sherins, R. J., and DeVita, V. T., Jr.: Effect of drug treatment of male reproductive capacity. Ann. Intern. Med., *79*:216, 1973.
145. Sherman, R. L., Susin, M., Weksler, M. E., and Becker, E. L.: Lipoid nephrosis in Hodgkin's disease. Am. J. Med., *52*:699, 1972.
146. Shimkin, M. B., Oppermann, K. C., Bostick, W. L., and Low-Beer, B. V. A.: Hodgkin's disease: an analysis of frequency, distribution, and mortality at the University of California Hospital, 1914–1951. Ann. Intern. Med., *42*:136, 1955.
147. Skarin, A. T., Pinkus, G. S., Myerowitz, R. L., Bishop, Y., and Moloney, W. C.: Combination chemotherapy of advanced lymphocytic lymphoma. Importance of histologic classification in evaluating response. Cancer, *34*:1023, 1974.
148. Smithers, Sir David: Hodgkin's Disease. Churchill, Livingstone, Edinburgh and London, 1973.
149. Sokal, J. E., and Shimaoka, K.: Pyrogen in the urine of febrile patients with Hodgkin's disease. Nature, *215*:1183, 1967.

150. Sparberg, M.: Diagnostically confusing complications of diphenylhydantoin therapy. Ann. Intern. Med., *59*:914, 1963.
151. Sparling, H. J., Jr., Adams, R. D., and Parker, F., Jr.: Involvement of the nervous system by malignant lymphoma. Medicine, *26*:285, 1947.
152. Spigel, S. C., and Coltman, C. A., Jr.: Therapy of mycosis fungoides with bleomycin. Cancer, *32*:767, 1973.
153. Spivack, S. D.: Drugs five years later: procarbazine. Ann. Intern. Med., *81*:795, 1974.
154. Straus, D. J., Vance, Z. B., Kasdon, E. J., and Robinson, S. H.: Atypical lymphoma with prolonged systemic remission after splenectomy. Am. J. Med., *56*:386, 1974.
155. Strum, S. B., and Rappaport, H.: The persistence of Hodgkin's disease in long-term survivors. Am. J. Med., *51*:222, 1971.
156. Stutzman, L., and Glidewell, O.: Multiple chemotherapeutic agents for Hodgkin's disease. J.A.M.A., *225*:1202, 1973.
157. Sugarbaker, E. D., and Craver, L. F.: Lymphosarcoma: a study of 196 cases with biopsy. J.A.M.A., *115*:17, 1940.
158. Symmers, D.: Follicular lymphadenopathy with splenomegaly. Arch. Pathol., *3*:816, 1927.
159. Symmers, D.: Giant follicular lymphadenopathy with or without splenomegaly. Its transformation into polymorphous cell sarcoma of the lymph follicles and its association with Hodgkin's disease, lymphatic leukemia and an apparently unique disease of the lymph nodes and spleen. A disease entity believed heretofore undescribed. Arch. Path., *26*:603, 1938.
160. Symposium: Staging in Hodgkin's disease. Cancer Res. *31*:1712, 1971.
161. Ultmann, J. E., Cunningham, J. K., and Gellhorn, A.: The clinical picture of Hodgkin's disease. Cancer Res., *26*:1047, 1966.
162. Variakojis, D., Rosas-Uribe, A., and Rappaport, H.: Mycosis fungoides: pathologic findings in staging laparotomies. Cancer, *33*:1589, 1974.
163. Vinciguerra, V., and Silver, R. T.: The importance of bone marrow biopsy in staging of patients with lymphosarcoma. Blood, *41*:913, 1973.
164. Wang, C. C.: Treatment of primary reticulum-cell sarcoma of bone by irradiation. N. Engl. J. Med., *278*:1331, 1968.
165. Ward, P. A., and Berenberg, J. L.: Defective regulation of inflammatory mediators in Hodgkin's disease. N. Engl. J. Med., *290*:76, 1974.
166. Warne, G. L., Fairley, K. F., Hobbs, J. B., and Martin, F. I. R.: Cyclophosphamide-induced ovarian failure. N. Engl. J. Med., *289*:1159, 1973.
167. Warnke, R. A., Kim, H., and Dorfman, R. F.: Malignant histiocytosis (histiocytic medullary reticulosis). 1. Clinicopathologic study: 29 cases. Cancer, *35*:215, 1975.
168. Webb, D. I., and Silver, R. T.: Hodgkin's disease: value of bone-marrow biopsy. N. Engl. J. Med., *279*:46, 1968.
169. Weick, J. K., Kiely, J. M., Harrison, E. G., Carr, D. T., and Scanlon, P. W.: Pleural effusion in lymphoma. Cancer, *31*:848, 1973.
170. Weiden, P. L., Lerner, K. F., Heywood, J. D., Fefer, A., and Thomas, E. D.: Pancytopenia and leukemia in Hodgkin's disease: report of three cases. Blood, *42*:571, 1973.
171. Weisberger, A. S., Levine, B., and Storaasli, J. P.: Use of nitrogen mustard in treatment of serous effusions of neoplastic origin. J.A.M.A., *159*:1704, 1955.
172. Wintrobe, M. M., Cartwright, G. E., Fessas, P., Haut, A., and Altman, S. J.: Chemotherapy of leukemia, Hodgkin's disease and related disorders. Ann. Intern. Med., *41*:447, 1954.
173. Wood, N. L., and Coltman, C. A.: Localized pulmonary extranodal Hodgkin's disease. Ann. Intern. Med., *73*:113, 1973.
174. Yam, L. T., and Crosby, W. H.: Early splenectomy in lymphoproliferative disorders. Arch. Intern. Med., *133*:270, 1974.
175. Young, R. C., Chabner, B. A., Canellos, G. P., Schein, P. S., and DeVita, V. T., Jr.: Maintenance chemotherapy for advanced Hodgkin's disease in remission. Lancet, *1*:1339, 1973.
176. Young, R. C., Corder, M. P., Haynes, H. A., and DeVita, V. T., Jr.: Delayed hypersensitivity in Hodgkin's disease: a study of 103 untreated patients. Am. J. Med., *52*:63, 1972.
177. Young, R. C., and DeVita, V. T., Jr.: Therapy of Hodgkin's disease. Ann. Intern. Med., *80*:274, 1974.
178. Young, R. C., DeVita, V. T., Jr., and Johnson, R. E.: Hodgkin's disease in childhood. Blood, *42*:163, 1973.
179. Ziegler, J.: Chemotherapy of Burkitts lymphoma. Cancer, *30*:1535, 1972.

CHAPTER 14

LYMPHOCYTES, PLASMA CELLS, AND THE IMMUNE SYSTEM

The immune system anatomically is composed of lymph nodes, lymphoid tissue in the gastrointestinal and respiratory tract, lymphatic channels, thymus, spleen, bone marrow, and blood. Although the lymphocyte is the predominant cellular element of this system, other cells such as the plasma cell, macrophage (monocyte, histiocyte), and the granulocyte serve vital roles. Other noncellular blood elements also are important functionally in the over-all defense of the host against foreign material; these include various activated components of the complement, clotting, fibrinolytic, and kinin systems.

DEVELOPMENT OF THE IMMUNE SYSTEM

Knowledge of the origin and differentiation of cells in the development of the immune system (Fig. 14–1) has come from phylogenetic, ontogenic, and other experimental studies in animals, and from elucidation of the various developmental immunodeficient disorders of man.

The concept of a pluripotential hemopoietic stem cell (hemangioblast) migrating from the yolk sac through the fetal liver, spleen, and bone marrow, and giving rise to all erythroid, myeloid, and lymphoid cellular elements, continues to gain support (Fig. 14–1).[7,50] Lymphoid stem cells which are derived from pluripotential stem cells in the yolk sac migrate to the fetal liver, spleen, and bone marrow (Fig. 14–1). From these sites lymphoid stem cells migrate to the thymus, where further differentiation occurs under the influence of the microenvironment of the thymus to produce circulating T-cells (thymus-dependent cells).[5,83,85] Other lymphoid stem cells, under the influence of the

521

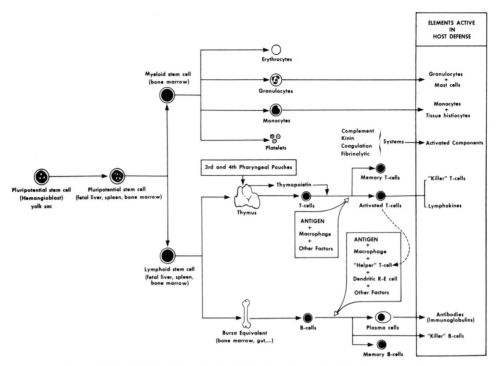

Figure 14–1 Cellular differentiation in the development of the immune system.

bursa of Fabricius in birds[9,84] or some mammalian equivalent (fetal liver, bone marrow, gut-associated lymphoid tissue), differentiate to become B-cells (bursa or bone marrow-dependent cells).[10,11,42,53] This stage of differentiation from lymphoid stem cells to T-cells and B-cells is antigen-independent. Further differentiation of T-cells to activated T-cells and B-cells to antibody-producing plasma cells is antigen-dependent and involves a complex interaction of many cellular and noncellular elements of the immune system (Fig. 14–1).

T-CELLS AND CELLULAR IMMUNITY

T-cells leave the thymus by way of the blood stream and are distributed to the thymus-dependent zones of lymph nodes, spleen, liver, and bone marrow. After migration from the thymus to the peripheral lymphoid structures, T-cells recirculate continuously from lymph nodes and other peripheral lymphatic tissues, either through the thoracic duct into the venous circulation, or directly into the venous circulation from organs such as the spleen. T-cells in the arterial blood are distributed not only to peripheral lymphoid structures, but also to tissues of nonlymphoid organs through the endothelial walls of the capillaries. Recirculation of T-cells to the thymus apparently does not occur. This pattern of lymphocyte circulation greatly increases the probability of contact between T-cells and foreign antigen.

Circulating T-cells and B-cells cannot be distinguished under the light microscope, nor probably under the electron microscope.[1,63] T-cells and B-cells are most readily separated by the nature of their membrane surface markers.[37,66] The property of human T-cells to form rosettes with sheep red blood cells is most often employed to identify these cells.[2] The nature of this sheep red blood cell receptor is not known. T-cells also react with nonspecific mitogens such as phytohemagglutinin (PHA) and concanavallin A (Con A). On exposure to these agents, T-cells transform from a small lymphocyte into a large pyroninophilic lymphoblast. Either by counting the morphologically transformed cells, or measuring tritiated thymidine uptake, or using autoradiography, the number and identity of T-cells can be assessed.[69] A highly specific mouse anti-T-cell serum is now available which is also employed to identify and study T-cells.[3]

Approximately 70 to 80 per cent of lymphocytes in the peripheral blood, and 90 per cent or more in the thoracic duct, show T-cell characteristics.[3] T-cells are also the predominant cell in the paracortical area of lymph nodes, in the periarterial lymphatic sheath of the spleen, and in other thymus-dependent areas of the peripheral lymphatic structures. Most circulating T-cells are long-lived lymphocytes. The average life span (intermitotic period) is approximately 4.4 years, and some cells survive for 20 years or more.[4,57] This compares to a life span of three days for short-lived lymphocytes, which are mostly B-cells.[91]

The mechanism of the initial cell-mediated immune response to antigen involves a complex series of events that is still poorly understood. It is currently believed that antigen is processed by macrophages or bound to the surface of macrophages prior to the interaction of antigen with specific antigenic receptors on T-cells (Fig. 14–1).[81] Others believe that antigen reacts with T-cells as the initial step.[19] As a result of these interactions, lymphocyte transformation and clonal proliferation of specific activated T-cells occur. These events usually take place in the thymus-dependent zones of lymph nodes and spleen. Little is known of the nature of the antigenic receptors on T-cells, but they are probably immunoglobulins. Some recent studies suggest that they may be related to antigens coded by the major histocompatibility gene complex (i.e., HL-A antigens in man or H-2 alloantigens in mice),[38,78] and may be related structurally to β-2 microglobulins.[13]

Activated T-cells are the effector cells ("killer cells") in cellular immunity (Fig. 14–1). In addition, some T-cells also function as "helper cells" in the antigen-dependent differentiation of B-cells to plasma cells,[19] and under some conditions other T-cells function as "suppressor cells" inhibiting B-cell response to antigen.[38] T-cells have other regulatory functions which also are important in the immune response.[38, 48] Finally, activated T-cells secrete many biologically-active substances (lymphokines) which may function as soluble mediators of immunity in the inflammatory response.[14] The lymphokines include macrophage migration inhibitory factor (MIF), macrophage, neutrophil, eosinophil, and lymphocyte chemotactic factors, macrophage activating factor, lymphotoxin, and factors that inhibit lymphocyte clone formation, lymphocyte proliferation, and DNA synthesis. Also secreted are mitogenic and skin reactive factors, immunoglobulins, interferon, and transfer factor.

Immune reactions involving T-cells (cellular immunity, delayed hypersensitivity reactions) develop more slowly than those mediated by antibodies (humoral immunity). Activated T-cells ("killer cells") have highly specific receptors which react with, and have the capacity to destroy, specific antigens or antigen-bearing target cells.[59] Other activated T-cells ("memory cells") (Fig. 14–1) react with antigen and undergo transformation and clonal proliferation. These in vitro observations probably correlate with delayed-type hypersensitivity reaction in vivo.[46,55,69] Clinical examples of immune responses involving delayed hypersensitivity include allograft rejection, graft versus host disease, contact allergy, delayed hypersensitivity skin reactions, some autoimmune diseases, immunity to most intracellular parasites and tumors, and immune surveillance in general.

The antigenic specificity responsible for eliciting a cell-mediated immune response is poorly understood. Antigens incorporated into adjuvants (e.g., killed tubercule bacilli in mineral oil) usually induce cellular immunity, as do intracellular parasites such as mycobacteria, Brucella organisms, and viruses.[82] The route of entry of antigens into the host is also important; antigens injected intradermally or subcutaneously are more likely to result in a cell-mediated response than those injected intravenously.[77]

B-CELLS, PLASMA CELLS, AND HUMORAL IMMUNITY

In man, the avian bursa of Fabricius equivalent (where lymphoid committed stem cells differentiate to become B-cells) is not well-defined anatomically.[10,42,53] The bone marrow, spleen, and gut-associated lymphoid tissue have been implicated most often as sites of B-cell differentiation. Recent evidence, however, suggests that none of these tissues is the exclusive bursa-equivalent.[42,53] More recent studies suggest that the fetal liver may be the bursa equivalent in mammals.[42,53] In adults animals, the bone marrow is a rich source both of pluripotential stem cells and of B-cells,[22,52,54,58,88] which suggests that the bone marrow possesses the microenvironment necessary to induce antigen-independent B-cell differentiation. Evidence for the existence of a similar microenvironment in other lymphoid structures in the adult animal is less convincing.

According to one hypothesis, the first detectable event to occur during this antigen-independent B-cell differentiation is the synthesis of IgM, followed sequentially by IgG and IgA synthesis.[42] It is not clear however, whether this scheme applies to all B-cells. The early synthesized IgM is monomeric in contrast to the pentameric IgM present in plasma; it is not secreted but is incorporated into the outer membrane of the lymphocyte.[42] Evidence now suggests that the sequential synthesis of IgM, IgG, and IgA during early B-cell differentiation represents a shift in synthesis of IgM to the production of IgG, and later to IgA, by the same clone of proliferating lymphocytes. This conclusion is based on the immunofluorescent staining pattern of surface immunoglobulins from serial biopsies of the bursa of Fabricius in chickens using fluorescin-tagged antibodies to IgM and IgG,[42] the suppressive effect of the administration of anti-μ (anti-IgM) antibodies on the synthesis of IgG and IgA,[39,65] and other studies.[66] Presumably, a similar switch occurs within the clone which leads to the proliferation of lymphocytes that synthesize IgD and IgE. Some recent evidence indicates that IgD is present on the surface of B-cells early in differentiation and may be synthesized before IgG or IgA.[78] The shift in synthesis of one immunoglobulin class to another is thought to represent a switch in expression of the gene for the constant region of the heavy chain. A similar switch in expression of the other three genes involved in immunoglobulin synthesis does not necessarily occur.

Upon completion of this antigen-independent clonal development under the inductive influence of the mammalian bursa-equivalent, B-cells are released to the bursa-dependent zones (i.e., germinal centers of lymph nodes and spleen) of the peripheral lymphoid tissues. Each clone of B-cells is committed to synthesize either IgM, IgG, IgA, IgD, or IgE.

Most B-cells are short-lived lymphocytes with a life span of approximately three days,[91] and circulate in a pattern similar to T-cells. B-cells are easily identified by the presence of membrane-bound immunoglobulins.[53,66] Monomeric IgM, IgD, and IgG are the most predominant immunoglobulins on the surface; membrane-bound IgA and IgE and found rarely. B-cells also are characterized by the presence of surface receptors for the third component of complement (C3) and probably the Fc portion of immunoglobulins.[53,66] The Fc receptor is closely associated with α–2–macroglobulins on the surface of B-cells, and is best demonstrated using aggregated immunoglobulins.[25] Some 10 to 20 per cent of peripheral blood lymphocytes have B-cell characteristics.[3]

The next step in B-cell differentiation is antigen-dependent. When B-cells are exposed to antigen, a complex sequence of events is initiated which involves interaction between antigen, macrophages, T-cells ("helper" or "suppressor" cells), dendritic reticulum cells, and B-cells. The B-cells proliferate to form memory cells and to undergo terminal differentiation to immunoglobulin-secreting plasma cells (Fig. 14–1).[19,38,48,81] The antigenic receptors on B-cells are immunoglobulins.[66,78]

The exact role of T-cells, macrophages, and dendritic reticulum cells in the initiation of a humoral immune response is still not clearly defined. Immunogenic response to haptens requires the presence of "helper" T-cells; T-cells probably recognize and bind to the carrier molecule of the hapten-carrier complex; the binding permits B-cells to react with the haptogenic determinants and mount an immune response. Some antigens such as pneumococcal polysaccharide do not require "helper" T-cells to elicit an immune response.[38] Under other conditions T-cells ("suppressor" T-cells) may actually inhibit the immune response by B-cells.[38] Most soluble antigens usually require macrophage processing before presentation to "helper" T-cells and B-cells, whereas tissue or cell antigens do not.[19,20,81] Macrophages also participate by removing excess antigen and thus potentiate the immune response. Other factors, such as the presence of opsonins and specific antibody, also are important.[79]

B-cells also may function as "killer cells" through the binding of antigen–antibody complexes by the Fc receptor (Fig. 14–1).

Antibodies produced in response to the initial exposure of a particular antigen to the immune system are heterogenous with regard to class of immunoglobulin, affinity of immunoglobulin for antigen, and specificity.[12,71] Factors that influence any given immune response include the physical state and dose of the antigen,[77] route of antigen entry into the host, antigen manipulation such as use of adjuvants,[1a] genetic factors,[48] and many others.[12,38,74,80] The initial immune response is often referred to as "primary immune response," and the response to second exposure to antigen (usually after an appropriate interval) as "secondary (anamnestic or "booster") response."

The first immunoglobulin detected in most primary immune responses is IgM, especially if the antigen is particulate. With very low doses of antigen, IgM may be the only antibody produced. If the initial dose is large, the IgM response is followed by the synthesis of IgG. Depending on the sensitivity of methods used, IgM may be detected in serum as early as eight to 16 hours (the usual lag period is two to four days) following intravenous injection of antigen.[79] IgG usually can be detected in the serum after four to seven days. Factors that determine the production of any specific class of immunoglobulin are still not well-defined. In the case of IgE, genetic factors and route of antigen administration are very important. Transmucosal administration of antigen frequently results in production of IgE.

The route of antigen administration, the nature and dose of antigen, and host factors also are important in the production of specific immunologic tolerance,[32] which is defined as nonreactivity to a substance that is ordinarily antigenic. Soluble monomeric antigens, very high and very low doses of certain antigens (serum proteins), and administration of antigen during fetal development all favor the induction of immunologic tolerance on subsequent exposures to that specific antigen.

Immunoglobulins: Nomenclature, Structure, and Function

Knowledge of the plasma proteins has increased as a direct result of improved methodology. As is usual in times of rapid technical advances, some overlapping in definition and confusion in terminology has resulted. The various techniques employed in the study of plasma proteins allow different views of the various fractions, and the technique employed in any given circumstance will therefore depend on the immediate aim of the investigator.

A 50 per cent saturation of plasma with ammonium sulfate will separate albumin from globulins. Tiselius later identified three globulin fractions which he termed alpha (α), beta (β), and gamma (γ).

In addition, plasma proteins can be separated by high centrifugal fields to give: (1) a 4S fraction with a molecular weight of 70,000 which is mostly albumin; (2) a 7S fraction with a molecular weight of 160,000 which is mostly gamma globulin; (3) a 19S fraction with a molecular weight of 1 million which is macroglobulin.

Electrophoresis, using a variety of quasisolid supporting media, is now employed clinically to characterize the plasma proteins. Serum may be separated into five components: albumin, α_1, α_2, β, and γ globulin. This technique has found widespread clinical application, and with careful control is easily reproduced (Fig. 14–2). Appropriate media include starch, filter paper, cellulose acetate, and agar gels. Starch gel electrophoresis allows separation on the basis both of the size and shape of the molecule and of the electrical charge, and

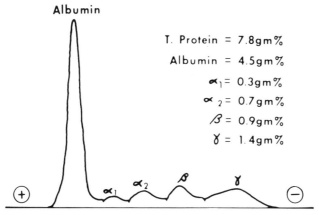

$$
\begin{aligned}
\text{T. Protein} &= 7.8\,\text{gm}\% \\
\text{Albumin} &= 4.5\,\text{gm}\% \\
\alpha_1 &= 0.3\,\text{gm}\% \\
\alpha_2 &= 0.7\,\text{gm}\% \\
\beta &= 0.9\,\text{gm}\% \\
\gamma &= 1.4\,\text{gm}\%
\end{aligned}
$$

Figure 14-2 Normal serum protein electrophoretic pattern.

permits a much greater subdivision of the major plasma proteins. The use of agar as supporting medium has the advantage that electrophoresis and immuno-diffusion may be carried out together in one process known as immunoelectro-phoresis.[90] With this technique, gamma globulin was found to be composed of three major fractions, γG, γA, γM, and two minor fractions, γD and γE (Fig. 14-3). These fractions are closely related chemically, immunologically, and functionally, and the term *immunoglobulins* has been applied to them.[30]

Several quantitative methods are now available to determine the concen-tration of the various classes of immunoglobulins and immunoglobulin subunits (i.e., light chains, heavy chains) in serum, urine, CSF, and external secretions (i.e., saliva).[31] Although the radial immunodiffusion technique is used most often,[21, 44] automated methods are now available.[68]

Immunoglobulin structure: Although functionally heterogenous, the five major immunoglobulin classes are structurally similar. The basic immuno-

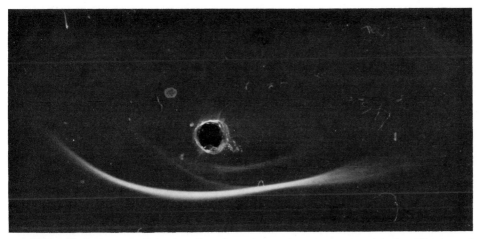

Figure 14-3 Immunoelectrophoretic pattern of normal serum gamma globulins. (Courtesy of Dr. David Normansell.)

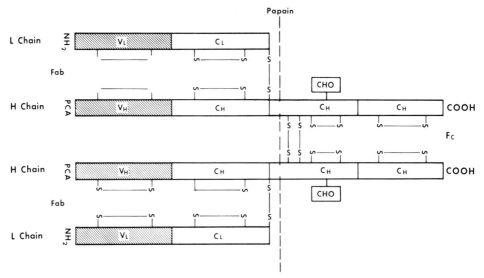

Figure 14–4   Schematic structure of 7S IgGl from data by Edelman et al.[15] NH₂, amino-terminal end; PCA, pyrrolidinecarboxylic acid; V$_L$, variable region of the light chain; C$_L$, constant region of the light chain; V$_H$, variable region of the heavy chain; C$_H$, constant region of the heavy chain; CHO, carbohydrate; Fab, antigen-binding fragment; Fc, crystallizable fragment.

globulin molecule is composed of two identical pairs of polypeptide chains held together by disulfide bonds and noncovalent interactions (Fig. 14–4).[15] The light (L) chains have a molecular weight of approximately 22,500 each; the molecular weight of each heavy (H) chain varies from 53,000 to 75,000, depending on the immunoglobulin class.[17, 47, 86] On the basis of antigenic differences of the H chains, the immunoglobulins may be subdivided into five major classes: IgG (immunoglobulin G), IgA, IgM, IgD, and IgE. The different H chains are designated by the Greek letters γ (gamma), α (alpha), μ (mu), δ (delta), and ϵ (epsilon), respectively. IgG, IgA, and IgM may be further divided into subclasses on the basis of other minor H chain antigenic determinants (Table 14–1).

Only two major types of L chains have been identified antigenically, and are referred to as κ (kappa) and λ (lambda). All immunoglobulins have either κ or λ light chains, but not both on the same molecule. Bence Jones proteins are free light chains, usually occurring as dimers of either κ or λ chains.[24, 67]

Much of our knowledge of the structure of the immunoglobulins has come from studies of the various subunits which result from enzymatic digestion,[33, 64] and of intact H and L chains which may be obtained by chemical cleavage of the disulfide bonds by reducing agents.[8, 17] Papain digestion of a 7S IgG molecule produces three fragments, two Fab fragments and one Fc fragment (Fig. 14–4). The two Fab fragments are identical and consist of one complete L chain and the amino-terminal end of one H chain. The antigen-binding activity resides in these two fragments. Each Fab piece has one antigen-binding site. The Fc fragment is a dimer of the carboxy-terminal ends of the H chains, and contains most of the carbohydrate portion of the molecule together with the class-specific antigenic determinants. This fragment also is responsible for the several im-

Table 14–1 *Structural and Biologic Properties of Human Immunoglobulins*

	IgG	IgA	IgM	IgD	IgE
Molecular weight	155,000	170,000	900,000	180,000	200,000
Heavy chain class	γ	α	μ	δ	ϵ
Number subclasses	4	2	2	?	?
Light chain type	κ or λ	κ or λ	κ or λ	κ or λ	κ or λ
Sedimentation coeff. ($S_{20,w}$)	7S	7S*	19S	7S	8S
J chain	0	+*	+	0	0
Transport piece	0	+*	0	0	0
Carbohydrate (%)	2.9	7.5	10.7	12.0	10.7
No. antigen-binding sites	2	2	5–10	2	2
Half-life (days)	21	6	5	2.8	2.2
Synthesis (mg./kg./day)	33	24	6.7	0.4	0.02
Mean serum conc. (mg.%)	1200	250	120	3	0.03
External secretions	+	++++	+	?	++
Intravascular (%)	45	42	75	75	50
Placental transfer	+	0	0	0	0
Reagenic activity	0	0	0	0	+
Complement fixation	+	0	+	?	?

*Polymers of IgA (9S, 11S, and 13S) may occur in serum. Secretory IgA is an 11S molecule composed of two 7S monomers of IgA, one J chain, and a glycoprotein (transport or secretory piece).

portant biologic properties of immunoglobulins including complement fixation, placental transfer, fixation to macrophages, lymphocytes, mast cells, and skin (Table 14–1).[72]

Both the L and H chains have variable regions (V_L and V_H, respectively) and constant regions (C_L and C_H, respectively) (Fig. 14–4). The variable regions are so named because of the marked variation in amino acid sequence that occurs in these areas, even among Ig molecules of a specific subclass such as IgG1.[15] Furthermore, there are three regions of hypervariability within each V_L and V_H region.[16, 89] The hypervariable regions of the L and H chains together form the two antigen-binding sites for each molecule.[6] It is this marked variability in the amino acid sequence in these regions that permits the production of specific antibodies to a large variety of antigens within any given class or subclass of immunoglobulins.

The amino acid sequence of the constant regions is much less variable, but minor differences do occur. A substitution of only one amino acid at position 191 in the C_L of the κ light chain accounts for the three allotypic markers (InV 1, InV 2, and InV 3) known to reside on this chain.[73] The OZ (+ and −) and Kern (+ and −) markers in the C_L of the λ light chain also result from single amino acid substitutions.[18, 26] Over 20 genetic markers (Gm factors) have been identified in the C_H of the γ heavy chain, and two (Am factors) in the C_H of the alpha heavy chain.[56]

IgG, IgD, IgE, and usually IgA circulate in the plasma as 7S monomers composed of two light chains, κ or λ, and two heavy chains, γ, δ, ϵ, or α.[86] IgM usually circulates as a 19S pentamer composed of five IgM monomers (each containing two light chains, κ or λ, and two μ chains) and another polypeptide called J chain (Fig. 14–5). The J chain is attached to the IgM monomers by disulfide bridges.[34, 40, 49] J chain is produced by plasma cells and has a molecular weight of approximately 23,000. The pentameric IgM molecule may have a

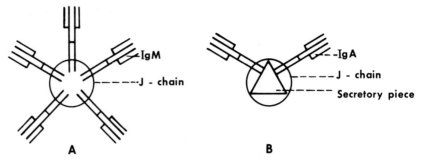

Figure 14-5   Schematic structure of IgM pentamer (A) and secretory IgA (B).

maximum of ten antigen-binding sites (two per monomer); with most antigens, however, only five can be demonstrated.

Although circulating IgA is mostly a 7S monomer, that found in external secretions (i.e., saliva, respiratory, and gastrointestinal secretions) is an 11S molecule referred to as secretory IgA.[72, 76] It is composed of two 7S IgA monomers, one J chain, and a glycoprotein known as secretory or transport piece (Fig. 14-5).[28, 34, 40, 49] The secretory piece has a molecular weight of 58,000, is synthesized by epithelial cells, and probably is attached to the IgA molecules during their transport across the mucosa.[75]

Function of immunoglobulins: The different classes and subclasses of immunoglobulins vary considerably in their biologic functions (Table 14-1).

IgG.   IgG constitutes approximately 75 per cent of the serum immunoglobulins. Four subclasses of IgG are now characterized (IgG1, IgG2, IgG3, and IgG4). Many of the biologic properties of IgG are subclass-specific.[72] For example, only IgG1 and IgG3 bind to macrophages and granulocytes, a process important in opsonization; the subclass IgG4 will not fix complement through the classical pathway.[23] Certain antibodies are also subclass-specific e.g., anti-Rh is either IgG1 or IgG3).[56] The significance of the small amount of IgG found in external secretions is not clear.[75]

IgA.   Secretory IgA is the predominant class of immunoglobulin present in external secretions such as saliva, tears, colostrum, nasal and bronchial secretions, seminal vesicles, cervix, urinary tract, and intestinal fluid. Most of the immunoglobulin portion of secretory IgA is synthesized by plasma cells that reside in the submucosa of these mucous membranes. In contrast, IgA in the serum and other internal secretions (e.g., CSF) is synthesized by plasma cells in the spleen, bone marrow, and lymph nodes. Although secretory IgA has antiviral and antibacterial activity, its importance in over-all host defense is unclear. Isolated deficiency of IgA is a frequent finding in population studies, as high as 0.03 per cent,[75] but is not necessarily associated with an increased susceptibility to infection; some individuals with a total absence of IgA in serum and secretions are completely asymptomatic.[27] (Chap. 18.)

IgM.   Circulating IgM is a pentamer (trace amounts of IgM monomer are detectable in normal human sera), and is essentially confined to the intravascular space (Table 14-1). IgM is often the first antibody synthesized in the primary immune response to most antigens.[51] In some instances IgM is the predominant antibody formed (e.g., heterophil antibody in infectious mononucleosis, Wasserman antibody in syphilis, cold agglutinins in mycoplasma infections and in idiopathic cold hemagglutinin disease). Only one molecule of IgM attached to a cell surface is necessary to fix complement; if this reaction occurs on the surface of red cells, intravascular hemolysis results. In contrast, two molecules of IgG, in close proximity on the cell surface, are necessary to fix complement.

IgD. The biologic properties of IgD are not well-defined. Recent evidence suggests that IgD may be important as a membrane receptor and is synthesized early in the antigen-independent differentiation of B-cells.[78]

IgE. IgE is the reagenic antibody and is the immunoglobulin responsible for mediating the Prausnitz-Küstner (P-K test) skin reaction and allergic (immediate hypersensitivity) reactions in atopic individuals.[35, 36, 43] Recent evidence indicates that most IgE, like IgA, is synthesized by plasma cells residing in secretory sites. Indeed, IgE is now classified as a secretory immunoglobulin, and is probably more concentrated in external secretions than in serum.[72, 75]

Circulating basophils and tissue mast cells have receptors for the Fc portion of the IgE. When antigen reacts with IgE that is membrane-bound, both basophils and mast cells release substances that are known to be important in immediate hypersensitivity reactions. These substances include histamine, slow-reacting substance (SRS), and eosinophil chemotactic factor (ECF).

OTHER ELEMENTS ACTIVE IN HOST DEFENSE

In addition to antibodies, lymphokines, and other noncellular mediators (e.g., histamine, SRS) of the inflammatory reaction, activated components of several plasma protein systems also are important in the over-all defense of the host against foreign material. These systems, which include the complement, clotting (Chapters 16 and 17), fibrinolytic (Chapters 16 and 17), and kinin systems, interact with each other at several steps during activation (Fig. 14–6).[70] Activation of Hageman factor (Factor XII) not only initiates the activation of the intrinsic clotting pathway, but also the fibrinolytic, kinin, and, through the action of plasmin, the complement system (Fig. 14–6).

Complement System

Complete activation of the complement system releases several components that are important not only in host defense against foreign material, but also in the pathogenesis of autoimmune disease such as autoimmune hemolytic anemia (Chapter 7).[23, 70] The complement system may be activated by two different pathways, the classic pathway and the alternate or properdin pathway (Fig. 14–7). The classic pathway is usually activated by antigen-antibody complexes which bind to the first component of complement (C1). This interaction activates C1, which in turn activates C4 and C2; C42 (activated C42) cleaves C3 into C3a and C3b. The complex C1423b then binds and cleaves C5, which results in sequential activation of C6 to C9. When the antigen is present on the red cell

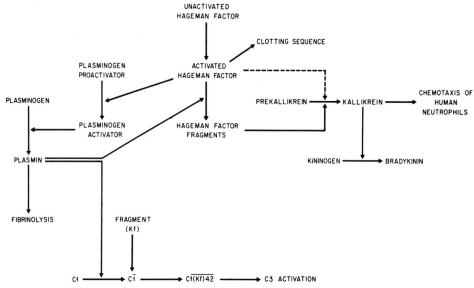

Figure 14-6 Interrelations between the coagulation, kinin, fibrinolytic, and complement systems. (Courtesy of Ruddy et al.[70] and the New England Journal of Medicine. Reprinted by permission from The New England Journal of Medicine, *287*:489, 1972.)

surface, as in the case in autoimmune hemolytic anemia, this reaction sequence often leads to lysis of the red cell.

Complement activation via the alternate pathway may be initiated not only by certain antibodies (aggregated IgA, IgE, and IgG4), but also by certain insoluble polysaccharides and cell wall lipopolysaccharides in the absence of antibody (Fig. 14–7). This pathway bypasses C1, C4, and C2, and proceeds directly to the activation of C3 and the latter components of complement. Properdin, a 5S α_2 glycoprotein, and other serum factors are necessary for the cleavage of C3 to C3b by this pathway.

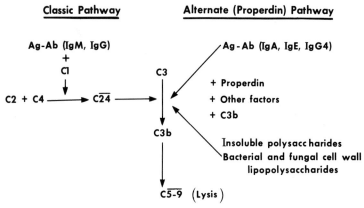

Figure 14–7 Pathways for activation of the complement system.

Cell lysis is only one of several biologic consequences of activation of the complement system. Many of the activated components possess other functions (i.e., C3b has opsonic properties and binds to complement receptors on B-cells, granulocytes and monocytes; C3a and C5a increase vascular permeability, and together with $\overline{C567}$ also have chemotactic properties; C1 and C4 result in viral neutralization).[23]

Kinin System

Activation of the kinin system results in the appearance of kallikrein which has chemotactic properties, bradykinin which is vasoactive, and a serum fragment, K_f, which enhances the capacity of $\overline{C1}$ (when complexed as $\overline{C1}K_f42$) to activate C3 (Fig. 14–6).

References

1. Alexander, E. L., and Wetzel, B.: Human lymphocytes: similarity of B and T cell surface morphology. Science, *188*:732, 1975.
1a. Allison, A. C.: Requirements of thymus-dependent lymphocytes for potentiation by adjuvants of antibody formation. Nature, *233*:330, 1971.
2. Bach, J. F.: Evaluation of T-cells and thymic serum factors in man using the rosette technique. Transplant Rev., *16*:196, 1973.
3. Bentwich, Z., and Kunkel, H. G.: Specific properties of human B and T lymphocytes and alterations in disease. Transplant Rev., *16*:29, 1973.
4. Buckton, K. E., Brown, W. M. C., and Smith, P. G.: Lymphocyte survival in men treated with x-rays for ankylosing spondylitis. Nature, *214*:470, 1967.
5. Cantor, H., and Weissman, I. L.: Development and function of subpopulations of thymocytes and T lymphocytes. Progr. Allergy. (In press.)
6. Capra, J. D., and Kehoe, J. M.: Hypervariable regions, idiotypy, and the antibody-combining site. Adv. Immunol., *20*:1, 1975.
7. Ciba Foundation Symposium 13 (new series). Haemopoietic Stem Cells. North-Holland Publ., Amsterdam, 1973.
8. Cohen, S.: Properties of the separated chains of human γ-globulin. Nature, *197*:253, 1963.
9. Cooper, M. D., Kincade, P. W., and Lawton, A. R.: Thymus and Bursal Function in Immunologic Development: A New Theoretical Model of Plasma Cell Differentiation. *In* Kagan, B. M., and Stiehm, E. R. (eds.): Immunologic Incompetence. Yearbook Publ., Chicago, Ill., 1971, p. 81.
10. Cooper, M. D., and Lawton, A. R.: The development of the immune system. Sci. Am., *231*:58, 1974.
11. Cooper, M. D., Lawton, A. R., and Kincade, P. W.: A developmental approach to the biological basis of antibody diversity. Contemp. Top. Immunobiol., *1*:33, 1972.
12. Cunningham, A. J.: The generation of antibody diversity: its dependence on antigenic stimulation. Contemp. Top. Mol. Immunol., *3*:1, 1974.
13. Cunningham, B., et al.: β_2-microglobulin and HL-A antigen. Transplant Rev., *21*:1, 1974.
14. David, J. R.: Lymphocyte mediators and cellular hypersensitivity. N. Engl. J. Med., *288*:143, 1973.
15. Edelman, G. M., Cunningham, B. A., Gall, W. E., Gottlieb, P. D., Rutishouser, U., and Waxdal, M. J.: The covalent structure of an entire γG immunoglobulin molecule. Proc. Natl. Acad. Sci., U.S.A., *63*:78, 1969.
16. Edelman, G. M., and Gall, W. E.: The antibody problem. Annu. Rev. Biochem., *38*:415, 1969.
17. Edelman, G. M., and Poulik, M. D.: Studies on structural units of the γ-globulins. J. Exp. Med., *113*:861, 1961.
18. Elin, D., and Fahey, J. L.: Two types of lambda polypeptide chains in human immunoglobulins. Science, *156*:947, 1967.
19. Feldman, M.: Cellular components of the immune system and their cooperation (T and B cells). Transplant Proc., *5*:43, 1973.

20. Fishman, M., Adler, F. L., and Rice, S. G.: Macrophage RNA in the in vitro immune response to phage. Ann. N. Y. Acad. Sci., *207*:73, 1973.
21. Fahey, J. L., and McKelvey, E. M.: Quantitative determination of serum immunoglobulins in antibody agar plates. J. Immunol., *94*:84, 1965.
22. Ford, C. E., Hamerton, J. L., Barnes, D. W. H., and Loutit, J. F.: Cytological identification of radiation chimeras. Nature, *177*:452, 1956.
23. Frank, M. M., and Atkinson, J. P.: Complement in clinical medicine. Dis. Month., Jan. 1975.
24. Friedman, H. P., Stavitsky, A. B., and Solomon, J. M.: Induction in vitro of antibodies to phage T2:antigens in the RNA extract employed. Science, *149*:1106, 1965.
25. Gelder, F., Hurtubise, P., Scillian, J., and Murphy, S.: The association of α_2–macroglobulin with the Fc receptor on B lymphocytes. Clin. Res., *23*:291A, 1975.
26. Gibson, D., Levanon, M., and Smithies, P.: Heterogeneity of normal human immunoglobulin light chains. Nonalleic variation in the constant region of λ chains. Biochem., *10*:3114, 1971.
27. Goldberg, L. S., Barnetti, E. V., and Fudenberg, H. H.: Selective absence of IgA. A family study. J. Lab. Clin. Med., *72*:204, 1968.
28. Halpern, M. S., and Koshland, M. E.: Novel subunit in secretory IgA. Nature, *228*:1276, 1970.
29. Hanna, M. G., and Hunter, R. L.: Localization of antigen and immune complexes in lymphatic tissue, with special reference to germinal centers. Adv. Exp. Med. Biol., *12*:257, 1971.
30. Heremans, J. F.: Immunochemical studies on protein pathology. The immunoglobulin concept. Clin. Chim. Acta, *4*:639, 1959.
31. Hobbs, J. R.: Immunoglobulins in clinical chemistry. Adv. Clin. Chem., *14*:219, 1971.
32. Howard, J. G., and Mitchison, N. A.: Immunological tolerance. Progr. Allergy, *18*:43, 1975.
33. Hsiao, S., and Putnam, F. W.: The cleavage of human γ-globulin by papain. J. Biol. Chem., *236*: 122, 1961.
34. Inman, F. P., and Mestecky, J.: The J chain of polymeric immunoglobulins. Contemp. Top. Mol. Immunol., *3*:111, 1974.
35. Ishizaka, K.: Human reagenic antibodies. Annu. Rev. Med., *21*:187, 1970.
36. Johansson, S. G. O., Bennich, H. H., and Berg, T.: The clinical significance of IgE. Progr. Clin. Immunol., *1*:157, 1972.
37. Jondal, M., Wigzell, H., and Aiuti, F.: Human lymphocyte subpopulations; classification according to surface markers and/or functional characteristics. Transplant Rev., *16*:163, 1973.
38. Katz, D. H., and Benacerrof, B.: The regulatory influence of activated T cells on B cell responses to antigen. Adv. Immunol., *15*:1, 1972.
39. Kincade, P. W., Lawton, A. R., Bockman, D. E., and Cooper, M. D.: Suppression of immunoglobulin G synthesis as a result of antibody-mediated suppression of immunoglobulin M in chicken. Proc. Natl. Acad. Sci., U.S.A., *67*:1918, 1970.
40. Koshland, M. D.: Structure and function of the J chain. Adv. Immunol., *20*:41, 1975.
41. Lawton, A. R., Asofsky, T., Hylton, M. B., and Cooper, M. D.: Suppression of immunoglobulin class synthesis in mice. I. Effects of treatment with antibody to mu-chain. J. Exp. Med., *135*:277, 1972.
42. Lawton, A. R., Kincade, P. W., and Cooper, M. D.: Sequential expression of germ line genes in development of immunoglobulin class diversity. Fed. Proc., *34*:33, 1975.
43. Lichtenstein, L. M.: Anaphylactic reactions to insect stings: a new approach. Hosp. Pract., *10*: 67, 1975.
44. Mancini, G., Carbonara, A. O., and Heremans, J. F.: Immunochemical quantitation of antigens by single radial immunodiffusion. Immunochemistry, *2*:235, 1965.
45. Manning, D. D., and Jutila, J. W.: Immunosuppression of mice injected with heterologous anti-immunoglobulin heavy chain antisera. J. Exp. Med., *135*:1316, 1972.
46. Marshall, W. H., Valentine, F. T., and Lawrence, H. S.: Cellular immunity in vitro. J. Exp. Med., *130*:327, 1969.
47. Mattioli, C., and Tomasi, T. B., Jr.: The human serum immunoglobulins. Dis. Month, April, 1970.
48. McDevitt, H. Q., and Benacerrof, B.: Genetic control of specific immune responses. Adv. Immunol., *11*:31, 1969.
49. Mestecky, J., Zikan, J., and Butler, W. T.: Immunoglobulin M and secretory immunoglobulin A: presence of a common polypeptide chain different from light chain. Science, *171*:1163, 1971.
50. Metcalf, D., and Moore, M. A. S.: Hematopoietic Cells: Their Origin, Migration, and Differentiation. North-Holland Publ., Amsterdam, 1971.

51. Metzger, H.: Structure and function of M macroglobulins. Adv. Immunol., *12*:57, 1970.
52. Micklem, H. S., Ford, C. E., Evans, E. P., and Gray, J.: Interrelationships of myeloid and lymphoid cells: studies with chromosome-marked cells transfused into laterally irradiated mice. Proc. Roy. Soc. London. [Biol.], *165*:78, 1966.
53. Miller, R. G., and Phillips, R. A.: Development of B lymphocytes. Fed. Proc., *34*:145, 1975.
54. Miller, R. G., and Phillips, R. A.: Sedimentation analysis of the cells in mice required to initiate an in vivo response to sheep erythrocytes. Proc. Soc. Exp. Biol. Med., *135*:63, 1970.
55. Mills, J. A.: The immunologic significance of antigen-induced lymphocyte transformation in vitro. J. Immunol., *97*:239, 1966.
56. Natvig, J. B., and Kunkel, H. G.: Human immunoglobulins: classes, subclasses, genetic variants, and idiotypes. Adv. Immunol., *16*:1, 1973.
57. Norman, A., Sasaki, M. S., Ottoman, R. E., and Fingerhut, A. G.: Lymphocyte lifetime in women. Science, *147*:745, 1964.
58. Nowell, P. C., Hirsch, B. E., Fox, D. H., and Wilson, D. B.: Evidence for the existence of multipotential lympho–hematopoietic stem cells. J. Cell. Physiol., *75*:151, 1970.
59. Paul, W. E.: Functional specificity of antigen binding receptors of lymphocytes. Transplant Rev., *5*:130, 1970.
60. Pierce, C. W., Asofsky, R., and Solliday, S. M.: Immunoglobulin receptors on B lymphocytes: shifts in immunoglobulin class during immune responses. Fed. Proc., *32*:41, 1973.
61. Pierce, C. W., Solliday, S. M., and Asofsky, R.: Immune response in vitro. IV. Suppression of primary γM, γG, and γA plaque-forming cell responses in mouse spleen cultures by class-specific antibody to mouse immunoglobulins. J. Exp. Med., *135*:675, 1972.
62. Pierce, C. W., Solliday, S. M., and Asofsku, R.: Immune response in vitro. V. Suppression of γM, γG, and γA plaque-forming cell responses in culture of primed mouse spleen cells by class-specific antibody to mouse immunoglobulins. J. Exp. Med., *135*:698, 1972.
63. Polliack, A., Lampen, N., Clarkson, B. D., Deharven, E., Bentwich, Z., Siegal, F. P., and Kunkel, H. G.: Identification of human B and T lymphocytes by scanning electron microscopy. J. Exp. Med., *138*:607, 1973.
64. Porter, R. R.: Hydrolysis of rabbit γ-globulin and antibodies with crystalline papain. Biochem. J., *73*:119, 1959.
65. Preud'homme, J. L., and Seligmann, M.: Primary immunodeficiency with increased numbers of circulating B lymphocytes contrasting with hypogammaglobulinemia. Lancet, *1*:442, 1972.
66. Preud'homme, J. L., and Seligmann, M.: Surface Immunoglobulins on Human-Lymphoid Cells. *In* Schwartz, R. S. (ed.): Prog. Clin. Immunol. Grune and Stratton, New York, 1974, p. 121.
67. Putman, F. W.: Structural relationships among normal human γ-globulin, myeloma globulins and Bence Jones proteins. Biochim. Biophys. Acta, *63*:539, 1962.
68. Ritchie, R. F., Alper, C. A., Graves, J., Pearson, N., and Larson, C.: Automated quantitation of proteins in serum and other biologic fluids. Am. J. Clin. Pathol., *59*:151, 1973.
69. Rocklin, R. E.: Clinical Applications of In Vitro Lymphocyte Tests. *In* Schwartz, R. S. (ed.): Prog. Clin. Immunol. Grune and Stratton, New York, 1974, p. 21.
70. Ruddy, S., Gigli, I., and Austen, K. F.: The complement system of man. N. Engl. J. Med., *287*: 489, 545, 592, 642, 1972.
71. Siskind, G. W., and Benacerrof, B.: Cell selection by antigen in the immune response. Adv. Immunol., *10*:1, 1969.
72. Spiegelberg, H. L.: Biological activities of immunoglobulins of different classes and subclasses. Adv. Immunol., *19*:259, 1974.
73. Steinberg, A. G.: Globulin polymorphism in man. Annu. Rev. Genet., *3*:25, 1969.
74. Taussig, M. J.: Antigenic competition. Curr. Top. Microbiol. Immunol., *60*:125, 1969.
75. Tomasi, T. B., and Grey, H. M.: Structure and function of immunoglobulin A. Progr. Allergy, *16*:81, 1972.
76. Tomasi, T. B., Jr.: Structure and function of mucosal antibodies. Annu. Rev. Med., *21*:281, 1970.
77. Uhr, J. W.: Delayed hypersensitivity. Physiol. Rev., *46*:359, 1966.
78. Uhr, J. W.: The membrane of lymphocytes. Hosp. Pract., *10*:113, 1975.
79. Uhr, J. W., and Finkelstein, M. S.: The kinetics of antibody formation. Progr. Allergy, *10*:37, 1967.
80. Uhr, J. W., and Moller, G.: Regulatory effect of antibody on the immune response. Adv. Immunol., *8*:81, 1968.
81. Unanue, E. R.: The regulatory role of macrophages in antigenic stimulation. Adv. Immunol., *15*:95, 1972.
82. Valentine, F. T., and Lawrence, H. S.: Cell mediated immunity. Adv. Intern. Med., *17*:51, 1971.

83. Warner, N. L.: Differentiation of immunocytes and the evolution of the immunological poten-
    tial. Front. Biol., 25:467, 1972.
84. Warner, N. L.: The immunological role of the avian thymus and bursa of Fabricius. Folia Biol.
    (Praha)., 13:1, 1967.
85. Weissman, I. L.: Thymus cell migration. J. Exp. Med., 126:291, 1967.
86. Wells, J. V., and Fudenberg, H. H.: Paraproteinemias. Dis. Month, Feb. 1974.
87. Wesley, W. B., and Möller, E.: The continuing carrier problem. Transplant Rev., 18:3, 1974.
88. Wu, A. M., Till, J. E., Siminovitch, L., and McCulloch, E. A.: A cytological study of the capacity
    for differentiation of normal hemopoietic colony-forming cells. J. Cell. Physiol., 69:177,
    1967.
89. Wu, T. T., and Kabat, E. A.: An analysis of the sequence of the variable regions of Bence Jones
    proteins and myeloma light chains and their implication for antibody complementarity.
    J. Exp. Med., 132:211, 1970.
90. Wunderly, C.: Immunoelectrophoresis: methods, interpretation, results. Adv. Clin. Chem.,
    4:207, 1961.
91. Yoffey, J. M., and Courtice, F. C.: Lymphatics, Lymph and the Lymphomyeloid Complex.
    Academic Press, New York, 1970, p. 714.

CHAPTER 15

MULTIPLE MYELOMA AND OTHER LYMPHOCYTE AND PLASMA CELL DYSCRASIAS

The spectrum of lymphocyte and plasma cell disorders in man is broad, and includes the congenital and hereditary immune deficiency defects, malignant neoplasms of lymphocytes and plasma cells, and many other acquired nonmalignant disorders.

ACQUIRED DISORDERS OF LYMPHOCYTES AND PLASMA CELLS ASSOCIATED WITH MONOCLONAL GAMMOPATHY

Malignant neoplasms of lymphocytes and plasma cells that are characterized by an increased production of a homogeneous immunoglobulin molecule or an immunoglobulin subunit (e.g., light chains, heavy chain fragments) are often referred to as primary malignant gammopathies (Table 15–1). The homogeneous proteins appear as a monoclonal spike ("M" spike) on serum or urinary electrophoresis (Fig. 15–1). These disorders include multiple myeloma, plasmacytoma, Waldenström's macroglobulinemia, the heavy chain diseases, and probably primary amyloidosis (Table 15–1). Occasionally, other malignant lymphocyte disorders (chronic lymphocytic leukemia and the malignant lymphomas) may be associated with an "M" spike in the serum (Chapters 12 and 13).

Many nonmalignant diseases also may be associated with increased numbers of plasma cells or lymphocytes in the bone marrow and an "M" spike in the

537

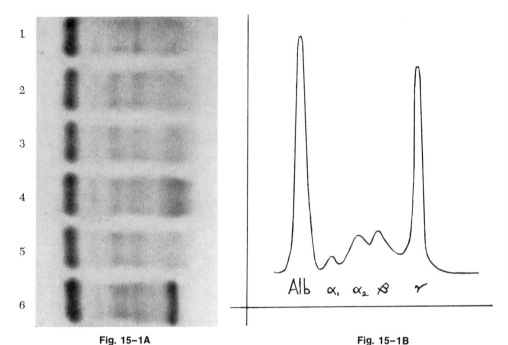

Fig. 15–1A   **Fig. 15–1B**

Figure 15–1A   Electrophoresis on cellulose acetate sheet. Note the heavy broad gamma fraction typical of a polyclonal gammopathy in no. 4, and compare to the heavy sharp gamma fraction in no. 6 which is typical of a monoclonal gammopathy.

Figure 15–1B   Quantitative analysis of the various fractions separated by electrophoresis may be obtained by the use of a densitometer, the main components of which are a photoelectric cell and galvanometer. This is the densitometer record of the electrophoretic pattern of serum no. 6 in *A*. The areas under the curves may be determined by planimetry, by weighing, or by an automatic integrator attached to the densitometer.

serum or urine (Table 15–1). Plasmacytosis on bone marrow examination and an "M" spike in the serum also are seen in the absence of any detectable underlying disease ("benign" monoclonal gammopathy) (Table 15–1).

MULTIPLE MYELOMA

Multiple myeloma is an unusual and interesting disease in many respects. Although the symptoms and findings on physical examination often are nonspecific, striking abnormalities are seen characteristically on roentgenologic and laboratory examination. Recent advances in diagnostic techniques have served to broaden the interest in multiple myeloma and related plasma cell and lymphocyte disorders. Intensive study has contributed both to a better understanding of the disease process, and to an understanding of the synthesis, structure, and genetics of normal gamma globulins.

Historic Aspects

Multiple myeloma was first reported in 1847 in a tradesman who presented with "mollities ossium" (soft bones) and urine containing large quantities of "animal matter." The patient was studied by Drs. MacIntyre and Watson, and a urine specimen was sent to Dr. Henry Bence Jones with the following note:[7]

Saturday, Nov. 1st, 1845

Dear Dr. Jones: The tube contains urine of very high specific gravity. When boiled it becomes slightly opaque. On the addition of nitric acid, it effervesces, assumes a reddish hue, and becomes quite clear; but as it cools, assumes the consistence and appearance which you see. Heat reliquefies it. What is it? . . .

Dr. Bence Jones described the peculiar properties of the unusual urinary protein which bears his name.[7] The name "multiple myeloma" was given to the disorder by von Rustizky in 1873.[6] Prior to 1900 it was thought that different cellular types were responsible for the tumor in different individuals. In 1900 Dr. James H. Wright established that the myeloma cell is related to the plasma cell, and concluded that the neoplasm arises from an abnormal proliferation of these cells.[136] These conclusions have been confirmed many times, particularly since the introduction of marrow aspiration by Arinkin in 1929.[3]

Pathogenesis and Pathologic Physiology

Many of the present concepts of the pathogenesis of multiple myeloma and other malignant plasma cell disorders have come from studies of the inducible immunoglobulin-secreting plasmacytomas in certain inbred strains of mice.[101] Most of the clinical features of the disease are attributable either to the infiltration of the bone marrow by the malignant plasma cells, to the effects of the tumor products (monoclonal immunoglobulins and subunits), or to abnormalities in host defense (e.g., hypogammaglobulinemia).[95] Although multiple myeloma appears to be primarily a diffuse disorder of the bone marrow, solitary intraosseous and extramedullary plasma cell tumors (plasmacytomas) do occur.[118]

The skeletal lesions characteristically are osteolytic, and involve sites of red marrow (e.g., ribs, sternum, vertebrae, skull, pelvic girdle). The patient usually will demonstrate multiple areas of involvement at time of diagnosis. In some patients, diffuse osteoporosis without discrete osteolytic lesions is seen; rarely, a patient will present with solitary or multiple osteosclerotic bone lesions.[118, 128] The mechanism of the bone resorption that leads to these osteolytic lesions was thought to be due to the pressure effect of the proliferating neoplastic plasma cells. Recent evidence, however, indicates that some malignant plasma cells secrete an osteoclast stimulating factor which probably contributes to the increased bone resorption.[90] Several of the clinical features of the disease are a direct result of the increased osteoclastic activity. These include bone pain, pathologic fractures, and a variety of symptoms secondary to hypercalcemia and hypercalciuria (e.g., nausea, vomiting, polyuria, polydipsia, lethargy, confusion, delirium, coma).

The monoclonal immunoglobulins or subunits that are synthesized and secreted by the neoplastic plasma cells are often referred to as abnormal proteins or paraproteins. Most studies, however, indicate that they are normal antibodies or subunits produced in excess by a clone of malignant plasma cells.[95] In the usual case of multiple myeloma, all the malignant plasma cells synthesize excessive amounts of only one of the two classes of L chains, and only one of the five

Table 15–1   *Acquired Disorders Associated with Monoclonal Gammopathy*

Clinical Disorders	Cytology of Cell Producing the Monoclonal Immunoglobulin	L-Chain Class	H-Chain Class	Urine Protein*	Serum M-Component	Relative Incidence‡
A. *Primary Malignant Monoclonal Gammopathies*						
1. Multiple Myeloma						
IgG	plasma cell	κ or λ	IgG	BJP (+) or (−)	IgG	50%
IgA	plasma cell	κ or λ	IgA	BJP (+) or (−)	IgA	22%
IgD	plasma cell	κ or λ	IgD	BJP (+) or (−)	IgD	<1%
IgE	plasma cell	κ or λ	IgE	BJP (+) or (−)	IgE	<1%
IgM	plasma cell	κ or λ	IgM	BJP (+)	IgM	<1%
Light Chain	plasma cell	κ or λ	none	BJP (+)	none	12%
Combined Monoclonal Gammopathies (biclonal, triclonal, etc.)	plasma cell	κ or λ	two or more	BJP (+) or (−)	two or more	<1%
2. Waldenström's Macroglobulinemia	Lymphocyte (Plasmacytoid)	κ or λ	IgM	BJP (+) or (−)	IgM	12%
3. Heavy Chain Disease						
IgG	plasma cell	none	IgG	IgG Fc-like fragment	IgG Fc-like fragment	<1%
IgA	plasma cell	none	IgA	IgA Fc-like fragment	IgA Fc-like fragment	<1%
IgM	plasma cell	none	IgM	κ–BJP§	IgM Fc-like fragment	<1%
IgD and IgE						not described to date
4. Plasmacytoma‖	plasma cell	κ or λ	either	BJP (+) or (−)	either	unknown
5. Amyloidosis¶	plasma cell	κ or λ	either	BJP (+) or (−)	either	unknown

6. Chronic Lymphocytic Leukemia	lymphocyte	κ or λ	either	BJP (+) or (−) usually (−)	either	unknown
7. Malignant Lymphoma	lymphocyte	κ or λ	either	"	either	unknown
B. *Secondary Monoclonal Gammopathies* 1. Associated with other Neoplasms (carcinomas, etc.)	**	κ or λ	either	BJP (+) or (−) usually (−)	either	unknown
2. Associated with Other Non-Neoplastic Disorders Cold Agglutinin Disease	plasma cell (lymphocyte ?)	κ	IgM	BJP (+) or (−) usually (−)	IgM	unknown
Lichen Myxedematous	"	λ	IgG	"	IgG	unknown
Pyoderma Gangrenosum	"	κ or λ	IgA	"	IgA	unknown
Gaucher's Disease	"	κ or λ	IgG	"	IgG	unknown
Connective Tissue Disorders	"	κ or λ	either	"	either	unknown
Autoimmune Disease	"	κ or λ	either	"	either	unknown
Others (chronic infections, liver disease, drug reactions, etc.)	"	κ or λ	either	"	either	unknown
C. *Benign Monoclonal Gammopathy*	plasma cell	κ or λ	either	BJP (+) or (−) usually (−)	either	1–2% (?)

*Normally 50–200 mg. of protein are excreted per 24 hours. Physical exercise may increase this sixfold. Only about 25% of the protein is albumin. The majority of the other proteins are immunoglobulins (IgG and IgA), light chains (κ or λ), Fc fragments, and probably other incomplete molecules.[103]

‡From Mattioli, C., and Tomasi, T. B., Jr.[82]

§An IgM Fc-like fragment has been demonstrated in the urine of only one of seven patients.[42]

||Solitary or multiple, intraosseous or extramedullary.

¶The major constituent of amyloid deposits in tissue in primary amyloidosis and in amyloidosis seen in association with multiple myeloma is a polypeptide with an amino acid sequence resembling the V_L region of κ or λ light chains. In secondary amyloidosis the major component is a polypeptide referred to as acid-soluble protein (A-protein) which is apparently of nonimmunoglobulin origin.[25, 45]

**In these secondary gammopathies it is not clear whether the M component is synthesized by the malignant cell involved or by the reactive plasmacytosis that often accompanies these neoplasms.

classes of H chains (Table 15–1). Most of the L and H chains are assembled by the malignant plasma cells and secreted as a complete immunoglobulin molecule. In more than 50 per cent of cases, however, the rate of synthesis of L chains exceeds that of H chains. These excess L chains are secreted by the cells as monomers or dimers. They usually do not accumulate in the serum, but are excreted by the kidney and appear in the urine as dimers of either κ or λ light chains (Bence Jones proteins). In approximately 12 per cent of cases, only L chains are synthesized and secreted by the malignant plasma cells ("Light chain" or "Bence Jones" myeloma) (Table 15–1). The prolonged excretion of Bence Jones protein in the urine, which may exceed 20 to 30 gm. per 24 hours in some patients, often results in renal failure ("myeloma kidney").[139] Apparently the light chains are not specifically toxic to the renal tissue but are precipitated in the tubular lumen, and result in the eventual loss of the proximal nephron unit. On histologic examination, the precipitated protein appears as intraluminal casts in the distal and convoluted renal tubules. The tubules are dilated and their epithelium is flattened; multinucleated giant cells may also be seen at the periphery of the casts. In addition to L chains, the casts also may contain amyloid fibrils,[75] a finding not too surprising in view of the molecular structure of amyloid seen in association with multiple myeloma.[25, 45] Whole immunoglobulin molecules also are frequently demonstrated in the casts. Renal tubular reabsorption defects like those seen in adult Fanconi syndrome probably are due to the renal casts.[36] Renal failure may also result from hypercalcemia, infection, and amyloid depostion in glomeruli, all of which are frequent findings in patients with multiple myeloma.[139]

The accumulation in the plasma of the monoclonal immunoglobulins and subunits also is responsible for many of the clinical features of the disease. The signs and symptoms seen in any given patient depend not only on the plasma concentration of the monoclonal proteins, but also on the physicochemical and antigenic properties of the particular immunoglobulin or subunit. The development of the hyperviscosity syndrome depends primarily on the plasma concentration of the monoclonal protein. However, the intrinsic viscosity and aggregation properties of the monoclonal immunoglobulin are also important. This syndrome is seen most frequently (85 to 90 per cent of cases) when the M-component is IgM, and is related to the high intrinsic viscosity property of this immunoglobulin.[12] The next most common class of immunoglobulin associated with the hyperviscosity syndrome is IgA, and is due to the tendency of IgA monomers to polymerize with increasing plasma concentration.[12,132] The hyperviscosity syndrome also is seen with IgG myeloma, and in most instances is the result of a very high plasma concentration of IgG. Some IgG subclasses (IgGl and IgG3), however, may have either a high intrinsic viscosity or an increased tendency to aggregate and be associated with the hyperviscosity syndrome at lower plasma concentrations.[16, 78, 104]

Other monoclonal immunoglobulins reversibly precipitate or gel at low temperatures and produce symptoms related to increased sensitivity to cold.[49] These proteins are referred to as cryoimmunoglobulins or cryoglobulins, and are usually IgM, IgG, or IgM-IgG complexes; monoclonal cold precipitable IgA and Bence Jones proteins also have been reported.[49] Symptoms related to these circulating cryoglobulins include purpura (particularly in those areas

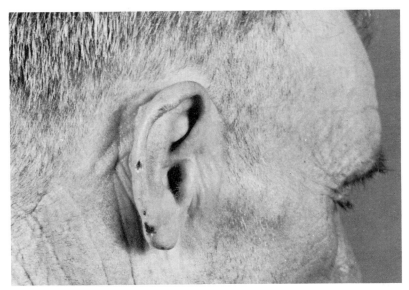

Figure 15–2 Ear of a patient with multiple myeloma complicated by cryoglobulinemia, showing ulceration and scarring.

where the temperature is low) (Fig. 15–2), acrocyanosis, Raynaud's phenomenon, cold urticaria, ulcer, and even gangrene of extremities.[49, 70]

Other hemostatic abnormalities occur frequently in multiple myeloma and are the result of several mechanisms.[72] Thrombocytopenia is a frequent finding, particularly late in the course of the disease and following chemotherapy. Impaired platelet aggregation and function may occur, and is thought to be secondary to coating of the platelet by the monoclonal immunoglobulins.[72] These monoclonal proteins have also been reported to complex with various coagulation factors (i.e., factors V, VII, VIII, prothrombin, fibrinogen) and cause bleeding. In some instances, the immunoglobulins have antigenic specificity for the coagulation factors (i.e., factor VIII, fibrin).[95]

Infection, especially with encapsulated bacteria (e.g., the pneumococcus), is a common complication and a major cause of death in multiple myeloma.[70, 123, 127] The increased susceptibility to infection is attributable to several factors which include low levels of normal immunoglobulins, impairment in the primary humoral immune response,[54] granulocytopenia, and defective granulocyte function.[99] The decrease in plasma concentration of normal immunoglobulins, which is a characteristic finding in myeloma, is due both to a decreased production and an increased catabolic rate of normal immunoglobulins.[53, 120] The granulocytopenia is secondary to a decrease in production in most instances, either the result of bone marrow replacement by malignant plasma cells or a complication of treatment. The frequent occurrence of pathologic fractures, particularly rib fractures which tend to impair ventilation, and the therapeutic use of immunosuppressive agents also contribute to the increased rate of infections in these patients.

The anemia in multiple myeloma may be the result of several mechanisms. A decreased red cell production is a factor in most patients, especially late in the course of the disease and following treatment.[23] Recently, another factor, dilution of the red cell mass, has been shown to be important.[11, 56, 57, 66] The colloid osmotic effect produced by the hyperglobulinemia appears to be the most likely cause of the increase in plasma volume and dilution of the red cell mass. Plasmapheresis produces a decrease in the "M" protein concentration, with a resultant decrease in plasma volume and an increase in the peripheral hematocrit.[57]

Amyloidosis is found in 6 to 15 per cent of patients with multiple myeloma. The distribution and structural characteristics of the amyloid material is similar to that seen in primary amyloidosis.[25, 45, 63, 75, 139] The deposition of amyloid is responsible for certain clinical features of the disease, e.g., renal failure, neuropathy.[8, 139] Amyloidosis is especially common in IgD myeloma.[64]

Clinical Manifestations

Multiple myeloma occurs in all races and has been reported from all parts of the world. The incidence in black Americans is twice that in Caucasians.[84, 85] Males probably are affected more frequently than females.[70, 96] The incidence of reported cases continues to rise, probably owing to the increased use of serum protein electrophoresis both as a screening and diagnostic test, and the wider use of bone marrow aspiration.[71, 85] Multiple myeloma accounts for approximately one per cent of malignant diseases and 10 per cent of hematologic malignancies.[70] The death rate from multiple myeloma in the United States is about two to three per 100,000 population.[70] It is characteristically a disease of older persons. Although cases have been reported in patients less than 20 years of age, 98 per cent of patients in one large series were over the age of 40 at diagnosis.[70]

The commonest presenting symptom is pain, which is due to the presence of the characteristic skeletal lesions; about 70 per cent of patients will present with bone pain as the initial symptom.[70] The vertebrae and ribs are the most frequent sites of involvement, and compression fractures of vertebrae and pathologic rib fractures are common.[118] Pathologic fractures of the femur, sternum, ilium, humerus, clavicle, and pubic bones occur less often. In some patients the discomfort is mild and poorly localized, but in others the occurrence of a fracture is accompanied by sudden onset of severe pain. Root symptoms secondary to compression fracture of vertebrae are common; cord compression and paraplegia also may develop. Pain without fracture occurs commonly in the low back, neck, hips, legs, shoulders, and arms, but headache secondary to osteolytic lesions in the skull, which are a hallmark of the disease, is rare.

Fever, secondary to bacterial infection, is the second most common presenting symptom. Pneumonia is the most frequent infection, although pyelonephritis, septicemia, and meningitis are not uncommon. The most frequent causative agents are the *Diplococcus pneumoniae*, *Staphylococcus aureus*, and *E. coli*;[38] a recent report indicates that gram-negative organisms are isolated most often in hospitalized patients with myeloma.[89]

Other presenting symptoms include those related to renal failure, anemia (i.e., weakness and easy fatigue), hemostatic abnormalities (i.e., easy bruising, bleeding), and weight loss.

Renal insufficiency is a common manifestation of multiple myeloma, occurring at some time during the course of the disease in at least 50 per cent of cases;[32, 80, 113, 128] 30 per cent of patients die as a result of renal failure. The onset of renal failure is usually insidious, but acute renal failure is not uncommon.[33] Pyelonephritis, hypercalcemia, and mechanical obstruction of the renal tubules by precipitated Bence Jones proteins are the most frequent causes of renal failure.[80, 113, 139] Other factors include amyloidosis, hyperviscosity, hyperuricemia, and plasma cell infiltration of the kidneys. Acute renal failure has been reported following intravenous pyelography; the etiology is unclear, but dehydration and the presence of Bence Jones protein in the urine are the most frequent common denominators.[73, 93] In a recent report hypercalcemia was the most common cause of acute renal failure.[33]

In addition to symptoms associated with nerve root or spinal cord compression (i.e., radicular pain, paraplegia), other clinical neurologic syndromes are seen and may dominate the clinical course of the disease. Encephalopathy secondary to hypercalcemia and/or hyperviscosity is one of the most striking manifestations encountered, and constitutes a medical emergency when present.[12, 37] Peripheral neuropathy (usually due to amyloid deposition), multifocal leukoencephalopathy, and many other neurologic complications have been reported.[118, 128]

The physical examination may disclose nothing more than is usually found in patients of the same age-group. Pallor and evidence of weight loss are the most common findings. Local swelling and tenderness on pressure over the areas of osseous involvement are important diagnostic signs. Palpation should be gentle in these patients. One of the authors once had the experience of producing a fracture of the sternum while testing for sternal tenderness, and then produced another in the humerus when he helped the patient change position. Also among the common signs are those associated with compression of the nerve roots or spinal cord. Palpable enlargement of the liver is reported to occur in from 26 to 40 per cent of patients, and splenomegaly in from 5 to 23 per cent.[1, 70, 119, 126] Lymphadenopathy is detected in approximately 4 per cent.[70] Other palpable tumor masses are seen only in a minority of patients, and then usually only in the later stages of the disease.[98, 118]

Laboratory Examination

Abnormalities of the skeleton demonstrable by x-ray constitute one of the most characteristic features of multiple myeloma. The most typical changes are the presence of multiple, clearly defined, punched-out lesions that involve several different bones (Fig. 15–3). The size of the lesions varies from a diameter of 1 or 2 mm. to areas as large as 10 to 12 cm.; the lesions are characterized by the absence of osteoblastic reaction.[55, 119] In some patients such definite lesions are absent and roentgenograms show only generalized demineralization, similar to that seen in senile or postmenopausal osteoporosis. In both types of lesions pathologic fractures, particularly compression fractures of the verte-

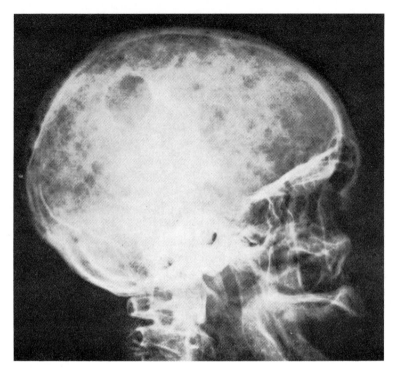

Figure 15–3 Roentgenogram of a patient with multiple myeloma showing the characteristic "punched-out" lesions.

bral bodies, are common. Lesions occur most commonly in the spine, ribs, skull, sternum, and clavicle; lesions of the distal extremities are less common. Since the advent of sternal puncture and more detailed study of the plasma proteins as diagnostic measures, it has become evident that some patients, perhaps 5 to 12 per cent, with undoubted myeloma have no demonstrable skeletal lesions at the time diagnosis is made.[6, 55, 74, 118, 119, 128, 131]

Many abnormalities occur in the peripheral blood in patients with multiple myeloma. Anemia, usually of moderate severity, is one of the commonest features and is rarely absent throughout the course of the disease; it is usually normochromic and normocytic. Occasionally, iron deficiency (secondary to blood loss) and folate deficiency (usually the result of poor nutrition) contribute to the anemia.[61] The initial leukocyte count is usually normal, but in a recent large series 16 per cent had leukopenia (leukocyte count less than 4000/mm.³) and 9 per cent had leukocytosis (leukocyte count greater than 10,000/mm.³).[70] The platelet count is normal in most patients but thrombocytopenia has been reported to occur in about 13 per cent and thrombocytosis in 1 per cent.[70] Examination of smear of the peripheral blood may suggest the diagnosis because of the presence of rouleaux formation of erythrocytes. Plasma cells are observed on differential count in approximately 15 per cent of patients;[70] the percentage probably is much higher if buffy coat preparations are studied.[44] The number of plasma cells in the peripheral blood may be so numerous that a diagnosis of "plasma cell leukemia" is made.[69, 105] Normoblasts and immature granulocytes (leukoerythroblastic changes) appear in the peripheral blood not infrequently, but are most likely to be seen in the advanced stage of the disease. These findings may signal the development of acute leukemia, which is being reported with increased frequency in patients whose survival is prolonged by treatment with alkylating agent therapy.[110]

Examination of bone marrow obtained by aspiration reveals a diagnostic or suspicious cell pattern in approximately 80 per cent of cases of multiple myeloma.[74] The most characteristic finding is the presence of "myeloma" cells, which may constitute from 4 to 90 per cent of the cells present.[19, 74] These cells, which vary from 15 to 40 μ in diameter, usually have a single eccentrically-placed nucleus. The chromatin pattern of the nucleus is finely divided, and often contains several small nucleoli or a single large nucleolus. Various types of inclusions are sometimes seen in the cytoplasm of myeloma cells. Some cells appear vacuolated (Mott cell) and others contain protein particles that are thought to originate in the cell. One such protein forms the Russell bodies, which appear eosinophilic with Wright's stain and sometimes resemble whole erythrocytes or fragments of erythrocytes. Other cells contain protein particles which have a bluish color when stained with Wright's stain; still others contain definite protein crystals (Fig. 15–4). In many patients the typical "myeloma" cells are not seen, but instead there is a large increase in cells that appear morphologically to be mature plasma cells. It is unusual to find more than 30 to 40 per cent plasma cells in the marrow in any disease other than multiple myeloma and primary amyloidosis. Less pronounced increases in the marrow plasma cells occur in other malignancies and in a number of nonmalignant disorders (Table 15–1).[20, 82, 132, 137]

A serum M-component demonstrable by electrophoresis or immunoelectrophoresis occurs in about 85 per cent of patients with myeloma.[60, 70] An additional 12 per cent have Bence Jones protein demonstrable in the urine, if urinary electrophoresis and immunoelectrophoresis are performed.[60, 70] The serum "M" spike usually is found in the γ region, but may occur in the β or α_2 region. Although a pattern of this type indicates the presence of a protein abnormality most likely to be associated with multiple myeloma, such changes are not diagnostic of multiple myeloma, since they have been described in patients with a wide spectrum of malignant and nonmalignant diseases (Table 15–1). An "M" spike may occur in the absence of any clinical disease and is referred to as "benign" monoclonal gammopathy (Table 15–1). Myeloma cannot be excluded by the failure to demonstrate a paraprotein either in the serum or in the urine; cases without an "M" spike in serum or urine have been reported, but the incidence is less than 1 %.[65, 70] The total protein is found to be over 8 gm. per 100 ml. in about 72 per cent of patients.[90] The increase occurs in the globulin fraction, and may amount to 10 or 11 gm. per 100 ml.; the albumin concentration is reduced in most cases. Cryoglobulinemia, although not diagnostic of multiple myeloma, should alert the physician to the possibility of the existence of one of the malignant gammopathies.

Other abnormalities, though nonspecific, are often helpful in diagnosis. The commonest of these is a greatly elevated sedimentation rate which occurs in the vast majority of patients with multiple myeloma, particularly if the serum protein is increased. When rouleaux formation is prominent on the blood smear, the sedimentation rate is usually greatly increased. Hypercalcemia

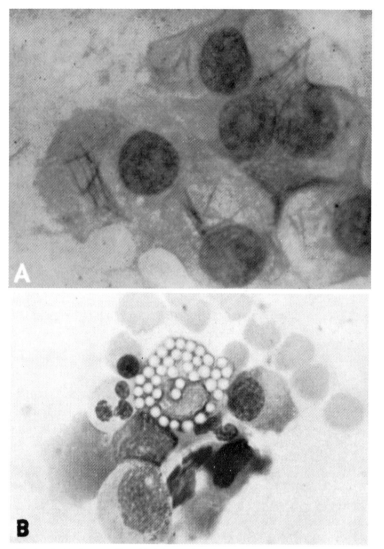

Figure 15-4 *A*, Myeloma cells with thin needle-shaped inclusion bodies which stained bright red with Wright's stain. *B*, Plasma cells containing Mott bodies; bone marrow aspiration, multiple myeloma.

is reported in from 20 to 39 per cent of patients.[6, 19, 70] Even when the calcium is markedly elevated, the levels of serum phosphorus and alkaline phosphatase are normal or only slightly elevated. Azotemia, elevated serum creatinine, and a low creatinine clearance are found initially in over 50 per cent of patients.[70] Hyperuricemia is also a frequent finding.

Diagnosis

The classic case of multiple myeloma is usually recognized without difficulty. In the middle-aged or elderly individual the occurrence of anemia and pain, particularly radicular pain associated with compression fractures of the spine, suggests the diagnosis. If increases in the level of serum globulin and Bence Jones proteinuria are demonstrated, the presence of multiple myeloma is very probable. The diagnosis is established if "myeloma" cells or greatly increased numbers of plasma cells are found in the bone marrow, together with an "M" spike on serum and/or urinary electrophoresis.

When many of the more common features of the disease are absent, or when some particular manifestation dwarfs the other features, the diagnosis may be more difficult. In older persons multiple myeloma must be considered in the differential diagnosis of any unexplained anemia, particularly if proteinuria is present. The diagnosis also should be considered in patients whose roentgenograms show osteoporosis or lytic lesions of the skeleton; the absence of osteoblastic changes, involvement of multiple vertebral bodies, involvement of the skull, and particularly the mandible, are all points that favor the diagnosis of multiple myeloma. Some patients with this disease come under observation first because of renal insufficiency, uremia, anemia, and proteinuria, and for this reason the diagnosis should be considered in all middle-aged or older persons with these manifestations. Not infrequently the patient consults a physician because of radicular pain, paraplegia, or some other neurologic difficulty, and attention may first be focused on the nervous system. The diagnosis of multiple myeloma is often missed in patients who present with recurrent infections (e.g., pneumonia). If the disease is present, the diagnosis can nearly always be established by careful study of the bone marrow and electrophoretic analysis of the serum and urine. All three of these examinations are usually abnormal if multiple myeloma is present; failure to demonstrate plasmacytosis on bone marrow examination and an "M" spike in the serum and/or urine practically excludes the disease from further consideration. The diagnosis is most difficult in those patients who present with generalized osteoporosis, an "M" spike in the serum or urine, and a mild degree of plasmacytosis in the bone marrow (less than 20 per cent mature plasma cells). Some of these patients have been followed for ten years or more without progression in symptoms or laboratory abnormalities, and have been referred to as "pseudomyeloma."[79] If the patient is symptomatic (i.e., there is bone pain), the decision to treat as a case of myeloma with radiotherapy, chemotherapy, or both becomes even more difficult. The differential diagnosis between "benign" monoclonal gammopathy and overt myeloma is also a difficult one, usually made only after a long period of observation.

Course and Prognosis

The course of multiple myeloma varies greatly. A small percentage of patients lead active lives relatively free from symptoms for a period of years without specific treatment.[118] Prior to the use of alkylating agents, however, the median survival from onset of symptoms was 15 to 17 months, and less than 12 months from time of diagnosis.[6, 70, 92, 118] With the use of alkylating agents alone or in combination with corticosteroids, the median survival has increased three to sevenfold from onset of therapy.[39] Approximately 70 per cent of patients will show an objective response to chemotherapy (i.e., a decrease of 50 per cent or more in the concentration of M-component in the serum or urine, a decrease in percentage of plasma cells in the bone marrow). The median survival for the responders is now between 24 and 50 months, but that of the non-responders is still less than 12 months.[9, 14, 39, 51, 125] Evidence also indicates that the "slow responders" have a much better prognosis than the "fast responders" (patients who demonstrate a rapid drop in concentration of the M-component with initiation of chemotherapy).[14, 51, 59, 125]

In most reports the single most important poor risk indicator is an elevated blood urea nitrogen or serum creatinine at the time of diagnosis.[59, 87, 21, 125] Other factors, including the amount of M-component present in the serum or urine, the degree of anemia, and the specific class of the M-component, may also be important in predicting prognosis.[48, 59, 132] Recently, a clinical staging system for multiple myeloma has been developed which is based primarily on a calculation of the mass of malignant plasma cells from serial measurements of the M-component concentration.[35] The approach is now being employed to plan and evaluate therapy, and predict prognosis.

Finally, an increasing number of long-term survivors who have received alkylating agents as maintenance are developing acute granulocytic leukemia.[110] Although other hematopoietic malignancies may occur more frequently in patients with multiple myeloma than in the general population, the long-term use of alkylating agents is thought to be an important etiologic factor.

Treatment

Treatment of multiple myeloma has improved greatly with the use of alkylating agents. A majority of patients can now expect a remission in their disease with prolongation of a comfortable and useful life. General measures such as maintenance of ambulation and adequate hydration, immobilization for painful skeletal lesions or pathologic fractures, employment of back braces for vertebral involvement, and the use of analgesics add greatly to the comfort of patients.

A variety of chemical agents have been used in the treatment of multiple myeloma in the past. Nitrogen mustard, TEM, radioactive phosphorus, stilbamidine, and urethan have all proved to be unsatisfactory.[19, 123]

Melphalan (L-phenylalanine mustard, Alkeran), alone or in combination with prednisone, has been highly effective in the treatment of multiple myeloma.[14, 39, 125] Melphalan may be given either continuously or intermittently. The response rate and median survival is probably the same with either method.[14, 39, 51, 83, 121, 125] When continuous therapy is employed, a loading dose of melphalan usually is given over a period of several days, and followed immediately or after a rest period by continuous maintenance therapy with melphalan at a reduced dose as tolerated.[39] The loading dose is usually 8 to 10 mg. per day for seven to ten days; the dose is then reduced to 2 mg. daily as tolerated for maintenace.

When used intermittently, melphalan is usually given in combination with prednisone.[39] We prefer the intermittent regimen; melphalan 0.25 mg./kg./day for four days and concurrent prednisone 2.0 mg./kg./day for four days are given by mouth every six weeks for six courses.[2] Maintenance usually consists of repeating the four-day course of melphalan and prednisone at lower doses every two or three months as tolerated. Bone marrow toxicity is usually the only major complication of melphalan therapy.[107]

Cyclophosphamide (Cytoxan), also an alkylating agent, is probably as effective as melphalan in the treatment of multiple myeloma.[39, 67, 86, 107] Intermittent and continuous therapy regimens are used. We usually give the drug in combination with prednisone on an intermittent schedule; cyclophosphamide, 250 mg./M²/day, and prednisone, 100 mg./M²/day, are given by mouth for four days every three weeks for six courses. Maintenance consists of repeating the four-day course of both drugs every one to two months.[9] In addition to bone marrow toxicity, hemorrhagic cystitis and bladder fibrosis are potential serious side-effects of cyclophosphamide therapy. In this regard, an adequate fluid intake is essential, especially when this treatment is given intermittently in high doses.

Although both melphalan and cyclophosphamide are alkylating agents, patients who fail to respond initially, or who become resistant to one drug after an initial good response, may achieve a good response to the other.[9, 10, 39]

Prednisone is not a very effective agent when used alone,[81] but intermittent high dose prednisone therapy may be helpful in patients who cannot tolerate alkylating agents because of bone marrow suppression.[112] When used in combination with an alkylating agent, it probably has a synergistic effect.[2, 39]

Other drugs such as BCNU and CCNU are now being tested in the treatment of multiple myeloma.[39]

Radiation therapy has an important place in the treatment of patients with multiple myeloma. When therapy is directed toward specific lesions, pain is often relieved promptly and spontaneous fractures may heal more rapidly. Most patients with the disease require local radiotherapy for painful bone lesions or pathologic fractures during its course. The use of radiation must be kept to a minimum to avoid the development of bone marrow suppression, which interferes with effective chemotherapy.

The management of hypercalcemia must be prompt and vigorous. A high parenteral fluid intake to promote a urinary output of at least 2000 ml./day is the most important therapeuic measure. In patients who fail to respond rapidly (within 24 hours) to parenteral fluids, the addition of prednisone, 50 to 100 mg./day, usually results in a prompt fall in serum calcium level. Diuretics such as thiazides and furosemide are helpful, but must be given in association with saline infusions to maintain fluid balance.[124] The intravenous infusion of phosphate may occasionally be necessary in resistant cases.[47] Although the hypocalcemic effect is usually prompt, this method of therapy should be used only in resistant cases; serum calcium levels must be measured frequently to prevent complications associated with hypocalcemia. Mithramycin also is an effective agent in the treatment of hypercalcemia and hypercalciuria.[121a]

Hyperuricemia should be treated with fluids and allopurinol (300 to 600 mg./day). Hyperviscosity is best treated by plasmapheresis and hydration. Infection should be treated promptly with appropriate antibiotic therapy. Prophylactic use of antibiotics and gamma globulin is of little, if any, value.[111] Acute renal failure has been successfully treated with dialysis while the effect of chemotherapy is awaited. When the plasma volume is expanded and the hematocrit is low, congestive heart failure may develop and necessitate plasmapheresis.

The effect of sodium fluoride on calcium metabolism in multiple myeloma has been under study recently to determine if it might have a place in the treatment of bone lesions. Following the administration of this salt, a coarsening of bone trabeculae has been noted by histologic and radiographic studies.[17] Calcium balance has become progressively more positive and the bone crystal appears to be more stable.[29, 91] Patients with severe bone pain may be relieved.[28] A recent report, however, indicated that no beneficial effect could be demonstrated with the administration of sodium fluoride.[52] Its use is not recommended.

Illustrative Case

CASE 1   MULTIPLE MYELOMA

A 56-year-old white man was admitted to the University of Virginia Hospital with a six-week history of pain in the mid-portion of his back.

Physical examination.   Vital signs were normal. There was tenderness to pressure in the mid-portion of the back with radiation of pain around the chest wall bilaterally, at about the level of D-8.

Laboratory studies.   Hematocrit was 36%; leukocyte, platelet, and differential counts were normal. Urinalysis was normal; results of the qualitative test for Bence Jones protein were negative. BUN was 14 mg. %, creatinine 0.9 mg. %, calcium 8.8 mg. %, phosphorus 3.6 mg. %, uric acid 5.8 mg. %, and alkaline phosphatase 2.8 Bodansky units. Total serum protein was 8.2 gm. %; serum protein electrophoresis revealed an albumin of 3.4 gm. %, α_1 globulin 0.3 gm. %, α_2 globulin 0.9 gm. %, β globulin 0.7 gm. %, and an "M" spike in the γ region of 2.9 gm. %. On immunoelectrophoresis a dense band was noted in the IgG region which measured 6000 mg. % (normal range 300 to 1600); IgA was 41 mg. % (normal range 150 to 400), and IgM 18 mg. % (normal range 50 to 200). Result of test for serum cryoglobulins was negative. Bone marrow aspiration revealed 18 % mature plasma cells. Roentgenograms of the vertebrae demonstrated a lytic process with a compression fracture of D-8.

Treatment and course.   The patient was fitted with a Taylor-type spine brace and given analgesics for pain. He was given 3500 rads to an area from D-5 to D-11 through a posterior port over a three-week period. At the end of two weeks he was ambulating without pain, and was able to discontinue the use of the back brace after three months. After completion of radiotherapy, the patient was placed on a chemotherapy regimen which consisted of oral Alkeran, 0.25 mg./kg./day, and oral prednisone, 2.0 mg./kg./day, for four days every six weeks for six courses. At completion of the six courses of Alkeran and prednisone, the monoclonal IgG level had dropped to 2200 mg. %. Maintenance therapy consisted of intermittent Alkeran and prednisone for four days every six to eight weeks. One year later the IgG level was 1400 mg. %.

The patient was asymptomatic and worked as an automobile salesman for the next 4½ years. He then developed progressive weakness, easy fatigue, and weight loss. On re-evaluation the hematocrit was 21%, WBC 2200/mm.³, and platelet count 101,000/mm.³ A repeat bone marrow aspiration and biopsy revealed a hypercellular marrow with an increase in all elements, but only 2.5 % mature plasma cells. Iron stain demonstrated many "ringed sideroblasts" diagnostic of sideroblastic anemia. Total serum protein was 6.9 gm. %; on electrophoresis the "M" spike had decreased to 1.3 gm. %.

The patient was thought to have a preleukemic condition and was given a two-month trial of oxymetholone, 100 mg./day, without benefit. During this two-month period he required packed red cell transfusions to maintain the hematocrit; WBC dropped to 1100/mm.³, and platelet count to 5000/mm.³; differential count (%): blast forms 3, promyelocytes 1, myelocytes 4, metamyelocytes 4, bands 5, segmented forms 48, lymphocytes 30, and 1 nucleated red blood cell. Bone marrow findings were unchanged except for megaloblastic changes in the red cell precursors. He also developed daily temperature elevations to 40° C. Studies failed to reveal an infectious etiology for the fever.

A regimen was started consisting of vincristine (Oncovin), 2.0 mg. intravenously weekly, and oral prednisone, 100 mg./day. Over the next four weeks he improved, and WBC increased to 3500/mm.³, hematocrit to 35%, and platelet count to 117,000/mm.³ Maintenance therapy will consist of daily 6'-mercaptopurine and weekly methotrexate; reinforcement therapy, consisting of one intravenous injection of vincristine and oral prednisone, 100 mg./day, for one week, will be given monthly.

Comments. This patient suffered back pain, which is the most frequent presenting symptom in multiple myeloma. Roentgenograms revealed a lytic process with compression fracture of D-8. There was mild anemia, and bone marrow aspiration revealed 18 % mature plasma cells. Serum protein was 8.2 gm. % and electrophoresis revealed an "M" spike in the gamma region which measured 2.9 gm. %. On immunoelectrophoresis a dense band was noted in the gamma region which measured 6000 mg. %, and was identified immunologically as IgG. No Bence Jones protein was found in the urine.

The patient showed an excellent objective response to intermittent Alkeran and prednisone therapy and has survived for a long time on maintenance Alkeran and prednisone. He has now developed a preleukemic condition, which is an increasingly frequent finding in patients treated with alkylating agents for multiple myeloma for long periods. Because of severe pancytopenia, fever, weight loss, and marked weakness he was treated according to an acute leukemia protocol, consisting of vincristine and prednisone, and has had a good initial response.

WALDENSTRÖM'S MACROGLOBULINEMIA

An increased serum concentration of a monoclonal IgM is seen with a number of clinical conditions (Table 15–1).[5] In 1944 Waldenström[129] described two patients with a malignant disorder characterized by lymphadenopathy, hepatosplenomegaly, infiltration of the bone marrow with "plasmacytoid" lymphocytes, and a marked elevation of a serum monoclonal macroglobulin.

Since then, many patients with this disorder (Waldenström's macroglobulinemia) have been described.[77, 128] The disease occurs most often in patients 50 to 70 years of age, and is somewhat more common in men. It represents about 12 per cent of the primary malignant gammopathies (Table 15–1).[82]

Clinical and Laboratory Manifestations

The clinical manifestations are very similar to those encountered in patients with chronic lymphocytic leukemia and lymphocytic lymphomas. A history of recent weight loss, weakness, lethargy, and lowered resistance to infections, and the finding of hepatosplenomegaly and slight-to-moderate lymphadenopathy, are common. Bleeding from the mucous membranes and retinal hemorrhage, usually secondary to hyperviscosity of the blood, is a frequent presenting symptom. Less commonly, Reynaud's phenomena and signs and symptoms of congestive heart failure are found.

Anemia is present in most patients at time of diagnosis, and is usually due to decreased red cell production and an increased plasma volume.[22, 57, 66] Leukocyte and platelet counts are usually normal.[77] Examination of the bone marrow aspirate reveals infiltration by cells which are difficult to classify and are frequently referred to as "lymphoplasmacytic" cells or "plasmacytoid" lymphocytes. The cells have cytoplasm like that of a plasma cell and a nucleus like that of a lymphocyte. Similar cells are seen in the lymph nodes, spleen, liver, and peripheral blood, particularly late in the course of the disease. Plasma cells and mast cells are also seen in the affected tissues. The total protein of the serum is almost always increased and associated with an elevated sedimentation rate and serum viscosity. A rather sharp peak in the beta or gamma region is found on serum electrophoresis. Immunoelectrophoresis reveals a dense IgM band.[94] On ultracentrifugation a characteristic sedimentation pattern is seen. The major component has a sedimentation coefficient of 19S with small amounts that sediment faster. The Sia water test is often positive, especially if the IgM is of γ mobility.[138] X-rays of the bones often reveal generalized demineralization, but punched-out lesions similar to those of multiple myeloma are rare.

Pathologic Physiology

The high concentration of macroglobulins in Waldenström's macroglobulinemia is the result of markedly increased synthesis of these proteins by the plasmacytoid lymphocytes found in the bone marrow, liver, lymph nodes, and spleen. Evidence suggests that Waldenström's macroglobulinemia represents an uninterrupted maturation of a malignant clone of cells from B-cells to IgM secreting plasma cells.[102, 133]

The frequent occurrence of the hyperviscosity syndrome is due to the high intrinsic viscosity properties of the circulating pentameric IgM molecules.[12] Hemorrhagic manifestations are the result of coating of platelets by the macroglobulins which interfere with platelet function[72] and the formation of complexes between macroglobulins and specific clotting factors (i.e., factor VIII).[72]

When the monoclonal IgM has properties of a cryoglobulin, symptoms and signs related to cold sensitivity develop.[49, 70] The decrease in normal gamma globulins contributes to the lowered resistance to infection.

Treatment and Prognosis

Alkylating agents (chlorambucil, melphalan, and cyclophosphamide) alone, or in combination with prednisone, are the drugs of choice in the treatment of Waldenström's macroglobulinemia.[77] The treatment schedules are similar to those employed in multiple myeloma. We prefer to use intermittent therapy which usually consists of melphalan or cyclophosphamide in combination with prednisone. An objective response (a decrease of 50 per cent or more in the serum "M" spike concentration) will occur in most patients. Plasmapheresis frequently is necessary to treat manifestations of the hyperviscosity syndrome.[12]

The median survival of patients who respond to chemotherapy is four years, compared to two years for nonresponders.[77]

HEAVY CHAIN DISEASES

The heavy chain diseases clinically are a heterogeneous group of malignant monoclonal gammopathies characterized by the presence of a monoclonal protein antigenically related to the Fc fragment of heavy chains in both the serum and urine. To date, γ-, α-, and μ- heavy chain diseases have been described.[41]

γ-Heavy Chain Disease (γ-HCD, Franklin's Disease)

Franklin described a patient with a malignant proliferative disorder of the reticuloendothelial system in whom asynchronous production of a protein which was antigenically like the Fc fragment of IgG was present as a monoclonal spike in both serum and urine.[43] Approximately 35 cases have now been reported.[41]

The clinical features resemble a malignant lymphoma rather than multiple myeloma. Lytic bone lesions have been demonstrated in only one patient. The disease appears to occur more commonly in males than in females, and only four patients have been under the age of 40 years.[41] Onset is usually insidious, with fever, lymphadenopathy, and anemia being the most common initial manifestations. Hepatosplenomegaly, marked swelling and erythema of the palate and uvula, recurrent infections, leukopenia, and thrombocytopenia also are frequent findings. Atypical lymphocytes and plasma cells often are seen in the blood smear.

The bone marrow aspirate usually reveals an increase in plasma cells, lymphocytes, and eosinophils; the bone marrow, however, may be normal.[41] Lymph node sections usually show a pleomorphic infiltration with plasma cells, lymphocytes, eosinophils, and histiocytes. Diagnosis is based on demonstration on immunoelectrophoresis of a monoclonal protein in the serum and urine which migrates in the $\gamma-\beta$ region. This protein is reactive with antisera to γ–heavy chains, but not with antisera to light chains.[41] Serum electrophoretic analysis usually reveals a broad spike in the $\gamma-\beta$ region, accompanied by hypo-gammaglobulinemia.

Treatment is unsatisfactory. The cellular infiltrates in lymph nodes and elsewhere respond temporarily to local radiotherapy. Prednisone also may be helpful. Combination drug therapy has not been evaluated adequately to date.

The length of survival is usually less than one year, but may be as long as five years. Infection is the most common cause of death.[41]

α–Heavy Chain Disease (α–HCD)

The initial patient with α–chain disease was a young Arab woman who had chronic diarrhea and malabsorption secondary to malignant lymphoma involving the entire small intestine ("Mediterranean lymphoma").[116] Fifty-nine cases have been reported.[41, 115] Unlike γ–HCD, α–HCD occurs in a younger age-group (cases have been reported in children).

In general the areas of involvement are limited to the intestine and abdominal lymph nodes; two children have been reported with involvement limited to the respiratory tract.[41, 122] The bone marrow, liver, spleen, and other lymphoid organs usually are not involved.[115] The characteristic histologic finding is a massive infiltration of the lamina propria of the intestine and abdominal lymph nodes with lymphocytes, plasma cells, and histiocytes. Clinical features are uniformly those of severe malabsorption (i.e., diarrhea, steatorrhea, hypocalcemia).

Diagnosis is made by the finding on immunoelectrophoresis of an α–heavy chain Fc-like fragment in the serum and/or urine.[41,115] The serum electrophoresis usually demonstrates marked hypogammaglobulinemia and no "M" spike. No Bence Jones protein is found in the urine.

Although complete remissions of the disease have been reported after treatment with antibiotics alone, treatment generally is unsatisfactory.[115] Responses have been reported with prednisone, cyclophosphamide, and radiotherapy.[115]

μ–Heavy Chain Disease (μ–HCD)

Seven cases of μ–HCD have been reported.[42] Six of the seven cases were patients with long-standing chronic lymphocytic leukemia (CLL). All were over the age of 40 years when the diagnosis was made. Hepatosplenomegaly was present in all seven cases; but, unlike most patients with CLL, only one had peripheral lymphadenopathy.

The disease should be suspected if vacuolated plasma cells are seen in the bone marrow, or if large amounts of κ-type Bence Jones protein are found in the urine. The serum protein electrophoresis is either normal or reveals only hypogammaglobulinemia. Diagnosis is made by the finding on immunoelectrophoresis of μ–chain Fc-like fragment in the serum (only the one patient who did not have CLL secreted this fragment in the urine).[42]

Therapeutic considerations generally do not differ from those usually encountered with CLL patients.

PLASMACYTOMA

Solitary plasma cell tumors (plasmacytomas) may be intraosseous or extramedullary.[93,117,118,128] Intraosseous plasmacytomas occur most often in the vertebrae, pelvis, and femur,[26, 118, 135] whereas 75 per cent of the extramedullary tumors occur in the submucosa of the upper respiratory tract.[114, 117, 135] These solitary tumors are generally thought to be early manifestations of multiple myeloma (2 to 10 per cent of patients with myeloma present with a solitary lesion as the only finding).[93] The interval between the appearance of the solitary tumor and the development of multiple myeloma is often many years;[26,88,117,118] in some patients dissemination has not occurred after 15 to 30 years of follow-up.[26, 88, 97] Other patients may develop multiple solitary lesions over a period of many years without dissemination to overt multiple myeloma.[118]

A thorough search for evidence of dissemination should be carried out in all patients who present with a solitary plasmacytoma. Studies should include a bone marrow aspiration, bone survey and scan, and a serum and urinary electrophoretic and immunoelectrophoretic analysis; the bone marrow aspiration should be from a site of radiographically normal bone. If no evidence of dissemination is found, the tumor should be irradiated with 4000 to 5000 rads. The patient must then be followed closely for an indefinite period. The presence of a monoclonal immunoglobulin or subunit in the serum or urine should not be considered evidence, alone, of dissemination. If the M-component fails to disappear with treatment of the solitary lesion, other solitary tumors are likely to be present, or dissemination probably has occurred.

AMYLOIDOSIS

The clinical manifestations of amyloidosis are secondary to the deposition of a homogeneous, eosinophilic material (amyloid) in various tissues throughout the body. The disease is seen most often in association with chronic infections (e.g., leprosy, tuberculosis, osteomyelitis, syphilis), and "autoimmune" disorders (e.g., rheumatoid arthritis), and is referred to as "secondary" amyloidosis.[24, 46] When amyloidosis occurs in the absence of any detectable underlying disease, it is referred to as "primary" amyloidosis. The amyloidosis which occurs in association with multiple myeloma resembles primary amyloidosis (see below). Heredofamilial forms of amyloidosis also occur. Finally, amyloid deposition, which is clinically inapparent, is seen with aging (senile amyloidosis).

The major constituent of the amyloid deposits in primary amyloidosis, and in amyloidosis seen in association with multiple myeloma, is a polypeptide with an amino acid sequence resembling the V_L region of κ or λ light chains.[45] These findings add considerable support to the concept that primary amyloidosis is a malignant plasma cell disorder.[63, 93] In secondary amyloidosis, the major component of the amyloid material is a polypeptide referred to as acid-soluble protein (A-protein), and is apparently not an immunoglobulin subunit.[25,45]

The clinical features of amyloidosis are quite variable and depend on the organs involved. The kidney is the most frequent site of involvement and potentially the most serious manifestation;[24] the nephrotic syndrome develops in 60 per cent or more of patients. Cardiac involvement is common (80 to 90 per cent), particularly in primary amyloidosis. The liver is involved in virtually all patients with both primary and secondary amyloidosis.[13] Involvement of the gastrointestinal tract, skin, and peripheral nervous system (especially in hereditary forms) is frequently seen. Purpura of eyelids, ear lobes, and periorbital areas is a particularly important diagnostic sign.

The length of survival usually is one to four years in both primary and secondary forms of the disease.[24] No effective therapy is available. In a rare case of secondary amyloidosis, the amyloid deposition may regress after successful treatment of the underlying disease.[68, 76] In a recent report, a combination of penicillamine, melphalan, prednisone, and fluoxymesterone resulted in the resolution of amyloid deposits in a patient with primary amyloidosis.[27]

SECONDARY MONOCLONAL GAMMOPATHIES

An "M" spike in the serum and/or urine is seen in association with many nonhematopoietic neoplasms (especially bowel and biliary tract neoplasms), and with many nonmalignant disorders (Table 15–1).[82, 137] The association with neoplasms may be coincidental; the "M" spike usually does not disappear with removal of the tumor. In the nonmalignant disorders the association is less likely to be coincidental. These disorders have as common features the presence of chronic inflammation and the tendency to develop hypergammaglobulinemia; a high concentration of rheumatoid factor in some patients with arthritis will appear as an "M" spike on serum electrophoresis.

BENIGN MONOCLONAL GAMMOPATHY

When an "M" spike is demonstrated on serum protein electrophoresis in the absence of any detectable underlying malignancy or chronic inflammation, the condition is referred to as "benign" monoclonal gammopathy.[128–130] In large random surveys of healthy populations, the incidence is about 1 per cent in subjects more than 25 years of age,[5] and 3 per cent in those over 70 years.[50] Others have reported an incidence of less than 0.5 per cent.[18, 40]

The diagnosis of "benign" monoclonal gammopathy usually depends on the absence of detectable skeletal lesions. Other findings that favor a benign course are a low level of M-component (less than 2 gm. per cent), little or no Bence Jones protein in the urine, normal serum levels of albumin and other immunoglobulins, and less than 20 per cent mature plasma cells in the bone marrow.[82, 100] Perhaps a better term to use initially is "idiopathic" monoclonal gammopathy. If the concentration of the M-component remains stable or decreases, and if no malignant disorder (e.g., multiple myeloma, Waldenström's macroglobulinemia) or inflammatory condition (e.g., rheumatoid arthritis) develops after many years of follow-up, the term "benign" monoclonal gammopathy is more appropriate. The percentage of patients who progress to overt malignant lymphocyte or plasma cell disorders, or who develop other malignant or nonmalignant diseases known to be associated with serum "M" spikes, is not yet known. Probably less than 25 per cent remain truly benign after five years.[30] Patients have been reported to develop multiple myeloma or Waldenström's macroglobulinemia 10 to 15 years later.[106]

HEREDITARY IMMUNE DEFICIENCY DEFECTS

Since the first report by Bruton in 1952[15] of a patient with an immunologic deficiency state associated with agammaglobulinemia, a great number of immune deficiency disorders have been described.[31, 109] The exact nature of the various defects is not completely understood, and the terminology remains confusing. In many instances, however, the approximate site of the defect in the development of the immune system is known (see Fig. 14–1 and Table 15–2).

PRIMARY STEM CELL DEFECTS

The prototype of a defect which occurs at the stem cell level is the Swiss-type agammaglobulinemia (alymphocytosis, thymic alymphoplasia).[58, 62] It is inherited both as an autosomal recessive and X-linked recessive disorder which, if untreated, usually results in death from infection during the first year of life. Patients with this disorder lack the ability to produce humoral antibody and have a marked decrease or absence of all immunoglobulins. They also have impaired cell-mediated immunity. There is usually a marked reduction of lymphocytes in the peripheral blood at varying times in the course of the illness. Examination of the bone marrow reveals a decrease in lymphocytes and an almost total absence of plasma cells. Germinal centers are not found in the lymph nodes. Tonsils, adenoids, Peyer's patches, and the plasma cell system of the lamina propria system are absent, as is the thymus.

Table 15–2 *Hereditary Immune Deficiency Defects*

1. Primary stem cell defects (i.e., Swiss-type agammaglobulinemia)

2. Primary B-cell defects (i.e., X-linked agammaglobulinemia)

3. Primary T-cell defects (i.e., congenital thymic aplasia)

PRIMARY B-CELL DEFECTS

Congenital agammaglobulinemia (X-linked agammaglobulinemia, Bruton's disease) represents a defect at the B-cell level. Patients with this disorder regularly demonstrate a marked decrease in IgG, IgM, and IgA. They either fail to form antibody, or form antibody poorly against a variety of antigens. Plasma cells are absent or markedly reduced, and germinal centers in lymphoid tissue are absent; in addition, there is absence of follicular structure in the poorly-developed Peyer's patches. The plasma cell system in the lamina propria of the intestinal tract and in the secretory glands is lacking. The number of B-cells, identifiable by surface markers, is markedly decreased in the peripheral blood and elsewhere. Thymic structure is normal, as is cell-mediated immunity.

Prompt and vigorous treatment of bacterial infections and regular injections of gamma globulin are essential.

PRIMARY T-CELL DEFECTS

Congenital thymic aplasia (DiGeorge's syndrome) is the prototype of a defect at the T-cell level.[34] In this disorder, there is a failure of development of the thymus and parathyroid glands (both derivatives of the third and fourth pharyngeal pouches). Patients develop symptoms of hypocalcemia early in life, and are unable to mount a cellular immune response. Although lymphoid stem cell precursors of T-cells are present, the antigen-independent differentiation to T-cells, which is thymus-dependent, does not occur. Thymus transplantation, which has been sucessful in some patients, results in rapid acquisition of T-cell function.[4, 21]

Familial defects also occur in the complement system,[109] and in granulocyte and monocyte function, all of which result in immune deficiency disorders (see Chapter 9).

References

1. Adams, W. S., Alling, E. L., and Lawrence, J. S.: Multiple myeloma. Am. J. Med., 6:141, 1949.
2. Alexanian, R., Haut, A., Khan, A. U., Lane, M., McKelvey, E. M., Migliore, P. J., Stucky, W. J., Jr., and Wilson, H. E.: Treatment for multiple myeloma. J.A.M.A., 208:1680, 1969.
3. Arinkin, M. L.: Die intravitale Untersuchungsmethodik des Knochenmarks. Folia Haematol., 38:233, 1929.
4. August, C. S., Rosen, F. S., Filler, R. M., Janeway, C. A., Markowski, B., and Kay, H. E. M.: Implantation of a fetal thymus, restoring immunological competence in a patient with thymic aplasia (DiGeorge's syndrome). Lancet, 2:1210, 1968.
5. Axelsson, U., Bachmann, R., and Hällen, J.: Frequency of pathological M-components in 6,995 sera from an adult population. Acta Med. Scand., 179:235, 1966.
6. Bayrd, E. D., and Heck, J. F.: Multiple myeloma: a review of eighty-three proved cases. J.A.M.A., 133:147, 1947.
7. Bence Jones, H.: Papers on chemical pathology. Lancet, 2:88, 1847.
8. Benson, M. D., Cohen, A. S., Brandt, K. D., and Cathcart, E. S.: Neuropathy, M components and amyloid. Lancet, 1:10, 1975.
9. Bergsagel, D. E.: Plasma cell myeloma. An interpretive review. Cancer, 30:1588, 1972.
10. Bergsagel, D. E., Cowan, D. H., and Hasselback, R.: Plasma cell myeloma: response of melphalan-resistant patients to high-dose intermittent cyclophosphamide. Can. Med. Assoc. J., 107:851, 1972.
11. Bjorneboe, M.: Gamma Globulin and Colloid-Osmotic Pressure. In Killander, J. (ed.): Gamma Globulins. Nobel Symposium. Interscience Publishers, Inc., New York, 1967, p. 545.

12. Bloch, K. J., and Maki, D. G.: Hyperviscosity syndromes associated with immunoglobulin abnormalities. Semin. Hematol., *10*:113, 1973.
13. Briggs, G. W.: Amyloidosis. Ann. Intern. Med., *55*:943, 1961.
14. Brook, J., Batemen, J. R., Gocka, E. F., Nakamura, E., and Steinfield, J. L.: Long-term low dose melphalan treatment of multiple myeloma. Arch. Intern. Med., *131*:545, 1973.
15. Bruton, O. C.: Agammaglobulinemia. Pediatrics, *9*:722, 1952.
16. Capra, J. D., and Kunkel, H. G.: Aggregation of γ G3 proteins: relevance to the hyperviscosity syndrome. J. Clin. Invest., *49*:610, 1970.
17. Carbone, P. P., Zipkin, I., Sokoloff, L., Frazier, P., Cook, P., and Mullins, F.: Fluoride effect on bone in plasma cell myeloma. Arch. Intern. Med., *121*:130, 1968.
18. Carrell, R. W., Colls, B. M., and Murray, J. T.: The significance of monoclonal gammopathy in a normal population. Aust. N. Z. J. Med., *4* 398, 1971.
19. Carson, C. P., Ackerman, L. V., and Malthy, J. D.: Plasma cell myeloma. A clinical, pathologic and roentgenologic review of ninety cases. Am. J. Pathol., *25*:849, 1955.
20. Clark, H., and Muirhead, E. E.: Plasmacytosis of bone marrow. Arch. Intern. Med., *94*:425, 1954.
21. Cleveland, W. W., Fogel, B. J., Brown, W. T., and Kay, H. E. M.: Foetal thymic transplant in a case of DiGeorge's syndrome. Lancet, *2*:1211, 1968.
22. Cline, J. C., Soloman, A., Berlin, N. I., and Fahey, J. L.: Anemia in macroglobulinemia. Am. J. Med., *34*:213, 1963.
23. Cline, M. J., and Berlin, I.: Studies of the anemia of multiple myeloma. Am. J. Med., *33*:510, 1962.
24. Cohen, A. S.: Amyloidosis. N. Engl. J. Med., *277*:522, 574, 628, 1967.
25. Cohen, A. S., and Cathcart, E. S.: Amyloidosis and immunoglobulins. Adv. Intern. Med., *19*:41, 1974.
26. Cohen, D. M., Svien, H. J., and Dahlin, D. C.: Long-term survival of patients with myeloma of the vertebral column. J.A.M.A., *187*:914, 1964.
27. Cohen, H. J., Lessin, L. S., Hallal, J., and Burkholder, P.: Resolution of primary amyloidosis during chemotherapy: studies in a patient with nephrotic syndrome. Ann. Intern. Med., *82*:466, 1975.
28. Cohen, P.: Fluoride and calcium therapy for myeloma bone lesions. J.A.M.A., *198*:583, 1966.
29. Cohen, P., Nichols, G. L., and Banks, H. H.: Fluoride treatment of bone rarefaction in multiple myeloma and osteoporosis. A review. Clin. Orthop., *64*:221, 1969.
30. Cooke, K. B.: Essential paraproteinemia. Proc. Roy. Soc. Med., *62*:777, 1969.
31. Cooper, M. D., Faulk, W. P., Fudenberg, H. H., et al.: Classification of primary immunodeficiencies. N. Eng. J. Med., *288*:966, 1973.
32. Dawson, A. A., and Ogstron, D.: Factors influencing the prognosis in myelomatosis. Postgrad. Med. J., *47*:635, 1971.
33. Defronzo, R. A., Humphrey, R. L., Wright, J. R., and Cooke, C. R.: Acute renal failure in multiple myeloma. Medicine, *54*:209, 1975.
34. DiGeorge, A. M.: Discussion of Cooper, M. D., Peterson, R. D. A., and Good, R. A.: A new concept of cellular basis of immunity. J. Pediatr., *67*:907, 1965.
35. Durie, B. G. M., and Salmon, S. E.: Cellular kinetics, staging, and immunoglobulin synthesis in multiple myeloma. Annu. Rev. Med.,*26*:283, 1975.
36. Engle, R. L., and Wallis, L. A.: Multiple myeloma and the adult Fanconi syndrome. I. Report of a case with crystal-like deposits in the tumor cells and in the epithelial cells of the kidney. Am. J. Med., *22*:5, 1957.
37. Evaldsson, U., Ertekin, C., Ingvar, D. H., and Waldenström, J. G.: Encephalopathia hypercalcemia. J. Chronic Dis., *22*:431, 1969.
38. Fahey, J. L., Scoggins, R., Utz, J. P., and Szwed, C. F.: Infection, antibody response and gamma globulin components in multiple myeloma and macroglobulinemia. Am. J. Med., *35*:698, 1963.
39. Farhangi, M., and Osserman, E. F.: Treatment of multiple myeloma. Semin. Hematol., *10*:149, 1973.
40. Fine, J. M., Lambin, P., and Leroux, P.: Frequency of monoclonal gammopathy (M-components) in 13,400 sera from blood donors. Vox Sang., *23*:336, 1972.
41. Frangione, B., and Franklin, E. C.: Heavy chain diseases: clinical features and molecular significance of the disordered immunoglobulin structure. Semin. Hematol., *10*:53, 1973.
42. Franklin, E. C.: μ–chain disease. Arch. Intern. Med., *135*:71, 1975.
43. Franklin, E. C., Lowenstein, J., Bigelow, B., and Meltzer, M.: Heavy chain disease. A new disorder of serum γ–globulins. Am. J. Med., *37*:332, 1964.
44. Ginsberg, D. M.: Circulating plasma cells in multiple myeloma. Ann. Intern. Med., *57*:843, 1962.
45. Glenner, G. G., and Terry, W. D.: Characterization of amyloid. Annu. Rev. Med., *25*:131, 1974.

46. Glenner, G. G., Terry, W. D., and Isersky, C.: Amyloidosis: its nature and pathogenesis. Semin. Hematol., *10*:65, 1973.

47. Goldsmith, R. S., and Ingbar, S. H.: Inorganic phosphate treatment of hypercalcemia of diverse etiologies. N. Engl. J. Med., *274*:1, 1966.

48. Gompels, B. M., Votaw, M. L., and Martel, W.: Correlation of radiological manifestations of multiple myeloma with immunoglobulin abnormalities and prognosis. Radiology, *104*:509, 1972.

49. Grey, H. M., and Kohler, P. F.: Cryoimmunoglobulins. Semin. Hematol., *10*:87, 1973.

50. Hällen, J.: Frequency of "abnormal" serum globulins (M-components) in the aged. Acta Med. Scand., *173*:737, 1963.

51. Hansen, O. P., Jessen, B., and Videbaek, A.: Prognosis of myelomatosis on treatment with prednisone and cytostatics. Scand. J. Haematol., *10*:282, 1973.

52. Harley, J. B., Schilling, A., and Oliver, G.: Ineffectiveness of fluoride therapy in multiple myeloma. N. Engl. J. Med., *286*:1283, 1972.

53. Harris, J., and Bagai, R.: Immune deficiency states associated with malignant disease in man. Med. Clin. North Am., *56*:501, 1972.

54. Harris, J. E., Alexanian, R., Hersh, E. M., and Miglione, P.: Immune function in multiple myeloma. Impaired responsiveness to keyhole limpet hemocyanin. Can. Med. Assoc. J., *104*:389, 1971.

55. Heiser, S., and Schwartzman, J.: Variations in the roentgen appearance of the skeletal system in myeloma. Radiology, *58*:178, 1952.

56. Herreman, G., et al.: L'hypervolemic de la macroglobulinemie de Waldenström. Nouv. Rev. Fr. Hematol., *8*:209, 1968.

57. Hess, C. E., Ayers, C. R., Wetzel, R. A., and Mohler, D. N.: Mechanism of dilutional anemia in multiple myeloma. Clin. Res., *18*:41, 1970 (Abstr.).

58. Hitzig, W. H., Biro, Z., Bosch, H., and Huser, H. J.: Agammaglobulinemie und Alymphocytose mit Schwund des lymphatischen Gewebes. Helvet. Paediatr. Acta, *13*:551, 1958.

59. Hobbs, J. R.: Growth rates and responses to treatment in human myelomatosis. Br. J. Haematol., *16*:607, 1969.

60. Hobbs, J. R.: Immunochemical classes of myelomatosis. Br. J. Haematol., *16*:599, 1969.

61. Hoffbrand, A. V., Hobbs, J. R., Kremenchuzky, S., and Mollin, D. L.: Incidence and pathogenesis of megaloblastic erythropoiesis in multiple myeloma. J. Clin. Pathol., *20*:699, 1967.

62. Hoyer, J. R., Cooper, M. D., Gabrielsen, M. A., and Good, R. A.: Lymphopenic forms of congenital immunologic deficiency diseases. Medicine, *47*:201, 1968.

63. Isobe, T., and Osserman, E. F.: Patterns of amyloidosis and their association with plasma-cell dyscrasia, monoclonal immunoglobulins and Bence-Jones proteins. N. Engl. J. Med., *290*:473, 1974.

64. Jancelewicz, Z., Takatsuki, K., Sugai, S., and Pruzanski, W.: IgD multiple myeloma. Arch. Intern. Med., *135*:87, 1975.

65. Kim, I., Harley, J. B., and Weksler, B.: Multiple myeloma without initial paraproteins. Am. J. Med. Sci., *264*:267, 1972.

66. Kopp, W. L., MacKinney, A. A., and Wasson, G.: Blood volume and hematocrit value in macroglobulinema and myeloma. Arch. Intern. Med., *23*:394, 1969.

67. Korst, D. R., Clifford, G. O., Fowler, W. M., Louis, J., Will, J., and Wilson, H. E.: Multiple myeloma. II. Analysis of cyclophosphamide therapy in 165 patients. J.A.M.A., *189*:758, 1964.

68. Kuhlback, B., and Wegelius, O.: Secondary amyloidosis: a study of clinical and pathological findings. Acta Med. Scand., *180*:737, 1966.

69. Kyle, R. A., Maldonade, J. E., and Bayrd, E. D.: Plasma cell leukemia: report on 17 cases. Arch. Intern. Med., *133*:813, 1974.

70. Kyle, R. A.: Multiple myeloma: review of 869 cases. Mayo Clin. Proc., *50*:29, 1975.

71. Kyle, R. A., Nobrega, F. T., and Kurland, L. T.: Multiple myeloma in Olmstead County, Minnesota, 1945–1964. Blood, *33*:739, 1969.

72. Lackner, H.: Hemostatic abnormalities associated with dysproteinemias. Semin. Hematol., *10*:125, 1973.

73. Lasser, E. C., Lang, J. H., and Zawadzki, Z. A.: Contrast media. Myeloma protein precipitates in urography. J.A.M.A., *198*:945, 1966.

74. Lichtenstein, L., and Jaffe, H. L.: Multiple myeloma. Arch. Pathol., *44*:207, 1947.

75. Limas, C., Wright, J. R., Matsuzaki, M., and Calkins, E.: Amyloidosis and multiple myeloma. Am. J. Med., *54*:166, 1973.

76. Lowenstein, J., and Gallo, G.: Remission of the nephrotic syndrome in renal amyloidosis. N. Engl. J. Med., *282*:128, 1970.

77. MacKenzie, M. R., and Fudenberg, H. H.: Macroglobulinemia: an analysis of forty patients. Blood, *39*:874, 1972.

78. MacKenzie, M. R., Fudenberg, H. H., and O'Reilly, R. A.: The hyperviscosity syndrome. I. In IgG myeloma. The role of protein concentration and molecular shape. J. Clin. Invest., *49*:15, 1970.
79. Maldonado, J. E., Riggs, B. W., and Bayrd, E. D.: Pseudomyeloma. Arch. Intern. Med., *135*: 267, 1975.
80. Martinez-Maldondo, M., Yium, J., Suki, W. N., and Eknoyam, G.: Renal complications in multiple myeloma: pathophysiology and some aspects of clinical management. J. Chronic Dis., *24*:221, 1971.
81. Mass, R. E.: A comparison of the effect of prednisone and a placebo in the treatment of multiple myeloma. Cancer Chemother. Rep., *16*:257, 1962.
82. Mattioli, C., and Tomasi, T. B., Jr.: The human serum immunoglobulins. Dis. Month., April, 1970.
83. McArthur, J. R., Athens, J. W., Wintrobe, M. M., and Cartwright, G. E.: Melphalan and myeloma: experience with a low-dose continuous regimen. Ann. Intern. Med., *72*:665, 1970.
84. McMahon, B., and Clark, D. W.: The incidence of multiple myeloma. J. Chronic Dis., *4*:508, 1956.
85. McPhedran, P., Heath, C. W., Jr., and Garcia, J.: Multiple myeloma incidence in metropolitan Atlanta, Georgia: racial and seasonal variations. Blood, *39*:866, 1972.
86. Medical Research Council: Myelomatosis: comparison of melphalan and cyclophosphamide therapy. Br. Med. J., *1*:640, 1971.
87. Medical Research Council: Report on the first myelomatosis trial. Part I. Analysis of presenting features of prognostic significance. Br. J. Haematol., *24*:123, 1973.
88. Meyer, J. E., and Schulz, M. D.: "Solitary" myeloma of bone. Cancer, *34*:438, 1974.
89. Meyers, B. R., Hirschman, S. Z., and Axelrod, J. A.: Current patterns of infection in multiple myeloma. Am. J. Med., *52*:87, 1972.
90. Mundy, G. R., Raisz, L. G., Cooper, R. A., Schechter, G. P., and Salmon, S. E.: Evidence for the secretion of an osteoclast stimulating factor in myeloma. N. Engl. J. Med., *291*:1041, 1974.
91. Neer, R. M., Zipkin, I., Carbone, P. P., and Rosenberg, L. E.: Effect of sodium fluoride therapy on calcium metabolism in multiple myeloma. J. Clin. Endocrinol., *26*:1059, 1966.
92. Osgood, E. E.: The survival time of patients with plasmacytic myeloma. Cancer Chemother. Rep., *9*:1, 1960.
93. Osserman, E. F.: Plasma cell myeloma: clinical aspects. N. Engl. J. Med., *261*:952, 1006, 1959.
94. Osserman, E. F., and Lawlor, D.: Immunoelectrophoretic characterization of serum and urinary proteins in plasma cell myeloma and Waldenström's macroglobulinemia. Ann N. Y. Acad. Sci., *94*:93, 1961.
95. Osterland, C. K., and Espinoza, L. R.: Biological properties of myeloma proteins. Arch. Intern. Med., *135*:32, 1975.
96. Owen, D. M.: Multiple myeloma. Geriatrics, *20*:1048, 1965.
97. Pankovich, A., and Griem, M.: Plasma cell myeloma. Radiology, *104*:521, 1972.
98. Pasmantier, N. W., and Azar, H. A.: Extraskeletal spread in multiple plasma cell myeloma. Cancer, *23*:167, 1969.
99. Penny, R., Castaldi, P. A., and Whitsed, H. M.: Inflammation and hemostasis in paraproteinemias. Br. J. Haematol., *20*:35, 1971.
100. Perry, M. C., and Kyle, R. A.: The clinical significance of Bence Jones proteinuria. Mayo Clin. Proc., *50*:234, 1975.
101. Potter, M.: The developmental history of the neoplastic plasma cell in mice: a brief review of recent developments. Semin. Hematol., *10*:19, 1973.
102. Preud'homme, J. L., and Seligmann, M.: Surface bound immunoglobulins as a cell marker in human lymphoproliferative diseases. Blood, *40*:777, 1972.
103. Pruzanski, W., and Ogryzlo, M. A.: Abnormal proteinuria in malignant diseases. Adv. Clin. Chem, *13*:335, 1970.
104. Pruzanski, W., and Watt, J. G.: Serum viscosity and hyperviscosity syndrome in IgG multiple myeloma. Ann. Intern. Med., *77*:853, 1972.
105. Pruzanski, W., Platts, M. E., and Ogryzlo, M. A.: Leukemic form of immunocytic dyscrasia (plasma cell leukemia): a study of ten cases and a review of the literature. Am. J. Med., *47*:60, 1969.
106. Ritzmann, S. E., Loukas, D., Sakai, H., Daniels, J. C., and Levin, W. C.: Idiopathic (asymptomatic) monoclonal gammopathies. Arch. Intern. Med., *135*:95, 1975.
107. Rivers, S. W., and Patno, M. E.: Cyclophosphamide vs. melphalan in treatment of plasma cell myeloma. J.A.M.A., *207*:1328, 1969.
108. Rosen, F. S.: The macroglobulins. N. Engl. J. Med., *267*:491, 546, 1962.
109. Rosen, F. S., Alper, C. A., and Janeway, C. A.: The Primary Immunodeficiencies and Serum Complement Defects. *In* Nathan, D. G., and Oski, F. A. (eds.): Hematology of Infancy and Childhood. W. B. Saunders Co., Philadelphia, 1974, p. 529.

110. Rosner, F., and Grunwald, H.: Multiple myeloma terminating in acute leukemia. Am. J. Med., *57*:927, 1974.

111. Salmon, S. E., Samal, B. A., Hayes, D. M., Hosley, H., Miller, S. P., and Schilling, A.: Role of gamma globulin for immunoprophylaxis in multiple myeloma. N. Engl. J. Med., *277*:1336, 1967.

112. Salmon, S. E., Shadduck, R. K., and Schilling, A.: Intermittent high-dose prednisone therapy for multiple myeloma. Cancer Chemother. Rep., *51*:179, 1967.

113. Schubert, G. E., Veigel, J., and Lennert, K.: Structure and function of the kidney in multiple myeloma. Virchows Arch. [Pathol. Anat.], *355*:135, 1972.

114. Schwartz, L.: Plasmacytoma of the upper respiratory tract and oral cavity. Arch. Otolaryngol., *60*:573, 1954.

115. Seligmann, M.: Immunochemical, clinical, and pathological features of α–chain disease. Arch. Intern. Med., *135*:78, 1975.

116. Seligmann, M., Danon, F., Hurez, D., Mihaesco, E., and Preud'homme, J. L.: Alpha chain disease: a new immunoglobulin abnormality. Science, *162*:1396, 1968.

117. Seltzer, A. P.: Plasmacytoma. J. Natl. Med. Assoc., *66*:217, 1974.

118. Snapper, I., and Kahn, A.: Myelomatosis: Fundamentals and Clinical Features. University Park Press, Baltimore, 1971.

119. Snapper, I., Turner, L. B., and Moscovitz, H. L.: Multiple Myeloma. Grune & Stratton, New York, 1953.

120. Solomon, A., Waldmann, T. A., and Fahey, J. L.: Metabolism of normal 6.6S gammaglobulin in normal subjects and in patients with macroglobulinemia and multiple myeloma. J. Lab. Clin. Med., *62*:1, 1963.

121. Southeastern Cancer Study Group: Treatment of myeloma. Arch. Intern. Med., *135* 157, 1975.

121a. Stamp, T. C. B., Child, J. A., and Walker, P. G.: Treatment of osteolytic myelomatosis with mithramycin. Lancet, *1*:719, 1975.

122. Stoop, J. W., Ballieux, R. E., Hijmans, W., and Zegers, B. J. M.: Alpha chain disease with involvement of the respiratory tract in a Dutch child. Clin. Exp. Immunol., *9*:625, 1971.

123. Study Committee of the Midwest Cooperative Chemotherapy Group. Multiple myeloma. J.A.M.A., *188*:741, 1964.

124. Suki, W. N., Yium, J. J., von Minden, M., Saller-Herbert, C., Eknoyan, G., and Martinez-Maldonado, M.: Acute treatment of hypercalcemia with furosemide. N. Engl. J. Med., *283*:836, 1970.

125. The Acute Leukemia Group B and the Eastern Cooperative Oncology Group. Melphalan and prednisone: an effective combination for the treatment of multiple myeloma. Am. J. Med., *54*:589, 1973.

126. Thomas, F. B., Clausen, K. P., and Greenbarger, N. J.: Liver disease in multiple myeloma. Arch. Intern. Med., *132*:195, 1973.

127. Twomey, J. J.: Infections complicating multiple myeloma and chronic lymphocytic leukemia. Arch. Intern. Med., *132*:562, 1973.

128. Waldenström, J.: Diagnosis and Treatment of Multiple Myeloma. Grune & Stratton, New York, 1970.

129. Waldenström, J.: Incipient myelomatosis or "essential" hyperglobulinemia with fibrinogenopenia—a new syndrome? Acta Med. Scand., *137*:216, 1944.

130. Waldenström, J.: The occurrence of benign essential monoclonal (M-type) non-macromolecular hyperglobulinemia and its differential diagnosis. Acta Med. Scand., *176*:345, 1964.

131. Wallerstein, R. S.: Multiple myeloma without demonstrable bone lesions. Am. J. Med., *10*:325, 1951.

132. Wells, J. V., and Fudenberg, H. H.: Paraproteinemias. Dis. Month., February, 1974.

133. Wernet, P., Feizi, T., and Kunkel, H. G.: Idiotypic determinants of immunoglobulin M detected on the surface of human lymphocytes by cytotoxicity assays. J. Exp. Med., *136*:650, 1972.

134. Whittaker, J. A., Tuddenham, E. G. D., and Bradley, J.: Hyperviscosity syndrome in IgA multiple myeloma. Lancet, *2*:572, 1973.

135. Wiltshaw, E.: Extramedullary plasmacytoma. Br. Med. J., *2*:327, 1971.

136. Wright, J. H.: A case of multiple myeloma. Tr. Assoc. Am. Physicians, *15*:137, 1900.

137. Zawadzki, Z. A., and Edwards, G. A.: Nonmyelomatous monoclonal immunoglobulinemia. Prog. Clin. Immunol., *1*:105, 1972.

138. Zinneman, H. H., and Seal, U. S.: Macroglobulins and the Sia water test. Am. J. Clin. Pathol., *45*:306, 1966.

139. Zlotnick, A., and Rosemmann, E.: Renal pathologic findings associated with monoclonal gammopathies. Arch. Intern. Med., *135*:40, 1975.

CHAPTER 16

HEMOSTASIS: THEORY AND CLINICAL APPLICATIONS

INTRODUCTION

It is not surprising that the events responsible for hemostasis have been studied so extensively. The process by which fluid blood becomes a solid clot has stirred the curiosity of many, and the dreadful consequences of failure to maintain hemostasis in a variety of disorders have lent further impetus to the study. New techniques for the investigation of these problems continue to be developed. Application of these techniques has made possible the development of useful concepts of blood coagulation and led to a better understanding of many of the blood dyscrasias which result in abnormal bleeding. Therapy continues to improve as a result and the clinician is now better able to cope with these distressing disorders.

NORMAL HEMOSTASIS

Hemostasis is the end result of a series of related but not necessarily interdependent events. Damage to a vessel wall is followed by immediate but temporary reflex vasoconstriction, and platelets accumulate at the site of injury and form a plug within seconds. The initial phase of hemostasis is followed by the formation of a fibrin clot which effectively seals the vessel and facilitates repair. The fibrin clot undergoes dissolution after repair of the vessel is complete. The defense mechanism of hemostasis can conveniently be divided into two phases, the initial vascular–platelet phase and the biochemical response.[312, 447]

THE VASCULAR–PLATELET PHASE OF HEMOSTASIS

Vascular

The response of the vessel wall to injury, the role of the vascular endothelium in repair, and the factors responsible for the maintenance of the functional efficiency of the vascular wall are little understood. The importance of the blood vessels in the maintenance of hemostasis is confirmed by the finding that acquired or hereditary disorders which affect their structural integrity or supportive tissue often result in hemorrhage. The interaction between the wall of the blood vessel, the formed elements, and the clotting factors in defense of hemostasis is less clear.[77, 103, 447, 488] This remains a promising area for research.[499]

Platelet

The platelet and its role in hemostasis have been extensively investigated in recent years.[202, 513] The vast majority of platelets are produced by the megakaryocytes in the bone marrow.[12, 34, 209, 563] However, small numbers of megakaryocytes are found to circulate in the blood of normal persons, and larger

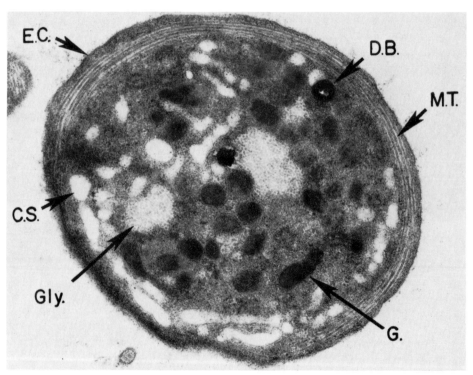

Figure 16–1 The appearance of a human platelet sectioned in the equatorial plane (×24,900). The structural elements noted include the exterior coat (EC), the circumferential band of microtubules (MT), granules (G), dense bodies (DB), the open canalicular system continuous with the cell surfaces (CS), and glycogen particles (Gly). (Reproduced by permission from White, J. G.: Blood, 32:324–335, 1968.)

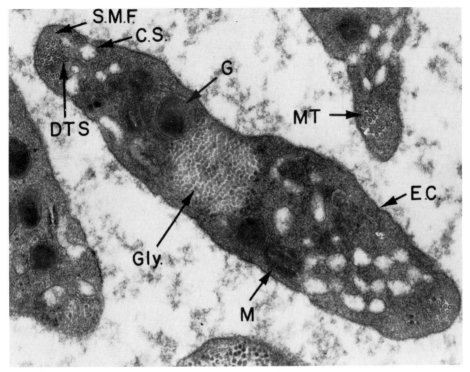

Figure 16-2 The anatomy of a human discoid platelet cut in cross section (×45,800). The structural elements noted include submembrane filaments (S.M.F.) and the dense tubular system (DTS), both of which are associated with the circumferential band of microtubules (MT), mitochondria (M), the exterior coat (E.C.), glycogen (Gly.), canalicular system (C.S.), and granules (G). (Reproduced by permission from White, J. G.: Blood, *31*:604–622, 1968.

numbers have been demonstrated in the venous blood of patients with malignancy.[238] The majority of these circulating megakaryocytes are trapped in the lungs, where they continue to release significant numbers of platelets.[265]

Some correlation of structure with function is now possible as a result of recent studies of the fine structure of the platelet (Fig. 16–1). The marginal bundle of microtubules appears to be composed of microfilaments which have a periodic substructure similar to that of isolated thrombosthenin.[549, 570, 572] Granules, numerous glycogen particles, mitochondria, and vacuoles have been identified.[549, 550] The matrix of the platelet is penetrated by an extensive canalicular system which is in continuity with the surface. Such a system provides the platelet with a large surface area and may bring the interior of the cell into closer proximity to the enveloping medium.[1] There is a fuzzy surface coating or "plasmatic atmosphere" of the platelet which is rich in carbohydrate material.[195] Three major classes of glycoproteins have been isolated from this surface coat by proteolytic digestion and distinguished by molecular weight, amino acids, and carbohydrate.[405]

The platelets are metabolically active and require a constant supply of ATP. Glucose is the principal source of energy and is metabolized anaerobically or aerobically. The platelet contains all of the enzymes of the glycolytic pathway, citric acid cycle, and the hexose monophosphate shunt; there is abundant glycogen which is available to the glycolytic pathway. Platelet aggregation coincides with stimulation of the hexose monophosphate shunt, later followed by an increase in Krebs cycle activity.[102] Marked stimulation of glucose oxidation occurs when the platelet is exposed to thrombin.[537] The concentration of platelets is an important variable in studies of platelet metabolism, and increased rates of glycogen degradation occur when the concentration is high, perhaps because the number of collisions between platelets would increase with increased concentration.[406]

Associated with the platelet are at least 15 different proteins, most of which also are found in the plasma, e.g., fibrinogen, albumin, prealbumin, globulins, plasminogen, and the coagulation Factors II, V, VIII, IX, X, XI, XII, and XIII.[271] Platelets retain Factors V and XI activity after repeated washing.[529a] Platelet fibrinogen appears to be different from plasma fibrinogen.[126] Specific platelet proteins are the contractile protein thrombosthenin, a specific thrombin-sensitive membrane glycoprotein,[406, 506, 518] and the platelet clotting factors.[45, 190, 370, 373]

Protein synthesis, which requires iron, has been demonstrated in young platelets.[63, 67, 186] Labeled amino acids may be incorporated into the contractile protein for at least 72 hours of platelet life span.[569] The platelet contains no DNA, and it has been postulated that stable mRNA is responsible for this activity; there is no RNA turnover.[67] Fatty acid and phospholipid synthesis is carried on by platelets.[112, 325] The platelet fatty acids are freely exchangeable with those in the plasma, and uptake is by an energy-independent mechanism.[503] The turnover rate of phospholipids is markedly stimulated by ADP.[299]

Platelets have classical D-type receptors which enable them to bind serotonin, which they incorporate against a concentration gradient.[358] The role of serotonin in hemostasis, if it has any, is unknown.[362] A reduction of 90 per cent of the normal serotonin activity of platelets has no significant effect on the bleeding time.[488] The amine appears to be concentrated in the electron dense granules of the platelet which also contain ADP, ATP, calcium, and PF-4.[226, 230, 340, 358, 550] Acid hydrolases and fibrinogen are stored in the alpha granules;[129, 226] catalase and lactic dehydrogenase are present in the soluble fraction.[331, 491]

Platelets release 50 per cent of their adenine nucleotides in response to certain stimuli such as exposure to collagen or thrombin.[125, 230, 398] Inasmuch as platelets require the presence and resynthesis of ATP in order to function as a living cell, such a loss would be catastrophic unless the cell was protected against the effect of nucleotide loss. The platelet has two different pools of adenine nucleotides; the storage pool is metabolically inert and is released while the metabolic pool actively participates in cellular metabolism. This pool is composed mainly of ATP and is constantly turning over.[227, 244]

Eighteen to 20 per cent of the extractable protein of the platelet is an actomyosin-like protein, thrombosthenin. This protein can be separated into two fragments, A and M. Thrombosthenin A has a molecular weight of 44,700 to 46,100 and resembles actin.[65] Thrombosthenin M resembles myosin and has a molecular weight of 542,700.[66] In vitro both thrombosthenin A and M are

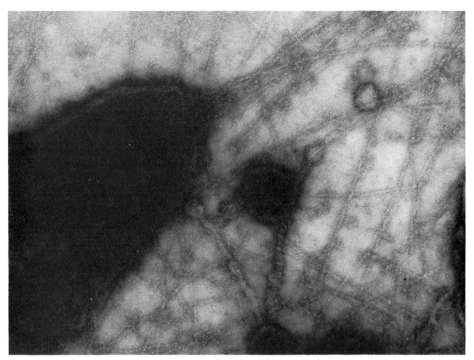

Figure 16–3 Micrograph of a thrombin-treated platelet which had been separated from plasma by gel filtration. The narrower extruded filaments are consistent with the actin moiety of thrombosthenin. ×280,000. (From Webber, A. J. and Budtz-Olsen, O. E.: Brit. J. Haemat., *26*:225, 1974.)

required for contraction which occurs in the presence of Mg^{++} and Ca^{++} concomitant with the splitting of ATP. The mechanism by which the interaction between the two filaments causes contraction is not understood.[43, 571] Electron microscopy has revealed that the extracted protein contains microfibrils which bear a striking resemblance to the actin and myosin of the smooth muscle, and may be responsible for the contractile properties of the platelet. Studies of the platelet under a variety of conditions have suggested that the microtubular structures represent different forms of the same substances.[549] The microtubules are formed when they are needed to maintain a rigid shape, whereas microfibrils are formed when contractile activity is needed.[572]

PLATELET CLOTTING FACTORS

Platelet clotting factors, by convention, are identified by Arabic numerals, in contrast to plasma clotting factors which are identified by Roman numerals.

Platelet factor 1 (PF-1). The "plasmatic atmosphere" of platelets has been shown to contain plasma clotting Factors I, II, V, VII, VIII, IX, XI, and XIII. Factors V and XI are tightly bound and resist repeated washings. Factor V has been demonstrated to be identical with platelet factor 1.[134]

Platelet factor 2 (PF-2). This is a heat-stable, relatively low molecular

weight protein which accelerates the conversion of fibrinogen (Factor I) to
fibrin (Factor Ia) by thrombin (Factor IIa). This increase in the reactivity of
fibrinogen to thrombin is associated with a release of nonprotein nitrogen,
suggesting that PF-2 has proteolytic activity. It will also produce platelet aggregation and neutralize antithrombin III.[382]

    Platelet factor 3 (PF-3). A liproprotein found in association with both the
platelet membrane and the platelet granules, PF-3 is required for the activation
of Factor VIII by activated Factor IX (IXa) and for the conversion of prothrombin (Factor II) to thrombin (IIa) by activated X (Xa) in the presence of
Factor V.[129] Both of these reactions require calcium ions. A close relationship
between the release reaction and the availability of PF-3 has been noted.[259]

    There is increasing evidence to support the concept that the platelet
membrane serves as a surface catalyst locally at the site of vessel injury and
probably represents PF-3 activity in vivo. The physiologic role of soluble platelet
phospholipids released during in vivo thrombus formation is uncertain.

    Platelet factor 4 (PF-4). Another low molecular weight, heat-stable pro-
tein, PF-4, neutralizes heparin and the antithrombin activity of fibrinogen
breakdown products (antithrombin IV).[370, 382] The major fraction of PF-4 is
found in the granules containing serotonin and nonmetabolic adenine nucleotides. A lesser amount is found in the cytoplasmic fraction.[130, 534]

FUNCTION OF THE PLATELET

    The platelet is chiefly important for the mechanical and chemical role it
plays in hemostasis and vascular repair.[311, 330] It acts mechanically to seal defects
in the vascular endothelium and to promote clot retraction by its interaction
with the strands of fibrin.[27, 260, 276, 519] It is important in blood coagulation because it provides an essential phospholipid. Interesting new data suggest that
platelets plus ADP will activate Factor XII.[532] PF-3 is not activated in this reaction. Platelets plus collagen will directly activate Factor XI without first activating Factor XII.[530] The ability of platelets plus collagen to bypass the activation of Factor XII provides an explanation for the usual benign course of
patients with Factor XII deficiency.[465, 531] Factor XIa continues to adhere to the
surface of the platelet, which affords protection against inactivation.[533] Platelets
also protect the biologic activity of Xa.[530]

    There is evidence that the platelet, like other formed elements in the blood,
may serve as part of a transport system that carries enzymes or other chemicals
from one part of the body to another. The avidity of platelets for serotonin
(5–hydroxytryptamine) is well-known, but no essential role in platelet metabolism or function has been identified for serotonin, and the platelet may serve
only as a storage site and transport mechanism for this amine.[358, 362]

    It has been noted that, in the presence of polystyrene particles or antigen–
antibody complexes, aggregation usually follows phagocytosis of the inducing agent by the platelet,[196, 398] and it has been suggested that platelets may
also have a role in rejection of organ transplants. Recently, a heat-stable nondialyzable cationic protein with a molecular weight of 30,000 which can markedly increase vascular permeability has been found in human platelet granules.[374]

Role in Hemostasis

PLATELET ADHESION

In vivo, circulating platelets adhere to exposed collagen in the area of injury to the vessel wall within one or two seconds, apparently the result of a specific biochemical reaction. The enzyme collagen:glucosyltransferase on the surface of the platelet may react with incomplete heterosaccharide chains of collagen. Platelet adhesion to collagen is inhibited by drugs which interfere with this enzymatic reaction.[74, 97, 253, 341, 502] Studies have indicated that microfibrillar collagen contains the minimal unit structure required to initiate platelet adhesion and aggregation.[251] Two binding sites on the platelet appear to be involved.[81, 419] Platelets may also adhere to the vascular basement membrane or to elastic fibers by a similar mechanism.[138, 251, 252, 507] Free carboxyl groups of collagen are not important for platelet adherence, but are critical for activation of Factor XII.[388]

The adhesion of platelets to collagen is restricted essentially to one layer of platelets. Following adherence to the collagen, the platelets release ADP, which results in further aggregation and a build-up of the platelet mass. In the presence of collagen or thrombin, the ADP-induced aggregation is accompanied by degranulation and the release of several platelet consituents.

In vitro, platelets adhere to glass, and a variety of methods have been developed to quantitate this phenomenon.[68, 218, 453, 454] Platelet adhesion to glass is different from platelet adhesion to collagen. Platelets from patients with thrombasthenia, for example, fail to demonstrate adhesion to glass but show normal adhesion to collagen. The in vitro tests are useful clinically and have demonstrated decreased adhesion to glass by platelets of patients with von Willebrand's disease, thrombopathia, chronic renal failure, and afibrinogenemia. It has been abundantly demonstrated that ADP and fibrinogen influence adhesiveness of platelets to glass beads, but the precise mechanism underlying the phenomenon remains to be elucidated.

PLATELET AGGREGATION IN VITRO

No aggregation of platelets occurs in static blood in vitro. Agitation must be sufficient to produce a minimal collision force before aggregation takes place, and platelets must be numerous enough for collisions to occur; little aggregation results if the concentration of platelets falls much below 50,000 per cu. mm.[263, 478] A wide variety of agents, including long-chain saturated fatty acids, thrombin, collagen, adenosine diphosphate (ADP), 5–hydroxytryptamine, and norepinephrine, are capable of inducing platelet aggregation in vitro.[212, 270, 362, 368, 408, 556, 573]

ADP plays a major role in platelet aggregation. Isolated platelet membranes have been shown to bind ADP reversibly in the presence of calcium ions. Each platelet membrane contained over 100,000 binding sites.[372] Platelet aggregation is not induced by ADP in the absence of Ca^{++}. Fibrinogen and at least one other protein co-factor are also required (Fig. 16–4).[86, 94, 120, 158, 347, 362, 371] If platelets aggregate in minimal concentrations of ADP, the aggre-

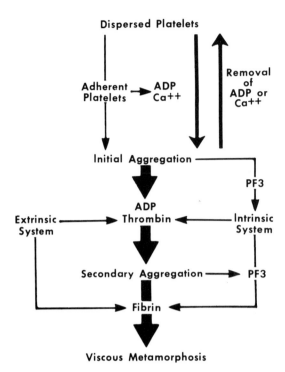

Figure 16-4 Adenosine diphosphate (ADP) appears to provide a common basis for the action of a variety of substances known to induce platelet aggregation. The action of ADP requires Ca^{++}, fibrinogen and one other protein co-factor. Removal of ADP or Ca^{++} results in dispersion of platelets.

gates will disperse after a period of time and the platelets will appear unaltered. Removal of Ca^{++} will also result in disaggregation. Thrombin or collagen increases the responsiveness of platelets to ADP-induced aggregation.[397] This initial reversible aggregation is known as primary aggregation. With higher concentrations of ADP, the initial primary aggregation is followed by a secondary irreversible aggregation in response to the ADP released from the platelets themselves.[207] Biochemical coagulation and platelet function are difficult to separate at this stage, and it has been suggested that thrombin is necessary for irreversible aggregation.[23]

There is much speculation as to the mechanism by which ADP induces platelet aggregation.[501] Serious objections have been raised to the suggestions that ADP–Ca^{++} complexes form an intercellular bridge, alter the charge of the platelet membrane, or act as an energy source.[457] It has been proposed that platelets require an active, constant source of energy to remain "unsticky," and that the source of this energy is ATP which is split by the ATPase on the platelet membrane. Addition of ADP would interfere with the reaction by product inhibition and would allow a change in the membrane, resulting in aggregation.[456] Another proposal has been that of a relaxation–contraction model which assumes that the normal "contracted" state of the platelet membrane is "relaxed" by the action of aggregating agents with the extrusion of thrombosthenin-rich cytogel. Cytogel between platelets interacts to bring about aggregation.[64, 538] Fibrinogen has also been proposed as the substance responsible for interplatelet bridging.[151]

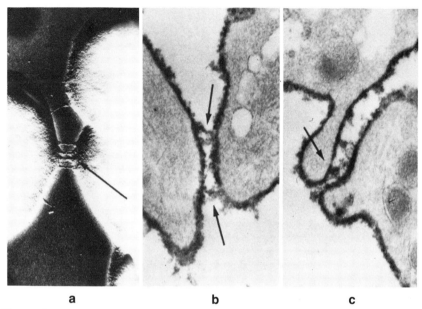

a   b   c

Figure 16–5 Interplatelet bonds formed after exposure of platelets to 10^{-7} M ADP. (a) Shadow casted interplatelet bonds × 16,291 (b, c). Interplatelet bonds stained with monospecific antihuman thrombosthenin rabbit serum × 29,620. Arrows indicate interplatelet bonds. From Booyse et al. Microvas. Res. 4:179, 1972.

Evidence indicates that, at any time, part of the platelet population may be temporarily refractory and not equally responsive to ADP. This refractory state may be related to the function of the contractile protein.[322, 448] The aggregation of platelets in vitro by ADP is inhibited by adenosine monophosphate (AMP), adenosine, and most strongly by 2–chloroadenosine,[70] each of which shows vasodilator activity in the human forearm. The nature of the receptor sites either on platelets or smooth muscle is unknown.[72] The mechanism by which these compounds interfere with the action of ADP is also unknown; it may relate to competition for bridging sites on the platelet or their participation in the synthesis of platelet ATP, which would favor the energy-producing reaction.[456, 457]

THE RELEASE REACTION

Exposure to ADP in vitro results in remarkable changes in the fine structure of the platelet.[548] The platelet loses its discoid shape, becomes irregularly swollen, and develops multiple pseudopods. "Stickiness" of the platelet occurs at this time, as aggregation is an associated phenomenon. The marginal microtubules crowd the organelles toward the center of the platelet, so that the granules come to lie in close apposition; some of the microtubules appear to have been replaced by microfibrils.[570] The contraction of the marginal microtubules moving the organelles to the center of the cell appears to be central to the process. The platelet canalicular system is altered, and

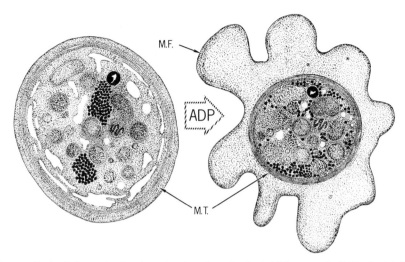

Figure 16–6 Schematic drawing showing the effect of ADP on an individual platelet. The circumferential band of microtubules contracts on exposure to ADP, forcing the organelles into close approximation. Swelling increases the cell size by some 15 per cent, and pseudopods containing microfilaments appear. These changes precede the platelet-release phenomena.

peripheral elements connected to the platelet surface become dilated and appear as deep clefts between the pseudopods.[548] The channels of the open canalicular system serve as conduits for carrying the products of the release reaction to the surface.[551, 552]

The platelet behaves as a secretory cell which, when stimulated, can empty substances stored in the granules into the external environment of the cell without loss of cytoplasmic enzymes, mitochondria, or damage to the membrane. The reaction is dependent on energy derived from glycolysis and from oxidative phosphorylation.[229] Emptying of the granules occurs with great rapidity. The content of the dense bodies is released in ten seconds and that of the alpha granules within 40 to 60 seconds. Following the reaction, morphologic studies reveal that many granules have disappeared, a complex vacuolar system has developed, and some of the remaining granules are less dense.[229] The membranes of the vacuoles appear to have fused with the surface-connecting system.[150] Stimuli such as ADP and epinephrine bring about the release of only the dense body contents: nonmetabolic ATP and ADP, serotonin, Ca^{++}, and PF-4. If the stimulus is an inducer such as thrombin, collagen, or latex particles, the alpha granules are emptied of fibrinogen and many lysosomal enzymes.[226] Although the concentration of fibrinogen and Ca^{++} is small compared to that in the plasma, both may be important between platelets in an aggregate to which the plasma has no access.[228]

The importance of ADP release is obvious, since it is the most powerful inducer of platelet aggregation available and, when degraded by adenyl kinase, becomes an inhibitor of further aggregation. ATP also contributes to the formation of adenosine, which is a potent inhibitor of platelet activity. The physiologic role played by the acid hydrolases is unknown, but it has been suggested that they participate in clot lysis.[228, 232, 312, 330] Those substances which are able to induce the platelet release reaction have no effect on isolated storage granules. It is believed that they exert their effect on the intact platelet by causing a conformational change in the membrane.[228]

There are two major types of specific inhibitors of the platelet release reaction; anti-inflammatory drugs, including aspirin and phenylbutazone, and membrane stabilizers, such as amitriptyline and imipramine. Vinca alkaloids appear to interfere with microtubular function and inhibit release.[172, 228]

Nonphysiologic stimuli such as phytohemagglutinin and phorbol myristate acetate from croton oil have been demonstrated to cause selective release from platelet storage granules.[550, 551, 552]

PLATELET AGGREGATION IN VIVO

ADP appears to be the stimulus responsible for platelet aggregation in vivo.[338, 478, 492] ADP has been successfully extracted from the vessel walls and from red cells, but the major source of ADP for initial hemostasis is the platelet. ADP must be present for thrombin to induce aggregation, but thrombin does alter platelet morphology in the absence of ADP.[204, 212] Recently, collagenase has been demonstrated in both the granules and membrane of the platelet. Collagenase activity can be detected in the early phase of aggregation. It is inhibited by α_1–antitrypsin in the plasma. Collagenase can destroy the ability

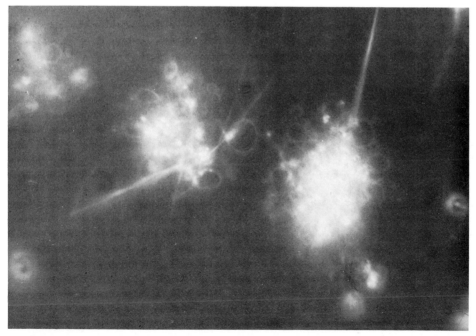

Figure 16–7 Viscous metamorphosis as observed through the phase microscope. Aggregation and fusion of platelets has occurred with formation of characteristic balloon-like structures. Needles of fibrin can be seen.

of collagen to aggregate platelets, and may act to limit the aggregation reaction.[104]

The formation of platelet plugs at the site of vessel damage in experimental animals is inhibited by a variety of enzyme poisons, suggesting dependence on metabolic activity. Anticoagulants do not inhibit platelet aggregation at the site of vessel injury, indicating probable independence of clotting factors.[231] The administration of ADP to experimental animals results in a fall in platelet concentration,[71] and the administration of adenosine and 2–chloroadenosine inhibits the formation of platelet thrombi and emboli in injured vessels.[73] The successful extraction of ADP from vessel walls lends further support to this concept.[362] The finding that intravascular platelet aggregations disperse, despite continued administration of ADP to experimental animals, suggests the presence of a mechanism that can limit the size and extent of platelet aggregation. It has been proposed that an enzyme system in the platelets and plasma constantly re-establish AMP : ADP ratios capable of inhibiting platelet aggregation, thus preventing a self-extending process.[269, 449]

CYCLIC AMP (cAMP) AND PROSTAGLANDINS

Cyclic AMP appears to play a role in the response of the platelet to a variety of stimuli. An elevation of cAMP levels in the platelet is associated with an inhibition of platelet aggregation and a tendency to disaggregation.[558] Adherence to collagen is also inhibited by agents which increase the level of cAMP.[98] Reduced levels of cAMP are associated with induction of aggregation.[337, 459]

The level of cAMP is determined by a balance between the activity of **adenyl cyclase** which catalyzes the conversion of ATP to cyclic 3'5' AMP and **phosphodiesterase** which carries the reaction to 5' AMP.[337, 460] As noted in Fig. 16–8, a number of agents will affect these reactions. Prostaglandins are synthesized and released by platelets, and PGE_1 has a profound inhibiting effect on platelet aggregation and adhesion. PGE_1 has been found to increase the level of cAMP by stimulating the activity of adenyl cyclase.[557] The action of PGE_2 has been variously reported to inhibit[91] or stimulate[496] adenyl cyclase activity. PGE_2 and $PGF_2\alpha$ are formed and released in response to thrombin or when aggregation occurs in response to ADP, collagen, or epinephrine.[495, 496]

Exposure of platelets to arachidonic acid induces the formation of prostaglandins and aggregation.[493, 497] An endoperoxide intermediate in the biosynthesis of prostaglandin is formed by the platelet one minute after exposure to this fatty acid and prior to aggregation. The appearance of this intermediate is closely correlated with the release of adenine nucleotides and 5–hydroxytryptamine (5–HT). Since PGE_2 and $PGF_2\alpha$ can not by themselves cause ADP release or aggregation, the endoperoxide was believed to be a trigger for the platelet release reaction.[497]

Most recently it has been demonstrated that prostaglandin endoperoxides (PG endoperoxides) are precursors of both prostaglandins and a new series of compounds, the thromboxanes. The thromboxanes, which have a half-life of about 30 seconds in aqueous solutions, appear to be potent regulators of the

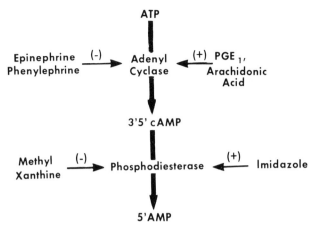

Figure 16–8 Substances affecting the level of cAMP in the platelet. Control is exercised through stimulation (+) or reduction (−) of activity of adenyl cyclase, which increases, or phosphodiesterase, which reduces, the levels or cAMP.

function of many cells. Thromboxane A_2 is a powerful platelet aggregating agent. Further study of these compounds should add much to our understanding of platelet functions.[274a]

Thrombin has been noted to reduce the cAMP of platelets by 70 to 90 per cent. Prostaglandins may serve to modulate the effect of thrombin through stimulation of adenyl cyclase activity.[87]

Epinephrine inhibits the effect of PGE_1 and basal adenyl cyclase activity. This appears to be an α–adrenergic mechanism and is blocked by the α–adrenergic antagonist phentolamine, but not by the β–adrenergic blocking activity of propanolol.[337] Evidence for the presence of β–adrenergic receptors effecting the disaggregation of platelets has been developed. Platelets exposed to the beta blocker propanolol are more susceptible to aggregation when exposed to epinephrine, which normally manifests both alpha and beta activity. The process may be mediated by cAMP.[1] Methyl xanthines appear to elevate cAMP levels by inhibiting phosphodiesterase activity. Imidazole enhances phosphodiesterase activity and reduces cAMP levels.[337]

THE BIOCHEMICAL PHASE OF HEMOSTASIS

Although much of our knowledge of blood coagulation is based on empiric laboratory tests, it nonetheless has found extensive clinical application. The theory of blood coagulation to be presented is but an expansion of the classic theory developed at the turn of the century. The various disorders of hemostasis will subsequently be presented within the same framework.

The system of nomenclature adopted by the International Committee for the Nomenclature of Blood Coagulation Factors[286, 316] and the commonly used synonyms are as follows:

COMMITTEE	SYNONYMS
Factor I	Fibrinogen
Factor II	Prothrombin
Factor III	Thromboplastin (tissue) (extrinsic prothrombin activator)
Factor IV	Calcium
Factor V	Accelerator globulin, labile factor, proaccelerin, co-factor of thromboplastin, AC globulin
Factor VI	No longer used
Factor VII	Serum prothrombin conversion accelerator (SPCA), proconvertin, stable factor, co-thromboplastin, prothrombin accelerator, autoprothrombin I
Factor VIII	Antihemophilic globulin (AHG), antihemophilic factor (AHF), thromboplastinogen A, platelet co-factor I, antihemophilic factor A
Factor IX	Plasma thromboplastin component (PTC), Christmas factor, autoprothrombin II, antihemophilic factor B, beta thromboplastin
Factor X	Stuart-Prower factor, Stuart factor
Factor XI	Plasma thromboplastin antecedent (PTA)
Factor XII	Hageman factor, contact factor
Factor XIII	Fibrin stabilizing factor, L-L factor, Laki-Lorand factor

Historic Aspects

The present concepts of the process of coagulation are better understood when viewed in historic perspective. For details of the early history of the study of coagulation, the reader is referred to the reviews by Gamgee in 1880[189] and Howell in 1935.[235]

In 1845 Buchanan[92] noted that a substance was formed during clotting which, when extracted from the clot, would cause the coagulation of serous fluids. The substance which Buchanan had discovered was thrombin. In 1859 Denis[189] demonstrated that a material which was the soluble precursor of the fibrin of the clot was present in the plasma. This protein was named fibrinogen. Schmidt,[467] working along similar lines in 1872, concluded that the formation of fibrin was due to the interaction of fibrinogen and serum globulin in the presence of thrombin. He noted that the clot-promoting substance, thrombin, could be extracted after a clot was formed, but no such substance could be demonstrated in the liquid state. From this observation he concluded that thrombin was present in the circulating blood in an inactive or precursor state, and the concept of prothrombin was evolved. In 1879 Hammarsten,[203] using a better method of preparation of fibrinogen, demonstrated that it could be converted to fibrin in the presence of thrombin without the participation of serum albumin or globulin.

In 1826 Joseph Jackson Lister, the father of Lord Lister, discovered that the spherical aberration of one lens could be neutralized by that of another, and the potential of light microscopy was vastly increased. As a result, George Gulliver in 1841 and William Addison in 1842 discovered and described the platelet.[441]

Osler described his studies of shed blood in 1874; he called attention to the granular masses of platelets, their pseudopods, and their intimate association with the formation of fibrin. "Mucoid degeneration" was the term Osler used to describe the morphologic changes in platelets in the early stages of coagulation known today as "viscous metamorphosis"[393, 441] (Fig. 16–7).

In 1872 the French hematologist Hayem began his studies of the platelet which established the cell as an entity and its role in coagulation.[216] In 1890 Arthus and Pagés[24] proved that calcium was essential for the coagulation of blood. It was shown that substances which bind or remove calcium from the blood prevent coagulation.

At the turn of the century Morawitz[364] was able to formulate the classic theory of coagulation. It is summarized as follows:

$$\text{Prothrombin} \xrightarrow{\text{Thrombokinase*}} \text{Thrombin}$$

$$\text{Fibrinogen} \xrightarrow[\text{Thrombin}]{\text{Ca}^{++}} \text{Fibrin}$$

The classic theory, which was simple and agreed with the known facts, remained unaltered until recently. As additional factors essential to the process of coagulation were discovered, expansion of the scheme became necessary, but the classic theory embodies the basic concept from which most of the modern theories of blood coagulation have evolved.

The most important contributions to the theory of coagulation have been concerned with the development of the substance activating prothrombin. For nearly 50 years after the introduction of the classic theory, research was hampered by the failure to realize that "thrombokinase" could derive not only from a tissue source but from the blood itself. The exact nature of the material responsible for the conversion of prothrombin to thrombin is unknown, and for purposes of discussion is designated as "thromboplastin activity." It is also known as prothrombinase.

Studies of patients with disorders of hemostasis have led to the discovery of new factors necessary for the development of normal thromboplastin activity. The general design of these investigations is simple. An in vitro test system is employed. The defect of the plasma, serum, or platelets of the patient under investigation is identified by successive substitutions of the corresponding fraction of normal blood until the coagulation defect is corrected. Thus localized to either the plasma, serum, or platelets, the defect is further identified by comparing the defective fraction with comparable fractions from patients

---

*Thromboplastin activity.

with known defects. In this way it can be determined whether the defect under study is the result of the deficiency of a known or previously unknown factor.

The result of such studies has been an expansion of the classic theory of coagulation.[316]

Present-Day Theories of Coagulation

For purposes of discussion the coagulation of blood may be considered to occur in three stages. During the first stage, thromboplastin activity develops as the result both of the coagulation factors in the blood and the admixture of tissue juices and plasma. The blood (intrinsic) and tissue (extrinsic) systems responsible for the development of thromboplastin activity may be separated in vitro and shown to be independent and equally potent. There seems little doubt that they both function in the physiologic defense of hemostasis. The second stage is the conversion of prothrombin to thrombin. The evolution of thrombin from prothrombin will occur in the presence of thromboplastin activity and calcium ions. The third stage is the conversion of fibrinogen to fibrin in the presence of thrombin. Each of these stages will be discussed separately.

The Development of Thromboplastin Activity

The first stage of blood coagulation may be outlined as shown in Figure 16–9.

This scheme indicates the factors unique to one or the other thromboplastin

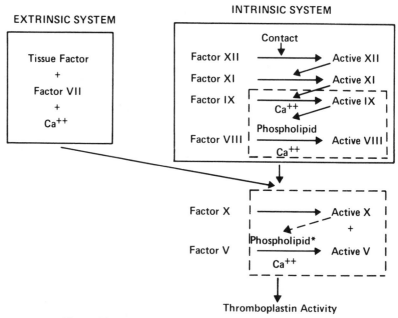

Figure 16–9   The development of thromboplastin activity.

activity generating system and those common to both. Each develops potent thromboplastin activity, though the rate of its development is more rapid in the extrinsic system.[50]

THE EXTRINSIC SYSTEM

Recent investigations have revealed that the formation of extrinsic thromboplastin activity involves two distinct steps.[152] The first reaction involves tissue factor (Factor III), Factor VII, Factor X, and calcium. The product of this reaction plus Factor V gives rise to thromboplastin activity.[509]

Tissue factor (Factor III). The extrinsic system requires a source of tissue factors. All tissues probably contain the factors essential to the development of thromboplastin activity and contribute to the physiologic defense of hemostasis. Brain or lung tissue is generally used as a tissue source in the performance of coagulation tests. The procoagulant activity of lymphocytes has been characterized as tissue factor, and tissue factor activity may develop in leukocytes during in vivo thrombin formation. A membrane-bound tissue factor which can be activated by a variety of stimuli may be present in many cells.[291, 438] For many years it was thought that these tissues contained one active principle, but investigation has now revealed that they contain a complex of heat-stable and heat-labile fractions.[316] Removal of 95 per cent of tissue factor phospholipid results in a loss of 98 per cent of its biologic activity.[379] The activity can be restored to the extracted tissue by the addition of brain phospholipid or highly purified phospholipid. Phosphatidyl ethanolamine was the most active phospholipid tested. Tissue factor appears to be a particle-bound lipoprotein, and its coagulant activity to be lipid-dependent.[410] It appears in highest concentration in the intima of blood vessels, particularly the plasma membranes of the endothelial cells.[568] The molecular weight of tissue factor is in doubt, but evidence suggests that the molecule may consist of aggregates of a single subunit of 20,000 daltons.[380] Peptidase activity has been demonstrated to be associated with the coagulant activity of tissue factor. Tissue factor may function biologically through a proteolytic mechanism.[411] It is well to recognize that the nature of this complex is not completely understood, and that it is in all probability the end result of a series of chemical and enzymatic reactions.

Marked quantitative and qualitative differences will appear in the results of laboratory tests if tissue extracts from various organs in the same species, or from the same organ from different species, are used. These results suggest that the mechanism of action of these materials is not the same and emphasize the need for careful control of reagents in laboratory studies.

Factor VII. Factor VII is one of the plasma factors essential for the development of thromboplastin activity from a tissue source. This factor is apparently formed in the liver and, like prothrombin, is dependent on vitamin K for its continued production. It is stable on storage under blood bank conditions. It behaves as an enzyme in the formation of thromboplastin activity and is found in both plasma and serum. It is adsorbed by inorganic adsorbent compounds and is relatively heat-stable.[396] It behaves as a beta globulin on electrophoresis. It is not considered to play any role in the production of thromboplastin activity by the intrinsic system,[7, 275, 396] but has been noted to be converted to an active form by XIIa.[19] Recent evidence suggests that Factor VII and Factor II are similar chemically.[225] Factor VII has been purified 330,000-fold from bovine plasma. The purified factor required tissue factor to develop proteolytic Factor X-activating capacity.[256] Following activation, Factor VII was isolated from the protein portion of tissue factor, and retained activity as long as phospholipid was undisturbed.[394]

The remaining factors necessary to the development of thromboplastin activity by the extrinsic system are essential to the intrinsic system as well. They will be discussed following a description of those factors unique to the intrinsic system.

THE INTRINSIC SYSTEM

The factors essential to the formation of intrinsic thromboplastin activity will be introduced in the order in which they are believed to react in vitro.

Factor XII (Hageman Factor). Factor XII was recognized when a patient was discovered whose blood did not coagulate in a normal period of time on contact with a glass surface.[336] The patient had no clinical disorder of hemostasis. Factor XII is not adsorbed by inorganic adsorbent compounds, nor is it consumed during coagulation;[318, 429] it behaves as a gamma globulin on electrophoresis and has a biologic half-time of between 50 and 70 hours.[524] Studies of purified factor XII indicate that it has a molecular weight of approximately 90,000 and is composed of three polypeptide chains of equal size held together by disulfide bridges.[110] It is activated on contact with glass and is thought to initiate clotting in vitro.[432] Activation of Factor XII is accompanied by a change in its physical properties,[144, 347a] and is believed to be the result of unfolding of the molecule with exposure of reactive sites. Subsequent loss of activity marks a return to its prior conformation, from which it can again be activated.[439, 504] Not all of Factor XII is activated in glass, since it must compete for binding sites with other plasma proteins which have affinity for glass.[201] Factor XII is also activated by ellagic acid,[76] cellulose sulfate, and ℓ-homocystine.[268, 430] It has been suggested that the frequency of thrombosis in patients with homocystinuria may be related to deposits of ℓ-homocystine in the walls of their blood vessels.[430]

Factor XII is also activated by collagen. Thermal denaturation or digestion of collagen blocks this effect, suggesting that the natural triple helical structure is important.[555] Esterification of 80 to 90 per cent of the free carboxyl groups of glutamic and aspartic acids reduced coagulant activity by over 90 per cent.[555] It appears that negatively charged sites are essential for the adsorption and activation of Factor XII, and that inhibition of Factor XII activity will result from their neutralization.[387, 388]

Factor XII may play a role in inflammation either directly or through the activation of a plasma kinin similar to or identical with bradykinin.[199, 268] Activation did not occur on exposure to immune complexes, but certain bacteria can cause activation in vitro.[111]

Factor XI (Plasma thromboplastin antecedent, PTA). Factor XI[446] was discovered, as was Factor IX, during investigation of persons with hemophilia-like states. It is thought to be a globulin and migrates electrophoretically with the beta globulins.[445] Since it is not consumed during coagulation, it is present in both plasma and serum. Unlike Factor IX, it is not adsorbed by inorganic precipitating compounds and is present in $Al(OH)_3$-absorbed plasma. Factor XI activity persists in fresh frozen plasma for at least two years, and for up to four months in plasma stored at room temperature.[114]

Highly purified Factor XI has been found to have a molecular weight of 210,000 on gel filtration.[464] Normal plasma contains natural inhibitors of activated XI; purified inhibitor of C1 esterase activity has been shown to inhibit XIa, and a second inhibitor with enzymatic properties has been identified.[183, 184] The importance of XIa inhibition is not clear. Patients with hereditary angioneurotic edema who have a reduced C1 inhibitor without a compensatory rise in the secondary inhibitors of XIa do not have a tendency to thrombosis.[22, 436] Inhibition of Factor XIa is reduced in pregnancy but any role in thrombosis is obscure.[22]

Factor XI can be activated by trypsin but not by a variety of other enzymes including chymotrypsin, thrombin, papain, ficin, plasmin, plasma kallikrein, tissue thromboplastin, and C1 esterase.[452] The activation of Factor XII, and subsequent activation of Factor XI, requires no Ca^{++} ions and is known as *the contact system*.[434] Studies of the product of the reaction between XII and XI have indicated that XIa is not a complex of XIIa and XIa.[431]

Factor IX (Plasma thromboplastin component, PTC, Christmas factor). Factor IX was discovered during the investigation of persons with hemophilia-like disorders.[9, 10, 51, 52] This factor, unlike Factor VIII, is not completely consumed in coagulation and is found in both plasma and serum. It is adsorbed by inorganic adsorbent compounds and is not present in $Al(OH)_3$-adsorbed plasma. Although Factor IX is relatively heat-labile, it fares somewhat better on storage at 4° C than does Factor VIII.[9] Factor IX activity can still be demonstrated in near normal amounts after two weeks of storage at 4° C, but may fall off rapidly thereafter.[79] Fresh-frozen plasma retains its Factor IX activity for long periods. Bovine Factor IX has been purified 22,000-fold from bovine plasma. It is a single polypeptide chain with 26 per cent carbohydrate and a molecular weight of $55,400 \pm 1300$.[188]

Factor IX is thought to be activated by activated Factor XI (XIa).[272, 433] Ca^{++} ions accelerate the reaction, but it has been recently reported that activated Factor IX can develop slowly in the absence of Ca^{++} ions.[466] The addition of calcium ions causes a reduction in the molecular size of both IX and IXa. The mechanism responsible for these changes is not clear.[109] Inactive Factor IX is the substrate for active Factor XI, and is proportionately reduced as active Factor IX develops.[386] The half-life of infused Factor IX has two phases, the first lasting 15.1 hours and the second 8.4 days.[8]

Factor VIII (Antihemophilic factor, AHF, antihemophilic globulin, AHG). Among the factors essential in the intrinsic system is Factor VIII,[51] originally termed antihemophilic factor because a deficiency of this factor was believed to be responsible for the bleeding diathesis in classic hemophilia. Factor VIII appears to be a relatively short-lived glycoprotein in vivo.[26, 78, 417] Evidence suggests that the site of its production may be the endothelial cells of the blood vessels.[236] Recently it was suggested that infused Factor VIII has a two-phase

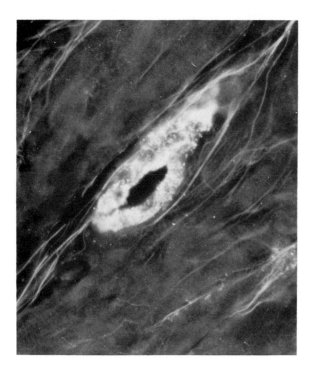

Figure 16–10 Immunofluorescent micrograph of small venule in human cardiac muscle section stained with rabbit anti-AHF antiserum. (×350). (From Hoyer, L. W. et al., J. Clin. Invest., 52:2737, 1973.)

survival in vivo, the first with a half-life of 3 to 4 hours followed by a longer phase with a nine- to 15-hour loss of activity. These studies were carried out in patients with hemophilia and little is known of its survival in normal humans.[223a] It is consumed during coagulation and therefore is found only in the plasma.[50] Factor VIII is not adsorbed by the inorganic adsorbent compounds and is present in Al(OH)$_3$-adsorbed plasma. Its activity in plasma or whole blood diminishes rapidly on storage under standard blood bank conditions, but will persist when fresh-frozen plasma is stored at $-30°$ C.[114] It is relatively heat-stable.

Factor VIII has not as yet been obtained in pure form, but has been concentrated 6300 times by agarose gel filtration.[264, 357, 435, 528]

Reduction of one highly purified Factor VIII protein of approximately 2×10^6 molecular weight with β mercaptoethanol resulted in a homogeneous single unit species with a molecular weight of 202,000 by sedimentation analysis. Low concentrations of thrombin initially increased Factor VIII activity threefold, and this was followed by complete loss of the activity in three hours.[35] Data suggest that activation and inactivation of the molecule by thrombin occurs as the result of cleavage of peptide bonds which produces fragments, the sum of which totals less than 10,000 molecular weight.[474] Carbohydrate analysis of a highly purified Factor VIII revealed 1 per cent sialic acid, 2.8 per cent hexosamine, and 1 to 2 per cent hexose (mannose, galactose, and fucose). Lipid content was less than 5 per cent of the protein content.[329, 541]

Studies have revealed more than one molecular form of Factor VIII in fresh human plasma. The major fraction sediments in the region of a γM immunoglobulin and has a molecular weight of approximately 2×10^6. A minor component, which sediments more slowly, may be associated with fibrinogen;[59] the rapidly sedimenting component, which is found in cryoprecipitates, is not so associated.[541] Factor VIII coagulant activity can be readily separated from Factor VIII antigen in the laboratory.[26a]

The activation of Factor VIII is believed to follow that of Factor IX and in turn to activate Factor X. Although activated Factor IX can activate Factor VIII, trace amounts of thrombin profoundly alter the reaction. Thrombin appears to make Factor VIII more reactive to the action of active IX, and may be responsible for the "autocatalytic reaction" in the blood clotting mechanism. The first traces of thrombin formed may catalyze the reaction of Factor VIII and speed more rapid generation of thromboplastin activity.[428] As the thrombin-activated Factor VIII is highly unstable, the process is self-limiting.[54, 474] It has been suggested that the extrinsic system may be the source of the first traces of thrombin generated in physiologic clotting, and if so it would play an important role in the development of intrinsic blood coagulation.[54]

Recently, human endothelial cells derived from umbilical veins have been propagated successfully in tissue culture for periods of up to five months.[249] The synthesis of antihemophilic factor antigen by the cultured cells has been demonstrated. No procoagulant activity has been demonstrated.

Factor VIII antigen has been demonstrated by immunofluorescent microscopy in the endothelial cells of arteries, capillaries, and veins, as well as in the cells lining the splenic and liver sinusoids.[236]

Platelet factor 3. The platelets play several important roles in hemostasis,[69, 208] among which is their contribution to the first stage of blood coagulation. The aggregation and fusion of platelets is known as viscous metamorphosis[38, 478] and is associated with the appearance of PF3 activity, which is probably unavailable until the platelets are disrupted (Fig. 16–7).[500] A number of phospholipids have been identified in the platelet, but those possessing the most marked coagulant activity appear to be phosphatidyl serine and phosphatidyl

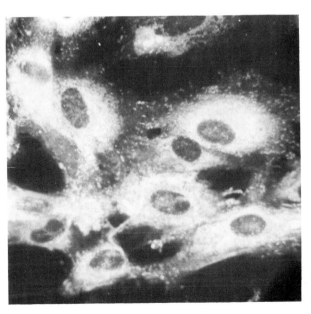

Figure 16–11 Immunofluorescence study of cultured human endothelial cells. Cells were stained with rabbit anti-AHF and then with fluorescein-conjugated goat anti-rabbit globulin. ×960. (Courtesy, Jaffe E. A. et al., J. Clin. Invest., 52:2757, 1973.)

ethanolamine. The activity of phosphatidyl serine is potentiated by lecithin but is not dependent on it.[61] Mixtures of phospholipids containing one negatively charged phospholipid have the most marked clot-promoting activity in vitro.[29, 122]

Additional factors.   Reports have appeared in the literature suggesting the possibility of additional factors important to the development of intrinsic thromboplastin activity. The Fletcher factor has been demonstrated to be identical to prekallikrein.[564] The Fitzgerald factor appears to play a role in fibrinolysis, kinin generation and vascular permeability as well as coagulation.[452a] The absence of the Passovoy factor results in a mild hemorrhagic diathesis. The partial thromboplastin time is prolonged, but levels of all known factors are normal. The prothrombin time is normal. The disorder is transmitted as an autosomal dominant.[234a] Further studies will be necessary before the significance of these clotting abnormalities can be assessed.[213, 402, 465]

FACTORS COMMON TO BOTH THE EXTRINSIC AND INTRINSIC SYSTEMS

Factor V.   Factor V is probably formed in the liver but is not vitamin K-dependent. It is found only in the plasma, as it is consumed during the coagulation of blood.[147] The time at which it enters the coagulation scheme has been investigated,[39, 51] and it seems to play an important part in the final phase of thromboplastin formation. Recent evidence indicates that Factor V acts as a co-factor with activated Factor X, phospholipid, and Ca^{++} to form the active prothrombin converting principle.[32, 359] It has been suggested that Factor V is bound to phospholipid together with factor Xa and prothrombin. Factor V may serve to orient factor Xa and prothrombin to one another so as to facilitate their reaction.[165, 166, 166a] Even after prolonged exposure to activated Factor X, Factor V alone is not able to activate any significant amount of prothrombin. Thrombin has been shown to increase the activity of Factor V possibly by increasing its phospholipid binding capacity.[166a]

Factor V is not adsorbed by inorganic adsorbent compounds and remains in $Al(OH)_3$–adsorbed plasma. It migrates between the beta and gamma globulins on filter paper electrophoresis and has a molecular weight of 290,000.[118, 168] It deteriorates rapidly on storage of blood under standard blood bank conditions. Several molecular forms of Factor V have been detected.[405a]

Factor X (Stuart factor).   Factor X[152, 198, 234, 381] is found in the plasma and serum, as it is not consumed during coagulation. It is adsorbed by inorganic adsorbent compounds, and is stable on storage for two months under standard blood bank conditions. It migrates on electrophoresis as an alpha globulin.[131] Factor X has been confused in the past with Factor VII, since the two have many properties in common.

Activated Factor X has been purified from human serum. Factor Xa has a molecular weight of 25,000 and contains 14 per cent carbohydrate. It appears to consist of one polypeptide chain. The molecular weight of Factor X prior to activation has been determined to be from 46,000 to 72,000.[42]

Bovine Factor X has been chromatographically separated into two forms, X_1 and X_2, which differ in carbohydrate composition. Both are made up of two unique polypeptide chains. The heavy chain contains all of the carbohydrate and has a molecular weight of 39,000. The light chain has a molecular weight of 15,000 and may be involved in the attachment of the molecule to lipid surfaces. The heavy chain is chemically similar to thrombin.[187, 246] Evidence also suggests that Factor X may occur as a single polypeptide chain with a molecular weight of 56,000.[339]

Bovine Factor X has been extensively studied. The activated factor is a proteolytic enzyme with an active serine site. Factor X may be activated by limited proteolysis. The esterase and coagulant activities of this serine enzyme are inhibited by diisopropylfluorophosphate (DFP).[245, 291]

Activated Factor X may be titrated with p–nitrophenyl–p′–guanidino-benzoate, which reacts at the site responsible for the coagulant activity. Such titrations indicate that bovine Factor X activated with Russell's viper venom has a single active site per 53,000 molecular weight.[495] Thrombin and two other polypeptides of 16,000 and 19,500 molecular weight were recovered after activation of Factor X with this venom. The heavy polypeptide may contain the original binding site and may exert some inhibitory action by competing for thrombokinase activity.[255]

Activated Factor X (Xa) appears to be the prime activator of prothrombin. At normal concentrations of Factor X, the reaction requires Ca^{++}, phospholipid, and Factor V as co-factor.[219] In very high concentration, Xa alone can activate prothrombin.[32, 565] Factor X probably undergoes some reorientation as the result of exposure to Factor V and phospholipid, which increases its activity. In the laboratory, prior to activation, Factor X is unaffected when perfused through an isolated rabbit liver, whereas activated Factor X is rapidly removed by such a procedure. Such a mechanism may function in vivo to assist the control of the level of activated products of blood coagulation.[135, 139]

Calcium (Factor IV). Calcium ions are necessary for the development of thromboplastin activity in concentrations of between 5 and 20 mg. per 100 ml. Marked prolongation of coagulation time occurs only when the calcium is below 2.5 mg. per 100 ml., and these levels are not seen clinically.[119] The effectiveness of oxalates and citrates as anticoagulants depends on their ability to bind calcium.

Conversion of Prothrombin to Thrombin

The second stage of blood coagulation may be outlined as follows:

$$\text{Prothrombin} \xrightarrow[\text{Ca}^{++}]{\text{Thromboplastin Activity}} \text{Thrombin}$$

Prothrombin (Factor II). The existence of prothrombin was suspected by Schmidt in 1892, and since that time this material has been extensively studied.[294, 471] Prothrombin has a molecular weight of approximately 75,000.[273, 282] Eighteen amino acids and hexosamine have been identified in the molecule. Glutamic acid, aspartic acid, and arginine make up approximately 33 per cent of the protein nitrogen.[281] Prothrombin biosynthesis has been shown to occur in microsomes and polysomes from rat livers.[257] Vitamin K may stimulate the de novo synthesis of prothrombin at the ribosomal level.[389] On electrophoresis, prothrombin behaves as an alpha–1 globulin. It is formed in the liver and is dependent for its production on adequate supply of vitamin K.

Recent work indicates that the activation of the proenzyme prothrombin (Factor II) by Factor Xa and Ca^{++} involves the splitting of prothrombin into two fractions.[165] One fraction has a molecular weight of 37,000 and is termed Intermediate 2. Factor Xa and Ca^{++} convert Intermediate 2 to thrombin. The reaction is accelerated by the presence of phospholipid and Factor V.[166, 166a, 247]

Phospholipids play a fundamental role in prothrombin activation. The protein components, prothrombin and Factors Xa and V, bind to phospholipid particle surfaces,[247] increasing their local concentration. The specificity of the binding appears to serve to orient the reactive components in the most optimum manner.[167]

Thrombin (Factor IIa).   This is quite similar to prothrombin in its amino acid content, and the amount formed in the presence of thromboplastin activity and Ca^{++} varies directly with the amount of prothrombin available.[156, 361] The conversion of bovine prothrombin by Factor Xa is accelerated 50 times in the presence of Ca^{++} and 90 times in the presence of Ca^{++} and phospholipid.[27] Thrombin is not present in circulating blood. It is the material found in shed blood which Buchanan in 1842 showed to be capable of clotting fluid from serous cavities. The species specificity of thrombin–fibrinogen reactions suggests an evolutionary adaptation of the two molecules to yield the most effective possible clotting process.[146] Recent studies indicate that some factor other than the amino acid sequence is responsible for the high level of specificity of the thrombin molecule for fibrinogen.[297] It has been suggested that thrombin has a primary binding site region for small molecule substrates which does not accommodate bulky substituent groups.[173] A unit of thrombin is defined as that amount of thrombin necessary to clot 1 ml. of standard fibrinogen solution in 15 sec. at 28° C. Thrombin has been highly purified. Some of the preparations contain 12,000 units per mg. of nitrogen.[472] Crystals of thrombin are tetragonal dipyramids.[523]

Several active thrombin molecules (α, β, and γ) of different molecular weights have been identified and are believed to result from autodigestion.[273, 283, 325, 395]

Conversion of Fibrinogen to Fibrin

The final stage of blood coagulation may be considered to occur as shown in Figure 16–12.

Fibrinogen (Factor I).   It will be recalled that the conversion of fibrinogen to fibrin in the final phase of coagulation was recognized in 1859 by Denis when he demonstrated the existence of fibrinogen.

Fibrinogen is formed in the liver and is present in the blood in a concentration of 300 mg. per 100 ml. It is a dimer consisting of two almost identical halves, each with three chains, α (A), β (B), and γ. Each chain has a free H_2N–terminal and COOH–terminal. The molecular weight of fibrinogen is 340,000 and that of the chains 64,000, 57,000 and 48,000 respectively. The two halves of the molecule and the chains are held together by disulfide bridges.[58, 60] The biologic half-life of fibrinogen determined by the I^{131} method is reported to be 109 ± 13 hrs.[211, 524]

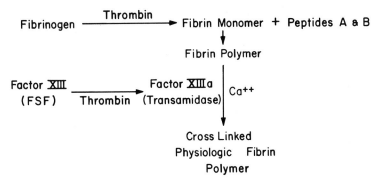

Figure 16–12 Final stage of blood coagulation.

Fibrin is formed when thrombin is added to fibrinogen.[157, 304, 316, 486] Thrombin has the ability to split arginylglycine bonds of the fibrinogen molecule to form a monomer of fibrin and two peptides, A and B.[44, 279] The fibrinopeptides are released from the H_2N–terminal end of the α (A) and β (B) chains. This reaction may lead to the unfolding of the molecule with exposure of polymerization sites.[60] Peptide A is apparently inert, but peptide B has been found to potentiate the contraction of smooth muscle.[194]

Careful physicochemical studies of bovine fibrinogen have revealed marked molecular heterogeneity in a single animal.[366] As new ways to study fibrinogen are developed, unusual (but not necessarily abnormal) fibrinogens may be found to be commonplace.[46]

Factor XIII (Fibrin stabilizing factor). End-to-end polymerization of the fibrin monomers, with one-third molecular length overlap between laterally adjacent fibrils, occurs independently of the presence of thrombin. There is evidence that polymerization may be delayed in the absence of Ca^{++}.[197, 266, 306, 335] Side-to-side bonding of these polymers occurs in the presence of activated Factor XIII (XIIIa), which is a transglutaminase.[181] The transglutaminases are widely distributed in animal tissues, and catalyze Ca^{++}–dependent acyl-transfer reactions in which the γ–carboxamide groups of peptide-bound glutamine residues are the acyl donors.

Activation of Factor XIII by thrombin does not require Ca^{++}, but the presence of the divalent cation does increase the rate of activation.[277, 304, 307, 482] In its active form (XIIIa), it will catalyze the formation of ϵ–(γ–glutamyl) lysine cross-links between fibrin monomers, causing the formation of an insoluble fibrin lattice.[145] The reaction in human and bovine plasma releases glucosylamine, and may account for the 20 per cent loss of carbohydrate from the clot if clotting takes place in the presence of Factor XIII.[82, 100, 301] No such release of carbohydrate has been found when rabbit blood is used, suggesting species variation.[424]

Factor XIII is a proenzyme found in the plasma, platelets, uterus, and placenta. It has a molecular weight of 350,000 and migrates in association with the

α-2 globulins. The molecule appears to be composed of four subunits composed of two types of chains with serine or histidine amino terminal residues.[512] Different subunit forms of the enzyme have been detected.[182] Factor XIII is nondialyzable and thermolabile.[302, 303, 461] Sulfhydryl inactivating compounds will inhibit its activity. It has a biologic half-life of between four and seven days, and very small amounts are required to cross-link fibrin. One milligram will stabilize 11,000 mg. of soluble fibrin.[11, 82]

Studies suggest that Factor XIII is not transported across the platelet membrane in vivo. Platelet Factor XIII is believed to originate in the megakaryocyte, and represent 30 to 50 per cent of whole blood Factor XIII activity.[342]

Venom Coagulant Systems

VENOM OF RUSSELL'S VIPER (STYPVEN)

Many snake venoms possess coagulant activity; of those tested, that of Russell's viper was the most potent.[267, 318] Study of the mode of action of this venom has contributed to the understanding of physiologic hemostasis and has led to its use as a local hemostatic agent. The venom has been purified,[553] and has been demonstrated to have esterase as well as coagulant activity. It behaves as an enzyme in the activation of a coagulation factor present in bovine serum. This factor has a molecular weight of 36,000, and is activated as a portion of the molecule is removed by the enzymatic action of the venom. The activated serum factor then reacts with Factor V, phospholipid, and Ca^{++} to form a product which can convert prothrombin to thrombin.[170] As this reaction does not occur when serum from patients deficient in Factor X is used, it is believed that the serum substrate for the venom is Factor X.[317]

VENOM OF THE MALAYAN PIT VIPER (*Agkistrodon rhodostoma*) (ARVIN, ANCROD, VENACIL)

The venom of the Malayan pit viper is of great interest, as it has the capacity to convert fibrinogen to fibrin directly without activation of any early coagulation factors.[15] The coagulant enzyme is a glycoprotein which has a single polypeptide chain containing 29 per cent carbohydrate by weight.[214] Unlike thrombin, this enzyme cleaves only fibrinopeptide A from fibrinogen. Fibrin monomers form rapidly despite the continued presence of fibrinopeptide B on the fibrin molecule.[414] The clot is friable since Factor XIII is not activated and cross-linking does not occur. The coagulant enzyme of the venom has now been shown to have a direct proteolytic effect on fibrin. It will progressively and totally digest the α chains of fibrin at a site different from that attacked by plasmin.[414] Platelet counts are unaffected.[89] Active fibrinolysis occurs locally and fibrin split products appear in the plasma. There are no massive clots and the small friable clots that form are removed by the reticuloendothelial system.[414] The fibrinogen converting fraction has been successfully separated from whole venom and has proved useful in anticoagulant therapy, since the blood is effectively defibrinated in two to four hours. The effect can be stopped with antivenom.[437] Conversion of fibrinogen to fibrin by the active principles of the venom of the Malayan pit viper is not impeded by heparin.[169] The clinical use of this material remains a subject for further investigation.

SUMMARY

In the light of recent evidence it is possible to draw the tentative scheme of blood coagulation shown in Figure 16–13.

Factor X now appears to be the pivotal substance activated by each of the mechanisms noted. This scheme fits known facts and contributes additional insights into the intrinsic system. Macfarlane has likened the intrinsic system to an electronic amplifier, and has pointed out that at each level a greater amount of proenzyme is activated, resulting in tremendous over-all gain.[318] The rapid disappearance of coagulant enzymes may serve to stop the system and protect the organism from widespread thrombosis.

No theory of blood coagulation may be considered fact until the responsible chemical reactions are elucidated. The one presented above is but an expansion of the classic theory and remains empiric. Deletions or additions must be made as old factors are reconsidered and new factors make their

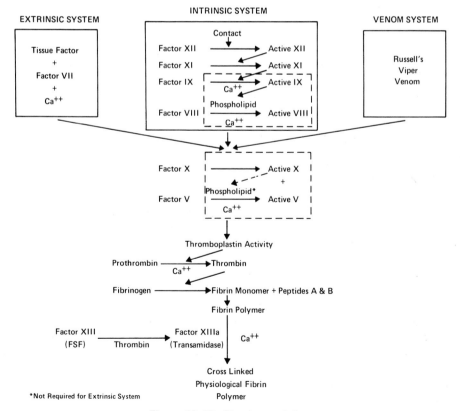

Figure 16–13 Blood coagulation.

appearance. Despite its defects, this theory serves as a useful clinical and laboratory guide.

FIBRINOLYSIS

PHYSIOLOGIC CLOT DISSOLUTION

The fibrinolytic system serves to remove superfluous fibrin after repair of a vessel is complete, and to protect the body from the effects of excess fibrin formation. Plasmin is the enzyme responsible for the digestion of fibrin. In health, only its precursor, plasminogen, is found in the plasma.[327]

Plasminogen

Human plasminogen is a globulin found in plasma fraction III of Cohn.[442, 485] It is a glycoprotein with a molecular weight of 89,000 ± 1500. Conversion to the active form, plasmin, is now believed to be due to cleavage of a single original valine bond by the activator. This cleavage results in a two-chain molecule held together by a single disulfide bond.[16, 440, 469] Sensitive radioimmunoassay has been developed to measure plasminogen and plasmin in the plasma.[423] Plasminogen has a strong affinity for fibrinogen, and their concentrations in most body fluids vary directly.

ACTIVATORS OF PLASMINOGEN

Plasminogen is converted to plasmin in the presence of "activators." Activators have been found in the plasma and in a variety of tissues, notably the uterus, thyroid, lung, prostate, and in the urine.[321] It is interesting to note that, by histologic techniques, plasminogen activator was consistently found associated with the vascular endothelium, particularly veins, venules, and pulmonary arteries.[41, 515, 516, 535] There was none in normal liver. In the liver of patients with cirrhosis, there was evidence of plasminogen activator around or in the veins.[515] Activator activity of the plasma is found to increase after exercise, and following the administration of epinephrine, nicotinic acid, or pyrogens.[95, 113, 280, 320] Recent evidence suggests that Factor XII (Hageman factor) and other products of the coagulation system may play a role in the activation of these proteolytic enzymes.[160, 215, 240, 349]

Urokinase is a plasminogen activator found in the urine.[274, 415] It is a proteolytic enzyme with broad substrate specificity[485] and wide temperature and pH stability. The conversion of plasminogen to plasmin by urokinase proceeds as a first order reaction with an optimum of about pH 9.[274] Urokinase appears to be produced in the kidney[40] and has a molecular weight of 53,000.[290] Investigations using an antiserum against pure urokinase have demonstrated that it is not identical with the activator found in human milk or tissue activators.[278] Preparations of urokinase suitable for intravenous administration are presently available for clinical investigation. Recent studies have shown them to have predictable thrombolytic activity.[176, 484] With continued improvement in purity and reduction in cost, urokinase may come to play an important role in thrombolytic therapy.[176, 479, 524]

Bacterial products capable of activating plasminogen have received intensive study.[108, 133] The best known is streptokinase, which has been highly purified in the hope of developing an effective thrombolytic agent..[106, 107] The mechanism of its action is not completely understood. Thus far no proteolytic or esterase activity of streptokinase has been reported. It requires a proactivator system in the plasma to function.[133, 202] Streptokinase cannot activate plasminogen directly. An activator is first generated by the action of streptokinase and plasminogen. The streptokinase – plasminogen complex can activate plasminogen to plasmin. Plasminogen thus appears to have a dual role as a proactivator and as substrate for the activator complex.[217, 480] Standardization of this agent has been difficult and pyrogenic reactions to its administration a frequent complication. Streptokinase is antigenic, and prior exposure to infection with streptococci will alter the dose requirements. Care must be exercised lest a coagulation defect be induced in the course of treatment.[18, 526]

INHIBITORS OF THE ACTIVATION OF PLASMINOGEN

The existence of naturally occurring inhibitors of plasminogen activators has not been proved.[485] A variety of synthetic substances have been reported to have antiplasmin activity or to inhibit the conversion of plasminogen to plasmin.[351]

The synthetic amino acid epsilon aminocaproic acid (EACA) is worthy of special note, as it has been demonstrated to be effective in inhibiting the conversion of plasminogen to plasmin both in vitro and in vivo. As it has but a weak antiplasmin effect, it is believed to inhibit the enzymatic conversion.[5, 149, 351, 479] It also inhibits the activation of plasminogen in the urine by urokinase[351] and has proved effective in the control of excessive hematuria following prostatectomy.[348, 450]

PLASMIN

Plasmin is the proteolytic enzyme that results from the enzymatic cleavage of the plasminogen molecule. It is an endopeptidase that can digest several proteins in the plasma, including a number of components of the coagulation and complement systems, certain trophic hormones, and others.[202, 400, 469] Under normal circumstances the action of plasmin in vivo is effectively specific for fibrin. Plasmin belongs to the same group of proteinases as trypsin, chymotrypsin, and thrombin. Human plasmin has the same molecular weight as plasminogen, $89,000 \pm 1500$.[181, 440]

The effect of plasmin on the subunit structure of human fibrin has been extensively studied. The lysis of fibrin or of fibrinogen proceeds through a series of steps beginning with formation of the initial X fragment. The X fragment is heterogeneous and contains extensively degraded α chains, partially digested β chains, and intact γ chains.

The X fragment is degraded to D and Y fragments with further digestion. Fragment D contains partially degraded β and γ chains and extensively degraded α chains held together by disulfide bridges.

The Y fragment is further degraded to another D fragment and an E fragment. The E fragment also contains extensively degraded α, β, and γ chains combined by disulfide bonds.[186, 332, 333]

The cleavages of fragments X and Y are considered to be asymmetric.[93]

Plasmin degradation of soluble fibrin is similar to that of fibrinogen, with the exception of the absence of fibrinopeptides A and B.[334]

The results of degradation of cross-linked fibrin by plasmin differ in that, instead of a D fragment, there is a derivative of approximately twice its size, D dimer or double D.[334]

ANTIPLASMIN

The plasma contains substances, which have not been adequately characterized, that appear to inhibit the action of plasmin.[485, 489, 490] Evidence has been presented for two inhibitors of plasmin in the plasma.[385] One substance was recently purified and found to be an α–1 globulin with a molecular weight of 55,000. This inhibitor has both slow and immediate antiplasmin activity.[473] The other reacts immediately, is more stable at extremes of pH, and resists high temperature. It appears to be an α–2 macroglobulin with the capacity to bind serine hydrolase enzymes like trypsin, thrombin, and plasmin to various degrees. The participation of plasma proteins in the fibrinolytic mechanism suggests that they function as a regulator and inhibitor of excessive fibrinolysis.[202]

Platelets also contain antiplasmin.[15] It has been shown that the antiplasmin of bovine platelets is separate from that of bovine plasma, though some of the latter may be adsorbed by the platelets.

PLASMINOGEN ACTIVATION TO PLASMIN

A schematic representation of the reactions believed to be responsible for the activation of plasminogen is shown in Figure 16–14.

A number of investigators have studied the various means by which the action of a proteolytic enzyme with so broad a potential substrate as plasmin is limited to fibrinolysis. At first, it was suggested that fibrin successfully competes with antiplasmin for plasmin. When plasmin forms in the circulation naturally, or as the result of an infusion of activator, it normally is bound to the excess of antiplasmin. In the presence of its preferred substrate fibrin, the complex dissociates and fibrinolysis ensues.[20]

Another concept emphasizes the biologic importance of the affinity of plasminogen for fibrinogen. When plasminogen is slowly converted to plasmin in the plasma, antiplasmin neutralizes its action and no proteolytic activity can be detected. Fibrin clots, however, contain relatively little antiplasmin, and when activators diffuse into the clot the plasmin activated is unopposed, and lysis of the clot results. There is therefore a dual response to the activation of plasmino-

I. In the Plasma as a general phenomenon.

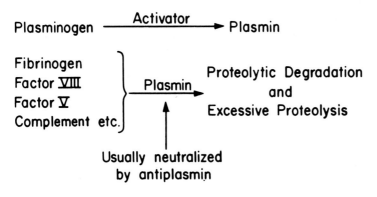

Plasminogen —— Activator ——→ Plasmin

Fibrinogen
Factor VIII
Factor V   Plasmin   Proteolytic Degradation
Complement etc.   and
                                   Excessive Proteolysis

                   Usually neutralized
                   by antiplasmin

II. Within the Fibrin Clot or on the wall of a vessel as a local phenomenon.

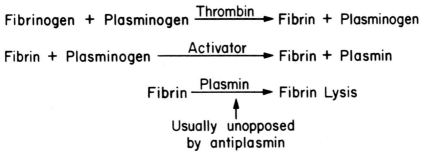

Fibrinogen + Plasminogen —— Thrombin ——→ Fibrin + Plasminogen

Fibrin + Plasminogen —— Activator ——→ Fibrin + Plasmin

Fibrin —— Plasmin ——→ Fibrin Lysis

                   Usually unopposed
                   by antiplasmin

Figure 16–14 Activation of plasminogen.

gen: plasmin which develops in the plasma is neutralized and plays little if any role in thrombolysis; plasmin which develops in the interstices of the clot is relatively unopposed and will effectively lyse the fibrin. In addition, certain tissues, especially the veins and pulmonary arteries, are rich in activator substances. The suggestion has been made that fibrin deposited on such tissues would lyse quickly and might do so without significant change in circulating plasmin.[479]

More recent studies indicate support for still another mechanism. This concept requires the binding or adsorption of induced activator by fibrin in the clot, which then activates the plasminogen carried to the clot by the plasma. Plasminogen is removed from the circulation and converted to plasmin within the thrombus and initiates fibrinolysis. The rate of lysis of an activator-rich clot is then a function of the circulating plasminogen.[102]

In terms of each of these proposals, the action of plasmin with broad digestive potential is limited by location and is biologically specific.[17]

PATHOLOGIC COAGULATION AND PROTEOLYSIS

Relationship to Thrombotic Disease

The possible relationship of some abnormality of the fibrinolytic mechanism to thrombotic disease remains of great interest.[413] Multiple thrombotic episodes were reported to be associated with an increase in an inhibitor of plasminogen activator in several patients.[80, 384] Thrombotic disorders have also been reported in two patients with high titers of antiplasmin and antiplasminogen.[375]

Relationship to Abnormal Hemostasis

The mechanisms responsible for keeping the blood fluid within the vascular systems have not been clearly defined. It seems reasonable to consider that there must be a delicate balance between those forces tending to produce coagulation and those tending to inhibit it. The body must have a mechanism for disposing of a clot once repair of a vessel is complete.

The Hypercoagulable State

Failure of the blood to remain fluid within the vascular system may result in a local thrombus, multiple thromboses, or diffuse intravascular coagulation (DIC).[369] Although thrombosis is an important defense mechanism, serious or fatal consequences may follow either a single thrombosis in an artery or vein or diffuse intravascular coagulation, which occurs in a number of different disorders.

When Virchow introduced the term thrombosis in 1856 he stated that stasis, changes in the walls of the vessels, and biochemical changes in the blood itself are the causes: concepts that have been extended since that time but have remained essentially valid.[508] Considerable effort has been devoted to the attempt to determine the factors that are responsible for nonphysiologic thrombosis and coagulation.[508] Factors such as changes in the vessel wall and stasis may be considered "local," whereas the biochemical aspect is a "general" one.

There is abundant clinical evidence that patients with certain conditions seem predisposed to intravascular thrombosis. The most often cited, but not uniformly supported, instance is that of the patient with malignancy.[296] Most reports indicate that the association is most common with mucin-producing tumors, particularly those arising in the body and tail of the pancreas, and have suggested a relationship between the frequency of thrombotic episodes and the grade of the malignancy.[345, 360, 494]

Other conditions thought to be associated with a hypercoagulable state appear to be examples of an inappropriate degree of response to a recognized stimulus, rather than a response to an ill-defined or unrecognized stimulus. Among these are pregnancy,[14] the postpartum and postoperative state,[536] prolonged bed rest,[542] atherosclerosis,[386] myocardial infarction, and congestive heart failure.[562] In each of these conditions, stasis or vessel wall injury might well be the precipitating cause of the thrombus. It is often difficult to decide whether the response is appropriate or inappropriate to the stimulus.

An association between oral contraceptives and thromboembolism has been recognized, and various abnormalities have been found in the blood or vascular system of patients taking contraceptives. The risk of hospital admission for venous thromboembolism is ninefold greater for women taking "the pill,"[527] and a convincing relationship has been demonstrated between the use of oral contraceptives and an increased incidence of death from pulmonary embolism or cerebral thrombosis;[416] no clear relationship to arterial thrombosis has been established. An increase in coagulation factors VII and X[416] and a decreased sensitivity to coumarin drugs have been reported.[161] There is an increase in platelet sensitivity to ADP,[162] which is thought to be secondary to an abnormality in the lecithin of the low density plasma lipoproteins.[62] An increased diameter of the veins at any given pressure has been clearly shown; this increased distensibility of the veins of the patient taking oral contraceptives results in a decrease in the velocity of venous blood flow, which is believed to be another factor contributing to thrombosis.[560] Oral contraceptives are contraindicated in patients with thromboembolism or a past history of any such disorder; their advantages must be carefully weighed against the dangers which have emerged from recent studies, before prescribing them for any patient. Further studies of these agents are urgently needed.

Although the hypercoagulable state is recognized clinically, laboratory evidence to support the concept is sparse. The levels of the various blood coagulation factors have been reported to be elevated in pregnancy,[14, 401] in the postpartum and postoperative states,[536] and in patients with atherosclerosis.[368] Recently, data have been presented which suggest that patients with a tendency to thrombosis have elevated levels of Factor VIII; in addition, experimental elevation of Factor VIII levels in the blood of dogs enhances intravascular coagulation.[404] Others have pointed out that it is not the absolute quantity of clotting factors present, but whether they circulate in an active form, that is important.[524] Large amounts of nonactivated Factor X fail to produce a thrombus in a laboratory animal, but a small amount of activated Factor X will; the addition of a small amount of phospholipid further reduces the small quantity of activated X required.[23, 524] Of great importance in maintaining the blood in a fluid state is the rate at which activated clotting factors can be removed from the blood by the reticuloendothelial system.[135, 153]

A variety of diseases have been associated with disseminated intravascular coagulation. In most instances the mediating mechanism has been shown to be intravascular hemolysis, tissue extracts, bacterial endotoxins, antigen-antibody complexes, chemical or physical agents, hypoxia, endothelial damage, fibrinolysin inhibitors, or thrombocythemia.[483]

Encouraging as recent advances in our knowledge of the hypercoagulable state have been, much work remains to be done before the specific biochemical changes responsible are understood.[115, 222, 344, 399]

Excessive Proteolysis

Study of iatrogenic proteolysis arising in the course of the therapeutic administration of thrombolytic agents has shed considerable light on the pathogenesis of these states.[181] If plasminogen is rapidly activated, antiplasmin cannot effectively neutralize the plasmin formed. Plasma fibrinogen, Factor VIII, and

Factor V levels fall, and a hemorrhagic diathesis may develop.[180] Studies of the effect of plasmin on fibrin and fibrinogen have revealed that the proteolytic products retain the antigenic identity of fibrin or fibrinogen. Initially, they tend to be large and have a significant antithrombin effect; the products of further proteolysis do not have a strong antithrombin effect, but are anticoagulant since they interfere with the polymerization of fibrin.[181] All interfere with platelet aggregation.[18, 28, 181, 284, 479] These products of proteolysis have also been found in patients with a hemorrhagic diathesis associated with fibrinolysis.[335, 377]

THE DEFIBRINATION SYNDROME (DISSEMINATED INTRAVASCULAR COAGULATION, CONSUMPTIVE COAGULOPATHY, PRIMARY PATHOLOGIC FIBRINOLYSIS, NONCONSUMPTIVE COAGULOPATHY)

The defibrination syndrome occurs in a large number of clinical conditions.[55, 137, 285, 343, 354, 367] The patient usually presents with symptoms of the underlying disease and, in addition, associated anemia, hypotension, hemorrhage, or thrombosis singly or in combination.[30, 205, 407, 451]

There are three major mechanisms which may be responsible for the syndrome of defibrination in clinical medicine (Fig. 16–15).

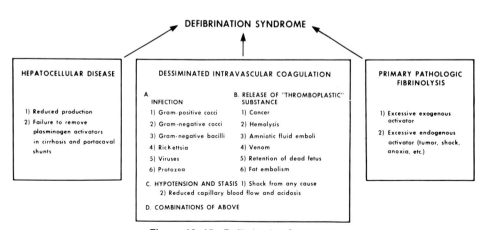

Figure 16–15 Defibrination Syndrome.

DISSEMINATED INTRAVASCULAR COAGULATION

The vast majority of patients have been found to have disseminated intra-vascular coagulation with secondary activation of the fibrinolytic system. Activation of the coagulation system has been reported in an ever-expanding variety of conditions which may be considered under four general categories: (1) infection; (2) release of "thromboplastic" material; (3) hypotension and stasis; and (4) a combination of the three.

Depending on the severity of the process, there is more, or less, consumption of Factors I, V, VIII, and X and the platelets; rarely, Factors II, IX, and XIII also are reduced. Activation of the fibrinolytic system may cause a further reduction of Factors I, V, and VIII as the result of proteolysis. Plasminogen is reduced and the products of proteolytic degradation of fibrinogen and fibrin appear in the circulating blood. Generally, little proteolytic activity can be demonstrated in the blood, and the presence of split products suggests fibrino-lytic activity at local sites of fibrin deposition.[355, 479] Since these split products are in themselves anticoagulant, they contribute significantly to the hemorrhagic diathesis.

PRIMARY PATHOLOGIC FIBRINOLYSIS

A minority of patients with defibrination syndrome have primary patho-logic fibrinolysis which can occur as the result of several mechanisms. In the presence of large amounts of plasminogen activator, much of the available plasminogen may be converted to plasmin and may overwhelm the antiplasmin system. This may occur as the result of the inadvertent administration of excessive amounts of exogenous plasminogen activator during thrombolytic therapy of thromboembolism. Large amounts of endogenous activator may be released from some activator-rich neoplastic tissue, such as found in metastatic carcinoma of the prostate, acute progranulocytic leukemia, or in the course of severe shock or hypoxia.[483] Impairment of the body's ability to remove plas-minogen activator from the circulation will also result in hyperplasminemia, which has been observed in cirrhosis of the liver and after portacaval shunting procedures.[178, 200] There is also the possibility that a fibrinolytic enzyme other than plasmin may gain access to the circulation.[179]

HEPATOCELLULAR DISEASE

Thirdly, the blood may be depleted of fibrinogen and other clotting factors as the result of severe hepatocellular disease (nonconsumptive coagulopathy). The most prominent result of the defect in synthesis is the reduction of the vitamin K–dependent factors, Factors II (prothrombin), VII, IX, and X. Vita-min K malabsorption, as the result of the disturbance in liver function, may further contribute to the decrease in synthesis[328] of these factors. Factors V and I (fibrinogen) may also be markedly reduced and XI and XIII variably reduced as the result of hepatocellular dysfunction.[116, 390, 428, 529] Thrombocytopenia may occur in the course of severe liver disease, and failure to remove activated clotting factors and plasminogen activator has been noted.[116, 137, 174, 443] The finding of normal or high levels of Factor VIII in the coagulopathy associated with severe liver disease is of value in separating this disorder from disseminated intravascular coagulation.[116] Generally, liver disease of a severity to produce these changes is easily recognized clinically.

Despite the advances made in the past few years toward the understanding of the defibrination syndromes which occur in many and varied disorders, much work remains before these syndromes can be clearly delineated and more adequately treated.[117, 124, 177, 179, 313, 352, 353, 409, 443, 483]

ANTICOAGULANTS

PHYSIOLOGIC ANTICOAGULANTS

Antithrombins

Thrombin has been noted to be an extremely potent proteolytic enzyme, and it must be removed or in some manner neutralized following physiologic coagulation, otherwise all of the blood in the body would soon be clotted.

A series of antithrombins have been described.[300, 314, 421, 470] In whole plasma, the two major mechanisms for the removal of thrombin appear to be the immediate adsorption and inactivation of most thrombin by fibrin, followed by a progressive inactivation of remaining thrombin by an antithrombin in the alpha globulin fraction of the serum.[314] When compared with two other naturally occurring thrombin inhibitors, α_2 macroglobulin and α_1 antitrypsin, antithrombin III appears to be the main inactivator of thrombin. When present in physiologic amounts, thrombin has a half-life of 40 seconds.[2] There is considerable evidence that antithrombin III, heparin cofactor, and anti-Factor Xa are functions of the same inhibitor and may inhibit other serine enzymes.[47, 123, 159, 447, 546] An α_2–macroglobulin also contributes to the inactivation of thrombin to a minor degree.[3, 192]

Several families have been reported whose members had repeated episodes of thrombosis and embolism associated with a decrease in antithrombin III activity.[159] In those studied, the levels of antithrombin III activity and levels of antithrombin III material measured immunologically were proportionally reduced.[462] Of interest is the recent report of another family with normal levels of antithrombin III when measured by immunologic techniques but depressed biologic activity, suggesting a qualitative molecular abnormality. The deficit appears to be inherited as an autosomal trait in both instances.[462]

Antithrombin activity has been reported to develop in the course of proteolysis of fibrinogen by plasmin in vitro.[277, 520]

PHARMACOLOGIC ANTICOAGULANTS

The major pharmacologic anticoagulants are heparin and the coumarin-indandione drugs. Their use has doubtless prevented many deaths from thrombosis and embolism and has made possible the rapid development of cardiovascular surgery and extracorporeal bypass procedures. However, they must be used with proper attention to laboratory control to prevent inadvertent hemorrhage.[13, 109a, 242]

Little or no controversy attends the use of pharmacologic anticoagulants to suppress the biochemical phase of blood coagulation in patients on cardiopulmonary bypass, during renal dialysis, after vascular reconstructive surgery, pulmonary embolism and in those with thrombophlebitis. There remains considerable disagreement over the indications for their use to prevent further thrombosis following myocardial infarction and cerebrovascular thrombosis. Further studies are needed to settle these issues.

Prior to the administration of these drugs the physician must determine by history, physical examination, and laboratory studies any actual or potential source of hemorrhage. He must then balance the risk of hemorrhage against that of thromboembolism for the particular patient under his care.

Anticoagulant therapy is usually contraindicated if the patient gives a history of hemorrhagic diathesis, active ulceration or bleeding from the gastrointestinal or genitourinary tract, recent trauma to the central nervous system, severe hepatic disease, or marked hypertension. The history of chronic ingestion of salicylates, phenylbutazone, or other agents which potentiate the action of the coumarin-indandione drugs might indicate a need to reduce the dosage of anticoagulant.[13] Broad-spectrum antibiotics which alter the bacterial flora of the intestinal tract and reduce bacterial synthesis of vitamin K may profoundly augment the response to coumarin-indandione anticoagulants. Malabsorption, biliary, or liver disease may also increase susceptibility to these medications.

Many drugs, such as phenobarbital, griseofulvin, and glutethimide, depress the effect of coumarin-like anticoagulants through their action as inducers of liver microsomal enzymes. Thus, the withdrawal of such drugs from patients stabilized on a given dose of these anticoagulants may precipitate a fall in Factors II, VII, IX, or X to dangerous levels. Other drugs, such as salicylates, phenylbutazone, and sulfonamides, which potentiate the effect of coumarin-like anticoagulants, may act by competitively displacing the anticoagulant from plasma proteins, thus making available more active anticoagulant.[310]

Heparin

Heparin is a mucopolysaccharide which is similar to the chondroitin-sulfuric acid of cartilage. It was isolated from the liver of dogs and contains large quantities of glucuronic acid (26 per cent) and glucosamine (23 per cent).[260] The natural occurrence of heparin in the tissues and circulating blood of man is disputed.

Heparin is a direct anticoagulant. Its effect is due to its chemical properties and it affects coagulation directly in vivo or in vitro. The action of heparin is preventive; there is little evidence to indicate any significant effect on a formed thrombus other than the prevention of extension.[136] Available evidence[49, 148, 323] indicates that heparin acts in vivo and in vitro by interfering with the development of thromboplastin activity. This is suggested by the fact that neither Factor VIII nor Factor V is consumed in its presence. There is also direct interference with thromboplastin activity at higher concentrations.

Heparin combines with a co-factor in plasma to inhibit thrombin. Recent evidence indicates that antithrombin III, activated Factor X inhibitor, and heparin co-factor are biologic activities which belong to a single plasma proteinase inhibitor.[47, 569] Heparin has been shown markedly to accelerate the rate of the reactions in which this inhibitor participates.[123] It appears that heparin binds antithrombin III, inducing an allosteric modification which renders the arginine-reactive site of antithrombin III more accessible to the serine in the active site of thrombin. The lysyl residues of the inhibitor probably serve as the binding site for heparin.[444]

The reaction of antithrombin III with activated Factor X is of great importance.[47, 567] One mg. of Xa inhibitor inhibits 32 units of Xa. This prevents the generation of 1600 NIH units of thrombin which otherwise would require 1000 mg. of inhibitor to neutralize.[546] Heparin dramatically increases the rate of this reaction, although it has no effect by itself on Xa.[566]

Evidence has now been presented which indicates that antithrombin III plays a role in the inhibition of activated Factor XI, and that heparin also accelerates that reaction.[123]

These findings suggest that other serine proteases in the coagulation sequence may be similarly inhibited.[123]

These reports have stimulated a great deal of interest in the use of heparin to prevent the occurrence of a hypercoagulable state without producing a hypocoagulable state. If heparin can augment the action of antithrombin III in neutralizing Xa and XIa, the explosive evolution of thrombin may be prevented.[546] Preliminary results of the use of low-dose heparin to prevent the evolution of thrombin, rather than the higher doses required after its formation, have been encouraging.[193, 262, 543, 547]

The clearance of heparin from the circulation is exponential at a rate dependent on the dose administered.[193] Twenty per cent is eliminated by the kidneys, and the rest is degraded by the liver. Patients vary widely in their response to the anticoagulant, however, and factors such as body weight, shock, fever, hepatic insufficiency and the presence of thrombosis may alter the amount necessary to achieve a therapeutic effect.[193] It is important to individualize control of heparin therapy.[171] Heparin does not cross the placenta, nor does it appear in the milk of a nursing mother.[136]

Heparin has several actions other than anticoagulation. It has a well-recognized lipemia-clearing activity mediated by its activation of endogenous lipoprotein lipase.[128, 493a]

Heparin is supplied in aqueous solution as the sodium salt. Since preparations vary in potency, it is well to order the number of units desired.[193]

ADMINISTRATION

Prevention of Thrombosis.   The use of heparin as a prophylactic agent is not new but has recently stimulated much interest.[443a, 475, 493a] One regimen suggests 5000 units subcutaneously two hours prior to surgery, continued every

12 hours for seven days.[262] Other regimens have been suggested.[193, 261, 288, 543] These levels rarely disturb the whole blood clotting time or the activated partial thromboplastin time.

Active Thrombosis. The intermittent or continuous intravenous administration of heparin is considered most satisfactory. When given intermittently the initial dose is 5000 to 10,000 units USP, and subsequent doses of 5000 units USP are given at four- to six-hour intervals depending on laboratory studies.

When continuous intravenous administration is employed, flow rates must be carefully monitored (preferably delivered by a constant infusion pump) to avoid inadvertant administration of excessive heparin. The average 24 hour requirement ranges from 25,000 to 30,000 units when heparin is administered continuously by the intravenous route. Again there is wide individual variation necessitating careful laboratory control.[193] Various different dosage schedules and methods of administration have been suggested.[136]

Control of anticoagulation is difficult as the administration of these drugs is largely on an empiric basis. It is not accurately known to what extent the clotting time should be prolonged to provide successful anticoagulation. The whole blood clotting time has been the test most widely used to control heparin therapy. Recent studies indicate that the activated whole blood partial thromboplastin time is also satisfactory.[56, 171, 193, 544, 575] It is usually desirable to administer sufficient heparin to prolong the whole blood clotting time or the activated partial thromboplastin time $1\frac{1}{2}$ to $2\frac{1}{2}$ times normal.[193] New methods to measure heparin effect are under development, and may prove useful in the control of anticoagulation but are not yet established.[132]

Heparin may also be given subcutaneously and concentrated solutions of heparin are available for this purpose. The subcutaneous injection of 10,000 units USP alters the whole blood clotting time for approximately eight hours. Long-acting "Depo" heparin preparations are also available. As the response to the subcutaneous administration of these preparations is not as predictable as when heparin is given by the intravenous route, and since the occurrence of large hematomas at the site of injection is a serious risk, the intravenous route is preferred. Intramuscular administration of heparin is not recommended because of the high risk of hematomas.

Aspirin should not be administered, as it interferes with platelet function, which is one of the few hemostatic defenses left to the patient receiving heparin.

Complications. The major complication is hemorrhage secondary to the anticoagulant effect. Trauma may be associated with serious hemorrhage; intramuscular medication should be avoided. Severe metabolic bone disease with osteoporosis and vetebral collapse has occurred following prolonged administration of doses of 10,000 units a day or more for over a year. Interference with aldosterone production, occasional alopecia, and transient thrombocytopenia have been reported. Hypersensitivity to heparin has been reported.[121, 136]

Antidote. The action of heparin may be quantitatively neutralized by protamine sulfate.[101] Protamine equivalence, however, varies with the source of heparin, the testing conditions, and, in vivo, with the amount of heparin in the circulation. The amount remaining in the circulation will depend on the time elapsed since the last dose, as well as the physiologic state of the patient.[254]

Protamine should be administered as a 1 per cent solution in an amount calculated to provide 1 to 1.25 mg. protamine per milligram of heparin but not in excess of 100 mg. over a 24-hour period. Excessive protamine may produce an anticoagulant effect.[543] The amount of heparin may be assumed to be approximately one-half the amount given one half-hour earlier.[193]

Protamine must be given slowly. If administered rapidly it will cause the release of histamine and will aggregate platelets.[254] It is interesting that the effect of protamine was discovered by investigators searching for a material to prolong the action of heparin. They chose protamine because of its action in slowing the release of insulin from subcutaneous depots.

Coumarin and Indandione Derivatives

At the time when the original investigations of vitamin K were being conducted, a number of workers were investigating the hemorrhagic sweet clover disease in cattle. Although first thought to be of infectious origin, it was soon recognized to result from the ingestion of spoiled sweet clover. The agent in spoiled sweet clover responsible for the hemorrhagic tendency was identified[237, 505] as 3,3'-methylene-bis (4'-hydroxycoumarin), and its effect on the prothrombin time demonstrated. This entire story is reviewed in excellent fashion by Link.[298]

A number of "coumarin drugs" have now been synthesized and are used in the prevention of thrombosis. The structural relationship between the coumarin drugs and synthetic vitamin K is striking, and it has been suggested that these anticoagulants may compete with vitamin K and substitute for it in reactions ordinarily leading to the formation of "prothrombin." They act as indirect anticoagulants. They do not alter clotting in vitro, but will impair coagulation in vivo by depressing the plasma levels of the vitamin K-dependent coagulation Factors II, VII, IX, and X. The coagulation factors disappear at different rates, depending on the half-life of each one. Factor VII has the shortest half-life and disappears first, followed by IX, X, and finally II. A circulating anticoagulant protein has been noted in patients with vitamin K deficiency. It is believed to be an analogue of Factor X.[220]

Despite much study, the precise manner in which these drugs affect the synthesis or cellular release of these factors remains unknown.[30, 155, 308, 309, 427, 511]

From 78 to 100 per cent of oral sodium warfarin is absorbed from the intestine in two hours.[84] Complexed to albumin, it is carried by the blood to the liver, where it is detoxified by enzymes in the microsomes. The biologic half-life is 42 ± 12 hours.[561] The drug is now believed to act after the synthesis of the protein component of the clotting factors.[378, 561] Studies of dicoumarol-induced bovine prothrombin have recently demonstrated a specific vitamin K-dependent peptide. The properties of this peptide, including its ability to bind calcium ions, appear to account for the differences between normal prothrombin and the biologically inactive form of the molecule which follows coumarin administration.[378, 561]

Following administration of coumarin drugs to man, an altered prothrombin molecule appears in the plasma which shares the main antigenic determinants with normal prothrombin, but is not activated by physiologic activators. It may be activated by staphylocoagulase in vitro to produce normal amounts of thrombin.[99, 221]

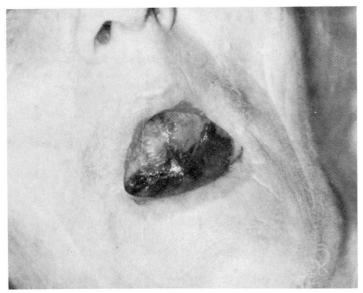

Figure 16–16 Large area of hemorrhage beneath the tongue of a patient who took salicylates for several days while on long-term anticoagulant therapy with coumarin compound.

Two groups of blood relatives have been reported in whom hereditary resistance to oral anticoagulant drugs has been documented. All were extremely sensitive to very small amounts of exogenous vitamin K. The abnormality is transmitted by a simple dominant effect on an autosomal chromosome.[391] The findings in these patients thus differ from those in the warfarin-resistant rats, which have been found to have 20 times the normal vitamin K requirement, suggesting a lowered binding capacity for both vitamin K and warfarin.[223]

Table 16–1 *Dosage Schedules for Coumarin and Indandione Drugs*

| | DRUG | DOSE (mg.)* | | RESPONSE (hrs.) | |
Class	Generic Name	Initial	Daily Maintenance	Onset of Activity After Initial Dose	Return to Normal After Last Dose
Coumarin	Bishydroxycoumarin	First day 300 Second day 200	25–100	48–96	48–96
	Warfarin	First day 40–60 Second day 0–15	5–10	30–48	72–110
Indandione	Phenindione	First day 200 Second day 100	25–100	24–48	48–72

*It is important to note that the doses given here represent a general approximation and that actual dosage required by an individual patient may vary widely in either direction from the figures given.

Coumarin and indandione derivatives are different chemical compounds which are closely related in structure and action and may be considered together.[239] These compounds are completely absorbed from the gastrointestinal tract, though in some individuals absorption is erratic. Peak plasma levels occur in from two to 13 hours and remain for variable periods. The duration of effect is related to persistence of the drug in the plasma, but it varies widely among various subjects. The response to these drugs is apt to be more pronounced in elderly or febrile patients. Anything which interferes with the availability of vitamin K, such as poor nutrition, malabsorption syndrome, oral antibiotics which alter normal bacterial flora, and biliary or liver disease will increase susceptibility to these drugs. The administration of salicylate, phenylbutazone, and oxyphenylbutazone may potentiate the effect of these anticoagulants. (Fig. 16–16).[295, 392, 468, 511, 539]

Increased resistance to the drugs has been noted following administration of liver microsomal enzyme inducers such as barbiturates.[155, 392]

The dosage schedule for these compounds must be developed for each patient. The figures given in Table 16–1 are intended only as general guide lines.

CONTROL OF THERAPY

In view of the variable effect of these drugs in different individuals, they cannot safely be used without access to a reliable laboratory in which their effect may be measured. The most widely used test to control anticoagulant therapy with the coumarin-indandione derivatives is the one-stage prothrombin time test.

The results of the test may be reported in a variety of ways, most of which relate the prothrombin time of the patient to that of a control plasma. The optimal range lies between one and one-half and two and one-half times normal, depending on the source of thromboplastin used.

The prothrombin and proconvertin (P and P) test and the thrombotest have also been used to control anticoagulant therapy with coumarin and indandione drugs with good results.

COMPLICATIONS

The most serious side-effect of these drugs is hemorrhage. Microscopic hematuria, epistaxis, or bleeding from the gums or rectum occurs in approximately 5 per cent of patients on short-term treatment. As many of these patients are not given long-term treatment, the incidence of hemorrhage is lower in the latter group. A rare complication is the occurrence of a sequence of petechiae, ecchymoses, hemorrhagic infarcts and progressive necrosis of the skin and underlying structures in random sites usually between the third and sixth day. The breast and penis have occasionally been involved. These lesions are believed to be due to a toxic reaction of the vascular system at the junction of the precapillary arteriole and capillary.[127, 365, 376] Of interest is the patient who will have significant gastrointestinal or genitourinary hemorrhage while in the "therapeutic range," focusing attention on the possible presence of otherwise unsuspected disease in these areas. Coumarin drugs pass the placental barrier and also appear in the milk. Infants may already be deficient in those factors affected by these drugs and their use is contraindicated in pregnancy or lactation.

Toxic reactions other than bleeding may occur but are quite rare. Nausea, vomiting, diarrhea, leukopenia, thrombocytopenia and leukemoid reactions, as well as hepatic and renal damage, have been reported to be somewhat more common with the indandione drugs than with those of the coumarin group.[13]

ANTIDOTES

Vitamin K administered intravenously, subcutaneously, intramuscularly, or orally, depending on the urgency, will reverse the effects of the coumarin-indandione drugs. The most active preparation is phytonadione (Vitamin K_1), which produces an effect in three to six hours, although the full effect is not apparent for 24 hours. Whole blood or plasma transfusion is used in addition to vitamin K if immediate correction is needed. Concentrates of vitamin K–dependent factors (Factors II, VII, IX, and X) (e.g., Konyne) also are effective. The use of such concentrates should be limited to those situations in which control cannot be effected by the above measures, since they are derived from pooled plasma and may transmit hepatitis. The factors involved are relatively stable, and ordinary bank blood or plasma will be effective. It should be noted that once vitamin K is given, the patient may be resistant to further anticoagulant therapy for a few days.

PLATELET INHIBITORS

Interest has markedly increased recently in the therapeutic use of agents which interfere with the role of platelets in thromboembolism. The two most promising drugs have been aspirin and dipyridamole.[85, 142]

Aspirin

Aspirin appears to inhibit the release of ADP from the platelet, thereby inhibiting secondary platelet aggregation. It does not inhibit primary ADP-induced aggregation.[540, 574] It may affect the occurrence and outcome of ischemic heart disease, but convincing data are not yet in hand.[75, 163] The benefits of its use in the prevention of venous thrombosis have not been striking.[458, 540]

Dipyridamole

This compound, first introduced as a vasodilator, has been shown to modify the uptake of adenosine by platelets. Like aspirin, dipyridamole does not inhibit the aggregation of platelets by ADP, but does appear to have a mild inhibitory effect on the platelet release reaction. There is evidence that it inhibits phosphodiesterase and enhances PGE_1, actions which tend to increase cAMP and inhibit platelet aggregation.[164, 455, 458]

Dipyridamole has been shown to be effective in reducing the incidence of thromboembolic incidents after cardiac valve replacement and the development of arterial thrombi in experimental animals.[140, 510] There has been no striking effect on the incidence of venous thrombotic disease.[90, 458]

The mechanisms by which these drugs affect platelet function are not clearly understood.[506, 540]

EXAMINATION OF THE PATIENT WITH HEMORRHAGIC DIATHESIS

The most accurate clinical diagnosis in the case of hemorrhagic diathesis is reached when a specific defect is demonstrated and its cause determined. To attain this goal, special laboratory techniques are often required in the course of the diagnostic examination which begins when the patient consults his physician because of abnormal bleeding. As with any diagnostic problem, however, the physician notes the character of the symptoms and signs, then proceeds in an orderly manner to a consideration of the various disorders known to produce such complaints. With constant review of the evidence collected during the course of his examination, the physician is able to exclude certain disorders while pursuing others with increased interest. Final identification of the cause of the complaint allows institution of rational therapy.

HISTORY

It is sometimes difficult to establish whether a particular patient has a hemorrhagic diathesis or not. The answer may be obvious if the patient presents with purpura or hemarthroses, but may be elusive when a patient with a history of "easy bruising" is to be evaluated prior to elective surgery. The presence of a hemorrhagic diathesis is best demonstrated by the history, as results of laboratory tests are often variable during the course of these disorders. A history of abnormal bleeding is far more significant than a battery of negative laboratory tests.

The history obtained from a patient suspected of having a bleeding diathesis should begin with a detailed review of the events of his birth and early childhood. Many disorders of hemostasis are hereditary and manifested soon after delivery. Specific inquiry should be made as to the occurrence of excessive bleeding from the umbilical cord or following circumcision. Prolonged bleeding or excessive bruising in the wake of minor trauma should be regarded with suspicion. Tonsillectomy and adenoidectomy are challenges to which many children are subjected and to which a child with a hemorrhagic diathesis may respond abnormally. Occasional epistaxis is not unusual in childhood, but repeated severe epistaxis is cause for concern. Loss of the first teeth during childhood is often accompanied by slight bleeding, but persistent bleeding is evidence in favor of a hemorrhagic diathesis.

On reaching adult life, the hemostatic defenses of the patient continue to be challenged. The female patient may note excessive menstrual bleeding; pregnancy and subsequent delivery further test hemostasis. If excessive bleeding occurs with delivery or menstruation, efforts should be made to determine whether some obstetric or endocrine condition, rather than a defect in hemostasis, could be responsible for the bleeding. Minor cuts and scratches sustained in the kitchen or garden constantly test the efficiency of hemostasis. Operative procedures constitute important diagnostic trials of hemostasis, and the result of each should be recorded. The oozing of blood from the gums after brushing the teeth occurs occasionally in normal persons, but is of significance if severe or persistent. Men are daily exposed to minor razor nicks and will remember excessive bleeding because of the inconvenience it causes. It is clear that the most important tests of hemostasis are those afforded by the stress of day-to-day life about the home or while at work. The results of these tests are available to the physician for the asking.

A careful history of drug ingestion must be obtained. The importance of the anticoagulants is obvious, but other drugs may also interfere with coagulation. Salicylates, phenylbutazone, and oxyphenylbutazone may potentiate anticoagulants, and salicylates alone can cause gastrointestinal hemorrhage; barbiturates may increase resistance to anticoagulants by induction of microsomal enzyme activity; dipyridamole and salicylates interfere with platelet aggregation and should be noted.

The family history is of paramount importance in determining if the defect is congenital or acquired. It is essential to discover whether any members of the patient's family are known to be "bleeders." If it appears likely that others do have a hemorrhagic diathesis, the physician should examine as many members of the family as are available. This is important not only to the patient at hand but for purposes of counseling members of the family group. Such studies will allow the physician the opportunity of contributing to the general understanding of the genetic mechanisms involved.

The onset of abnormal bleeding at birth or during infancy is strong evidence that the disorder was genetically transmitted, and a negative family history does not rule out this possibility. Some disorders of coagulation are transmitted by genes that are autosomal recessive, and the patient must be homozygous for the abnormal gene in order that its presence be clinically apparent. The child in question may be the first member of the family homozygous for the abnormal gene or may represent a mutation. The patient may be assumed to have an acquired hemorrhagic diathesis if he has reached adult life before the onset of abnormal bleeding and has a negative family history.

PHYSICAL EXAMINATION

Once it is established that the patient has a defect in hemostasis, it is important to determine what phase of hemostasis is defective and, if the hemorrhagic diathesis is of the acquired type, the nature of the underlying disease. The physical examination, with particular reference to the characteristics of the abnormal bleeding, will usually provide helpful information.

A disorder of the vascular phase of hemostasis is suggested by the finding of petechiae, ecchymoses, and superficial bruising. Characteristically these lesions are found in the skin of the extremities and over pressure points. The most common sites are the lower legs and ankles, but the forearms, wrists, and buttocks are frequently involved. Petechiae may also be seen in the mucous membranes of the mouth and on ophthalmoscopic examination of the retina. The ecchymotic lesions of senile purpura are located over the dorsum of the hands and feet where there is but scant subcutaneous tissue to provide support for the vessels. The occurrence of purpuric lesions only in the skin of the hands, feet, and ears suggests the presence of a cold precipitable protein or cold agglutinin, as these areas are most subject to exposure to the elements. Petechial hemorrhages widely scattered over the trunk as well as the extremities may be the result of a rickettsial, bacterial, or viral infection. A clue to the etiology of the purpura may be found in the associated dermatologic lesions. The Schönlein-Henoch syndrome is characteristically associated with a variety of skin lesions, and erythema, edema, and necrosis of the skin have all been noted. The presence of eczema, hives or wheals may indicate that an allergy is the inciting cause of the purpura; the finding of purplish-red infiltrations of the skin associated with petechiae and ecchymoses might point to a leukemic process.

A disorder of blood coagulation is suspected in the presence of joint hemorrhage, large hematomas, post-traumatic hemorrhage and delayed hemorrhage. The joint into which bleeding has occurred is painful and swollen, and the presence of fluid is usually demonstrable. Later there may be ankylosis and residual bone destruction. All joints should be carefully examined for evidence of prior hemorrhage. Hematomas may develop at any site but occur most frequently in those parts of the body exposed to trauma. Truly spontaneous hemorrhage is very rare, but the amount of trauma necessary to produce hemorrhage may be slight indeed. It has been reported, for example, that hemorrhage into a vocal cord may occur while a patient is singing. Common locations of deep hematomas are the tongue, neck, buttocks, and extremities. The persistence of bleeding following operative or accidental trauma, or its recurrence, should alert the physician to the possibility of a bleeding dyscrasia.

Other details of the physical examination are also important. Ophthalmoscopic examination of the retina may reveal retinopathy compatible with the presence of leukemia, thrombocytopenia, anemia, or polycythemia. Of these, only the lesions of leukemia are specific. The perivascular sheathing of the retinal veins seen in this disorder is thought to represent collections of leukocytes. Subhyaloid, flame-shaped, or punctate hemorrhages may be seen in patients with severe anemia or thrombocytopenia. Distention of the veins and a diffuse plethora of the retina are often present in polycythemia. The presence of hemorrhagic lesions with pale centers is suggestive of endocarditis, though similar lesions may occur in anemia and in tuberculosis.

The gums of patients with leukemia may be swollen and oozing blood. Ulcerations of the buccal mucosa and posterior pharynx are also commonly associated with this disease. The mouth is also a frequent site of the lesions of hereditary hemorrhagic telangiectasia.

LABORATORY EXAMINATION

Following completion of the clinical examination of the patient, the physician must turn to the laboratory for further information as to the nature of any defect in hemostasis which he has uncovered. It is important that he understand just what information laboratory tests do and do not afford. The tests which are used to identify defects in hemostasis are empiric. The reagents used in the performance of the tests are not pure and the reactions involved are largely unknown. Their usefulness is directly related to the experience of the technical staff who must perform the tests and the ability of the physician to interpret them.

The technical staff must be familiar with the range of normal results in their own laboratory. Results considered to be within the normal range in one laboratory may not be so considered in another. The constant use of normal controls is essential if meaningful results are to be obtained. The physician should become thoroughly familiar with the laboratory tests available to him. He should know something of the nature and purity of the reagents used, the technique of performing the tests, and the calculations used to derive the results recorded in the chart. He will then be able to interpret correctly the results of these empiric procedures and so obtain much useful information.

The platelet count, bleeding time, tourniquet test, and estimation of retraction all measure the adequacy of the vascular phase of hemostasis. The *platelet count* is quantitative and affords information as to the number of circulating platelets.[83] The factor used in calculating the result of the indirect count is from 2500 to 5000, and that used in the direct count from 1000 to 1500. A variation of 10 platelets counted by either method may result in a difference of 10,000 to 50,000 platelets per cu. mm. being recorded in the chart. A careful examination of the peripheral blood smear often affords as much information as the quantitative enumeration of the platelets.

The *bleeding time* is designed to test the response of small vessels to injury.[154] It is immediately apparent that variations in the thickness of the skin and the distribution of the vessels combine to prevent uniformity of the test from patient to patient, or indeed in the same patient from day to day. It is likely that the Ivy method of obtaining the average bleeding time of three uniform punctures of the skin of the inner surface of the forearm has some advantage over that obtained from the single ear lobe puncture. Again it should be pointed out that the reliability of this test is directly related to the experience of the person doing it. False positive as well as false negative results may be obtained.

The *tourniquet test* is less reliable than either the platelet count or the bleeding time. Designed to test the response of the small vessels to stress, its reproducibility is depressingly rare. Minor variations from normal are unreliable and major variations can in many instances be predicted in advance. When it seems obvious that the tourniquet test will be positive, the performance of the test with the attendant discomfort to the patient is perhaps unwise.

Both the speed and completeness of *clot retraction* have been correlated with the quantity and quality of the platelets in the blood. In addition to reflecting alterations in platelet number and function, clot retraction is affected by the red blood cell volume.[6, 315]

The *one-stage prothrombin time* test is used to reveal deficiencies of those factors essential to the conversion of prothrombin to thrombin in the presence of *tissue* thromboplastin activity. The factors which influence the results of the test are Factor V, Factor X, Factor VII, and prothrombin. Since the end point of the test is the formation of a fibrin clot, a deficiency of fibrinogen will also be revealed. This test, despite its lack of specificity, is of great clinical importance.[420]

The *coagulation time* is another nonspecific test which measures the over-all effectiveness of blood coagulation.[287] It is a rather insensitive test and moderate abnormalities of the first stage of blood coagulation may go undetected. It is most accurately performed by the Lee and White four tube method. Care should be taken that an admixture of tissue juices with the blood does not occur during venipuncture.

The *partial thromboplastin time* is an excellent test which has proved valuable in the detection of deficiencies in the intrinsic system. It is simpler to perform and less time-consuming than the thromboplastin generation test, and it has had widespread acceptance. The crucial aspect of this test is the use of a "partial," rather than a "complete," thromboplastin, as is used in the one-stage prothrombin time test. The partial thromboplastin will not react with Factor VII of the extrinsic system but does allow activation of the intrinsic system, and clinically important clotting deficiencies of Factors XII, XI, IX, VIII, X, V, as well as II and I, can generally be excluded if the results are normal. Defects in Factor VII, Factor XIII, and platelets will not be detected.

The test is sometimes difficult to interpret since mild deficiencies may not be detected. Usually deficiencies will be detected if the levels are below 35 per cent, but occasionally a patient with a deficiency at the 20 per cent level will have test results in the upper range of normal. Rarely, apparently normal individuals with no detectable clotting abnormality may have values slightly above the normal range.[37]

Estimations of the *split products* of proteolytic digestion of fibrinogen and fibrin have been made by a number of methods.[96, 175, 179, 355, 521] One of the most sensitive is the hemagglutination immunoassay. Serially diluted serum is incubated with antifibrinogenic rabbit serum. The quantity of split products present in the serum determines the residual antibody, which can be measured using tanned fibrinogen-coated red cells. Normal serum is found to contain up to 6 μg/ml.; that of patients with defibrination syndromes has up to 200 μg/ml.[356]

The *thromboplastin generation test* has proved to be one of the most important tests of blood coagulation.[8] It will reveal any deficiency of the coagulation factors essential to the development of thromboplastin activity in the intrinsic (blood) system. The test is based on the fact that potent thromboplastin activity develops during the incubation at 37° C of normal $Al(OH)_3$ adsorbed plasma (containing Factor VIII, Factor XI, Factor XII, and Factor V), normal serum (containing Factor X, Factor XI, Factor XII, and Factor IX), platelets or a platelet substitute such as cephalin, together in the presence of calcium ions. The rate of development of the thromboplastin activity in normal platelet-free citrated plasma is measured by adding a sample of the incubation mixture and a source of calcium ions at one-minute intervals and measuring the time required for it to produce a clot. The rate of development of thromboplastin activity in incubation mixtures using normal components is then compared with the rates obtained when the patient's plasma, serum, or platelets are substituted serially for their normal counterparts in three additional incubation mixtures. Each of the three mixtures contains two normal components and one from the patient. Thus the defect may be localized in the serum, adsorbed plasma, or platelets.

If the development of thromboplastin activity is abnormal when the patient's serum is substituted for the normal serum in the incubation mixture, the defect should be considered to be any one of the factors found in normal serum (Factor X, Factor XI, Factor XII, or Factor IX). Both Factor XI and Factor XII are also present in $Al(OH)_3$ adsorbed plasma and, as they would be contributed by the normal adsorbed plasma in the mixture, their absence in the patient's serum would not be revealed. Thus the defect must be considered to be either of Factor IX or Factor X. As Factor X is essential to the one-stage prothrombin time test and Factor IX is not, they can be separated by this test.

Should the development of thromboplastin activity be decreased when the patient's $Al(OH)_3$ adsorbed plasma is substituted for normal adsorbed plasma in the incubation mixture, the defect will be considered due to a deficiency of one of the factors contained in normal adsorbed plasma (Factor VIII, Factor V, Factor XI, or Factor XII). A deficiency of Factor XI or Factor XII is ruled out, as they would be contributed by the normal serum in the incubation mixture. The defect must then be one of Factor VIII or Factor V. Once again the one-stage prothrombin time test serves to differentiate the two, as Factor V is essential for the normal evaluation of thrombin in the test and Factor VIII is not.

Factor XI and Factor XII are present both in normal serum and in $Al(OH)_3$ adsorbed plasma. Should the patient have a deficiency of either factor it will not be revealed if normal adsorbed plasma or normal serum is in the incubation mixture. However, when the patient's serum and $Al(OH)_3$ adsorbed plasma are used together in the incubation mixture in place of their normal counterparts, the thromboplastin generation will be abnormal.[425, 426] There remains the task of separating Factor XII deficiency from that of Factor XI. This can usually be done on clinical grounds as patients with Factor XII deficiency have no hemorrhagic diathesis. Furthermore, the addition of Factor XI–deficient plasma or serum will correct the clotting defect of Factor XII deficiency and vice versa. This, however, requires the availability of abnormal serum or plasma.

Circulating anticoagulants may produce abnormal results in the thromboplastin generation test when either the patient's serum or adsorbed plasma is substituted in the incubation mixture. If the titer of circulating anticoagulant is sufficiently high, both the patient's serum and adsorbed plasma will produce abnormal results. As circulating anticoagulants are not adsorbed by inorganic precipitating agents, the use of 50 per cent normal and 50 per cent patient's adsorbed plasma and normal serum in the incubation mixture will also produce abnormal results. As the results of the thromboplastin generation test in the case of Factor V or Factor VIII deficiency would be corrected by such an addition of normal adsorbed plasma, this maneuver may be used to identify the presence of circulating anticoagulants.

Should the platelets of the patient be deficient in factors necessary for the development of thromboplastin activity, it will be apparent when appropriate dilutions of platelets from the patient and from a normal donor are compared under conditions of the test.

Prothrombin, Factor VII, fibrinogen, Factor V, and Factor X are all essential for the normal evolution of thrombin from prothrombin in the presence of *tissue* thromboplastin activity. A deficiency of any of these factors results in a prolonged one-stage prothrombin time. If a patient has a prolonged one-stage prothrombin time and results of the thromboplastin generation test are normal, Factor V deficiency and Factor X deficiency are removed from consideration. A thrombin titer will determine whether a fibrinogen deficiency is responsible for the abnormal results of the test. To separate Factor VII deficiency from prothrombin deficiency, a modification of the thromboplastin generation test may be employed. The patient's plasma is used as a substrate to test the thromboplastin activity of a normal incubation mixture. It has been shown that the substrate clotting time in the presence of normal intrinsic thromboplastin activity depends on the concentration in the substrate of prothrombin and fibrinogen. A normal clotting time precludes a prothrombin deficiency.[234]

FIBRINOGEN CONCENTRATION

The thrombin time and fibrinogen titer are used to estimate the concentration of fibrinogen in a patient's plasma. The thrombin used is that which is commercially available. It is made up according to the manufacturer's instructions and should be adjusted so that 0.1 ml. of thrombin will give a clotting time of 10 to 12 seconds when added to 0.25 ml. normal plasma. Platelet-free citrated plasma from the patient and a normal control are prepared by centrifuging citrated whole blood at 2000 rpm for 15 minutes. Serial dilutions of both normal and patient's plasma are made, and the highest dilution which contains a visible clot after addition of 0.1 ml. of thrombin is determined. Normal plasma should still contain a clot when diluted $\frac{1}{64}$ or $\frac{1}{128}$. The thrombin time is the thrombin clotting time of the $\frac{1}{2}$ dilution of patient's plasma compared to that of a normal. The objection to using whole blood for these determinations is that it is difficult to see the clot. This test also has the advantage over those which estimate the quantity of fibrinogen biochemically in that what is tested is reactive fibrinogen, whereas the biochemical assay may include inert fibrinogen or other protein.[481]

Acquired hypofibrinogenemia often presents as an obstetrical or surgical emergency, and the equipment necessary to perform the simple tests required for the diagnosis should be convenient to the operating and delivery rooms. Failure of shed blood to form a firm clot should immediately alert the attending physician to this emergency. As acquired hypofibrinogenemia also may be associated with Factor V and Factor VIII deficits, treatment must remedy these defects as well as replace the fibrinogen.

CHOICE OF LABORATORY TESTS

These laboratory tests are sufficient to obtain the information needed to identify the particular defect responsible for disordered hemostasis in the vast majority of patients. There are many excellent laboratory procedures available which might serve to augment or extend the results obtained by those presented, but space does not permit their inclusion. For details of other methods the reader is referred to texts devoted entirely to the subject of blood coagulation.[53, 233, 422, 514]

The physician must determine which of these tests is necessary on the basis of his clinical findings. If the clinical examination gives no clue as to which phase of hemostasis is at fault, the platelet count, bleeding time, tourniquet test, partial thromboplastin time, and one-stage prothrombin time should be obtained. This group of tests affords information concerning both phases of hemostasis, and if the results of each are normal it is unlikely that the patient has a

Table 16–2   *Tests of Hemostasis*

		SCREENING TESTS					SOME ADDITIONAL TESTS		THROMBOPLASTIN GENERATION				MODIFIED THROMBO-PLASTIN GENERA-TION TEST	FIBRINO-GEN ASSAY	CLOT SOLU-BILITY
Phase	NAME	PLATELET COUNT	BLEEDING TIME	CLOT RETRAC-TION	ONE STAGE PRO-THROM-BIN	PTT	TOURNI-QUET TEST	CLOTTING TIME	Serum	Plasma	Platelets	Serum and Plasma			
Vascular Phase of Hemostasis	Thrombocytopenic Purpura	A	A	A	N	N	A	N	N	N	N	N	N	N	N
	Non-thrombocytopenic Purpura	N	A	N	N	N	A	N	N	N	N	N	N	N	N
	Hereditary Hemorrhagic Telangiectasia	N	N	N	N	N	N	N	N	N	N	N	N	N	N
Biochemical — First Stage of Clotting	Factor VIII Deficiency	N	N	N	N	A	N	N/A	N	A	N	A	N	N	N
	Factor IX Deficiency	N	N	N	N	A	N	N/A	A	N	N	A	N	N	N
	Factor XI Deficiency	N	N	N	N	A	N	N/A	N	N	N	A	N	N	N
	Factor XII Deficiency	N	N	N	N	A	N	A	N	N	N	A	N	N	N
	Circulating Anticoagulants	N	N	N	N/A	N/A	N	N/A	N/A	N/A	N	N/A	N/A	N	N
First and Second Stage of Clotting	Factor X Deficiency	N	N	N	A	A	N	N/A	A	N	N	N	N	N	N
	Factor V Deficiency	N	N	N	A	A	N	N/A	N	N	N	A	N	N	N
First or Second Stage of Clotting	Prothrombin Deficiency	N	N	N	A	A	N	N/A	N	N	N	N	A	N	N
	Factor VII Deficiency	N	N/A	N	A	N	N	N	N	N	N	N	N	N	N
Third Stage of Clotting	Congenital Afibrinogenemia	N	N/A	A	A	A	N	A	N	N	N	N	A	A	N
	Acquired Hypofibrinogenemia	N/A	N/A	A	A	A	N	A	N/A	N	N	N/A	A	A	N
	Factor XIII Deficiency	N	N	N	N	N	N	N	N	N	N	N	N	N	A
Vascular and Biochemical Phase of Hemostasis	von Willebrand's Disease	N	A	N	N	N/A	N	N	N	N	A	N	A	N	N

N = Normal.   A = Abnormal.   N/A = Inconstant.

disorder of hemostasis. The thromboplastin generation test will be needed to detect a mild abnormality of the first stage of coagulation.

If the results of the clinical examination suggest a disorder of the vascular phase of hemostasis, the platelet count, tourniquet test, bleeding time, measurement of clot retraction, partial thromboplastin time, and one-stage prothrombin time should be obtained. The partial thromboplastin time and one-stage prothrombin time should be within normal limits if only the vascular phase of coagulation is abnormal. The tourniquet test should be positive and the bleeding time prolonged. The platelet count may be depressed, and clot retraction may be poor or not occur at all. If the bleeding time alone is abnormal, a Factor VIII assay and platelet function study should be obtained. If the platelet count is quantitatively normal but there is a prolonged bleeding time and poor clot retraction, special biochemical studies of the platelets may be necessary to identify the defect.[206] The platelet may also be at fault when, despite a strong history of abnormal hemostasis, all the tests of coagulation are normal. Comparative dilution of the patient's platelets and platelets from a normal donor in the thromboplastin generation test may reveal a defect in platelet Factor 3.

If the physician feels that the biochemical phase of hemostasis is at fault, the platelet count, bleeding time, one-stage prothrombin time, and thromboplastin generation test should be obtained. The platelet count and bleeding time should be normal. If the one-stage prothrombin time is prolonged and the thromboplastin generation test reveals no deficiency of Factor V or Factor X, it must be determined if diminished prothrombin, fibrinogen, or Factor VII is responsible. A thrombin time and fibrinogen titer will establish the adequacy of fibrinogen concentration, and a modification of the thromboplastin generation test will separate Factor VII and prothrombin.

Table 16–2 notes the results of various laboratory tests in disorders of hemostasis.

References

1. Abdulla, Y. H.: B adrenergic receptors in human platelets. J. Athero. Res., 9:171, 1969.
2. Abildgaard, U.: Inhibition of the thrombin-fibrinogen reaction by antithrombin III studied by N-terminal analysis. Scand. J. Clin. Lab. Invest., 20:207, 1967.
3. Abildgaard, U.: Inhibition of the thrombin-fibrinogen reaction by α_2-macroglobulin studied by N-terminal analysis. Thromb. Diath. Haemorrh., 21:173, 1969.
4. Abildgaard, U., Fagerhol, M. K., and Egeberg, O.: Comparison of progressive antithrombin activity and the concentration of three thrombin inhibitors in human plasma. Scand. J. Clin. Lab. Invest., 26:349, 1970.
5. Ablondi, F. B., Hagan, J. J., Philips, M., and DeRenzo, E. C.: Inhibition of plasmin, trypsin and streptokinase activated fibrinolytic system by epsilon animocaproic acid. Arch. Biochem. Biophys., 82:153, 1959.
6. Ackroyd, J. F.: A simple method of estimating clot retraction with a survey of normal values and the changes that occur with menstruation. Clin. Sci., 7:231, 1949.
7. Ackroyd, J. F.: Function of factor VII. Br. J. Haematol., 2:397, 1956.
8. Adelson, E., Rheingold, J. J., Parker, O., Steiner, M., and Kirby, J. C.: The survival of factor VIII (antihemophilic globulin) and factor IX (plasma thromboplastin component) in normal humans. J. Clin. Invest., 42:1040, 1963.
9. Aggeler, P. M., Spaet, T. H., and Emery, B. F.: Purification of plasma thromboplastin factor B (plasma thromboplastin component) and its identification as a beta globulin. Science, 119:806, 1954.
10. Aggeler, P. M., White, S. G., Glendening, M. B., Pope, E. W., Leake, T. B., and Bates, G. B.: Plasma thromboplastin component (PTC) deficiency: a new disease resembling hemophilia. Proc. Soc. Exp. Biol. Med., 79:692, 1952.
11. Alami, S. Y., Hampton, J. W., Race, G. J., and Speer, R. J.: Fibrin stabilizing factor (factor XIII). Am. J. Med., 44:1, 1968.
12. Albrecht, M.: Studies on the evolution of thrombocytes, experiences with megakaryocytes in vitro. Int. Soc. Hematol., 437:346, 1956. (Abstr.)
13. Alexander, B.: Anticoagulant therapy with coumarin congeners. Am. J. Med., 33:679, 1962.
14. Alexander, B., Meyers, L., Kenny, J., Goldstein, R., Gurewich, V., and Grinspoon, L.: Blood coagulation in pregnancy. Proconvertin and prothrombin and the hypercoagulable state. N. Engl. J. Med., 254:358, 1956.
15. Alkjaersig, N.: The Antifibrinolytic Activity of Platelets. In Blood Platelets. Henry Ford Hospital Symposium. Little, Brown & Co., Boston, 1961.
16. Alkjaersig, N., Fletcher, A. P., and Sherry, S.: The activation of human plasminogen II. A kinetic study of activation with trypsin, urokinase and streptokinase. J. Biol. Chem., 233:86, 1958.

17. Alkjaersig, N., Fletcher, A. P., and Sherry, S.: The mechanism of clot dissolution by plasmin. J. Clin. Invest., *38*:1086, 1959.
18. Alkjaersig, N., Fletcher, A. P., and Sherry, S.: Pathogenesis of the coagulation defect developing during pathological plasma proteolytic ("fibrinolytic") states. II. The significance, mechanism and consequences of defective fibrin polymerization. J. Clin. Invest., *41*:917, 1962.
19. Altman, R., and Hemker, H. C.: Contact activation in the extrinsic blood clotting system. Thromb. Diath. Haemorrh., *18*:525, 1967.
20. Ambrus, C. M., and Markus, G.: Plasmin–antiplasmin complex as a reservoir of fibrinolytic enzyme. Am. J. Physiol., *199*:491, 1960.
21. Amir, J., Pensky, J., and Ratnoff, O. D.: Plasma inhibition of activated plasma thromboplastin antecedent (Factor XIa) in pregnancy. J. Lab. Clin. Med., *79*:106, 1972.
22. Amir, J., Ratnoff, O. D., and Pensky, J.: Partial purification and some properties of a plasma inhibitor of activated plasma thromboplastin antecedent (factor XI). J. Lab. Clin. Med., *80*:786, 1972.
23. Ardlie, N. G., and Han, P.: Enzymatic basis for platelet aggregation and release: the significance of the 'platelet atmosphere' and the relationship between platelet function and blood coagulation. Br. J. Haematol., *26*:331, 1974.
24. Arthus, M., and Pagés, C.: Nouvelle théorie chimique de la coagulation du sang. Arch. Physiol. Norm. Pathol., *2*:739, 1890.
25. Ashford, T. P., and Freiman, D. G.: Platelet aggregation at sites of minimal endothelial injury. An electron microscopic study. Am. J. Pathol., *53*:599, 1968.
26. Austen, D. E. G., and Bidwell, E.: Carbohydrate structure in factor VIII. Thromb. Diath. Haemorrh., *28*:464, 1972.
26a. Austen, D. E. G., Carey, M., and Howard, M. A.: Dissociation of factor VIII-related antigen into subunits. Nature, *253*:55, 1975.
27. Bajaj, S. P., and Mann, K. G.: Simultaneous purification of bovine prothrombin and factor X. Activation of prothrombin by trypsin-activated factor X. J. Biol. Chem., *248*:7729, 1973.
28. Bang, N. U., Fletcher, A. P., Alkjaersig, N., and Sherry, S.: Pathogenesis of the coagulation defect developing during pathological plasma proteolytic ("fibrinolytic") states. III. Demonstration of abnormal clot structure by electron microscopy. J. Clin. Invest., *41*: 935, 1962.
29. Bangham, A. D.: A correlation between surface charge and coagulant action of phospholipids. Nature, *192*:1197, 1961.
30. Barnhart, M. I., Anderson, R. F., and Bernstein, M. H.: Liver ultrastructure after coumadin and vitamin K. Fed. Proc., *23*:520, 1964.
31. Barrocas, A.: Disseminated intravascular coagulation. Milit. Med., *138*:9, 1973.
32. Barton, P. G., Jackson, C. M., and Hanahan, D. J.: Relationship between factor V and activated factor X in the generation of prothrombinase. Nature, *214*:923, 1967.
33. Barton, P. G., Yin, E. T., and Wessler, S.: Reactions of activated factor X-phosphatide mixtures in vitro and in vivo. J. Lipid Res., *11*:87, 1970.
34. Bedson, S. P., and Johnston, M. E.: Further observations on platelet genesis. J. Pathol. & Bacteriol., *28*:101, 1925.
35. Bell, R. G., and Matschinger, J. T.: A possible mechanism for the action of warfarin. Fed. Proc., *29*:381, 1970.
36. Bennett, B., Forman, W. B., and Ratnoff, O. D.: Studies on the nature of antihemophilic factor (factor VIII). Further evidence relating the AHF-like antigens in normal and hemophilic plasmas. J. Clin. Invest., *52*:2191, 1973.
37. Bennington, J. L., Fonty, R. A., and Hougie, C.: Laboratory Diagnosis. The Macmillan Company, New York, 1970, p. 669.
38. Bergsagel, D. E.: Viscous metamorphosis of platelets. Br. J. Haematol., *2*:130, 1956.
39. Bergsagel, D. E., and Hougie, C.: Intermediate stages in the formation of blood thromboplastin. Br. J. Haematol., *2*:113, 1956.
40. Bernik, M. B., and Kwaan, H. C.: Origin of fibrinolytic activity in cultures of the human kidney. J. Lab. Clin. Med., *70*:650, 1967.
41. Bernik, M. B., and Kwaan, H. C.: Plasminogen activator activity in cultures from human tissues. An immunological and histochemical study. J. Clin. Invest., *48*:1740, 1969.
42. Berre, A. G., Osterud, B., Christensen, T. B., Holm, T., and Prydz, H.: Some characteristics of the coagulation factor Xa purified from human serum. Biochem. J., *135*:791, 1973.
43. Bettex-Galland, M., Lüsher, E. F., and Weible, E. R.: Thrombosthenin—electron microscopical studies on its localization in human blood platelets and some properties of its subunits. Thromb. Diath. Haemorrh., *22*:431, 1969.
44. Bettleheim, F. R.: The clotting of fibrinogen II. Fractionation of peptide material liberated. Biochem. Biophys. Acta, *19*:121, 1956.

45. Bezkorvaing, A., and Rafelson, M. E., Jr.: Characterization of some proteins from normal human platelets. J. Lab. Clin. Med., *64*:212, 1964.
46. Biggs, R.: Dysfibrinogenaemia. Thrombosis et Diathesis Haemorrhagica, *29*:523, 1973.
47. Biggs, R., Denson, K. W. E., Akman, N., Borrett, R., and Hadden, M.: Antithrombin III, antifactor Xa and heparin. Br. J. Haematol., *19*:283, 1970.
48. Biggs, R., and Douglas, A. S.: The thromboplastin generation test. J. Clin. Pathol., *6*:23, 1953.
49. Biggs, R., Douglas, A. S., and Macfarlane, R. G.: The action of thromboplastic substances. J. Physiol., *122*:554, 1953.
50. Biggs, R., Douglas, A. S., and Macfarlane, R. G.: The formation of thromboplastin in human blood. J. Physiol., *119*:89, 1953.
51. Biggs, R., Douglas, A. S., and Macfarlane, R. G.: The initial stages of blood coagulation. J. Physiol., *122*:538, 1953.
52. Biggs, R., Douglas, A. S., Macfarlane, R. G., Dacie, J. V., Pitney, W. R., Merskey, C., and O'Brien, J. R.: Christmas disease. Br. Med. J., *2*:1378, 1952.
53. Biggs, R., and Macfarlane, R. G.: Human blood Coagulation. 2nd. Ed. Charles C Thomas, Springfield, Ill., 1957.
54. Biggs, R., Macfarlane, R. G., Denson, K. W. E., and Ash, B. J.: Thrombin and the interaction of factors VIII and IX. Br. J. Haematol., *11*:276, 1965.
55. Bisno, A. L., and Freeman, J. C.: The syndrome of asplenia, pneumococcal sepsis and disseminated intravascular coagulation. Ann. Intern. Med., *72*:389, 1970.
56. Blakely, A. A.: A rapid bedside method for the control of heparin. Can. Med. Assoc., *99*:1072, 1968.
57. Blix, S.: Anticoagulant treatment of the defibrination syndrome. Acta Med. Scand., *181*:597, 1967.
58. Blombäck, B., Gröndahl, M. J., Hessel, B., Iwanaga, S., and Wallén, P.: Primary structure of human fibrinogen and fibrin. II. Structural studies on NH_2-terminal part of γ chain. J. Biol. Chem., *248*:5806, 1973.
59. Blombäck, M., and Blombäck, B.: Fractions rich in factor VIII. Bibli. Haematol., *29*(part 4): 1116, 1969.
60. Blombäck, M., Blombäck, B., Gröndahl, N. J., Gårdlund, B., Hessel, B., Kowalska-Loth, B., and Reuterby, J.: On the molecular structure of fibrinogen. Thromb. Diath. Haemorrh. (Suppl.), *54*:117, 1973.
61. Blomstrand, R., Nakayama, F., and Nilsson, I. M.: Identification of phospholipids in human thrombocytes and erythrocytes. J. Lab. Clin. Med., *59*:771, 1962.
62. Bolton, C. H., Hampton, J. R., and Mitchell, J. R. A.: Effect of oral contraceptive agents on platelets and plasma phospholipids. Lancet, *1*:1336, 1968.
63. Booyse, F. M., Hoveke, T. P., and Rafelson, M. E., Jr.: Studies on human platelets. II. Protein synthetic activity of various platelet populations. Biochem. Biophys. Acta., *157*:660, 1968.
64. Booyse, F. M., Hoveke, T. P., Kisieleski, D., and Rafelson, M. E., Jr.: Mechanism and control of platelet–platelet interaction. Microvasc. Res., *4*:179, 199, 207, 1972.
65. Booyse, F. M., Hoveke, T. P., and Rafelson, M. E., Jr.: Human platelet actin. Isolation and properties. J. Biol. Chem., *248*:4083, 1973.
66. Booyse, F. M., Hoveke, T. P., Zschocke, D., and Rafelson, M. E., Jr.: Human platelet myosin. Isolation and properties. J. Biol. Chem., *246*:4291, 1971.
67. Booyse, F. M., and Rafelson, M. E., Jr.: Studies on human platelets. I. Synthesis of platelet protein in a cell free system. Biochim. Biophys. Acta, *145*:188, 1967.
68. Borchgrevink, C. F.: Platelet adhesion in vivo in patients with bleeding disorders. Acta Med. Scand., *170*:231, 1961.
69. Bordet, D. J., and Delange, L.: La coagulation du sang et la genèse de la thrombine. Ann. Inst. Pasteur, *9*:42, 1912.
70. Born, G. V. R.: Strong inhibition by 2-chloroadenosine of the aggregation of blood platelets by adenosine diphosphate. Nature, *202*:95, 1964.
71. Born, G. V. R., and Cross, M. J.: Effect of adenosine diphosphate on concentration of platelets in circulating blood. Nature, *197*:974, 1963.
72. Born, G. V. R., Haslam, R. J., Goldman, M., and Lowe, R. D.: Comparative effectiveness of adenosine analogues as inhibitors of blood-platelet aggregation and as vasodilators in man. Nature, *205*:678, 1965.
73. Born, G. V. R., Honour, A. J., and Mitchell, J. R. A.: Inhibition by adenosine and by 2-chloroadenosine of the formation and embolization of platelet thrombi. Nature, *202*:761, 1964.
74. Bosman, H. B.: Platelet adhesiveness and aggregation. II. Surface sialic acid, glycoprotein: N–acetyl–neuraminic acid transferase, and neuraminidase of human blood platelets (BBA 26962). Biochim. Biophys. Acta, *279*:456, 1972.
75. Boston Collaborative Drug Surveillance Group. Regular aspirin intake and acute myocardial infarction. Br. Med. J., *1*:440, 1974.

76. Botti, R. E., and Ratnoff, O. D.: Studies on the pathogenesis of thrombosis: an experimental "hyper-coagulable" state induced by the intravenous injection of ellagic acid. J. Lab. Clin. Med., *64*:385, 1964.

77. Bowie, E. J. W., Cooper, H., Fuster, V., Kazmier, F., and Owen, C. A., Jr.: The diagnosis of intravascular coagulation. Thromb. Diath. Haemorrh. (Suppl.),*56*:137, 1973.

78. Bowie, E. J., Thompson, J. H., Jr., Didisheim, P., and Owen, C. A., Jr.: Disappearance rates of coagulation factors: transfusion studies in factor-deficient patients. Transfusion, *7*:174, 1967.

79. Brafield, A. J., Madras, M. B., and Case, J.: The stability of Christmas factor. A guide to the management of Christmas disease. Lancet, *2*:867, 1956.

80. Brakman, P., Mohler, E. R., Jr., and Astrup, T.: A group of patients with impaired plasma fibrinolytic system and selective inhibition of tissue activator-induced fibrinolysis. Scand. J. Haematol., *3*:389, 1966.

81. Brass, L. F., and Bensusan, H. B.: Role of collagen quaternary structure in platelet–collagen interaction. J. Clin. Invest., *54*:1480, 1974.

82. Bray, B. A., and Laki, K.: Glycopeptides from fibrinogen and fibrin. Biochemistry, *7*:3119, 1968.

83. Brecher, G., and Cronkite, E. P.: Morphology and enumeration of human blood platelets. J. Appl. Physiol., *3*:365, 1950.

84. Breckenridge, A., and Orme, M.: Kinetics of warfarin adsorption in man. Clin. Pharmacol. Ther., *14*:955, 1973.

85. Breddin, K.: Prophylaxis of arterial and venous thrombosis by inhibitors of platelet aggregation. Thromb. Diath. Haemorrh. (Suppl.), *59*:240, 1974.

86. Brinkhous, K. M., Read, M. S., and Mason, R. G.: Plasma thrombocyte-agglutinating activity and fibrinogen. Synergism with adenosine diphosphate. Lab. Invest., *14*:335, 1965.

87. Brodie, G. N., Baenziger, N. L., Chase, L. R., and Majerus, P. W.: The effects of thrombin on adenyl cyclase activity and a membrane protein from human platelets. J. Clin. Invest., *51*:81, 1972.

88. Brodsky, I., and Siegel, N. H.: The diagnosis and treatment of disseminated intravascular coagulation. Med. Clin. North Am., *54*:555, 1970.

89. Brown, C. H., III, Bell, W. R., Shreiner, D. P., and Jackson, D. P.: Effects of Arvin on blood platelets. In vitro and in vivo studies. J. Lab. Clin. Med., *79*:758, 1972.

90. Browse, N. L., and Hull, J. H.: Effects of dipyridamole on the incidence of clinically detectable deep-vein thrombosis. Lancet, *2*:718, 1969.

91. Bruno, J. J., Taylor, L. A., and Droller, M. J.: Effects of prostaglandin E_2 on human platelet adenyl cyclase and aggregation. Nature, *251*:721, 1974.

92. Buchanan, A.: On the coagulation of the blood and other fibriniferous liquids. J. Physiol., *2*:158, 1879–1880.

93. Budzynski, A. Z., Marder, V. J., and Shainoff, J. R.: Structure of plasmic degradation products of human fibrinogen. Fibrinopeptide and polypeptide chain analysis. J. Biol. Chem., *249*:2294, 1974.

94. Caen, J. P.: Is fibrinogen the plasma co-factor in ADP-induced human platelet aggregation? Nature, *205*:1120, 1965.

95. Cash, J. D., and Woodfield, D. G.: Fibrinolytic response to moderate, exhaustive and prolonged exercise in normal subjects. Nature, *215*:628, 1967.

96. Catt, K. J., Hirsh, J., Castelan, D. J., Niall, H. D., and Tregear, G. W.: Radioimmunoassay of fibrinogen and its proteolysis products. Thromb. Diath. Haemorrh., *20*:1, 1968.

97. Cazenave, J.-P., Packham, M. A., Guccione, M. A., and Mustard, J. F.: Inhibition of platelet adherence to a collagen-coated surface by non-steroidal anti-inflammatory drugs, pyrimido–pyrimidine and tricyclic compounds, and lidocaine. J. Lab. Clin. Med.,*83*:797, 1974.

98. Cazenave, J.-P., Packham, M. A., Guccione, M. A., and Mustard, J. F.: Inhibition of platelet adherence to a collagen-coated surface by agents that inhibit platelet shape change and clot retraction. J. Lab. Clin. Med., *84*:483, 1974.

99. Cesbron, N., Boyer, C., Guillin, M-C., and Ménaché, D.: Human coumarin prothrombin—chromatographic, coagulation and immunologic studies. Thromb. Diath. Haemorrh., *30*:437, 1973.

100. Chandrasekhar, N., Osbahr, A., and Laki, K.: The mode of action of the Laki-Lorand factor in the clotting of fibrinogen. Biochem. Biophys. Res. Commun., *15*:182, 1964.

101. Chargaff, E., and Olson, K. B.: Studies on the chemistry of blood coagulation. VI. Studies on the action of heparin and other anticoagulants. J. Biol. Chem., *122*:153, 1938.

102. Chaudhry, A. A., Sagone, A. L., Jr., Metz, E. N., and Balcerzak, S. P.: Relationship of glucose oxidation to aggregation of human platelets. Blood, *41*:249, 1973.

103. Chen, T. I., and Tsai, C.: The mechanism of haemostasis in peripheral vessels. J. Physiol., *107*:280, 1940.

104. Chesney, C. Mcl., Harper, E., and Colman, R. W.: Human platelet collagenase. J. Clin. Invest., *53*:1647, 1974.
105. Chesterman, C. N., Allington, M. J., and Sharp, A. A.: Plasminogen activator – relationship to fibrin. Nature [New Biol.], *238*:15, 1972.
106. Chesterman, C. N., and Biggs, J. C.: Thrombolytic therapy with streptokinase. Med. J. Aust., *2*:839, 1970.
107. Chesterman, C. N., and Sharp, A. A.: Arterial thrombolysis. Lancet, *2*:264, 1971.
108. Christensen, L. R.: Streptococcal fibrinolysis: a proteolytic reaction due to a serum enzyme activated by streptococcal fibrinolysin. J. Gen. Physiol., *28*:363, 1944–1945.
109. Chuang, T. F., Sargeant, R. B., and Hougie, C.: The effect of calcium ions on the properties of factor IX and its activated form. Br. J. Haematol., *27*:281, 1974.
109a. Clagett, G. P., and Salzman, E. W.: Current concepts: prevention on venous thromboembolism in surgical patients. N. Engl. J. Med., *290*:93, 1974.
110. Cochrane, C. G., Sitzer, S. D., and Aikin, B. S.: Hageman factor: its structure and activation. Fed. Proc., *31*:623, 1972. (Abstr.)
111. Cochrane, C. G., Wuepper, K. D., Aiken, B. S., Revak, S. D., and Speigelberg, H. L.: The interaction of Hageman factor and immune complexes. J. Clin. Invest., *51*:2736, 1972.
112. Cohen, P., and Wittels, B.: Energy substrate metabolism in fresh and stored human platelets. J. Clin. Invest., *49*:119, 1970.
113. Cohen, R. J., Epstein, S. E., Cohen, L. S., and Dennis, L. N.: Alterations of fibrinolysis and blood coagulation induced by exercise, and the role of beta-adrenergic-receptor stimulation. Lancet, *2*:1264, 1968.
114. Collins, I. S.: The stability of coagulation factors in stored blood. Med. J. Aust., *2*:718, 1955.
115. Conner, W. E.: The acceleration of thrombus formation by certain fatty acids. J. Clin. Invest., *41*:1199, 1962.
116. Corrigan, J. J., Jr., Bennett, B. B., and Bueffel, B.: The value of factor VIII levels in acquired hypofibrinogenemia. Am. J. Clin. Pathol., *60*:897, 1973.
117. Corrigan, J. J., Jr., and Jordan, C. M.: Heparin therapy in septicemia with disseminated intravascular coagulation. N. Engl. J. Med., *283*:778, 1970.
118. Cox, F. M., Lanchantin, G. F., and Ware, A. G.: Chromatographic purification of human serum accelerator globulin. J.Clin. Invest., *35*:106, 1956.
119. Crane, M. M., and Sanford, H. H.: The effect of variations in total calcium concentration upon the coagulation time of blood. Am. J. Physiol., *118*:703, 1937.
120. Cross, M. J.: Effect of fibrinogen on the aggregation of platelets by adenosine diphosphate. Thromb. Diath. Haemorrh., *12*:524, 1964.
121. Curry, N., Bardana, E. J., and Pirofsky, B.: Heparin sensitivity. Arch. Intern. Med., *132*:744, 1973.
122. Daemen, F. J. M., van Arkel, C., Hart, H. C., van der Drift, C., and van Deenen, L. L. M.: Activity of synthetic phospholipids in blood coagulation. Thromb. Diath. Haemorrh., *13*:194, 1965.
123. Damus, P. S., Hicks, M., and Rosenberg, R. D.: Anticoagulant action of heparin. Nature, *246*:355, 1973.
124. Damus, P. S., and Salzman, E. W.: Disseminated intravascular coagulation. Arch. Surg., *104*:262, 1972.
125. Davey, M. G., and Löscher, E. F.: Release reactions of human platelets induced by thrombin and other agents. Biochim. Biophys. Acta, *165*:490, 1968.
126. Davey, M. G., and Lüscher, E. F.: Platelet Proteins. *In* Kowalski, E., and Niewiarowski, S. (eds.): The Biochemistry of Blood Platelets. Academic Press, New York, 1967, p. 9.
127. Davis, C. E., Jr., Wiley, W. B., and Faulconer, R. J.: Necrosis of the female breast complicating oral anticoagulant treatment. Ann. Surg., *175*:647, 1972.
128. Davis, H. L., and Davis, N. L.: Heparin and lipid metabolism. Lancet, *2*:651, 1969.
129. Day, H. J., and Solum, N. O.: Fibrinogen associated with sub-cellular platelet particles. Scand. J. Haematol., *10*:136, 1973.
130. Day, H. J., Stormorken, H., and Holmsen, H.: Subcellular localization of platelet factor 3 and platelet factor 4. Scand. J. Haematol., *10*:254, 1973.
131. Denson, K. W.: Electrophoretic studies of the Prower factor: a blood coagulation factor which differs from factor VII. Br. J. Haematol., *4*:313, 1958.
132. Denson, K. W. I., and Bonnar, J.: The measurement of heparin. Thromb. Diath. Haemorrh., *30*:471, 1973.
133. DeRenzo, E. C., Boggiano, E., Barg, W. F., Jr., and Buck, F. F.: Interaction of streptokinase and human plasminogen. IV. Further gel electrophoretic studies on the combination of streptokinase with human plasminogen or human plasmin. J. Biol. Chem., *242*:2428, 1967.
134. Deutsch, E., and Lechner, K.: Platelet Clotting Factors. *In* Kowalski, E., and Niewiarowski, S. (eds.): The Biochemistry of Blood Platelets. Academic Press, New York, 1967, p. 23.

135. Deykin, D.: The role of the liver in serum-induced hypercoagulability. J. Clin. Invest., *45*:256, 1966.
136. Deykin, D.: Current concepts: the use of heparin. N. Engl. J. Med., *280*:937, 1969.
137. Deykin, D.: The clinical challenge of disseminated intravascular coagulation. N. Engl. J. Med., *283*:636, 1970.
138. Deykin, D.: Emerging concepts of platelet functions. N. Engl. J. Med., *290*:144, 1974.
139. Deykin, D.: Cochios, F., DeCamp, G., and Lopez, A.: Hepatic removal of activated factor X by the perfused rabbit liver. Am. J. Physiol., *214*:414, 1968.
140. Didisheim, P.: Inhibition by dipyridamole of arterial thrombosis in rats. Thromb. Diath. Haemorrh., *20*:257, 1968.
141. Didisheim, P.: The intravascular coagulation and fibrinolysis (ICF) syndrome. Thromb. Diath. Haemorrh., *46*:119, 1971.
142. Didisheim, P., Kazmier, F. J., and Fuster, V.: Platelet inhibition in the management of thrombosis. Thromb. Diath. Haemorrh., *32*:21, 1974.
143. Didisheim, P., Kazmier, F. J., and Fluster, V.: Platelet inhibition in the management of thrombosis. Thromb. Diath. Haemorrh., *32*:21, 1974.
144. Donaldson, V. H., and Ratnoff, O. D.: Hageman factor: alterations in physical properties during activation. Science, *150*:754, 1965.
145. Doolittle, R. F.: Structural details of fibrin stabilization: implication for fibrinogen structure and initial fibrin formation. Thromb. Diath. Haemorrh., *54*:155, 1973.
146. Doolittle, R. F., Oncley, J. L., and Surgenor, D. M.: Species differences in the interaction of thrombin and fibrinogen. J. Biol. Chem., *237*:3123, 1962.
147. Douglas, A. S.: Factor-V consumption during blood coagulation. Br. J. Haematol., *2*:153, 1956.
148. Douglas, A. S.: The action of heparin in the prevention of prothrombin conversion. J. Clin. Invest., *35*:533, 1956.
149. Douglas, A. S., and McNicol, G. P.: Thrombolytic therapy. Br. Med. Bull., *20*:228, 1964.
150. Droller, M. J.: Ultrastructure of the platelet release reaction in response to various aggregating agents and their inhibitors. Lab. Invest., *29*:595, 1973.
151. Droller, M. J., and Fox, M. C.: Ultrastructural visualization of the thrombin-induced platelet release reaction. Scand. J. Haematol., *11*:35, 1973.
152. Duckert, F., Flückiger, P., Matter, M., and Koller, F.: Clotting factor X. Physiologic and physiochemical properties. Proc. Soc. Exp. Biol. Med., *90*:17, 1955.
153. Duckert, F., and Streuli, F.: Role of coagulation in thrombosis. Thromb. Diath. Haemorrh. (Suppl.), *21*:185, 1966.
154. Duke, W. W.: The relation of blood platelets to hemorrhagic diseases. J.A.M.A., *55*:1185, 1910.
155. Dulock, M. A., and Kolmen, S. N.: Influence of vitamin K on restoration of prothrombin complex proteins and fibrinogen in plasma of depleted dogs. Thromb. Diath. Haemorrh., *20*:136, 1968.
156. Eagle, H.: The role of prothrombin and of platelets in the formation of thrombin. J. Gen. Physiol., *18*:531, 1934–1935.
157. Eagle, H.: The formation of fibrin from thrombin and fibrinogen. J. Gen. Physiol., *18*:547, 1934–1935.
158. Egberg, N., and Johnsson, H.: Platelet aggregation induced by ADP and thrombin in reptilase defibrinated dogs. Thromb. Res., *1*:95, 1972.
159. Egeberg, O.: Inherited antithrombin deficiency causing thrombophilia. Thromb. Diath. Haemorrh., *13*:516, 1965.
160. Eisen, V.: Fibrinolysis and formation of biologically active polypeptides. Br. Med. Bull., *20*:205, 1964.
161. Elgee, N. T.: Medical aspects of oral contraceptives. Ann. Intern. Med., *72*:409, 1970.
162. Elkeles, R. S., Hampton, J. R., and Mitchell, J. R. A.: Effect of oestrogens on human platelet behavior. Lancet, *2*:315, 1968.
163. Elwood, P. C., Cochrane, A. L., Burr, M. L., Sweetnam, P. M., Williams, G., Welsby, E., Hughes, S. J., and Renton, R.: A randomized controlled trial of acetyl salicylic acid in the secondary prevention of mortality from myocardial infarction. Br. Med. J., *1*:436, 1974.
164. Emmons, P. R., Harrison, M. J. G., Honour, A. J., and Mitchell, J. R. A.: Effect of dipyridamole on human platelet behaviour. Lancet, *2*:603, 1965.
165. Esmon, C. T., and Jackson, C. M.: The conversion of prothrombin to thrombin. III. The factor X_a–catalyzed activation of prothrombin. J. Biol. Chem., *249*:7782, 1974.
166. Esmon, C. T., and Jackson, C. M.: The conversion of prothrombin to thrombin. IV. The function of the fragment 2 region during activation in the presence of factor V. J. Biol. Chem., *249*:7791, 1974.
166a. Esmon, C. T., Owen, W. G., Duiquid, D. L., and Jackson, C. M.: The action of thrombin on blood clotting factor V: conversion of factor V to a prothrombin-binding protein. Biochim. Biophys. Acta, *310*:289, 1973.

167. Esmon, C. T., Owen, W. G., and Jackson, C. M.: The conversion of prothrombin to thrombin. V. The activation of prothrombin by factor X_a in the presence of phospholipid. J. Biol. Chem., 249:7798, 1974.

168. Esnouf, M. P., and Jobin, F.: The isolation of factor V from bovine plasma. Biochem. J., 102: 660, 1967.

169. Esnouf, M. P., and Tunnah, G. W.: The isolation and properties of the thrombin-like activity from Ancistrodon rhodostoma venom. Br. J. Haematol., 13:581, 1967.

170. Esnouf, M. P., and Williams, W. J.: The isolation and purification of a bovine-plasma protein which is a substrate for the coagulant fraction of Russell's-viper venom. Biochem. J., 84:62, 1962.

171. Estes, J. W.: Kinetics of the anticoagulant effect of heparin. J.A.M.A., 212:1492, 1970.

172. Evans, G., Packham, M. A., Nishizawa, E. E., Mustard, J. F., and Murphy, E. A.: Effect of acetylsalicylic acid on platelet function. J. Exp. Med., 128:877, 1968.

173. Fasco, M. J., and Fenton, J. W., II: Specificity of thrombin. I. Esterolytic properties of thrombin, plasma, trypsin, and chymotrypsin with NB–substituted guanidino derivatives of P–nitrophenyl–P'–guanidinobenzoate. Arch. Biochem. Biophys., 159:802, 1973.

174. Finkbiner, R. B., McGovern, J. J., Goldstein, R., and Bunker, J. P.: Coagulation defects in liver disease and response to transfusion during surgery. Am. J. Med., 26:199, 1959.

175. Fisher, S., Fletcher, A. P., Alkjaersig, N., and Sherry, S.: Immunoelectrophoretic characterization of plasma fibrinogen derivatives in patients with pathological plasma proteolysis. J. Lab. Clin. Med., 70:903, 1967.

176. Fletcher, A. P.: Pharmacology of thrombolysis: urokinase. J. Clin. Pathol., 25:633, 1972.

177. Fletcher, A. P., and Alkjaersig, N.: Plasma fibrinogen and hemostatic functions. Progr. Hemat., 5:246, 1966.

178. Fletcher, A. P., Biederman, O., Moore, D., Alkjaersig, N., and Sherry, S.: Abnormal plasminogen-plasmin system activity (fibrinolysis) in patients with hepatic cirrhosis: its cause and consequences. J. Clin. Invest., 43:681, 1964.

179. Fletcher, A. P., Alkjaersig, N., Fisher, S., and Sherry, S.: The proteolysis of fibrinogen by plasmin: the identification of thrombin clottable fibrinogen derivatives which polymerize abnormally. J. Lab. Clin. Med., 68:780, 1966.

180. Fletcher, A. P., Alkjaersig, N., and Sherry, S.: Fibrinolytic mechanisms and the development of thrombolytic therapy. Am. J. Med., 33:738, 1962.

181. Fletcher, A. P., Alkjaersig, N., and Sherry, S.: Pathogenesis of the coagulation defect developing during pathological plasma proteolytic ("fibrinolytic") states. I. The significance of fibrinogen proteolysis and circulating fibrinogen breakdown products. J. Clin. Invest., 41:896, 1962.

182. Folk, J. E., and Chung, S. I.: Molecular and catalytic properties of transglutaminases. Adv. Enzymol., 38:109, 1973.

183. Forbes, C. D., Pensky, J., and Ratnoff, O. D.: Inhibition of activated Hageman factor and activated plasma thromboplastin antecedent by purified serum $C\bar{I}$ inactivator. J. Lab. Clin. Med., 76:809, 1970.

184. Forbes, C. D., and Ratnoff, O. D.: Studies on plasma thromboplastin antecedent (factor XI), PTA deficiency and inhibition of PTA by plasma: pharmacologic inhibitors and specific antiserum. J. Lab. Clin. Med., 79:113, 1972.

185. Freedman, M. L., and Karpatkin, S.: Requirement of iron for platelet protein synthesis. Biochem. Biophys. Res. Commun., 54:475, 1973.

186. Furlan, M., and Beck, E. A.: Plasmic degradation of human fibrinogen. 1. Structural characterization of degradation products. Biochim. Biophys. Acta, 263:631, 1972.

187. Fujikawa, K., Legaz, M. E., and Davie, E. W.: Bovine factor X_1 and X_2 (Stuart factor) isolation and characterization. Biochemistry, 11:4882, 1972.

188. Fujikawa, K., Thompson, A. R., Legaz, M. E., Meyer, R. B., and Davie, E. W.: Isolation and characterization of bovine factor IX (Christmas Factor). Biochemistry, 12:4938, 1973.

189. Gamgee, A.: Physiological Chemistry of the Animal Body. Vol. 1. Macmillan and Co., London, 1880.

190. Ganguly, P., and Moore, R.: Studies on human platelet proteins. Clin. Chim. Acta, 17:153, 1967.

191. Ganrot, P. O.: Electrophoretic separation of two thrombin inhibitors in plasma and serum. Scand. J. Clin. Lab. Invest., 24:11, 1969.

192. Ganrot, P. O., and Niléhn, J.-E.: Competition between plasmin and thrombin for α_2-macroglobulin. Clin. Chim. Acta, 17:511, 1967.

193. Gentin, E.: Guidelines for heparin therapy. Ann. Intern. Med., 80:77, 1974.

194. Gladner, J. A., Murtaugh, P. A., Folk, J. E., and Laki, K.: Nature of peptides released by thrombin. Ann. N. Y. Sci., 104:47, 1963.

195. Glynn, M. F.: The role of the platelet membrane in platelet function. I. Blood coagulation. Am. J. Clin. Pathol., *60*:309, 1973.

196. Glynn, M. F., Movat, H. Z., Murphy, E. A., and Mustard, J. F.: Study of platelet adhesiveness and aggregation with latex particles. J. Lab. Clin. Med., *65*:179, 1965.

197. Godal, H. C.: Delayed fibrin polymerization due to removal of calcium ions. Scand. J. Clin. Lab. Invest., *24*:29, 1969.

198. Graham, J. B., Barrow, E. M., and Hougie, C.: Stuart clotting defect. II. Genetic aspects of a "new" hemorrhagic state. J. Clin. Invest., *36*:497, 1957.

199. Graham, R. C., Ebert, R. H., Ratnoff, O. S., and Moses, J. M.: Pathogenesis of inflammation. II. In vivo observations of the inflammatory effects of activated Hageman factor and bradykinin. J. Exp. Med., *121*:807, 1965.

200. Grossi, C. E., Moreno, A. H., and Rousselot, L. M.: Studies on spontaneous fibrinolytic activity in patients with cirrhosis of the liver and its inhibition by epsilon amino caproic acid. Ann. Surg., *153*:383, 1961.

201. Haanen, C., Morselt, G., and Schoenmakers, J.: Contact activation of Hageman factor and the interaction of Hageman factor and plasma thromboplastin antecedent. Thromb. Diath. Haemorrh., *17*:307, 1967.

202. Hamberg, U.: The fibrinolytic activation mechanism in human plasma. Proc. Roy. Society, Series B, Biol. Sci., *173*:293, 1969.

203. Hammarsten, O.: Über das Fibrinogen. Pflügers Arch., *19*:563, 1879.

204. Han, P., and Ardlie, N. G.: Platelet aggregation and release by ADP and thrombin: evidence for two separate effects of ADP on platelets, involvement of fibrinogen in release, and mechanism of inhibitory action of acetylsalicylic acid. Br. J. Haematol., *26*:357, 1974.

205. Hardaway, R. M., III: Disseminated intravascular coagulation. Thromb. Diath. Haemorrh. (Suppl.), *46*:209, 1971.

206. Hardisty, R. M., Dormandy, K. M., and Hutton, R. A.: Thrombasthenia. Study of three cases. Brit. J. Haematol., *10*:371, 1964.

207. Hardisty, R. M., Hutton, R. A., Montgomery, D., Rickard, S., and Trebilcock, H.: Secondary platelet aggregation: a quantitative study. Br. J. Haematol., *19*:307, 1970.

208. Hardisty, R. M., and Pinniger, J. L.: Congenital afibrinogenaemia: further observations on the blood coagulation mechanism. Br. J. Haematol., *2*:139, 1956.

209. Harker, L. A.: Megakaryocyte quantitation. J. Clin. Invest., *47*:452, 1968.

210. Harker, L. A.: Kinetics of thrombopoiesis. J. Clin. Invest., *47*:458, 1968.

211. Hart, H. C.: The biological half-life of I^{131}–fibrinogen. Thromb. Diath. Haemorrh. (Suppl.), *17*:121, 1965.

212. Haslam, R. J.: Role of adenosine diphosphate in the aggregation of human blood platelets by thrombin and by fatty acids. Nature, *202*:765, 1964.

213. Hathaway, W. E., Belhasen, L. P., and Hathaway, H. S.: Evidence for a new plasma thromboplastin factor. I. Case report coagulation studies and physiochemical properties. Blood, *26*:521, 1965.

214. Hatton, M. W. C.: Studies on the coagulant enzyme from agkistrodon rhodostoma venom. Isolation and some properties of the enzyme. Biochem. J., *131*:799, 1973.

215. Hawkey, C.: Activation product and the fibrinolytic system. Nature, *197*:162, 1963.

216. Hayem, G.: Sur la formation de la fibrin du sang, études au microscope. C. R. Acad. Sci. [D] (Paris), *86*:58, 1878.

217. Heimburger, N.: The mechanism of action of streptokinase. J. Clin. Pathol., *25*:632, 1972.

218. Hellum, A. J.: The adhesiveness of human platelets in vitro. Scand. J. Clin. Lab. Invest., *12*: Suppl. 51, 1. 1960.

219. Hemker, H. C., Esnouf, M. P., Hemker, P. W., Swart, A. C. W., and Macfarlane, R. G.: Formation of prothrombin converting activity. Nature, *215*:248, 1967.

220. Hemker, H. C., and Muller, A. D.: Kinetic aspects of the interaction of blood-clotting enzymes. VI. Localization of the site of blood coagulation inhibition by the protein induced by vitamin K absence (PIVKA). Thromb. Diath. Haemorrh., *20*:78, 1968.

221. Hemker, H. C., Muller, A. D., and Loeliger, E. A.: Two types of prothrombin in vitamin K deficiency. Thromb. Diath. Haemorrh., *23*:633, 1970.

222. Henderson, E. S., and Rapaport, S. I.: The thrombotic activity of activation product. J. Clin. Invest., *41*:235, 1962.

223. Hermodson, M. A., Suttie, J. W., and Link, K. P.: Warfarin metabolism and vitamin K requirement in the warfarin-resistant rat. Am. J. Phys. Med., *217*:1316, 1969.

223a. Hershgold, E. J.: Properties of factor VIII. In Progress in Hemostasis and Thrombosis. Spaet, T. H. (ed.), New York, Grune and Stratton, 1974, p. 99.

224. Hiraki, K.: The function of the megakaryocyte: observations both in idiopathic thrombocytopenic purpura and normal adults. Int. Soc. Hematol., *436*:345, 1956. (Abstr.)

225. Hogenauer, E., Lechner, K., and Deutsch, E.: Isolation and characterization of blood clotting factors VII and X. Thromb. Diath. Haemorrh., *19*:304, 1968.

226. Holme, R., Sixma, J. J., Mürer, E. H., and Hovig, T.: Demonstration of platelet fibrinogen secretion via the surface connecting system. Thromb. Res., *3*:347, 1973.

227. Holmsen, H.: Adenine Nucleotide Metabolism in Platelets and Plasma. *In* Kowalski, E., and Niewiarowski, S. (eds.): Biochemistry of Blood Platelets. Academic Press. New York, 1967, p. 81.

228. Holmsen, H.: The platelet: its membrane physiology and biochemistry. Clin. Haematol., *1*:235, 1972.

229. Holmsen, H., Day, H. J., and Stormorken, H.: The blood platelet release reaction. Scand. J. Haematol. (Suppl.), 8, 1969.

230. Holsen, H., and Day, H. T.: Thrombin-induced platelet release reaction and platelet lysosomes. Nature, *219*:760, 1968.

231. Honour, A. J., and Mitchell, J. R. A.: Platelet clumping in injured vessels. Br. J. Exp. Pathol., *45*:75, 1964.

232. Horowitz, H. I., and Papayoanou, M. F.: Release of nonsedimentable platelet factor 3 during coagulation. J. Lab. Clin. Med., *169*:1003, 1967.

233. Hougie, C.: Fundamentals of Blood Coagulation in Clinical Medicine. McGraw-Hill, New York, 1963.

234. Hougie, C., Barrow, E. M., and Graham, J. B.: Stuart clotting defect. I. Segregation of an hereditary hemorrhagic state from the heterogeneous group heretofore called "stable factor" (SPCA, proconvertin, Factor VII) deficiency. J. Clin. Invest., *36*:485, 1957.

234a. Hougie, C. McPherson, R. A., and Aronson, L.: Passovoy factor: a hitherto unrecognized factor necessary for haemostasis. Lancet, *2*:290, 1975.

235. Howell, W. H.: Theories of blood coagulation. Physiol. Rev., *15*:435, 1935.

236. Hoyer, L. W., de los Santos, R. P., and Hoyer, J. R.: Antihemophilic factor antigen. Localization in endothelial cells by immunofluorescent microscopy. J. Clin. Invest., *52*:2737, 1973.

237. Huebner, C. F., and Link, K. P.: Studies on the hemorrhagic sweet clover disease. VI. The synthesis of the δ-diketone derived from the hemorrhagic agent through alkaline degradation. J. Biol. Chem., *138*:529, 1941.

238. Hume, R., West, J. T., Malmgren, R. A., and Chu, E. A.: Quantitative observations of circulating megakaryocytes in the blood of patients with cancer. N. Engl. J. Med., *270*:111, 1964.

239. Hunter, R. B., and Shepherd, D. M.: Chemistry of coumarin anticoagulant drugs. Br. Med. Bull., *11*:56, 1955.

240. Iatridis, S. G., and Ferguson, J. H.: Effect of physical exercise on blood clotting and fibrinolysis. J. Appl. Physiol., *18*:337, 1963.

241. Inceman, S., Caen, J., and Bernard, J.: La "métamorphose visqueuse" des plaquettes de thrombasthénie de Glanzmann. Nouv. Rev. Fr. Hematol., *3*:575, 1963.

242. Ingram, G. I. C.: Anticoagulant therapy. Pharmacol. Rev., *13*:279, 1961.

243. Inman, W. H. W., and Vessey, M. P.: Investigation of deaths from pulmonary, coronary and cerebral thrombosis and embolism in women of child-bearing age. Br. Med. J., *2*:193, 1968.

244. Ireland, D. M.: Effect of thrombin on the radioactive nucleotides of human washed platelets. Biochem. J., *103*:857, 1967.

245. Jackson, C. M.: Carbohydrate moiety differences between two forms of bovine factor X. Fed. Proc., *31*:241, 1972.

246. Jackson, C. M.: Characterization of two glycoprotein variants of bovine factor X and demonstration that the factor X zymogen contains two polypeptide chains. Biochemistry, *11*:4873, 1972.

247. Jackson, C. M., Owen, W. G., Gitel, S. N., and Esmon, C. T.: The chemical role of lipids in prothrombin conversion. Thromb. Diath. Haemorrh. (Suppl.), *57*:273, 1974.

248. Jacobson, R. J., and Jackson, D. P.: Microangiopathic hemolytic anemia in defibrination syndrome. Ann. Intern. Med., *72*:794, 1970.

249. Jaffe, E. A., Hoyer, L. W., and Nachman, R. L.: Synthesis of antihemophilic factor antigen by cultured human endothelial cells. J. Clin. Invest., *52*:2757, 1973.

249a. Jaffe, E. A., Hoyer, L. W., and Nachman, R. L.: Synthesis of von Willebrand factor by cultured human endothelial cells. Proc. Natl. Acad. Sci. U.S.A., *71*:1906, 1974.

250. Jaffe, E. A., Nachman, R. L., Becker, C. G., and Minick, C. R.: Culture of human endothelial cells derived from umbilical veins. Identification by morphologic and immunologic criteria. J. Clin. Invest., *52*:2745, 1973.

251. Jaffe, R., and Deykin, D.: Evidence for a structural requirement for the aggregation of platelets by collagen. J. Clin. Invest., *53*:875, 1974.

252. Jamieson, G. A., and Barber, A. J.: Biochemistry of platelet membranes. Thromb. Diath. Haemorrh. (Suppl.), *54*:239, 1973.

253. Jamieson, G. A., Urban, C. L., and Barber, A. J.: Enzymatic basis for platelet:collagen adhesion as the primary step in haemostasis. Nature [New Biol.], *234*:5, 1971.
254. Jaques, L. B.: Protamine—antagonist to heparin. Can. Med. Assoc. J., *108*:1291, 1973.
255. Jesty, J., and Esnouf, M. P.: The preparation of activated factor X and its action on prothrombin. Biochem. J., *131*:791, 1973.
256. Jesty, J. and Nemerson, Y.: Purification of factor VII from bovine plasma. Reaction with tissue factor and activation of factor X. J. Biol. Chem., *249*:509, 1974.
257. Johnson, A. H.: Platelets and Thrombosis: Interaction with Components of the Vessel Wall. *In* The Platelet. Brinkhous K. M., Shermer, R. W., and Mustofi, F. K. (eds.) Williams and Wilkins, Baltimore, 1971.
258. Johnston, M., and Olson, R. E.: Studies of prothrombin biosynthesis in cell-free systems. II. Incorporation of L-(U-^{14}C) leucine into prothrombin by rat liver microsomes and ribosomes. J. Biol. Chem., *247*:3994, 1972.
259. Joist, J. H., Dolezel, G., Lloyd, J. V., Kinlough–Rathbone, R-L., and Mustard, J. F.: Platelet factor 3 availability and the platelet release reaction. J. Lab. Clin. Med., *84*:474, 1974.
260. Jorpes, J. E.: The origin and the physiology of heparin: the specific therapy in thrombosis. Ann. Intern. Med., *27*:361, 1947.
261. Kakkar, V. V., Corrigan, T. P., and Fossard, D. P.: Prevention of fatal pulmonary embolism using low doses of subcutaneous heparin. Eur. Surg. Res. 5(Suppl.), *2*:25, 1973.
262. Kakkar, V. V., Corrigan, T., Spindler, J., Fossard, D. P., Flute, P. T., Drelin, R. Q., Wessler, S., and Yin, E. T.: Efficacy of low doses of heparin in prevention of deep-vein thrombosis after major surgery. Lancet *2*:101, 1972.
263. Karpatkin, S., Charmatz, A., and Langer, R. M.: Glycogenesis and Glyconeogenesis in human platelets. Incorporation of glucose, pyruvate and citrate into platelet glycogen, glycogen synthetase and fructose–1,6 diphosphatase activity. J. Clin. Invest., *49*:140, 1970.
264. Kass, L., Ratnoff, O. D., and Leon, M. A.: Studies on the purification of antihemophilic factor (factor VIII). J. Clin. Invest., *48*:351, 1969.
265. Kaufman, R. M., Airo, R., Pollack, S., Crosby, W. H., and Doberneck, R.: Origin of pulmonary megakaryocytes. Blood, *25*:767, 1965.
266. Kay, D., and Cuddigan, B. J.: The fine structure of fibrin. Br. J. Haematol., *13*:341, 1967.
267. Kellaway, C. H.: Snake venoms. Bull. Johns Hopkins Hosp., *60*:1, 1937.
268. Kellermeyer, W. F., Jr., and Kellermeyer, R. W.: Hageman factor activation and kinin formation in human plasma induced by cellulose sulfate solutions. Proc. Soc. Exp. Biol. Med., *130*:1310, 1969.
269. Kerby, G. P., and Taylor, S. M.: The role of human platelets and plasma in the metabolism of adenosine diphosphate and monophosphate added in vitro. Thromb. Diath. Haemorrh., *12*:510, 1964.
270. Kerr, J. W., Pirrie, R., MacAulay, I., and Bronte-Stewart, B.: Platelet-aggregation by phospholipids and free fatty acids. Lancet, *1*:1296, 1965.
271. Kiesselbach, T., and Wagner, R.: Fibrin stabilizing factor: a thrombin-labile platelet protein. Am. J. Phys. Med., *211*:1472, 1966.
272. Kingdon, H. S., and Davie, E. W.: Further studies on the activation of factor IX by activated factor XI. Thromb. Diath. Haemorrh. (Suppl.), *17*:15, 1965.
273. Kisiel, W., and Hanahan, D. J.: The action of Factor Xa, thrombin and trypsin on human factor II. Biochim. Biophys. Acta, *329*:221, 1973.
274. Kjeldgaard, N. O., and Ploug, J.: Urokinase, an activator of plasminogen from human urine. II. Mechanism of plasminogen activation. Biochim. Biophys. Acta, *24*:283, 1957.
274a. Kolata, G. B.: Thromboxanes: the power behind the prostaglandins? Science, *190*:770, 1975.
275. Koller, F., Loeliger, A., and Duckert, F.: Experiments on a new clotting factor (factor VII). Acta Haematol., *6*:1, 1951.
276. Kopéc, M., Budzynski, A. Z., Latallo, Z. S., Lipinski, B., Stachurska, J., Wegrzynowicz, Z., and Kowalski, G.: Interaction of Platelet and Fibrinogen Degradation Products in Hemostasis. *In* Kowalski, E., and Niewiarowski, S. (eds.): The Biochemistry of Blood Platelets. Academic Press, New York, 1967. p. 147.
277. Kowalski, E.: Fibrinogen derived inhibitors of blood coagulation. New blood clotting factors. Thromb. Diath. Haemorrh. (Suppl.), *4*:211, 1960.
278. Kucinski, C. S., Fletcher, A. P., and Sherry, S.: Effect of urokinase antiserum on plasminogen activators: demonstration of immunologic dissimilarity between plasma plasminogen activator and urokinase. J. Clin. Invest., *47*:1238, 1968.
279. Kwaan, H. C., McFadzean, A. J. S., and Cook, J.: Plasma fibrinolytic activity in cirrhosis of the liver. Lancet, *1*:132, 1956.
280. Laki, K., Gladner, J. A., and Folk, J. E.: Some aspects of the fibrinogen fibrin transition. Nature, *187*:758, 1960.

281. Laki, K., Kominz, D. R., Symonds, P., Lorand, L., and Seegers, W. H.: The amino acid composition of bovine prothrombin. Arch. Biochem. Biophys., *49*:276, 1954.
282. Lamy, F., and Waugh, D. F.: Certain physical properties of bovine prothrombin. J. Biol. Chem., *203*:489, 1953.
283. Lanchantin, G. F., Friedmann, J. A., and Hart, D. W.: Two forms of human thrombin. Isolation and characterization. J. Biol. Chem., *248*:5956, 1973.
284. Latallo, Z. S., Fletcher, A. P., Alkjaersig, N., and Sherry, S.: Inhibition of fibrin polymerization by fibrinogen proteolysis products. Am. J. Physiol., *202*:681, 1962.
285. Latour, J. G., MaKay, D. G., and Parrish, M. H.: Activation of Hageman factor by cardiac arrest. Thromb. Diath. Haemorrh., *27*:543, 1972.
286. Laurell, C. B.: Synonyms for components influencing blood coagulation. Blood, *7*:555, 1952.
287. Lee, R. I., and White, P. D.: A clinical study of the coagulation time of blood. Am. J. M. Sci., *145*:495, 1913.
288. Le Quesne, L. P.: Current concepts: deep-vein thrombosis and pulmonary embolism. N. Engl. J. Med., *291*:1292, 1974.
289. Lerner, R. G., Goldstein, R., and Cummings, G.: Synthesis of tissue factor by leukocytes during in vitro thrombosis formation. Fed. Proc., *31*:197, 1972.
290. Lesuk, A., Terminiello, L., and Traver, J. H.: Crystalline human urokinase: some properties. Science, *147*:880, 1965.
291. Levenson, J. E., and Esnouf, M. P.: The inhibition of activated factor X with diisopropyl fluorophosphate. Br. J. Haematol., *17*:173, 1969.
292. Lewis, J. H.: Separation and molecular weight estimation of coagulation and fibrinolytic proteins by Sephadex gel filtration. Proc. Soc. Exp. Biol. Med., *116*:120, 1964.
293. Lewis, J. H., and Doyle, A. P.: Effects of epsilon aminocaproic acid on coagulation and fibrinolytic mechanisms. J.A.M.A., *188*:56, 1964.
294. Lewis, J. H., Ferguson, J. H., Spaugh, E., Fresh, J. W., and Zucker, M. B.: Acquired hypoprothrombinemia. Blood, *12*:84, 1957.
295. Lewis, R. J., Trager, W. F., Chan, K. K., Breckenridge, A., Orme, M., Roland, M., and Schary, W.: Warfarin, Stereochemical aspects of its metabolism and the interaction with phenylbutazone. J. Clin. Invest., *53*:1607, 1974.
296. Lieberman, J. S., Borrero, J., Urdaneta, E., and Wright, I. S.: Thrombophlebitis and cancer. J.A.M.A., *177*:542, 1961.
297. Liem, R. K. H., and Scheraga, H. A.: Mechanism of action of thrombin on fibrinogen. IV. Further mapping of the active sites of thrombin and trypsin. Arch. Biochem. Biophys., *160*:33, 1974.
298. Link, K. P.: The anticoagulant from spoiled sweet clover hay. Harvey Lect., *39*:162, 1944.
299. Lloyd, J. V., Nishizawa, E. E., Halder, J., and Mustard, J. F.: Changes in ^{32}P–labeling of platelet phospholipids in response to ADP. Br. J. Haematol., *23*:571, 1972.
300. Loeliger, A., and Hers, J. F. P.: Chronic antithrombinemia (antithrombin V) with hemorrhagic diathesis in a case of rheumatoid arthritis with hypergammaglobulinemia. Thromb. Diath. Haemorrh., *1*:499, 1957.
301. Loewy, A. G., Dahlberg, J. E., Dorwart, W. V., Jr., Weber, M. J., and Eisele, J.: A transamidase mechanism for insoluble fibrin formation. Biochem. Biophys. Res. Commun., *15*:177, 1964.
302. Loewy, A. G., Dahlberg, A., Dunathan, K., Kriel, R., and Wolfinger, H. L., Jr.: Fibrinase. II. Some physical characteristics. J. Biol. Chem., *236*:2634, 1961.
303. Loewy, A. G., Veneziale, C., and Forman, M.: Purification of the factor involved in the formation of urea-insoluble fibrin. Biochim. Biophys. Acta, *26*:670, 1957.
304. Lorand, L.: Interaction of thrombin and fibrinogen. Physiol. Rev., *34*:742, 1954.
305. Lorand, L., Downey, J., Gotoh, T., Jacobsen, A., and Tokura, S.: The transpeptidase system which crosslinks fibrin by γ-glutamyl-ε-lysine bond. Biochem. Biophys. Res. Commun., *31*:222, 1968.
306. Lorand, L., Urayama, T., Atencio, A. C., and Hsia, D. Y. Y.: Inheritance of deficiency of fibrin-stabilizing factor. Am. J. Hematol. Genet., *22*:89, 1970.
307. Lorand, L., Urayama, T., deKiewiet, J. W. C., and Nossel, H. L.: Diagnostic and genetic studies on fibrin-stabilizing factor with a new assay based on amine incorporation. J. Clin. Invest., *48*:1054, 1969.
308. Lowenthal, J., and Birnbaum, H.: Vitamin K and coumarin anticoagulants: dependance of anticoagulant effect on inhibition of vitamin K transport. Science, *164*:181, 1969.
309. Lowenthal, J., and Macfarlane, J. A.: Nature of the antagonism between vitamin K and coumarin anticoagulants. Thromb. Diath. Haemorrh., *19*:611, 1968.
310. Lubran, M.: The effects of drugs on laboratory values. Med. Clin. North Am., *53*:211, 1969.
311. Lüscher, E. F.: Platelets in hemostasis and thrombosis. Br. J. Haematol., *13*:1, 1967.

312. Lüscher, E. F.: Report of subcommittee on current concepts of hemostasis. Thromb. Diath. Haemorrh. (Suppl.), *26*:323, 1967.
313. Lüscher, E. F., and Pfueller, S. L.: Disseminated intravascular coagulation from an immunological viewpoint. Thromb. Diath. Haemorrh. (Suppl.), *45*:129, 1971.
314. Lyttleton, J. W.: The antithrombin activity of human plasma. Biochem. J., *58*:8, 1954.
315. Macfarlane, R. G.: A simple method for measuring clot retraction. Lancet, *1*:1199, 1939.
316. Macfarlane, R. G.: Blood coagulation with particular reference to the early stages. Physiol., Rev., *36*:479, 1956.
317. Macfarlane, R. G.: The coagulant action of Russell's viper venom: the use of antivenom in defining its reaction with a serum factor. Br. J. Haematol., *7*:496, 1961.
318. Macfarlane, R. G.: An enzyme cascade in the blood clotting mechanism, and its function as a biochemical amplifier. Nature, *202*:498, 1964.
319. Macfarlane, R. G., and Ash, B. J.: The activation and consumption of factor X in recalcified plasma. The effect of added factor VIII and Russell's viper venom. Br. J. Haematol., *10*:217, 1964.
320. Macfarlane, R. G., and Biggs, R.: Fibrinolysis: its mechanism and significance. Blood, *3*:1167, 1948.
321. MacKay, A. C. P., Das, P. C., Myerscough, P. R., and Cash, J. D.: Fibrinolytic components of human uterine arterial and venous blood. J. Clin. Pathol., *20*:227, 1967.
322. Macmillan, D. C.: Secondary clumping effect in human citrated platelet rich plasma produced by adenosine diphosphate and adrenaline. Nature, *211*:140, 1966.
323. MacMillan, R. L., and Brown, K. W. G.: Heparin and thromboplastin. J. Lab. Clin. Med., *44*:378, 1954.
324. Maekawa, T., Arai, H., and Kobayashi, N.: The effects of aspirin on platelets and experimental thrombosis. Thromb. Diath. Haemorrh. (Suppl.), *60*:363, 1974.
325. Majerus, P. W., Smith, M. B., and Clamon, G. H.: Lipid metabolism in human platelets. I. Evidence for complete fatty acid synthesizing protein. J. Clin. Invest., *48*:156, 1969.
326. Mann, K. G., Yip, R., Heldebrant, C. M., and Fass, D. N.: Multiple active forms of thrombin. III. Polypeptide chain location of active site serine and carbohydrate. J. Biol. Chem., *248*:1868, 1973.
327. Mann, R. D.: Effect of age, sex and diurnal variation on the human fibrinolytic system. J. Clin. Pathol., *20*:223, 1967.
328. Mant, M. J., Hirsh, J., Pineo, G. F., and Luke, K. H.: Prolonged prothrombin time and partial thromboplastin time in disseminated intravascular coagulation not due to deficiency of factors V and VIII. Br. J. Haematol., *24*:725, 1973.
329. Marchesi, S. L., Shulman, N. R., and Gralnick, H. R.: Studies on the purification and characterization of human factor VIII. J. Clin. Invest., *51*:2151, 1972.
330. Marcus, A. J.: Platelet function. N. Engl. J. Med., *280*:1213, 1278, 1330, 1969.
331. Marcus, A. J.: Zucker-Franklin, D., Safier, L. B., and Ullman, H. L.: Studies on human platelet granules and membranes. J. Clin. Invest., *45*:14, 1966.
332. Marder, V. J.: The structure–function relationship of fibrinogen. Thromb. Diath. Haemorrh. (Suppl.), *54*:135, 1973.
333. Marder, V. J.: Identification and purification of fibrinogen degradation products produced by plasmin. Consideration on the structure of fibrinogen. Scand. J. Haematol. (Suppl.), *13*:21, 1971.
334. Marder, V. J., and Budzynski, A. Z.: Degradation products of fibrinogen and crosslinked fibrin-projected clinical applications. Thromb. Diath. Haemorrh., *32*:49, 1974.
335. Marder, V. J., and Shulman, N. R.: Molecular weight derivatives of human fibrinogen produced by plasmin. II. Mechanism of their anticoagulant activity. J. Biol. Chem., *244*:2120, 1969.
336. Margolius, A., and Ratnoff, O. D.: Observations on the hereditary nature of Hageman trait. Blood, *11*:565, 1956.
337. Marquis, N. R., Becker, J. A., and Vigdahl, R. L.: Platelet aggregation. III. An epinephrine-induced decrease in cyclic AMP synthesis. Biochem. Biophys. Res. Commun., *39*:783, 1970.
338. Marr, J., Barboriak, J. J., and Johnson, S. A.: Relationship of appearance of adenosine diphosphate, fibrin formation and platelet aggregation in the haemostatic plug in vivo. Nature, *205*:259, 1965.
339. Mattock, P., and Esnouf, M. P.: A form of bovine factor X with single polypeptide chain. Nature [New Biol.], *242*:90, 1973.
340. Maynert, E. W., and Issac, L.: Uptake and binding of serotonin by platelet and its granules. Adv. Pharmacol., *6*:113, 1968.

341. McChesney, C. Mcl., Harper, E., and Colman, R. W.: Critical role of the carbohydrate side chains of collagen in platelet aggregation. J. Clin. Invest., *51*:2693, 1972.
342. McDonagh, J., McDonagh, R. P., Delâge, J.-M., and Wagner, R. H.: Factor XIII in human plasma and platelets. J. Clin. Invest., *48*:940, 1969.
343. McKay, D. G.: Disseminated Intravascular Coagulation: An Intermediary Mechanism of Disease. Harper & Row. New York, 1965.
344. McKay, D. G.: Progress in disseminated intravascular coagulation. Calif. Med., *3*:186, 279, 1969.
345. McKay, D. G., Mansell, H., and Hertig, A.: Carcinoma of the body of the pancreas with fibrin thrombosis and fibrinogenopenia. Cancer, *6*:862, 1953.
346. McKay, D. G., and Müller-Bergnaus, E. G.: Therapeutic implication of disseminated intravascular coagulation. Am. J. Cardiol., *20*:392, 1967.
347. McLean, J. R., Maxwell, R. E., and Hertler, D.: Fibrinogen and adenosine diphosphate-induced aggregation of platelets. Nature, *202*:605, 1964.
347a. McMillin, C. R., Saito, H., Ratnoff, O. D., and Walton, A. G.: Secondary structure of human Hageman Factor (factor XII) and its alteration by activating agents. J. Clin. Invest., *54*: 1312, 1974.
348. McNicol, G. P.: Disordered fibrinolytic activity and its control. Scott. Med. J., *7*:266, 1962.
349. McNicol, G. P.: The mechanism of fibrinolysis. Proc. Roy. Soc., Series B, Biol. Sci., *173*:285, 1969.
350. McNicol, G. P., and Douglas, A. S.: ϵ-Aminocaproic acid and other inhibitors of fibrinolysis. Br. Med. Bull., *20*:233, 1964.
351. McNicol, G. P., Fletcher, A. P., Alkjaersig, N., and Sherry, S.: Use of epsilon aminocaproic acid in management of postoperative hematuria. J. Urol., *86*:829, 1961.
352. Merskey, C.: Editorial: defibrination syndrome or . . . ? Blood, *41*:599, 1973.
353. Merskey, C.: Diagnosis and treatment of intravascular coagulation. Br. J. Haematol., *15*:523, 1968.
354. Merskey, C., Johnson, A. J., Kleiner, G. J., and Wohl, H.: The defibrination syndrome: clinical features and laboratory diagnosis. Br. J. Haematol., *13*:528, 1967.
355. Merskey, C., Kleiner, G. J., and Johnson, A. J.: Quantitative estimation of split products of fibrinogen in human serum. Relation to diagnosis and treatment. Blood, *28*:1, 1966.
356. Mertins, B. F., McDuffie, F. C., Bowie, E. J. W., and Owen, C. A., Jr.: Rapid sensitive method for measuring fibrinogen split products in human serum. Mayo Clin. Proc., *44*:114, 1969.
357. Michael, S. E., and Tunnah, G. W.: The purification of factor VIII (antihaemophilic globulin). Br. J. Haematol., *9*:236, 1963.
358. Michal, F.: Blood platelets—platelet 5–HT receptors are of the classical D type. Nature, *221*: 1253, 1969.
359. Milestone, J. H.: Thrombokinase as prime activator of prothrombin: historical perspectives and present status. Fed. Proc. *23*:742, 1964.
360. Miller, J. R., Baggenstoss, A. H., and Comfort, M. W.: Carcinoma of the pancreas: effect of histological type and grade of malignancy on its behavior. Cancer, *4*:233, 1951.
361. Miller, K. D., Brown, R. K., Casillas, G., and Seegers, W. H.: The amino acid composition of thrombin preparations. Thromb. Diath. Haemorrh., *3*:362, 1959.
362. Mitchell, J. R. A., and Sharp, A. A.: Platelet clumping in vitro. Br. J. Haematol., *10*:78, 1964.
363. Mitchell, J. S.: Metabolic effects of therapeutic doses of X and gamma radiations. Br. J. Radiol., *16*:339, 1943.
364. Morawitz, P., Trans. by Hartmann, R. C., and Guenther, P. F.: The Chemistry of Blood Coagulation. Charles C Thomas, Springfield, Ill., 1958.
365. Moses, R. G., and Warren, J. R.: Coumarin necrosis. Med. J. Austr., *2*:76, 1973.
366. Mosher, D. F., and Blout, E. R.: Heterogeneity of bovine fibrinogen and fibrin. J. Biol. Chem., *248*:6896, 1973.
367. Müller-Berghaus, G., and Schneberger, R.: Hageman factor activation in the generalized Shwartzman reaction induced by endotoxin. Br. J. Haematol., *21*:513, 1971.
368. Murphy, E. A., and Mustard, J. F.: Coagulation tests and platelet economy in atherosclerotic and control subjects. Circulation, *25*:114, 1962.
369. Mustard, J. F., Murphy, E. A., Rowsell, H. C., and Downie, H. G.: Factors influencing thrombus formation in vivo. Am. J. Med., *33*:621, 1962.
370. Nechman, R. L.: Platelet proteins. Semin. Hemat., *5*:18, 1968.
371. Nachman, R. L.: Immunologic studies of platelet protein. Blood, *25*:703, 1965.
372. Nachman, R. L., and Ferris, B.: Binding of adenosine diphosphate by isolated membranes from human platelets. J. Biol. Chem., *249*:704, 1974.
373. Nachman, R. L., Marcus, A. J., and Safier, L. B.: Platelet thrombosthenin, subcellular localization and function. J. Clin. Invest., *46*:1380, 1967.

374. Nachman, R. L., and Weksler, B.: The platelet as an inflammatory cell. Ann. N. Y. Acad. Sci., *201*:131, 1972.

375. Naeye, R. L.: Thrombotic disorders with increased levels of antiplasmin and antiplasminogen. N. Engl. J. Med., *265*:867, 1961.

376. Nalbardian, R. M., Mader, I. J., Barrett, J. L., Pearce, J. F., and Rupp, E. C.: Petechiae, ecchymoses, and necrosis of skin induced by coumarin congeners. J.A.M.A., *192*:107, 1965.

377. Nanninga, L. B., and Guest, M. M.: Preparation and properties of anticoagulant split product of fibrinogen and its determination in plasma. Thromb. Diath. Haemorrh., *17*:440, 1967.

378. Nelsestuen, G. L., and Suttie, J. W.: The mode of action of vitamin K. Isolation of a peptide containing the vitamin K-dependent portion of prothrombin. Proc. Natl. Acad. Sci. U.S.A., *70*:3366, 1973.

379. Nemerson, Y.: Phospholipid requirement of tissue factor in blood coagulation. J. Clin. Invest., *47*:72, 1968.

380. Nemerson, Y., and Pitlick, F. A.: Extrinsic Clotting Pathways. *In* Spaet, T. (ed.): Progress in Hemostasis and Thrombosis. Vol. I. Grune and Stratton, New York, 1972.

381. Niemetz, J.: Factors influencing the consumption of factor X (Stuart-Prower factor) during intrinsic coagulation. Thromb. Diath. Haemorrh., *18*:332, 1967.

382. Niewiarowski, S., Farbiszewski, R., and Poplawski, A.: Studies on Platelet Factor 2 (PF$_2$–fibrinogen activating factor) and platelet Factor 4 (PF$_4$-antiheparin factor). *In* Kowalski, E., and Niewiarowski, S. (eds.): Biochemistry of Blood Platelets. Academic Press, New York, 1967, p. 35.

383. Nilsson, I. M., Anderson, L., and Bjorkman, S. E.: Epsilon-amino caproic acid (EACA) as a therapeutic agent based on 5 years clinical experience. Acta Med. Scand. (Suppl.), *448*:1, 1966.

384. Nilsson, I., Krook, H., Sternby, N.-H., Söderberg, E., and Söderström, N.: Severe thrombotic disease in a young man with bone marrow and skeletal changes and with a high content of an inhibitor in the fibrolytic system. Acta Med. Scand., *169*:323, 1961.

385. Norman, P. S., and Hill, B. M.: Studies of the plasmin system. III. Physical properties of the two plasmin inhibitors in plasma. J. Exp. Med., *108*:639, 1958.

386. Nossel, H. L.: The activation and consumption of factor IX. Thromb. Diath. Haemorrh., *12*:505, 1964.

387. Nossel, H. L., Drillings, M., and Hsieh, R.: Inhibition of Hageman factor activation. J. Clin. Invest., *47*:1172, 1968.

388. Nossel, H. I., Wilner, G. D., and LeRoy, E. C.: Blood polar groups important for initiating coagulation and aggregating platelets. Nature, *221*:75, 1969.

389. Olson, R. E., Kipfer, R. K., Morrissey, J. J., and Goodman, S. R.: Function of vitamin K in prothrombin synthesis. Thromb. Diath. Haemorrh. (Suppl.), *57*:31, 1974.

390. Olson, J. P., Miller, L. L., and Troup, S. G.: Synthesis of clotting factors by the isolated perfused rat liver. J. Clin. Invest., *45*:690, 1966.

391. O'Reilly, R. A.: The second reported kindred with hereditary resistance to oral anticoagulant drugs. N. Engl. J. Med., *282*:1448, 1970.

392. O'Reilly, R. A.: Hazards of anticoagulant treatment: other drugs, other diseases. Thromb. Diath Haemorrh. (Suppl.), *56*:211, 1973.

393. Osler, W.: On certain problems in the physiology of the blood corpuscles. Med. News, *48*: 365, 393, 421, 1886. Br. Med. J., *1*:807, 861, 917, 1886. (Abstr.)

394. Østerud, B., Berre, A., Otnaess, A-B, Bjørklid, E., and Prydz, H.: Activation of the coagulation factor VII by tissue thromboplastin and calcium. Biochemistry, *11*:2853, 1972.

395. Owen, W. G., Esmond, C. T., and Jackson, C. M.: The conversion of prothrombin to thrombin. I. Characterization of the reaction products formed during the activation of bovine prothrombin. J. Biol. Chem., *249*:594, 1974.

396. Owren, P. A.: Proconvertin, the new clotting factor. Scand. J. Clin. Lab. Invest., *3*:168, 1951.

397. Packham, M. A., Guccione, M. A., Chang, P.-L., and Mustard, J. F.: Platelet aggregation and release: Effects of low concentrations of thrombin or collagen. Am. J. Physiol., *225*:38, 1973.

398. Packham, M. A., Nishizawa, E. E., and Mustard, J. F.: Response of platelets to tissue injury. Biochem. Pharmacol. (Suppl.), *17*:171, 1968.

399. Pascuzzi, C. A., Spittel, J. A., Jr., Thompson, J. H., Jr., and Owen, C. A., Jr.: Thromboplastin generation accelerator. A newly recognized component of the blood coagulation mechanism present in excess in certain thrombotic states. J. Clin. Invest., *40*:1006, 1961.

400. Pasquini, R., and Hershgold, E. J.: Effects of plasmin on human factor VIII (AHF). Blood, *41*:105, 1973.

401. Pechet, L., and Alexander, B.: Increased clotting factors in pregnancy. N. Engl. J. Med., *265*: 1093, 1961.

402. Pechet, L., Cochios, F., and Deykin, D.: Further studies on the Dynia clotting abnormality. Thromb. Diath. Haemorrh., *17*:365, 1967.

403. Penick, G. D.: Blood States that Predispose to Thrombosis. *In* Sherry, S. (ed.): Thrombosis. Proc. Natl. Acad. Sci. 553, 1969.

404. Penick, G. D., Dejanov, I. I., Reddick, R. L., and Roberts, H. R.: Predisposition to intravascular coagulation. Thromb. Diath. Haemorrh., (Suppl.), *21*:543, 1966.

405a. Philip, G., Moran, J., and Colman, R. W.: Dissociation and association of the oligomeric forms of factor V. Biochem., *9*:2212, 1970.

405. Pepper, D. S., and Jameson, G. A.: Isolation of a macroglycopeptide from human platelets. Biochemistry, *9*:3706, 1970.

406. Phillips, D. R., and Agin, P. P.: Thrombin interaction with human platelets potentiation of thrombin-induced aggregation and release by inactivated thrombin. Thromb. Diath. Haemorrh., *32*:207, 1974.

407. Pierce, L. E.: Disseminated intravascular coagulation. Am. Fam. Physician, *7*:118, 1973.

408. Pilkington, T. R. E.: The effect of fatty acids and detergents on the calcium clotting time of human plasma. Clin. Sci., *16*:269, 1957.

409. Pineo, G. F., Regoeczi, E., Hatton, M. W. C., and Brain, M. C.: The activation of coagulation by extracts of mucus: a possible pathway of intravascular coagulation accompanying adenocarcinoma. J. Lab. Clin. Med., *82*:255, 1973.

410. Pitlick, F. A., and Nemerson, Y.: Binding of the protein component of tissue factor to phospholipids. Biochemistry, *9*:5105, 1970.

411. Pitlick, F. A., and Nemerson, Y., Gottlieb, A. J., Jordan, R. B., and Williams, W. J.: Peptidase activity associated with the tissue factor of blood coagulation. Biochemistry, *10*:2650, 1971.

412. Pitney, W. R.: Heparin therapy and its laboratory control. Brit. J. Haematol., *18*:499, 1970.

413. Pizzo, S. V., Schwartz, M. L., Hill, R. L., and McKee, P. A.: The effect of plasmin on the subunit structure of human fibrin. J. Biol. Chem., *247*:636, 1972.

414. Pizzo, S. V., Schwartz, M. L., Hill, R. L., and McKee, P. A.: Mechanism of ancrod anticoagulation. A direct proteolytic effect on fibrin. J. Clin. Invest., *51*:2841, 1972.

415. Ploug, J., and Kjeldgaard, N. O.: Urokinase, an activator of plasminogen from human urine. I. Isolation and properties. Biochim. Biophys. Acta, *24*:278, 1957.

416. Poller, L., Tabiowo, A., and Thomson, J. M.: Effect of low-dose oral contraceptives on blood coagulation. Br. Med. J., *3*:218, 1968.

417. Pool, J. G., Cohen, T., and Creger, W. P.: Biological half-life of transfused antihemophilic globulin (factor VIII) in normal man. Br. J. Haematol., *13*:822, 1967.

418. Prentice, C. R. M., and Ratnoff, O. D.: The action of Russell's viper venom on factor V and the prothrombin-converting principle. Br. J. Haematol., *16*:291, 1969.

419. Puett, D., Wasserman, B. K., Ford, J. D., and Cunningham, L. W.: Collagen–mediated platelet aggregation. Effects of collagen modification involving the protein and carbohydrate moieties. J. Clin. Invest., *52*:2495, 1973.

420. Quick, A. J.: The prothrombin in hemophilia and in obstructive jaundice. J. Biol. Chem., *109*:73, 1935.

421. Quick, A. J.: The normal antithrombin of the blood and its relation to heparin. Am. J. Physiol., *123*:712, 1938.

422. Quick, A. J.: The Physiology and Pathology of Hemostasis. Lea & Febiger, Philadelphia, 1951.

423. Rabiner, S. F., Goldfine, I. D., Hart, A., Summaria, L., and Robbins, K. C.: Radioimmunoassay of human plasminogen and plasmin. J. Lab. Clin. Med., *74*:265, 1969.

424. Raisys, V., Molner, J., and Winzler, R. J.: Study of carbohydrate release during the clotting of fibrinogen. Arch. Biochem., *113*:457, 1966.

425. Ramot, B., Angelopoulos, B., and Singer, K.: Plasma thromboplastin antecedent deficiency. Arch. Intern. Med., *95*:705, 1955.

426. Ramot, B., Singer, K., Heller, P., and Zimmerman, H. J.: Hageman factor (HF) deficiency. Blood, *11*:745, 1956.

427. Ranhotra, G. S., and Johnson, B. C.: Vitamin K and the synthesis of factor VII by isolated rat liver cells. Proc. Soc. Exp. Biol. Med., *132*:509, 1969.

428. Rapaport, S. I.: Plasma thromboplastin antecedent levels in patients receiving coumarin anticoagulants and in patients with Laennec's cirrhosis. Proc. Soc. Exp. Biol. Med., *108*:115, 1961.

429. Ratnoff, O. D.: A familial trait characterized by deficiency of a clot-promoting fraction of plasma. J. Lab. Clin. Med., *44*:915, 1954.

430. Ratnoff, O. D.: Activation of Hageman factor by L-homocystine. Science, *162*:1007, 1968.

431. Ratnoff, O. D.: Studies on the product of the reaction between activated Hageman factor (factor XII) and plasma thromboplastin antecedent (factor XI). J. Lab. Clin. Med., *80*:704, 1972.

432. Ratnoff, O. D., Botti, R. E., Crum, J. D., and Donaldson, V. H.: The activation of PTA (factor XI) and Hageman (factor XII). Thromb. Diath. Haemorrh., *17*:7, 1965.

433. Ratnoff, O. D., and Davie, E. W.: The activation of Christmas factor (factor IX) by activated plasma thromboplastin antecedent (activated factor XI). Biochemistry, *1*:677, 1962.

434. Ratnoff, O. D., Davie, E. W., and Mallett, D. L.: Studies on the action of Hageman factor: evidence that activated Hageman factor in turn activates plasma thromboplastin antecedent. J. Clin. Invest., *40*:803, 1961.

435. Ratnoff, O. D., Kass, L., and Lang, P. D.: Studies on the purification of antihemophilic factor VIII. J. Clin. Invest., *48*:957, 1969.

436. Ratnoff, O. D., Pensky, J., and Donaldson, V. H.: The inhibitory properties of plasma against activated plasma thromboplastin antecedent (factor XIa) in hereditary angioneurotic edema. J. Lab. Clin. Med., *80*:803, 1972.

437. Reid, H. A., and Chan, K. E.: The paradox in therapeutic defibrination. Lancet, *1*:485, 1968.

438. Rickles, F. R., Hardin, J. A., Pitlick, F. A., Hoyer, L. W., and Conrad, M. E.: Tissue factor activity in lymphocyte cultures from normal individuals and patients with hemophilia A. J. Clin. Invest., *52*:1427, 1973.

439. Ridgway, H., and Speer, R. J.: The formation and "decay" of XIIa. Thromb. Diath. Haemorrh., *18*:259, 1967.

440. Robbins, K. C., Summaria, L., Hsieh, B., and Shah, R. J.: The peptide chains of human plasmin. J. Biol. Chem., *242*:2333, 1967.

441. Robb-Smith, A. H. T.: Why the platelets were discovered. Br. J. Haematol., *13*:618, 1967.

442. Roberts, P. S., and Burkat, R. K.: Purification of human plasminogen. Thromb. Diath. Haemorrh., *17*:423, 1967.

443. Rodriguez-Erdmann, F.: The syndrome of intravascular coagulation. Clotting system derangement may result in ischemic necrosis and severe hemorrhagic diathesis. Postgrad. Med. J., *55*:91, 1974.

443a. Rosenberg, R. D.: Actions and interactions of antithrombin and heparin. N. Engl. J. Med., *292*:146, 1975.

444. Rosenberg, R. D., and Damus, P. S.: The purification and mechanism of action of human antithrombin–heparin cofactor. J. Biol. Chem., *248*:6490, 1973.

445. Rosenthal, R. L.: Properties of plasma thromboplastin antecedent (PTA) in relation to blood coagulation. J. Lab. & Clin. Med., *45*:123, 1955.

446. Rosenthal, R. L.: Dreskin, O. H., and Rosenthal, N.: New hemophilia-like disease caused by deficiency of third plasma thromboplastin factor. Proc. Soc. Exp. Biol. Med., *82*:171, 1953.

447. Roskam, J.: Hemostasis and homeostasis. Thromb. Diath. Haemorrh., *18*:553, 1967.

448. Rozenberg, M. C., and Holmsen, H.: Adenosine nucleotide metabolism of blood platelets. IV. Platelet aggregation response to exogenous ATP and ADP. Biochim. Biophys. Acta, *157*:280, 1968.

449. Rutty, D. A.: A mechanism to limit platelet aggregation in vivo. Nature, *206*:1263, 1965.

450. Sack, E., Spaet, T. H., Gentile, R. L., and Hudson, P. B.: Reduction of postprostatectomy bleeding by epsilon-aminocaproic acid. N. Engl. J. Med., *266*:541, 1962.

451. Salmon, J., Lambert, and Louis, J.: Pathogenesis of the intravascular coagulation syndrome induced by immunological reactions. Thromb. Diath. Haemorrh. (Suppl.), *45*:161, 1971.

452. Saito, H., Ratnoff, O. D., Marshall, J. S., and Pensky, J.: Partial purification of plasma thromboplastin antecedent (factor XI) and its activation by trypsin. J. Clin. Invest., *52*:850, 1973.

452a. Saito, H., Ratnoff, O. D., Waldmann, R., and Abraham, J. P.: Fitzgerald trait. J. Clin. Invest., *55*:1082, 1975.

453. Salzman, E. W.: Measurement of platelet adhesiveness. A simple in vitro technique demonstrating an abnormality in von Willebrand's disease. J. Lab. Clin. Med., *62*:724, 1963.

454. Salzman, E. W.: Measurement of platelet adhesiveness: progress report. Thromb. Diath. Haemorrh. (Suppl.), *26*:323, 1967.

455. Salzman, E. W.: Prostaglandins, cyclic AMP and platelet function. Thromb. Diath. Haemorrh. (Suppl.), *60*:311, 1974.

456. Salzman, E. W., Chambers, D. A., and Neri, L. L.: Possible mechanism of aggregation of blood platelets by adenosine diphosphate. Nature, *210*:167, 1966.

457. Salzman, E. W., Chambers, D. A., and Neri, L. L.: Incorporation of labelled nucleotides and aggregation of human blood platelets. Thromb. Diath. Haemorrh., *15*:52, 1966.

458. Salzman, E. W., Harris, W. H., and DeSanctis, R. W.: Reduction in venous thromboembolism by agents affecting platelet function. N. Engl. J. Med., *284*:1287, 1971.

459. Salzman, E. W., Kensler, P. C., and Levine, L.: Cyclic 3′, 5′–adenosine monophosphate in human blood platelets. IV. Regulatory role of cyclic AMP in platelet function. Ann. N. Y. Acad. Sci., *201*:61, 1972.

460. Saltzman, E. W., Rubino, E. B., and Sims, R. V.: Cyclic 3′, 5′–adenosine monophosphate in

human blood platelets. III. The role of cyclic AMP in platelet aggregation. Ser. Haematol., *3*:100, 1970.

461. Samih, Y. A., Hampton, J. W., Race, G. J., and Speer, R.: The relationship of plasma fibrinogen (factor I) level to fibrin stabilizing factor (factor XIII) activity. Blood, *31*:93, 1968.

462. Sas, G., Blaskó, G., Bánhegyi, D., Jákó, J., and Pálos, L. Á.: Abnormal antithrombin III (antithrombin III 'Budapest') as a cause of a familial thrombophilia. Thromb. Diath. Haemorrh., *32*:105, 1974.

463. Sawyer, W. D., Fletcher, A. P., Alkjaersig, N., and Sherry, S.: Studies on the thrombolytic activity of human plasma. J. Clin. Invest., *39*:426, 1960.

464. Schiffman, S., and Lee, P.: Preparation, characterization, and activation of a highly purified factor XI: evidence that a hitherto unrecognized plasma activity participates in the interaction of factors XI and XII. Br. J. Haematol., *27*:101, 1974.

465. Schiffman, S., Rapaport, S. I., and Chong, M. M. Y.: Platelets and initiation of intrinsic clotting. Br. J. Haematol., *24*:633, 1973.

466. Schiffman, S., Rapaport, S. I., and Patch, M. J.: The identification and synthesis of activated plasma thromboplastin component (PTC). Blood, *22*:733, 1963.

467. Schmidt, A.: Neue Untersuchungen über die Faserstoffgerinnung. Pflügers Arch., *6*:413, 1872.

468. Schulert, A. R., and Weiner, M.: The physiologic disposition of phenylindanedione in man. J. Pharmacol. Exp. Ther., *110*:451, 1954.

469. Schulman, S., Alkjaersig, N., and Sherry, S.: Physicochemical studies on human plasminogen (profibrinolysin) and plasmin (fibrinolysin). J. Biol. Chem., *233*:91, 1958.

470. Seegers, W. H., Johnson, J. F., and Fell, C.: An antithrombin reaction related to prothrombin activation. Am. J. Physiol., *176*:97, 1954.

471. Seegers, W. H., McClaughry, R. I., and Fahey, J. L.: Some properties of purified prothrombin and its activation with sodium citrate. Blood, *5*:421, 1950.

472. Seegers, W. H., and McGinty, D. A.: Further purification of thrombin: probable purity of products. J. Biol. Chem., *146*:511, 1942.

473. Shamash, Y., and Rimon, A.: The plasmin inhibitors of human plasma. III. Purification and partial characterization. Biochim. Biophys. Acta, *121*:35, 1966.

474. Shapiro, G. A., Andersen, J. C., Pizzo, S. V., and McKee, P. A.: The subunit structure of normal and hemophilic factor VIII. J. Clin. Invest., *52*:2198, 1973.

475. Sharnoff, J. G.: Results in the prophylaxis of postoperative thromboembolism. Surg. Gynecol. Obstet., *123*:303, 1966.

476. Sharp. A. A.: Pathological fibrinolysis. Br. Med. Bull., *20*:240, 1964.

478. Sharp. A. A.: Present status of platelet aggregation. N. Engl. J. Med., *272*:89, 1965.

479. Sharp. A. A.: The significance of fibrinolysis. Proc. Roy. Soc. Series B. Biol. Sci., *173*:311, 1969.

480. Sharp. A. A., Allington, M. J., and Chesterman, C. N.: Thrombolytic therapy: pharmacology. J. Clin. Pathol., *25*:630, 1972.

481. Sharp. A. A., Howie, B., Biggs, R., and Methuen, D. T.: Defibrination syndrome in pregnancy. Value of various diagnostic tests. Lancet, *2*:1309, 1958.

482. Sheltaway, M. J., Miloszewski, K., and Losowsky, M. S.: Studies on the activation of human factor XIII. Thromb. Diath. Haemorrh., *28*:473, 1972.

483. Sherry, S.: Fibrinolysis. Annu. Rev. Med., *19*:247, 1968.

484. Sherry, S.: Urokinase. Annols. Intern. Med., *69*:415, 1968.

485. Sherry, S., Fletcher, A. P., and Alkjaersig, N.: Fibrinolysis and fibrinolytic activity in man. Physiol. Rev., *39*:343, 1959.

486. Sherry, S., Troll, W., and Glueck, H.: Thrombin as a proteolytic enzyme. Physiol. Rev., *34*:736, 1954.

487. Shirasawa, K., Barton, B. P., and Chandler, A. B.: Localization of ferritin-conjugated antifibrin fibrinogen in platelet aggregates produced in vitro. Am. J. Pathol., *66*:379, 1972.

488. Shore, P. A., Pletscher, A., Tomich, E. G., Kuntzman, R., and Brodie, B. B.: Release of blood platelet serotonin by reserpine and lack of effect on bleeding time. J. Pharmacol. Exp. Ther., *117*:232, 1956.

489. Shulman, N. R.: Studies on the inhibition of proteolytic enzymes by serum. I. The mechanism of the inhibition of trypsin, plasmin and chymotrypsin by serum using fibrin tagged with I^{131} as a substrate. J. Exp. Med., *95*:571, 1952.

490. Shulman, N. R.: Studies on the inhibition of proteolytic enzymes by serum. II. Demonstration that separate proteolytic inhibitors exist in serum: their distinctive properties and the specificity of their action. J. Exp. Med., *95*:593, 1952.

491. Siegel, A., and Lüscher, E.: Non-identity of the α granules of human blood platelets with typical lysosomes. Nature, *215*:745, 1967.

492. Silver, M. D., Stehbens, W. E., and Silver, M. M.: Platelet reaction to adenosine diphosphate in vivo. Nature, *205*:91, 1965.

493. Silver, M. J., Smith, J. B., Ingerman, C., and Kocsis, J. J.: Arachidonic acid–induced human platelet aggregation and prostaglandin formation. Prostaglandins, 4:863, 1973.
493a. Silverglade, A. (ed.): A heparin symposium. Cur. Therapeut. Res. 18:1, 1975.
494. Sise, H. S., Moschos, C. B., and Becker, R.: On the nature of hypercoagulability. Am. J. Med., 33:667, 1962.
495. Smith, J. B., Ingerman, C., Kocsis, J. J., and Silver, M. J.: Formation of prostaglandins during the aggregation of human blood platelets. J. Clin. Invest., 52:965, 1973.
496. Smith, J. B., Ingerman, C., Kocsis, J. J., and Silver, M. J.: Prostaglandins in platelet function. Thromb. Res. (Suppl. 1) 4:49, 1974.
497. Smith, J. B., Ingerman, C., Kocsis, J. J., and Silver, M. J.: Formation of an intermediate in prostaglandin biosynthesis and its association with the platelet release reaction. J. Clin. Invest., 53:1468, 1974.
498. Smith, R. L.: Titration of activated bovine factor X. J. Biol. Chem., 248:2418, 1973.
499. Spaet, T. H.: Vascular factors in the pathogenesis of hemorrhagic syndromes. Blood, 7:641, 1952.
500. Spaet, T. H., and Cintron, J.: Studies on platelet factor-3 availability. Br. J. Haematol., 11:269, 1965.
501. Spaet, T. H., and Lejnieks, I.: Studies on the mechanism whereby platelets are clumped by adenosine diphosphate. Thromb. Diath. Haemorrh., 15:36, 1966.
502. Spaet, T. H., and Stemerman, M. B.: Platelet Adhesion. Ann. N. Y. Acad Sci., 201:13, 1972.
503. Spector, A. A., Hoak, J. C., Warner, E. D., and Fry, G. L.: Uptake of free fatty acids by human platelets. J. Clin. Invest., 49:1489, 1970.
504. Speer, R. J., Ridgway, H., and Hill, J. M.: Activated human Hageman factor (XII). Thromb. Diath. Haemorrh., 14:1, 1965.
505. Stahmann, M. A., Huebner, C. F., and Link, K. P.: Studies on the hemorrhagic sweet clover disease. V. Identification and synthesis of the hemorrhagic agent. J. Biol. Chem., 138:513, 1941.
506. Steiner, M.: Effect of thrombin on the platelet membrane (BBA 71187). Biochim. Biophys. Acta, 323:653, 1973.
507. Stemerman, M. B.: Vascular Intimal Components: Precursors of Thrombosis. In Spaet, T. H. (ed.): Progress in Hemostasis and Thrombosis. Grune & Stratton, New York, 1974.
508. Straub, P.: Chronic intravascular coagulation: localized or generalized? Thromb. Diath. Haemorr. (Suppl.), 56:1, 1973.
509. Straub, W., and Duckert, F.: The formation of extrinsic prothrombin activator. Thromb. Diath. Haemorrh., 5:402, 1961.
510. Sullivan, J. M., Harken, D. E., and Gorlin, R.: Pharmacologic control of thromboembolic complications of cardiac valve replacement. N. Engl. J. Med., 284:1391, 1971.
511. Suttie, J. W.: Control of clotting factor biosynthesis by vitamin K. Fed. Proc., 28:1696, 1969.
512. Takagi, T., and Konishi, K.: Purification and some properties of fibrin stabilizing factor. Biochim. Biophys. Acta, 271:363, 1972.
513. Tocantins, L. M.: The mammalian blood platelets in health and disease. Medicine, 17:155, 1938.
514. Tocantins, L. M.: The Coagulation of Blood. Methods of Study. 1st Ed. Grune & Stratton, New York, 1955.
515. Todd, A. S.: The histological localisation of fibrinolysin activator. J. Pathol. Bacteriol., 78:281, 1959.
516. Todd, A. S.: Localisation of fibrinolytic activity in tissues. Br. Med. Bull., 20:210, 1964.
517. Tollefsen, D. M., Feagler, J. R., and Majerus, P. W.: Induction of the platelet release reaction by phytohemagglutinin. J. Clin. Invest., 53:211, 1974.
518. Tollefsen, D. M., Feagler, J. R., and Majerus, P. W.: The binding of thrombin to the surface of human platelets. J. Biol. Chem., 249:2646, 1974.
519. Tranzer, J. P., and Baumgartner, H. R.: Filling gaps in the vascular endothelium with blood platelets. Nature, 216:1126, 1967.
520. Triantaphyllopoulos, D. C.: Nature of thrombin-inhibiting effect of incubated fibrinogen. Am. J. Physiol., 197:575, 1959.
521. Triantaphyllopoulos, E., and Triantaphyllopoulos, D. C.: Fibrinogenolysis: the micromolecular derivatives. Br. J. Haematol., 15:337, 1968.
522. Truman, W. H. W., and Vessey, M. P.: Investigation of deaths from pulmonary, coronary and cerebral thrombosis and embolism in women of child-bearing age. Br. Med. J., 2:193, 1968.
523. Tsernoglou, D., Walz, D. A., McCoy, L. E., and Seegers, W. H.: An x-ray crystallographic study of thrombin. J. Biol. Chem., 249:999, 1974.
524. Veltkamp, J. J., Loeliger, E. A., and Hemker, H. C.: The biological half-time of Hageman factor. Thromb. Diath. Haemorrh., 13:1, 1965.

525. A Cooperative Study (Original Contributions): Urokinase–streptokinase embolism trial. J.A.M.A., *229*:1606, 1974.
526. Verstraete, M., Amery, A., and Vermylen, J.: Feasibility of adequate thrombolytic therapy with streptokinase in peripheral arterial occlusions. I. Clinical and arteriographic results. Br. Med. J., *1*:1499, 1963.
527. Vessey, M. P., and Doll, R.: Investigation of the relation between use of oral contraceptives and thromboembolic disease. Br. Med. J., *2*:199, 1968.
528. Wagner, R. H., Cooper, H. A., and Owen, W. G.: Dissociation of antihemophilic factor and separation of a small active fragment. Thromb. Diath. Haemorrh. (Suppl.), *54*:185, 1973.
529. Walls, W. D., and Losowsky, M. S.: Plasma fibrin stabilizing factor (FSF) activity in normal subjects and patients with chronic liver disease. Thromb. Diath. Haemorrh., *21*:134, 1969.
529a. Walsh, P. N.: Albumin density gradient separation and washing of platelets and the study of platelet coagulant activities. Br. J. Haematol., *22*:205, 1972.
530. Walsh, P. N.: Platelet coagulant activities and hemostasis: a hypothesis. Blood, *43*:597, 1974.
531. Walsh, P. N.: The effects of collagen and kaolin on the intrinsic coagulant activity of platelets. Evidence for an alternative pathway in intrinsic coagulation not requiring factor XII. Br. J. Haematol., *22*:393, 1972.
532. Walsh, P. N.: The role of platelets in the contact phase of blood coagulation. Br. J. Haematol., *22*:237, 1972.
533. Walsh, P. N., and Biggs, R.: The role of platelets in intrinsic factor-Xa formation. Br. J. Haematol., *22*:743, 1972.
534. Walsh, P. N., and Biggs, R.: Release of heparin-neutralizing activity by platelets. Fed. Proc., *32*:844, 1973.
535. Warren, B. A.: Fibrinolytic activity of vascular endothelium. Br. Med. Bull., *20*:213, 1964.
536. Warren, R.: Postoperative thrombophilia. N. Engl. J. Med., *249*:99, 1953.
537. Warshaw, A. L., Laster, L., and Shulman, W. R.: The stimulation by thrombin of glucose oxidation in human platelets. J. Clin. Invest., *45*:1923, 1966.
538. Webber, A. J., and Budtz-Olsen, O. E.: Thrombin-stimulated release of platelet microfibrils. Br. J. Haematol., *26*:255, 1974.
539. Weiner, M., Shapiro, S., Axelrod, J., Cooper, J. R., and Brodie, B. B.: The physiological disposition of dicumarol in man. J. Pharmacol. Exp. Ther., *99*:409, 1950.
540. Weiss, H. J.: The pharmacology of platelet inhibition. Progr. Hemost. Thromb., *1*:199, 1972.
541. Weiss, H. J., and Kochwa, S.: Molecular forms of antihaemophilic globulin in plasma, cryoprecipitate and after thrombin activation. Br. J. Haematol., *18*:89, 1970.
542. Wessler, S.: Thrombosis in the presence of vascular stasis. Am. J. Med., *33*:648, 1962.
543. Wessler, S.: Anticoagulant therapy — 1974. J.A.M.A., *228*:757, 1974.
544. Wessler, S., and Deykin, D.: Regulating heparin therapy. J.A.M.A., *225*:319, 1973.
545. Wessler, S., and Yin, E. T.: The experimental hypercoagulable state induced by factor X. A comparison of the non-activated and activated forms. J. Lab. Clin. Med., *72*:256, 1968.
546. Wessler, S., and Yin, E. T.: Theory and practice of minidose heparin in surgical patients: a status report. Circulation, *47*:671, 1973.
547. Wessler, S., and Yin, E. T.: On the antithrombotic action of heparin. Thromb. Diath. Haemorrh., *32*:71, 1974.
548. White, J. G.: Five structure alterations induced in platelets by adenosine disphosphate. Blood, *31*:604, 1968.
549. White, J. G.: The substructure of human platelet microtubules. Blood, *32*:638, 1968.
550. White, J. G.: The dense bodies of human platelets: inherent electron opacity of the serotonin storage particles. Blood, *33*:598, 1969.
551. White, J. G.: Exocytosis of secretory organelles from blood platelets incubated with cationic polypeptides. Am. J. Pathol., *69*:41, 1972.
552. White, J. G., Rao, G. H. R., and Estensen, R. D.: Investigation of the release reaction in platelets exposed to phorbol myristate acetate. Am. J. Pathol., *75*:301, 1974.
553. Williams, W. J., and Esnouf, M. P.: The fractionation of Russell's-viper venom (vipera russellii) with special reference to the coagulant protein. Biochem. J., *84*:52, 1962.
554. Willis, A. L.: An enzymatic mechanism for the antithrombotic and antihemostatic actions of aspirin. Science, *183*:325, 1974.
555. Wilner, G. D., Nossel, H. L., and LeRoy, E. C.: Activation of Hageman factor by collagen. J. Clin. Invest., *47*:2608, 1968.
556. Wilner, G. D., Nossel, H. L., and LeRoy, E. C.: Aggregation of platelets by collagen. J. Clin. Invest., *47*:2616, 1968.
557. Wolfe, S. M., and Shulman, N.-R.: Adenyl cyclase activity in human platelets. Biochem. Biophys. Res. Commun., *35*:265, 1969.
558. Wolfe, S. M., and Shulman, N.-R.: Inhibition of platelet energy production and release reaction by PGE_1, theophylline and cAMP. Biochem. Biophys. Res. Commun., *41*:128, 1970.

559. Wood, E. H., Prentice, C. R. M., McGrouther, D. A., Sinclair, J., and McNicol, G. P.: Trial of aspirin and RA 233 in prevention of postoperative deep-vein thrombosis. Thromb. Diath. Haemorrh., *30*:18, 1973.

560. Wood, J. E.: Oral contraceptives, pregnancy and the veins. Circulation, *38*:627, 1968.

561. Woolf, I. L., and Babior, B. M.: Vitamin K and warfarin. Metabolism, function & interaction. Am. J. Med., *53*:261, 1972.

562. Wright, I. S.: Pathogenesis and treatment of thrombosis. Circulation, *5*:161, 1952.

563. Wright, J. H.: The histogenesis of the blood platelets. J. Morphol., *21*:263, 1910.

564. Wuepper, K. D.: Prekallikrein deficiency in man. Clin. Res., *21*:248, 1973.

565. Yin, E. T., and Wessler, S.: Investigation of the apparent thrombogenicity of thrombin. Thromb. Diath. Haemorrh., *20*:465, 1968.

566. Yin, E. T., and Wessler, S.: Heparin-accelerated inhibition of activated factor X by its natural inhibitor. Biochim. Biophys. Acta, *201*:387, 1970.

567. Yin, E. T., Wessler, S., and Stall, P. J.: Biological properties of the naturally occurring plasma inhibitor to activated factor X. J. Biol. Chem., *246*:3712, 1971.

568. Zeldis, S. M., Nemerson, Y., Pitlick, F. A., and Lentz, T. L.: Tissue factor (thromboplastin); localization to plasma membranes by peroxidase-conjugated antibodies. Science, *175*:766, 1972.

569. Zieve, P. D., and Soloman, H. M.: Uptake of amino acids by the human platelet. Am. J. Physiol., *214*:58, 1968.

570. Zucker-Franklin, D.: Microfibrils of blood platelets: their relationship to microtubules and the contractile protein. J. Clin. Invest., *48*:165, 1969.

571. Zucker-Franklin, D., and Grusky, G.: The actin and myosin filaments of human and bovine blood platelets. J. Clin. Invest., *51*:419, 1972.

572. Zucker-Franklin, D., Nachman, R., and Marcus, A. J.: Ultrastructure of thrombosthenin, the contractile protein of human blood platelets. Science, *157*:945, 1967.

573. Zucker, M. B., and Borrelli, J.: Platelet clumping produced by connective tissue suspensions and by collagen. Proc. Soc. Exp. Biol. Med., *109*:779, 1962.

574. Zucker, M. B., and Peterson, J.: Effect of acetyl salicylic acid, other non-steroidal anti-inflammatory agents, and dipyridamole on human blood platelets. J. Lab. Clin. Med., *76*:66, 1970.

575. Zucker, S., Cathy, M. H., and Wylie, R. L.: Control of heparin therapy. Sensitivity of the activated partial thromboplastin time for monitoring the antithrombotic effects of heparin. J. Lab. Clin. Med., *73*:320, 1969.

CHAPTER **17**

DISORDERS OF HEMOSTASIS

The various clinical syndromes which occur as the result of disordered hemostasis have been defined largely by application of a series of empiric laboratory tests.

Incomplete understanding of the biochemical reactions involved in these tests makes impossible a definitive classification of the disorders of hemostasis at this time. For purposes of discussion, they will be presented within the framework of theory presented in Chapter 16 and grouped according to the results of the major laboratory tests.

CLASSIFICATION

I. Vessel and/or platelet abnormalities
   A. Purpura
      1. Thrombocytopenic purpura
         a. Secondary
         b. Idiopathic
         c. Neonatal
         d. Thrombotic
         e. Hereditary
      2. Nonthrombocytopenic purpura
         a. Thromboasthenia, thrombocytopathy, and platelet release abnormality
         b. Allergic
         c. In association with infection
         d. Other
   B. Hereditary telangiectasia
II. Abnormalities of blood coagulation
   A. Disorders affecting predominantly the first stage of blood coagulation and resulting in an abnormal thromboplastin generation test
      1. Factor XII (Hageman trait) deficiency
      2. Factor VIII (Antihemophilic factor, AHF) deficiency

3. Factor IX (Plasma thromboplastin component PTC) deficiency (Christmas disease)
4. Factor XI (plasma thromboplastin antecedent, PTA) deficiency
5. Circulating anticoagulants

B. Disorders affecting both the first and second stage of blood coagulation and resulting in an abnormality of both the thromboplastin generation test and the one-stage prothrombin time
1. Factor V deficiency
2. Factor X (Stuart factor) deficiency

C. Disorders affecting predominantly the first or second stage of blood coagulation and resulting in an abnormal one-stage prothrombin time with a normal thromboplastin generation test
1. Factor VII deficiency
2. Prothrombin deficiency (Factor II deficiency)

D. Disorders affecting the third stage of blood coagulation resulting in qualitative or quantitative changes in fibrinogen or fibrin
1. Hereditary quantitative fibrinogen deficiency
2. Hereditary qualitative fibrinogen deficiency
3. Acquired hypofibrinogenemia
4. Factor XIII (fibrin-stabilizing factor) deficiency

III. Disorders affecting vessel and/or platelet function and blood coagulation — Von Willebrand's disease

VESSEL AND/OR PLATELET ABNORMALITIES

THE PURPURAS

The term purpura originated from the Greek word *porphyra*, which was the name of the mollusk from which a purple dye was obtained.[261] Prior to the eighteenth century, purpuric lesions were thought to occur only during the course of "fevers" such as plague or typhus. From that time, however, it has been recognized that purpura may occur in the absence of a febrile illness.

The conventional classification of the purpuras into those associated with thrombocytopenia and those with quantitatively normal platelets seems justified. The difference is striking.

Thrombocytopenic Purpura

The relationship between a decrease in the number of platelets in the peripheral blood and the occurrence of spontaneous bleeding is well-known. The level below which the platelets must fall before bleeding occurs varies from person to person. Bleeding is rare when the platelet count is above 50,000 per cu.mm., but it may not occur when the platelets fall below this level. The life span of the platelet has been variously estimated at from three to ten days. If a strict balance between production and destruction is to be maintained, 10 to 30 per cent of the circulating platelets must be replaced daily.

Thrombocytopenia, like anemia or fever, should be considered as a symptom of disease, not as a disease in itself. Every effort must be made to determine the cause.

PATHOLOGIC PHYSIOLOGY OF THROMBOCYTOPENIA

The physiologic function of the platelets has been extensively investigated, and knowledge of their role in hemostasis continues to accumulate.[251, 266, 352, 408, 460, 482, 507] Platelets are known to participate in both the vascular and biochemical defense of hemostasis.[81, 82, 320] They mechanically plug rents in the wall of a vessel by their agglutination and thrombus formation. Evidence is growing that adenosine diphosphate (ADP) released from injured tissue or from the platelets themselves is the substance responsible for aggregation of platelets at the site of vessel injury.[28, 76, 165, 437, 554] The rate of removal or neutralization of ADP is likely to be important in the control of the extent of the thrombus.[219] Platelets are essential to the normal evolution of thromboplastin activity in the intrinsic or blood system, and in the final phase of coagulation they influence clot retraction by their interaction with fibrin. The capacity of the platelets to bring about clot retraction depends on their contractile protein, which in turn is dependent on the presence of adenosine triphosphate as an energy source.[58, 199] They have also been demonstrated to contain a heparin-neutralizing factor.

It is apparent that a quantitative decrease in cells which play an important mechanical role in hemostasis and participate in at least two of the three major stages of blood coagulation would represent a serious hazard to the organism. It is not readily apparent, however, why relatively comparable degrees of thrombocytopenia are associated with such variability in clinical findings. It has been speculated that the plasma may contain a factor that is essential to the maintenance of vascular integrity and is complementary to the mechanical role of the platelet. The importance of such a factor in hemostasis would be enhanced if the platelets were diminished.[6]

The disturbed laboratory tests and clinical findings presented by patients with thrombocytopenic purpura may be ascribed to a defect in hemostasis resulting from a quantitative decrease in platelets in association with some as yet undefined change in the vascular endothelium.

CLINICAL EXAMINATION

Characteristically, the clinical manifestations of thrombocytopenic purpura from any cause develop over a period of several days or weeks, though the onset may on occasion be sudden, particularly in children. Bruising or prolonged bleeding from minor trauma, menorrhagia, or epistaxis may be noted before the appearance of petechiae, which are the hallmark of thrombocytopenia. Petechiae vary in size from those too small to see with the unaided eye to those approximately $1/16$ inch in diameter. They are the result of tiny extravasations of blood from the arteriolar end of the capillary loop in the skin or mucous membranes.[250] A coalescence of petechiae results in larger lesions of varied size which are referred to as ecchymoses.

Purpuric lesions may occur anywhere in the body. Those located in the mucous membranes are not as well supported as those in the skin, and free bleeding into the genitourinary tract or the gastrointestinal tract is common. The total amount of blood found in the urine or feces is more likely the result of multiple tiny hemorrhages than of a large hemorrhage from a single petechia. The occurrence of bleeding within the central nervous system presents the most serious threat. Once again it appears that the failure of the supporting tissues to contain the petechial hemorrhage allows its progression to serious proportions. The occurrence of bleeding in the optic fundus is not infrequent and may result in permanent impairment of vision.

The physical findings will vary, depending on the organ system involved and the magnitude of the blood loss.

LABORATORY EXAMINATION

Thrombocytopenia is the sine qua non of this condition. The degree of depression of the platelet count varies and is not always related to the severity of the clinical manifestations. If symptoms are present, however, the platelet count is usually below 50,000 per cu.mm. Anemia is not commonly noted in these patients. If present, the type and degree of the anemia usually reflects the magnitude of the bleeding or the effect of an underlying disease. The total and differential leukocyte counts almost invariably are normal in patients with idiopathic thrombocytopenic purpura; significant abnormalities occur in nearly all varieties of the secondary forms. The clotting time is normal. The bleeding time is prolonged, but may vary from day to day. The results of the test may return to normal during the course of the disease, though the platelet level remains depressed. Clot retraction is poor and, indeed, there may be no retraction of the clot after 24 hours. The degree of clot retraction is usually directly proportional to the number of platelets present. The tourniquet test is positive, but the performance of the test is usually unnecessary and unwarranted in the presence of thrombocytopenic purpura. Increased peripheral destruction of platelets may be detected by following their survival after tagging with ^{51}Cr.[1, 371]

Examination of smears made from bone marrow aspirates may be valuable in establishing the diagnosis. The megakaryocytes in idiopathic thrombocytopenic purpura are often increased in number but immature. Many will contain but two or four nuclei rather than the characteristic polyploid nucleus of the mature megakaryocyte (Fig. 17–1). The cytoplasm is reduced, vacuolated and contains few granules. Only rare platelets are seen forming at the edge of the cytoplasm. Similar findings are often present in thrombocytopenic purpura which occurs in certain susceptible persons on exposure to a particular drug, food, or chemical.

CLINICAL SYNDROMES

Thrombocytopenic purpura will be discussed under four headings: (1) secondary thrombocytopenic purpura; (2) idiopathic thrombocytopenic pur-

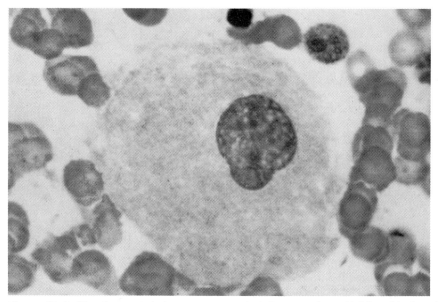

Figure 17–1 Megakaryocyte in bone marrow aspirate from a patient with idiopathic thrombocytopenic purpura. Note the immaturity of the nucleus, the reduction in cytoplasm, and the absence of platelets forming at the edge of the cytoplasm.

pura; (3) neonatal thrombocytopenic purpura; and (4) thrombotic thrombocytopenic purpura.

As there is considerable variation in the etiology, course, prognosis, and treatment of these disorders, they will be discussed separately.

Secondary thrombocytopenic purpura. Secondary thrombocytopenic purpura bears a clear and identifiable relationship to some etiologic agent or disease. Some of the diseases and chemical and physical agents that may result in this condition are listed in Table 17–1. Although thrombocytopenic purpura per se is a serious condition, the ultimate prognosis for any given patient with the secondary form of the disorder depends largely on the underlying cause. Thrombocytopenic purpura following measles, threatening as it may be, does not carry so grave a prognosis as that associated with a malignancy.

Mechanisms. Thrombocytopenia is the end result of decreased production of platelets, increased destruction of platelets, a combination of the two, or abnormal pooling. The means through which this result is reached vary with the inciting cause.

A plasma factor required for normal platelet production has been described. Absence of this factor has been demonstrated to result in thrombocytopenia, and thrombopoiesis is stimulated in these patients by infusions of normal plasma.[447, 448]

The decrease in platelets which occurs as the result of the invasion of the bone marrow by tumor cells, granuloma, the reticuloendothelioses, lipoidoses, and micro-organisms is thought to be the result of (a) physical crowding of normal megakaryocytes; (b) competitive utilization of nutrient substrate by the invading cells; or (c) production of metabolic end products by the invading cells which are toxic to the normal marrow elements. Thrombocytopenia that follows exposure to ionizing radiation and those chemicals which universally depress bone marrow function is believed to be due to the interference of those agents with cellular division, perhaps through inhibition of deoxyribonucleic acid synthesis.[346] Vitamin B_{12}, folic acid, and severe iron deficiencies may result in thrombocytopenia.

The possibility has been considered that the spleen may also produce a humoral factor which depresses megakaryocytic function.[216] Thrombocytopenic purpura may be the presenting problem of patients with disseminated lupus erythematosus; the responsible mechanism probably is immunologic.[92, 125]

Increased destruction of platelets occurs when they are sequestered in hemangioblastoma.[33, 184, 216] During hypothermia they are sequestered in the spleen, the liver, and possibly the intestinal tract and marrow; the sequestered platelets return to the circulation with rewarming.[520] Increased permeability of the capillaries during heat stroke is thought to be responsible for a decrease in the number of platelets.[552]

Table 17–1   *Causes of Secondary Thrombocytopenic Purpura*

1. *Invasion of the marrow cavity with subsequent suppression or destruction of the normal marrow elements by:*
   a. Malignant cells: carcinoma, sarcoma, leukemia, lymphoma
   b. Granuloma: sarcoid, tuberculosis
   c. Lipoidosis: Gaucher's disease, reticuloendotheliosis
   d. Microorganisms: bacteremia, viremia
2. *Direct suppression of marrow elements by:*
   a. Physical agents: roentgen rays, radioactive isotopes
   b. Chemical agents:
      (1) Universal susceptibility: urethan, alkylating agents (nitrogen mustard, busulfan, chlorambucil, TEM), benzol, antimetabolites (amethopterin, aminopterin, 6-MP)
      (2) Individual susceptibility:
         (a) Drugs: any from the group of analgesics, antipyretics, antibiotics, chemotherapy, antihistamines, hormones
         (b) Food
         (c) Insecticides: DDT
         (d) Dyes: organic
         (e) Other: any new agents to which the patient has been exposed must be suspected
3. *Peripheral destruction of platelets by:*
   a. Excessive demands from abnormal coagulation:
      (1) Widespread intravascular clotting
      (2) Burns
   b. Hypersplenism: enlarged spleen from any cause
   c. Hypothermia and heat stroke
   d. Hemangioendothelioma
   e. Blood transfusions:
      (1) Incompatible: immunologic incompatibility of platelets as well as red cells, trapping and stasis, intravascular coagulation
      (2) Compatible: after large numbers of transfusions; perhaps the result of immunologically incompatible platelets
   f. Viremia and bacteremia
   g. Collagen disorders

Several different platelet serologic types have been demonstrated,[216, 466] and thrombocytopenia may occur secondary to blood transfusions as the result of incompatibility of platelet types. Stasis due to sludging, or excessive utilization of platelets in those cases of incompatible transfusion accompanied by intravascular clotting, may result in thrombocytopenia.[216] The mechanism responsible for thrombocytopenia which may occur following massive transfusions is obscure;[287] dilution with platelet-poor bank blood and stimulation of an iso-antibody response by incompatible platelets may be factors. In a recent study of post-transfusion purpura, platelet antibodies were found in plasma and serum, and microaggregation and lysis of platelets demonstrated. The patient developed severe thrombocytopenia with lingual and buccal hemorrhagic bullae and purpura seven days after transfusion of whole blood.[4]

An enlarged spleen may trap large numbers of platelets. Normally the cardiovascular system contains approximately two-thirds of the platelets, and one-third are in the spleen. Without any change in total numbers of platelets, a large spleen could harbor one-half of the platelets; a very large spleen might contain nine-tenths of the platelets. A large spleen may alter the peripheral platelet count without any deviation of total platelet mass, life span, or production.[29, 473] Increased plasma volume and hemodilution may be important.

Viremia and bacteremia are thought to cause agglutination and destruction of platelets in vivo.[107, 187, 216, 343] Recent studies indicate that trypanosomes and trypanosome-free supernatant of disrupted organisms caused agglutination of rat, rabbit, and human platelets. The agglutination was not complement-, ADP-, or kinin-dependent and appears to represent a new mechanism.[129] Megakaryocytes may appear inactive and diminished in number as well.[481]

The manner in which certain drugs, foods, or chemicals induce thrombocytopenia in susceptible individuals has been the subject of extensive investigations.[6, 24, 216, 485, 486] Thrombocytopenia in alcoholics has been attributed in the past to folic acid deficiency or hypersplenism, but there have been reports of thrombocytopenia in chronic alcoholics in the absence of cirrhosis, splenomegaly, or folic acid deficiency. The platelet counts returned to normal on withdrawal from alcohol. It has been suggested that alcohol acts directly on the megakaryocyte or platelet, just as it affects erythropoiesis and leukopoiesis.[222, 300, 394] Abnormal platelet function also is seen in patients with cirrhosis of the liver.[503]

Whether increased destruction or decreased production is responsible for drug-induced thrombocytopenia has been for many years the subject of a lively debate. It is now known that immunologic factors can affect both the rate of destruction and of production of platelets.[7, 8, 10] According to one concept, a drug and platelet together act as a hapten and exhibit weakly antigenic properties. Antibodies may be formed which will destroy the platelets on the next exposure to that particular drug. The four factors necessary to demonstrate agglutination and lysis of platelets are: (1) platelets; (2) the drug; (3) serum from the drug-sensitive patient; and (4) complement. Agglutination alone may occur without complement.[8] The factor responsible for the lysis of platelets is in the serum of the affected patient. Lysis and complement fixation may be demonstrated in vitro using serum from an affected patient, the drug, and his own or normal platelets, but will not occur if normal serum is used.

Other evidence suggests that platelets as well as red cells and leukocytes react with antibody because their membranes are capable of nonspecific adsorption of certain drug-antibody complexes. According to this "innocent bystander" concept, the complete antigen is not a cellular constituent but a noncellular substance complexed with the drug. The antibody against the complete antigen is capable of reacting against the drug alone as well. The size, configuration, and charge on the antigen (drug)-antibody complex, rather than the characteristics of the antigen (drug) alone, determine the target cell with which it can react; the physical-chemical characteristics of the target cell determine its *accidental* participation in the reaction. The attachment of the antigen (drug)-antibody complex to the cell then leads to aggregation of the cells or complement fixation.[465] The site of destruction of the aggregated platelets appears to relate to the size of the aggregates; large aggregates are removed by the liver, whereas smaller ones are trapped in the spleen.[30]

Whichever concept proves to be correct, the immunologic basis for this form of thrombocytopenia has been amply demonstrated,[8] and the responsible plasma factor has been passively transferred.[56, 489] As the administration of minute amounts of the offending drug after recovery may cause severe thrombocytopenia to recur in these patients, it is best not to test the drug in vivo to confirm the suspicion of sensitivity.

Management. It is clear in the light of the foregoing discussion that a searching history must be obtained from any patient presenting with thrombocytopenia. Precipitating causes are legion. Exposure to any new drug, chemical, or foodstuff must be suspect, and the possible association with recent infection should be kept in mind. Accidental as well as therapeutic exposure to ionizing radiation must be looked for in view of the widespread use of nuclear fission products in industry and medicine. A careful history and physical examination will often reveal the underlying disease.

Treatment of secondary thrombocytopenic purpura will depend in large measure on the nature of the underlying disorder. In addition to therapy directed at the precipitating cause, therapy to relieve the bleeding diathesis may be indicated and will be discussed under idiopathic thrombocytopenic purpura.

Idiopathic thrombocytopenic purpura. The separation by Werlhof of the "morbus maculosus hemorrhagicus" from the infectious diseases in 1735 was the first recognition of this disorder as a distinct entity. It was not until 1883 that Krauss recognized that the platelets of these patients were deficient in number.[261] Kaznelson suggested the use of splenectomy in the treatment of these patients in 1916. As the term "idiopathic" indicates, knowledge of the etiology of this disorder is still incomplete and the diagnosis is made only after exclusion of the many causes of secondary thrombocytopenic purpura. Rare instances of congenital and familial idiopathic thrombocytopenia have been reported.[70, 216, 443, 452]

Adult patients meeting the diagnostic criteria for idiopathic thrombocytopenic purpura seen at the University of Virginia Hospital from 1945 through 1970 numbered 66. They ranged in age from 14 to 80 years at the time of initial examination, and approximately one-quarter were below 21 years of age. Sixty-eight per cent of the patients were female, a sex proportion also noted in other studies.[506]

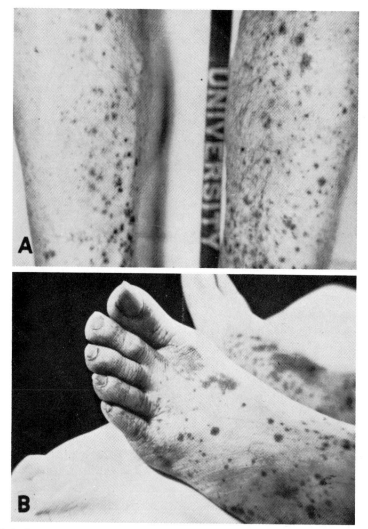

Figure 17–2 Petechiae and ecchymoses in a patient with idiopathic thrombocytopenic purpura.

Mechanism. A great deal of effort has been made to elucidate the factors responsible for the development of idiopathic thrombocytopenic purpura. The finding that an altered immunologic response was the basis of some of the drug-induced secondary thrombocytopenic purpuras spurred efforts to demonstrate a similar mechanism in connection with the idiopathic variety.

The evidence indicates that an abnormal immunologic mechanism may be responsible for the low platelet count in many patients with this disorder.[215, 217] The infusion of plasma from patients with this disorder will cause a transient thrombocytopenia in normal recipients. Infants born of mothers with idiopathic thrombocytopenic purpura may have neonatal thrombocytopenia. Normal platelets infused into patients with idiopathic thrombocytopenic purpura frequently have a short survival. The platelet-depressing factor in the serum of these patients has been found to affect autologous as well as homologous platelets, to be species-specific, to be adsorbed by platelets, and to be present in the

7S immunoglobulin fraction of the plasma.[469] Despite such evidence for a humoral platelet-depressing factor, efforts to develop an in vitro test to demonstrate antiplatelet antibodies in the blood of these patients have been repeatedly frustrated.[120] The platelet-aggregating properties of serum from patients with idiopathic thrombocytopenic purpura, at first thought indicative of platelet antibodies,[217, 485] appear now to be due to thrombin arising from the prothrombin remaining after coagulation of the thrombocytopenic blood.[255] The substrate for the action of thrombin is a clottable protein similar to or identical with fibrinogen which is adsorbed on the surface of the platelet.[444] More recently-introduced methods for the in vitro detection of platelet antibodies, under conditions which rule out the possibility of thrombin or thrombin-generating agents being responsible, appear promising. The antiplatelet factor measured by these techniques is an IgG immunoglobulin.[234, 268] Recent studies indicate that the bone marrow increases platelet production in response to low peripheral platelet count in the same manner as it responds to thrombopheresis. Platelet production was measured in 35 patients with idiopathic thrombocytopenic purpura and in 21 normal controls. The mean platelet production was $2.3 \times$ normal with values as high as $3-5 \times$ normal. There was a highly significant negative correlation with the peripheral platelet count. When the platelet count remained at or above 50,000 mm[3], the platelet production remained in the high normal range but progressively increased as the platelet count fell.[91]

It is not always possible to demonstrate increased platelet destruction; hence a decrease in the production of platelets may be responsible for thrombocytopenia in some instances,[396] although thrombopoietin activity is detectable.[108, 325]

Sensitized platelets may be removed from the circulation by the spleen or the liver. The spleen has been demonstrated to be the major site for removal of platelets when they are lightly coated with antibodies, but when the disorder is more severe the liver also participates. The site of destruction therefore depends on the intensity of the immunologic process at any particular point in the course of the illness.[29, 31, 469, 470] The spleen may also contribute to the production of platelet agglutinins and in some manner suppress megakaryocyte function in the bone marrow.[216, 328] Recent data demonstrate that in vitro immunoglobulin synthesis by human splenic tissue from a patient with idiopathic thrombocytopenic purpura is five times that of normal splenic tissue. The immunoglobulins produced by one such sample showed binding to autologous and homologous platelets.[328] Qualitative platelet abnormalities which appear to be the result of an antiplatelet antibody[119] have been reported in patients with idiopathic thrombocytopenic purpura.

Clinical examination. The disease may begin insidiously with an increased tendency to bruise, followed in days or weeks by the appearance of petechiae on the skin or mucous membranes. In other patients, there may be a sudden onset with the appearance of petechiae and moderate-to-severe bleeding from the gastrointestinal or genitourinary tract. Neurologic defects or death may be the result if bleeding occurs in the central nervous system. The historic account of the illness and the results of the physical examination will depend largely on the site and extent of the bleeding.

Course and prognosis. The disease may pursue an unremitting and fulminant course to death in a few days or stop as suddenly as it began, within days or weeks of onset. The designation of idiopathic thrombocytopenic purpura as being of the acute or chronic variety must be retrospective, and is of little help in handling the new patient. The vast majority of patients with acute idiopathic thrombocytopenia have a complete and permanent recovery within two to three months. If they fail to recover within six months they are considered as having chronic idiopathic thrombocytopenic purpura. Death may result in either the acute or chronic type, and there may be recurrences after many years of remission.

Treatment. Evaluation of the various forms of treatment used in this disorder is made difficult by its unpredictable course.[112, 464, 483] The major therapeutic modalities used have been splenectomy, adrenocortical steroids, and immunosuppressive drugs.

Splenectomy was first suggested by a third-year medical student named Kaznelson in 1916.[261] Its effect is to remove the major site of sequestration of lightly sensitized platelets. When it can be demonstrated that the spleen is the predominant site of platelet destruction, a rise in platelet count is to be expected after splenectomy, and the long-term result is usually good. The effect of splenectomy on the production of platelet antibodies remains to be demonstrated.[329] Failure of splenectomy occurs as the result of high titers of platelet–antibody with heavily-coated platelets and more hepatic sequestration.[469] The high incidence of systemic lupus erythematosus following splenectomy in one series does not appear to be commonplace.[406]

The rationale for the use of adrenocortical steroids lies in the observation that they decrease antigen–antibody reactions and protect the vascular endothelium in some fashion as yet not understood.[285, 424, 483] They also appear to inhibit the sequestration of sensitized platelets by the reticuloendothelial system of the spleen and liver.[483] The last appears to be the most important mechanism concerned. Reports have emphasized the low percentage of sustained remission in patients treated with steroids, compared to those treated by splenectomy.[102, 106, 340, 530, 547]

There have been reports on the use of immunosuppressive agents in the treatment of those patients refractory to adrenocortical steroids and splenectomy.[85, 155, 496] One review indicates that, in some patients with chronic ITP refractory to adrenocortical steroids and splenectomy, these agents have a successful response. In most patients, however, the response is of short duration, and in some the course of the disease was of such short duration that the "response" may have been a spontaneous remission. The response to immunosuppressive therapy is much greater after splenectomy. Azathioprine and cyclophosphamide appear to be the drugs of choice.[85, 155, 496] The immunosuppressive effect of cyclophosphamide is better but the complications are more serious.[153] Such treatment should be used only for those patients who have failed to respond to adrenocortical steroids and splenectomy, or who are a poor risk for splenectomy. A response rate of 15 to 35 per cent has been reported. This form of therapy remains experimental and carries uncertain risks; it is not recommended for general use.[153]

Supportive therapy consists mainly of whole blood and platelet transfusions. Packed red cells should be used when indicated to restore oxygen-carrying capacity. Platelet transfusions may be of value immediately prior to emergency splenectomy,[295] in retinal hemorrhage and in suspected cerebral hemorrhage. Platelet concentrates prepared from freshly donated blood are usually employed. Unfortunately, the response to platelet transfusion is poor since the platelets are damaged by antibody and rapidly sequestered.[555] They should not be used unless there is significant hemorrhage, since routine use may lead to the development of isoantibodies.[181, 555]

In reviewing our experience it was apparent that the initial response to treatment with adrenocortical steroids was a more specific and reliable indicator of prognosis than was the duration of symptoms prior to treatment. Remission could not be consistently correlated with the duration of symptoms except in those instances which followed acute infectious disease. A good response to adrenocortical steroids could be taken to indicate a similar response to be expected from splenectomy, but duration of symptoms was of little or no use as a prognostic guide.

On the basis of these observations the following general plans of therapy seem indicated.

When first seen, these patients, whether "acute" or "chronic," are started on prednisone, 40 to 60 mg. daily by mouth. When the higher dosage is used initially it is normally reduced over the next several days to 40 mg. daily. An increase in platelet count may be expected in from 75 to 87 per cent of patients, but remission is sustained in less than 44 per cent.[106, 340, 506]

In those patients whose platelet count rises to normal and is maintained for several weeks, the dosage is tapered. If the platelet count falls, the original dose of the drug is reinstituted. If a response ensues, this dosage is maintained for several additional weeks, depending on the clinical situation, prior to tapering.

A second course of adrenocortical steroid therapy seems justified prior to consideration of splenectomy in those patients who suffer a relapse after having responded to the initial course of adrenocortical therapy. Splenectomy is recommended if it is not possible to obtain a remission with steroids. The decision as to just when a splenectomy should be performed must be made for each patient individually, depending on the course of disease. It is important to note that idiopathic thrombocytopenic purpura may recur months or even years after splenectomy, and may be related to the presence of an accessory spleen.[217, 514] The effectiveness of further corticosteroid therapy in patients who have relapsed after splenectomy is variable, and its use needs to be individualized.

Neonatal thrombocytopenic purpura.   Thrombocytopenic purpura occurring at the time of delivery may affect both the mother and baby, the baby alone, or the mother alone.[201, 216, 217, 514] The infant usually appears normal at the time of delivery but develops purpura several hours later. The hemorrhagic manifestations may disappear after a few days but the thrombocytopenia often persists for weeks.

Mechanisms.   Investigators have now established that several mechanisms may result in neonatal thrombocytopenia purpura.

Isoimmune neonatal thrombocytopenia.   Isoimmune neonatal thrombocytopenia has been likened to that of Rh sensitization.[217, 384, 514] Several platelet types have now been identified, and, should the mother and fetus have different platelet types, maternal isoagglutinins may form, cross the placenta, and destroy the platelets of the fetus. Maternal immunization against antigens on fetal platelets has been demonstrated in both megakaryocytic and amegakaryocytic neonatal thrombocytopenic purpura. The antibody disappears from the infant's plasma in approximately two weeks and recovery ensues.[466]

A similar mechanism is believed to operate in instances of neonatal thrombocytopenic purpura occurring in infants of mothers with idiopathic thrombocytopenic purpura. The platelet-depressing factor present in the mother's plasma is thought to gain access to the circulation of the fetus, and thrombocytopenia results. The thrombocytopenia may persist longer than that seen in association with demonstrated maternal isoagglutinins.[466, 467] Most infants with isoimmune neonatal thrombocytopenic purpura recover without sequelae. However, severe complications or death may occur. In one review an immediate mortality of 12.7 per cent was noted. Intracranial hemorrhage was the most common cause of death.[384]

Neonatal purpura and the rubella syndrome. Thrombocytopenic purpura may be one manifestation of the congenital rubella syndrome. It appears most commonly in those infants whose mothers were infected during the fourth to eighth week of gestation. Rubella virus was recovered from 83 per cent of infants with purpura in one study. The clinical picture may vary from that of an apparently healthy infant with a few scattered petechiae to that of a moribund infant with extensive purpuric lesions. Often platelets are but slightly reduced on the first day or two of life, but may drop over the next few days to low levels. Recovery occurs at a variable rate. Severe hemorrhage may occur but is unusual.[5]

Associated abnormalities may include retarded intrauterine growth, hepatomegaly, splenomegaly, congenital heart disease, eye defects, bone lesions, hepatitis, and anemia. Bone marrow specimens contain a reduced number of megakaryocytes.[116] A variety of mechanisms have been suggested to account for the occurrence of purpura in the course of viral illness. The virus may alter the platelets so that they become antigenic and stimulate antibody formation; a virus-antibody complex may "accidentally" attach to the platelets and cause their destruction; or the virus could damage the platelet or megakaryocyte directly and cause their destruction.[354, 370a] Vascular damage may result from direct virus attachment, the presence of virus-antibody complexes, or from the development of intravascular thrombi.[45] The damaged vessel walls may allow the escape of blood. The precise mechanism is not known.[45, 354]

Neonatal purpura and maternal ingestion of drugs. There have been several reports of neonatal thrombocytopenic purpura occurring in infants delivered of mothers without thrombocytopenia or detectable antiplatelet antibody in their serum. It was suggested but not proved that the thrombocytopenia in the infant was the result of the mother's having received one of the thiazides during the prepartum period. The precise mechanism of action by which these drugs may cause thrombocytopenia is not known, but there are reports of adults developing thrombocytopenia after taking thiazides.[170, 428]

Therapy. Most infants with isoimmune neonatal purpura recover without sequelae, but serious complications or death may occur. The aim of therapy is to tide the infant over the days or weeks until recovery occurs. Steroid therapy is used because it may suppress antibody formation, interfere with antigen-antibody complexes, and reduce reticuloendothelial activity. Steroids also have a salutary effect on the vascular endothelium.

Blood transfusions should be used if indicated. Evidence suggests that platelet transfusions of the mother's platelets, washed with normal plasma to remove iso-antibody, are effective.[11] Exchange transfusions have been advocated in an effort to remove the circulating antibody.[384]

Splenectomy is not indicated unless there is a failure to control symptoms with steroids and platelet transfusions.

Infants born to mothers who have idiopathic thrombocytopenic purpura generally recover without serious sequelae. Steroid therapy may be very helpful. Once again, splenectomy is not indicated unless steroid therapy fails and the situation is life-threatening.

Infants with the congenital rubella syndrome should be isolated because they shed virus and are contagious for a variable period of time. There is no specific therapy for congenital rubella, and the thrombocytopenia is treated in the same manner as other forms of neonatal purpura.[5, 117, 249] The value of steroids in the treatment of the thrombocytopenia must be carefully weighed against their potential depression of the immunologic mechanism.

Thrombotic thrombocytopenic purpura (TTP, Thrombohemolytic thrombocytopenic purpura). Thrombotic thrombocytopenic purpura is an unusual malady first described by Moschowitz in 1925.[348] The syndrome is now being recognized more frequently prior to death.[437, 502] It occurs most commonly in the female in the 10-to-40 age-group and may develop during pregnancy.[475] It has been reported in one newborn infant.[347] The course of the disease is marked by the occurrence of fever, hemolytic anemia, thrombocytopenic purpura, changing neurologic signs, and renal disease.[22, 314]

Mechanism. The relationship of this disorder to the collagen diseases was pointed out quite early, and the suggestion that it is primarily the result of a vascular lesion has received support.[175, 186, 294] The characteristic pathologic lesion of thrombotic thrombocytopenic purpura is partial or complete occlusion of many small arterioles and capillaries (rarely venules).[186] These lesions are widespread in the body, and any organ may be involved. The most commonly involved organs are the heart, adrenals, kidneys,[314] pancreas, and brain. The occlusive material is acidophilic, amorphous, and hyalin-like.[186, 502] A recent study noted lesions due to platelet aggregates with variable amounts of fibrin. Less common lesions were secondary to loose platelet aggregates.[357] A vasculitis secondary to an infectious or immunologic process may be responsible for the aggregation of platelets.[214, 318, 529] The thromboses may result in aneurysmal dilatation of the vessel and subsequent rupture.

The hemolytic anemia that occurs in patients with this disorder is of an extracorpuscular type. The Coombs antiglobulin test is usually negative. It has been suggested that the characteristic red cell distortion, shistocytes, helmet cells, and burr cells, may result from direct contact of either the patient's or transfused normal red cells, with fibrin or with diseased small blood vessels.[22, 89]

The purpuric manifestations of the disorder are characteristic, but the mechanism by which the platelets are reduced has been the source of much debate.[175, 186] There is little evidence of diffuse intravascular coagulation though fibrin split products may be slightly elevated.[294] A shortened survival time of normal platelets in these patients has been described, but infusions of plasma from patients with thrombotic thrombocytopenic purpura did not diminish the number of platelets in a normal recipient, indicating an absence of platelet antibodies. No platelet agglutinins have yet been described. There is evidence of alteration in megakaryocytic function in some patients, the megakaryocytes being immature.

The neurologic lesions are secondary to vascular lesions in the brain.

It has been pointed out that renal disease with hematuria, proteinuria, casts, and azotemia may be a prominent feature of thrombotic thrombocytopenic purpura;[314] azotemia may occur without demonstrable red cells, casts, or protein in the urine. The marked endothelial proliferation of the small arteries and arterioles of the kidney may be associated with thrombi and may contain "foamy" macrophages.

It has been suggested that thrombotic thrombocytopenic purpura is not a disease but a syndrome with diverse etiologies, including vasculitis and infection, but the manner in which the lesions are produced remains obscure.[214, 258, 357, 383, 511, 521]

Clinical aspects. Although chronic or relapsing forms have been noted in the literature, most patients present with a dramatic and fulminating disease resulting in death in a few days or weeks.[175, 180] The diagnosis is suspected in a young person critically ill with fever, renal disease, hemolytic anemia with fragmented red cells, thrombocytopenic purpura, and changing neurologic signs. Positive diagnosis has been made following the finding of characteristic lesions in small vessels removed by bone marrow or lymph node biopsy.[259] Muscle biopsy may also be helpful.[119]

Occult vascular disease and infection with agents as varied as Microtatobiotes,[337] Aspergillus,[511] and meningococcus[336] have been implicated in thrombotic thrombocytopenic purpura and should be searched for in any patient with the disorder.

Treatment. Recent reports of prolonged survival of patients with thrombotic thrombocytopenic purpura lend some urgency to the need for early diagnosis.[229, 314] Massive doses of steroids and splenectomy have been noted to prevent the rapid deterioration of these patients. Transfusions should be used to replace blood loss from hemorrhage or hemolysis. Anticoagulation has been used with variable success, but may prevent damage to vital organs.[57, 280] Efforts to interfere with platelet aggregation by the use of dextran,[294] and more recently with dipyridamole and aspirin[21, 172, 259, 436] have been reported to be successful despite failure, in one instance, of splenectomy, steroid therapy, and anticoagulation with heparin.[21]

Hereditary thrombocytopenias with associated defects in platelet function. The *Bernard–Soulier* syndrome is a rare autosomal recessive trait characterized by giant platelets, modest thrombocytopenia, and decreased PF3 activity. The nature of the platelet defect is unclear; a fundamental membrane defect has been suggested.[71]

An *inherited thrombocytopenia* associated with a shortened platelet life span transmitted as an autosomal dominant has been reported.[353] Platelets from healthy persons had normal survival in these patients.

The *May–Hegglin* anomaly may be associated with a hemorrhagic diathiasis. This rare condition, with giant platelets, mild thrombocytopenia, and Döhle inclusion bodies in the polymorphonuclear leukocytes, is transmitted as an autosomal dominant trait. There may be mild thrombocytopenia and diminished PF3 activity.[309]

The *Wiskott–Aldrich* syndrome appears to be transmitted as a sex-linked recessive trait. Female carriers have been reported to have mild-to-moderate thrombocytopenia. Patients with this disorder have eczema, thrombocytopenia, and repeated infections. Most die in infancy or childhood of hemorrhage or infection, and those who survive often develop malignant disease in later childhood.[118,248] Autologous platelets have a shortened survival due to intrinsic defect. A defect in oxidative phosphorylation common to both platelets and macrophages has been suggested.[288] Platelets are reduced in size and are of various shapes. Studies of their ultrastructure has revealed reduced numbers of dense bodies and large numbers of tubules. A decrease in aggregation in response to collagen and ADP has been noted, together with a decrease in storage pool ADP. It is postulated that the abnormal platelets are recognized by the reticuloendothelial system and phagocytized. Splenectomy is associated with an excessive mortality rate and is contraindicated.[200]

Illustrative Cases

SECONDARY THROMBOCYTOPENIC PURPURA

A 14-year-old white girl had been well until three or four days prior to admission when she contracted measles, which was epidemic in her community and present in her home. Eighteen hours before admission she had a sudden epistaxis and later vomited blood and passed tarry stools. Her mother, who had raised 14 children and "knew the measles," stated that she had noted a change in the character of the rash during the 24 hours prior to admission.

Careful questioning failed to reveal any history of a hemorrhagic diathesis in the patient or in her family. There had been no known exposure to chemicals, and she had received no drugs.

Physical examination.   There were many petechiae over the lower legs and back, and subconjunctival hemorrhages were noted in both eyes. There was a small amount of blood in the posterior pharynx and mild oozing from the nares. There were small nodes in both the posterior cervical triangles and the suboccipital area, but the spleen was not palpable. The remainder of the examination was noncontributory.

Laboratory examination.   This showed a hematocrit of 26% and a white blood cell count of 11,000 per cu.mm. Urinalysis was negative but the stool examination was positive for occult blood. The bleeding time was 12 minutes, and clot retraction poor after two hours. There were no platelets seen on examination of multiple smears. Prothrombin time and coagulation time were normal. Preparations made to demonstrate the lupus erythematosus cell phenomena were negative on three occasions. Bone marrow megakaryocytes were diminished in number and immature in appearance. Atypical lymphocytes and young plasma cells were seen on examination of the bone marrow smear and the smear of the peripheral blood. A diagnosis of thrombocytopenia secondary to measles was made.

Course. Because of continued bleeding and low hematocrit, the patient was transfused with 500 ml. of fresh whole blood. Prednisone was administered orally in a dosage of 25 mg. three times a day. The patient's nose was packed and bleeding was controlled adequately, though there was slight oozing for the first four days. Platelets, seen for the first time on a smear made on the sixth hospital day, numbered 216,000 by the 11th hospital day. At that time the bleeding time had returned to 2½ minutes. The prednisone was reduced gradually. Her platelets remained at normal levels for the four months she was followed after steroid therapy had been discontinued.

Comments. This girl presents the classic clinical and laboratory findings of thrombocytopenic purpura. In addition to the failure to find platelets in the peripheral blood, the megakaryocytes seen in the marrow preparation were immature and may not have been forming platelets. L.E. preparations were obtained, because purpuric lesions may be the presenting complaint of patients subsequently found to have disseminated lupus erythematosus. The presence of the atypical lymphocytes and young forms of plasma cells suggested a virus disease. In view of the history of measles, it was felt that this represented *secondary thrombocytopenic purpura* occurring as the result of measles.

Thrombocytopenia is a rare sequela of measles. The appearance of the purpuric rash has been reported[217] as occurring from the third day of the measles rash to as long as two weeks subsequent to its disappearance. Contrary to popular opinion, purpura does not follow only severe attacks of measles, and the accompanying infection may be but a mild one.

Steroids were used to sustain the patient through what proved to be self-limited acute thrombocytopenia secondary to an infectious viral disease.

The prognosis is good in this case, and it is doubtful if the patient will have a recurrence, but she was instructed to return immediately if symptoms returned.

IDIOPATHIC THROMBOCYTOPENIC PURPURA

History. A 24-year-old white married mother had been in good health until four months prior to admission, when she noted bruising without recognized trauma. Bruising continued, and when she sought medical attention three months prior to admission she was told that "her platelets were less than 10,000." Intramuscular injections of ACTH gel were given with improvement. The platelets returned to normal levels and bruising ceased. After an interval of two or three weeks excessive bruising was again noted, and upon examination platelets once more were found to be low. With the onset of excessive menstrual bleeding she was referred for further treatment. No significant family or personal history could be elicited. There had been no exposure to toxins nor had there been any recent infections.

Physical examination. There were many ecchymoses over the upper and lower extremities. Several petechiae were noted on the buccal mucosa. The remainder of the examination was negative. No lymph nodes were enlarged and the spleen was not palpable.

Laboratory examination. This revealed a hematocrit of 41% and a white blood cell count of 10,300 per cu.mm. Differential white count was normal. Urinalysis was normal and examination of the feces was negative for occult blood. The platelet count was 22,000 and bleeding time 18 minutes. Coagulation time and prothrombin time were both normal. A diagnosis of idiopathic thrombocytopenia purpura was made.

Course. Since the patient had responded once to adrenocortical steroid therapy, it was decided to attempt once again to control her bleeding with these compounds. Oral prednisone, 15 mg. every six hours (60 mg. a day), was begun. After four days the platelet count was 150,000 per cu.mm., and bruising had ceased. The dose of prednisone was reduced to 10 mg. every six hours (40 mg. a day), and improvement continued. On the sixth day the platelet count was 409,000 per cu.mm., and the dosage of prednisone was reduced to five mg. four times a day. The patient was discharged in the care of her physician and was instructed to take 5 mg. prednisone three times a day.

The dosage of prednisone was decreased gradually and after two months was discontinued. Immediately the platelets fell to less than 10,000. In view of the two relapses following withdrawal of steroid therapy, it was decided that splenectomy should be performed. Prednisone was restarted in preparation for operation and continued through the postoperative period. The platelet count at time of operation was 748,000 per cu.mm., and on the first postoperative day was 898,000. The patient was discharged with instructions to reduce the prednisone gradually over an eight-day period. She continued well during the following year without the support of adrenocortical steroid therapy.

Comment. Careful search failed to reveal any primary etiology, and a diagnosis of idiopathic thrombocytopenic purpura was made. Laboratory findings confirmed the diagnosis.

Splenectomy was performed because adrenocortical steroid administration could not be discontinued without relapse after a six-month trial period. The good response to splenectomy was anticipated in view of the earlier temporary response to steroids. The increase in thrombocytes after splenectomy is but one of the characteristic changes in the peripheral blood after this operation. Others include the appearance of target cells. Howell-Jolly bodies, leukocytosis, and nucleated red blood cells. The removal of the spleen decreases the peripheral destruction of these elements. A relapse may occur in this patient as long as 20 to 25 years after splenectomy. If this happens, a decision must then be made as to whether an accessory spleen may be present.

Nonthrombocytopenic Purpura

Patients with nonthrombocytopenic purpura may have all the hemorrhagic lesions noted for those with thrombocytopenic purpura. They differ in that their platelet count remains within the normal range. Characteristic lesions include petechiae, ecchymoses, hematomas or spontaneous bleeding from the genitourinary tract or gastrointestinal tract.

THROMBASTHENIA, THROMBOCYTOPATHY, AND PLATELET RELEASE ABNORMALITY

A hemorrhagic diathesis has been attributed to qualitative as well as quantitative changes in the platelets.[260, 289, 476, 512] As the platelets play so broad a role in the defense of hemostasis, altered platelet function may affect the vascular or biochemical phase of hemostasis or both. It is not surprising to find a wide range of abnormal tests reported in the literature, since individual platelet functions are difficult to assess and more than one function may be altered.

In addition to the disorders described below, rare patients have been described in whom there is spontaneous bruising which seems to be associated with a failure of the platelets to adhere to collagen in vivo and in vitro.[230, 231]

The study of these disorders is complicated by confusing and overlapping terminology. In general, the term *thrombasthenia* is applied to platelet disorders characterized by abnormal clot retraction and deficient primary ADP-induced platelet aggregation. The term *thrombocytopathy* is applied to those conditions in which abnormalities of Platelet Factor 3 appear to be the major finding. Platelet release abnormality indicates a condition in which the platelet fails to release normal amounts of ADP in response to aggregating agents.[231, 320]

Thrombasthenia

Hereditary thrombasthenia (Glanzmann's disease) is a disorder characterized by a prolonged bleeding time, poor clot retraction, and the failure of platelets to aggregate in the presence of ADP. The disorder appears to be transmitted by an autosomal recessive defect and is manifested in childhood by easy bleeding from mucous membranes and skin. There is evidence of some improvement in hemostasis with age. Transfusions of fresh whole blood or platelets alone are usually helpful. Platelet life span is normal.[103] Platelets from patients with thrombasthenia have been reported to have a decreased ability to activate the intrinsic contact system and an immunologic defect or absence of the surface-localized thrombosthenin (S–thrombosthenin).[75, 526] A variety of biochemical abnormalities have been reported; none has been consistent.

Patients have been reported[199] in whom a deficiency of glyceraldehyde-3–phosphate dehydrogenase and pyruvate kinase resulted in a 50 per cent reduction of platelet ATP. As the contractile protein of the platelet is dependent on ATP as an energy source,[58, 308] any interference with the formation or function of ATP might result in abnormal platelet function.

Other patients have a normal platelet glycolytic cycle and normal platelet ATP levels. It was suggested that reduced Mg^{++} and ATPase levels were perhaps responsible for nonutilization of platelet ATP. One report noted a failure of these platelets to make platelet phospholipid available in vitro, and suggested that the defects may be attributable to a single abnormality of the platelet membrane.[291]

Reduction in glutathione reductase activity has been reported in two patients.[349] More recently a separate kindred with deficient glutathione peroxidase activity and increased levels of glutathione was reported. These findings suggest a defect in the reductive capacity of the platelets of some of these patients. Additional studies are needed.[269, 349] Reduced levels of platelet fibrinogen have been reported in some patients.[541, 556]

Thrombocytopathy (Platelet Factor 3 Deficiency)

Platelet Factor 3 (PF-3) may be quantitatively reduced or unavailable to participate in hemostasis. The specific nature of the defect is unknown in either.[87, 326, 538] Special studies are necessary to distinguish between these patients and those with thrombasthenia or von Willebrand's disease.[441, 539]

Patients have a mild-to-moderate hemorrhagic diathesis characterized by epistaxis, spontaneous bruising, menorrhagia, and an unpredictable amount of bleeding during surgery; in a few patients severe symptoms occur, but visceral hemorrhage and hemarthrosis are rarely seen.

Both primary and secondary forms of the disorder have been reported, but the primary form is rare.[88] The secondary or acquired disorder has been reported in multiple myeloma, idiopathic thrombocytopenic purpura, disseminated lupus erythematosus, uremia, chronic liver disease, and chronic lymphocytic leukemia. The major defect in all forms may be the result of defective ADP release affecting the availability of PF-3 and interfering with its clot-promoting function.

Platelet Release Abnormality (Thrombopathia)

Platelet release abnormality is the term applied to a disorder characterized by a failure to release normal amounts of ADP from the platelets in response to aggregating agents, although the platelets themselves can respond to extrinsic ADP by normal aggregation.[105, 211, 320, 537] Disaggregation is rapid; it occurs in two to three minutes.[124, 534, 539]

Platelet aggregation is associated with an increase in PF-3 availability.[210] Failure to release platelet ADP and maintain aggregation reduces the availability of this important substance despite its presence in the platelets. Aggregation induced by thrombin, collagen, and epinephrine is absent or deficient. The defect in the majority of patients now appears to be a deficiency in the nonmetabolic pool of adenine nucleotides normally present in platelet dense bodies. This nucleotide is normally extruded from the platelets by way of the canalicular system during the release reaction. Low platelet serotonin and epinephrine levels have also been noted. There is a decrease in platelet dense bodies on electron microscopy. A similar defect has been noted in some patients with albinism.[212, 546] In other patients, no defect in the storage pool could be detected and it was suggested that the defect may be similar to that produced by aspirin.[220, 241, 542]

The disorder, which may be inherited or acquired, is characterized by mild bleeding, mainly spontaneous bruising, and a prolonged bleeding time in the presence of a normal number of platelets. The abnormalities found in this group of patients are similar to those which occur after the ingestion of aspirin.[539]

It is probable that various types of platelet dysfunction can arise from a number of different causes. Considerable work is needed to clarify these problems and, in view of studies on ADP storage and release phenomenon, to reassess much of the earlier work on platelet dysfunction.

ALLERGIC PURPURA

This disorder, known also as the Schönlein-Henoch syndrome, was extensively studied by Osler,[373] and his reports are the basis of much of our present-day knowledge of the variability of the clinical findings. It occurs most commonly in male children, but is also found in adults.[17, 27]

Mechanism. The etiology of this disorder remains unknown. There is increased capillary permeability which allows the escape of elements of the blood into the surrounding tissue, but the nature of the capillary lesion is not clear. In some cases infection may play a role. Streptococcal infection of the throat has been implicated by some,[388] but the evidence is weak.[7, 35, 519] Hypersensitivity to certain foods has been implicated in some instances, and recovery has followed avoidance of the offending agent. Some have pointed to a resemblance between the lesions of allergic purpura and those of the collagen diseases, but again the evidence is incomplete.[136] Recent studies which revealed an elevated IgA level in some patients with this disorder have prompted comparison with immune complex disease.[79, 509] Again, the evidence is inconclusive.

Clinical examination. The presenting complaints will depend on the site and extent of the involvement. Osler[373] remarked that the two outstanding clinical features were recurrence, at long or short intervals, and marked variability of the skin lesions. The syndrome characteristically recurs several times before final remission. The recurrences may appear over a period of weeks, months, or in some cases, years. There are skin lesions of great variability. There may be only purpura, with petechiae and ecchymoses, or there may be associated effusion, erythema, or necrosis of the skin. Gastrointestinal involvement is marked by colicky abdominal pain which is often of great severity and occurs chiefly at night. Diarrhea and vomiting are frequent, and both the vomitus and stools may contain blood.[7, 373] Intussusception or perforation may occur.[17, 427] Gastrointestinal x-rays may reveal edema of the mucosa early in the course of the illness and evidence of submucosal hemorrhage and mucosal ulceration later. These changes are reversible.[27] Hematuria and proteinuria occur in from 12 to 49 per cent of the reported series.[227] In most cases they are transient findings. In some the hematuria and proteinuria may persist for months or years unaccompanied by azotemia or hypertension. A few develop azotemia, hypertension, and occasionally the nephrotic syndrome early in the course of their illness. These patients may die of rapidly progressive renal failure over a period of months or as the result of slowly developing renal failure over a period of years.[7, 42, 136, 167, 227, 331, 378] Joint symptoms may be the presenting complaint. Several joints are usually involved by pain at one time, and there may or may not be associated swelling.

The prognosis for life is generally good unless the patient develops progressive renal disease, uncontrolled gastrointestinal hemorrhage, edema of the glottis, or unrecognized intussusception or perforation.[17, 42] The disease is marked by repeated attacks which may extend over months or years, though most recover after a month or so.

There is no consistent laboratory finding. There may be an anemia if the bleeding has been extensive enough, but this is rare. Platelets, of course, are normal or only slightly reduced. The capillary fragility test is positive in some cases but not all.[7]

Treatment. The treatment of this syndrome is largely supportive. A careful search should be made for an offending food in chronic cases. Throat culture should be made and dealt with as indicated. The frequency with which the syndrome is accompanied by nephritis makes it imperative to pay close attention to the cultures. Ackroyd feels the patients should be kept in bed in the hope of reducing the incidence and severity of nephritis.[7]

Steroids alone have not proved effective in the management of skin manifestations or renal involvement, but are useful in the control of joint involvement, soft tissue swelling, and gastrointestinal symptoms.[17, 179, 488] The likelihood of intussusception or perforation should be kept in mind in order that surgical intervention can be performed immediately if it should become necessary.[17]

Immunosuppressive agents and steroids have been used in the successful management of progressive renal failure.[179, 340]

PURPURA IN ASSOCIATION WITH INFECTION

Purpura in association with infection has been known since ancient times.[261] It is a recognized and expected clinical finding in such disorders as Rocky Mountain spotted fever, typhus, meningococcemia, and bacterial endocarditis. In each of these disorders an escape of blood elements into the surrounding tissue follows damage to the vascular endothelium.

There are instances in which purpura is associated with severe forms of viral exanthems, such as chickenpox or smallpox. In these instances the purpura seems to occur because of the unusual severity of the disease, which causes damage to the vascular endothelium.[262]

In the presence of such vascular damage and/or hypotension, diffuse intravascular coagulation may occur and be responsible for the thrombocytopenia.

Finally, purpura may be associated with infection in certain patients who exhibit what appears to be individual susceptibility. The purpura may be thrombocytopenic or nonthrombocytopenic. Both types have occurred in association with scarlet fever, varicella, measles, tuberculosis, infectious mononucleosis, and infectious hepatitis.[7] These diseases need not be particularly severe for purpura to be a complication. The natural history of the purpura in these instances is similar to that of idiopathic thrombocytopenic purpura. The mechanism responsible for the purpura in these instances is not clear. No histologic change in the vascular system has been demonstrated.

Treatment. Although treatment with appropriate antibiotics is directed at the underlying disease, care should be taken to tide the patient over the hemorrhagic episode. Adrenocortical steroids may be helpful, but caution must be observed in the light of reports of the extraordinary severity and frequent deaths from varicella in children who have been on steroid therapy.[203]

Such steroids should be used with caution in varicella, if at all, and with caution in other virus exanthems. In patients with thrombocytopenia the use of platelet transfusions should be considered. Splenectomy would not be indicated except possibly in chronic cases, for example, those associated with tuberculosis involving the spleen.

Purpura Fulminans

Purpura fulminans is a rare, severe, usually fatal illness which occurs most often in children and young adults. The disorder is marked by the sudden appearance of large areas of cutaneous gangrene and hemorrhage during the convalescent period of a variety of infectious diseases such as streptococcus pharyngitis, scarlet fever, varicella, meningococcemia, and rubella. Associated with the skin manifestations are chills, fever, shock, coma, and death. The mortality rate has been 90 per cent in the past. The pathogenesis of the disorder is not completely clear. There is extensive intravascular coagulation and stasis. There is a marked similarity to the Shwartzman phenomenon.

The Shwartzman reaction is produced in rabbits by two intravenous injections of toxin from gram-negative bacteria administered 24 hours apart. Each injection activates the clotting system, but the reticuloendothelial system is able to clear the activated coagulation factors, fibrin, and endotoxin after the first injection. The second injection finds the reticuloendothelial system blocked as a result of the first injection, and produces massive precipitation of fibrin which results in severe vascular disturbances.[235] In recent years an increasing number of patients have been recognized with clinical course and laboratory studies resembling the generalized Shwartzman reaction.[425]

The Shwartzman reaction in the experimental animal can be blocked by the administration of anticoagulants,[327, 425] and these agents have been successfully employed in the treatment of purpura fulminans. Heparin is usually the agent of choice and may be needed for a prolonged period.[26, 122, 140, 425, 459] The use of low molecular weight dextran has been advocated and may reduce the tendency to thrombosis.[283, 354, 380] The administration of fibrinogen is usually contraindicated since the intravascular deposition of fibrin may be increased. Late in the course of the disorder enhancement of fibrinolysis may be indicated.[426] Since necrotic lesions resembling purpura fulminans may be seen in other conditions not involving intravascular coagulation, the diagnosis of intravascular coagulation must be carefully substantiated prior to treatment.

Other Types

Nonthrombocytopenic purpura may occur following exposure to chemicals or drugs to which the individual is susceptible,[7] in vitamin C deficiency,[228] as the result of certain snake bites,[275] and in disorders characterized by the presence of abnormal serum proteins. In the last-named disorders, deposition of abnormal proteins in the small vessels alters their permeability and allows escape of fluid content. This is seen in multiple myeloma, in association with cryoglobulins or para-amyloid and Waldenström's macroglobulinemia,[524] and the "benign"

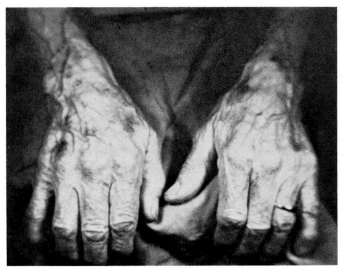

Figure 17–3 Senile purpura.

(polyclonal) hypergammaglobulinemic purpura also described by Waldenström.[524a] In the latter disorder, seen predominently in women, purpura occurs particularly over the lower extremities.[289a] The IgG is usually elevated and immune complexes are noted. Many of these patients develop Sjögren's syndrome and various disorders of connective tissue.[289a] Purpura may also occur in association with cold agglutinins, for example, following viral pneumonia. Nonthrombocytopenic purpura may be a feature of old age, presumably as the result of loss of support to the small vessels.

Ingestion of aspirin and other anti-inflammatory compounds can cause abnormal bleeding associated with a prolonged bleeding time in the presence of a normal number of platelets.[402, 536] These drugs interfere with platelet–collagen reaction and block the secondary wave of platelet aggregation; aggregation induced by ADP or epinephrine, the release of serotonin, and activation of PF-3 are abnormal. These effects, which follow the ingestion of small doses of aspirin, may be detected for from four to seven days, although salicylate is no longer demonstrable in the plasma.[539]

Both normal[130] and abnormal[263] platelet collagen reactions have been reported in Ehlers–Danlos syndrome.

HEREDITARY HEMORRHAGIC TELANGIECTASIA

This hereditary vascular anomaly was first described in 1896 by Rendu.[372] In 1901 Osler[372] reported several cases in detail and noted most of the clinical findings known today. Weber[531] reported an extensive family study in 1907, and two years later Hanes[207] made further contributions on the subject and suggested the name by which the disorder is known today.

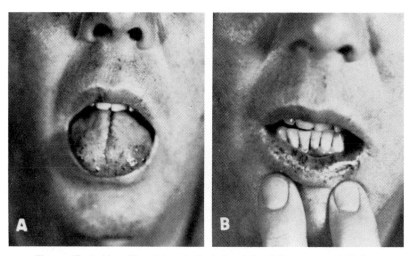

Figure 17–4   Hereditary telangiectasia involving (A) tongue and (B) lips.

PATHOLOGIC PHYSIOLOGY

Hereditary hemorrhagic telangiectasia is genetically transmitted by either sex as an autosomal dominant. Often the disease may not become apparent until the second or third decade when the lesions develop and gradually increase in number. Abnormal bleeding may not occur until middle- or old age and often grows more severe with advancing years.[207] Some patients are unaffected by the presence of telangiectasia, and hemorrhage does not occur. These lesions are composed of greatly dilated, thin-walled vessels which are reported to lack adequate smooth muscle and elastic tissues.[207] The fine structure of these vessels has been studied, and large vascular channels were found lined with a single layer of endothelial cells on a continuous basement membrane.[257]

In recent years angiographic studies have provided evidence of extensive involvement of larger vessels of the vascular system in this disorder.[80] Pulmonary arteriovenous fistulas have been reported which may lead to erythrocytosis, cyanosis, and clubbing and may be associated with a significant incidence of central nervous system complications, including sterile embolism and brain abscess.[55, 141, 183] Shunting may be so extensive in the liver that portosystemic encephalopathy may occur in the absence of cirrhosis.[342] Vascular abnormalities have also been reported to involve the spleen, eye,[551] central nervous system, and bone.[205]

An interesting syndrome of calcinosis, Reynaud's phenomena, sclerodactyly, and telangiectasia (CRST) has been reported.[131, 549] The telangiectases seen in these patients appear somewhat later and there is less tendency to episodes of hemorrhage. The gross and microscopic appearance of these lesions as well as their distribution is similar to that found in hereditary hemorrhagic telangiectasia, but the lack of a family history of hemorrhagic diathesis or similar telangiectases serves to distinguish this syndrome from hereditary hemorrhagic telangiectasia. The CRST syndrome is classified as a collagen disorder. It is slowly progressive as compared with diffuse systemic sclerosis.

CLINICAL EXAMINATION

The characteristic vascular lesions are pinpoint in size or several millimeters in diameter. They are red or purple in color and slightly raised from the surrounding surface. They may blanch slightly with pressure. The lesions, which may occur anywhere on the surface of the body or in any organ, are most frequently found on the skin of the face, the ears, the hands or feet, at the base of the fingernails, or on the mucous membranes of the nose and mouth.

The diagnosis must be suspected in cases of recurrent hemorrhage associated with telangiectasia and a family history of abnormal bleeding. The most common complaints are those of hemorrhage and anemia. Hemorrhage may occur as the result of slight trauma to one of the vascular lesions anywhere on the body, or may be spontaneous. Hemorrhage from the nose or mouth is common, but bleeding may occur from the respiratory tract, gastrointestinal tract, or genitourinary tract as well.

The importance of finding the lesions of hereditary hemorrhagic telangiectasia is enhanced by the recently-established associations with significant large vessel abnormalities in various parts of the body.

The chief laboratory findings are those of anemia. There may be iron deficiency with low serum iron and high iron-binding capacity if bleeding has been chronic. Coagulation studies and platelets are completely normal.

TREATMENT

The use of electrocoagulation and skin grafts has been successful in controlling some of the accessible lesions.[442] One of Osler's patients used a small balloon which he inserted into his nose in a deflated condition and then inflated to control nasal hemorrhage. This procedure is used with success today. The management of hemorrhage from the lesions of hereditary hemorrhagic telangiectasia presents a difficult problem when they are located in the gastrointestinal tract. They are difficult if not impossible to localize by x-ray but occasionally may be demonstrated by endoscopy.[548] Although resection may remove one source of hemorrhage the future development of similar lesions remains a constant threat.

The management of large vessel abnormalities must depend on individual evaluation of their hemodynamic significance, the prognosis, and the risk involved.

ABNORMALITIES OF BLOOD COAGULATION

An inherited deficiency of the appropriate activity of each of the clotting factors has been recorded. The deficiencies were all believed to be quantitative until recently, when it was demonstrated that the plasma of patients with a deficiency of Factors I, II, VIII, IX, or X may also contain functionally inactive molecular forms of these factors. Additional qualitative, quantitative, or combination defects will undoubtedly be detected. The familial occurrence of a deficiency of more than one clotting factor has also been noted.

Acquired deficiency of each of the clotting factors has also been reported. Such deficiencies may result from impaired synthesis, as in the course of liver disease, the development of circulating anticoagulants in association with any of a wide variety of disorders, as the result of the intended action of medicinal agents such as the anticoagulant drugs, or the toxic effect of a variety of drugs or chemical or physical agents. Deficiency of various clotting factors may also arise in the course of the defibrination syndrome as the result of over-utilization or proteolysis.

DISORDERS AFFECTING PREDOMINANTLY THE FIRST STAGE OF BLOOD COAGULATION

Factor XII (Hageman Trait) Deficiency

The existence of Factor XII was discovered as the result of studies undertaken to explain the unexpected finding of a greatly prolonged clotting time of the blood of a patient with no personal or family history of hemorrhagic diathesis.[410]

PATHOLOGIC PHYSIOLOGY

Hageman trait is the inherited deficiency of the specific plasma protein Factor XII.[270, 409] The plasma of affected kindred is deficient in Factor XII antigen and in its procoagulant, inflammatory, and fibrinolysis-inducing activities. This disorder represents a true quantitative deficiency of Factor XII rather than a qualitative variation in the molecule.[51, 410, 414] In the majority of instances the disorder is transmitted as an autosomal recessive defect. A kindred has been described recently in which the trait is transmitted as an autosomal dominant.[51] Heterozygotes have from 25 to 60 per cent of the normal concentration of Factor XII, whereas the homozygotes have less than 1 per cent.[409, 414]

Factor XII circulates in an inert form, but once a sample of blood is removed from the body and placed in contact with glass or other active surfaces it undergoes physical and chemical changes which initiate the intrinsic clotting sequence.[480] The mechanism of Factor XII activation in vivo is not completely understood, but contact with exposed collagen fibers may play a role.[411] Factor XII participates in a number of the biologic activities of the body. It plays a role in the process of inflammation and activation of the kallikrein-kinin system, the fibrinolytic system, and the complement system.[196, 333, 411, 413] It may also play a role in the pathogenesis of acute gouty arthritis.[276, 277, 499]

CLINICAL MANIFESTATIONS

With very few exceptions, these patients have no personal or family history of a hemorrhagic diathesis. The exceptions have included patients with menorrhagia or mild bleeding following significant trauma.[73, 163, 410] The clotting time is prolonged and the generation of thromboplastin activity abnormal. Direct comparison of the patient's plasma or serum with that of a patient known to have the defect is the only way to establish a firm diagnosis.

The several reports of thrombosis in patients with Factor XII deficiency[178, 238] may relate to the role of this factor in the initiation of fibrinolysis.

TREATMENT

There is no need to treat patients with classic Factor XII deficiency if they have no hemorrhagic diathesis. The atypical patient with hemorrhagic diathesis would probably respond to treatment with plasma.[68]

Disorders of Factors VIII, IX, and XI

The following disorders are grouped together because of the similarity of their clinical and laboratory findings. Each results in a delay in the development of blood thromboplastin activity to a greater or less extent[96, 478] but produces no alteration in the one-stage prothrombin time.

"Hemophilia" is one of the oldest recognized bleeding disorders and affected members of several of the ruling houses in Europe.[434] It has been recognized in recent years that the clinical findings of classic "hemophilia" may result from any one of three distinct genetic defects or from acquired circulating anticoagulants. These disorders can be differentiated only by appropriate laboratory tests, since they present similar clinical findings. It is for this reason that accurate classification of the cases presented in the older literature as "hemophilia" is not possible. The three genetic disorders now recognized, with their relative incidence in two series,[162, 429, 430] are as follows:

1. Factor VIII (Antihemophilic factor, AHF) deficiency, 80 to 82 per cent
2. Factor IX (Plasma thromboplastin component, PTC) deficiency (Christmas disease), 11 to 15 per cent
3. Factor XI (Plasma thromboplastin antecedent, PTA) deficiency, 5 to 7 per cent

Factor VIII (Antihemophilic Factor, AHF) Deficiency

PATHOLOGIC PHYSIOLOGY

Factor VIII deficiency is passed from one generation to the next as a sex-linked recessive. Ordinarily the female is a carrier and manifests no clinical signs or symptoms of the disorder.

The genetic possibilities inherent in this and similar disorders are best indicated by the use of symbols and diagrams. By common usage the male is designated as XY, and the female XX. In order for a male to be conceived, the male parent must contribute the Y chromosome; the female contributes the X. Specific genes are usually referred to by superscript letters. A dominant gene is designated by a capital letter and a recessive by a lower case letter.

The abnormal gene responsible for Factor VIII deficiency is recessive and is designated by the lower case letter h. The normal gene, which is dominant, is designated by a capital H. A normal female would thus be designated $X^H X^H$. The carrier female would be $X^H X^h$. In the case of the carrier female, expression will depend on which X chromosome is functional in the somatic cells. The carrier usually has no symptoms, since random distribution would result in at least 50 per cent of the X chromosomes being X^H in the somatic cells.[279] The Y chromosome of the male does not carry this gene and has neither H nor h. Whether a male child has Factor VIII deficiency or not depends entirely on the character of the X chromosome he must receive from the female. If the female carrier contributes the normal X^H to the male offspring, the male is normal. If, however, the X chromosome contributed by the female to her male offspring, is that which carries the abnormal gene, it finds expression as there is no normal gene (H) to suppress it.

The accompanying diagrams will illustrate the possibilities. The male in each instance is designated by the rectangle and the female by the circle.

Figure 17–5 represents a normal family with no factor deficiency. All offspring are normal.

Figure 17–6 indicates that a mating of a normal male and a carrier female may result in a hemophilic male or a carrier female as well as normal children of both sexes. Unfortunately, there is no way to establish with complete certainty whether a female is a carrier or not. The degree of recessiveness may vary because of random suppression of the abnormal X chromosome in accordance with the Lyon hypothesis. Carrier females may have normal or markedly depressed procoagulant activity. Normal Factor VIII levels do not rule out the carrier state, though markedly reduced levels would be highly suggestive of the presence of the abnormal chromosome. Recently it has been demonstrated that carrier females have a discrepancy between the level of Factor VIII coagulant activity and that measured by immunologic assay. 90 per cent of carriers can be detected in this manner. Such assays should prove to be of great importance to suspected carriers.[49, 50, 147]

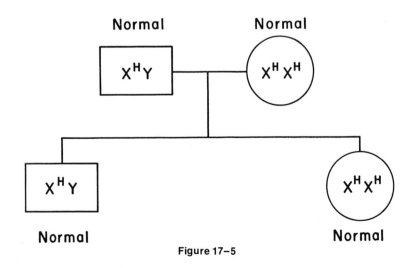

Figure 17–5

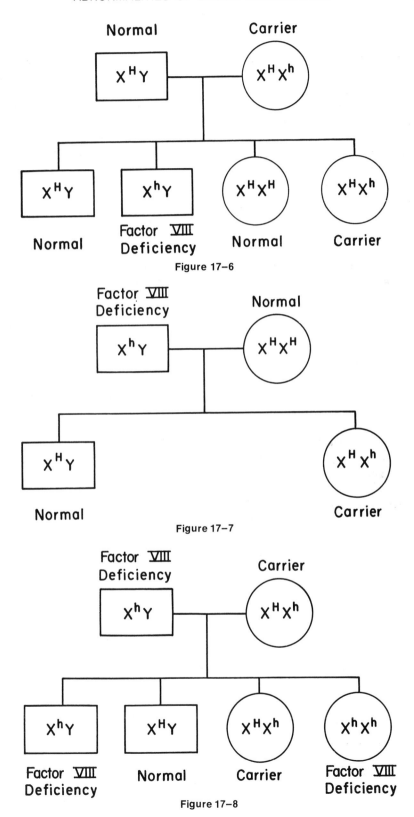

Figure 17–6

Figure 17–7

Figure 17–8

Figure 17–7 indicates the results of a mating of a Factor VIII-deficient male with a normal female. All their female children *must* be carriers, since the only X chromosome the male has to contribute carries the abnormal gene. On the other hand, none of the male offspring can have hemophilia, since a male must receive the lone X chromosome from the normal mother.

In Figure 17–8 we see the results of the mating of a Factor VIII-deficient male and a carrier female. For many years the possibility that a female could have a Factor VIII deficiency was not accepted, but several well-documented cases have now been reported.[334, 545] The female offspring of the mating noted here would receive an X^h from the Factor VIII-deficient male, and the second X^h from the carrier mother.

In Figure 17–9 we see the result of a mating between a normal male and a Factor VIII-deficient female. All male progeny would receive X^h from the mother, and all female would receive an X^H from the father in addition to the X^h from the mother. All males would then be Factor VIII-deficient and all females would be carriers.

The mating of a male and a female both deficient in Factor VIII has probably never occurred except in laboratory animals. All the offspring of such a mating would be Factor VIII-deficient (Fig. 17–10).

As there are patients with hemophilia who have no family history of the disorder, the rate of mutation is thought to be high.

Although the defect in classic hemophilia is transmitted as a sex-linked recessive mendelian characteristic, there is evidence that at least one and possibly two autosomal loci are involved in Factor VIII production as well. Von Willebrand's disease, characterized by a prolonged bleeding time and decreased Factor VIII level, is transmitted by an autosomal dominant gene, and one report has appeared in which Factor VIII deficiency alone appears to have been transmitted as an autosomal dominant trait.[37, 226]

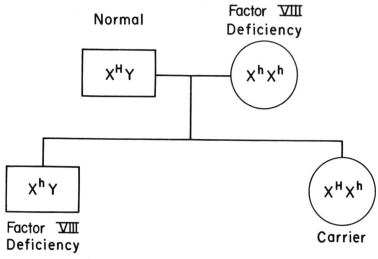

Figure 17–9

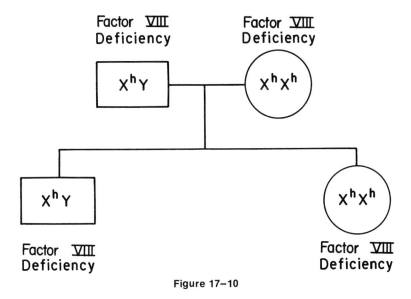

Figure 17–10

The result of the genetic defect is now known to be a reduction in the coagulant activity of Factor VIII, a globulin first described by Patek and Taylor.[379] In the absence of this activity, the first phase of coagulation is retarded. Since the platelets and the capillaries are unaffected, the bleeding time is normal but the coagulation time is often prolonged. The more severe the deficiency of Factor VIII activity, the more severe the bleeding problem. Levels of below 3 per cent are usually found in symptomatic patients, though a bleeding diathesis may be found in patients with levels as high as 20 per cent. A recent study suggests that variation in platelet coagulant function from patient to patient with the same level of Factor VIII coagulant activity may be responsible for the differences in clinical behavior.[540] The level of Factor VIII activity in any one patient is remarkably constant throughout his life.

Data indicate that reduced Factor VIII coagulant activity occurs as the result of qualitative change in the Factor VIII molecule rather than a quantitative deficiency of the globulin.[151, 247] Using a naturally-occurring human antibody against Factor VIII, investigators found that the plasma of a small percentage of patients with classic hemophilia would neutralize the antibody. Hemagglutination-inhibition tests using rabbit antibody to highly purified Factor VIII from normal humans have revealed the presence of a protein antigenically related to, or identical with, Factor VIII in similar amounts in both normal and hemophilic plasma and serum.[491] The evidence suggests the presence in the plasma of hemophilic patients of a molecule with the same antigenic determinants as Factor VIII but lacking Factor VIII coagulant activity.[134] Similar information has been developed concerning Factor IX deficiency.[245, 421]

Factor VIII coagulant activity is needed in the development of blood thromboplastin activity, and in its complete absence the only effective hemostatic defense left to the patient is that supplied by the vascular and platelet phase of hemostasis and the extrinsic system. In the event of a defect in the larger vessels, these defenses are not sufficient to maintain hemostasis, and extensive bleeding may occur.

The structure of Factor VIII-related antigen is poorly understood. It probably has a high molecular weight (approximately 2×10^6) and is composed of multiples of a single subunit of 180,000 to 190,000 daltons. It may circulate as a nonhomogeneous molecular population.[240] A single theory to account for recently developed data in this field is lacking.[34, 191, 239, 278, 417]

CLINICAL ASPECTS

In the past, many born with Factor VIII deficiency died in infancy or in the first five years, but with modern therapy there has been marked improvement in the prognosis. The availability of adequate transfusion service has probably been the most important factor in the reduction of mortality from this disorder.

Mildly affected hemophiliacs may reach adult life before serious bleeding occurs. The more severely affected individuals generally have repeated episodes of bleeding from the skin, the serous surfaces, the gastrointestinal tract, the genitourinary tract, or into joint spaces. Bleeding does not often, if ever, occur in the absence of trauma. Recurrent hemarthroses often result in permanent ankylosis and deformity.

Until recently conditions which made surgery imperative were considered to be catastrophic. Now it is possible to manage such emergencies with a good chance of success.[313]

For many years the diagnosis of "hemophilia" was made when it could be demonstrated in vitro that plasma from the patient in question did not correct clotting defect of a patient with known "hemophilia." The diagnostic difficulties previously encountered are now recognized to have occurred because any one of several defects can produce clinical findings of classic hemophilia. These defects may be identified only by proper laboratory tests. The platelet count, tourniquet test, and bleeding time are unaffected, as they depend on capillary integrity and platelets, both of which are normal in Factor VIII deficiency.[403] Clot retraction is likewise normal, since there is adequate fibrin and normal platelet function. The prothrombin time is normal, since this test system bypasses the factor deficient in hemophilia.

The coagulation time may be prolonged owing to a decrease in the formation of thromboplastin activity. It is important to note, however, that the coagulation time may be normal despite relatively severe Factor VIII deficiency. The thromboplastin generation test and the partial thromboplastin time can be used to identify the specific defect in any of these disorders.[64] Modifications may be made in these tests which enable the percentage of Factor VIII activity present in the suspect plasma to be determined.

TREATMENT

The treatment of patients with hemophilia has improved considerably in recent years. Modern blood banking methods have made available large quantities of whole blood and plasma; high potency preparations of Factor VIII from animal blood are in use in Europe[312] and concentrates of human Factor VIII are available in this country and in Europe.[391] Although none of these materials provides "the answer" for hemophilia, as does vitamin B_{12} for pernicious anemia, they have nonetheless proved a great boon to the hemophiliac. Hemostasis is more quickly secured and blood loss is more quickly replaced. If the patient is properly prepared, major surgery, though still hazardous, is feasible.

Normal plasma. The use of normal human plasma as a source of Factor VIII has been successful in controlling most hemorrhage into soft tissues, hematuria, and the bleeding which follows tooth extraction in those hemophilic patients with a mild deficiency. It must be freshly prepared, for it loses over 50 per cent of its activity in four days if stored at usual blood bank temperatures of 2 to 4° C.[274] Plasma which has been quickly separated and frozen at −30° C retains its activity for 30 days or more, and is an excellent product to have available. The relatively low concentration and short half-life of Factor VIII in normal plasma are inherent limitations, and it is difficult to maintain patients free of bleeding following major surgery or severe trauma without the danger of overloading the circulatory system.

Heterologous concentrates. The need for a source of concentrated Factor VIII has long been recognized. The first successful preparation of high potency material was from animal blood[60, 312] and made it possible to give to the patient an amount of Factor VIII equivalent to that found in 8 liters of human blood in a single infusion of small volume. However, as these preparations are of heterologous protein, they are antigenic and thus limited in their usefulness. It has proved possible to give a single course of therapy to a patient over a period of eight to ten days, but the response to the infusions often progressively diminishes. A second course may be given but carries the risk of anaphylactic reaction. Since there are only two animal preparations available (bovine and porcine), they are reserved for more serious episodes of bleeding and major surgery in those countries where they are used. They are not available in the United States.

Human factor VIII concentrates. The rapid improvement in concentrates of human Factor VIII over the past few years has had a major impact on the treatment of patients with hemophilia. For many years, the only concentrate available was that prepared by a modification of the Cohn procedure of plasma fractionation.[274] Starting with pooled plasma, the final preparation contained a tenfold concentration of Factor VIII.

This concentrate has not been widely accepted in the treatment of hemophilia because the use of pooled plasma as a starting material makes the risk of serum hepatitis high, and the potency, although better than that of fresh plasma, is still so low that circulatory overload may occur. Hemolysis has been noted during the administration of this material to some patients and has been attributed to the presence of high titer anti-A or -B isoantibodies contaminating the concentrate.[322]

An important breakthrough occurred when it was recognized that Factor VIII could be separated from plasma by cryoprecipitation.[156, 324, 384, 391, 395] When previously-frozen plasma is thawed at icebox temperature, most Factor VIII remains as a precipitate and can be separated from the rest of the plasma by centrifugation.[393] After extraction of the precipitate containing the Factor VIII, the remaining plasma may be used for other purposes.[368] This process results in a concentration of Factor VIII some 10 to 15 times that of normal plasma, but the danger of transmitting serum hepatitis remains a problem.[115] The great advantage of this technique has been its practicality. Cryoprecipitated antihemophilic factor can be produced and stored in any well-equipped blood bank laboratory.

A second major advance occurred when it was found that Factor VIII would precipitate in the presence of certain amino acids. One glycine-precipitated fraction has been developed which contains a 100-400 X concentration of Factor VIII.[97]

The Factor VIII level of a patient with hemophilia may be brought to hemostatic levels with a small volume of such material administered by syringe. If the cost of such preparations can be reduced and the possibility of the transmission of hepatitis is eliminated, continued improvement in the concentration of Factor VIII will make it practical to treat more patients with hemophilia prophylactically.[61, 272, 412, 423, 455] One carefully controlled program of supervised patient management of hemophilia has resulted in definite improvements. Compared with the previous year there were impressive decreases in absenteeism, days in hospital, and out-patient visits. Health care costs were reduced 45 per cent and use of concentrates slightly reduced. The major hazard appeared to be an increase in the risk of hepatitis for the family caring for the patient.[296, 297] Further studies of prophylactic and home care treatment programs are indicated.[95, 233, 405, 407]

Since the use of human plasma concentrates carries the risk of hepatitis, some make it a practice to administer prophylactic gamma globulin while the Factor VIII level is being maintained.

Recent evidence strongly suggests that the endothelial cells of the blood vessels are the site of production of Factor VIII. This probably accounts for the transient elevation of Factor VIII levels reported to occur following transplantation of the spleen[221, 364] and liver.[319]

Proper dental hygiene should not be neglected. Dental extractions have been rendered more safe by the use of dental splints of acrylic resin.[550] These splints protect the gum and prevent the dislodgment of a clot once it has formed, thus avoiding the use of sutures. If gum margins are sutured there is a constant danger that bleeding may continue beneath the suture and dissect into the fascial planes of the neck, causing respiratory obstruction. Calcium-alginate gauze soaked in Russel viper venom may be placed between the splint and the gum to act as a local hemostatic agent. Fresh plasma or one of the available concentrates[97] is given these patients an hour before the extraction and thereafter as indicated. The use of high doses of steroids has been reported to reduce bleeding after dental extraction in patients with hemophilia.[508] Hemorrhage-free dental extraction, without the use of plasma or blood, using protective splints and carefully packing the sockets with the patient under hypnosis, has also been reported.[307]

Hemorrhage in the tissue of the throat, at the base of the tongue, or in the neck is usually controlled by the infusion of concentrate. The possibility of respiratory obstruction should be appreciated in time to enable an endotracheal tube to be passed. Tracheostomy should be avoided if possible as it increases the danger of serious hemorrhage. The blood in these tissues does not localize and the surgeon should not attempt drainage, as such efforts result only in further bleeding and increased danger to the patient. The hemorrhage will cease and the blood will be absorbed quickly if an adequate concentration of Factor VIII is obtained. Superficial hemorrhage in accessible sites is controlled by the immediate application of local pressure while the infusion of fresh plasma or concentrate is started. After an elevation of the Factor VIII level in the recipient is obtained, the pressure should be released to allow blood with adequate Factor VIII to replace the Factor VIII-deficient blood in the vessels, and then reapplied.

Fresh joint hemorrhage continues to be treated as conservatively as possible. Infusion of fresh plasma or concentrates to raise the levels of Factor VIII is of great importance and, if started early, may abort the episode.[16] Bed rest, ice bags, and compression bandages on the affected joint during the acute phase all offer relief. Many feel that aspiration and lavage of the joint should be avoided as it may lead to further bleeding or infection,[487] others believe it to be of value.[135] Cautious activity with good physiotherapy as improvement occurs seems indicated. It is desirable to have the joint in the most functional position should ankylosis occur.

With the increased availability of antihemophilic factor concentrates surgical procedures to correct hemophilic arthropathy can be pursued more vigorously. Some have reported that synovectomy results in better joint function and reduces the frequency of hemorrhage.[271, 274, 359, 492] A five-day course of steroid therapy has been reported to be of benefit in the management of these patients.[282]

Surgery should be avoided if possible. Should major surgery be essential, a concentration of not under 35 per cent Factor VIII must be obtained. Since this is not possible using plasma alone, animal or human Factor VIII concentrates must be available. It is essential that surgery on these patients be carried out in centers where careful laboratory control can be exercised.[115, 313]

Interpersonal problems may develop between the physician and the patient with hemophilia during long-term management. In a recent study, patients with hemophilia were found to complain most about delays in institution of infusion therapy, inadequate analgesia, and inept venipuncture by hospital staff personnel. These patients become quite expert at the diagnosis of bleeding and resent any delay in treatment.[16, 164]

Aspirin should not be given to patients with hemophilia, as it causes defective platelet function, and together with the Factor VIII deficiency may aggravate the bleeding difficulty with serious or even catastrophic results.[264]

Illustrative Case

An 18-year-old white male was seen for the first time when he entered the University to continue his education. He was the only child born to his parents. His maternal uncle was known to have hemophilia.

Hemophilia was first suspected in infancy when he was noted to have repeated soft tissue hematomas in response to trivial injury. Painful hemorrhages into the major joints became commonplace as he became more active. He lived on a farm, distant from medical facilities, and treatment was often delayed. By the time he reached high school age, increasing deformity and limitation of motion of his knees and ankles required that he use a wheelchair.

School attendance was always irregular, and he was never able to attend for more than three weeks without interruption. Despite these handicaps, he completed the work of high school, largely through work at home.

Physical Examination. The patient was a bright, alert, young man in no distress. His outlook was excellent and he was anxious to undertake the work of college. The major findings included moderate limitation of extension of the left elbow, flexion contractures of both knees, and marked limitation of motion of his right ankle. There was marked muscle wasting of the lower extremities.

Laboratory studies. Coagulation studies revealed a normal platelet count, bleeding time, and prothrombin time. Partial thromboplastin time was prolonged and assays revealed less than 1% Factor VIII. There were no circulating anticoagulants detected.

X-rays revealed subchondral cystic changes with irregularities of the articulating surfaces of both knees and the right ankle. Marked demineralization of the bone was noted.

Course. This patient had severe hemophilia with less than 1% Factor VIII activity. He was treated with cryoprecipitates whenever he felt that joint hemorrhage had occurred. Arrangements were made for him to be brought to the emergency room at the onset of hemorrhage and 8 to 10 units of cryoprecipitate were administered intravenously. As a result he received cryoprecipitate every six to 10 days; treatment which raised his Factor VIII levels from > 1% prior to infusion to approximately 20% immediately after. During the four years of college he had no major hemorrhage and lost no time from school. When at home on vacations, arrangements were made for him to receive one of the commercial concentrates whenever necessary.

Comment. This case history demonstrates several features of importance. It is a classic example of the devastating effect of hemophilia prior to the availability of modern treatment. In the patient's early years concentrates were not available; in addition, he lived in a rural area where medical care was not immediately available.

The use of Factor VIII assays clearly identified the deficiency of Factor VIII and was used as a guide to therapy. The normal bleeding time served to rule out von Willebrand's disease. Plasma concentrates and cryoprecipitates were of immense value to this young man and their use enabled him to complete his college education without interruption; they may make remedial orthopedic surgery possible in the future.

This patient's family recognized the genetic risk of hemophilia but prior to the patient's birth his mother had no way of knowing whether she was a carrier. The recent development of new techniques for detection of carriers is of great importance. The relationship between the patient and his family was excellent. The parents showed wisdom in allowing the patient to pursue his education away from home despite the increased risk of trauma. As a result he will now be able to support himself and lead an independent life.

Factor IX (Plasma Thromboplastin Component, PTC) Deficiency (Christmas Disease, Hemophilia B)

The practice of comparing the coagulation characteristics of plasma from patients with undiagnosed hemorrhagic disease with those of plasma from clinically accepted cases of hemophilia in order to establish the diagnosis of hemophilia has in the past led to considerable confusion.[478] In 1947 Pavlosky[38] reported that the addition of blood from one hemophilic patient to that of another in vitro occasionally resulted in a normal coagulation time. Aggeler et al.[12] and Biggs et al.[65] later recognized that the existence of a heretofore unrecognized factor must be postulated and that the absence of this factor would produce a syndrome clinically indistinguishable from hemophilia. Factor IX has now been extensively investigated. Many patients thought to have Factor VIII deficiency have now been recognized to have a deficiency of this factor.

PATHOLOGIC PHYSIOLOGY

This defect is transmitted as a sex-linked recessive with genetic possibilities similar to those described above under Factor VIII deficiency. Hemorrhagic symptoms, however, may occur more frequently in female Factor IX heterozygotes. Recent reports suggest that deficiency of Factor IX activity may result from qualitative as well as quantitative changes in Factor IX.[245, 421] Multiple genetic forms have been reported. In one variant there is no detectable protein that cross-reacts with human anti-factor IX antibody designated negative for cross-reacting material (CRM−). There is another which reacts as does normal plasma designated as positive for cross-reacting material (CRM+). There is still a third which has reduced cross-reacting material which correlates with the coagulant activity.[338, 356]

Some of the patients with functionally inactive Factor IX have been shown to have a grossly prolonged prothrombin time if ox-brain thromboplastin is used. The functionally inactive Factor IX molecule interferes in some way with the reaction involving Factor VII and brain and provides a third way to classify patients with Factor IX deficiency (hemophilia B_m).[99, 245, 345] Another genetic variant has been reported in which the patient has a striking decrease in the hemorrhagic symptoms with advancing age. Young children average a 1 per cent Factor IX level; in older adults the level is 20 to 60 per cent. Longitudinal studies in two patients have noted an increase in Factor IX levels from 1 per cent to about 20 per cent with the sharpest rise at puberty.[516] Detection of additional genetic variants appears likely.

Like Factor VIII, Factor IX takes part in the first phase of the coagulation of blood. A deficiency of this factor retards the development of thromboplastin activity. The platelets and capillaries are unaffected and repair of small capillary defects proceeds normally.

The severity of the hemorrhagic diathesis appears to vary directly with the level of Factor IX activity. Variation in severity occurs more commonly between families than within the same family. Studies of a large kindred have revealed an increase in the number of children born into those families whose members have a hemorrhagic diathesis.[525]

CLINICAL FINDINGS

These patients may present any of the hemorrhagic manifestations found in Factor VIII deficiency. Manifestations of the hemorrhagic diathesis may appear at birth with bleeding from the umbilical cord, or following circumcision. Excessive bleeding will follow minor trauma and surgical procedures throughout the life of the patient.

The laboratory findings in this disorder follow the same general pattern as those in Factor VIII deficiency. The platelet count, capillary fragility, clot retraction, bleeding time, and prothrombin time are normal. The coagulation time is often prolonged, since the development of thromboplastin activity is retarded. As in Factor VIII deficiency, however, Factor IX-deficient patients may have normal coagulation times. As Factor IX is not consumed during coagulation it is present in normal serum. As a consequence, the coagulation of Factor IX-deficient plasma may be brought to normal in vitro by the addition of normal serum. The defect will not be corrected by the addition of $Al(OH)_3$-treated normal serum or plasma since $Al(OH)_3$ adsorbs Factor IX completely. This disorder may be identified by the thromboplastin generation test or by the partial thromboplastin time, which are based on these facts. Substitution in the incubation mixture of the patient's serum for the normal serum will retard the normal evolution of thromboplastin activity.

Hemizygous males are most severely affected, but this gene appears to be less completely recessive than that responsible for Factor VIII deficiency, and finds expression in some female heterozygotes. Female carriers may have symptoms of abnormal bleeding as well as depressed levels of Factor IX.

TREATMENT

Patients with Factor IX deficiency may have a clinical course as severe as that in those with Factor VIII deficiency. The infusion of fresh-frozen plasma at a dose of 15 to 20 ml./kg. will usually result in a rise in the patient's Factor IX level of only 5 to 10 per cent. For major surgery or severe post-traumatic hemorrhage, a Factor IX level greater than 25 per cent should be maintained until healing is complete.[418] These levels cannot be maintained using plasma alone, and concentrates are necessary.[237, 418] Development of concentrated preparations of Factor IX has been a boon for patients requiring therapy for control of major hemorrhage.[62, 67] They have been recommended for management of those patients whose required level of Factor IX could not be maintained with infusions of plasma alone. Since the concentrates are prepared from pooled plasma they may transmit hepatitis.[94, 171, 237, 477, 510]

Factor IX is stable on storage at blood bank temperatures for two or three weeks.[168, 195, 430] The results of plasma transfusions as measured by the assay of Factor IX are often disappointing and the clinical response can be better than expected from the assay level. The comments that have been made on the clinical management of Factor VIII deficiency apply equally to the management of this disorder.

Factor XI (Plasma Thromboplastin Antecedent, PTA) Deficiency

Factor XI deficiency was described by Rosenthal in 1953.[432] The clinical findings are similar to those of mild Factor VIII and Factor IX deficiency, the hemostatic defect being less severe.

PATHOLOGIC PHYSIOLOGY

Factor XI deficiency was earlier believed to be transmitted as an autosomal dominant trait with a high degree of penetrance and variable expression.[293, 446] Later studies suggest inheritance as an incompletely recessive trait. A level of less than 20 per cent of Factor XI has been found in the homozygotes, and between 20 and 70 per cent among the heterozygotes.[293] Recent immunologic investigation studies indicate that the synthesis of Factor XI is impaired since no antigen related to this factor can be found in patients with a deficiency.[157]

Factor XI deficiency, like Factor IX or Factor VIII deficiency, retards the development of adequate thromboplastin activity during the first phase of coagulation. Factor XI activity has been reported to increase in the plasma four to five hours following a fat-rich meal.[143]

CLINICAL ASPECTS

Patients of either sex present with a bleeding diathesis. The bleeding episodes are neither so frequent nor so severe as those encountered in patients with severe Factor VIII and Factor IX deficiency, and there appear to be periods when bleeding does not occur despite major trauma. Menorrhagia may be a serious feature. The bleeding diathesis is usually of equal severity in various members of the family. Rarely, epistaxis or post-traumatic bleeding may be life-threatening. There is no absolute relationship between the Factor XI level and the occurrence of bleeding.[193] An asymptomatic patient with less than 1 per cent Factor XI activity has been reported.[142]

The laboratory findings follow the same general pattern as that described for Factor VIII or Factor IX deficiency. The platelet count, capillary fragility test, bleeding time, clot retraction, and fibrinogen assay are all normal. The coagulation time may reflect the impaired evolution of thromboplastin activity.[365] The partial thromboplastin time and thromboplastin generation test are usually abnormal.

Unlike Factor VIII, Factor XI is not consumed during coagulation, and with Factor IX is present in both plasma and serum. Factor XI, however, is not adsorbed from normal plasma by $Al(OH)_3$; Factor IX is adsorbed. Consequently, the clotting time of Factor XI-deficient plasma is corrected by $Al(OH)_3$-treated normal plasma, which does not correct the clotting time of Factor IX-deficient plasma. It is also corrected by the addition of normal serum, which would not correct the clotting time of Factor VIII-deficient plasma. The three disorders may be separated by the thromboplastin generation test, the design of which makes use of these facts. No defect is apparent when the patient's adsorbed plasma or serum is incubated with normal serum or adsorbed plasma respectively. The defect is discovered when the patient's adsorbed plasma and serum are tested together.

TREATMENT

There is no clear relationship between the level of Factor XI and the severity of hemorrhagic symptoms.[293] Replacement is usually required only in the event of severe injury or surgery. If surgery cannot be avoided, these patients should be carefully prepared. It has been suggested that levels of 50 per cent Factor XI are necessary to maintain hemostasis if extensive surgery is contemplated.[400] It was found that 4.5 ml. of fresh or fresh-frozen plasma per kg. body weight raised the level of Factor XI by 10 per cent. The half-life of the infused activity was up to 60 hours.[400, 431, 433] There is a tendency for secondary bleeding to occur two to three days after surgery and smaller amounts of plasma may be indicated at intervals following surgery.[387] Others have suggested giving one liter of plasma daily until healing is complete.[418] A recent report noted a large amount of Factor XI in commercial prothrombin concentrate and its successful use during hip surgery in a patient with severe deficiency. The considerable risk of hepatitis would appear to preclude its use in all but the most exceptional circumstances.[59]

Circulating Anticoagulants

Severe hemorrhagic symptoms may be caused by a variety of circulating anticoagulants. Some of the circulating anticoagulants are antibodies; the nature of the others is poorly understood. They may interfere with coagulation at several points and produce any of the findings noted to occur as the result of deficiencies of specific coagulation factors.

When specific antibodies occur in patients with an inherited hemorrhagic diathesis, treatment is made far more difficult. Although there may be no increase in the number of hemorrhagic episodes, the treatment of each episode is complicated by the need to overcome the effect of the circulating antibody as well as to treat the original defect.

Antibodies to coagulation factors developing during or subsequent to pregnancy may produce a severe hemorrhagic diathesis which persists for months or years.[369] There have been reports of circulating anticoagulants occuring in association with a heterogeneous group of disorders including syphilis, disseminated lupus erythematosus,[93] chronic nephritis, tuberculous lymphadenopathy, and the collagen diseases.[163, 292, 306, 330, 382] Rarely they may develop spontaneously in persons without known disease.

The anticoagulants associated with lupus erythematosus (the lupus anticoagulants) are poorly understood.[151a]

CLINICAL FINDINGS

Patients with circulating anticoagulants may have any of the physical findings associated with their underlying disorder as well as those affecting blood coagulation. Once again it is in the laboratory that positive identification of the disorder is made. Since the vascular phase of hemostasis is unaffected, the platelet count, bleeding time, tourniquet test, and, if fibrinogen is unaffected, clot retraction are normal. Fibrinogen assay is abnormal if the anticoagulant is directed against fibrinogen. Interference by the circulating anticoagulant with the formation of thromboplastin activity results in an abnormal partial thromboplastin time and thromboplastin generation test. Diminished formation of thromboplastin activity occurs when the patient's serum or adsorbed plasma is substituted in the incubation mixture. The use of 50 per cent normal and 50 per cent patient's adsorbed plasma with normal serum in the incubation mixture results in diminished formation of thromboplastin activity. The presence of a circulating anticoagulant is thereby suspected, as any genetic defect likely to be confused with it would have been corrected by the addition of 50 per cent normal adsorbed plasma. Assays of specific factors before and after incubation will identify the factor which is the target of the inhibitor. Some of the antibodies are slow-acting and the incubation period should be at least one hour.[54]

The lupus anticoagulant does not cause a progressive lengthening of the partial thromboplastin time; a finding which serves to distinguish the lupus anticoagulant from the specific antibodies.[151a] The lupus anticoagulant may be associated with marked abnormalities in laboratory tests in the absence of clinical findings of a hemorrhagic diathiasis.[183a]

Heparin-like compounds may be differentiated from circulating anticoagulants by the addition to the plasma of protamine sulfate or toluidine blue which neutralizes the heparin-like compounds and leaves circulating anticoagulants unaffected.

PATHOLOGIC PHYSIOLOGY

The circulating anticoagulants have been shown to interfere with the reactions leading to the formation of thromboplastin activity in the intrinsic system, thrombin-fibrinogen reactions, fibrin polymerization, and fibrin stabilization.[74, 161, 242, 254, 363a] Others have suggested they may interfere with the action of formed thromboplastin.[150, 163, 292, 330]

The circulating anticoagulants are believed to result from some immunologic mechanism.[208, 242, 292, 528] They are present in the gamma fraction of the plasma and several recent reports have identified them in the IgG_4 subclass in acquired hemophilia.[25, 495, 513] The finding of circulating anticoagulants in patients treated repeatedly with blood or blood products, following pregnancy, and in association with diseases known to have deranged immunologic mechanisms, particularly in disseminated lupus erythematosus, has lent substance to this theory. In one study the level of the inhibitor rose sharply four to five days after plasma infusion, peaked at 10 to 14 days, and slowly declined. The magnitude and timing of the inhibitor varied among the patients studied and was used as a guide in therapy.[493, 495] There are, however, instances in which such a mechanism does not seem to operate and the mechanism is unclear.[113, 242]

Circulating anticoagulants are relatively heat-stable and fare well on storage at 0 to 4° for long periods of time. Specific inhibitors against Factor VIII are most common, but have been demonstrated against Factors IX, V, II, XI, XII, XIII, and fibrinogen (Factor I). In those instances when circulating anticoagulants interfere with Factor V, or thromboplastin activity itself, the one-stage prothrombin time will of course be prolonged.

The lupus anticoagulant appears to inhibit the action of formed prothrombin activator (thromboplastin activity); perhaps by reaction with the phospholipid component of the prothrombin activator complex. Normal plasma contains a cofactor which potentiates its activity. The lupus anticoagulant has been associated with IgG protein in the plasma of some patients and the IgM proteins in others. It may play a role in the thrombocytopenia often associated with lupus erythematosus and may also be associated with prothrombin deficiency.[151a]

TREATMENT

Treatment of these patients is the same as that employed in other disorders interfering with the formation of blood thromboplastin activity. Occasionally massive transfusions of fresh blood effect a response when smaller ones do not. The deficiency of specific clotting factors secondary to circulating anticoagulants should be treated with specific factor concentrates if they are available, using the level of inhibitor activity as a guide to therapy.[419, 495]

Constant infusion of Factor VIII concentrates, which takes advantage of the time-dependent antigen-antibody reaction seen in acquired hemophilia, has been shown to be helpful in some cases. However, porcine and bovine Factor VIII are probably the best therapy in life-threatening hemorrhages.[468] Adrenocortical steroids have been used with success in the treatment of patients with the lupus anticoagulant but have shown little efficacy against specific inhibitors.[46, 151a, 183a]

Immunosuppressive therapy has been reported to be effective in the treatment of nonhemophilic patients with circulating anti-Factor VIII who were unresponsive to conventional therapy.[382, 461]

DISORDERS AFFECTING BOTH THE FIRST AND SECOND STAGES OF BLOOD COAGULATION

The disorders to be discussed in this section affect the first and second stages of blood coagulation. The thromboplastin generation test and the one-stage prothrombin time test are abnormal. Both disorders may be hereditary or acquired.

Factor V Deficiency (Parahemophilia)

Factor V deficiency was first demonstrated to be a distinct clinical entity by Owren[375] in 1947. The young woman whose disorder he reported suffered from epistaxis, easy bruising, and excessive menstrual bleeding. The one-stage prothrombin time was prolonged and was not shortened by the addition of prothrombin. It was corrected, however, by the addition of a prothrombin-free plasma fraction obtained from a normal source. Thus it was demonstrated that a deficiency of a factor other than prothrombin could not only prolong the one-stage prothrombin time but also could produce a serious clinical disorder.

PATHOLOGIC **PHYSIOLOGY**

Factor V deficiency may be congenital or acquired. The congenital form is thought to be transmitted as an autosomal recessive, although the abnormal gene has a potency roughly equal to the normal counterpart. There is a high degree of variation in expressivity, which is thought responsible for the finding of some heterozygotes with hemorrhagic symptoms, although in others the carrier state is not detectable.[281] Consanguinity has been noted to be a feature of some of the family pedigrees. Studies indicate that there is decreased synthesis of Factor V in the congenital form rather than production of a defective molecule.[152, 159] Congenital Factor V deficiency has been reported to occur in association with congenital Factor VIII deficiency.[453] One study suggests an autosomal inheritance of this double defect with a marked degree of penetrance in heterozygotes with varying degrees of expressivity. The defect must be regarded as a distinct entity, and needs further study.[191]

The acquired form of the disorder has been reported in association with a variety of diseases.[484] Notably the level of Factor V is depressed in association with fibrinolysis and certain instances of acquired fibrinogen deficiency. As Factor V is essential to the first phase of blood coagulation, its deficiency will result in the inadequate production of thromboplastin activity. Fantl[149] has reported that abnormal bleeding will occur when the level of Factor V falls below 30 per cent of normal. Serum does not contain Factor V because it is consumed during the process of blood coagulation.

Factor V can be synthesized by the isolated perfused rat liver. The synthesis was unaffected by the addition of coumarin. Indirect evidence also points to the liver, as the normal source of Factor V and acquired deficiencies have been reported in severe liver disease.[376] The factor is not vitamin K-dependent, and deficiency of Factor V does not occur secondary to biliary tract obstruction or during the administration of coumarin drugs.

A specific inhibitor of Factor V has been reported in the plasma and serum of an elderly female under treatment for tuberculosis.[302]

CLINICAL FINDINGS

In a review of the reported cases of congenital Factor V deficiency,[149] it was noted that bleeding occurs in the first few years of life. Bleeding from accidental or operative trauma was excessive and spontaneous bleeding into the genitourinary tract and the gastrointestinal tract was noted. Hemarthrosis was not common. Menstrual bleeding is found to be excessive and may be life-threatening. The clincial findings of the acquired form of the disorder are similar to those of the congenital variety, complicated of course by the underlying disease.

The vascular phase of hemostasis is unaffected. Platelets are normal in number and function, and the bleeding time and tourniquet test are normal. There is no quantitative or qualitative defect in fibrinogen. Since Factor V deficiency affects the first stage of coagulation, it is reflected in an abnormal thromboplastin generation test and partial thromboplastin time. The one-stage prothrombin time is prolonged since Factor V is essential for the normal evolution of thrombin from prothrombin under the conditions of the test. Inadequate formation of thromboplastin activity is responsible for the abnormal coagulation time.

The laboratory findings in the acquired form of the disorder will of course be modified by the associated disease.

TREATMENT

Treatment consists of the administration of fresh plasma by the intravenous route. Studies indicate that hemostasis is satisfactory if the Factor V level is 10 to

15 per cent of normal. Such levels may be obtained by the infusion of 10 to 15 ml./kg. of body weight of fresh or fresh-frozen plasma,[77, 149] and should be repeated as laboratory studies indicate and the clinical condition allows. The half-life of the infused Factor V activity appears to be 12 to 20 hours.

Factor X (Stuart Factor) Deficiency

In 1957, Hougie, Barrow, and Graham[243] restudied a patient thought to suffer from a deficiency of Factor VII. Their careful work established the heterogeneity of the coagulation defects in the patients in this group. A new blood clotting factor was uncovered and its properties detailed in their report.

PATHOLOGIC PHYSIOLOGY

Factor X deficiency is transmitted by an incompletely recessive autosomal gene.[192] Although most severe in the homozygote, bleeding tendencies have been noted in the heterozygote, and carriers can often be detected with appropriate tests. Factor X deficiency, like that of Factors II, VIII, IX, and fibrinogen, can result from a qualitative as well as a quantitative abnormality. The plasma of some patients with Factor X deficiency has been demonstrated to have a protein antigenically similar to Factor X though functionally inactive.[132, 173]

Factor X deficiency is more commonly an acquired defect. With the other vitamin K-dependent factors (II, VII, and IX), Factor X will be reduced by anything which interferes with the metabolic function of vitamin K. It may also be one of a variety of proteins whose synthesis is affected by liver disease.

Rarely, an isolated deficiency of Factor X may develop. A temporary deficiency of Factor X developed in one patient presumably as the result of contact with a farm insecticide.[194] In another report, a 10-year-old boy suddenly developed a severe hemorrhagic diathesis as the result of an acquired deficiency of Factor X. The defect persisted for six months, after which Factor X reappeared. No inhibitor could be detected and no cause was discovered despite extensive studies.[44] Factor X deficiency may also occur in association with amyloidosis.[56a]

Factor X is essential in the first phase of blood coagulation, and a deficiency of the factor is demonstrated by the thromboplastin generation test and the partial thromboplastin time. The defect is apparent when the patient's serum is substituted for normal serum in the incubation mixture. Factor X is adsorbed by $Al(OH)_3$ from plasma. As $Al(OH)_3$-treated plasma is used in performance of the test, the defect is not detectable when the patient's $Al(OH)_3$-treated plasma is substituted for normal. Both normal and patient plasma are deficient in Factor X under conditions of the test. Factor X is present in normal serum, as it is not consumed in coagulation and substitution of the patient's serum for normal serum in the incubation mixture reveals the defect. The one-stage prothrombin time is prolonged since Factor X, as well as Factors II, V, and VII, is essential for optimal development of thromboplastin activity from the usual tissue sources and platelets.[316]

Factor X has been shown to be vitamin K-dependent and is reduced after several days of administration of coumarin drugs.[189, 420] The average intra-vascular half-life of Factor X has been reported to be 32.5 hours in one study[420] and to vary from 48 to 60 hours in another.[63] Extravascular diffusion occurs, as demonstrated by the appearance of the factor in the lymph of a patient with Factor X deficiency following transfusion of normal plasma.[189, 420]

CLINICAL FINDINGS

The patients described have had a moderate bleeding diathesis. Though hemorrhagic symptoms may occur in childhood, clinical manifestation of the disorder may not appear until later in life. Frequent epistaxis and the formation of hematomas have been most disturbing. Hemarthrosis has been reported but is mild and infrequent. Although the defect is most severe in the homozygote, it is important to note that heterozygotes with hemorrhagic symptoms have been reported. These patients, usually female, have been noted to be bad operative risks and to have persistent anemia, presumably secondary to menor-rhagia.

The bleeding time, tourniquet test, and platelets are normal. Fibrinogen is quantitatively and qualitatively normal. The whole blood clotting time, partial thromboplastin time, and thromboplastin generation test are abnormal, owing to deficient formation of blood thromboplastin activity. One-stage prothrombin time is prolonged, as Factor X is required for evolution of optimal extrinsic thromboplastin activity.

TREATMENT

Transfusion with whole blood or plasma is effective in the treatment of hemorrhage. As Factor X is relatively stable, it is not necessary to use freshly-prepared blood or plasma. The general management of these patients is similar to that of those with antihemophilic factor deficiency.

Factor X has an in vivo half-life of 48 to 60 hrs, and a level of 10 to 20 per cent of normal levels must be maintained for hemostasis.[418] Plasma is usually sufficient, but if adequate levels cannot be maintained concentrates can be used. They should be used only if hemostatic levels of Factor X cannot be maintained with plasma alone, as some of the material is reported to transmit hepatitis.[94, 171, 477, 510]

DISORDERS AFFECTING PREDOMINANTLY THE FIRST OR SECOND STAGE OF BLOOD COAGULATION

The following disorders affect predominantly the first or second stage of blood coagulation and result in an abnormal one-stage prothrombin time test. Although congenital prothrombin deficiency is recognized, it is extremely rare. Many cases formerly thought to represent congenital deficiency of prothrombin have on retesting in the light of present knowledge proved to be deficiencies of Factor V, Factor X, or Factor VII.

Factor VII Deficiency

In 1951, Alexander, Goldstein, Landwehr, and Cook reported the first patient recognized to have a congenital deficiency of Factor VII.[14, 182] The characteristic defect noted was a prolonged one-stage prothrombin time corrected by normal plasma or serum but not by $Al(OH)_3$-treated plasma. Since the two-stage prothrombin time was consistently normal, it was recognized that the defect could not be due to a prothrombin deficiency. As $Al(OH)_3$-treated plasma contains Factor V, its failure to correct the prolonged one-stage prothrombin time also established the syndrome as distinct from Factor V deficiency.

Since 1951, a number of case reports described as Factor VII deficiency have appeared in the literature. All had prolonged one-stage prothrombin times uncorrected by $Al(OH)_3$-treated plasma, but results of other coagulation tests varied. A third factor (Factor X) has been shown to be necessary for optimum development of thromboplastin activity under the conditions of one-stage prothrombin time test.[150] Some of the cases formerly designated Factor VII deficiency have now been re-examined and found to be deficient not in Factor VII but in Factor X. Much of the confusion in the literature prior to 1957 relative to Factor VII deficiency can now be resolved.

PATHOLOGIC PHYSIOLOGY

Factor VII deficiency may be inherited or acquired. Homozygotes have a hemorrhagic diathesis and have Factor VII levels of 10 per cent or less. Heterozygotes usually have no clinical symptoms and have Factor VII levels of about 50 per cent.[188, 204, 223, 321, 374]

Evidence has been presented for two types of defect: one with Factor VII antigen, the other without.[185, 399] Factor VII levels have been noted to be similar in men, and in women not on birth control pills. There is a significant increase in Factor VII levels in some women on low estrogen birth control pills.[100] Factor VII activity in plasma stored at $0°$ C for 16 hrs increases five- to tenfold. This cold promoted activation of Factor VII is dependent on the presence of Factor XII and the kallikreinogen–kallikrein system.[176] Neither synthetic nor natural estrogens induced cold activation of Factor VII in vitro.[177]

It seems clear from the studies carried out on the blood of patients with Factor VII deficiency that this factor, although necessary for optimal development of extrinsic thromboplastin activity, is not required for the development of intrinsic thromboplastin activity. Normal clotting time, partial thromboplastin time, and thromboplastin generation test are therefore understandable. The presence of hemorrhagic symptoms in these patients attests to the importance of the development of optimal extrinsic thromboplastin activity in the physiologic defense of hemostasis.[3]

Factor VII is thought to be formed in the liver and is vitamin K-dependent. An acquired Factor VII deficiency may occur in severe liver disease and during the administration of coumarin drugs. There is evidence that the administration of coumarin drugs results in the production of a Factor VII molecule without clotting activity.[185] A two-component decay curve has been reported following rapid infusion of a Factor VII concentrate into patients with hereditary Factor VII deficiency.[321] The first component, with a half-life of 35 minutes, probably represents equilibration with the extravascular space, and the second, with a half-life of 300 minutes, the metabolic decay phase.

The clinical and laboratory findings in acquired Factor VII deficiency would of course reflect the primary disorder in addition to presenting those of the congenital deficiency. The acquired form is usually complicated by additional acquired coagulation defects.

CLINICAL FINDINGS

Patients with Factor VII deficiency may have the onset of abnormal bleeding in infancy, and hemorrhage from the cord has been noted. Gastrointestinal hemorrhage, easy bruising, and frequent epistaxis are common. These patients may also have mild hemarthroses. The tourniquet test and platelets are normal. In most patients bleeding time is normal but in as many as one-third it may be prolonged. This finding cannot be explained at present. The thromboplastin generation test and partial thromboplastin time are normal in Factor VII deficiency but abnormal in Factor X deficiency. The one-stage prothrombin time is prolonged and not corrected by the addition of $Al(OH)_3$-treated plasma (containing Factor V). In the Stypven time test the venom of the Russell's viper will correct the prothrombin time of Factor VII-deficient plasma, but not that of Factor X-deficient plasma.

The laboratory findings of acquired Factor VII deficiency will of course also reflect the underlying pathology.

TREATMENT

Fresh, stored, or supernatant plasma after removal of cryoprecipitate, all contain Factor VII and may be used for replacement. The effects are short-lived and the prothrombin time returns to pretransfusion levels within 24 hours;[182] the half-life is on the order of 4 hours.[140, 176a, 182, 236] Maintenance of a Factor VII concentration of 10 to 20 per cent by the infusion of plasma or plasma concentrates to patients with congenital Factor VII deficiency has been reported to be sufficient to control spontaneous as well as postoperative hemorrhage.[321]

Factor VII deficiency secondary to anticoagulant coumarin drug therapy will respond to vitamin K_1 administration.

One of the concentrates of Factors II, VII, IX, and X may be needed in the treatment of patients with this defect who fail to respond to other measures. Unfortunately these concentrates carry a high risk of hepatitis.[94, 171, 237, 477, 510]

Factor II Deficiency (Prothrombin Deficiency)

In 1934 Dam and Schonheyder[20, 128] noted that chicks raised on an artificial diet had a hemorrhagic diathesis unaffected by ascorbic acid. The following year Dam[127] proposed the name vitamin K for the antihemorrhagic factor deficient in the diet and noted that it was fat-soluble. Many compounds have been found to have vitamin K activity. All these compounds are essentially derivatives of 2-methyl, 1, 4-naphthoquinone. They differ from the synthetic menadione by having a group substituted in the 3-position, and from each other by the nature of the group. Vitamin K_1, which is 2-methyl, 3-phytyl, 1, 4-naphthoquinone, was isolated from alfalfa, and Vitamin K_2 from putrefying fish meal.[18, 98] Vitamin K_1 and menadione are both used clinically.

PATHOLOGIC PHYSIOLOGY

Congenital hypoprothrombinemia exists but is extremely rare.[78, 273, 392] It is inherited as an autosomal trait and is usually a mild disorder. The severity of the symptoms seems to reflect the level of prothrombin activity. Patients have been identified with immunologically-active Factor II material with decreased coagulant activity.[264, 457] A deficiency of both coagulant and immunologic activity has also been described.[41, 273] The homozygotes in one family had coagulant levels of approximately 5 per cent. Each had 100 per cent levels of prothrombin by immunoassay.[264] Another family had no homozygotes. The heterozygotes had 50 per cent coagulant activity.[457] In one instance, the immunologically detectable abnormal molecule underwent some change during activation but was unable to release the active enzyme thrombin; in another, the molecule was slowly activated.[264, 457]

The acquired form of the deficiency is vastly more common and usually the result of liver disease or some disturbance in vitamin K metabolism.

It is not possible to produce a significant dietary deficiency of vitamin K in man as the intestinal bacteria produce sufficient vitamin to cover the daily needs. A deficiency will become apparent in any situation wherein the vitamin cannot be absorbed from the intestinal tract, however. Vitamin K is fat-soluble and its absorption from the intestinal tract is impaired by disorders (such as biliary tract obstruction) which result in a decrease in bile acids and consequent decrease in fat absorption.[401] Loss of large quantities of fat in the stool will likewise lead to loss of the vitamin. The occurrence of vitamin K deficiency in patients receiving wide-spectrum antibiotics over long periods of time with sterilization of the intestinal tract and loss of vitamin K-producing bacteria has been reported when associated with a vitamin K-deficient diet.

Severe liver disease may also result in prothrombin deficiency. In these cases there is an adequate amount of the vitamin, but the reactions in which it takes part in the liver are impaired.

The administration of anticoagulant drugs may produce the same effects as vitamin K deficiency. Anything which interferes with the availability of vitamin K, such as poor nutrition, malabsorption syndrome, oral antibiotics which alter normal bacterial flora, or biliary or liver disease, will increase susceptibility to these drugs. The administration of salicylate, phenylbutazone and oxyphenylbutazone, quinine, or quinidine can reduce the vitamin K-dependent coagulation factors of normal people or of patients with liver disease, and can act to potentiate the effect of oral anticoagulants.[38, 284, 301, 498] Rarely, isolated prothrombin deficiency may be acquired.[267, 299]

In the absence of vitamin K, a prothrombin molecule may be found in the plasma which is immunologically similar to normal prothrombin but converts far more slowly to thrombin.[133, 223] Evidence suggests that vitamin K is needed in the attachment of some noncarbohydrate prosthetic group which contains the Ca^{++} binding sites.[358] Studies of plasma from dicoumarol-treated cows have suggested that normal prothrombin has calcium-dependent antigenic determinants lacking in the abnormal molecule.[491] The variant molecules may be precursors of the normal molecule.[315]

Prothrombin, Factor VII, Factor IX, and Factor X levels are below normal during the first six weeks of life.[273, 523] Although most investigators have found a rise in these factors following the administration of vitamin K to the mother in labor or to the newborn infant, others[160] have failed to achieve this result. It has been suggested[273, 523] that the low concentration of these factors in the neonatal period could be responsible for some instances of hemorrhagic disease of the newborn.[2, 3] Though this point is not yet settled,[160] it is common practice to administer a routine prophylactic dose of 0.5 to 1.0 mg. vitamin K_1 to all infants at birth. Since human milk contains less vitamin K than cow's milk, this appears to be of particular importance to breast-fed infants.[497] Some types of soy bean protein formula have been found to have lower concentrations of vitamin K than others and may contribute to the problem.[351] Large doses of vitamin K (over 5 mg.) have been reported to increase serum bilirubin levels and the risk of kernicterus in premature infants, and should be avoided.[339]

CLINICAL EXAMINATION

Hypoprothrombinemia may result in a hemorrhagic diathesis manifested by bleeding from the gums, nose, or gastrointestinal tract. Hemarthrosis is rare. Hematemesis and soft tissue bleeding have been recorded; there may be severe hemorrhage after surgical trauma. Excessive menstrual flow is also a common finding.

A prolongation of the one-stage prothrombin time and partial thromboplastin time is found in these disorders. The thromboplastin generation tests should be normal and the modified thromboplastin generation test will indicate a deficiency of prothrombin. Fibrinogen assays are normal.

TREATMENT

Patients with congenital prothrombin deficiency may be treated with stored plasma or the supernatant remaining after removal of cryoprecipitate from plasma. In the event of serious trauma or surgery, the desired level of 40 per cent of normal activity may be difficult to achieve with plasma, and concentrates may be required.[418] Since the concentrates are prepared from pooled plasma there is the danger of the transmission of hepatitis.[171, 224, 440, 477]

In those patients with acquired prothrombin deficiency, blood transfusions should be given in emergency situations and will serve to treat shock, correct anemia, and aid in restoration of missing coagulation factors. In nonemergency situations vitamin K may be used. It has been found,[404] contrary to the original report.[19] that natural vitamin K_1 (2-methyl, 3-phytyl, 1, 4-naphthoquinone) (phytonadione) is more effective than the synthetic vitamin K (menadione).

Vitamin K_1 may be given by the intramuscular, subcutaneous, or intravenous route. It is given slowly by the intravenous route in severe deficiencies when bleeding is imminent or has occurred. The time needed for a response to the drug to be demonstrable depends on the cause of the deficiency and the amount of vitamin administered. Generally, bleeding is controlled in three to six hours. If the intravenous route is unavoidable, it is recommended that 10 to 25 mg. be administered slowly at a rate not exceeding 1 mg. per min., as severe toxic reactions have occurred with rapid intravenous administration.

Vitamin K_1 is also available in 5 mg. tablets for oral administration in non-emergency situations. Five to 10 mg. is given initially and the dosage adjusted depending on the clinical situation. In the presence of obstructive jaundice or biliary fistula, the concomitant administration of bile salts is necessary when the drug is given by mouth.

Synthetic vitamin K (menadione), supplied as the sodium salt of 2-methyl, 1, 4-naphthohydroquinone, is a water-soluble compound. It is supplied in 0.5 ml. ampules containing 2.5 mg. and in 1 ml. ampules containing 5 or 10 mg. It may be administered subcutaneously, intramuscularly, or intravenously. A 10 ml. ampule containing 72 mg. is available for intravenous administration in emergency situations.

Patients with hepatic insufficiency and associated hypoprothrombinemia usually have significant deficiencies in Factor V, Factor XIII, and fibrinogen in addition to having fibrinolysis and thrombocytopenia. The prothrombin complex concentrate contains Factors II, VII, IX, and X, but has no effect on the other coagulation defects associated with hepatic insufficiency. In consideration of the limited hemostatic benefits in patients with hepatic disease and the current high risk of hepatitis, the concentrates are presently contraindicated in these patients.[440]

In patients with vitamin K deficiency secondary to overdosage with coumarin anticoagulants, the concentrates containing the prothrombin complex have a dramatic effect. However, a similar, immediate response can be achieved with fresh single-donor plasma or within four to twelve hours after the use of intravenous vitamin K. The high risk of hepatitis must be weighed in individual circumstances.[167, 224, 440, 477]

Illustrative Case

CASE 1

This 10-year-old child was admitted to the hospital for investigation of a hemorrhagic diathesis. At birth she had a severe hemorrhage from the umbilicus, and over the succeeding years recurrent episodes of epistaxis, gastrointestinal hemorrhages, and multiple hematomas. Excessive bleeding often followed minor trauma but hemarthroses had not occurred.

Physical examination revealed only the presence of multiple bruises on the lower legs.

Laboratory examination. Erythrocyte count 4.58 mil. per cu.mm., leukocyte count 9880 per cu.mm., hemoglobin 10.5 gm. per 100 ml. Tourniquet test, bleeding time, clot retraction, and coagulation time were normal. Platelet count (indirect) 261,000 per cu.mm. Quick one-stage prothrombin time was 54 seconds with a control of 14 seconds.

On the patient's first admission at the age of 5 years, it was thought that she had idiopathic hypoprothrombinemia on the basis of the data then available.

During a subsequent admission, it was found that, when normal plasma was mixed with that of the patient, the prothrombin time was reduced but did not return to normal. The addition of "purified" prothrombin did not result in a normal one-stage prothrombin time. One part of serum when mixed with three parts of the patient's plasma resulted in a normal one-stage prothrombin time. On the basis of these studies it was felt that she probably had a Factor V deficiency.

The patient was then followed at another hospital where it was realized that she could not represent a Factor V deficiency since the one-stage prothrombin time was corrected by the addition of normal serum and not by normal plasma. Factor VII was described at that time, and it was noted that the clinical and laboratory findings of this patient fitted well with those of the Factor VII deficiency state. She was then carried as a Factor VII deficiency until the thromboplastin generation test became available. Once again she was re-evaluated. It was concluded that a deficiency of Factor X was responsible for her hemorrhagic diathesis.

Comment.   This case illustrates the growth of our knowledge of the first and second stage of blood coagulation. The patient was known to have abnormal bleeding which was not related to platelet or vessel factors. She was studied extensively with all the tests available during each hospitalization. A diagnosis of idiopathic hypoprothrombinemia was made when she was first admitted on the basis of the one-stage prothrombin time test. It was not until the thromboplastin generation test became available, and it was found that the substitution of this patient's serum for normal serum in the incubation mixture resulted in a reduction in thromboplastin activity, that she could be identified as having a Factor X defect.

DISORDERS AFFECTING THE THIRD STAGE OF BLOOD COAGULATION

Fibrinogen deficiency may be either congenital or acquired. The congenital variety is quite rare. Acquired fibrinogen deficiencies are more common, usually present as complications of certain surgical procedures or obstetric accidents, and are of grave importance.

Hereditary Quantitative Fibrinogen Deficiency

PATHOLOGIC PHYSIOLOGY

Congenital fibrinogen deficiency appears to be genetically transmitted as an autosomal recessive. In many of the reported cases the family history revealed consanguineous marriages in parents or grandparents.[15, 174, 310, 397]

In these cases the absence of fibrinogen prevents the coagulation process from completing its final phase, i.e., the conversion of fibrinogen to the fibrin clot. Thus a clot does not form. The arrest of small vessel hemorrhage is normal as it is brought about by vasoconstriction and platelet thrombi.[213] Lack of platelet fibrinogen results in abnormal adhesion of platelets to glass and decreased aggregation in response to small amounts of ADP. Platelet aggregation induced by high levels of ADP and connective tissue is normal, as is ADP release.[202, 252] These platelets behave normally in normal plasma. Menstrual bleeding is normal and seems to be controlled by vasoconstriction of endometrial arterioles.[298] These patients have been shown to have a decrease in synthesis of fibrinogen rather than an increase in its destruction. Minute traces of fibrinogen have been detected immunochemically in the blood and connective tissues of some of these patients, and the defect may not be absolute in all instances.[174] Others have been unable to detect fibrinogen by any method.[213]

CLINICAL EXAMINATION

The disorder is often manifested at birth by the occurrence of bleeding from the umbilical cord.[213, 310, 397, 451] The condition resembles Factor VIII deficiency clinically but usually is less severe.[15] Persistent bleeding may occur, however, in the wake of minor trauma, and spontaneous bleeding may occur into joint spaces or soft tissues. Crippling hemarthroses are extremely rare in this disorder.[310, 397] The thromboplastin generation test is normal since there is no defect in the early stage of clotting. Platelet count and tourniquet test are normal. In one-third of the reported cases the bleeding time has been variably prolonged, secondary to the lack of platelet fibrinogen.[202] The whole blood clotting time, one-stage prothrombin time, and thrombin time all require a fibrin clot as an end-point and are abnormal in the absence of fibrinogen. Fibrinogen assay reveals only minute traces or a complete absence of fibrinogen.

TREATMENT

The hemostatic defect in patients with congenital fibrinogen deficiency can be corrected by the administration of fibrinogen. One-half of the fibrinogen administered intravenously to patients with congenital afibrinogenemia has been reported to leave the circulation in 48 hours, and that remaining disappears with a half-life of approximately four days.[298] The early loss of one-half of the administered fibrinogen is thought to represent equilibration with the extravascular compartment.[174] The mass of plasma protein located in extravascular spaces is approximately equal to the mass of plasma protein circulating within the blood vessels, and the two are in dynamic equilibrium. As the extravascular deficit must be made up as well as that of the intravascular compartment, the first dose of fibrinogen administered will have less effect on the plasma fibrinogen level than will subsequent doses of comparable size. The level of fibrinogen required for hemostasis is reported to be 50 to 100 mg. per 100 ml. which can be obtained using fresh or stored plasma.[418] Transfusions of whole blood should be given to replace blood loss if need be.[397]

Hereditary Qualitative Fibrinogen Abnormalities

There have been many reports of inherited qualitative abnormalities in plasma fibrinogen.[158, 317, 332, 350, 522] These abnormal fibrinogens are named for the city in which they are discovered: e.g., fibrinogen Cleveland. Most of the reported individuals had no personal or family history of hemorrhagic diathesis. A few reports indicate a mild hemorrhagic diathesis, others, problems with wound healing, and some of the reported patients had thrombosis.[144, 158]

The defect is characterized in some by delayed aggregation of fibrin monomers.[198, 290] In others there is a defect in the release of the fibrinopeptides.[126] None has been reported that interfered with cross-linking by Factor XIII.[333] The defect is transmitted as an autosomal dominant, and in the heterozygotes a normal fibrinogen fraction can be identified.[522] A specific amino acid substitution has been identified in the plasma fibrinogen of one patient.[317]

Acquired qualitative fibrinogen abnormalities have been reported in various liver diseases; hepatocellular cancer, acute liver failure, and chronic hepatitis. The main abnormality in these instances was abnormal fibrin monomer aggregation.[333]

Acquired Fibrinogen Deficiency*

PATHOLOGIC PHYSIOLOGY

The mechanism by which the blood becomes depleted of fibrinogen in these conditions has been extensively studied. The fibrinogen level may be reduced as the result of deficient production (as in severe liver disease), excessive utilization (as in intravascular coagulation), increased destruction (as occurs in primary pathologic fibrinolysis), or some combination of these mechanisms.[40, 114, 398, 415, 416, 445, 462, 532] Separation of excessive utilization from excessive destruction is difficult but clinically important.

Liver injury has been known for many years to result in a decrease in plasma fibrinogen,[544] and some patients with severe hepatocellular disease have been found to have low levels of fibrinogen. It has been emphasized that the liver disease must be severe for the hypofibrinogenemia to occur, and that when it occurs the association is seldom in doubt.[335]

Widespread intravascular coagulation may stimulate fibrinolysis, which further reduces clotting Factors I, V, VIII, and X as the result of proteolysis.[328, 391, 445, 459] Proteolytic digestion of fibrinogen and fibrin results in split products, which are in themselves anticoagulant since they interfere with thrombin activity, platelet function, and fibrin polymerization.[459]

Primary pathologic fibrinolysis may occur as the result of the administration of excessive amounts of exogenous activator during thrombolytic therapy,[462] the release of excessive endogenous activator from neoplastic tissue,[500] or severe shock or anoxia.[462] Failure of the liver to remove circulating activators may also result in excessive proteolysis.[40, 415, 416, 462, 532] The syndrome of primary pathologic fibrinolysis is now considered to be rarely responsible for hypofibrino-

---

*See also p. 598, Ch. 16.

genemia.[458] The disturbance in hemostasis is not so profound as that associated with diffuse intravascular coagulation.

CLINICAL EXAMINATION

Acquired hypofibrinogenemia may be seen in association with diffuse hepatocellular disease, diffuse intravascular coagulation, or primary pathologic fibrinolysis. The clinical and laboratory findings are those of anemia, thrombosis, hemorrhage, and the underlying disease. Hepatocellular disease, anoxia, or shock of a severity to produce these findings is seldom in clinical doubt.

The development of hypofibrinogenemia in the course of disseminated intravascular coagulation, however, may be remarkably sudden. The occurrence of hypocoagulable or incoagulable blood in a patient previously free of hemorrhagic diathesis is dramatic in the acute form; in the subacute or chronic form it may go on for days or weeks.[36, 335]

Severe hemorrhage has been noted primarily in obstetric patients with the acute form of the syndrome. It may develop suddenly during labor or shortly thereafter, and is manifested by generalized bleeding and incoagulability of the blood. The acute form has been seen most frequently following abruptio placenta,[336, 445, 532] in association with amniotic fluid emboli,[415] and in septic abortion.[336] A similar syndrome has also been reported following pulmonary resections, allergic reactions, purpura fulminans, incompatible blood transfusions, septicemia, and severe burns.[32, 500, 501]

Patients with neoplastic disease and women with retained dead fetus generally have the subacute or chronic form, with excessive bruising, bleeding from the gums and nose, and thrombosis of superficial or deep veins.

The differential diagnosis between disseminated intravascular coagulation with secondary fibrinolysis, primary pathologic fibrinolysis, and the coagulopathy of severe liver disease is difficult because of overlapping laboratory findings. The level of clotting factors must always be considered in relation to the underlying disorder. In septicemia, for example, the plasma levels of fibrinogen and Factor VIII often are elevated. The finding of "normal" levels may represent the result of utilization of these factors in disseminated intravascular coagulation. There is no practical reliable way to detect intermediate products of coagulation or those which initiate intravascular coagulation.

Certain laboratory tests may be helpful. In *disseminated intravascular coagulation* the peripheral blood smear may show a reduction in platelets and schistocytes. These fragmented red blood cells, however, occur in fewer than 50 per cent of these patients.[255a] Fibrinogen and Factor VIII may be reduced relative to the level of these factors that would be expected in view of the underlying disorder. Prothrombin also is reduced and fibrin split products are present.

In the syndrome of *primary pathologic fibrinolysis*, the blood smear usually is normal. Fibrinogen and Factors V and VIII often are reduced as the result of degradation of these proteins by plasmin. Fibrin split products are present.

The *coagulation defects secondary to liver disease* are infrequently associated with reduced platelets. Blood coagulation factors, especially the Vitamin K-dependent factors may be reduced; Factor VIII is often normal or elevated. Fibrin split products are absent or present in small amounts. Clinical judgment and careful evaluation of the laboratory results will usually resolve the question.

TREATMENT

Once the diagnosis of disseminated intravascular coagulation is made, the underlying disease should be treated and appropriate supportive therapy instituted. Many episodes of defibrination are of short duration and no specific therapy is indicated in the absence of bleeding or anticipated surgery if the inciting cause can be controlled. If the defibrination is secondary to disseminated intravascular coagulation with associated fibrinolysis, anticoagulation with heparin may be indicated. Heparin therapy has often been useful in the management of chronic disseminated intravascular coagulation particularly that associated with the entrance of "thromboplastic" material into the circulation. When the syndrome is associated with sepsis or shock, the use of heparin remains controversial.[71a, 121a, 335a, 335, 463a]

If bleeding is a major manifestation of the syndrome, transfusion may be necessary. Packed red cells may be used to replace red cell loss. Fresh-frozen plasma contains Factors V and VIII, and may be helpful in this syndrome. These factors usually are present in low concentrations in stored plasma. Thrombocytopenia rarely requires specific therapy, but platelet transfusion is occasionally necessary.

Administration of purified fibrinogen is contraindicated if the coagulant agent is still present and active, since it might increase the propensity to thrombosis.[328] It may be indicated after the coagulation process is controlled, if the patient continues to bleed due to residual incoagulable blood. Since fibrinogen is prepared from pooled plasma, its administration is accompanied by a high risk of hepatitis.[386]

When primary pathologic fibrinolysis has resulted in defibrination, the treatment of choice is epsilon aminocaproic acid (EACA).[328, 335, 459, 462] EACA is one of several synthetic amino acids that are effective inhibitors of plasminogen activation.[297a, 360, 459] If this drug is given to a patient with disseminated intravascular coagulation without first controlling the coagulation process, there is always the potential hazard of further vascular occlusion as the result of inhibition of fibrinolysis.[175, 153a, 329a, 350, 458]

The severity of the process of disseminated intravascular coagulation depends on the amount and potency of the clot-promoting agent, the condition of the vascular endothelium, the rate of activation of the fibrinolytic system, the functional capacity of the hepatocellular system and the reticuloendothelial system.[98a] Once the mechanism responsible for the disorder is controlled, the split products formed during digestion of fibrinogen and fibrin are removed from the circulation by the reticuloendothelial system over a period of several hours. Since the severity of the disorder is critically dependent on the levels of fibrinogen and fibrin split products, their rapid removal contributes to the control of the hemorrhagic diathesis.

The clinical and hematologic problems presented by the defibrination syndrome vary so much from patient to patient that no standard therapy is possible. Acquired hypofibrinogenemia must be controlled to allow time to discover and treat the primary disease process. The differential diagnosis of the defibrination syndrome is often so difficult that the careful use of heparin and epsilon-aminocaproic acid together has been suggested.[328, 462]

Illustrative Case

History. In December, 1963 this 45-year-old housewife was admitted to the University Hospital for the second time because of migratory phlebitis of seven months' duration.

She first developed superficial thrombophlebitis in April, 1963 while in another hospital under observation for intermittent hypertension. Recurrent episodes of superficial and deep phlebitis over the next few weeks, despite the use of oral anticoagulants, prompted her first University of Virginia Hospital admission in May, 1963. At that time her left leg was edematous to the buttock and there was induration of the skin over the calf. Homans' sign was negative. The leg was cool and pale and unaffected by position. Physical examination was otherwise negative. Laboratory studies at that time were: hematocrit 36%, hemoglobin 10.1 gm.%, leukocyte count 12,200 per cm., and platelet count 377,000 per cu.mm.; stool examination for occult blood was negative three times. X-ray examination of the chest, gall bladder, and upper and lower gastrointestinal tract was negative. Consultation with the gynecologist and surgeon failed to reveal any evidence of malignancy. She was treated with Butazolidin, ferrous sulfate, and Coumadin, and discharged to the care of her physician.

Anticoagulation was continued, but in August, 1963 she again had thrombophlebitis in the right leg and required admission to her local hospital for five days.

Two weeks prior to the admission in December, 1963, the patient again developed swelling and redness with minimal pain in the calves of both legs despite continued oral anticoagulation, and was readmitted to her local hospital. In the week prior to admission she noted mild epistaxis and painful areas over the dorsum of her left hand and left neck; the ends of her toes became black and very painful two days prior to transfer to the University Hospital.

Physical examination. This revealed a moderately obese female in moderate distress. Blood pressure was 130/80, pulse 86, and temperature 99.2° F. There was a superficial bleeding point in the anterior nares on the nasal septum on the left. The liver edge extended the width of two fingers below the right costal margin and the upper border was in the seventh interspace. The spleen was not palpable. There was a large, firm, non-tender, moveable, irregular mass arising from the left side of the pelvis and extending into the lower abdomen to the level of the umbilicus. A tender, firm cord was noted in the course of a superficial vein on the dorsum of the left hand and another on the left side of the neck, thought to be in the external jugular vein. Both legs were swollen. The skin was slightly erythematous over the dorsum of the feet, and the distal portion of the toes was black. Blisters were noted on the dorsal surface of the great toes. The dorsalis pedis pulses were palpable bilaterally. Pelvic examination revealed a large, firm, irregular mass on the left which appeared to be attached to the fundus of the uterus.

Laboratory examination. Hematocrit was 32%, leukocyte count 9900 per cu.mm., and differential count normal. A thromboplastin generation test was performed using barium sulfate—absorbed plasma diluted $1/_{50}$ rather than $1/_{10}$ in order to delay the generation of thromboplastin activity; the minimal clotting time of eight minutes with a control of 14 minutes suggested more rapid development of thromboplastin activity.

Course.   The patient was transferred to surgery where a 10 × 15 cm. cystic tumor of the left ovary was removed. The tumor was not adherent to the surrounding structures, and there was no evidence of intraperitoneal metastatic disease. Intravenous and subcutaneous heparin therapy was begun and continued for the duration of her hospital stay. On the first postoperative day, 15 microcuries of radioactive chromic phosphate was installed intraperitoneally. The toes were treated by careful debridement of necrotic tissue. A staphylococcus aureus infection of the abdominal lesion, discovered on the 14th day, was successfully treated with penicillin. On the 21st hospital day, oral anticoagulation with coumarin was substituted for heparin therapy. The patient's feet continued to improve and she was discharged to the care of her physician.

No evidence of accelerated generation of thromboplastin activity could be detected in the patient's plasma when she returned in three months, and there was no clinical evidence of intravascular coagulation before her death from metastasis two years later.

Comment.   This patient with chronic disseminated intravascular coagulation demonstrates several points of interest. She had migratory phlebitis for seven months prior to the discovery of the tumor despite extensive

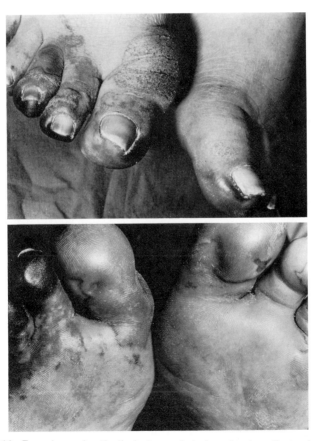

Figure 17–11 Two views of patient's feet on admission showing effects of vascular insufficiency, ranging from bleb formation to well demarcated areas of dry gangrene.

investigation for a malignant tumor. Severe hemorrhage was not a feature of the illness but modest epistaxis had occurred. The gangrene of the toes appeared quite similar to that seen with frostbite in which capillary circulation is bypassed by shunting; the presence of microthrombi in the small vessels cannot be excluded, however. Oral anticoagulants were not effective in preventing the continual thrombotic process before treatment of the malignancy.

Factor XIII (Fibrin Stabilizing Factor) Deficiency

The fibrin clot formed as the result of coagulation in whole blood or plasma is insoluble in 5 M urea, whereas the fibrin clot formed when purified fibrinogen in saline is exposed to thrombin is soluble in 5 M urea. This difference is due to the presence in whole blood and plasma of a factor capable of forming stabilizing covalent bonds between the fibrin filaments. Without this factor, the fibrin clot is held together only by hydrogen bonds and dissolves in a number of solvents which do not affect normal clots. The factor is known as Factor XIII, the fibrin stabilizing factor (FSF), or the L-L factor.[139, 303]

CLINICAL ASPECTS

Reports of patients with congenital deficiency of Factor XIII have emphasized the occurrence of umbilical hemorrhage 12 to 14 days after birth, repeated hematomas, and slow wound healing.[39, 252] Bleeding generally occurs 24 to 36 hours after injury. Family studies are compatible with an incompletely recessive autosomal inheritance of the trait.[145]

The acquired form may occur in association with multiple myeloma, lead poisoning, pernicious anemia, or cirrhosis of the liver.[304, 305, 367]

Patients with a deficiency of Factor XIII lack the capacity to form ϵ-(γ-glutamyl) lysine bridges between fibrin monomers and the normal insoluble fibrin lattice does not form.[154, 450]

New techniques for the identification of Factor XIII deficiency have been developed which allow study of heterozygotes and the effect of transfusions. Following transfusion of fresh plasma, the level of Factor XIII fell to pretransfusion levels in five or six days.[305, 344]

Fibrin stabilizing activity has been reported to be decreased in a variety of acquired disorders.[367]

TREATMENT

The defect is corrected by the administration of transfusions of small amounts of whole blood. The half-life of the factor appears to be about three days. Fresh plasma or cryoprecipitate is a good source of Factor XIII and has been used in the prophylactic treatment of patients with severe deficiency of this proenzyme.[23]

DISORDERS AFFECTING VESSEL AND/OR PLATELET FUNCTION AND BLOOD COAGULATION

Von Willebrand's Disease (Inherited Autosomal Hemorrhagic Diathesis with Antihemophilic Factor Deficiency and Prolonged Bleeding Time)

In 1926 von Willebrand described a hemorrhagic diathesis found in members of a family living on the Åland Islands off the coast of Finland. He designated the condition pseudohemophilia and felt that it resulted from abnormal platelet function. Several reports of cases of pseudohemophilia have since appeared in the literature. Generally, the patients reported have had clinical findings similar to those of the family described by von Willebrand, but the results of the laboratory tests have varied greatly. It now seems apparent that the term pseudohemophilia as used in the literature is not specific. Reassessment of the patients originally described by von Willebrand has made clear the nature of their defect[362] and it seems reasonable to refer to their disorder as von Willebrand's disease.

PATHOLOGIC PHYSIOLOGY

Von Willebrand's disease is inherited and transmitted as an autosomal dominant with varying degrees of expressivity.[86, 362, 363] Although the underlying cause of the defect in hemostasis is not understood, the disorder is manifested by a prolonged bleeding time and a decrease in Factor VIII. A defect in platelet function has been suspected since the original description of the disorder. Studies have indicated that Platelet Factor 3 (PF-3) is normal; the platelets have a normal surface charge and adhere normally to connective tissue.[541] Release of ADP by the platelets and their aggregation proceeds normally.[479]

A marked decrease in platelet adhesiveness to collagen has been demonstrated in vivo.[76] Decreased retention of platelets in columns of glass beads are often seen in vitro. A failure of the platelets of most patients to aggregate on exposure to the antibiotic ristocetin has been demonstrated in most cases. This drug causes aggregation of normal platelets.[246, 540, 542] The relationship of these defects to the prolonged bleeding time is not clear. Family studies have revealed that asymptomatic relatives of patients with von Willebrand's disease may have normal bleeding time and Factor VIII levels with abnormal platelet adhesiveness in vitro.[494]

A report has noted the association of intermittent thrombocytopenia with von Willebrand's disease.[359] In 1941 Macfarlane[311] demonstrated that the capillaries in the nail beds of some of these patients appeared bizarre and failed to constrict normally.

The abnormal bleeding time of these patients has been corrected by the infusion of normal or hemophilic plasma fraction 1–0.[121, 362, 385] This "bleeding time factor" in plasma fraction 1–0 is labile and lost on contact with glass. It is reported to correct abnormal platelet adhesiveness and ristocetin aggregation in vitro.[439, 540] The "bleeding time factor" is present in cryoprecipitate but not in commercially prepared Factor VIII concentrates.[385]

The Factor VIII level may be raised and the bleeding time simultaneously corrected by the administration of fraction 1-0 of normal plasma.[359, 362] Of immense interest is the report that improvement in Factor VIII levels and bleeding time could be obtained equally well using plasma from patients with classic hemophilia.[359, 362] Since such plasma contains little or no Factor VIII procoagulant, it must in some manner stimulate the release or synthesis of endogenous Factor VIII activity in patients with von Willebrand's disease.[53, 72, 121] The substances responsible for stimulating these patients to produce their own Factor VIII have not been completely identified. It appears to be concentrated in the fibrinogen fraction of the plasma, even in that prepared from "outdated" plasma. The serum contains this substance in good concentration, and it is present in cryoprecipitates.[53] Albumin and globulin contain no such activity.[69] It is not absorbed by $Ca_3(PO_4)_2$.

The decrease in Factor VIII levels found in many patients with von Willebrand's disease indicates that the regulation of Factor VIII is controlled by at least two genes: the X-chromosome gene which is abnormal in classic hemophilia and an autosomal gene which is abnormal in von Willebrand's disease.[190, 193, 535]

At the time of the original studies Factor VIII could be assayed only by its biologic activity in coagulation tests. Increased use of immunologic techniques has now allowed the recognition of the Factor VIII molecule independent of its coagulant activity and has provided interesting new information.[553] Patients with classic hemophilia have been shown to have normal plasma levels of Factor VIII antigen despite low levels of Factor VIII procoagulant.[146, 191, 197] The majority of patients with von Willebrand's disease have a Factor VIII antigen level which parallels the level of Factor VIII procoagulant.[48, 505] The rise in Factor VIII antigen which occurs following infusion of Factor VIII concentrate to patients with classical hemophilia remains elevated two to three times as long as does the Factor VIII procoagulant.[49] However, the rise in Factor VIII procoagulant in the plasma of patients with von Willebrand's disease, after the infusion of normal or hemophilic plasma, continues after the Factor VIII antigen has returned to preinfusion base line.[52]

Such studies indicate that the antigenic site and the site of biologic coagulant activity are not identical and may be dissociated in vivo. They appear to be metabolized differently in the two disorders.

Several variants of von Willebrand's disease have been reported.[278, 505] In one kindred the patients have proportionally normal or near-normal Factor VIII antigen and procoagulant levels with abnormal ristocetin-induced aggregation.[278, 504, 505] The relationship between reduced ristocetin-induced platelet aggregation, decreased platelet adhesiveness, and the long bleeding time in von Willebrand's disease is not yet established. Some studies suggest that they are all closely-related manifestations of a deficiency of Factor VIII antigen.[83, 84, 540, 543] If verified, the data would suggest that the von Willebrand's disease variant may be associated with a molecular abnormality of Factor VIII antigen affecting those functions.[505]

Von Willebrand's disease now appears to be a heterogeneous disorder which results from one or more qualitative or quantitative abnormalities in the Factor

VIII molecule. The reported variations in the laboratory and clinical findings in these patients suggest that Factor VIII procoagulant activity, Factor VIII-related antigen, and the factor responsible for correcting platelet function (ristocetin aggregation and bleeding time) may all vary independently.[43, 84, 244] The nature of von Willebrand's disease will not be completely understood until more is learned about the synthesis of Factor VIII and the molecular configuration that determines its biologic and immunologic characteristics.

It is of interest that a disorder resembling von Willebrand's disease has been reported in pigs and in dogs.[138] Acquired von Willebrand's disease occurring in the course of systemic lupus erythematosus has been reported in one patient.[472]

CLINICAL FEATURES

This disorder is often apparent in the first few weeks of life when spontaneous bleeding from the nose or gums may occur. Excessive bleeding often follows minor trauma. Uterine bleeding may be excessive and pregnancy is often complicated by bleeding episodes.[101, 121, 291, 363] Mucosal bleeding from the gastrointestinal tract may occur.[90] Neither petechiae nor hemarthroses are common in this disease. The great variability in the bleeding tendency in the same patient from time to time makes the clinical course difficult to anticipate, but it is rare for these patients to succumb during an episode of bleeding.

The hemorrhagic diathesis in these patients relates most clearly to the degree of Factor VIII deficiency,[69, 494] and adequate hemostatic control for surgery is usually maintained when adequate levels of Factor VIII are attained, though the Ivy bleeding time may not be shortened. In those patients with spontaneous bleeding, however, hemostatic control may not be adequate unless the Ivy bleeding time is also corrected.

The diagnosis of von Willebrand's disease can usually be established by the demonstration of a prolonged bleeding time and a decrease in Factor VIII level. The new ristocetin-induced platelet aggregation test appears to be very helpful, particularly in establishing the diagnosis in mildly affected heterozygotes.[246, 540, 543] The Ivy bleeding time has been shown to be more sensitive than the Duke bleeding time but both are useful. Tests of platelet adhesiveness are under continuing study but are not yet standardized.[206, 218, 232, 390, 438] The laboratory findings in this group of patients are not consistent from patient to patient or indeed in the same patient from one examination to the next.[13, 66, 361, 363, 449] Repeated testing may be necessary in order to establish the diagnosis.

TREATMENT

The fact that more than one disorder has been included under the name von Willebrand's disease in the past may be responsible for the wide variation reported in response to therapy.

Appropriate transfusion therapy can accomplish several important effects for these patients. The bleeding time may be corrected, Factor VIII levels restored, and the patient stimulated to produce his own Factor VIII for a period of one to two hours. The stimulation of endogenous Factor VIII makes it easier to raise and maintain adequate levels of Factor VIII in these patients than in patients with classic hemophilia. The use of fresh plasma and fresh-frozen plasma has been effective in the control of Factor VIII levels. The bleeding time is more difficult to correct, since the "bleeding time factor" is labile and lost on contact with glass. The finding that the "bleeding time factor" is present in cryoprecipitate makes it possible to correct the Factor VIII level and the bleeding time simultaneously.[53, 385] There was one report of a patient who became unresponsive to plasma following a large number of transfusions necessitated by persistent gastrointestinal bleeding. Neither the bleeding time nor the Factor VIII level would respond any longer to infusions of fresh plasma. An anti-Factor VIII inhibitor could not be demonstrated.[90]

The natural history of this disorder is extremely variable and it is difficult to interpret the efficacy of a particular therapeutic maneuver. Surgery may be a major hazard to these patients and should be avoided if possible. If surgery is unavoidable, the patient should be prepared by the administration of fresh or fresh-frozen plasma or cryoprecipitate, and these infusions should be repeated every second day until healing is complete.

Illustrative Case

History. A 50-year-old white married woman was admitted to the hospital for the extraction of several teeth. She had been known to be a "bleeder" all her life. Minor cuts and abrasions were followed by excessive bleeding in childhood, and there had been repeated epistaxis, subcutaneous hemorrhages, and oozing from the gums. At 18 years of age she had a severe hemorrhage which continued for two to three days following the extraction of a tooth. Following a miscarriage at the age of 33 she had intermittent bleeding for six months. Bleeding was finally controlled by the administration of a number of whole blood transfusions. There were, however, long intervals of freedom from any evidence of bleeding tendency.

She began to have severe pain as the result of dental caries while in her late thirties. Dental extractions were denied her on several occasions because of her history of a hemorrhagic diathesis. She was 42 years of age when Gelfoam and topical thrombin became available, and an extraction was successfully carried out using these agents. She was now admitted for further dental work, having had but one nosebleed of any significance in seven years and only rare vaginal spotting.

The patient's mother and father were first cousins. There was no history of any abnormal bleeding in either the parents or grandparents. Two brothers had died following hemorrhage in infancy, another brother died following uncontrollable epistaxis, and a fourth brother bled to death during an appendectomy. A fifth committed suicide. The remaining five siblings were alive and well without historic evidence of abnormal bleeding.

A review of the old record revealed marked variability of the bleeding time and the fact that the coagulation time was somewhat prolonged occasionally. Prothrombin time, platelet counts, and clot retraction were consistently normal. The results of the tourniquet test varied and from time to time were slightly positive. On one occasion the bleeding time was noted to be 17½ minutes from one ear lobe while at the same time it was 180 minutes in the other. There was also striking evidence that the infusion of whole blood affected the bleeding time. On one occasion the capillaries were visualized directly, and it was noted that they did not retract properly after being punctured with a needle.

Physical examination.   In addition to dental caries for which the patient was admitted, the only positive physical finding was very slight hepatomegaly.

Laboratory findings.   The red blood cell count was 3.5 mil. per cu.mm.; hemoglobin 9.6 gm. per 100 ml., hematocrit 29%, and platelets 364,000 per cu.mm. The bleeding time was discontinued at 15 minutes, the coagulation time was 13 mintues, and the thromboplastin generation test revealed a depression of Factor VIII.

Course.   The patient was given prednisone and 3 units of fresh (four to six hours' old) blood. The bleeding time and thromboplastin generation test returned to normal and she tolerated the removal of three teeth without excessive bleeding. Within 48 hours the bleeding time was again prolonged despite continued administration of prednisone. Five hundred ml. of fresh plasma was given, and once again the bleeding time was returned to normal. She tolerated the removal of two more teeth without excessive bleeding.

Comment.   The history presented indicates the variability of the clinical manifestations of this disorder. There is clear evidence that the bleeding time was affected both by whole blood transfusions and plasma transfusions. The patient's platelets were normal in the thromboplastin generation test. The decreased Factor VIII and prolonged bleeding time indicates the similarity of this patient's disorder to those described by von Willebrand, though this patient's defect may have been inherited as an autosomal recessive. The clinical course was favorably altered by the administration of fresh plasma. The administration of adrenocortical steroids was not considered to have played a role in the correction of the bleeding time, since it was prolonged again 48 hours after administration of fresh whole blood despite their continued administration. In retrospect, the use of dental splints as described under the treatment of Factor VIII deficiency may have obviated some of this patient's difficulty with extraction.

References

1. Aas, K. A., and Gardner, F. H.: Survival of blood platelets labeled with Chromium[51]. J. Clin. Invest.,*37*:1257, 1958.
2. Aballi, A. J., Banus, V. L., deLamerens, S., and Rozengvaig, S.: Coagulation studies in the newborn period. III. Hemorrhagic disease of the newborn. Am. J. Dis. Child., *97*:524, 1959.
3. Aballi, A. J., Banus, V. L., deLamerens, S., and Rozengvaig, S.: Coagulation studies in the newborn period. IV. Deficiency of Stuart-Prower factor as a part of the clotting defect of the newborn. Am. J. Dis. Child., *97*:549, 1959.
4. Abramson, N., Eisenberg, P. D., and Aster, R. H.: Post-transfusion purpura: immunologic aspects and therapy. N. Engl. J. Med.,*291*:1163, 1974.
5. Ackerman, B. D., Taylor, W. F., Ingman, M. J., and O'Loughlin, B. J.: Diagnosis and treatment of congenital rubella. G. P., *40*:137, 1969.

6. Ackroyd, J. F.: The pathogenesis of thrombocytopenic purpura due to hypersensitivity to Sedormid (allyl-isopropyl acetylcarbamide). Clin. Sci., 7:249, 1949.
7. Ackroyd, J. F.: Allergic purpura, including purpura due to foods, drugs, and infection. Am. J. Med., 14:605, 1953.
8. Ackroyd, J. F.: The role of Sedormid in the immunologic reaction that results in platelet lysis in Sedormid purpura. Clin. Sci., 13:409, 1954.
9. Ackroyd, J. F.: Function of factor VII. Br. J. Haematol., 2:397, 1956.
10. Ackroyd, J. F.: The immunological basis of purpura due to drug hypersensitivity. Proc. Roy. Soc. Med., 55:30, 1962.
11. Adner, M. M., Fisch, G. R., Starobin, S. B., and Aster, R. N.: Use of compatible platelet transfusions in treatment of congenital iso-immune thrombocytopenic purpura. N. Engl. J. Med., 280:244, 1969.
12. Aggeler, P. M., White, S. G., Glendening, M. B., Pope, E. W., Leake, T. B., and Bates, G. B.: Plasma thromboplastin component (PTC) deficiency: a new disease resembling hemophilia. Proc. Soc. Exp. Biol. Med., 79:692, 1952.
13. Alexander, B., and Goldstein, R.: Dual hemostatic defect in pseudohemophilia. J. Clin. Invest. 32:551, 1953. (Abstr.)
14. Alexander, B., Goldstein, R., Landwehr, G., and Cook, C. D.: Congenital SPCA deficiency: a hitherto unrecognized coagulation defect with hemorrhage rectified by serum and serum fractions. J. Clin. Invest., 30:596, 1951.
15. Alexander, B., Goldstein, R., Rich, L., LeBolloc'h, A. G., and Diamond, L. K.: Congenital afibrinogenemia. Blood, 9:843, 1954.
16. Ali, A. M., Gandy, R. H., Britten, M. L., and Dormandy, K. M.: Joint hemorrhage in haemophilia: is full advantage taken of plasma therapy? Br. Med. J., 3:828, 1967.
17. Allen, D. M., Diamond, L. K., and Howell, D. A.: Anaphylactoid purpura in children (Schönlein-Henoch syndrome). Am. J. Dis. Child., 99:833, 1960.
18. Almquist, H. J.: Purification of the antihemorrhagic vitamin. J. Biol. Chem., 114:241, 1936.
19. Almquist, H. J., and Klose, A. A.: Antihemorrhagic activity of 2-methyl-1,4-naphthoquinone. J. Biol. Chem., 130:787, 1939.
20. Almquist, H. J., and Stokstad, E. L. R.: Hemorrhagic chick disease of dietary origin. J. Biol. Chem., 111:105, 1935.
21. Amir, J., and Krauss, S.: Treatment of thrombotic thrombocytopenic purpura with antiplatelet drugs. Blood, 42:27, 1973.
22. Amorosi, E. L., and Ultman, J. E.: Thrombotic thrombocytopenic purpura. Medicine, 45:139, 1966.
23. Amris, C. J., and Hilden, M.: Treatment of Factor XIII deficiency with cryoprecipitate. Thromb. Diath. Haemorrh., 20:528, 1968.
24. Ancona, G. C., Ellenhorn, W. J., and Falconer, E. H.: Purpura due to food sensitivity. J. Allergy, 22:487, 1951.
25. Andersen, B. R., and Terry, W. D.: Gamma G4-globulin antibody causing inhibition of clotting Factor VIII. Nature, 217:174, 1968.
26. Antley, M., and McMillan, C. W.: Sequential coagulation studies in purpura fulminans. N. Engl. J. Med., 276:1287, 1967.
27. Arcomano, J. P., and Eskes, P. W. H.: "Schönlein-Henoch syndrome." Am. J. Dis. Child., 114:674, 1967.
28. Ashford, T. P., and Freiman, D. G.: The role of the endothelium in the initial phases of thrombosis: electron microscopic study. Am. J. Pathol., 50:257, 1967.
29. Aster, R. H.: Pooling of platelets in the spleen: role in the pathogenesis of "hypersplenic" thrombocytopenia. J. Clin. Invest., 45:645, 1966.
30. Aster, R. H., and Jandle, J. H.: Platelet sequestration in man. I. Methods. II. Immunological and clinical studies. J. Clin. Invest., 43:843, 856, 1964.
31. Aster, R. H., and Keene, W. R.: Site of platelet destruction in idiopathic thrombocytopenic purpura. Br. J. Haematol., 16:61, 1969.
32. Astrup, T.: Fibrinolysis in the organism. Blood, 11:781, 1956.
33. Atkins, H. J., Wolff, J. A., and Sitarz, A.: Giant hemangioma in infancy with secondary thrombocytopenic purpura. Am. J. Roentgenol., 89:1062, 1963.
34. Austen, D. E. G.: Factor VIII of small molecular weight and its aggregation. Br. J. Haematol., 27:89, 1974.
35. Ayoub, E. M., and Hoyer, J.: Anaphylactoid purpura: streptococcal antibody titers and B gammaglobulin levels. J. Pediatr., 75:193, 1969.
36. Baker, L. R. I., Rubenberg, M. L., Dalie, J. V., and Brain, M. C.: Fibrinogen catabolism in microangiopathic haemolytic anaemia. Br. J. Haematol., 14:617, 1968.

37. Barrow, E. M., Heindel, C. C., Roberts, H. R., and Graham, J. B.: Heterozygosity and homozygosity in von Willebrand's disease. Proc. Soc. Exp. Biol. Med., *118*:684, 1965.

38. Barrow, M. V., Quick, D. T., and Cunningham, R. W.: Salicylate hypoprothrombinemia in rheumatoid arthritis with liver disease. Arch. Intern. Med., *120*:620, 1967.

39. Barry, A., and Delâge, J. M.: Congenital deficiency of fibrin-stabilizing factor: observation of a new case. N. Engl. J. Med., *272*:943, 1965.

40. Barry, A. P., Geoghegan, F., and Shea, S. M.: Acquired fibrinopenia in pregnancy. Br. Med. J., *2*:287, 1955.

41. Baudo, F., de Cataldo, F., Josso, F., Silvello, L., and Tarallo, P.: Hereditary hypoprothrombinaemia. True deficiency of Factor II. Acta Haematol., *47*:243, 1972.

42. Ballard, H. S., Eisinger, R. P., and Gallo, G.: Renal manifestations of the Henoch–Schönlein syndrome in adults. Am. J. Med., *49*:328, 1970.

43. Baugh, R., Brown, J., Sargent, R., and Hougie, C.: Separation of human Factor VIII activity from the von Willebrand's antigen and ristocetin platelet aggregating activity. Biochem. Biophys. Acta, *371*:360, 1974.

44. Bayer, W. L., Dario, C. C., Szeto, I. L. F., and Lewis, J. H.: Acquired Factor X deficiency in a Negro boy. J. Pediatr., *44*:1007, 1969.

45. Bayer, W. L., Sherman, F. E., Michaels, R. H., Szeto, I. L. F., and Lewis, J. H.: Purpura in congenital and acquired rubella. N. Engl. J. Med., *273*:1362, 1965.

46. Beck, P., Giddings, J. C., and Bloom, A. L.: Inhibitor of Factor VIII in mild haemophilia. Br. J. Haematol., *17*:283, 1969.

47. Bennett, B.: Annotation: anti-haemophilic factor, normal and abnormal. Br. J. Haematol., *26*:1, 1974.

48. Bennett, B., and Ratnoff, O. D.: Studies on the response of patients with classic hemophilia to transfusion with concentrates of antihemophilic factor. J. Clin. Invest., *51*:2593, 1972.

49. Bennett, B., and Ratnoff, O. D.: Functional deficiencies of antihemophilic factor (AHF, Factor VIII). Thromb. Diath. Haemorrh. (Suppl.), *54*:197, 1973.

50. Bennett, B., and Ratnoff, O. D.: Detection of the carriers of hemophilia. N. Engl. J. Med., *288*:342, 1973.

51. Bennett, B., Ratnoff, O. D., Holt, J. B., and Roberts, H. R.: Hageman trait (Factor XII deficiency): a probable second genotype inherited as an autosomal dominant characteristic. Blood, *40*:412, 1972.

52. Bennett, B., Ratnoff, O. D., and Levin, J.: Immunologic studies in von Willebrand's disease. J. Clin. Invest., *51*:2597, 1972.

53. Bennett, E., and Dormandy, K.: Pool's cryoprecipitate and exhausted plasma in the treatment of von Willebrand's disease and Factor XI deficiency. Lancet, *2*:731, 1966.

54. Bennington, J. L., Fonty, R. A., and Hougie, C.: Laboratory Diagnosis. Collier-Macmillan, Ltd., London, 1970, p. 522.

55. Beresford, O. D.: Hereditary haemorrhagic telangiectasia with pulmonary arteriovenous fistula. Br. J. Dis. Chest, *61*:219, 1967.

56. Berger, H.: Cause of drug-induced thrombocytopenic purpura identified by the passive transfer reaction. Ann. Intern. Med., *56*:618, 1962.

56a. Bernhardt, B., Valletta, M., Brook, J., and Lejneiks, I.: Amyloidosis with Factor X deficiency. Am. J. Med. Sci., *264*:411, 1972.

57. Bernstock, L., and Herson, C.: Thrombotic thrombocytopenic purpura. Remission on treatment with heparin. Lancet, *1*:28, 1960.

58. Bettex-Galland, M., and Lüscher, E. F.: Extraction of an actomyosin-like protein from human thrombocytes. Nature, *184*:276, 1959.

59. Bick, R. L., Adams, T., and Radack, K.: Surgical hemostasis with a Factor XI-containing concentrate. J.A.M.A., *229*:163, 1974.

60. Bidwell, E.: The purification of bovine antihaemophilic globulin. Br. J. Haematol., *1*:35, 1955.

61. Biggs, R.: Fractions rich in Factor VIII. Bibl. Haematol., *29*:1122, 1968.

62. Biggs, R., Bidwell, E., Handley, D. A., Macfarlane, R. G., Trueta, J., Elliot-Smith, A., Dike, G. W. R., and Ash, B. J.: The preparation and assay of a Christmas-factor (factor IX) concentrate and its use in the treatment of two patients. Br. J. Haematol., *7*:349, 1961.

63. Biggs, R., and Denson, K. W. E.: The fate of prothrombin and Factors VIII, IX and X transfused to patients deficient in these factors. Br. J. Haematol., *9*:532, 1963.

64. Biggs, R., and Douglas, A. S.: The thromboplastin generation test. J. Clin. Pathol., *6*:23, 1953.

65. Biggs, R., Douglas, A. S., Macfarlane, R. G., Dacie, J. V., Pitney, W. R., Merskey, C., and O'Brien, J. R.: Christmas disease. Br. Med. J., *2*:1378, 1952.

66. Biggs, R., and Macfarlane, R. G.: Haemophilia and related conditions. Br. J. Haematol., *4*:1, 1958.

67. Biggs, R., and Macfarlane, R. G.: Christmas disease. Postgrad. Med. J., *38*:3, 1962.
68. Biggs, R., and Macfarlane, R. G.: Treatment of Haemophilia and Other Coagulation Disorders. F. A. Davis Co., Philadelphia, 1966, p. 246.
69. Biggs, R., and Matthews, J. M.: The treatment of haemorrhage in von Willebrand's disease and the blood level of factor VIII (AHG). Br. J. Haematol., *9*:203, 1963.
70. Bithell, T. C., Didisheim, P., Cartwright, G. E., and Wintrobe, M. M.: Thrombocytopenia inherited as an autosomal dominant trait.Blood, *25*:231, 1965.
71. Bithell, T. C., Parekh, S. J., and Strong, R. R.: Platelet-function studies in the Bernard–Soulier syndrome. Am. N. Y. Acad. Sci., *201*:145, 1972.
71a. Blix, S.: Anticoagulant treatment of the defibrination syndrome. Acta Med. Scand., *181*:597, 1967.
72. Blombäck, M., Jorpes, J. E., and Nilsson, I. M.: Von Willebrand's disease. Am. J. Med., *34*:236, 1963.
73. Bok, J., Veltkamp, J. J., and Loeliger, E. A.: Moderate Factor XII deficiency. Thromb. Diath. Haemorrh., *13*:8, 1965.
74. Bonnin, J. A., Cohen, A. K., and Hicks, N. D.: Coagulation defects in a case of systemic lupus erythematosus with thrombocytopenia. Br. J. Haematol., *2*:168, 1956.
75. Booyse, F., Kisieleski, D., Seeler, R., and Rafelson, M., Jr.: Possible thrombosthenin defect in Glanzmann's thrombasthenia. Blood, *39*:377, 1972.
76. Borchgrevink, C. F.: Platelet adhesion in vivo in patients with bleeding disorders. Acta Med. Scand., *170*:231, 1961.
77. Borchgrevink, C. F., and Owren, P. A.: Surgery in a patient with Factor V (proaccelerin) deficiency. Acta Med. Scand., *170*:743, 1961.
78. Borchgrevink, C. F., Egeberg, O., Pool, J. G., Skulason, T., Stormorken, H., and Waaler, B.: A study of a case of congenital hypoprothrombinemia. Br. J. Haematol., *5*:294, 1959.
79. Borges, W. H.: Anaphylactoid purpura. Med. Clin. North Am., *56*:201, 1972.
80. Borman, J. B., and Schiller, M.: Osler's disease with multiple large vessel aneurysms. Angiology, *20*:113, 1969.
81. Born, G. V. R.: Changes in the distribution of phosphorus in platelet-rich plasma during clotting. Biochem. J., *68*:695, 1958.
82. Born, G. V. R., and Esnouf, M. P.: Appearance of a phosphorus compound in platelet-rich plasma on clotting. Nature, *183*:478, 1959.
83. Bouma, B. N., van Mourik, J. A., Sixma, J. J., Mochtar, I. A., Wiegerinck, Y., and de Graaf, S.: Von Willebrand factor and antihemophilic Factor A (Factor VIII). Thromb. Diath. Haemorrh. (Suppl.), *54*:191, 1973.
84. Bouma, B. N., Wiegerinck, Y., Sixma, J. J., van Mourik, J. A., and Mochtar, J. A.: Immunological characterization of purified anti-haemophilic Factor A (Factor VIII) which corrects abnormal platelet retention in von Willebrand's disease. Nature (New Biol.), *236*:104, 1972.
85. Bouroncle, B. A., and Doan, C. A.: Treatment of refractory idiopathic thrombocytopenic purpura. J.A.M.A., *207*:2049, 1969.
86. Bowie, E. J., Didisheim, P., Thompson, J. H., Jr., and Owen, C. A.: The spectrum of von Willebrand's disease. Thromb. Diath. Haemorrh., *18*:40, 1967.
87. Bowie, E . J. W., and Owen, C. A., Jr.: Thrombopathy. Semin. Hematol., *5*:73, 1968.
88. Bowie, E. J. W., Thompson, J. H., Jr., and Owen, C. A., Jr.: The blood platelet (including a discussion of the qualitative platelet diseases). Proc. Mayo Clinic, *40*:625, 1965.
89. Brain, M. C., Dacie, J. V., and Hourihane, D. O'B.: Microangiopathic haemolytic anaemia: the possible role of vascular lesions in pathogenesis. Br. J. Haematol., *8*:358, 1962.
90. Brandstaetter, S., Scharf, J., Salomon, H., and Tatarsky, I.: Gastrointestinal bleeding in von Willebrand's disease. Arch. Intern. Med., *118*:108, 1966.
91. Branehög, I., Kutti, J., and Weinfeld, A.: Platelet survival and platelet production in idiopathic thrombocytopenic purpura. Br. J. Haematol., *27*:127, 1974.
92. Breckenridge, R. T., Moore, R. D., and Ratnoff, O.: A study of thrombocytopenia. New histologic criteria for the differentiation of idiopathic thrombocytopenia and thrombocytopenia associated with disseminated lupus erythematosus. Blood, *30*:39, 1967.
93. Breckenridge, R. T., and Ratnoff, O. D.: Studies on the site of action of a circulating anticoagulant in disseminated lupus erythematosus. Am. J. Med., *35*:813, 1963.
94. Breen, F. A., and Tullis, J. L.: Prothrombin concentrates in treatment of Christmas disease and allied disorders. J.A.M.A., *208*:1848, 1969.
95. Brinkhous, K. M., Carnery, C. N., and Shermer, R. W.: Use of high-potency antihemophilia factor concentrates in prophylaxis. Thromb. Diath. Haemorrh. (Suppl.), *43*:139, 1971.
96. Brinkhous, K. M., Langdell, R. D., Penick, G. D., Graham, J. B., and Wagner, R. H.: Newer approaches to the study of hemophilia and hemophilioid states. J.A.M.A., *154*:481, 1954.
97. Brinkhous, K. M., Shanbrom, E., Roberts, H. R., Webster, W. P., Fekete, L., and Wagner,

R. N.: A new high-potency glycine-precipitated antihemophilic factor (AHF) concentrate. J.A.M.A., *205*:613, 1968.

98. Brinkley, S. B., MacCorquodale, D. W., Thayer, S. A., and Doisy, E. A.: The isolation of vitamin K₁. J. Biol. Chem., *130*:219, 1939.

98a. Brodsky, I., and Siegel, N. H.: The diagnosis and treatment of disseminated intravascular coagulation. Med. Clin. North Am., *54*:555, 1970.

99. Brown, P. E., Hougie, C., and Roberts, H. R.: The genetic heterogeneity of hemophilia B. N. Engl. J. Med., *283*:61, 1970.

100. Brozovic, M., Stirling, Y., Harricks, C., North, W. R. S., and Meade, T. W.: Factor VIII in an industrial population. Br. J. Haematol., *28*:381, 1974.

101. Buchanan, J. C., and Leavell, B. S.: Pseudohemophilia: report of 13 new cases and statistical review of previously reported cases. Ann. Intern. Med., *44*:241, 1956.

102. Bunting, W. L., Kiely, J. M., and Campbell, D. C.: Idiopathic thrombocytopenic purpura. Arch. Intern. Med., *108*:733, 1961.

103. Caen, J., Castaldi, P. A., Leclerc, J. C., Inceman, S., Larrieu, M. J., Probst, M., and Bernard, J.: Congenital bleeding disorders with long bleeding time and normal platelet count. I. Glanzmann's thrombasthenia (report of 15 patients). Am. J. Med., *41*:4, 1966.

104. Caen, J., and Cousin, C.: Le trouble d'adhésivité "in vivo" des plaquettes dans la maladie de Willebrand et les thrombasthénies de Glanzmann. Nouv. Rev. Fr. Hematol., *2*:685, 1962.

105. Caen, J. P., Sultan, Y., and Larrieu, M. J.: New familial platelet disease. Lancet, *1*:203, 1968.

106. Carpenter, A. F., Wintrobe, M. M., Fuller, E. A., Hunt, A., and Cartwright, G. E.: Treatment of idiopathic thrombocytopenic purpura. J.A.M.A., *171*:1911, 1959.

107. Casey, T. P., and Matthews, J. R. D.: Thrombocytopenic purpura in infectious mononucleosis. N. Z. Med. J., *77*:318, 1973.

108. Choi, S. F., McClure, P. D., and Vranic, M.: Thrombopoietin activity in idiopathic thrombocytopenic purpura. Br. J. Haematol., *15*:345, 1968.

109. Clancy, R., Jenkins, E., and Firkin, B.: Qualitative platelet abnormalities in idiopathic thrombocytopenic purpura. N. Engl. J. Med., *286*:622, 1972.

110. Cohen, P., and Gardner, F. H.: The thrombocytopenic effect of sustained high-dosage prednisone therapy in thrombocytopenic purpura. N. Engl. J. Med., *265*:611, 1961.

111. Coldwell, B. B., and Zawidzka, Z.: Effect of acute administration of acetylsalicylic acid on the prothrombin activity of bishydroxycoumarin-treated rats. Blood, *32*:945, 1968.

112. Conley, C. L., Evans, R. S., Harrington, W. J., Schwartz, S. O., and Dameshek, W.: Panels in therapy. X. Treatment of acute ITP. Blood, *11*:384, 1956.

113. Conley, C. L., Rathbun, H. K., Morse, W. I., II, and Robinson, J. E., Jr.: Circulating anticoagulant as a cause of hemorrhagic diathesis in man. Johns Hopkins Hosp. Bull., *83*:288, 1948.

114. Connor, W. E., Hoak, J. C., and Warner, E. D.: Massive thrombosis produced by fatty acid infusion. J. Clin. Invest., *42*:860, 1963.

115. Cooke, J. V., Holland, P. V., and Shulman, N. R.: Cryoprecipitate concentrates of Factor VIII for surgery in hemophiliacs. Ann. Intern. Med., *68*:39, 1968.

116. Cooper, L. Z., Green, R. H., Krugman, S., Giles, J. P., and Mirick, G. S.: Neonatal thrombocytopenic purpura and other manifestations of rubella contracted in utero. Am. J. Dis. Child., *110*:416, 1965.

117. Cooper, L. Z., Ziring, P. R., Ockerse, A. B., Fedun, B. A., Kiely, B., and Krugman, S.: Rubella: clinical manifestations and management. Am. J. Dis. Child., *118*:18, 1969.

118. Cooper, M. D., Chase, H. P., Lowman, J. T., Krivit, W., and Good, R. A.: Immunologic defects in patients with Wiskott–Aldrich syndrome. Birth Defects., *4*:378, 1968.

119. Cooper, T., Stickney, J. M., Pease, G. L., and Bennett, W. A.: Thrombotic thrombocytopenic purpura. Am. J. Med., *13*:374, 1952.

120. Corn, M., and Upshaw, J. D.: Evaluation of platelet antibodies in idiopathic thrombocytopenic purpura. Arch. Intern. Med., *109*:157, 1962.

121. Cornu, P., Larrieu, M. J., Caen, J., and Bernard, J.: Transfusion studies in von Willebrand's disease. Effect on bleeding time and Factor VIII. Br. J. Haematol., *9*:189, 1963.

121a. Corrigan, J. J., Jr., and Jordan, C. M.: Heparin therapy in septicemia with disseminated intravascular coagulation. N. Engl. J. Med., *283*:778, 1970.

122. Cram, D. L., and Soley, R. L.: "Purpura fulminans." Brit. J. Dermatol., *80*:323, 1963.

123. Cream, J. J., Gumpel, J. M., and Peachey, R. D. G.: Schönlein–Henoch purpura in the adult. Q. J. Med., *39*:461, 1970.

124. Cronberg, S., and Nilsson, I. M.: Investigation of patients with mild thrombasthenia–a haemorrhagic disorder with prolonged bleeding time probably due to a primary platelet defect. Acta Med. Scand., *183*:163, 1968.

125. Cronberg, S., and Nilsson, I. M.: Circulating anticoagulant against Factors XI and XII together with massive spontaneous platelet aggregation. Scand. J. Haematol., *10*:309, 1973.

126. Crum, E. D., Shainoff, J. R., Graham, R. C., and Ratnoff, O. D.: Fibrinogen Cleveland. II. An abnormal fibrinogen with defective release of fibrinopeptide A. J. Clin. Invest., *53*:1308, 1974.
127. Dam, H.: The antihemorrhagic vitamin of the chick. Biochem. J., *29*:1273, 1935.
128. Dam, H., and Schonheyder, F.: A deficiency disease in chicks resembling scurvy. Biochem. J., *28*:1355, 1934.
129. Davis, C. E., Robbins, R. S., Weller, R. D., and Braude, A. I.: Thrombocytopenia in experimental trypanosomiasis. J. Clin. Invest., *53*:1359:1974.
130. Deliyannis, A. A., Kontopoulou-Griva, I., and Tsevrenis, H. V.: Normal platelet aggregating properties of Ehlers–Danlos syndrome "collagen." Thromb. Diath. Haemorrh., *32*:203, 1974.
131. Dellipiani, A. W., and George, M.: Syndrome of sclerodactyly, calcinosis. Reynaud's phenomenon and telangiectasia. Br. Med. J., *4*:334, 1967.
132. Denson, K. W. E.: Abnormal forms of Factor X. Lancet, *2*:1256, 1969.
133. Denson, K. W. E.: The levels of Factors II, VII, IX, and X by antibody neutralization techniques in the plasma of patients receiving phenindione therapy. Br. J. Haematol., *20*:643, 1971.
134. Denson, K. W. E., Biggs, R., Borrett, H. R., and Cobb, K.: Two types of haemophilia (A$^+$ and A$^-$): a study of 48 cases. Br. J. Haematol., *17*:163, 1969.
135. DePalma, A.: Hemophilic arthropathy. Clinical orthopedics and related research. 52:145, 1967.
136. Derham, R. J., and Rogerson, M. M.: The Schönlein-Henoch syndrome and collagen disease. Arch. Dis. Child., *27*:139, 1952.
137. Djerassi, I., Farber, S., and Evans, A. E.: Transfusions of fresh platelet concentrates to patients with secondary thrombocytopenia. N. Engl. J. Med., *268*:221, 1963.
138. Dodds, W. J.: Canine von Willebrand's disease. J. Lab. Clin. Med., *76*:713, 1970.
139. Duckert, F., Jung, E., and Shmerling, D. H.: A hitherto undescribed congenital haemorrhagic diathesis probably due to fibrin stabilizing factor deficiency. Thromb. Diath. Haemorrh., *5*:179, 1961.
140. Dudgeon, D. L., Kellogg, D. R., Gilchrist, G. S., and Woolley, M. W.: Purpura fulminans. Arch. Surg., *103*:351, 1971.
141. Dyer, N. H.: Cerebral abscess in hereditary haemorrhagic telangiectasia: report of two cases in a family. J. Neurol. Neurosurg. Psychiatry, *30*:563, 1967.
142. Edson, J. R., White, J. G., and Krivit, W.: The enigma of severe Factor XI deficiency without hemorrhagic symptoms. Thromb. Diath. Haemorrh., *18*:342, 1967.
143. Egeberg, O.: Blood Factor XI after fat-rich meals. Thromb. Diath. Haemorrh., *15*:390, 1966.
144. Egeberg, O.: Inherited abnormality causing thrombophilia. Thromb. Diath. Haemorrh., *17*:176, 1967.
145. Egeberg, O.: New families with hereditary hemorrhagic trait due to deficiency of fibrin stabilizing factor (F. 13). Thromb. Diath. Haemorrh., *20*:534, 1968.
146. Ekert, H., Helliger, H., and Muntz, R. H.: Antihaemophilic-factor-like protein in haemophilia. Med. J. Aust., *2*:210, 1973.
147. Ekert, H., Helliger, H., and Muntz, R. H.: Detection of carriers of haemophilia. Thrombosis, *30*:255, 1973.
148. Evensen, S. A., Solum, N. O., Grøttum, A., and Hovig, T.: Familial bleeding disorder with a moderate thrombocytopenia and giant blood platelets. Scand. J. Haematol., *13*:203, 1974.
149. Fantl, P.: Parahemophilia (proaccelerin deficiency) occurrence and biochemistry. *In* Brinkhous, K. M. (ed.): Hemophilia and Hemophilioid Diseases. University of North Carolina Press, Chapel Hill, 1957, p. 79.
150. Fantl, P., and Nance, M. H.: An acquired haemorrhagic disease in a female due to an inhibitor of blood coagulation. Med. J. Aust., *2*:125, 1946.
151. Feinstein, D., Chong, M. N. Y., Kasper, C. K., and Rapaport, S. I.: Hemophilia A: polymorphism detectable by a Factor VIII antibody. Science, *163*:1071, 1969.
151a. Feinstein, D. I., and Rapaport, S. I.: Acquired inhibitors of blood coagulation. *In* Progress in Hemostasis and Thrombosis. Spaet, T. H. (ed.) Grune and Stratton, New York, 1972, p. 75.
152. Feinstein, D. I., Rapaport, S. I., McGehee, W. G., and Patch, M. J.: Factor V anticoagulants: clinical biochemical and immunological observations. J. Clin. Invest., *49*:1578, 1970.
153. Finch, S. C., Castro, O., Cooper, M., Covey, W., Erichson, R., and McPhedran, P.: Immunosuppressive therapy of chronic idiopathic thrombocytopenic purpura. Am. J. Med., *56*:4, 1974.
153a. Fisher, S., Fletcher, A. P., Alkjaersig, N., and Sherry, S.: Immunoelectrophoretic characterization of plasma fibrinogen derivatives in patients with pathological plasma proteolysis. J. Lab. Clin. Med. *70*:903, 1967.

154. Folk, J. E., and Chung, S. I.: Molecular and catalytic properties of transglutaminases. Adv. Enzymol., *38*:109, 1973.
155. Fontein, D. L., Waldring, M. C., and Nieweg, H. O.: Management of idiopathic thrombocytopenic purpura. Br. J. Haematol., *17*:301, 1969.
156. Forbes, C. D., Hunter, J., Barr, R. D., Davidson, J. F., Short, D. W., McDonald, G. A., McNicol, G. P., Wallace, J., and Douglas, A. S.: Cryoprecipitate therapy in haemophilia. Scot. Med. J., *14*:1, 1969.
157. Forbes, C. D., and Ratnoff, O. D.: Studies on plasma thromboplastin antecedent (factor XI) PTA deficiency and inhibition of PTA by plasma, pharmacologic inhibitors and specific antiserum. J. Lab. Clin. Med., *79*:113, 1972.
158. Forman, W. B., Ratnoff, O. D., and Boyer, M. N.: An inherited qualitative abnormality in plasma fibrinogen: fibrinogen Cleveland. J. Lab. Clin. Med., *72*:455, 1968.
159. Fratantoni, J. C., Hilgartner, M., and Nachman, R. L.: Nature of the defect in congenital Factor V deficiency: study in a patient with an acquired circulating anticoagulant. Blood, *39*:751, 1972.
160. Fresh, J. W., Ferguson, J. H., Stamey, C., Morgan, F. M., and Lewis, J. H.: Blood prothrombin. proconvertin and proaccelerin in normal infancy: questionable relationships to vitamin K. Pediatrics, *19*:241, 1957.
161. Frick, P. G.: Hemophilia-like disease following pregnancy. Blood, *8*:598, 1953.
162. Frick, P. G.: Relative incidence of anti-hemophilic globulin (AHG), plasma thromboplastin component (PTC), and plasma thromboplastin antecedent (PTA) deficiency. J. Lab. Clin. Med., *43*:860, 1954.
163. Frick, P. G.: Acquired circulating anticoagulants in systemic "collagen disease": autoimmune thromboplastin deficiency. Blood, *10*:691, 1955.
164. Frommer, E., and Ingram, G. I. C.: Haemophiliacs and their doctors. Practitioner, *202*:413, 1969.
165. Gaarder, A., Jonsen, J., Laland, S., Hellem, A., and Owren, P. A.: Adenosine diphosphate in red cells as a factor in the adhesiveness of human blood platelets. Nature, *192*:531, 1961.
166. Ganguly, P.: Studies on human platelet proteins. II. Effect of thrombin. Blood, *33*:590, 1969.
167. Gary, N. E., Mazzara, J. T., and Holfelder, L.: The Schönlein-Henoch syndrome. Ann. Intern. Med., *72*:229, 1970.
168. Geratz, J. D., and Graham, J. B.: Plasma thromboplastin component (Christmas factor, factor IX) levels in stored human blood and plasma. Thromb. Diath. Haemorrh., *4*:376, 1960.
169. Genton, E., and Pechet, L.: Thrombolytic agents: a perspective. Ann. Intern. Med., *69*:625, 1968.
170. Gesink, M. H., and Bradford, H. A.: Thrombocytopenic purpura associated with chlorothiazide therapy. J.A.M.A., *172*:556, 1960.
171. Gilchrist, G. S., Ekert, H., Shanbrom, E., and Hammond, D.: New concentrate for treatment of Factor IX deficiency. N. Engl. J. Med., *280*:291, 1969.
172. Giromini, M., Bouvier, C. A., Dami, R., Denizot, M., and Jeannet, M.: Effect of dipyridamole and aspirin in thrombotic microangiopathy. Br. Med. J., *1*:545, 1972.
173. Girolami, A., Sticchi, A., and Bareggi, G.: Crossover electrophoresis (electrosyneresis) visualization of the abnormal Factor X (Factor X Friuli). J. Lab. Clin. Med., *80*:740, 1972.
174. Gitlin, D., and Borges, W. H.: Studies on the metabolism of fibrinogen in two patients with congenital afibrinogenemia. Blood, *8*:679, 1953.
175. Gitlow, S., and Goldmark, C.: Generalized capillary and arteriolar thrombosis. Ann. Intern. Med., *13*:1046, 1939.
176. Gjønnaess, H., and Stormorken, H.: Activation of Factor VII in oral contraception. Thromb. Diath. Haemorrh. (Suppl.), *50*:109, 1972.
177. Gjønnaess, H.: Cold promoted activation of Factor VII occurrence and relation to sex hormones and antifertility compounds. Gynecol. Invest., *4*:61, 1973.
178. Glueck, H. I., and Roehll, W., Jr.: Myocardial infarction in patient with Hageman (Factor XII) defect. Ann. Intern. Med., *64*:390, 1966.
179. Goldbloom, R. B., and Drummond, K. N.: Anaphylactoid purpura with massive gastrointestinal hemorrhage and glomerulonephritis. Am. J. Dis. Child., *116*:97, 1968.
180. Goldenfarb, P. B., and Finch, S. T.: Thrombotic thrombocytopenic purpura. J.A.M.A., *226*:644, 1973.
181. Goldfinger, D., and McGinnis, M. H.: Rh-incompatible platelet transfusions—risks and consequences of sensitizing immunosuppressed patients. N. Engl. J. Med., *284*:942, 1971.
182. Goldstein, R., and Alexander, B.: Further Studies on Proconvertin Deficiency and the Role of Proconvertin. *In* Brinkhous, K. M. (ed.): Hemophilia and Hemophilioid Disease. University of North Carolina Press, Chapel Hill, 1957, p. 93.
183. Gomes, M. R., Bernatz, P. E., and Dines, D. E.: Pulmonary arteriovenous fistulas. Am. J. Thorac. Surg., *7*:582, 1969.

183a. Gonyea, L., Herdman, R., and Bridges, R. A.: The coagulation abnormalities in systemic lupus erythematosus. Thromb. Diath. Haemorrh., *20*:457, 1968.

184. Good, T. A., Carnazzo, S. F., and Good, R. A.: Thrombocytopenia and giant hemangioma in infants. Am. J. Dis. Child., *90*:260, 1955.

185. Goodknight, M. S. H., Feinstein, D. I., Østerud, B., and Rapaport, S. I.: Factor VII antibody neutralizing material in hereditary and acquired factor VII deficiency. Blood, *38*:1, 1971.

186. Gore, I.: Disseminated arteriolar and capillary platelet thrombosis. A morphologic study of its histogenesis. Am. J. Pathol., *26*:155, 1950.

187. Graham, D. Y., Brown, C. H., III, Benrey, J., and Butel, J. S.: Thrombocytopenia. A complication of mumps. J.A.M.A., *227*:1162, 1974.

188. Graham, J. B.: Genetic Problems: Hemophilia and Allied Diseases. *In* Brinkhous, K. M. (ed.): Hemophilia and Hemophilioid Diseases. University of North Carolina Press, Chapel Hill, 1957, p. 137.

189. Graham, J. B.: Stuart clotting defect and Stuart factor. Thromb. Diath. Haemorrh. (Suppl.), *1*:22, 1960.

190. Graham, J. B.: Biochemical genetic speculations provoked by considering the enigma of von Willebrand's disease. Thromb. Diath. Haemorrh. (Suppl.), *11*:119, 1963.

191. Graham, J. B.: The nature of antihemophilic factor (AHF): introduction and overview. Thrombosis, *54*:177, 1973.

192. Graham, J. B., Barrow, E. M., and Hougie, C.: Stuart clotting defect. II. Genetic aspects of a "new" hemorrhagic stage. J. Clin. Invest., *36*:497, 1957.

193. Graham, J. B., Barrow, E. M., and Roberts, H. R.: Possible implications of the autosomal and x-linked hemophilia phenotypes. Thromb. Diath. Haemorrh. (Suppl.), *17*:151, 1965.

194. Graham, J. B., Barrow, E. M., and Wynne, T. R.: Stuart Clotting Defect. III. An Acquired Case with Complete Recovery. *In* Brinkhous, K. M. (ed.): Hemophilia and Other Hemorrhagic States. University of North Carolina Press, Chapel Hill, 1959, Chapter 18.

195. Graham, J. B., and Geratz, J. D.: Recent Experiences with Transfusion Therapy in PTC-Deficiency. *In* Holländer, L. (ed.): Trans. VII Congr. Int. Soc. Blood Trans., Basel, 1959.

196. Graham, R. C., Jr., Ebert, R. H., Ratnoff, O. S., and Moses, J. M.: Pathogenesis of inflammation. II. In vivo observations of the inflammatory effects of activated Hageman factor and bradykinin. J. Exp. Med., *121*:807, 1965.

197. Gralnick, H. R., Coller, B. S., and Marchesi, S. L.: Factor VIII—immunological studies in haemophilia and von Willebrand's disease. Nature (New Biol.), *244*:281, 1973.

198. Gralnick, H. R., Givelber, H. M., and Finlayson, J. S.: A new congenital abnormality of human fibrinogen—Fibrinogen Bethesda II. Thromb. Diath. Haemorrh., *29*:562, 1973.

199. Gross, R.: Metabolic Aspects of Normal and Pathological Platelets. *In* Blood Platelets. Little, Brown & Co., Boston, 1961, p. 407.

200. Gröttum, K. A., Hovig, T., Holmsen, H., Abrahamsen, A. F., Jeremic, M., and Seip, M.: Wiskott–Aldrich syndrome: qualitative platelet defects and short platelet survival. Br. J. Haematol., *17*:373, 1969.

201. Gröttum, K. A., and Solum, N. O.: Congenital thrombocytopenia with giant platelets: a defect in the platelet membrane. Br. J. Haematol., *16*:277, 1969.

202. Gugler, E., and Luscher, E. F.: Platelet function in congenital afibrinogenemia. Thromb. Diath. Haemorrh., *14*:361, 1965.

203. Haggerty, R. J., and Eley, R. C.: Varicella and cortisone. Pediatrics, *18*:160, 1956.

204. Hall, C. A., Rapaport, S. I., Ames, S. B., DeGroot, J. H., Allen, E. S., and Ralston, M. A.: A clinical and family study of hereditary proconvertin (factor VII) deficiency. Am. J. Med., *37*:172, 1964.

205. Halpern, M., Turner, A. F., and Citron, B. P.: Angiodysplasias of the abdominal viscera associated with hereditary hemorrhagic telangiectasia. Am. J. Roentgenol., *102*:783, 1968.

206. Hampton, J. R.: The study of platelet behaviour and its relevance to thrombosis. J. Atherosclerosis Res., *7*:729, 1967.

207. Hanes, F. M.: Multiple hereditary telangiectases causing hemorrhage. Bull. Johns Hopkins Hosp., *20*:63, 1909.

208. Hardisty, R. M.: Acquired haemophilia-like disease. J. Clin. Pathol., *7*:26, 1954.

209. Hardisty, R. M., Dormandy, K. M., and Hutton, R. A.: Thrombasthenia. Br. J. Haematol., *10*:371, 1964.

210. Hardisty, R. M., and Hutton, R. A.: Platelet aggregation and the availability of Platelet Factor 3. Br. J. Haematol., *12*:764, 1966.

211. Hardisty, R. M., and Hutton, R. A.: Bleeding tendency associated with "new" abnormality of platelet behaviour. Lancet, *1*:983, 1967.

212. Hardisty, R. M., and Mills, D. C. B.: The platelet defect associated with Albinism. Ann. N.Y. Acad. Sci., *201*:429, 1972.

213. Hardisty, R. M., and Pinniger, J. L.: Congenital afibrinogenaemia: further observations on the blood coagulation mechanism. Br. J. Haematol., *2*:139, 1956.

214. Harker, L. A., and Slichter, S. J.: Platelet and fibrinogen consumption in man. N. Engl. J. Med., *287*:999, 1972.
215. Harrington, W. J.: The clinical significance of antibodies for platelets. Sang, *25*:712, 1954.
216. Harrington, W. J.: The purpuras. D.M., July, 1957.
217. Harrington, W. J., Sprague, C. C., Minnich, V., Moore, C. V., and Dubach, R.: Immunologic mechanisms in idiopathic and neonatal thrombocytopenic purpura. Ann. Intern. Med., *38*:433, 1953.
218. Hartman, R. C.: Tests of platelet adhesiveness and their clinical significance. Semin. Hematol., *5*:60, 1968.
219. Haslam, R. J.: Role of adenosine diphosphate in the aggregation of human blood platelets by thrombin and by fatty acids. Nature, *202*:765, 1964.
220. Hathaway, W. E.: Bleeding disorders due to platelet dysfunction. Am. J. Dis. Child., *121*:127, 1971.
221. Hathaway, W. E., Mull, M. M., Githens, J. H., Groth, C. G., Marchioro, T. L., and Starzl, T. E.: Attempted spleen transplant in classical hemophilia. Transplantation, *7*:73, 1969.
222. Haut, M. J., and Cowan, D. H.: The effect of ethanol on hemostatic properties of human blood platelets. Am. J. Med., *56*:22, 1974.
223. Heikinheimo, R., and Reinikainen, M.: Congenital Factor VII deficiency—two cases in children of cousins. Thromb. Diath. Haemorrh., *21*:245, 1969.
224. Hellerstein, L. J., and Deykin, D.: Hepatitis after Konyne administration. N. Engl. J. Med., *284*:1039, 1971.
225. Hemker, H. C., Muller, A. D., and Loeliger, E. A.: Two types of prothrombin in vitamin K deficiency. Thromb. Diath. Haemorrh., *23*:633, 1970.
226. Hensen, A., Mattern, M. J., and Loeliger, E. A.: Hemophilia A with apparently autosomal dominant inheritance—evidence for a second autosomal locus involved in Factor VIII production. Thromb. Diath. Haemorrh., *14*:341, 1965.
227. Heptinstall, R. H.: Pathology of the Kidney. Little, Brown and Co., Boston, 1966, p. 335.
228. Hess, A. F., and Fish, M.: Infantile scurvy: the blood, the blood-vessels and the diet. Am. J. Dis. Child., *8*:385, 1914.
229. Hill, J. M., and Loeb, E.: Massive hormonal therapy and splenectomy in acute thrombotic thrombocytopenic purpura. J.A.M.A., *173*:778, 1960.
230. Hirsh, J., Castelan, D. J., and Loder, P. B.: Spontaneous bruising associated with a defect in the interaction of platelets and connective tissue. Lancet, *2*:18, 1967.
231. Hirsh, J., and Doery, J. C. G.: Platelet function in health and disease. Progr. Haematol., *7*:185, 1972.
232. Hirsh, J., and McBride, J. A.: Increased platelet adhesiveness in recurrent venous thrombosis and pulmonary embolism. Br. Med. J., *2*:797, 1965.
233. Hirschman, R. J., Itscoitz, S. B., and Shulman, N. R.: Prophylactic treatment of Factor VIII deficiency. Blood, *35*:189, 1970.
234. Hirschman, R. J., and Shulman, N. R.: The use of platelet serotonin release as a sensitive method for detecting anti-platelet antibodies and a plasma anti-platelet factor in patients with idiopathic thrombocytopenic purpura. Br. J. Haematol., *24*:793, 1973.
235. Hjort, P. F., and Rapaport, S. I.: The Shwartzman reaction: pathogenic mechanisms and clinical manifestations. Am. Rev. Med., *16*:135, 1965.
236. Hoag, M. S., Aggeler, P. M., and Fowell, A. H.: Disappearance rate of concentrated proconvertin extract in congenital and acquired hypoproconvertinemia. J. Clin. Invest., *39*:554, 1960.
237. Hoag, M. S., Johnson, F. F., Robinson, J. A., and Aggeler, P. M.: Treatment of hemophilia B with a new clotting-factor concentrate. N. Engl. J. Med., *280*:581, 1969.
238. Hoak, J. C., Seanson, L. W., Warner, E. D., and Connor, W. E.: Myocardial infarction associated with severe Factor XII deficiency. Lancet, *2*:884, 1966.
239. Holmberg, L., and Nilsson, I. M.: Immunologic studies of Haemophilia A. Scand. J. Haematol., *10*:12, 1973.
240. Holmberg, L., and Nilsson, I. M.: AHF-Related protein in clinical praxis. Scand. J. Haematol., *12*:221, 1974.
241. Holmsen, H., and Weiss, H. J.: Further evidence for a deficient storage pool of adenine nucleotides in platelets from some patients with thrombocytopathia—"storage pool disease." Blood, *39*:197, 1972.
242. Hougie, C.: Circulating anticoagulants. Br. Med. Bull., *11*:16, 1955.
243. Hougie, C., Barrow, E. M., and Graham, J. B.: Stuart clotting defect. I. Segregation of an hereditary hemorrhagic state from the heterogeneous group heretofore called "stable factor" (SPCA, proconvertin, Factor VII) deficiency. J. Clin. Invest., *36*:485, 1957.
244. Hougie, C., Sargeant, R. B., Brown, J. E., and Baugh, R. F.: Evidence that Factor VIII and the ristocetin aggregating factor (VIII [Rist]) are separate molecule entities. Proc. Soc. Exp. Biol. Med., *147*:58, 1974.

245. Hougie, C., and Twomey, J. J.: Hemophilia B in a new type of Factor IX deficiency. Lancet, *1*:698, 1967.
246. Howard, M. A., and Firkin, B. G.: Ristocetin — a new tool in the investigation of platelet aggregation. Thromb. Diath. Haemorrh., *26*:362, 1971.
247. Hoyer, L. W., and Breckenridge, R. T.: Immunologic studies of antihemophilic factor (AHF, Factor VIII): cross-reacting material in a genetic variant of hemophilia A. Blood, *32*:962, 1968.
248. Huber, J.: Experience with various immunologic deficiencies in Holland. Birth Defect., *4*:53, 1968.
249. Hughes, D. W. O. G., Parkinson, R., Beveridge, J., Reid, R. R., and Murphy, A. M.: The expanded congenital rubella syndrome: report of two cases with   onatal purpura and review of the recent literature. Med. J. Aust., *1*:420, 1967.
250. Humble, J. G.: The mechanism of petechial hemorrhage formation. Blood, *4*:69, 1949.
251. Iatridis, P. G., and Ferguson, J. H.: The plasmatic atmosphere of blood platelets. Evidence that only fibrinogen, AcG, and activated Hageman factor are present on the surface of platelets. Thromb. Diath. Haemorrh., *13*:114, 1965.
252. Ikkala, E., and Nevanlinna, H. R.: Congenital deficiency of fibrin stabilizing factor. Thromb. Diath. Haemorrh., 7:567, 1962.
253. Inceman, S., Caen, J., and Bernard, J.: Aggregation, adhesion and viscous metamorphosis of platelets in congenital fibrinogen deficiencies. J. Lab Clin. Med., *68*:21, 1966.
254. Ingram, G. I. C.: Observations in a case of multiple hemostatic defects. Br. J. Haematol., *2*:180, 1956.
255. Jackson, D. P., Schmid, H. J., Zieve, P. D., Levin, J., and Conley, C. J.: Nature of a platelet-agglutinating factor in serum of patients with idiopathic thrombocytopenic purpura. J. Clin. Invest., *42*:383, 1963.
255a. Jacobson, R. J., and Jackson, D. P.: Microangiopathic hemolytic anemia in defibrination syndrome. Ann. Intern. Med., *72*:794, 1970.
256. Jaffe, E. A., Nachman, R. L., and Merskey, C.: Thrombotic thrombocytopenic purpura — coagulation parameters in twelve patients. Blood, *42*:499, 1973.
257. Jahnke, V.: Ultrastructure of hereditary telangiectasia. Arch. Ololaryngol., *91*:262, 1970.
258. JiJi, R. M., Firozvi, T., and Spurling, C. L.: Chronic idiopathic thrombocytopenic purpura. Arch. Intern. Med., *132*:380, 1973.
259. Jobin, F., and Delâge, J. M.: Aspirin and prednisone in microangiopathic hemolytic anemia. Lancet, *2*:208, 1970.
260. Johnson, S. A., Monto, R. W., and Caldwell, M. J.: A new approach to the thrombocytopathies. Thrombocytopathy A. Thromb. Diath. Haemorrh., *2*:279, 1958.
261. Jones, H. W., and Tocantins, L. M.: The history of purpura hemorrhagica. Ann. M. History, *5*:349, 1933 (N.S.).
262. Jorpes, J. E.: The origin and the physiology of heparin: the specific therapy in thrombosis. Ann. Intern. Med., *27*:361, 1947.
263. Josso, F., Monasterio de Sanchez, J., Lavergne, J. M., Menache, D., and Soulier, J. P.: Congenital abnormality of the prothrombin molecule (Factor II) in four siblings: prothrombin Barcelona. Blood, *38*:9, 1971.
264. Kaneshiro, M. M., Mielke, C. H., Jr., Kasper, C. K., and Rapaport, S. I.: Bleeding time after aspirin in disorders of intrinsic clotting. N. Engl. J. Med., *281*:1039, 1969.
265. Karaca, M., Cronberg, L., and Nilsson, I. M.: Abnormal platelet–collagen reaction in Ehlers–Danlos syndrome. Scand. J. Haematol., *9*:465, 1972.
266. Karpatkin, S.: Heterogeneity of human platelets. II. Functional evidence suggestive of young and old platelets. J. Clin. Invest., *48*:1083, 1969.
267. Karpatkin, S., Ingram, F. I. C., and Graham, J. B.: Severe isolated prothrombin deficiency: an acquired state with complete recovery. Thromb. Diath. Haemorrh., *8*:221, 1962.
268. Karpatkin, S., and Siskind, G. W.: In vitro detection of platelet antibody in patients with idiopathic thrombocytopenic purpura and systemic lupus erythematosus. Blood, *33*:795, 1969.
269. Karpatkin, S., and Weiss, J.: Deficient glutathione peroxidase with elevated reduced glutathione in thrombasthenia. N. Engl. J. Med., *287*:1062, 1972.
270. Kasper, C. K., Buechy, D. Y. E. W., and Aggeler, P. M.: Hageman factor (Factor XII) in an affected kindred and normal adults. Br. J. Haematol., *14*:543, 1968.
271. Kasper, C. K., and Southgate, M. T.: The many facets of hemophilia. J.A.M.A., *228*:85, 1974.
272. Kass, L. Ratnoff, O. D., and Leon, M. A.: Studies on the purification of antihemophilia factor (Factor VIII). J. Clin. Invest., *48*:351, 1969.
273. Kattlove, H. E., Shapiro, S. S., and Spivack, M.: Hereditary prothrombin deficiency. N. Engl. J. Med., *282*:57, 1970.
274. Kekwick, R. A., and Wolf, P.: A concentrate of human antihaemophilic factor — its use in six cases of haemophilia. Lancet, *1*:647, 1957.

275. Kellaway, C. H.: Snake venom. Bull. Johns Hopkins Hosp., *60*:1, 1937.

276. Kellermeyer, R. W.: Inflammatory process in acute gouty arthritis. III. Vascular permeability-enhancing activity in normal human synovial fluid: induction by Hageman factor activators; and inhibition by Hageman factors antiserum. J. Lab. Clin. Med., *70*:365, 1967.

277. Kellermeyer, R. W.: Hageman factor and acute gouty arthritis. Arthritis Rheum., *11*:452, 1968.

278. Kernoff, P. B. A., Gruson, R., and Rizza, C. R.: A variant of Factor VIII-related antigen. Br. J. Haematol., *26*:435, 1974.

279. Kerr, C. B., Preston, A. E., Barr, A., and Biggs, R.: Inheritance of Factor VIII. Thromb. Diath. Haematol. (Suppl.), *17*:173, 1965.

280. Kibel, M. A., and Barnard, P. J.: Treatment of acute hemolytic-uremic syndrome with heparin. Lancet, *2*:259, 1964.

281. Kingsley, C. S.: Familial Factor V deficiency: the pattern of heredity. Q. J. Med., *23*:323, 1954.

282. Kisker, C. T., and Burke, C.: Use of steroids in treatment of acute hemarthrosis in patients with hemophilia. N. Engl. J. Med., *282*:639, 1970.

283. Kisker, C. T., Glueck, H., and Kander, E.: Anaphylactoid purpura progressing to gangrene and its treatment with heparin. J. Pediatr., *73*:748, 1968.

284. Koch-Weser, J.: Quinidine-induced hypoprothrombinemic hemorrhage in patients on chronic warfarin therapy. Ann. Intern. Med., *68*:511, 1968.

285. Kramar, J.: Stress and capillary resistance (capillary fragility). Am. J. Physiol., *175*:69, 1953.

286. Krause, W. H., Heene, D. L., and Lasch, H. G.: Congenital dysfibrinogenemia (fibrinogen Giessen). Thromb. Diath. Haemorrh., *29*:547, 1973.

287. Krevans, J. R., and Jackson, D. P.: Hemorrhagic disorder following massive whole blood transfusions. J.A.M.A., *159*:171, 1955.

288. Kuramoto, A., Steiner, M., and Baldini, M. G.: Lack of platelet response to stimulation in the Wiskott–Aldrich syndrome. N. Engl. J. Med., *282*:475, 1970.

289. Kurstjens, R., Bolt, C., Vossen, M., and Haanan, C.: Familial thrombopathic thrombocytopenia. Br. J. Haematol., *15*:305, 1968.

289a. Kyle, R. A., Gleich, G. J., and Bayrd, E. D.: Benign hypergammaglobulinemic purpura of Waldenstrom. Medicine, *50*:113, 1971.

290. Lacombe, M., Soria, J., Soria, C., d'Angelo, G., Lavallee, R., and Bonny, Y.: Fibrinogen Montreal—a new case of congenital dysfibrinogenemia with defective aggregation of monomers. Thromb. Diath. Haemorrh., *29*:536, 1973.

291. Larrieu, M. J., Caen, J., Lelong, J. C., and Bernard, J.: Maladie de Glanzmann. Nouv. Rev. Fr. Hematol., *1*:662, 1961.

292. Lee, S. L., and Sanders, M.: A disorder of blood coagulation in systemic lupus erythematosus. J. Clin. Invest., *34*:1814, 1955.

293. Leiba, H., Ramot, B., and Many, A.: Heredity and coagulation studies in ten families with Factor XI (plasma thromboplastin antecedent) deficiency. Br. J. Haematol., *11*:654, 1965.

294. Lerner, R. G., Rapaport, S. I., and Meltzer, J.: Thrombotic thrombocytopenic purpura. Ann. Intern. Med., *66*:1180, 1967.

295. Levin, R. H., Pert, J. H., and Freireich, E. J.: Response to transfusion of platelets pooled from multiple donors and the effects of various technics of concentrating platelets. Transfusion, *5*:54, 1965.

296. Levine, P. H., and Britten, A. F. H.: Supervised patient-management of hemophilia. Ann. Intern. Med., *78*:195, 1973.

297. Levine, P. H.: Efficacy of self-therapy in hemophilia. N. Engl. J. Med., *291*:1381, 1974.

297a. Lewis, J. H., and Doyle, A. P.: Effects of epsilon aminocaproic acid on coagulation and fibrinolytic mechanisms. J.A.M.A., *188*:56, 1964.

298. Lewis, J. H., and Ferguson, J. H.: Afibrinogenemia. Report of a case. Am. J. Dis. Child., *88*:711, 1954.

299. Lewis, J. H., Ferguson, J. H., Spaugh, E., Fresh, J. W., and Zueker, M. B.: Acquired hypoprothrombinemia. Blood, *12*:84, 1957.

300. Lindenbaum, J., and Hargrave, R. L.: Thrombocytopenia in alcoholics. Ann. Intern. Med., *68*:526, 1968.

301. Link, K. P.: The anticoagulant from spoiled sweet clover hay. Harvey Lect., *39*:162, 1944.

302. Lopez, V., Pflugshaupt, R., and Bütler, R.: A specific inhibitor of human clotting Factor V. Acta Haematol., *40*:275, 1968.

303. Lorand, L.: Properties and significance of the fibrin stabilizing factor (FSF). Thromb. Diath. Haemorrh. (Suppl.), *1*:238, 1962.

304. Lorand, L., Urayama, T., Atencio, A. C., and Hsia, D. Y-Y.: Inheritance of deficiency of fibrin-stabilizing factor. Am. J. Hematol. Genet., *22*:89, 1970.

305. Lorand, L., Urayama, T., deKiewiet, J. W. C., and Nossel, H. L.: Diagnostic and genetic studies on fibrin-stabilizing factor with a new assay based on amine incorporation. J. Clin. Invest., *48*:1054, 1969.

306. Lozner, E. L., Jolliffe, L. S., and Taylor, F. H. L.: Hemorrhagic diathesis with prolonged coagulation time associated with a circulating anticoagulant. Am. J. Med. Sci., *199*:318, 1940.
307. Lucas, O. N., Finkelman, A., and Tocantins, L. M.: Management of tooth extraction in hemophiliacs by the combined use of hypnotic suggestion, protective splints and packing of sockets. J. Oral Surg., *20*:488, 1962.
308. Lüscher, E. F.: Retraction activity of the platelets: biochemical background and physiological significance. *In* Blood Platelets. Henry Ford Hospital Symposium. Little, Brown & Co., Boston, 1961, p. 445.
309. Lusher, J. M., Schneider, J., Mizukami, I., and Evans, R. K.: The May–Hegglin anomaly: platelet function ultrastructure and chromosome studies. Blood, *32*:950, 1968.
310. Macfarlane, R. G.: A boy with no fibrinogen. Lancet, *1*:309, 1938.
311. Macfarlane, R. G.: Critical review: the mechanism of haemostasis. Q. J. Med., *10*:1, 1941 (N.S.).
312. Macfarlane, R. G., Biggs, R., and Bidwell, E.: Bovine antihaemophilic globulin in the treatment of haemophilia. Lancet, *1*:1316, 1954.
313. Macfarlane, R. G., Mallan, P. C., Wills, L. J., Bidwell, E., Biggs, R., Fraenkel, F. J., Honey, G. E., and Taylor, K. B.: Surgery in haemophilia. Lancet, *2*:251, 1957.
314. MacWhinney, J. B., Jr., Packer, J. T., Miller, G., and Greendyke, R. M.: Thrombotic thrombocytopenic purpura in childhood. Blood, *19*:181, 1962.
315. Malhotra, O. P.: Plasma prothrombin — induction of atypical prothrombins by Dicoumarol. Nature (New Biology), *239*:59, 1972.
316. Malhotra, O. P., and Carter, J. R.: Prothrombin in Factor X deficiency. J. Lab. Clin. Med., *75*:120, 1970.
317. Mammen, E. F., Prasad, A. S., Barnhart, M. I., and Au, C. C.: Congenital dysfibrinogenemia: fibrinogen Detroit. J. Clin. Invest., *48*:235, 1969.
318. Mant, M. J., Cauchi, M. N., and Medley, G.: Thrombotic thrombocytopenic purpura: report of a case with possible immune etiology. Blood, *40*:416, 1972.
319. Marchiora, T. L., Hougie, C., Ragde, H., Epstein, R. B., and Thomas, E. D.: Hemophilia: role of organ homografts. Science, *163*:188, 1968.
320. Marcus, A. J.: Platelet function. N. Engl. J. Med., *280*:1213, 1278, 1330, 1969.
321. Marder, V. J., and Shulman, N. R.: Clinical aspects of congenital Factor VII deficiency. Am. J. Med., *37*:182, 1964.
322. Marder, V. J., and Shulman, N. R.: Major surgery in classic hemophilia using Fraction I. Am. J. Med., *41*:56, 1966.
323. Margolis, J.: Hageman factor and capillary permeability. Aust. J. Exp. Biol. Med. Sci., *37*:239, 1959.
324. Masure, R.: Human Factor VIII prepared by cryoprecipitation. Vox Sang., *16*:1, 1969.
325. McClure, P. D., and Choi, S. I.: Thrombopoietin and erythropoietin levels in idiopathic thrombocytopenic purpura and iron-deficiency anaemia. Br. J. Haematol., *15*:351, 1968.
326. McClure, P. D., Ingram, G. I. C., Stacey, R. S., Glass, U. H., and Matchett, M. O.: Platelet function tests in thrombocythemia and thrombocytosis. Br. J. Haematol., *12*:478, 1966.
327. McKay, D. G.: Progress in disseminated intravascular coagulation. II. California Medicine, *3*:186, 279, 1969.
328. McKay, D. G., and Müller-Berghaus, G.: Therapeutic implications of disseminated intravascular coagulation. Am. J. Cardiol., *20*:392, 1967.
329. McMillan, R. M., Longmire, R. L., Yelenosky, R., Smith, R. S., and Craddock, C. G.: Immunoglobulin synthesis in vitro by splenic tissue in idiopathic thrombocytopenic purpura. N. Engl. J. Med., *286*:681, 1972.
329a. McNicol, G. P., and Douglas, A. S.: E–Aminocaproic acid and other inhibitors of fibrinolysis. Br. Med. Bull., *20*:233, 1964.
330. Meacham, G. C., and Weisberger, A. S.: Unusual manifestations of disseminated lupus erythematosus. Ann. Intern. Med., *43*:143, 1955.
331. Meadow, S. R., Glasgow, E. F., White, R. H. R., Moncrieff, M. W., Cameron, J. S., and Ogg, C. S.: Schönlein–Henoch nephritis. Q. J. Med., *41*:241, 1972.
332. Ménaché, D.: Constitutional and familial abnormal fibrinogen. Thromb. Diath. Haemorrh., (Suppl.), *13*:173, 1963.
333. Ménaché, D.: Abnormal fibrinogens — a review. Thrombosis, *29*:525, 1973.
334. Merskey, C.: The occurrence of haemophilia in the human female. Q. J. Med., *20*:299, 1951 (N.S.).
335. Merskey, C.: Diagnosis and treatment of intravascular coagulation. Br. J. Haematol., *15*:523, 1968.
335a. Merskey, C.: Editorial: defibrination syndrome or . . . ? Blood, *41*:599, 1973.

336. Merskey, C., Johnson, A. J., Kleiner, G. J., and Wohl, H.: The defibrination syndrome: clinical features and laboratory diagnosis. Br. J. Haematol., *13*:528, 1967.

337. Mettler, N. E.: Isolation of a microtatobiote from patients with hemolytic-uremic syndrome and thrombotic thrombocytopenic purpura and from mites in the United States. N. Engl. J. Med., *281*:1023, 1969.

338. Meyer, D., and Larrieu, M. J.: Factor VIII and IX variants. Relationship between hemophilia Bm and hemophilia B+. Eur. J. Clin. Invest., *1*:425, 1971.

339. Meyer, T. C., and Angus, J.: The effect of large doses of "Synkavit" in the newborn. Arch. Dis. Child., *31*:212, 1956.

340. Meyers, M. C.: Results of treatment in 71 patients with idiopathic thrombocytopenic purpura. Am. J. Med. Sci., *242*:295, 1961.

341. Michael, A. F., Vernier, R. L., Drummond, K. N., Levitt, J. I., Herdman, R. C., Fish, A. J., and Good, R. A.: Immunosuppressive therapy of chronic renal disease. N. Engl. J. Med., *276*:817, 1967.

342. Michaeli, D., Ben-Bassat, I., Miller, H. I., and Deutsch, V.: Hepatic telangiectasis and porto-systemic encephalopathy in Osler-Weber-Render disease. Gasteroenterology, *54*:929, 1968.

343. Mills, S. D.: Purpuric manifestations occurring in measles in childhood. J. Pediatr., *36*:35, 1950.

344. Miloszewski, K., Walls, W. D., and Losowsky, M. S.: Absence of plasma transamidase activity in congenital deficiency of fibrin stabilizing factor (Factor XIII). Br. J. Haematol., *17*:159, 1969.

345. Minami, G. R., Kasper, C. K., and Rapaport, S. I.: Incidence of hemophilia B variants. Clin. Res., *17*:116, 1969.

346. Mitchell, J. S.: Metabolic effects of therapeutic doses of X and gamma radiations. Br. J. Radiol., *16*:339, 1943.

347. Monnens, L. A. H., and Retera, R. J. M.: Thrombotic thrombocytopenic purpura in a neonatal infant. J. Pediatr., *71*:118, 1967.

348. Moschowitz, E.: An acute febrile pleiochromic anemia with hyaline thrombosis of the terminal arterioles and capillaries. An undescribed disease. Arch. Intern. Med., *36*:89, 1925.

349. Moser, K., Lechner, K., and Vinazzer, H.: A hitherto not described enzyme defect in thrombasthenia: glutathionreductase deficiency. Thromb. Diath. Haemorrh., *19*:46, 1968.

350. Mosesson, M. W., and Beck, E. A.: Chromatographic, ultracentrifugal, and related studies of fibrinogen "Baltimore." J. Clin. Invest., *48*:1656, 1969.

351. Moss, M. H.: Hypoprothrombinemic bleeding in a young infant. Am. J. Dis. Child., *117*:540, 1969.

352. Mürer, E. H.: Thrombin-induced release of calcium from blood platelets. Science, *166*:623, 1969.

353. Murphy, S., Oski, F. A., and Gardner, F. H.: Hereditary thrombocytopenia with an intrinsic platelet defect. N. Engl. J. Med., *281*:857, 1969.

354. Myllylä, G., Vaheri, A., Vesikari, T., and Penttinen, K.: Interaction between human blood platelets, viruses and antibodies. Clin. Exp. Immunol., *4*:323, 1969.

355. Najean, Y., Ardaillou, N., Dresch, C., and Bernard, J.: The platelet destruction site in thrombocytopenic purpuras. Br. J. Haematol., *13*:409, 1967.

356. Neal, W. R., Tayloe, D. T., Jr., Cederbaum, A. I., and Roberts, H. R.: Detection of genetic variants of haemophilia B with an immunosorbent technique. Br. J. Haematol., *25*:63, 1973.

357. Neame, P. B., Lechago, J., Ling, E. T., and Koval, A.: TTP: report of a case with disseminated intravascular platelet aggregation. Blood, *42*:805, 1973.

358. Nelsestuen, G. L., and Suttie, J. W.: The mode of action of vitamin K. Isolation of a peptide containing the vitamin K-dependent portion of prothrombin. Proc. Natl. Acad. Sci., U.S.A., *70*:3366, 1973.

359. Nilsson, I. M.: Treatment of haemophilia A and von Willebrand's disease. Bibl. Haematol., *23*:1307, 1965.

360. Nilsson, I. M., Anderson, L., and Bjorkman, S. E.: Epsilon-aminocaproic acid (EACA) as a therapeutic agent based on 5 years clinical experience. Acta Med. Scand. (Suppl.), *448*:1, 1966.

361. Nilsson, I. M., and Blombäck, M.: Von Willebrand's disease in Sweden. Occurrence, pathogenesis and treatment. Thromb. Diath. Haemorrh. (Suppl.), *2*:102, 1963.

362. Nilsson, I. M.: Blombäck, M., Jorpes, E., Blombäck, B., and Johansson, S.-A.: Von Willebrand's disease and its correction with human plasma fraction 1-0. Acta Med. Scand., *159*:179, 1957.

363. Nilsson, I. M., Blombäck, M., and von Francken, I.: On an inherited autosomal hemorrhagic

diathesis and antihemophilic globulin (AHG) deficiency and prolonged bleeding time. Acta Med. Scand., *159*:35, 1957.

363a. Nilsson, I. M., Hedner, U., Ekberg, M., and Denneberg, T.: A circulating anticoagulant against factor V. Acta Med. Scand., *195*:73, 1974.

364. Norman, J. C., Covelli, V. H., and Sise, H. S.: Transplantation of the spleen: experimental cure of hemophilia. Surgery, *64*:1, 1968.

365. Nossel, H. L., Niemitz, J., Mibashan, R. S., and Schulze, W. G.: The measurement of Factor XI (plasma thromboplastin antecedent): diagnosis and therapy of the congenital deficiency state. Br. J. Haematol., *12*:133, 1966.

366. Nussbaum, M., and Dameshek, W.: Transient hemolytic and thrombocytopenic episode (? acute transient thrombohemolytic thrombocytopenic purpura) with probable meningococcemia. N. Engl. J. Med., *256*:448, 1957.

367. Nussbaum, M., and Morse, B. S.: Plasma fibrin stabilizing factor activity in various diseases. Blood, *23*:669, 1964.

368. Oberman, H. A., and Penner, J. A.: Utilization of residual plasma following preparation of Factor VIII cryoprecipitate. J.A.M.A., *205*:819, 1968.

369. O'Brien, J. R.: An acquired coagulation defect in a woman. J. Clin. Pathol., *7*:22, 1954.

370. O'Brien, J. R., and Heywood, J. B.: Some interactions between human platelets and glass: von Willebrand's disease compared with normal. J. Clin. Pathol., *20*:56, 1967.

370a. Oski, F. A., and Naiman, J. L.: Effect of Live Measles Vaccine on the Platelet Count. N. Engl. J. Med., *275*:352, 1966.

371. Oski, F. A., Naiman, J. L., and Diamond, L. K.: Use of the plasma acid phosphatase value in the differentiation of thrombocytopenic states. N. Engl. J. Med., *268*:1423, 1963.

372. Osler, W.: On a family form of recurring epistaxis, associated with multiple telangiectases of the skin and mucous membranes. Johns Hopkins Hosp. Bull., *12*:333, 1901.

373. Osler, W.: The visceral lesions of purpura and allied conditions. Br. Med. J., *1*:517, 1914.

374. Owen, C. A., Amundsen, M. A., Thompson, J. H., Jr., Spittell, J. A., Bowie, E. J. W., Stilwell, G. G., Hewlett, J. S., Mills, S. D., Sauer, W. G., and Page, R. P.: Congenital deficiency of Factor VII (hypoproconvertinemia). Am. J. Med., *37*:71, 1964.

375. Owren, P. A.: The coagulation of blood—investigation on a new clotting factor. Acta Med. Scand. (Suppl.), 194, 1947.

376. Owren, P. A.: The diagnostic and prognostic significance of plasma prothrombin and factor V levels in parenchymatous hepatitis and obstructive jaundice. Scand. J. Clin. Lab. Invest., *1*:131, 1949.

377. Packham, M. A., Nishizawa, E. E., and Mustard, J. F.: Response of platelets to tissue injury. Biochem. Pharmacol., *17*:171, 1968.

378. Panner, B.: Nephritis of Schönlein-Henoch syndrome. Arch. Pathol., *74*:230, 1962.

379. Patek, A. J., Jr., and Taylor, F. H. L.: Hemophilia. II. Some properties of a substance obtained from normal human plasma effective in accelerating the coagulation of hemophilic blood. J. Clin. Invest., *16*:113, 1937.

380. Patterson, J. H., Pierce, R. B., Amerson, J. R., and Watkins, W. L.: Dextran therapy of purpura fulminans. N. Engl. J. Med., *273*:734, 1965.

381. Pavlosky, A.: Contribution to the pathogenesis of hemophilia. Blood, *2*:185, 1947.

382. Payne, R. W., and Harris, M. C.: Factor VIII inhibitor: acquired haemostatic defect in a non-haemophiliac patient with rheumatoid arthritis. Scott. Med. J., *17*:310, 1972.

383. Paz, R. A., Elijovich, F., Barcat, J. A., and Sanchez–Avalos, J. C.: Fatal simultaneous thrombocytopenic purpura in siblings. Br. Med. J., *4*:727, 1969.

384. Pearson, H. A., Shulman, N. R., Marder, V. J., and Cone, T. E., Jr.: Iso-immune neonatal thrombocytopenic purpura: clinical and therapeutic considerations. Blood, *23*:154, 1964.

385. Perkins, H. A.: Brief report: correction of the hemostatic defects in von Willebrand's disease. Blood, *30*:375, 1967.

386. Phillips, L. L.: Homologous serum jaundice following fibrinogen administration. Surg. Gynecol. Obstet., *121*:551, 1965.

387. Phillips, L. L., Hyman, G. A., and Rosenthal, R. L.: Prolonged postoperative bleeding in a patient with Factor XI (PTA) deficiency. Ann. Surg., *162*:37, 1965.

388. Philpott, M. G.: The Schönlein-Henoch syndrome in childhood with particular reference to the occurrence of nephritis. Arch. Dis. Child., *27*:480, 1952.

389. Pike, I. M., Yount, W. J., Puritz, E. M., and Roberts, H. R.: Immunochemical characterization of a monoclonal γ G4, γ human antibody to Factor IX. Blood, *40*:1, 1972.

390. Pitney, W. R., and Potter, M.: Retention of platelets by glass bead filters. J. Clin. Pathol., *20*:710, 1967.

391. Pool, J. G.: The effect of several variables on cryoprecipitated Factor VIII (AHG) concentrates. Transfusion, *7*:165, 1967.

392. Pool, J. G., Desai, R., and Kropatkin, M.: Severe congenital hypoprothrombinemia in a Negro boy. Thromb. Diath. Haemorrh., *8*:235, 1962.

393. Pool, J. G., Hershgold, E. J., and Pappenhagen, A. R.: High potency antihemophilic factor concentrate prepared from cryoglobulin precipitate. Nature, *203*:312, 1964.

394. Post, R. M., and Desforges, J. F.: Thrombocytopenia and alcoholism. Ann. Intern. Med., *68*:1230, 1968.

395. Prentice, C. R. M., Breckenridge, R. T., Forman, W. B., and Ratnoff, O. D.: Treatment of hemophilia (Factor VIII deficiency) with human antihemophilic factor prepared by the cryoprecipitate process. Lancet, *1*:457, 1967.

396. Presley, S. J., Best, W. R., and Limarzi, L. R.: Bone marrow in idiopathic thrombocytopenic purpura. J. Lab. Clin. Med., *40*:503, 1952.

397. Prichard, R. W., and Vann, R. L.: Congenital afibrinogenemia. Am. J. Dis. Child., *88*:703, 1954.

398. Pritchard, J. A., and Wright, M. R.: Studies to determine the cause of hypofibrinogenemia in placental abruption. Am. J. Med., *27*:321, 1959.

399. Prydz, H.: Studies on Proconvertin (factor VII). VI. The production in rabbits of an anti-serum against factor VII. Scand. J. Clin. Lab. Invest., *17*:66, 1965.

400. Purcell, G., Jr., and Nossel, H. L.: Factor XI (PTA) deficiency: surgical and obstetrical aspects. Obstet. Gynecol., *35*:69, 1970.

401. Quick, A. J.: The prothrombin in hemophilia and in obstructive jaundice. J. Biol. Chem., *109*:73, 1935.

402. Quick, A. J.: Salicylates and bleeding: aspirin tolerance test. Am. J. Med. Sci., *252*:265, 1966.

403. Quick, A. J.: Clinical course in hemophilia. J.A.M.A., *210*:1, 1969.

404. Quick, A. J., and Collentine, G. E.: The role of vitamin K in the synthesis of prothrombin. Am. J. Physiol., *164*:716, 1951.

405. Rabiner, S. F., and Telfer, M. C.: Home transfusions for patients with hemophilia A. N. Engl. J. Med., *283*:1011, 1970.

406. Rabinowitz, Y., and Dameshek, W.: Systemic lupus erythematosus after "idiopathic" thrombocytopenic purpura: a review. Ann. Intern. Med., *52*:1, 1960.

407. Ramsay, D. M., and Parker, A. C.: A trial of prophylactic replacement therapy in haemophilia and Christmas disease. J. Clin. Pathol., *26*:243, 1973.

408. Rand, M., and Reid, G.: Source of "serotonin" in serum. Nature, *168*:385, 1951.

409. Ratnoff, O. D., Busse, R. J., Jr., and Sheon, R. P.: The demise of John Hageman. N. Engl. J. Med., *279*:760, 1968.

410. Ratnoff, O. D., and Colopy, J. E.: Familial hemorrhagic trait associated with deficiency of clot promoting fraction of the plasma. J. Clin. Invest., *34*:602, 1955.

411. Ratnoff, O. D., and Colopy, J. E.: Biology and pathology of initial stages of blood coagulation. Progr. Hematol., *5*:204, 1966.

412. Ratnoff, O. D., Kass, L., and Lang, P. D.: Studies on the purification of antihemophilic factor, Factor VIII. J. Clin. Invest., *48*:957, 1969.

413. Ratnoff, O. D., and Miles, A. A.: Induction of permeability-increasing activity in human plasma by activated Hageman factor. Br. J. Exp. Pathol., *45*:328, 1964.

414. Ratnoff, O. D., and Steinberg, A. G.: Further studies on inheritance of Hageman trait. J. Lab. Clin. Med., *59*:980, 1962.

415. Reid, D. E., Weiner, A. E., and Roby, C. C.: Intravascular clotting and afibrinogenemia: the presumptive lethal factors in the syndrome of amniotic fluid embolism. Am. J. Obstet. Gynecol., *66*:465, 1953.

416. Reid, D. E., Weiner, A. E., Roby, C. C., and Diamond, L. K.: Maternal afibrinogenemia associated with long-standing intrauterine fetal death. Am. J. Obstet. Gynecol., *66*:500, 1953.

417. Rick, M. E., and Hoyer, L. W.: Immunologic studies of antihemophilic factor (AHF, Factor VIII). V. Immunologic properties of AHF subunits produced by salt dissociation. Blood, *42*:737, 1973.

418. Rizza, C. R.: The Management of Patients with Coagulation Factor Deficiencies. *In* Biggs, R. (ed.): Human Blood Coagulation, Haemostasis and Thrombosis. Oxford, Blackwell Scientific Publ., 1972.

419. Rizza, C. R., and Biggs, R.: The treatment of patients who have factor VIII antibodies. Br. J. Haematol., *24*:65, 1973.

420. Roberts, H. R., Lechler, E., Webster, W. P., and Penick, G. D.: Survival of transfused Factor X in patients with Stuart disease. Thromb. Diath. Haemorrh., *13*:305, 1965.

421. Roberts, H. R., Grizzle, J. E., McLester, W. D., and Penick, G. D.: Genetic variants of hemophilia B: detection by means of a specific PTC inhibitor. J. Clin. Invest., *47*:360, 1968.

422. Robinson, A. J., Aggeler, P. M., McNicol, G. P., and Douglas, A. S.: An atypical genetic haemorrhagic disease with increased concentration of a natural inhibitor of prothrombin consumption. Br. J. Haematol., *13*:510, 1967.

423. Robinson, P. M., Tittley, P., and Smalley, R. K.: Prophylactic therapy in classical hemophilia: a preliminary report. Can. Med. Assoc. J., 97:559, 1967.
424. Robson, H. N., and Duthie, J. J. R.: Further observations on capillary resistance and adrenocortical activity. Br. Med. J., 1:994, 1952.
425. Rodriguez-Erdmann, F.: Treatment of the Shwartzman reaction. N. Engl. J. Med., 271:632, 1964.
426. Rodriguez-Erdmann, F.: Bleeding due to increased intravascular blood coagulation, hemorrhagic syndromes caused by consumption of blood-clotting factors (consumption-coagulopathies). N. Engl. J. Med., 273:1370, 1965.
427. Rodriguez-Erdmann, F., and Levitan, R.: Gastrointestinal and roentgenological manifestations of Henoch-Schoenlein purpura. Gastroenterology, 54:260, 1968.
428. Rodriguez, S. U., Leikin, S. L., and Hiller, M. C.: Neonatal thrombocytopenia associated with anti-partum administration of thiazide drugs. N. Engl. J. Med., 270:881, 1964.
429. Rosenthal, M. C.: Deficiency in plasma thromboplastin component. II. Its incidence in hemophilic population. Critique of methods for identification. Am. J. Clin. Pathol., 24:910, 1954.
430. Rosenthal, M. C., and Sanders, M.: Plasma thromboplastin component deficiency. Am. J. Med., 16:153, 1954.
431. Rosenthal, R. L.: Properties of plasma thromboplastin antecedent (PTA) in relation to blood coagulation. J. Lab. Clin. Med., 45:123, 1955.
432. Rosenthal, R. L., Dreskin, O. H., and Rosenthal, N.: New hemophilia-like disease caused by deficiency of a third plasma thromboplastin factor. Proc. Soc. Exp. Biol. Med., 82:171, 1953.
433. Rosenthal, R. L., and Sloan, E.: PTA (Factor XI) levels and coagulation studies after plasma infusions in PTA-deficiency patients. J. Lab. Clin. Med., 66:709, 1965.
434. Rosner, F.: Medical history: hemophilia in the Talmud and rabbinic writings. Ann. Intern. Med., 70:833, 1969.
435. Rossi, E. C., and Green, D.: Disorders of platelet function. Med. Clin. North Am., 56:35, 1972.
436. Rossi, E. C., Redondo, D., and Borges, W. H.: Thrombotic thrombocytopenic purpura. J.A.M.A., 228:1141, 1974.
437. Ruffolo, E. H., Pease, G. L., and Cooper, T.: Thrombotic thrombocytopenic purpura. Arch. Intern. Med., 110:78, 1962.
438. Salzman, E. W.: Measurement of platelet adhesiveness: progress report. Thromb. Diath. Haemorrh. (Suppl.), 26:323, 1967.
439. Salzman, E. W., and Britten, A.: In vitro correction of defective platelet adhesiveness in von Willebrand's disease. Fed. Proc., 23:239, 1964.
440. Sandler, S. G., Rath, C. E., and Ruder, A.: Prothrombin complex concentrates in acquired hypoprothrombinemia. Ann. Intern. Med., 79:485, 1973.
441. Sanfelippo, M. J., and Hussey, C. V.: Thrombopathy. Identification and distribution. Am. J. Clin. Pathol., 61:628, 1974.
442. Saunders, W. H.: Hereditary hemorrhagic telangiectasia. Arch. Otolaryngol., 76:245, 1962.
443. Schaar, F. E.: Familial idiopathic thrombocytopenic purpura. J. Pediatr., 62:546, 1963.
444. Schmid, H. J., Jackson, D. P., and Conley, C. L.: Mechanism of action of thrombin on platelets. J. Clin. Invest., 41:543, 1962.
445. Schneider, C. L.: Fibrin embolism (disseminated intravascular coagulation) with defibrination as one of the end-results during placenta abruptio. Surg. Gynecol. Obstet., 92:27, 1951.
446. Schneider, C. L.: Rapid estimation of plasma fibrinogen concentration and its use as a guide to therapy of intravascular defibrination. Am. J. Obstet. Gynecol., 64:141, 1952.
447. Schulman, I., Abildgaard, C. F., Cornet, J., Simone, J. V., and Currimbhoy, Z.: Studies on thrombopoiesis. II. Assay of human plasma thrombopoietic activity. J. Pediatr., 66:604, 1965.
448. Schulman, I., Pierce, M., Lukens, A., and Currimbhoy, Z.: Studies on thrombopoiesis. I. A factor in normal human plasma required for platelet production: chronic thrombocytopenia due to its deficiency. Blood, 16:943, 1960.
449. Schulman, I., Smith, G. H., Erlandson, M., and Fort, E.: Vascular hemophilia. Am. J. Dis. Child., 90:526, 1955.
450. Schwartz, M. L., Pizzo, S. V., Hill, R. L., and McKee, P. A.: The effect of fibrin-stabilizing factor on the subunit structure of human fibrin. J. Clin. Invest., 50:1506, 1971.
451. Scott, J. S.: Blood coagulation failure in obstetrics, effects of dextran and plasma. Br. Med. J., 2:290, 1955.
452. Seip, M.: Hereditary hypoplastic thrombocytopenia. Acta Paediatr., 52:370, 1963.
453. Seligsohn, U., and Ramot, B.: Combined Factor V and Factor VIII deficiency: report of four cases. Br. J. Haematol., 16:475, 1969.
454. Serpick, A. A.: Platelet transfusion therapy. J.A.M.A., 192:625, 1965.

455. Shanbrom, E., and Thelin, G. M.: Experimental prophylaxis of severe hemophilia with a Factor VIII concentrate. J.A.M.A., *208*:1853, 1969.

456. Shapiro, C. M., Texidor, T. A., Robbins, K. C., and Rabiner, S. F.: Clinical remission of purpura hyperglobulinemia. Arch. Intern. Med., *124*:81, 1969.

457. Shapiro, S. S., Martinez, J., and Halburn, R. R.: Congenital dysprothrombinemia: an inherited structural disorder of human prothrombin. J. Clin. Invest., *48*:2251, 1969.

458. Sharp, A. A.: Pathological fibrinolysis. Br. Med. Bull., *20*:240, 1964.

459. Sharp, A. A.: The significance of fibrinolysis. Proc. Roy. Soc., Series B. Biol. Sci., *173*:311, 1969.

460. Sharp, A. A., Howie, B., Biggs, R., and Methuen, D. T.: Defibrination syndrome in pregnancy. Value of various diagnostic tests. Lancet, *2*:1309, 1958.

461. Sherman, L. A., Goldstein, M. A., and Sise, H. S.: Circulating anticoagulant (antifactor VIII) treated with immunosuppressive drugs. Thromb. Diath. Haemorrh., *21*:249, 1969.

462. Sherry, S.: Fibrinolysis. Annu. Rev. Med., *19*:247, 1968.

463. Sherry, S.: Thrombolysis by urokinase. J. Atherosclerosis Res., *9*:1, 1969.

463a. Sherry, S., Troll, W., and Glueck, H.: Thrombin as a proteolytic enzyme. Physiol. Rev., *34*:736, 1954.

464. Shulman, I.: Diagnosis and treatment: management of idiopathic thrombocytopenic purpura. Pediatrics, *33*:979, 1964.

465. Shulman, N. R.: Mechanism of blood cell destruction in individuals sensitized to foreign antigens. Tr. Assoc. Am. Physicians, *76*:72, 1963.

466. Shulman, N. R., Aster, R. H., Leitner, A., and Hiller, M. C.: Immunoreactions involving platelets. V. Post-transfusion purpura due to a complement-fixing antibody against a genetically controlled platelet antigen. A proposed mechanism for thrombocytopenia and its relevance in "autoimmunity." J. Clin. Invest., *40*:1597, 1961.

467. Shulman, N. R., Aster, R. H., Pearson, H. A., and Hiller, M. C.: Immunoreactions involving platelets. VI. Reactions of maternal isoantibodies responsible for neonatal purpura. Differentiation of a second platelet antigen system. J. Clin. Invest., *41*:1059, 1962.

468. Shulman, N. R., and Hirschman, R. J.: Acquired hemophilia. Tr. Assoc. Am. Physicians, *82*:388, 1969.

469. Shulman, N. R., Marder, V. J., and Weinrack, R. S.: Similarities between known antiplatelet antibodies and the factor responsible for thrombocytopenia in idiopathic purpura. Physiologic, serologic, and isotopic studies. Ann. N. Y. Acad. Sci., *124*:499, 1965.

470. Shulman, N. R., Weinrach, R. S., Libre, E. P., and Andrews, H. L.: The role of the reticuloendothelial system in the pathogenesis of idiopathic thrombocytopenic purpura. Tr. Assoc. Am. Physicians, *78*:374, 1965.

471. Sibinga, C. T., Gökemeyer, J. D. M., ten Kate, L. P., and Bos-van Zwol, F.: Combined deficiency of Factor V and Factor VIII: report of a family and genetic analysis. Br. J. Haematol., *23*:467, 1972.

472. Simone, J. V., Cornet, J. A., and Abildgaard, C. F.: Acquired von Willebrand's syndrome in systemic lupus erythematosus. Blood, *31*:806, 1968.

473. Skudowitz, R. B., Katz, J., Lurie, A., Levin, J., and Metz, J.: Mechanisms of thrombocytopenia in malignant tertian malaria. Br. Med. J., *2*:515, 1973.

474. Smith, H.: Purpura fulminans complicating varicella: recovery with low molecular weight dextran and steroids. Med. J. Aust., *2*:685, 1967.

475. Soloman, W., Turner, D. S., Block, C., and Posner, A. C.: Thrombotic thrombocytopenic purpura in pregnancy. J.A.M.A., *184*:587, 1963.

476. Soulier, J. P.: Syndromes hémorrhagiques avec atteinte isolée de la résistance capillaire. Sang, *21*:801, 1950.

477. Soulier, J. P., Josso, F., Steinbuch, M., and Cosson, A.: The therapeutical use of Fraction P.P.S.B. Bibl. Haematol., *29*:1127, 1968.

478. Soulier, J. P., and Larrieu, M. J.: Differentiation of hemophilia into two groups. A study of thirty-three cases. N. Engl. J. Med., *249*:547, 1953.

479. Spaet, T. H., and Zucker, M. B.: Mechanism of platelet plug formation and role of adenosine diphosphate. Am. J. Phys. Med., *206*:1267, 1964.

480. Speer, R. J., Ridgway, H., and Hill, J. M.: Activated human Hageman Factor (XII). Thromb. Diath. Haemorrh., *14*:1, 1965.

481. Staub, H. P.: Postrubella thrombocytopenic purpura. A report of eight cases with discussion of hemorrhagic manifestations of rubella. Clin. Pediatr., *7*:350, 1968.

482. Stefanini, M.: Basic mechanisms of hemostasis. Bull. N. Y. Acad. Med., *20*:239, 1954.

483. Stefanini, M.: Management of thrombocytopenic states. Arch. Intern. Med., *95*:543, 1955.

484. Stefanini, M.: Activity of plasma labile factor in disease. Lancet, *1*:606, 1951.

485. Stefanini, M., and Chatterjea, J. B.: Studies on platelets. IV. A thrombocytopenic factor in normal human blood plasma or serum. Proc. Soc. Exp. Biol. Med., *79*:623, 1952.

486. Stefanini, M., Chatterjea, J. B., Dameshek, W., Zannos, L., and Santiago, E. P.: The effect of

transfusion of platelet-rich polycythemic blood on the platelets and hemostatic function in "idiopathic" and "secondary" thrombocytopenic purpura. Blood, 7:53, 1952.

487. Stefanini, M., and Dameshek, W.: The Hemorrhagic Disorders. Grune and Stratton, New York, 1955.

488. Stefanini, M., Roy, C. A., Zannos, L., and Dameshek, W.: Therapeutic effect of pituitary adrenocortotropic hormone (ACTH) in a case of Henoch-Schönlein vascular (anaphylactoid) purpura. J.A.M.A., 144:1372, 1950.

489. Steinkamp, R., Moore, C. V., and Doubek, W. G.: Thrombocytopenic purpura caused by hypersensitivity to quinine. J. Lab. Clin. Med., 45:18, 1955.

490. Stenflo, J., and Ganrot, P. -O.: Vitamin K and the biosynthesis of prothrombin. J. Biol. Chem., 247:8160, 8167, 1972.

491. Stites, D. P., Hershgold, G. J., Perlman, J. D., and Fudenberg, H. H.: Factor VIII: Detection by hemagglutination inhibition. Hemophilia and von Willebrand's disease. Science, 171:196, 1971.

492. Storti, E., Traldi, A., Tosatti, E., and Davoli, P. G.: Synovectomy, a new approach to haemophilic arthropathy. Acta Haematol., 41:193, 1969.

493. Strauss, H. S.: Acquired circulating anticoagulants in hemophilia A. N. Engl. J. Med., 281:866, 1969.

494. Strauss, H. E., and Bloom, G. E.: Von Willebrand's disease. N. Engl. J. Med., 273:171, 1965.

495. Strauss, H. S., and Merler, E.: Characterization and properties of an inhibitor of Factor VIII in the plasma of patients with hemophilia A following repeated transfusions. Blood, 30:137, 1967.

496. Sussman, L. N.: Azathioprine in refractory thrombocytopenic purpura. J.A.M.A., 202:259, 1967.

497. Sutherland, J. M., Glueck, H. I., and Gleser, G.: Hemorrhagic disease of the newborn. Am. J. Dis. Child., 113:524, 1967.

498. Suttie, J. W.: Control of clotting factor biosynthesis by vitamin K. Fed. Proc., 28:1696, 1969.

499. Szpilmanowa, H., and Stachurska, J.: Hageman factor (Factor XII) activity in synovial fluid of rheumatoid arthritis patients and its possible pathogenic significance. Experientia, 24:784, 1968.

500. Tagnon, H. J., Schulman, P., Whitmore, W. F., and Leone, L. A.: Prostatic fibrinolysin. Am. J. Med., 15:875, 1953.

501. Tagnon, H. J., Whitmore, W. F., and Shulman, N. R.: Fibrinolysis in metastatic cancer of the prostate. Cancer, 5:9, 1952.

502. Talbot, J. H., and Ferrandis, R. M.: Collagen Diseases. Grune and Stratton, New York, 1956.

503. Thomas, D. P., Ream, V. J., and Stuart, R. K.: Platelet aggregation in Laennec's cirrhosis. N. Engl. J. Med., 276:1344, 1967.

504. Thomson, C., Forbes, C. D., and Prentice, C. R. M.: Abnormal Factor VIII in von Willebrand's disease. Scott. Med. J., 19:58, 1974.

505. Thompson, C., Forbes, C. D., and Prentice, C. R. M.: Evidence for a qualitative defect in Factor VIII-related antigen in von Willebrand's disease. Lancet, 1:594, 1974.

506. Thompson, R. L., Moore, R. A., Hess, C. E., Wheby, M. S., and Leavell, B. S.: Idiopathic thrombocytopenic purpura. Arch. Intern. Med., 130:730, 1972.

507. Tocantins, L. M.: Platelets and the structure and physical properties of blood clots. Am. J. Physiol., 114:709, 1936.

508. Trieger, N., and McGovern, J. J.: Evaluation of corticosteroids in hemophilia. N. Engl. J. Med., 266:432, 1962.

509. Trygstad, C. W., and Stiehan, E. R.: Elevated serum IgA globulin in anaphylactoid purpura. Pediatrics, 47:1023, 1971.

510. Tullis, J. L., and Melin, M.: Management of Christmas disease and Stuart-Prower deficiency with a prothrombin-complex concentrate (Factors II, VII, IX, and X). Bibl. Haematol., 29:1134, 1968.

511. Umlas, J., and Kaiser, J.: Thrombohemolytic thrombocytopenic purpura (TTP): a disease or a syndrome? Am. J. Med., 49:723, 1970.

512. Van Creveld, S., Ho, L. K., and Veder, H. A.: Thrombopathia. Acta Haematol., 19:199, 1958.

513. Van Creveld, S., Mochtar, I. A., Van Charantevan Der Meulen, C. C. M., Pascha, C. N., and Stibbe, J.: Investigation of circulating anticoagulants against AHF (Factor VIII) in three patients with hemophilia A. Acta Haematol., 39:214, 1968.

514. Vandenbroucke, J., and Verstraete, M.: Thrombocytopenia due to platelet agglutinins in the newborn. Lancet, 1:593, 1955.

515. van Itterbeek, H., Vermylen, J., and Verstraete, M.: High obstruction of urine flow as a complication of the treatment with fibrinolysis inhibitors of haematuria in haemophiliacs. Acta Haematol., 39:237, 1968.

516. Veltkamp, J. J., Meilof, J., Remmelts, H. G., Van der Vlerk, D., and Loeliger, E. A.: Another genetic variant of haemophilia B; hemophilia B Leyden. Scand. J. Haematol., 7:82, 1970.
517. Veltkamp, J. J., and van Tilburg, N. C.: Detection of heterozygotes for recessive von Wille-brand's disease by the assay of antihemophilic factor-like antigen. N. Engl. J. Med., 289:882, 1973.
518. Veltkamp, J. J., and van Tilburg, N. H.: "Autosomal hemophilia": a variant of von Wille-brand's disease. Br. J. Haematol., 26:141, 1974.
519. Vernier, R. L., Worthen, H. B., Peterson, R. D., Colle, E., and Good, R. A.: Anaphylactoid purpura: pathology of the skin and kidney and frequency of streptococcal infection. Pediatrics, 27:181, 1961.
520. Villalobus, T. J., Adelson, E., and Barila, T. J.: Hematologic changes in hypothermic dogs. Proc. Soc. Exp. Biol. Med., 89:192, 1955.
521. Vitsky, B., Suzuki, Y., Strauss, L., and Churg, J.: The hemolytic-uremic syndrome. Am. J. Pathol., 57:627, 1969.
522. Von Felten, A., Frick, P. G., and Straub, P. W.: Studies on fibrin monomer aggregation in congenital dysfibrinogenemia fibrin fraction. Br. J. Haematol., 16:353, 1969.
523. Waddell, W. W., Jr., Guerry, D., III, Bray, W. E., and Kelley, O. R.: Possible effects of vitamin K on prothrombin and clotting time in newly-born infants. Proc. Soc. Exp. Biol. Med., 40:432, 1939.
524. Waldenström, J.: Incipient myelomatosis or "essential" hyperglobulinemia with fibrinogeno-penia—a new syndrome? Acta Med. Scand., 117:216, 1944.
524a. Waldenström, J.: Three new cases of purpura hyperglobulinemia: study in long-lasting benign increase in serum globulin. Acta Med. Scand., 142(Suppl. 266):931, 1952.
525. Wall, R. L., McConnell, J., Moore, D., Macpherson, C. R., and Marson, A.: Christmas disease, color blindness and blood group Xg. Am. J. Med., 43:214, 1967.
526. Walsh, P. N.: Platelet coagulant activities in thrombasthenia. Br. J. Haematol., 23:553, 1972.
527. Walsh, P. N., Rainsford, S. G., and Biggs, R.: Platelet coagulant activities and clinical severity in haemophilia. Thromb. Diath. Haemorrh., 29:722, 1973.
528. Wardle, E. N.: Immunoglobulins and immunological reactions in hemophilia. Lancet, 2:233, 1967.
529. Watson, C. G., and Cooper, W. M.: Thrombotic thrombocytopenic purpura: concomitant occurrence in husband and wife. J.A.M.A., 215:1821, 1971.
530. Watson-Williams, E. J., Macpherson, A. I., and Davidson, S.: The treatment of idiopathic thrombocytopenic purpura; a review of ninety-three cases. Lancet, 2:221, 1958.
531. Weber, F. P.: Multiple hereditary developmental angiomata (telangiectases) of the skin and mucous membranes associated with recurring hemorrhages. Lancet, 2:160, 1907.
532. Weiner, A. E., Reid, D. E., and Roby, C. C.: Incoagulable blood in severe premature separation of the placenta. A method of management. Am. J. Obstet. Gynecol., 66:475, 1953.
533. Weiss, H. J.: Abnormalities in platelet function due to defects in the release reaction. Ann. N. Y. Acad. Sci., 201:161, 1972.
534. Weiss, H. J.: Platelet aggregation, adhesion and adenosine diphosphate release in thrombo-pathia (platelet Factor 3 deficiency) comparison with Glanzmann's thrombasthenia and von Willebrand's disease. Am. J. Med., 43:570, 1967.
535. Weiss, H. J.: Analytic review: von Willebrand's disease—diagnostic criteria. Blood, 32:4, 1968.
536. Weiss, H. J., Aledort, L. M., and Kochwa, S.: Effect of salicylates on hemostatic properties of platelets in man. J. Clin. Invest., 47:2169, 1968.
537. Weiss, H. J., Chervenick, P. A., Zalusky, R., and Factor, A.: A familial defect in platelet function associated with impaired release of adenosine diphosphate. N. Engl. J. Med., 281:1264, 1969.
538. Weiss, H. J., and Eichelberger, J. W., Jr.: The detection of platelet defects in patients with mild bleeding disorders. Am. J. Med., 32:872, 1962.
539. Weiss, H. J., and Eichelberger, J. W., Jr.: Secondary thrombocytopathia: platelet Factor 3 in various disease states. Arch. Intern. Med., 112:827, 1963.
540. Weiss, H. J., Hoyer, L. W., Rickles, F. R., Varma, A., and Rogers, J.: Quantitative assay of a plasma factor deficient in von Willebrand's disease that is necessary for platelet aggrega-tion. J. Clin. Invest., 52:2708, 1973.
541. Weiss, H. J., and Kochwa, S.: Studies of platelet function and proteins in 3 patients with Glanz-mann's thrombasthenia. J. Lab. Clin. Med., 71:153, 1968.
542. Weiss, H. J., and Rogers, J.: Thrombocytopathia due to abnormalities in platelet release reac-tion—studies on six unrelated patients. Blood, 39:187, 1972.
543. Weiss, H. J., Rogers, J., and Brand, H.: Defective ristocetin-induced platelet aggregation in von Willebrand's disease and its correction by factor VIII. J. Clin. Invest., 52:2697, 1973.

544. Whipple, G. H.: Fibrinogen. I. An investigation concerning its origins and destruction in the body. Am. J. Phys. Med., *33*:50, 1914.
545. Whissell, D. Y., Hoag, M. S., Aggeler, P. M., Kropatkin, M., and Garner, E.: Hemophilia in a woman. Am. J. Med., *38*:119, 1965.
546. White, J. G., Edson, J. R., Desnick, S. J., and Witkop, C. J.: Studies of platelets in a variant of the Hermansky–Pudlak syndrome. Am. J. Pathol., *63*:319, 1971.
547. Wilde, C., Ellis, D., and Cooper, W. M.: Splenectomy for chronic idiopathic thrombocytopenic purpura. Arch. Surg., *95*:344, 1967.
548. Williams, G. A., and Brick, I. B.: Gastrointestinal bleeding in hereditary hemorrhagic telangiectasia. Arch. Intern. Med., *95*:41, 1955.
549. Winterbauer, R. H.: Multiple telangiectasia, Reynaud's phenomenon, sclerodactyly, and subcutaneous calcinosis: a syndrome mimicking hereditary hemorrhagic telangiectasia. Bull. Johns Hopkins Hosp., *114*:361, 1964.
550. Wishart, C., Smith, A. C., Honey, G. E., and Taylor, K. B.: Dental extraction in haemophilia. Lancet, *2*:363, 1957.
551. Wolper, J., and Laibson, R. R.: Hereditary hemorrhagic telangiectasis (Rendu-Osler-Weber disease) with filamentary keratitis. Arch. Ophthalmol., *81*:272, 1969.
552. Wright, D. O., Reppert, L. B., and Cuttino, J. T.: Purpuric manifestations of heat-stroke. Arch. Intern. Med., 77:27, 1946.
553. Zimmerman, T. S., and Edgington, T. S.: Molecular immunology of Factor VIII. Annu. Rev. Med., *25*:303, 1974.
554. Zucker, M. B.: In vitro abnormality of the blood in von Willebrand's disease correctable by normal plasma. Nature, *197*:601, 1963.
555. Zucker, M. B., and Lundberg, A.: Platelet transfusion. Anesthesiology, *27*:385, 1966.
556. Zucker, M. B., Pert, J. H., and Hilgartner, M. W.: Platelet function in a patient with thrombasthenia. Blood, *28*:524, 1966.

CHAPTER **18**

TRANSFUSION THERAPY

Increased knowledge of the numerous blood groups, improved techniques in cross-matching the donor and recipient, and the development of more efficient methods of preserving and storing blood have all combined to make progress in blood transfusion one of the foremost accomplishments of modern medicine. The important technical details related to this broad subject are thoroughly covered in several monographs.[35, 99] Publications prepared by the American Association of Blood Banks and by the Committee on Transfusion and Transplantation (American Medical Association) give authoritative and concise statements concerning minimal standards for processing donors and general principles of blood transfusion.[27, 28] The current status of red cell preservation has been reviewed extensively in the proceedings of two recent scientific conferences.[26]

The development of the new national blood policy[104, 129] has identified four important goals for an improved national blood service:

(1) to assure a supply of blood and blood products adequate to meet all the treatment and diagnostic needs of our population;

(2) to attain the highest standard of blood transfusion therapy through full application of currently available scientific knowledge and advancement of the scientific base;

(3) to assure access to the national supply of blood and blood products by everyone in need, regardless of economic status;

(4) to establish and maintain efficient collection, processing, storage, and utilization of the national supply of blood and blood products.

The extent to which these important goals can be realized relates not only to the efforts of those involved in procurement, processing, and distribution of blood and blood products, but also to the habits, practices, and perceptions of practicing physicians and their patients.[25]

HISTORY

The early history of blood transfusions has been summarized by several authors.[42, 75, 140] Authentic references to blood transfusions date from the middle of the seventeenth century. In 1667 Lower transfused blood of a lamb into a "mildly melancholy insane" man and this was considered successful. In the same year Jean Baptist Denis transfused 9 ounces of lamb's blood into a youth, and the lad made a remarkable recovery from an obscure fever. Denis repeated the procedure in other patients until he encountered a fatal hemolytic reaction in a man who was given lamb's blood for insanity. This patient had received two previous transfusions; the first had no untoward effect, but black urine accompanied the second. Denis was charged with murder, but was exonerated after a prolonged legal battle. Transfusion was forbidden by Parliament and Papal Bull, and little interest was shown in the subject for the next 150 years. In 1818 James Blundell, a London physiologist and obstetrician, used indirect blood transfusions in ten patients with postpartum hemorrhage, and five of these were successful. Interest in this field increased, and by 1875 at least 347 transfusions of human blood had been recorded.

The modern era of blood transfusions began in 1900 when Landsteiner described the presence of isoagglutinating and isoagglutinable substances in human blood.[80] In 1936 the first blood bank in the United States was organized at Cook County Hospital in Chicago by Fantus.[44] The operation of blood banks has led to an increasing use of blood transfusion. The availability and safety of whole blood and its components have made possible many operations and other treatments that otherwise would have been impossible. The easy availability of blood transfusion also has led to its use in situations in which it is not necessary, a procedure that subjects the patient to an unnecessary hazard.

BLOOD GROUPS

Blood groups are important in clinical medicine primarily because of their relationship to hemolytic transfusion reactions and hemolytic disease of the newborn. Blood group antigens, which are located on the cell membrane, also provide gene markers that are utilized in the study of human population genetics and in anthropology. Further study can be expected to identify the relationship of the different blood groups to differences in susceptibility to certain diseases such as duodenal ulcer, pernicious anemia, and carcinoma of the stomach, and the role of this relationship to natural selection. Determination of the blood groups is important also in legal questions concerning parentage. Excellent summaries of this complex and rapidly expanding field are available.[6, 72, 91, 100, 103, 116, 119, 142]

The important discovery that human erythrocytes belong to several different antigenic systems was made in 1900 by Landsteiner, who identified the ABO blood groups.[80] Over 250 antigens have now been identified on red blood cells, and the end is not in sight. Mollison lists 15 different antigenic systems that have been recognized: ABO (A_1A_2BO); MNSs; P; Rh; Lutheran; Kell; Lewis; Duffy; Kidd; Diego; Yt, I, Xg, Dombrock, and Colton. The blood group systems in which naturally-occurring antibodies are most often found are ABO, MNSs, P, Lewis, and Wright.[100] The antigens (other than those that belong to these systems) which have been identified are classed as "public" (found almost universally) or "private" (limited to one or several families). Further investigation may prove that some of these really belong to already-recognized systems and that others are examples of new systems not yet established as such. The ABO and

Rh systems are of particular importance in clinical medicine because they are responsible for nearly all instances of hemolytic transfusion reactions and hemolytic disease of the newborn. The other antigens may be responsible for severe instances of these disorders, but they occur only rarely.

The ABO system consists of four main blood groups: A, B, AB, and O. The antigens, A and B, occur on the erythrocytes, and the agglutinins, anti-A and anti-B, occur in the serum in a reciprocal fashion. Thus a person who belongs to the AB blood group will have the antigens A and B on the erythrocytes and no agglutinins in the serum. A person with group O blood has neither A nor B antigen on the red cells but has both anti-A and anti-B agglutinins in the serum. A person with group A blood has A antigen on the cells and anti-B agglutinins in the serum; a patient with group B blood has B antigen on the cells and anti-A agglutinins in the serum. It is thus possible to determine the blood group of an unknown blood by noting the reactions of the red cells to anti-A and anti-B sera.

Table 18–1 *The ABO Blood Groups*

Name Of Blood Group	Antigens In Red Cells (Agglutinogens)	Antibodies In Serum (Agglutinins)	Incidence In Whites (%)
O	none	anti-A and anti-B	45
A	A	anti-B	41
B	B	anti-A	10
AB	A and B	none	4

It has been demonstrated that several subgroups of A exist. The most important are A_1 and A_2. Accordingly, subgroups A_1, A_2, A_1B, and A_2B are recognized. About 80 per cent of persons in group A belong to subgroup A_1 and 20 per cent belong to subgroup A_2; about 60 per cent of persons in group AB belong to subgroup A_1B and 40 per cent belong to A_2B.[97] The erythrocytes of subgroup A_1 are agglutinated more strongly by anti-A sera than are cells of subtype A_2. For this reason, cells containing the A_2 antigen may be missed unless anti-A serum that is known to produce a strong reaction with A_2 cells is used when the blood group is determined.

About 85 per cent of persons who possess the A or B substance in their tissues secrete the substance in the saliva, urine, tears, semen, gastric juice, and milk.[35] Such persons are termed "secretors"; those who do not possess this faculty are termed "non-secretors." The ability to secrete the group-specific substance is inherited as a Mendelian dominant character.[35, 97]

The MNS blood system was discovered by Landsteiner and Levine in 1927.[81] These blood group factors, which are found in the blood of every person, occur independently of factors of the ABO blood groups. The MNS system is of little importance in clinical medicine because it is very rarely associated with hemolytic transfusion reactions or hemolytic disease of the newborn. These reactions are almost nonexistent because agglutinins for the MNS agglutinogens are rarely found, either as so-called "natural antibodies" or as a response to the injection of blood of a different type.

Antibodies to erythrocytes are usually either γG (IgG) or γM (IgM) immunoglobulins. Antigens representing the phenotypes of all of the systems noted above are present in very large numbers on the red cell. The number of any one of these antigens varies from as few as 25,000 per red cell in the case of the Rh (D) system to as many as 1 million per red cell for the ABO system.

Red cells repel one another, since they are negatively charged, and in order for agglutination to occur this charge must be overcome or reduced. γM (IgM) antibodies are large, and as few as ten antibodies per red cell can actually bridge the "charge gap" between cells and cause visible agglutination. γG (IgG) antibodies are smaller and do not bridge the "charge gap" unless there are several thousand antibodies per cell. This heavy coat of γG antibodies mitigates the inherent negative charge of the cells, allowing them to move close enough for the smaller γG antibodies to bridge the gap and cause agglutination. Agglutination therefore requires several thousand more γG antibodies than γM antibodies. If there are relatively few antigens on the red cell, direct agglutination does not occur no matter how high a concentration of γG antibody is introduced, since there will be an insufficient coating of antigen-antibody complexes to change the charge of the cell. The presence of these small numbers of γG antigen-antibody complexes can be detected, however, if the "charge gap" can be overcome. This may be accomplished in several ways. The charge itself may be dispersed by lowering the ionic strength of the supporting medium, or may be reduced by enzymatic removal of the neuraminic acid residues responsible for the negative charge. High-speed centrifugation may be used to overcome physically the "charge gap" and force the cells into close proximity. The "charge gap" may also be bridged by adding an intermediate antibody attachment, as in the Coombs test, which uses a rabbit anti-human γG to agglutinate γG coated cells.[100]

Specific isoimmune antibodies which occur in human serum may be of the "immune antibody" or "natural antibody" type. Immune antibodies arise as the result of transfusions from a blood donor or, in the case of a pregnant female, from a fetus. Natural antibodies may be present in the serum of an individual with no history of transfusion, pregnancy, or other specific opportunities for immunization. The natural antibodies are assumed to form in response to "accidental" immunization by cross-reacting antigens from the environment. A and B antigens, for example, are ubiquitous in nature. Since they are present in dust and many foods, virtually all individuals lacking one of these antigens will have formed an antibody to it by the end of the first year of life. Antibodies of a single specificity may occur as a mixture of γM and γG immunoglobulins or as either type alone. Generally, natural antibodies are of the γM type and immune antibodies are of the γG type, but there are numerous exceptions. An extensive discussion of this subject may be found in the book by Mollison.[100]

The Rh factor was discovered by Landsteiner and Wiener in 1940.[82] They observed that serum from rabbits that had been injected with erythrocytes of the rhesus monkey caused agglutination of the red cells from about 85 per cent of human beings without relation to their other blood groups. The new system was termed the Rh system. The rapid discovery of several different antigens in this system and the introduction of different terminologies for the antigens have led to some confusion. The equivalent gene symbols used by Wiener[142] and by Fisher and Race[116] and the approximate incidence of each are shown in Table 18–2, prepared by Dr. O. B. Bobbitt. According to the Fisher-Race concept, there are three sets of closely linked allelic genes, C and c, D and d, E and e; every person inherits one gene from each pair, a total of three genes from each parent. Everyone has paired chromosomes of eight possible types that result from different combinations of the genes. According to the Fisher-Race nomen-

Table 18–2 *The Rh Blood Types*

SYMBOL	GENOTYPES (SYNONYMS)		APPROX. INCIDENCE (%)	
	Wiener	English	White	Black
	R^1R^0	CDe/cDe ⎱	34	23
	R^1r	CDe/cde ⎰		
	R^1R^1	CDe/CDe	18	4
	R^2R^0	cDE/cDe ⎱	12	12
	R^2r	cDE/cde ⎰		
Rh₀(D) Positive	R^1R^2	CDe/cDE	13	3
	R^0R^0	cDe/cDe ⎱	2	48
	R^0r	cDe/cde ⎰		
	R^2R^2	cDE/cDE	2	2
		Others	< 2	< 2
		Total Rh₀(D) pos.	83	93
Rh₀(D) Negative	rr	cde/cde	16	6
	r'r	Cde/cde ⎱	< 2	< 2
	r''r	cdE/cde ⎰		
		Total Rh₀(D) neg.	17	7

clature these are designated as follows: cde; Cde; cdE; CdE; cDe; CDe; cDE; CDE. The corresponding symbols according to the Wiener nomenclature are r, r', r'', r^y, R^0, R^1, R^2, R^z. Wiener feels that these antigens are controlled by a single gene.[142]

The importance of the Rh system in clinical medicine, particularly in erythroblastosis fetalis, was first demonstrated by Levine and Stetson.[85] The natural occurrence of iso-antibody for the Rh factor is exceedingly rare. However, the introduction of erythrocytes from an Rh-positive person into an Rh-negative person may stimulate the production of the corresponding antibodies. Although there are as many different Rh antibodies as there are Rh antigens, the Rh₀(D) antigen is by far the most potent and thus the most important in clinical medicine. Persons who have the Rh₀(D) antigen are referred to as "Rh-positive," and those who lack the Rh₀(D) antigen are referred to as "Rh-negative." About 83 per cent of American whites and 93 per cent of American blacks are Rh-positive. Immunization may result from the introduction of the Rh₀(D) antigen by the transfusion of Rh-positive blood into an Rh-negative recipient or by the passage of erythrocytes from an Rh-positive fetus into the circulation of an Rh-negative mother. When Rh-positive blood is transfused into the Rh-negative recipients, about 50 to 75 per cent of the recipients become immunized, but only about 5 per cent of Rh-negative mothers are immunized by pregnancies.[97]

The isoimmunization of an Rh-negative mother by her Rh-positive fetus can now be prevented.[36, 47] Since most fetal cells gain access to the maternal circulation at the time of delivery, there is time to determine the infant's blood type and to intervene to prevent isoimmunization if necessary. If the infant is Rh-positive, concentrated gamma globulin obtained from persons hyperimmune to the D antigen is injected into the mother; the Rh immunoglobulin must be administered intramuscularly since intravenous administration of gamma globulin is unsafe. A rapid removal of fetal Rh-positive cells is effected by the Rh-immunoglobulin. The precise mechanism by which passive antibody is able to effect specific immunosuppression of the active immunity that follows injection of an antigen is not completely understood, but is believed to relate to the "walling off" of the antigen by circulating antibody so that it either fails to reach immunologically competent cells at all, or reaches them only in an inactive state.

RED CELL STORAGE

LIQUID RED-CELL STORAGE

When fresh, normal erythrocytes are transfused into a compatible recipient, the donated cells have a half-life of 60 days. When blood is stored in ACD or CPD mixture at 4° C and then transfused, a portion of the cells leave the circulation within the first 24 hours, but the remainder survive fairly well. After 14 days of storage, 90 per cent of the cells survive for more than 24 hours and the survival time of these cells is almost normal; after storage for 28 days, only 70 per cent of the cells survive for 24 hours, and all have disappeared by 80 days.[100]

A variety of blood additives are in use in other countries, or under study here and abroad, that improve the viability of red cells and reduce the rate of decline of $2,3-DPG$.[25]

FROZEN RED-CELL STORAGE

Red cells may be frozen in the presence of a variety of cryoprotective agents, stored for at least ten years, and recovered in high yield. Eighty per cent of red cells stored under these conditions will survive and function normally after transfusion. The multiple entries needed to remove the cryoprotective agent after thawing create a considerable hazard of bacterial contamination and necessitate a brief post-thaw shelf life of 24 hours.[25]

The process is currently more expensive than liquid storage and does not appear to offer sufficient advantage to justify its routine use at present. The limited use of frozen red cells does assure the availability of rare blood types for transfusion and can provide storage of blood for autologous transfusion. It may also prevent sensitization by histocompatibility antigens of candidates for organ transplants by removal of white blood cells. Frozen blood storage would also provide for emergency military and civil defense needs by allowing the development of large stockpiles.[25]

INDICATIONS FOR BLOOD COMPONENT THERAPY

Whole blood is a mixture of erythrocytes, leukocytes, and platelets suspended in plasma. Plasma is largely water, but it contains important electrolytes and proteins. The techniques available in modern blood banks now allow the physician to administer to his patient whole blood or some component of whole blood. The physician must assess the requirements of each patient individually and use only those components indicated. If the growing needs for blood and blood products are to be met, the best possible use must be made of each donated unit of blood.

To increase oxygen-carrying capacity of blood and expand volume. Whole blood transfusion is used when the oxygen-carrying capacity of the blood and the circulating blood volume must be restored simultaneously. It is indicated in the treatment of acute severe hemorrhage, and the criteria for adequate transfusion rest primarily on the evaluation of the clinical condition of the patient, though measurement of blood volume and hematocrit may be of assistance. Seldom, if ever, is complete replacement of the lost blood necessary.[32]

To increase oxygen-carrying capacity of blood with little or no volume expansion. Packed red cells should be administered to those patients who require an increase in the oxygen-carrying capacity of their blood to prevent acute hypoxia or invalidism, but who are not in need of increased blood volume. Transfusion is probably advisable for patients with severe chronic anemia if the hemoglobin level is less than 6.0 gm. per cent.[100] The use of packed red cells in transfusing patients of this type, and also those with cardiac disease, allows an increase in oxygen-carrying capacity of the blood with as small an increment in blood volume as possible. In patients with heart disease, 250 ml. of packed cells should be administered slowly over a period of about four hours and the patient should be watched carefully for any evidence of heart failure. The transfusion can be repeated in 24 hours if indicated, as long as no untoward event has occurred. However, many patients with chronic anemia who require blood transfusions can be given 500 ml. of packed cells in one day.

Packed red cells which have been properly prepared by sedimentation or centrifugation have a post-transfusion survival equivalent to those in whole blood.[69] The reduction in the amount of plasma transfused with the packed cells is believed to account for the reported reduction in the incidence of hepatitis transmitted by packed red cells.[76]

To expand circulatory volume without an increase in oxygen-carrying capacity. Blood plasma has been used for many years to expand the circulatory volume. The increasing evidence of hepatitis transmission and the availability of products such as dextran and albumin have served to reduce its use for this purpose. Fresh-frozen plasma and stored plasma are both useful sources of certain blood clotting factors.

Plasma protein fraction U.S.P. is a by-product of the commercial preparation of fibrinogen and gamma globulin. It contains 5 gm. per cent protein, nearly all of which is albumin, and has been useful as a plasma expander. The material is held at 60° C for ten hours to inactivate the hepatitis virus. It is not a source of clotting factors.

Human serum albumin is fractionated from blood plasma. Its administration carries no risk of hepatitis. It contains no blood group antibody and it fares well on storage. Serum albumin is available as a 5 per cent or 25 per cent solution. The 5 per cent solution is iso-osmotic and can be used to expand the blood volume; the 25 per cent solution is often used to treat hypoproteinemia with little risk of circulatory overload, but will result in expansion of the blood volume in patients who are not dehydrated.

To provide needed components of plasma.   Plasma and fractions of plasma have long been used in the treatment of blood coagulation defects.[2] The effective treatment of deficiencies of specific coagulation factors has been difficult because their low concentration in normal plasma makes circulatory overload a constant threat; their short survival time in vivo, often necessitates repeated transfusions, and the short survival of some coagulation factors during storage makes fresh preparation a necessity.

Fibrinogen was one of the first materials to become available in relatively pure form. It is prepared as a dry powder in an ampule and must be carefully mixed with distilled water before infusion; too much agitation may cause denaturation of the protein and loss of biologic activity. The administration of fibrinogen is accompanied by a high risk of hepatitis.[108]

For many years, fresh-frozen plasma or fresh plasma was the only source of the labile blood clotting factors V and VIII. A number of techniques for the concentration of Factor VIII have now been developed,[14, 29, 92, 117] but the most significant improvement has been the development of cryoprecipitation by Pool.[34, 109] The technique is simple and inexpensive and can be carried out in any well-equipped blood bank. The material prepared is an excellent source of Factor VIII, concentrated 10 to 15 times, and contains Factor V, Factor I, Factor XIII, and the bleeding-time factor and Factor VIII–stimulating factor missing in von Willebrand's disease,[5, 12, 18, 94, 107, 109, 110] but the risk of hepatitis transmission remains.

Although Factor IX is relatively stable on storage, treatment of patients with Factor IX deficiency has posed problems similar to those encountered in the treatment of Factor VIII deficiency. Recently, potent, highly stable concentrates have been prepared which contain Factors II, VII, IX, and X.[17, 49, 66, 132] The activity of these factors in 10 ml. of the concentrate is equivalent to that found in 250 ml. of normal plasma. This development represents a great advance in the treatment of patients with single or multiple deficiencies of these factors that cannot be managed with whole plasma. This material is prepared from pooled plasma and its use is accompanied by a high risk of hepatitis.[49]

The relatively long biologic half-life and low levels required for hemostasis make it possible to treat Factor XI deficiency with whole plasma. Although Factor XI is relatively stable on storage, fresh or fresh-frozen plasma is generally used.[113]

Platelet transfusion.   The use of platelet transfusions has grown in recent years because of the more vigorous treatment of leukemia and generalized neoplasia. Platelet transfusions continue to be of great importance in the treatment of bone marrow failure with thrombocytopenia, and neonatal thrombocytopenia and thrombocytopenia secondary to drugs, radiation, or infection. The recent use of intensive cancer chemotherapy would not have been possible without the availability of platelet transfusions.[38]

Reduction of platelet numbers may occur as the result of increased destruction, reduced production, or some combination of the two. Clinically significant bleeding rarely occurs with platelet counts above 50,000 mm^3 if platelet function is normal. Platelet transfusions have been most useful in the treatment of thrombocytopenia secondary to reduced production.[39]

Platelets may be given in fresh whole blood to those patients who also need red cells and plasma; if red cells are not needed, platelet-rich plasma may be prepared by proper centrifugation. Platelet concentrates are the best means of delivering platelets without the attendant risk of circulatory overload. With proper centrifugation of the platelet-rich plasma, a platelet concentrate with a yield equal to that of the original plasma can be prepared which can be administered in 20 to 30 ml. of plasma.[69]

Platelets are usually collected for transfusion in CPD anticoagulant. Clumping of platelets may occur if the blood is refrigerated prior to processing.[20] Recently it has been reported that the addition of prostaglandin E_1 will inhibit the aggregation of platelets and allow 50 per cent recovery after as long as six days' storage at $4°$ C.[10] Such an additive remains investigational at present,

Platelets are prepared for transfusion by low-gravity centrifugation which separates the red cells and most white cells from the platelet-rich plasma. In a normal unit of whole blood the platelet-rich plasma will contain approximately 1.1×10^{11} platelets.[21] If used for transfusion, the plasma must be ABO-compatible with the recipient. Usually, platelet-rich plasma is used to prepare platelet concentrates which have the advantage of providing large numbers of platelets in small volumes of plasma. There has been argument concerning the need for ABO-compatible platelets. A and B blood group antigens have been shown to exist on the platelet membrane, but their importance remains unclear.[7] The presence of small numbers of red cells in platelet concentrates, however, does expose recipients to red cell antigens. Rh sensitization may be of consequence to females at the child-bearing age, and the use of Rh immunoglobulin should be considered.[20]

Multiple transfusions from random donors usually result in alloimmunization of the patient.[60, 131]

Antiplatelet antibodies are difficult to detect even when these patients no longer respond to platelet transfusions.[143] Such patients, however, will often respond to platelets from siblings or unrelated donors whose lymphocytes were genotypically identical for the HL-A antigens. It would appear that the most important determinants of platelet compatibility are closely related to the HL-A loci.[143] Such testing should be more widely available in the future. Once a compatible donor is identified, the technique of plateletpheresis makes possible the recovery of large numbers of platelets from a single donor.[57, 133]

Efforts are continuing to discover better ways of storing platelets. If not used when processed, they are usually stored at $4°$ C or $22°$ C. Platelets stored at $22°$ C. survive better after transfusion than those stored at $4°$ C., but the higher temperature has been shown to increase the risk of the growth of bacteria inadvertently introduced during phlebotomy or processing, and may present a risk to patients with reduced host defenses.[52, 74, 141] Recently, a functional defect has been appreciated in platelets stored at $22°$ C. Aggregation in response to ADP, epinephrine, and collagen has been reported to be decreased.[11, 63] The clinical significance of the difference in post-transfusion survival of platelets stored at $4°$ C. and $22°$ C. respectively appears to be small, whereas the preservation of function and reduction in bacterial proliferation at

4° C. seems appreciable. Further studies of the problems of short-term storage of platelets are needed. Long-term storage of platelets in the frozen state is under investigation in a number of centers, and offers promise of more efficient use of this blood component if better recoveries can be obtained.[41, 64, 73, 139]

Persons who have ingested aspirin within 36 hours, or other drugs known to interfere with platelet function, should not be used as donors.[128]

Granulocyte transfusion. Infection is now the major cause of death of patients whose bone marrow function has been compromised as the result of neoplastic disease or its treatment.[15] Patients with neutropenia are at high risk of acquiring infection. Diagnosis and treatment is often delayed, as they may fail to demonstrate the usual signs of inflammation or systemic symptoms. Granulocyte transfusion has long been considered to be of potential therapeutic usefulness in the treatment of these infections, but the difficulties attending the harvesting of sufficient numbers of viable granulocytes have been discouraging.[33, 101, 127]

Recent development of new methods for the collection of granulocytes has stimulated further interest in granulocyte transfusion.[96]

Granulocytes collect in the upper red blood cell layer near the plasma interface when whole blood is spun in a low-gravity centrifuge.[21, 57] This fact has allowed development of the continuous-flow centrifuge with which granulocytes may be semi-selectively removed from whole blood while plasma and most of the red cells are returned to the donor.[48] A second method is that of filtration leukapheresis.[40] Blood, anticoagulated with heparin, is passed through one or more nylon wool filters which selectively retain granulocytes, some platelets, and monocytes. Other formed elements of the blood pass through the filter and are returned to the donor. The retained cells may then be eluted from the filters and transfused into leukopenic patients.

Function of granulocytes processed by filtration leukapheresis and continuous-flow centrifugation appears comparable to that of those obtained directly from the peripheral blood.[65, 123]

Repeated donations have proved to be possible with both systems; higher numbers of granulocytes are generally collected by filtration leukapheresis.[21] A variety of techniques are under study to increase the yield of both systems.[86, 95] Donor red cell loss appears to be the major limiting factor at present, but platelet counts as well as hematocrit or hemoglobin must be carefully monitored.

Attempts to preserve leukocytes by freezing have not yet proved successful.[90]

ABO compatibility should be assured, not only because these antigens occur on leukocytes but because a substantial number of red cells also are transfused. Careful selection of an HL-A–matched donor appears to reduce reactions and increase the number of circulating transfused leukocytes. Since they must share at least two HL-A loci, siblings, and to a lesser degree parents or children, appear to represent the most likely donors for the neutropenic patient.[15] The percentage recovery of normal neutrophils one hour after their transfusion into neutropenic patients was clearly related to the number of donor-recipient HL-A–matched loci.[15, 65, 123, 134]

Leukocyte alloantibodies causing leukoagglutination or lymphocyte toxicity may be present in spite of an HL-A match, and tests should be performed to detect their presence.[15, 54]

The usual precautions against viral hepatitis and other blood-borne infections must be carried out.[15]

Recipients of granulocyte transfusions are reported to have a variety of reactions. Mild fever and chills occured in 60 per cent in one study[65] and 25 per cent in another.[134] Severe reactions manifested by arrhythmias, chest pain, cyanosis, and dyspnea have been seen in a small minority of recipients, and may be related to the rate of infusion of cells and the sequestration of leukocytes in the lungs.[65, 123, 134]

Results of a recently-reported randomized trial of conventional therapy alone versus conventional therapy plus granulocyte transfusion support claims for the efficacy of the latter form of therapy.[65] Granulocytes used in this study were collected by filtration leukapheresis, and the authors recommend that more than 2×10^{10} granulocytes should be given with each granulocyte transfusion and that it be administered extremely slowly. Several transfusions were needed to effect a good result.[65] Vigorous conventional therapy should be continued.

COMPLICATIONS OF BLOOD TRANSFUSIONS

Blood transfusions have sometimes been given for reasons that appear questionable at best. Among these are its use as a "tonic," as an aid to convalescence from some infection, or as a routine preoperative or postoperative measure. Transfusion in these circumstances is of doubtful value and every transfusion is potentially dangerous.[30, 31]

Even under the best circumstances blood transfusion is associated with some risk; for this reason the procedure should be employed only when the danger of withholding the transfusion exceeds the attendant risk of complications therefrom. The complications that can follow blood transfusions are hemolytic, febrile, and allergic reactions, and the transmission of disease. The incidence and severity of the various types of reactions are difficult to state with exactness, and probably vary from one institution to another. The mortality rate has been quoted as 0.16 per 1000 in 1949,[35] and in 1960 was estimated to be as low as one in 250,000 or 350,000 transfusions.[71] In the University of Virginia Hospital between 1955 and 1958 there was one fatal reaction in 25,465 transfusions, an incidence of about 0.04 per 1000. In the period 1958 to 1964 there were three fatal reactions in 59,441 transfusions, an incidence of about 0.05 per 1000. Three of these four deaths followed hemolytic reactions that were caused by clerical errors made by personnel in or out of the blood bank; the other fatality was the result of serum hepatitis.

Hemolytic transfusion reactions. One of the most serious complications of transfusions is the occurrence of intravascular hemolysis that results from the administration of incompatible blood. Although any antigen-antibody may be involved in these reactions, those involved in the ABO, Rh, and Kell systems are of greatest significance clinically.[144] In the most severe reactions, the antigen is on the donor's red cell and the antibody is in the recipient's plasma; usually, less severe reactions occur when an antibody in the donor's plasma reacts with an antigen on the recipient's red cells or on other donor red cells transfused to the patient. Hemolytic transfusion reactions are usually manifested by burning along the course of the vein being used for infusion, flushing of the face, pain in the lumbar region, a sense of constriction in the chest, chills, hemoglobinemia, and hemoglobinuria, but serious hemolytic reactions can be manifested by nothing more than urticaria or low-grade fever, especially if the patient is under an anesthetic. Any unusual reaction in a patient receiving a transfusion must be considered a hemolytic reaction and treated accordingly, until it is proved otherwise.

Symptoms of this type do not occur if a similar amount of hemolyzed compatible blood is injected, and for this reason it is assumed that the symptoms are caused by some substance that is released by the combination of antigen and antibody.[100] Following acute intravascular hemolysis, free hemoglobin is released and bound by serum haptoglobin. The hemoglobin-haptoglobin complex is cleared by the reticuloendothelial system. If the amount of hemoglobin released exceeds the capacity of the plasma haptoglobin, free hemoglobin will appear in the plasma. As an early step in the catabolism of hemoglobin, the iron–porphyrin compound heme is cleaved from globin. Methemalbumin may be formed by the binding of hematin by albumin and can be observed from five to 24 hours after the hemolytic episode.[43]

Hemoglobin appears in the urine after the reabsorption capacity of the proximal renal tubules is exceeded. Some of the hemoglobin reabsorbed by the renal tubules is deposited as hemosiderin. As these renal tubular cells are sloughed for the next several days, they can be identified in a centrifuged specimen of urine. The finding of hemosiderin indicates that intravascular hemolysis has taken place. The appearance of jaundice is generally delayed for more than 12 hours. A significant increase in the serum bilirubin level within 24 hours after the transfusion is good evidence of a rapid (one to two hours) release of a large amount of hemoglobin, whereas a rise of 1 mg. in the bilirubin level within four to six hours can be considered to be within the range usually seen after the administration of 500 ml. of blood.

Some patients develop renal failure following a hemolytic transfusion reaction. The precise mechanism responsible for this serious turn of events is not known, but it is believed to be related to the occurrence of tubular ischemia resulting from vasoconstriction of cortical microcirculation, stasis, and fibrin thrombi, mediated through release of substances activated by the antigen–antibody reaction.

Intravascular hemolysis may also result in diffuse intravascular coagulation, with excessive utilization of blood clotting factors, and secondary fibrinolysis. This condition, known as the defibrination syndrome (DIC), may first be manifested by abnormal bleeding and requires immediate treatment.[77, 144] See Ch. 17 p. 691.

Management of hemolytic transfusion reaction. When a hemolytic transfusion reaction is suspected, the blood transfusion should be stopped immediately. The seriousness of the reactions is often directly related to the amount of incompatible blood administered. Serious renal damage is infrequent in adults if less than 200 ml. of incompatible blood is given.[35]

Osmotic diuresis should be initiated with mannitol.[9] An intravenous infusion of 10 per cent mannitol at a rate titrated to give a urine output of 100 ml. per hour has proved effective. One thousand ml. mannitol infusions may be alternated with 1000 ml. Ringer's lactate or 5 per cent glucose and water. Diuresis should be maintained until free hemoglobin is no longer visible in the patient's plasma. Vasopressor drugs should not be given, as they have not proved effective and may produce further vasoconstriction in the kidneys. Some have suggested the use of ethacrynic acid or furosemide to produce increased renal blood flow and diuresis, especially in those patients who fail to respond to mannitol.[53, 83a] Toxic effects of ethacrynic acid and furosemide have included transient and permanent hearing loss, tinnitus, and vertigo.[54, 83a] Laboratory studies of coagulation should be closely monitored. Intravascular coagulation may contribute significantly to the development of renal failure and may be judiciously treated with heparin if present.[120, 121]

If the patient does not respond and urine output decreases, excessive fluid administration must be avoided. Fluids are restricted to 500 ml. plus visible output in a 24-hour period. One hundred gm. of carbohydrate should be given daily at a constant rate to avoid periods of hypoglycemia and to decrease catabolism.[9] The serum electrolytes must be followed closely, and if marked derangement occurs despite the use of ion exchange resins, particularly in the potassium level, dialysis should be performed. Measures such as renal decapsulation, spinal anesthesia, intravenous procaine hydrochloride, and aklalinization are probably of no value.[91]

Mollison has listed indications for hemodialysis as follows: (1) blood urea more than 400 mg. per 100 ml., (2) plasma bicarbonate less than 12 mEq. per liter; (3) plasma potassium more than 7.5 mEq. per liter; (4) electrocardiographic evidence of intraventricular block, widening of QRS complexes from hyperkalemia; (5) uremic stupor, vomiting, cough, or fits.[100] Indications for dialysis vary somewhat from hospital to hospital. At the University of Virginia Hospital the same guides are followed in general, but usually dialysis is performed if the blood urea level is 300 mg. per 100 ml.; a potassium level of 6.5 mEq. per liter, despite the use of ion exchange resins, is considered another indication. Also an effort is made to perform dialysis before the clinical features of the uremic syndrome become prominent.

An important part of the management of a hemolytic transfusion reaction is the effort to determine the cause of hemolysis. Investigation of the reaction is facilitated if a sample of blood is drawn from each patient immediately before transfusion and a few ml. of blood from each transfusion bottle is saved for several days. The following procedures are followed at the University of Virginia Hospital:

1. The patient and blood container are checked for clerical error, and the blood container is returned to the blood bank for retyping and bacteriologic investigation (stain of uncentrifuged plasma for bacteria and culture of specimen);

2. Typing and cross-matching are repeated using the patient's pretransfusion blood;

3. A direct antiglobulin (Coombs) test is performed on the patient's post-transfusion blood;

4. An immediate check of patient's plasma for free hemoglobin is made; one-hour and 24-hour post-transfusion urine specimens are examined for hemoglobin, and determinations of bilirubin are made on six-hour and 24-hour sera;

5. Specimens of blood from the donor and recipient are held for six days after transfusion; the patient can be tested for immune response (i.e., high titers of anti-A or anti-B or for other acquired antibody).

Febrile reactions. Febrile reactions, which are reported to have an incidence of 18 per 1000 transfusions,[35] may develop from pyrogens, or from the lysis of erythrocytes or leukocytes. Pyrogens, which are bacterial polysaccharides, are contaminants introduced in the chemical substances used in the preparation of the solutions or the apparatus. The use of disposable transfusion sets has greatly reduced the incidence of this type of reaction. A febrile reaction usually accompanies a severe hemolytic reaction and may occur after hemolysis of mild degree. Since a febrile reaction may herald the onset of a hemolytic reaction, the transfusion must be stopped and an investigation undertaken. A frequent cause of febrile reactions in patients who receive repeated transfusions over a long period is the development of leukocyte or platelet alloantibodies.[19] The reactions, which may be severe, usually occur only in patients with a history of repeated transfusions or pregnancies. Patients who have repeated febrile reactions to transfusions should be studied for this type of reaction. Such reactions usually can be prevented if the buffy coat is removed by centrifugation. After a febrile reaction has occurred, aspirin, 1.0 gm., is usually effective treatment.

Allergic reactions. Allergic reactions, such as urticaria, asthma, or facial edema, occur as the result of abnormal reactions on the part of the patient. An incidence of about 3 per cent has been reported.[126] The transfusion is stopped as soon as the reaction occurs, as it may become more severe or may be a sign of an impending hemolytic reaction. The patient should be given an antihistamine drug intramuscularly. In patients who have frequent allergic reactions, administration of an antihistaminic drug one hour before the transfusion usually suppresses the reaction. It is poor practice to add antihistamine drugs to the blood to be transfused.

Infection. **Syphilis.** Syphilis is transmitted only rarely by blood which has been stored. The use of the blood bank has probably been the greatest single factor in the reduction of the transmission of this disease by transfusion. Storage of blood at 4° to 6° C for four to five days is usually sufficient to render it noninfectious. The chance of transmission of the disease by fresh blood and fresh blood products remains.[69]

Malaria. The possibility of the accidental transmission of malaria by the transfusion of fresh or stored blood has long been recognized. Storage of blood at 4° to 6° C for days or even weeks fails to destroy the malarial parasite. Most of the reported cases have been due to *P. malariae* and *P. vivax*, but a few cases caused by *P. falciparum* have been recorded. In each instance, the donors of the blood had been residents for a period of time in malarious areas. Some had lived outside these areas for as long as 20 years without symptoms of the disease, and in many no parasites could be detected in their blood.[13, 56]

The return of many servicemen from areas with endemic malaria and the increase in worldwide civilian travel will make prevention of transfusion malaria more difficult. All persons who have traveled or lived in such areas must be considered potential carriers.[56] Of importance is the fact that malaria has been transmitted by fresh plasma, which usually contains some red cells.[37]

The incubation period of transfusion malaria has been reported to vary between five and 74 days.[135] Malarial infection should be considered a possibility if fever of uncertain origin occurs following transfusion.[105]

Viral hepatitis. Probably the greatest single problem of blood transfusion at the present time is the transmission of viral hepatitis. This is known to occur as the result of infection with the virus of infectious hepatitis (hepatitis A) which has an incubation period of 15 to 50 days, or the virus of serum hepatitis (hepatitis B) which has an incubation period of 50 to 160 days. There is increasing evidence that additional viruses may be involved as etiologic agents in viral hepatitis.[46, 51, 111]

The incidence of post-transfusion hepatitis may vary in different localities and from one blood bank to another. The over-all frequency of post-transfusion hepatitis in one study from 1967 to 1969 was 20 cases per 1000 units. The exclusion of commercial and Hb_sAg-positive donors resulted in a hepatitis rate of 3.7 cases per 1000.[4] The reason for the residual cases of post-transfusion hepatitis may be related to the failure of current methods to detect low titer Hb_sAg which was still infective, or to the presence of other viruses.[4] The recent development of a method for detection of hepatitis A virus by immune electron microscopy should aid the identification of the residual hepatitis-producing agents.[45] Agents other than hepatitis A and B, cytomegalic virus, and Epstein-Barr virus may remain to be identified.[46, 111]

The incidence of hepatitis rises with the number of transfusions given, and the death rate from hepatitis increases dramatically in the older age-groups.[55] In one study, all deaths occurred in patients over 35 years of age.[3]

The prevention of viral hepatitis remains a problem, and careful screening of donors for a past history of hepatitis is essential. The discovery of an antigenic lipoprotein associated with virus-like particles in the serum of some patients with hepatitis and some carriers of the infection has resulted in the development of a variety of laboratory screening tests which have allowed elimination of some asymptomatic carriers as donors, reducing the incidence of transfusion hepatitis by about one-third.[51, 122] The virus-like particles in the serum samples of patients with hepatitis appear to be identical with the Australia, SH, or hepatitis-associated antigen.[8] They have been shown to persist for long periods in the serum of patients following clinical or subclinical infection, and appear to be capable of transmitting disease in concentrations too low to be detected by current methods.[8] The solid-phase radioimmunoassay test, although not sufficiently sensitive to detect all infectious samples, is more sensitive than other methods.[4, 50] Recent modifications of the test seem to have reduced the incidence of false positive results.[68, 114] The limited ability of current laboratory techniques to detect all infectious samples probably results from the heterogeneity of agents capable of producing hepatitis.[8, 46, 51, 111]

One study indicated that the administration of 10 ml. of gamma globulin within one week after transfusion, and again one month later, prevented three-

quarters of the expected icteric post-transfusion hepatitis but did not change
the incidence of nonicteric hepatitis.[99] Minor variations in this regimen did not
show the same results.[67, 89] More recently, a specific hepatitis B–immune serum
has been developed which has been reported to modify or prevent viral hepatitis
type B after parenteral exposure under controlled conditions in 70 per cent of
subjects.[50, 78, 112] These encouraging results offer hope of developing effective
prophylactic therapy in the future. The exclusion of commercial and Hb$_s$Ag-
positive blood donors in one study has produced a dramatic decrease in post-
transfusion hepatitis.[4] The recent discovery of a virus-like antigen in the stools
of patients with hepatitis A, and the development of a serologic technique with
which to detect antibody to it, may provide a means of detection of this virus in
blood and blood products. Continued search is needed for additional agents
which may cause post-transfusion hepatitis as well as for means by which all
these agents might be inactivated or removed from blood.[4, 46]

Bacterial infection.   Transmission of bacterial infection by transfusion is
seldom seen at present. However, certain saprophytic bacteria may enter the
blood to be transfused. The gram-positive organisms, such as diphtheroids, have
produced only fever with no serious constitutional symptoms. The gram-
negative organisms have been responsible for a type of overwhelming shock that
is almost invariably fatal. The syndrome is characterized by chills, fever, hypotension, severe pain in the abdomen and extremities, and dryness and flushing
of the skin. Symptoms usually occur within 30 minutes of the start of the transfusion and may follow the administration of only 50 ml. of blood. Treatment
with broad spectrum antibiotics, vasopressors, and massive doses of steroids
must begin as soon as the syndrome is recognized. The outlook for these patients is poor.[16] Scrupulous care must be taken in collection, storage, and
administration of blood and blood products in order that they may not become
contaminated.[69]

Microaggregates.   Microaggregates of leukocytes and platelets accumulate
in stored blood and will pass through the standard 170 micron pore filter used
in transfusion sets.[125, 130] They have been suspected of causing postperfusion or
shock lung when filtered by the capillaries of the lungs of patients on pulmonary
bypass or receiving large amounts of stored blood.[93, 118] The use of filters with a
pore size of 25 to 40μ has been shown effectively to remove microaggregates.[106, 118]

REACTIONS DUE TO ANTI–IgA PROTEIN

Reactions beginning soon after the start of a transfusion and characterized
by a variable symptom complex which may include urticaria, flushing, abdominal
pain, vomiting, diarrhea, chills, fever, edema, bronchospasm, and hypotension,
have been reported to occur in patients with anti-IgA antibodies.[83, 98, 124, 136, 138]
The antibodies are of the IgG class and fix complement.[124]

Persons with a total lack of IgA protein develop class-specific IgA antibodies
of broad reactivity. Immunization may occur on exposure to IgA as the result

of transfusion or pregnancy. Anti-IgA antibodies may occur as the result of exposure to maternal IgA in utero and may be responsible for reactions in individuals with no prior history of transfusion or pregnancy.[61, 136]

Individuals with normal levels of IgA appear to develop anti-IgA antibodies of limited specificity against some IgA component missing from their serum. Such antibodies generally occur in multitransfused patients.[136-138]

Individuals who lack IgA and have developed class-specific antibodies appear to have the highest titer and are subject to the most severe reactions. Reactions in either group may be alarming, and should be treated as any anaphylactoid reaction, with fluids (not blood products), vasopressors, steroids, oxygen, epinephrine, and other supportive measures.[59]

Reactions of this type may be avoided by using blood or blood products from donors deficient in IgA. These patients have also been successfully transfused with red cells which have been washed several times.[59, 83]

OTHER PROBLEMS

Pulmonary edema may occur as the result of circulatory overload. Tourniquets should be applied at the upper portion of the four extremities without delay and should be rotated in such a manner that none remains in place longer than 15 minutes. Phlebotomy with the removal of 500 ml. of blood is advisable, and the administration of morphine may be desirable. Even if the patient responds well to these measures he should be observed carefully, and any other necessary treatment should be given. Pulmonary edema, which is most likely to occur in elderly patients with severe chronic anemia and in those with heart disease, can be avoided if the patient is transfused slowly with packed red cells. Whole blood is to be avoided.

When a large number of units of stored blood are given, citrate and potassium toxicity are potential hazards. Citrate toxicity results in a depression of ionization of the divalent cations, such as Ca^{++}. The excitable tissues of the body are susceptible to such depression, the effect on the cardiac muscle being most important. Hypothermia or liver disease may augment the problems by slowing the metabolism of citrate. Citrate toxicity may be treated by the administration of appropriate solutions of calcium chloride or calcium gluconate intravenously.[87, 144]

Since the plasma potassium gradually increases on storage as the result of the breakdown of red cells, the transfusion of stored blood may result in an acute rise in serum potassium in the recipient. This is particularly hazardous to patients already hyperkalemic, and can be avoided by the administration of fresh blood to such patients.[144]

Massive transfusions of blood may result in the development of thrombocytopenia. This is probably a dilution effect that is the result of using large quantities of blood that contain no viable platelets.[70] The administration of 500 ml. of fresh blood, not more than three to four hours' old, for each three or four units of bank blood may prevent this complication.[144]

References

1. Adner, M. M., Fisch, G. R., Starobin, S. G., and Aster, R. N.: Use of "compatible" platelet transfusions in treatment of congenital isoimmune thrombocytopenic purpura. N. Engl. J. Med., *280*:244, 1969.
2. Aggler, P. M.: Physiological basis for transfusion therapy in hemorrhagic disorders: a critical review. Transfusion, *1*:71, 1961.
3. Allen, J. G., and Sayman, W. A.: Serum hepatitis from transfusions of blood: epidemiologic study. J.A.M.A., *180*:1079, 1962.
4. Alter, H. J., Holland, P. V., Purcell, R. H., Lander, J. L., Feinstone, S. M., Morrow, A. G., and Schmidt, P. J.: Post-transfusion hepatitis after exclusion of commercial and hepatitis-B antigen-positive donors. Ann. Intern. Med., 77:691, 1972.
5. Amris, C. J., and Hilden, M.: Treatment of factor XIII deficiency with cryoprecipitate. Thromb. Diath. Haemorrh., *20*:528, 1968.
6. Andresen, P. H.: The Human Blood Groups. Charles C Thomas, Springfield, Ill., 1952.
7. Aster, R. H.: Effect of anticoagulant and ABO incompatibility on recovery of transfused human platelets. Blood, *26*:732, 1965.
8. Barker, L. F., Shulman, N. R., Murray, R., Hirschman, R. J., Ratner, F., Diefenbach, W. C. L., and Geller, H. M.: Transmission of serum hepatitis. J.A.M.A., *211*:1509, 1970.
9. Barry, K. G., and Crosby, W. H.: The prevention and treatment of renal failure following transfusion reactions. Transfusion, *3*:34, 1963.
10. Becker, G. A., Junicki, T., and Aster, R. H.: Effect of prostaglandin E$_1$, on harvesting of platelets from refrigerated whole blood. J. Lab. Clin. Invest., *83*:304, 1974.
11. Becker, G. A., Tuccelli, M., Kunicki, T., Chalos, M. K., and Aster, R. H.: Studies of platelet concentrates stored at 22° and 4° C. Transfusion, *13*:61, 1973.
12. Biggs, R.: Fractions rich in factor VIII. Bibl. Haematol., *29*:1122, 1968.
13. Black, R. H.: Investigation of blood donors in accidental transfusion of malaria-*Plasmodium vivax, falciparum* and *malariae* infections. Med. J. Aust., *2*:446, 1960.
14. Bloom, A. L., and Emmanuel, J. H.: Use of cryoprecipitate antihaemophilic factor for the treatment of haemophilia. J. Med., *37*:(N.S.)291, 1968.
15. Boggs, D. R.: Transfusion of neutrophils to prevent or treat infection in neutropenic patients. N. Engl. J. Med., *290*:1055, 1974.
16. Braude, A. L.: Transfusion reactions from contaminated blood. N. Engl. J. Med., *258*:1289, 1958.
17. Breen, F. A., and Tullis, J. L.: Prothrombin concentrates in treatment of Christmas disease and allied disorders. J.A.M.A., *208*:1848, 1969.
18. Brinkhous, K. M., Shanbrom, E., Roberts, H. R., Webster, W. P., Fekete, L., and Wagner, R. H.: A new high-potency glycine-precipitated antihemophilic factor (AHF) concentrate. J.A.M.A., *205*:613, 1968.
19. Brittingham, T. E., and Chaplin, H., Jr.: Febrile transfusion reactions caused by sensitivity to donor leukocytes and platelets. J.A.M.A., *165*:819, 1957.
20. Buchholz, D. H.: Blood transfusion: merits of component therapy. 1. The clinical use of red cells, platelets and granulocytes. J. Pediatr., *84*:1, 1974.
21. Buchholz, D. H., Schiffer, C. A., Wiernik, P. H., Betts, S. W., and Reilly, J. A.: Granulocyte harvest for transfusion: Donor response to repeated leukapheresis. Transfusion, *15*:96, 1975.
22. Buchholz, D. H., Young, V. M., Friedman, N. R., Reilly, J. A., and Mardiney, M. R., Jr.: Bacterial proliferation in platelet products stored at room temperature — transfusion-induced enterobacter sepsis. N. Engl. J. Med., *285*:429, 1971.
23. Buchholz, D. H., Young, V. M., Friedman, N. R., Reilly, J. A., and Mardiney, M. R., Jr.: Detection and quantitation of bacteria in platelet products stored at ambient temperature. Transfusion, *13*:268, 1973.
24. Cash, J. D.: Platelet transfusion therapy. Clin. Haematol., *1*:395, 1972.
25. Chaplin, H., Jr., Beutler, E., Collins, J. A., Giblett, E. R., and Polesky, H. F.: Current status of red-cell preservation and availability in relation to the developing national blood policy. N. Engl. J. Med., *291*:68, 1974.
26. Chaplin, H., Jr., Jaffe, E. R., Lenfant, C., and Valeri, C. R.: Preservation of red blood cells: proceedings of a conference, June 5–6, 1972. Washington D. C., Natl. Acad. Sci., 1973.
27. Committee of the Joint Blood Council and American Association of Blood Banks: Standards for a Blood Transfusion Service. Joint Blood Council, Washington, D. C., and American Association of Blood Banks, Chicago, Ill., 1958.
28. Committee on Transfusion and Transplantation (American Medical Association): General Principles of Blood Transfusion. American Medical Association, Chicago, Ill., 1970.

29. Cooke, J. V., Holland, P. V., and Shulman, N. R.: Cryoprecipitate concentrates of factor VIII for surgery in hemophiliacs. Ann. Intern. Med., *68*:39, 1968.

30. Crosby, W. H.: Misuse of blood transfusion. Blood, *13*:1198, 1958.

31. Crosby, W. H.: The single unit transfusion. Transfusion, *4*:329, 1964.

32. Crosby, W. H., and Howard, J. M.: The hematologic response to wounding and to resuscitation accomplished by large transfusions on stored blood. A study of battle casualties in Korea. Blood, *9*:439, 1954.

33. Dale, D. C., Reynolds, H. Y., Pennington, J. E., Elin, R. J., Pitts, R. J., Pitts, T. W., and Graw, R. G., Jr.: Granulocyte transfusion therapy of experimental pseudomonas pneumonia. J. Clin. Invest., *54*:664, 1974.

34. Dallman, P. R., and Pool, J. G.: Treatment of hemophilia with factor VIII concentrates. N. Engl. J. Med., *278*:199, 1968.

35. DeGowin, E. L., Hardin, R. C., and Alsever, J. B.: Blood Transfusion. W. B. Saunders Co., Philadelphia, 1949.

36. Diamond, L. K.: Protection against Rh sensitization and prevention of erythroblastosis fetalis. Pediatrics, *41*:1, 1968.

37. Dike, A. E.: Two cases of transfusion malaria. Lancet, *2*:72, 1970.

38. Djerassi, I.: The role of platelet administration in a blood transfusion service. Transfusion, *6*:55, 1966.

39. Djerassi, I., and Farber, S.: Control and prevention of hemorrhage: platelet transfusion. Cancer Res., *25*:1499, 1965.

40. Djerassi, I., Kim, J. S., Mitrakul, C., Suvansri, U., and Ciesielka, W.: Filtration leukapheresis for separation and concentration of transfusable amounts of normal human granulocytes. J. Med. Exp. Clin, (Basel), *1*:358, 1970.

41. Djerassi, I., Roy, A., Kim, J., and Cavins, J.: Dimethylacetamide, a new cryoprotective agent for platelets. Transfusion, *11*:72, 1971.

42. Editorial: Blood banks. Va. Med. Mon., *78*:275, 1951.

43. Fairley, N. H.: Methaemalbumin. Q. J. Med., *10*:95, 1941.

44. Fantus, B.: The therapy of the Cook County Hospital: blood preservation. J.A.M.A., *109*:128, 1937.

45. Feinstone, S. M., Kapikian, A. A., and Purcell, R. H,: Hepatitis A: detection by immune electron microscopy of a virus-like antigen associated with acute illness. Science, *182*:1026, 1973.

46. Feinstone, S. M., Kapikian, A. Z., Purcell, R. H., Alter, H. J., and Holland, P. V.: Transfusion-associated hepatitis not due to viral hepatitis type A or B. N. Engl. J. Med., *292*:767, 1975.

47. Freda, V. J., Gorman, J. G., Pollack, W., Robertson, J. G., Jennings, E. R., and Sullivan, J. F.: Prevention of Rh isoimmunization: progress report of the clinical trial in mothers. J.A.M.A., *199*:390, 1967.

48. Freireich, E. J., Judson, G., and Levin, R. H.: Separation and collection of leukocytes. Cancer Res., *25*:1516, 1965.

49. Gilchrist, G. S., Ekert, H., Shanbrom, E ., and Hammond, D.: New concentrate for treatment of factor IX deficiency. N. Engl. J. Med., *280*:291, 1969.

50. Ginsberg, A. L., Conrad, M. E., Bancroft, W. H., Ling, C. M., and Overby, L. R.: Prevention of endemic HAA–positive hepatitis with gamma globulin. N. Engl. J. Med., *286*:562, 1972.

51. Gocke, D. J.: A prospective study of post-transfusions hepatitis. The role of Australia antigen. J.A.M.A., *219*:1165, 1972.

52. Goddard, D., Jacobs, S. I., and Manohitharajah, S. M.: The bacteriological screening of platelet concentrates stored at 22° C. Transfusion, *13*:103, 1973.

53. Goldfinger, D.: Complications of hemolytic transfusion reactions: pathogenesis and therapy. *In* New approaches to transfusion reactions. Technical workshop. Am. Assoc. Blood Banks, 15, 1974.

54. Goldstein, I. M., Eyre, H. J., Terasaki, P. I., Henderson, E. S., and Graw, R. G., Jr.: Leukocyte transfusions: role of leukocyte alloantibodies in determining transfusion response. Transfusion, *11*:19, 1971.

55. Grady, G. F., Chalmers, T. C., and the Boston Inter-Hospital Liver Group: Viral hepatitis in a group of Boston hospitals. N. Engl. J. Med., *272*:657, 1965.

56. Grant, D. B., Perinpanayagam, M. S., Shute, P. G., and Zeitlin, R. A.: A case of malignant tertian (*Plasmodium falciparum*) malaria after blood transfusion. Lancet, *2*:469, 1960.

57. Graw, R. G., Jr., Herzig, G. P., Eisel, R. J., and Perry, S.: Leukocyte and platelet collection from donors with the continuous-flow blood cell separator. Transfusion, *11*:94, 1971.

58. Graw, R. G., Jr., Herzig, G., Perry, S., and Henderson, E. S.: Normal granulocyte transfusion therapy: treatment of septicemia due to gram-negative bacteria. N. Engl. J. Med., *287*:367, 1972.

59. Greenwalt, T. J., and Jamieson, G. A.: The Human Red Cell in Vitro. 5th Am. Red Cross-Scient. Symp. May 7–8, 1973. Grune & Stratton, New York,

60. Grumet, F. C., and Yankee, R. A.: Long-term platelet support for patients with aplastic anemia. Effect of splenectomy and steroid therapy. Ann. Intern. Med., *73*:1, 1970.

61. Grumet, F. C., and Yankee, R. A.: Non-red cell reactions. *In* New approaches to transfusion reactions. A technical workshop. Am. Assoc. Blood Banks, 39, 1974.

62. Hampers, C. L., Prager, D., and Senior, J. R.: Post-transfusion anicteric hepatitis. N. Engl. J. Med., *271*:747, 1964.

63. Handin, R. I., and Valeri, C. R.: Hemostatic effectiveness of platelets stored at 22° C. N. Engl. J. Med., *285*:538, 1971.

64. Handin, R. I., and Valeri, C. R.: Improved viability of previously-frozen platelets. Blood, *40*: 509, 1972.

65. Higby, D. J., Yates, J. W., Henderson, E. S., and Holland, J. F.: Filtration leukapheresis for granulocyte transfusion therapy. N. Engl. J. Med., *292*:761, 1975.

66. Hoag, M. S., Johnson, F. F., Robinson, J. A., and Aggeler, P. M.: Treatment of hemophilia B with a new clotting-factor concentrate. N. Engl. J. Med., *280*:581, 1969.

67. Holland, P. V., Rubinson, R. M., Morrow, A. G., and Schmidt, P. J.: γ-globulin in the prophylaxis of post-transfusion hepatitis. J.A.M.A., *196*:471, 1966.

68. Hollinger, F. B., Aach, R. D., Gitnick, G. L., Roche, J. K., and Melnick, J. L.: Limitations of solid-phase radioimmunoassay for HB Ag in reducing frequency of post-transfusion hepatitis. N. Engl. J. Med., *289*:385, 1973.

69. Huestis, D. W., Bove, J. R., and Busch, S.: Practical Blood Transfusion. Little, Brown and Co., Boston, 1969.

70. Jackson, D. P., Krevans, J. R., and Conley, C. L.: Mechanism of the thrombocytopenia that follows multiple whole blood transfusions. Tr. Assoc. Am. Physicians, *69*:155, 1956.

71. Joseph, J. H.: Mortality due to blood transfusion. Lancet, 2:709, 1960.

72. Kabat, E. A.: Blood Group Substances. Their Chemistry and Immunochemistry. Academic Press, Inc., New York, 1955.

73. Kahn, R. A., and Flinton, L. J.: Evaluation of ethylene glycol as a cryoprotective agent for blood platelets. Cryobiology, *10*:148, 1973.

74. Katz, A. J., and Tilton, R. C.: Sterility of platelet concentrates stored at 25° C. Transfusion, *10*:329, 1970.

75. Kilduffe, R. A., and DeBakey, M.: The Blood Bank and the Technique and Therapeutics of Transfusion. C. V. Mosby Co., St. Louis, 1942, p. 1.

76. Kliman, A.: Low risk of hepatitis after packed red cells. N. Engl. J. Med., 277:1320, 1967.

77. Krevans, J. R., Jackson, D. P., Conley, C. L., and Hartman, R. C.: The nature of the hemmorrhagic disorder accompanying hemolytic transfusion reactions in man. Blood, *12*:834, 1957.

78. Krugman, S., Giles, J. P., and Hammond, J.: Viral hepatitis, type B (MS–2 strain). J.A.M.A., *218*:1665, 1971.

79. Kunin, C. M.: Serum hepatitis from whole blood: incidence and relation to source of blood. Am. J. Med. Sci., *237*:293, 1959.

80. Landsteiner, K.: Zur Kenntnis der antifermentativen, lytischen und agglutinierenden Wirkungen des Bluxserums und der Lymphe. Zentralbl., *27*:357, 1900.

81. Landsteiner, K., and Levine, P.: A new agglutinable factor differentiating individual human bloods. Proc. Soc. Exp. Biol. Med., *24*:600, 1927.

82. Landsteiner, K., and Wiener, A. S.: An agglutinable factor in human blood recognized by immune sera for rhesus blood. Proc. Soc. Exp. Biol. Med., *43*:223, 1940.

83. Leikola, J., Koistinen, J., Lehtinen, M., and Virolainen, M.: IgA-induced anaphylactic transfusion reactions: a report of four cases. Blood, *42*:111, 1973.

83a. Levin, N. W.: Furosemide and ethacrynic acid in renal insufficiency. Med. Clin. North Am., *55*:107, 1971.

84. Levin, R. H., Freireich, E. J., and Chappell, W.: Effect of storage up to 48 hours on response to transfusions of platelet rich plasma. Transfusion, *4*:251, 1964.

85. Levine, P., and Stetson, R. E.: An unusual case of intragroup agglutination. J.A.M.A., *113*:126, 1939.

86. Lowenthal, R. M., and Park, D. S.: The use of dextran as an adjunct to granulocyte collection with the continuous-flow blood cell separator. Transfusion, *15*:23, 1975.

87. Ludbrook, J., and Wynn, V.: Citrate intoxication. A clinical and experimental study. Br. Med. J., 2:523, 1558.

88. MacKay, I. R.: Chronic hepatitis: effect of prolonged suppressive treatment and comparison of azathioprine with prednisolone. Q. J. Med., *37*:379, 1968.

89. Mainwaring, R. L., and Brueckner, G. G.: Fibrinogen-transmitted hepatitis. J.A.M.A., *195*:437, 1966.

90. Malinin, T. I.: Injury of human polymorphonuclear granulocytes frozen in the presence of cryoprotective agents. Cryobiology, 9:123, 1972.
91. Manuila, A.: Blood groups and disease. Hard facts and delusions. J.A.M.A., 167:2047, 1958.
92. Marder, V. J., and Shulman, N. R.: Major surgery in classic hemophilia using fraction I. Am. J. Med., 41:56, 1966.
93. Marshall, B. E., Soma, L. R., Harp. J. R., Neufeld, G. R., Wurzel, H. A., and Dodd, D. C.: Pulmonary function after exchange transfusion of stored blood in dogs. Am. Surg., 179:46, 1974.
94. Masure, R.: Human factor VIII prepared by cryoprecipitation. Vox Sang., 16:1, 1969.
95. McCredie, K. B., and Freireich, E. J.: The use of etiocholanolone to increase collection of granulocytes with the IBM blood cell separator. J. Clin. Invest., 49:63a, 1970.
96. McCredie, K. B., Freireich, E. J., Hester, J. P., and Vallejos, C.: Leukocyte transfusion therapy for patients with host-defense failure. Transplant Proc., 5:1285, 1973.
97. Miller, S. E.: Textbook of Clinical Pathology. 5th Ed. Williams and Wilkins Co., Baltimore, 1955, p. 296.
98. Miller, W. V., Holland, P. V., Sugarbaker, E., Strober, W., and Waldmann, T. A.: Anaphylactic reaction to IgA: a difficult transfusion problem. Am. J. Clin. Pathol., 54:618, 1970.
99. Mirick, G. S., Ward, R., and McCollum, R. W.: Modification of post-transfusional hepatitis by gamma globulin. N. Engl. J. Med., 273:59, 1965.
100. Mollison, P. L.: Blood Transfusion in Clinical Medicine. Blackwell Scientific Publications, Oxford, 1972.
101. Morse, E. E., Bronson, W., Carbonne, P. P., and Freireich, E. J.: Effectiveness of granulocyte transfusions from donors with chronic myelocytic leukemia to patients with leukopenia. Clin. Res., 9:332, 1961.
102. Morse, E. E., Freireich, E. J., Carbone, P. P., Bronson, W., and Frei, E., III: The transfusion of leukocytes from donors with chronic myelocytic leukemia to patients with leukopenia. Transfusion, 6:183, 1966.
103. Mourant, A. E.: The Distribution of the Human Blood Groups. Charles C Thomas, Springfield, Ill., 1954.
104. National Blood Policy. Fed. Registr., 39(47):9329, 1974.
105. Pantelakis, S. N., Karaklis, A., and Doxiadis, S. A.: Transfusion malaria. Clin. Pediatr., 5:543, 1966.
106. Patterson, R. H., and Twitchell, J. B.: Disposable filter for microemboli. J.A.M.A., 215:76, 1971.
107. Perkins, H. A.: Brief report: correction of the hemostatic defects in von Willebrand's disease. Blood, 30:375, 1967.
108. Phillips, L. L.: Homologous serum jaundice following fibrinogen administration. Surg. Gynecol. Obstet., 121:551, 1965.
109. Pool, J. G., Hershgold, E. J., and Pappenhagen, A. R.: High potency antihemophilic factor concentrate prepared from cryoglobulin precipitate. Nature, 203:312, 1964.
110. Prentice, C. R. M., Breckenridge, R. T., Foreman, W. B., and Ratnoff, O. D.: Treatment of hemophilia (Factor VIII deficiency) with human antihemophilic factor prepared by the cryoprecipitate process. Lancet, 1:457, 1967.
111. Price, A. M., Brotman, B., Grady, G. F., Kuhns, W. J., Hazzi, C., Levine, R. W., and Millian, S. J.: Long-incubation post-transfusion hepatitis without serological evidence of exposure to hepatitis–B virus. Lancet, 2:241, 1974.
112. Price, A. M., Szmuness, W., Woods, K. R., and Grady, G. F.: Antibody against serum–hepatitis antigen. N. Engl. J. Med., 285:933, 1971.
113. Purcell, G., Jr., and Nossel, H. L.: Factor XI (PTA) deficiency—surgical and obstetric aspects. Obstet. Gynecol., 35:69, 1970.
114. Purcell, R. H., Wong, D. C., Alter, H. J., and Holland, P. V.: Microtiter solid–phase radio–immunoassay for hepatitis B antigen. Appl. Microbiol., 26:478, 1973.
115. Race, R. R., and Sanger, R.: The inheritance of blood groups. Br. Med. Bull., 15:99, 1959.
116. Race, R. R., and Sanger, R.: Blood Groups in Man. 5th Ed., Blackwell Scientific Publications. Oxford, 1968.
117. Ratnoff, O. D., Kass, L., and Lang, P. D.: Studies on the purification of antihemophilic factor. Factor VIII. J. Clin. Invest., 48:957, 1969.
118. Reul, G. J., Jr., Greenberg, S. D., Lefrak, E. A., McCollum, W. B., Beall, A. C., Jr., and Jordan, G. L., Jr.: Prevention of post-traumatic pulmonary insufficiency. Arch. Surg., 106:386, 1973.
119. Roberts, J. A. F.: Some associations between blood groups and disease. Br. Med. Bull., 15:129, 1959.
120. Rock, R. C., Bove, J. R., and Nemerson, Y.: Heparin treatment of intravascular coagulation accompanying hemolytic transfusion reactions. Transfusion, 9:57, 1969.

121. Sacks, E. S., and Nepa, O. M.: Fibrinogen and fibrin degradation products in hemolytic trans-fusion reactions. Transfusion, *10*:317, 1970.

122. Saravis, C. A., Trey, C., and Grady, G. F.: Rapid screening test for detecting hepatitis-associated antigen. Science, *169*:298, 1970.

123. Schiffer, C. A., Buchholz, D. H., Aisner, J., Betts, S. W., and Wiernik, P. H.: Clinical experi-ence with transfusion of granulocytes obtained by continuous-flow filtration leukapheresis. Am. J. Med., *58*:373, 1975.

124. Schmidt, A. P., Taswell, H. F., and Gleich, G. J.: Anaphylactic transfusion reactions associated with anti–IgA antibody. N. Engl. J. Med., *280*:188, 1969.

125. Solis, R. T.: Microembolization and blood transfusions. In seminar on current technical topics. Am. Assoc. Blood Banks, 31, 1974.

126. Stephen, C. R., Martin, R. C., and Bourgeois-Gavardin, M.: Antihistamine drugs in treatment of nonhemolytic transfusion reactions. J. Am. Med. Assoc., *158*:525, 1955.

127. Straumia, M. M.: The effect of leukocytic cream injections in the treatment of the neutropenias. Am. J. Med. Sci., *187*:527, 1934.

128. Stuart, M. J., Murphy, S., Oski, F. A., Evans, A. E., Donaldson, M. H., and Gardner, F. H.: Platelet function in recipients of platelets from donors ingesting aspirin. N. Engl. J. Med., *287*:1105, 1972.

129. Surgenor, D. MacN.: Progress toward a national blood system. New Engl. J. Med., *291*:17, 1974.

130. Swank, R. L., and Porter, G. A.: Disappearance of microemboli transfused into patients during cardiopulmonary bypass. Transfusion, *3*:192, 1963.

131. Tejada, F., Bias, W. B., Santos, G. W., and Zieve, P. D.: Immunologic response of patients with acute leukemia to platelet transfusions. Blood, *42*:405, 1973.

132. Tullis, J. L., and Melin, M.: Management of Christmas disease and Stuart-Prower deficiency with a prothrombin-complex concentrate. (Factor II, VII, IX & X.) Bibl. Haematol., *29*: 1134, 1968.

133. Tullis, J. L., Tinch, R. J., Baudanza, P., Gibson, J. G., II, Diforte, S., Conneely, G., and Murphy, K.: Plateletpheresis in a disposable system. Transfusion, *11*:368, 1971.

134. Vallejos, C., McCredie, K. B., Bodey, G. P., Hester, J. P., and Freireich, E. J.: White blood cell transfusions for control of infections in neutropenic patients. Transfusion, *15*:28, 1975.

135. Vartan, A. E.: Transfusion malaria in a man with Christmas disease. Br. Med. J., *4*:466, 1967.

136. Vyas, G. N., and Fudenberg, H. H.: Isoimmune anti–IgA causing anaphylactoid transfusion reactions. N. Engl. J. Med., *280*:1073, 1969.

137. Vyas, G. N., Levin, A. S., and Fudenberg, H. H.: Intrauterine isoimmunization caused by maternal IgA crossing the placenta. Nature (Lond.), *225*:275, 1970.

138. Vyas, G. N., Perkins, H. A., and Fudenberg, H. H.: Anaphylactoid transfusion associated with anti–IgA. Lancet, *2*:312, 1968.

139. Weatherbee, L., Starkweather, W. H., Knorpp, C. T., Schinitzer, B., and Spencer, H. H.: An approach to the long-term preservation of platelets. Cryobiology, *8*:393, 1971.

140. Wedgwood, R. J., and Riese, G. R.: Touching a cure of an inverterate phrensy by the trans-fusion of blood. N. Engl. J. Med., *248*:902, 1953.

141. Wrenn, H. E., and Speicher, C. E.: Platelet concentrates: sterility of 400 single units stored at room temperature. Transfusion, *14*:171, 1974.

142. Wiener, A. S., and Wexler, I. B.: Heredity of the Blood Groups. Grune and Stratton, New York, 1958.

143. Yankee, R. A., Graff, K. S., Dowling, R., and Henderson, E. S.: Selection of unrelated com-patible platelet donors by lymphocyte HL–A matching. N. Engl. J. Med., *288*:760, 1973.

144. Young, L. E.: Complications of blood transfusions. Ann. Intern. Med., *61*:136, 1964.

INDEX

Tests (*Continued*)
  Kahn, in infectious mononucleosis, 357
  liver function, in infectious mononucleosis, 357
  monospot, 358
  osmotic fragility, in hereditary sphero-cytosis, 206–207
  Paul-Bunnell, in infectious mononucleosis, 356
  prothrombin and proconvertin (P and P), 606
  Schilling, in pernicious anemia diagnosis, 106
  Sia, in macroglobulinemia, 554
Thalassemia (Cooley's anemia), 231–238
Thalassemia-C disease, 239
Thalassemia–hemoglobin E disease, 239
Thalassemia-sickle cell disease, 238
Thrombasthenia, 654
Thrombin
  chemistry, 588
  conversion from Factor II, 588
  history, 578
  time, 614
Thrombocyte (platelet), 16
Thrombocythemia, idiopathic, 379
  in iron deficiency, 143
Thrombocytic series, 15–16
Thrombocytopenia, 637–651
Thrombokinase, 579
Thromboplastin, 580
Thromboplastin generation test, 612
Thrombosis, in hypercoagulable state, 596
  in polycythemia vera, 392
Thrombosthenin, 568
Thrombotic thrombocytopenic purpura, 649
Thymoma, in erythrocytic hypoplasia, 184
Tissue thromboplastin, 581
Tooth extractions, in Factor VIII deficiency, 670
Tourniquet test, in hemorrhagic diathesis, 611
Toxic granulation, 11
Transcobalamin I, 94
Transcobalamin II, 93
Transfer RNA, 34–35
Transferrin
  function, 130
  molecular weight, 131
  variations in disease, 133
Transfusion(s)
  complications of, 729
  exchange, in erythroblastosis fetalis, 245
   indications, 245
  hepatitis and, 733
  history of, 719
  in sickle cell anemia, 227–228
  indications for, 724
  intrauterine, in erythroblastosis fetalis, 246
  of blood components, 724–729
   granulocytes, 728
   plasma, 726
   platelets, 726
   red cells, 724–726
   survival of, 724

Transfusion(s) (*Continued*)
  reactions
   allergic, 732
   anti-IgA protein, 734–735
   cause of, determination of, 731
   chemical, citrate toxicity, 735
    potassium toxicity, 735
   febrile, 732
   hemolytic, 729
    management, 730
   infection, 732
    viral hepatitis, 733
   pulmonary edema, 735
   thrombocytopenia and, 735

Ulcer(s), of legs, chronic, in hereditary spherocytosis, 205
  in sickle cell disease, 220, 221
Uremia, anemia of, 297–300
Urokinase, 592
Uroporphyrin, 36

van den Bergh reaction, 40
Vascular lesions, as factors in secondary poly-cythemia, 398
Vena cavogram, inferior, in Hodgkin's disease, 478
Venesection, in polycythemia vera, 395
Verodoperoxidase, 12
Virocytes, 356
Viruses, role in leukemia, 416–417
Vitamin B$_6$. See *Pyridoxine.*
Vitamin B$_{12}$, 49, 86
  absorption of, 87
  deficiency, 93–107
  formula, 86
  in nucleic acid synthesis, 90–92
  metabolism of, 86–107
  serum levels, in chronic granulocytic leu-kemia, 500
  transport, 88
Vitamin E, 49
Vitamin K, 686
  as antidote to coumarin-indanedione drugs, 607
von Willebrand's disease, 695–699

Waldenström's macroglobulinemia, 553–555
  clinical findings, 554
  hyperviscosity syndrome in, 554
  treatment, 555
Wassermann test, in infectious mononu-cleosis, 357

Xanthine oxidase, and iron absorption, 127

Pg 212 6-6-PD DEFICIENCY 10-13% AMERICAN BLACKS
SICKLE CELL = 9% AMERICAN BLACKS
SEVERE ANEMIA INDUCED BY Pg 213 VIT K DIURETICS
many more.